Handbook of Pesticide Toxicology

Handbook of Pesticide Toxicology

VOLUME 2

CLASSES OF PESTICIDES

EDITED BY

Wayland J. Hayes, Jr.
Vanderbilt University
School of Medicine
Nashville, Tennessee

Edward R. Laws, Jr.
Department of Neurological Surgery
George Washington University School of Medicine
Washington, D.C.

Academic Press, Inc.
Harcourt Brace Jovanovich, Publishers
San Diego New York Boston London Sydney Tokyo Toronto

Academic Press, Inc.
San Diego, California 92101

United Kingdom Edition published by
Academic Press Limited
24–28 Oval Road, London NW1 7DX

Library of Congress Cataloging-in-Publication Data

Handbook of pesticide toxicology / Wayland J. Hayes, Jr., Edward R.
  Laws, Jr., editors.
      p.   cm.
    Includes bibliographical references.
    Contents: v. 1. General principles -- v. 2-3. Classes of
  pesticides.
     ISBN 0-12-334161-2   (v. 1 : alk. paper) -- ISBN   0-12-334162-0
  (v. 2 : alk. paper) -- ISBN   0-12-334163-9   (v. 3 : alk. paper)
     1. Pesticides--Toxicology.   I. Hayes, Wayland J., Date.
  II. Laws, Edward R.
  RA1270.P4H36   1991
  615.9'02--dc20   90-313
                                                        CIP

Printed in the United States of America
90 91 92 93   9 8 7 6 5 4 3 2 1

To Philip Theophrastus Bombast von Hohenheim
called PARACELSUS who said

Was ift das nit gifft ift: alle ding find
gifft/vnd nichts ohn gifft/Allein die dofis macht
das ein ding kein gift ift.

or in more familiar language
Dosage Alone Determines Poisoning

Contents of the Handbook

Contents of Volume 2

14 Solvents, Fumigants, and Related Compounds

P. J. Gehring, R. J. Nolan, P. G. Watanabe, and A. M. Schumann

15 Chlorinated Hydrocarbon Insecticides

Andrew G. Smith

16 Organic Phosphorus Pesticides

Michael A. Gallo and Nicholas J. Lawryk

Inorganic and Organometal Pesticides

Thomas W. Clarkson
University of Rochester

There are at least 18 elements that characterize one or more inorganic pesticides. Of these elements, ten (chromium, copper, zinc, phosphorus, sulfur, tin, arsenic, selenium, fluorine, and chlorine) have been shown to be essential for normal growth. In these instances, the toxic effects clearly do not depend on the element *per se* but on the specific properties of one form of the element or one of its compounds, or merely on an inordinately high dosage. The other eight elements (barium, cadmium, mercury, thallium, lead, bismuth, antimony, and boron) have not been shown to be essential to growth of animals, although there is evidence that some may be. In any event, experience has shown that toxicity is not an argument against essentiality. Some highly toxic elements such as iron, selenium, arsenic, and fluorine certainly are essential to normal development.

In the following sections, representative inorganic pesticides are arranged with reference to the periodic classification of the elements. In some instances this has involved sequential consideration of the members of a periodic group, such as the halides. In other instances, a series of elements, such as the heavy metals, have been considered in the order of their atomic numbers. This arrangement of the elements helps to explain the chemistry and toxicology of their compounds.

A final section is composed of miscellaneous elements either because the compounds involved are not important as pesticides or as toxicants for mammals, or for both reasons.

The organometals and organometalloids have been described in connection with the corresponding inorganic compounds because, even though organic combination usually changes the absorption and distribution of a toxic metal and thus changes the emphasis of its effects, the basic mode of action remains the same. The poisoning produced by the highly toxic alkyl mercury compounds is mercury poisoning. This is in contrast to organic compounds of nonmetals, which often show no trace of any characteristic effect of a "toxic" atom. Thus the effects of the highly toxic monosodiumfluoroacetate show no real resemblance to poisoning by inorganic fluorides.

12.1 BARIUM

Barium is an alkaline earth metal in the same group as magnesium, calcium, strontium, and radium. Its valence is two. All water- and acid-soluble compounds of this element are poisonous. The intravenous LD 50 values of three of these compounds expressed as Ba^{2+} in two strains of mice ranged from 8.12 to 23.31 mg/kg, the toxicity being approximately the same as that of magnesium and greater than that of strontium (Syed and Hosain, 1972).

12.1.1 BARIUM CARBONATE

12.1.1.1 Identity, Properties, and Uses

Chemical Name Barium carbonate.

Structure $BaCO_3$.

Synonyms Barium carbonate occurs in nature as the mineral witherite. A code designation for commercial barium carbonate is C.I.-77,099. The CAS registry no. is 513-77-9.

Physical and Chemical Properties Barium carbonate has the empirical formula $CBaO_3$ and a molecular weight of 197.37. It is a tasteless, odorless, heavy white powder with a density of 4.2865. At about 1300°C it decomposes into BaO and CO_2. Its vapor pressure is negligible. Barium carbonate is almost insoluble in water. It is slightly soluble (1 : 1,000) in water saturated with carbon dioxide, soluble in dilute hydrochloric or nitric acids or in acetic acid, and soluble in solutions of ammonium chloride nitrate.

Formulations and Uses Barium carbonate is a rat poison. It also is used in ceramics, paints, enamels, rubber, and certain plastics. The technical product is 98–99% pure. Rodenticidal baits contain 20–25% of the compound.

12.1.1.2 Toxicity to Laboratory Animals

Basic Findings The oral LD 50 of a suspension of barium carbonate for wild Norway rats is 1480 mg/kg. The animals survive 1–8.5 days (Dieke & Richter, 1946). Strain differences in LD 50 values have been reported in mice (Syed and Hosain, 1972).

Apparently no study has been made of the effects of repeated doses of barium carbonate. However, the much more soluble and somewhat more toxic barium chloride has been studied. Rabbits given subcutaneous doses at rates as high as 10 mg/kg day showed no clinical effects. Rabbits given two daily doses at the rate of 10 mg/kg developed weakness, urination, defecation, difficult breathing, bradycardia, extrasystoles, and other signs lasting 2–4 hr following each dose (Fazekas *et al.*, 1953).

Absorption, Distribution, Metabolism, and Excretion Barium carbonate is highly insoluble in water. It is partially solubilized by acid in the stomach. The only real danger of the rodenticide is through ingestion. Various barium compounds can cause pneumoconiosis, but no form of poisoning by barium has been of much significance in industry.

Using ^{131}Ba, it was shown that absorption from the gastrointestinal tract of the rat was rapid and complete. The form of the curves of stomach, small intestine, and large intestine suggested a period of excretion by way of the gastrointestinal tract that followed the period of absorption and reached its maximum at about 48 hr. This excretion into the gastrointestinal tract was confirmed by other studies in which barium was administered by the intravenous route. Storage in bone increased for about 48 hr following oral administration and then decreased far more slowly than storage in other tissues. From the sixth day onward nearly all the barium remaining in the body was in the bone (Castagnou *et al.*, 1957). Several animal studies suggest that barium is incorporated into the bone matrix in a similar fashion to calcium (Bauer *et al.*, 1956; Bligh and Taylor, 1963; Dencker *et al.*, 1976; Taylor *et al.*, 1962). The uptake into bone decreases with age of the animal.

Study of rats injected intraperitoneally with ^{140}Ba indicated that excretion was most rapid during the first 4 hr and reached 7% in the urine and 20% in the feces in 24 hr (Bauer *et al.*, 1956).

Experiments in dogs showed that barium can be actively reabsorbed by the kidney tubules. Its clearance was correlated with calcium clearance. Protein binding of barium averaged 54% and was of the same order of magnitude as that of other alkaline earths. The data did not exclude a common transport mechanism with calcium (Rahill and Walser, 1965).

Mode of Action Barium stimulates striated, cardiac, and smooth muscle, regardless of innervation. It is antagonistic to all muscle depressants, no matter whether they act primarily on nerve or muscle. Initial stimulation of contraction leads to vasoconstriction through direct action on arterial muscle, peristalsis through action on smooth muscle, tremors and cramps through action on the skeletal muscles, and various arrhythmias through action on the heart. If the dose is sufficient, stimulation is followed by weakness and eventually by paralysis of the different kinds of muscle. Some effects such as hypertension, violent tremors, and convulsions are uncommon following ingestion of barium carbonate. They are more likely to follow absorption of more soluble barium compounds. If death does occur, it is caused by failure of muscular contraction leading to respiratory failure or cardiovascular collapse (Sollmann, 1957).

12.1.1.3 Toxicity to Humans

Experimental Exposure A solution of ^{140}BaCl$_2$ was injected intramuscularly into five children and intravenously into two adults, all with normal skeletal metabolism. Three of the children and one adult also received ^{45}CaCl$_2$ in the same injection. Following injection, the concentration of barium in the serum fell rapidly for about 0.6 day and then more slowly; even so, the amount detected on day 6 was less than 0.0002% of the dose. The pattern of excretion of calcium was similar, but both the initial and final rates were slower. Bone took up barium more rapidly than calcium under the same conditions, but, because of the more rapid excretion of barium, less of it was available to the bone. However, skeletal metabolism of the two elements was closely similar. Therefore, barium-140, which has a half-life of only 12.8 days, can be used for the study of skeletal metabolism in people (Bauer *et al.*, 1957).

Therapeutic Use Although barium carbonate has not been used as a drug, something can be learned from the use of the far more soluble barium chloride. The latter compound was formerly used in treating complete heart block. The degree of block was not changed, but even when the ventricular rate was not increased, the periods of marked bradycardia and asystole often were prevented. The usual dose was 30 mg three or four times a day or about 1.7 mg/kg/day. Use of the drug was abandoned, largely because of its toxicity.

Accidental Poisoning Apparently the major accident involving barium carbonate was one in which 85 British soldiers were poisoned by eating pastry made from flour accidentally contaminated by the compound intended for use as rat poison. The clinical picture was basically the same in all patients. In spite of some individual variation, three poorly defined stages could be recognized: (1) an acute gastroenteritis with mild sensory disturbance, (2) loss of deep reflexes and the onset of muscle paralysis, and (3) progressive muscular paralysis.

The first symptoms, which appeared 45–90 min after the contaminated food was eaten, were tingling around the mouth and in the neck, vomiting, and precipitate action of the bowels. Often the bowel action preceded the vomiting. Vomiting persisted, and later specimens contained flecks of blood. The stools became fluid and diarrheic, but contained nether blood nor mucus. Some patients complained of midabdominal colic, but this was not severe. Others had giddiness and palpitations.

The pupils, at first dilated, returned to normal within 2 hr; they reacted to light, but accommodation-convergence was impaired or lost. The heart rate varied from normal to rapid, but because of extrasystoles and perhaps variation in force, the pulse rate was always slower and sometimes only half as fast. Usually the rhythm was restored to normal in 2–3 hr. There was no staining of the lips or mouth, no rash, and no sweating. The patients complained of coldness; the temperatures were normal or subnormal.

Symptoms typical of the second stage usually were noticed 2 to 3 hr after the onset of illness. The tingling of the face and neck disappeared; instead tingling was experienced in the hands and feet. Vomiting and diarrhea continued in several cases throughout the first 24 hr, but this was no guide to the severity of the poisoning. The pupils responded rather sluggishly to light, accommodation was poor, and convergence was lost completely. In three cases there was some incoordination of the soft palate, but no true paralysis. The triceps jerks were absent; the biceps and supinator reflexes were sluggish and later absent. The knee jerks were lost in many cases, but the ankle jerks were consistently present. Varying degrees of motor paralysis developed. The extensor groups of muscles were affected before the flexor; the arms were affected before the legs; the muscle paralysis followed the same sequence as the loss of tendon reflexes. This sequence or pattern did not conform to a segmental or peripheral nerve distribution. There was no cranial nerve palsies, only minor disturbances of sight or hearing, and no defects of speech. The abdominal and plantar reflexes were normal. Sensation was unaffected, and there was no deep muscle tenderness.

Often improvement in all affected systems began 3–4 hr after onset, and recovery was complete within 24–36 hr. Only a few of the most severely affected patients proceeded to the third stage. In these few, general muscle paralysis began on the second day of the illness and lasted for a further 24 hr. There was complete muscle paralysis of arms and legs, and in one case the paralysis affected the muscles of respiration, but function of the diaphragm was sufficiently spared that the patient survived. Even these dangerously ill patients remained mentally clear, and recovery was surprisingly rapid; by the fourth day all affected muscles had regained their full power. There were no deaths.

Many of the patients with severe early diarrhea recovered much more rapidly than those with delayed bowel action (Morton, 1945).

Another major outbreak was caused by the substitution of barium carbonate for potato flour used in turkey sausage. There were over 100 cases but only 19 required hospitalization. In general, the findings were similar to those just described, but there were some additional ones. The blood pressure of patients was normal. Gastrointestinal bleeding for 4 days reduced the hemoglobin of one patient from 12.8 to 7.2 gm/100 ml. Muscular twitching was observed, especially in the more seriously ill patients. Maintenance in a respirator was required for 2.5 days in one case and for a shorter period in another. Testicular pain without objective sign was present in three

cases. It was of particular interest that no children became sick—or at least not sick enough to be brought to hospital— even though they had eaten the same food that made normal adults sick. Three adults who had had gastrectomies were unaffected also. Normal stomach acidity is required to solubilize barium carbonate (Lewi and Bar-Khayim, 1964).

A few additional signs and symptoms (thirst, sweating, blurred vision, a desire to urinate, and a moderately increased blood pressure) were recorded in an outbreak caused by substitution of barium carbonate for barium sulfate in preparation of a barium meal. Some of these cases illustrated the benefit of prompt administration of sodium or magnesium sulfate (Dean, 1950).

Electrocardiographic changes considered characteristic of hypokalemia have been reported by several authors in cases of poisoning by barium carbonate. Diengott *et al.* (1964) apparently were first to demonstrate hypokalemia (2.0–2.4 mEq/liter). Vomiting and diarrhea had not been sufficient in every instance to explain the low potassium levels, and exactly how barium produced hypokalemia was unexplained. It was the judgment of the attending physicians that infusion of as much as 9 gm of potassium chloride changed the clinical course or at least accelerated recovery. (One 75-year-old patient treated with KCl died suddenly 12 hr after developing right facial paresis and left hemiplegia. Autopsy was inadequate to explain the cause of death, but it seems likely he had a stroke unrelated to treatment and related only secondarily if at all to poisoning.)

Chronic effects in humans have not been well established. Brenniman *et al.* (1979) reported on approximately 150,000 people exposed to barium in drinking water at concentrations about 2 mg/liter (in excess of the federal standard) compared with communities having low levels in drinking water (less than 0.2 mg/liter) and noted that higher rates of cardiovascular disease were associated with higher barium concentrations. The study has two weaknesses—it depended on death certificates, which are known to lack accuracy on cause of death, and it did not take into account the use of home water softeners.

Dosage Response When barium carbonate was mistakenly used as an x-ray contrast medium, six patients survived 133 gm each (about 1900 mg/kg) but another died after only 53 gm. The author cited earlier reports indicating that as little as 4 gm (about 57 mg/kg) has proved fatal (Dean, 1950). However, such incidents must be rare, for in one large outbreak with no deaths among 85 cases, it was estimated, on the basis of analysis of the contaminated food, that the most severe cases received about 15 gm of barium carbonate (about 214 mg/kg). This rate is less than the LD 50 for the rat but sufficient to kill some rats. It seems likely that vomiting is important in protecting people who ingest barium carbonate.

Although the calculation must be viewed with caution, one might (by taking the ratio of the LD 50 values into account) conclude that a dosage of 28 mg/kg/day for barium carbonate is equivalent to what many years ago was a usual but often toxic dosage of 1.7 mg/kg/day for barium chloride.

The permissible occupational intake of soluble barium salts (as Ba^{2+}) is 0.07 mg/kg/day.

Laboratory Findings Hypokalemia may occur in severe poisoning. Apparently there is no report of the concentration of barium in a case of poisoning.

Following a single substantial dose, barium is deposited in bone (Bauer *et al.*, 1956). However, under practical conditions it does not act as a bone seeker. The concentration in normal human bone ash is only 7 ppm compared to average concentrations of 2.3–28 ppm in the ash of different organs (Snowden and Stitch, 1957; Snowden, 1958). Tipton and Cook (1963) reported that (except for skin, lung, and intestine, which may be environmentally exposed) the median value for barium in tissue ash did not exceed 7 ppm in the United States. Much higher concentrations of barium usually are found in Africa, the Near East, and the Far East (Tipton *et al.*, 1965). On a wet weight basis, the concentration of barium in normal plasma does not exceed 0.44 ppm (Gofman *et al.*, 1964).

Treatment of Poisoning Emptying of the stomach by vomiting or gastric lavage should be followed by sodium or magnesium sulfate (30 gm). These compounds act not only as purgatives but as detoxifying antidotes because they precipitate the toxic barium ion as insoluble barium sulfate. On the basis of both experimental studies and clinical experience, Lydtin *et al.* (1965) recommended that magnesium sulfate and calcium chloride be administered intravenously as early as possible in barium intoxication. They found this treatment effective even when administered several hours after intake of the poison.

The fluid and salt balance should be followed with particular attention to potassium and replacement therapy carried out as required. Be sure to have a respirator available. It may be lifesaving.

Atropine sulfate has been recommended for cramps and quinidine sulfate to prevent extrasystoles. The rationale of using these drugs in barium poisoning is not clear.

12.2 CHROMIUM

Chromium is a metal somewhat like iron and separated from it in the periodic table only by manganese. Chromium has valences of two, three, and six, but only hexavalent chromium compounds (chromates) are important as pesticides. They are also the most toxic.

Chromium in its trivalent state is an essential element. It is thought to be a necessary part of the glucose tolerance factor of the liver and required for certain other aspects of carbohydrate metabolism (Mertz, 1967).

12.2.1 SODIUM DICHROMATE

12.2.1.1 Identity, Properties, and Uses

Chemical Name Sodium dichromate.

Structure $Na_2Cr_2O_7 \cdot 2H_2O$.

Synonyms Other names for the compound are bichromate of soda and sodium bichromate. The CAS registry no. is 10588-01-9.

Physical and Chemical Properties Anhydrous sodium dichromate has the empirical formula $Cr_2Na_2O_7$ and a molecular weight of 261.96. The dihydrate forms reddish to bright orange elongated prismatic crystals with a density of 2.348 at 25°C. The anhydrous salt melts at 356.7°C and begins to decompose at about 400°C. It is very soluble in water.

Use Sodium dichromate is used as a defoliant of cotton and other plants and as a wood preservative.

12.2.1.2 Toxicity to Laboratory Animals

Basic Findings The lethal intravenous dosages of sodium dichromate for several species are in the range of 37–417 mg/kg. The toxicity of the potassium salt is of the same order of magnitude and its lethal oral dosage for the dog is 2829 mg/kg (Spector, 1955). Although one report (Schroeder, 1973) indicated that prolonged administration of 5 ppm hexavalent chromium in drinking water produced a slight decrease in growth, other studies indicate that concentrations up to 10,000 ppm may be given without ill effect (MacKenzie *et al.*, 1958; Gross and Heller, 1946).

Absorption, Distribution, Metabolism, and Excretion Chromate is absorbed by the lung (Baetjer *et al.*, 1959), gastrointestinal tract (MacKenzie *et al.*, 1959; Ogawa, 1976), and skin (Wahlberg, 1965). It can also be absorbed from skin injured by it, and when the burn covers as much as 10% of the body surface the absorption may be sufficient to cause fatal poisoning.

Normal male rats have average chromium concentrations of 0.05 ppm in the liver, 0.28 ppm in the kidney, 0.77 ppm in the bone, and 0.91 ppm in the spleen. The values for females are slightly higher for some tissues, reflecting greater food intake. Male rats fed hexavalent chromium in their drinking water for a year at a rate of 25 ppm were uninjured, but they stored chromium at average concentrations of 3.2 ppm in liver, 10.47 ppm in kidney, 4.07 ppm in bone, and 23.85 ppm in spleen. Trivalent chromium was stored much less when fed at the same rate (MacKenzie *et al.*, 1958).

Effects on Organs and Tissues Acute poisoning may produce death rapidly through shock or after several days through renal tubular damage and uremia. In most cases, the primary effect of acute exposure is kidney failure (Mathur *et al.*, 1977; Evan and Dail, 1974). Berry *et al.* (1978) noted that chromium was localized within the proximal renal tubules specifically within the lysosomes. It was retained throughout the study period of 8 months and was eliminated only when the entire cytoplasm underwent necrosis. Kirschbaum *et al.* (1981) have postulated that the initial effect is on specific elements of the microfilamentous system that is responsible for directing intracellular flow of reabsorbed solutes. The liver and other organs may be involved but generally to a lesser degree.

In at least some countries, workers heavily exposed to chrome compounds have shown an excess of bronchiogenic cancer, and this has led to attempts to duplicate the findings in animals. A 1973 World Health Organization (WHO) review (where references may be found) concluded that "In many experiments, various chromium compounds have been shown to induce tumors in mice and rats." Six squamous cell carcinomas and two adenocarcinomas were found in 100 rats that had had pellets of calcium chromate implanted intrabronchially. One squamous cell carcinoma was found among 100 other rats that received chromium "process residue." Other chromium compounds were negative (Laskin *et al.*, 1970). An increase of pulmonary adenomas but no squamous cell carcinomas appeared in mice that inhaled calcium chromate dust throughout their lives (Nettesheim *et al.*, 1971). Several authors have reported sarcomas at the site of injection or implantation. However, the relevance of such sarcomas is questionable. A number of studies involving oral or respiratory exposure have been negative (Steffee and Baetjer, 1965). All in all, evidence for the carcinogenicity of chromium in animals is weak.

12.2.1.3 Toxicity to Humans

Use Experience Significant injury to the liver, gastrointestinal system, and blood has been reported rarely in connection with industrial exposure. However, many cases of industrial injury to the skin and to the nasal and respiratory mucous membranes have been produced by hexavalent chromium compounds (Browning, 1969). A small part of this involved chromates intended for use in pesticides. Contact dermatitis was reported in men who handled timber treated with chromium (Behrbohm, 1957).

Most concern about the toxicology of chromates was the result of a high incidence of bronchiogenic cancer among men with heavy occupational, respiratory exposure in Germany (Pfeil, 1935); the United States (Machle and Gregorius, 1948; Baetjer, 1950a,b; Mancuso and Hueper, 1951; Koven *et al.*, 1953; Brinton *et al.*, 1952; Taylor, 1966; Hayes *et al.*, 1979); Norway (Langard and Norseth, 1975); and the United Kingdom (Bidstrup and Case, 1956; Royle, 1975). In most of the studies, smoking data were inadequate to evaluate smoking as a confounding variable. However, the reported relative risks— in the range of 23 to 32—are higher than what would normally be due to smoking, where relative risks are about 10-fold (U.S. Department of Health and Human Services, 1982). Overall, despite some negative findings (Okubo and Tsuchiya, 1979), there is sufficient evidence to classify chromium as a human carcinogen according to the definitions of the International Agency for Research on Cancer (IARC) (1980).

The exact form of chromium responsible for lung cancer in chromate workers is not clear (WHO, 1973). Certainly the condition occurred when exposure to a wide range of chrome compounds was high. Workroom concentrations as high as 3.27, 5.6, or even 50 mg/m^3 have been reported. New cases apparently do not occur in new plants where it is possible to enforce a threshold limit of 0.1 mg/m^3 expressed as CrO_3 (Stokinger, 1963). In order to give an even greater margin of safety, the threshold limit value recently has been reduced to 0.05 mg/m^3 expressed as chromium ion.

There is no evidence that the use of chromates as wood preservatives offers any hazard of cancer.

Dosage Response Judging from urinary excretion, absorption of chromium at a rate of not less than 0.02 mg/kg/day led to serious illness; twice that rate of absorption also produced liver injury in other workers, although no symptoms appeared. Recommended occupational standards are 500 µg/m^3 for soluble and 1000 µm/m^3 for insoluble forms of chromium [Occupational Safety and Health Administration (OSHA), (1978)].

Laboratory Findings Chromium can be detected in almost every sample of normal tissue. For most organs, the median value for concentration is close to the limits of detection. For example, the median concentration in the liver ash is 0.7 ppm or about 0.009 ppm, wet weight. The concentration in plasma does not exceed 0.04 ppm (Gofman *et al.*, 1964). The lung and skin, however, have median concentrations in the order of 0.17 and 0.22 ppm, wet weight, presumably because of their direct exposure to contamination. Most investigators have found similar results in the United States (Tipton and Cook, 1963). However, men of the same age from the Near East and Far East have significantly higher values for all tissues except lung (Tipton *et al.*, 1965).

Investigations by Guthrie *et al.* (1978), Kayne *et al.* (1978), and Andersen (1981) indicate that measurements of chromium by atomic absorption in normal blood and urine before 1978 were probably too high due to inadequate background correction. Kayne *et al.* (1978) reported a mean value in human serum in nonexposed adults as 0.14 ppb. These findings agree with those of Versieck *et al.* (1968) who, in 20 adult subjects, found a range of 0.04 to 0.35 ppb with a mean value of 0.16 ppb. Some previous measurements are in good agreement with these figures (Hambridge, 1971; Pekarek *et al.*, 1974). The most recent figures for normal urinary concentrations of chromium indicate values less than 1 ppb with mean values between 0.3 and 0.4 ppb (Guthrie *et al.*, 1978; Kayne *et al.*, 1978; Veillen *et al.*, 1979). Chromium concentrations have been reported in human hair (Schroeder and Tipton, 1968; Hambridge *et al.*, 1972; Hambridge and Droegnueller, 1974), but it is not clear to what extent hair concentrations represent tissue chromium or the degree of external exposure of the hair.

Urinary concentrations in occupational exposures are several orders of magnitude higher than normal values. Tandon *et al.* (1977) reported values in the range of 91 to 1116 ppb in electroplaters and polishers having 2–10 years of exposure. Values did not correlate with length of exposure. Pascale *et al.*

(1952) reported urinary concentrations in the range of 180 to 2880 ppb in clinically asymptomatic workers with a moderate disturbance in liver function.

Treatment of Poisoning Chromium is chelated by dimercaprol and by calcium disodium edetate, of which the latter is preferred (Hayes, 1975). Otherwise treatment is symptomatic (Hayes, 1975). Chelating agents are also valuable for treating chrome ulcers of the skin. A 10% calcium disodium edetate ointment was effective in treating all of 54 chrome skin ulcers. In about 90% of cases, the complex chrome salts adherent to the base of the ulcer could be removed painlessly after the ointment had been applied for 24 hr. In the remaining cases, removal of the adherent chrome could be carried out after 48 or at most 72 hr. Once its base had been cleared of chrome salts, the ulcer healed promptly (Maloof, 1955).

12.3 COPPER

Copper compounds are not an important source of poisoning [for a recent general review, see U.S. Environmental Protection Agency (USEPA), 1987]. With few exceptions, those used as pesticides owe their mammalian toxicity to a massive overdose of copper ions, especially the cupric ion. Because many of the compounds do not dissolve readily, their toxicity is low. However, copper sulfate is a soluble, ionizable compound. It has been the cause of the majority of cases of poisoning involving copper compounds, and its effects are typical of those involving an excess of copper ions.

The toxicities of copper acetoarsenite and copper arsenate are related to their arsenic content (see Section 12.12).

Copper is an essential element. It is closely associated with the absorption and metabolism of iron. Zinc and molybdenum also interact with copper. Copper is necessary for the formation of hemoglobin, although it is not part of the molecule. When copper is deficient, hemoglobin is not formed at the normal rate even though there is a reserve of iron in the liver. Copper is also required for bone formation. The element is also essential for carbohydrate metabolism, catecholamine biosynthesis, and the cross-linking of collagen, elastin, and hair keratin. Copper is an integral part of more than 12 specific proteins including cytochrome oxidase, tyrosinase, ascorbic acid oxidase, uricase, catalase, and peroxidase.

Deficiency of copper occurs occasionally in domestic animals and is easily produced experimentally. Signs of copper deficiency include anemia, gastrointestinal disturbances, depressed growth, dystrophy of bone, depigmentation of hair or wool, impaired reproduction, and heart failure (Underwood, 1977). Copper deficiency has not been described in humans, probably because adequate copper occurs in such a wide variety of human food.

Many vegetables, cereals, and meats contain between 1 and 10 ppm of copper, but liver contains about 24 ppm and oysters about 36 ppm. The normal dietary intake of copper usually does not exceed 5 mg/day but usually does exceed 2 mg/day

(Davies and Bennett, 1983). Kehoe *et al.* (1940a) reported an average intake of 2.32 mg/day. Additional intake such as that from occupational exposure leads to little increase in the retention of copper. Drinking water is not an important source of copper except in rare cases where soft water has been contained in copper piping for long periods (Piscator, 1979). The existence of a hereditary disease (hepatolenticular degeneration or Wilson's disease) characterized by abnormal absorption and retention of copper from a normal diet calls attention to the precision with which copper metabolism is regulated in healthy persons. Some information on the concentration of copper in different normal tissues is given in Section 12.3.1.3.

12.3.1 COPPER SULFATE

12.3.1.1 Identity, Properties, and Uses

Chemical Name Cupric sulfate.

Structure $CuSO_4$.

Synonyms Copper sulfate also is known as blue copperas, bluestone, blue vitrol, Roman vitrol, and Salzburg vitrol. It occurs in nature as the mineral hydrocyanite. The CAS registry no. is 7758-98-7.

Physical and Chemical Properties Copper sulfate occurs as the anhydride, a monohydrate, and the pentahydrate, which is the form used as a fungicide or algacide. The molecular weight for the anhydride is 159.61, and that for the pentahydrate is 267.6. The pentahydrate forms a blue, crystalline, odorless solid with a metallic taste. It occurs in nature as the mineral chalcanthite. Its density at 15.6°C is 2.286. Most formulations of copper sulfate contain 98–99% pure salt. The compound is soluble in water (316 g/liter at 0°C) but insoluble in ethanol and most organic solvents. Copper sulfate solutions are strongly corrosive to iron and galvanized iron. The crystals are slightly efflorescent in air.

History, Formulations, and Uses The fungicidal activity of soluble copper salts was discovered in 1807 by B. Prévost. The algicidal properties of the salts came into practical use about 1895. Copper sulfate is used as a fungicide for control of downy mildew, blights, leaf spots, apple scab, bitter rot, and peachleaf curl. It also is used as an herbicide for the control of algae in water. Bordeaux mixture, formed from $CuSO_4$ and $Ca(OH)_2$, is used as a fungicide and seed treatment.

12.3.1.2 Toxicity to Laboratory Animals

Basic Findings The oral LD 50 of copper sulfate for the rat is 960 mg/kg (Stokinger, 1981) and in mice is 87 mg/kg (Jones *et al.*, 1980). The reason for large species differences is not known. Poisoned animals show violent retching, muscular spasms, and collapse. The onset is within a few minutes of dosing, and many rats die within an hour. However, some survive the gastrointestinal irritation only to die several days later of systemic effects (Lehman, 1951, 1952).

Rats fed copper sulfate for 4 weeks at a dietary level of 500 ppm as copper (about 25 mg/kg/day) showed slightly decreased food intake and a slight decrease in growth rate but appeared entirely normal. Higher dietary levels of copper led to progressively greater food refusal. Rats fed 4000 ppm ate less than one-fifth the normal amount of food, lost weight, and died within a week. Part of their trouble was starvation, for they ingested less copper (7.6 mg/rat/day) than rats that survived 4 weeks when fed 2000 ppm (9.8 to 11.8 mg/rat/day) (Boyden *et al.*, 1938). Pigs maintained on diets supplemented with copper sulfate (250–425 ppm) for 48–79 days exhibited a gradual development of anemia, jaundice, hepatic necrosis, gastrointestinal hemorrhage, and decreased weight gain (Suttle and Mills, 1966a,b). Pigs exposed to 100–500 ppm of copper sulfate in the diet for 54–88 days experienced reductions in hemoglobin and hematocrit and reduced weight gain (Kline *et al.*, 1971). Data are not available for long-term toxicity in experimental animals.

Two inhalation studies (Johansson *et al.*, 1984; Lundborg and Camner, 1984) found no toxic effects in the lungs of rabbits exposed to 0.6 mg/m³ of copper chloride 6 hr/day, 5 days/week for up to 6 weeks. Pimentel and Marques (1969) exposed 12 guinea pigs to a saturated atmosphere of Bordeaux mixture for 6.5 months, three times daily (the duration of each exposure was not reported), and found micronodular lesions and hysticocytic granulomas. In a brief report, Eckert and Jerochin (1982) claim that copper sulfate is the principal toxic agent in Bordeaux mixtures.

Absorption, Distribution, Metabolism, and Excretion The normal uptake of copper is outlined in Section 12.3 and its normal storage in Section 12.3.1.3. Rats fed copper for 4 weeks at the rate of about 22 mg/kg/day showed only a slightly increased concentration in the blood or spleen but about a 14-fold greater concentration in the liver. Rats fed copper for the same period at a rate of about 46 mg/kg/day showed a maximal increase of 2–5 times in the copper content of the blood and spleen but an increase as great as 300 times in the liver (Boyden *et al.*, 1938).

Copper absorption after an oral dose occurs in the upper gastrointestinal tract in mammals (Evans, 1973). Two mechanisms are involved. One is an energy-dependent process involving copper–amino acid complexes (Kirchgessner *et al.*, 1967) and the other involves an inducible carrier protein (Evans and Johnson, 1978). Absorbed copper is predominantly bound to albumin and is transported to the liver, which is the main storage organ. Copper is incorporated into a number of enzymes. It is secreted in bile and also incorporated into ceruloplasm, an alpha globulin that accounts for about 90% of all copper in plasma. Ceruloplasmin is a major regulator of copper retention and storage. The major route of excretion is the feces via secretion in bile. Urinary excretion is a minor route (Underwood, 1977).

Mode of Action The corrosive effect of large doses of copper sulfate in the gastrointestinal tract leads to shock, which may be the cause of death. Damage to the erythrocytes, liver, and kidney may combine to kill patients who survive the initial effects. The biochemical mechanism of excessive doses of copper is not well understood.

12.3.1.3 Toxicity to Humans

Therapeutic Use Copper sulfate (300 mg in 100 ml of water) has been used as an emetic in cases of known or suspected poisoning by other compounds. If vomiting did not occur, intestinal colic, diarrhea, and systemic symptoms often appeared (Sollmann, 1957).

Although copper is essential for life, it is questionable whether people ever fail to get enough in their diet. Be that as it may, some preparations now on the market supply not only iron and often vitamins but also copper. This may be in the form of 1 mg of copper sulfate per tablet.

Accidental and Intentional Poisoning At least until recently, practically all systemic illness attributed to copper sulfate was the result of accidental or suicidal ingestion. Although such acute poisoning is uncommon in the United States, it is common in some countries (Chawla and Mehta, 1973).

The corrosive action of the copper may produce a characteristic stain of the mucous membranes of the mouth and pharanyx and will certainly produce severe painful gastrointestinal irritation, nausea, and diarrhea. The repeated vomiting of bluegreen masses is common. The stools are profuse and watery at first and later contain blood. Patients often die in shock 2 or 3 hours after ingestion of the poison. If they survive, the absorption of copper produces severe hemolysis so that hemoglobinuria and anemia are present in 5–6 hours, and icterus appears soon after. If the patient survives a few days, signs of liver damage and renal tubular damage may appear. A fatal case was described in detail by Chugh *et al.* (1975). In one series of cases, 11 of 29 patients developed acute renal failure. Intravascular hemolysis appeared to be the chief factor responsible for the renal lesions. Although uremia was controlled adequately by dialysis, only 6 of the 11 patients recovered. Septicemia was responsible for death in three, hepatic failure in one, and methemoglobinemia in another (Chugh *et al.*, 1977). Katoh *et al.* (1977) reported a case that was typical in showing the usual initial signs followed by severe anemia, icterus, and kidney failure but very unusual in that the patient died after surviving 40 days.

Two unusual cases attributed to residues were reported from Hungary. A 9-year-old boy died 10 hr after eating three bunches of grapes and a 5-year-old died 24 hr after eating two bunches. Much of the poison was expelled by vomiting, which began soon after the grapes were eaten. Expressed as $CuSO_4$, a total of 572 mg, equivalent to 22 mg/kg, was recovered from all tissues in the first case. A total of 463 mg, equivalent to 28.9 mg/kg, was recovered in the second case (Fazekas, 1964). In view of the large amount of copper found in the tissues and the fact that it represented only a fraction of that originally present on the grapes, one can only conclude that the residues were massive. The fruit must have been encrusted with copper sulfate.

A disease known as Indian childhood cirrhosis has been associated with high intakes of copper (Sharda, 1984). The disease is characterized by hepatic necrosis, Mallory's hyaline inclusions in many hepatocytes, intralobular fibrosis, and very high copper content in liver (Pundit and Bhave, 1983). It is generally believed that water and milk stored in copper or brass vessels lead to high intakes in children.

Use Experience   Ordinary occupational exposure may lead to an itching, papulovesicular eczema. Contact with the eye by copper sulfate dust or even strong solutions may produce conjunctivitis or ulceration of the cornea.

Two cases of pneumoconiosis were described in spraymen who had applied Bordeaux mixture to vineyards for several years. Symptoms included shortness of breath, weakness, loss of weight, and cough productive of a thick, yellow sputum. Although no tubercle bacilli were found, tuberculosis was diagnosed on the basis of diffusely abnormal chest x-rays. In hospital, both patients improved slowly, both clinically and radiologically. However, recovery was incomplete, and symptoms recurred as soon as the men were reexposed to Bordeaux mixture spray (Pimentel and Marques, 1969). The account indicated that the condition responded to cessation of exposure and may have been improved by rest, but there was no evidence that drugs intended for tuberculosis are beneficial against copper pneumoconiosis. Later study showed that some patients presented not with characteristic respiratory symptoms but with chills, fever, joint and muscular pain, weakness, and/or anorexia that became severe enough to cause hospitalization only 2 or 3 weeks after onset. Although no pathological organism was identified, it was assumed that persons suffering from vineyard sprayer's lung were unusually susceptible to infection. Regardless of the exact mechanism, the condition certainly was the cause of death in many in whom it was recognized (Pimentel and Menezes, 1975, 1976). Apparently no evaluation of the hazard of using Bordeaux mixture sprays has been made. One paper (Pimentel and Menezes, 1976) was based on 30 autopsies, but there was no indication of the size of the population of workers with similar exposure from whom this sample was drawn. Be that as it may, it is astonishing that so serious a disease was recognized so recently in connection with a kind of occupational exposure that began in 1882. In fact the recent recognition of the condition and the restricted geographical distribution of cases recognized so far forces one to consider the possibility that some unrecognized factor may be critical to development of the condition. Epidemiological study certainly is needed.

Dosage Response   The fatal dose for humans is difficult to estimate because of vomiting, but it is about 10 gm for adults or 140 mg/kg. This estimate of the fatal ingested dosage is not inconsistent with the observed fatal retained dosage mentioned

earlier. An 18-month-old boy narrowly survived a dosage estimated at 262 mg/kg that was reduced to an unknown degree by vomiting and gastric lavage (Walsh et al., 1977). The usual emetic dose of copper sulfate is 4.3 mg/kg or slightly more. However, an accidental dosage probably no more than half as large as regards copper ion may cause vomiting, diarrhea, and abdominal cramps (Pennypacker et al., 1975). The average normal intake of copper ion is about 0.03 mg/kg/day. The permissible occupational respiratory intake is 0.143 mg/kg/day.

Laboratory Findings   The peak blood copper level in a fatal case was 82.67 ppm (Chugh et al., 1975). A child who narrowly survived had an initial serum level of 16.5 ppm (Walsh et al., 1977).

The milk of female vineyard workers, who were exposed to copper sulfate and a variety of other pesticides, contained 6.2 times as much copper as the milk of milkmaids who did equally hard work but were not exposed to pesticides. Placentas from the vineyard workers contained 4.7 times more copper than those from milkmaids (Nikitina, 1974).

Copper is essential to life and occurs in all tissues. Kehoe et al. (1940a) reported that the concentrations in blood, muscle, and most of the viscera range from 0.85 to 1.90 ppm. Values for plasma lie in the narrow range of 1.16 to 1.42 ppm (Gofman et al., 1964). The concentrations in the brain (2.2–6.8 ppm), liver (7.1 ppm in adults and 24 ppm in infants), and bone (3.7–4.7 ppm in rib and 6.8 ppm in long bones) are higher. The concentration in erythrocytes is slightly greater than that in the plasma. The values reported by Tipton and Cook (1963) and by Liebscher and Smith (1968) are basically similar but expressed on a different basis. The organs of Orientals frequently contain more copper than those of Americans (Tipton et al., 1965). The concentration of copper in the urine varies from 0.01 to 0.08 and averages about 0.034 ppm (Kehoe et al., 1940a). Fecal excretion is greater than urinary excretion and averages 1.96 mg/day according to Kehoe et al. (1940a). A review of the literature on the concentration of copper in normal tissue and excreta was prepared by Kehoe et al. (1940b).

Pathology   Persons who die soon after ingestion of copper sulfate show on autopsy a characteristic staining of the lining of the digestive tract and fatty degeneration of the liver, kidney, and to some degree other organs. Persons who develop acute renal failure as part of acute poisoning by copper sulfate may or may not show well established acute tubular necrosis. In those who survive long enough, granulomatous lesions of the kidney may develop (Chugh et al., 1977).

Biopsy revealed nodules containing copper in the lungs of men who developed pneumoconiosis following years of exposure to Bordeaux mixture (Pimentel and Marques, 1969). Later study of biopsy and autopsy material from workers exposed to Bordeaux mixture sprays for 3 to 35 years revealed that many rural workers who developed pulmonary granulomas developed liver granulomas also, and in some the liver was enlarged. The liver granulomas varied, with all transitional forms, from those consisting entirely of histiocytic cells to those consisting of clusters of epithelioid cells perfectly organized in sarcoid-type follicles. No giant cells or lymphocytic borders were observed. A finely granular material in the granuloma cells and in prominent Kupffer cells did not stain for ferric iron but was positive for copper when stained with rubeanic acid. No copper was demonstrable in the hepatocytes. Thus the distribution of copper in the liver was entirely different from that in any previously described granulomatosis of whatever origin. Some of the patients also had micronodular cirrhosis or fatty change of the liver, but it was thought that this might be due to alcoholism. Angiosarcoma and idiopathic portal hypertension also were seen (Pimentel and Menezes, 1975, 1976).

Treatment of Poisoning   Treatment should include a prompt effort to prevent absorption and later the use of a chelating agent. The protein of milk or egg white combines with copper to form an insoluble copper proteinate. However, the product must be removed by vomiting or lavage before it is digested and the copper released. Copper may also be precipitated by potassium ferrocyanide given in a dose of 600 mg in a glass of water.

BAL, dicalcium EDTA, and penicillamine are all effective in binding copper. Penicillamine is definitely the drug of choice in Wilson's disease. There is less experience on which to base a choice in the treatment of acute poisoning.

12.4 ZINC

Zinc follows copper in the periodic table, and, like copper, it is an essential element. More than 20 metalloenzymes containing zinc have been identified. These include alcohol dehydrogenase, alkaline phosphatase, carbonic anhydrase, and DNA polymerase [National Research Council (NRC), 1979]. Zinc forms a necessary part of carbonic anhydrase, carboxypeptidase, alcohol dehydrogenase, lactic acid dehydrogenase, glutamic dehydrogenase, and alkaline dehydrogenase molecules (Vallec, 1959, 1962).

It has been known for some time that a deficiency of zinc leads to testicular atrophy and failure of body growth in animals. Recently, zinc deficiency, complicated only by iron deficiency, has been found in patients from villages in the Middle East who exhibited severe growth retardation and sexual hypofunction. In adolescent patients, zinc supplementation alone resulted in body growth, gonadal development, and the appearance of secondary sexual characteristics. Some of the dwarfs who received reagent grade iron but no zinc failed to develop sexually, and their growth rate was less than that following zinc (Prasad, 1966). Dermatitis also is seen in zinc deficiency. Animal experiments indicate that simultaneous administration of cadmium will exacerbate the effects of zinc deficiency (Petering et al., 1971). Poor intestinal absorption of

zinc is believed to be a factor in the familial disease acrodermatitis enterohepatica (Moynahan, 1974).

Zinc is a normal constituent of food, and only rarely is it possible to avoid an adequate intake. The average daily intake of zinc in different areas of the world ranges from 5 to 22 mg in adults (Halsted et al., 1974). Protein-rich foods, especially marine organisms such as oysters, have the highest levels (10–50 mg/kg wet weight), whereas concentrations in grains, vegetables, and fruits are relatively low, usually less than 5 mg/kg fresh weight (Great Britain Ministry of Agriculture, Fisheries and Food, 1981). The concentration in drinking water is usually the same as in freshwater and seawater (1–10 μg/liter) but may be much higher if the water is passed through zinc-coated pipes (Sharrett et al., 1982). Information on the concentration of zinc in normal human tissue is given in Section 12.4.1.3.

Pesticides containing zinc may be divided into four classes: (a) Most inorganic and certain organic compounds of zinc that are toxic because sufficient doses supply an excess of zinc ions. Examples include zinc chloride and zinc acetate. These compounds are discussed in the following section. (b) Complexes of zinc with other elements, the greater toxicity of which predominates in the effect of the complex regardless of the exact chemical combination. An example is zinc arsenate. (c) Zinc phosphide, which owes its toxicity to the phosphine (PH_3) it produces (see Sections 12.4.2 and 14.6.2). (d) Certain organic compounds of zinc, the toxicity of which is not essentially different from those of similar compounds that are salts of other metals. An example is zineb (see Section 21.12.5).

12.4.1 ZINC CHLORIDE

12.4.1.1 Identity, Properties, and Uses

Chemical Name   Zinc chloride.

Structure $ZnCl_2$.

Synonyms   Other names include butter of zinc and zinc dichloride. The CAS registry no. is 7646-85-7.

Physical and Chemical Properties   Zinc chloride has the empirical formula Cl_2Zn and a molecular weight of 136.29. It forms white, odorless, very deliquescent granules with a density of 2.907. It has a melting point of approximately 290°C and a boiling point of 732°C. One gram of zinc chloride dissolves in 0.5 ml water, 1.3 ml ethanol, or 2 ml glycerol. The compound is freely soluble in acetone. Zinc oxychloride is formed in the presence of water.

Formulations and Uses   Technical grade is at least 95% pure, the remainder being mostly water and oxychloride. Zinc chloride may be used with copper and chromium compounds as a wood preservative.

12.4.1.2 Toxicity to Laboratory Animals

Basic Findings   Zinc chloride may be taken as typical of those compounds that owe their toxicity to the zinc ion. However, in order to gain a reasonably complete picture of the toxicity of the ion it is necessary to refer to other compounds also. The small differences in toxicity between most zinc compounds are explained by differences in their solubility and degree of ionization.

The intraperitoneal lethal dose of zinc chloride for the mouse is 31 mg/kg (Franz, 1962). The oral lethal dose of the equally soluble zinc sulfate for both rats and rabbits is in the range of 1914 to 2200 mg/kg (Spector, 1955).

It requires repeated intake of massive amounts of zinc to cause injury. Even when they were fed zinc carbonate at a dietary level of 7000 ppm of zinc (about 350 mg/kg/day), young rats survived, although they developed marked anemia in 4 weeks and grew poorly. A dietary level of 10,000 ppm killed up to 75% of rats in 3–5 weeks. For rats on either of these diets, the additional feeding of copper maintained the hemoglobin at significantly higher levels. A mixture of iron, copper, and cobalt maintained hemoglobin at essentially normal levels, although iron or cobalt supplements alone had no effect. Iron, copper, and cobalt had no effect on subnormal growth of rats fed zinc, but supplements of liver extract produce a highly significant growth response (Smith and Larson, 1946). Certain of these results have been retested and confirmed, and it was found that repression of growth is linear over the dietary range of 3000 to 7000 ppm (Van Reen and Pearson, 1953). Mice given 500 mg Zn/liter as zinc sulfate in drinking water exhibited hypertrophy of the adrenal cortex and of the pancreatic islets (Aughey *et al.*, 1977).

Absorption, Distribution, Metabolism, and Excretion   Early studies (Drinker *et al.*, 1927a,b) indicate that animals can regulate zinc absorption such that large oral doses produce minimal change in tissue levels. Thus intestinal absorption is highly variable (10–90%), depending on zinc status and the magnitude of the oral dose. Also, calcium and phytates in food interfere with zinc absorption (Becker and Hoekstra, 1971). Metallothionein may play a role in regulation of zinc absorption (Richards and Cousins, 1976). In humans, absorption of zinc in fish food is about 35% (Honstead and Brady, 1967).

Zinc is highest in bone, liver, and kidney in mice 2 weeks after a single trace dose (Ansari *et al.*, 1975). Levels in human tissues are reported in Section 12.4.1.3.

Zinc is secreted in bile (Barrowman *et al.*, 1973) and fecal excretion is considerably greater than urinary excretion in both animals (Schryver *et al.*, 1980) and humans (Aamodt *et al.*, 1979). In humans in normal zinc studies, the biological half-time is in the range 160–500 days (Aamodt *et al.*, 1975). Bone and muscle, which contain the major amount of the body zinc, have longer biological half-times than other tissues, e.g., liver (NRC, 1979).

Mode of Action   A sufficient dose of a soluble zinc salt can produce shock and lead to rapid death. The mechanism of delayed mortality is poorly understood. The toxicity of prolonged high intake of zinc consists, at least in part, of a relative deficiency of other trace metals and nutrients (Smith and Larson, 1946) and is not caused by inhibition of catalase or cytochrome oxidase (Van Reen and Pearson, 1953). Campbell and Mills (1979) have shown that copper deficiency caused by excessive zinc intake may play a role in zinc toxicity.

Treatment of Poisoning in Animals   By using ^{65}Zn injected intravenously as the chloride, it was shown that the intramuscular injection of British Anti-Lewisite (BAL) doubled the concentration of zinc in the red cells, increased urinary excretion as much as 20 times (from a level of 4% or less of the administered dose), and decreased fecal excretion (from a level of 31% to 42% of the administered dose in rats that received no BAL). Total excretion of zinc was increased. Under the conditions used, the injection of BAL completely eliminated acute toxicity but did not prevent death 72–96 hours after injection. In fact, BAL seemed to accentuate the renal damage caused by sufficient zinc (Bruner, 1950). The study throws no light on the question of whether BAL would divert a harmful amount of zinc through the kidneys under practical conditions of accidental poisoning.

12.4.1.3 Toxicity to Humans

Therapeutic Use   Zinc oxide and zinc carbonate, which are highly insoluble, are applied liberally to inflamed skin in the form of powder, calamine lotion, and the like. Zinc chloride, sulfate, and acetate have been used for their antiseptic, astringent, or caustic properties. Their use is limited by difficulty of local control, not by systemic effects. Zinc sulfate has been used as an emetic at an oral dose of 1000 or 2000 mg in a glass of water (Sollmann, 1957). This dose intentionally produces a concentration in the water well above the threshold (675–2280 ppm) that may lead to vomiting if taken on an empty stomach, as sometimes happens accidentally when fruit juice or other acid drinks are stored in galvanized vessels.

Accidents and Use Experience   Zinc chloride is caustic. Stokinger (1963) recorded without detail or reference that it has caused dermatitis in men working with railroad crossties treated with the compound as a fungicide. More direct contact with zinc chloride, as in its use as a soldering flux, may cause ulceration of the fingers, hands, and forearms. Respiratory exposure to a sufficient concentration of zinc chloride smoke is highly irritating to the mucous membranes of the nasopharynx, trachea, and bronchi and may be fatal (Evans, 1945). Schaidt *et al.* (1979) have proposed that the high toxicity of $ZnCl_2$ in the lung is due to the formation of hydrochloric acid.

Zinc chloride intended for use as a pesticide apparently has not led to injury other than dermatitis. Ingestion undoubtedly would produce illness similar to that caused by copper sulfate. In several instances, the preparation or storage of an acid food in a galvanized or zinc-plated vessel has led to severe vomiting and to headache and discomfort in the chest (Hegsted *et al.*, 1945).

Dosage Response The lethal dose in humans is unknown but has been estimated at 3000–5000 mg (43–71 mg/kg). The emetic dosage is 14–28 mg/kg. Zinc intake from food and water is usually at the rate of about 0.14–0.21 mg/kg/day but in some communities it may reach 0.75 mg/kg/day without injury. To prevent respiratory irritation and other effects of fumes from $ZnCl_2$, the American Conference of Governmental Industrial Hygienists (ACGIH) (1981) have set a threshold limit value of 1 mg/m^3 and a short-term exposure limit of 2 mg/m^3.

Laboratory Findings There is only moderate variation between the normal concentrations of zinc in different tissues; in most organs it is about 20 to 30 ppm; in liver, bone, and voluntary muscle it is from 60 to 180 ppm. Higher concentrations are found in the prostate (860 ppm) and the retina (500–1000 ppm), while blood contains 6.6–8.8 ppm, of which the greater part is in the red cells. The plasma contains only 0.93–1.03 ppm (Gofman et al., 1964), but whole blood contains 0.60–19.87 ppm with a mean of 5.30 ppm (Kubota et al., 1968). Excretion of zinc is chiefly via the feces (Vallee, 1959). The daily urinary output is about 0.5 mg (Halsted et al., 1974; Elinder et al., 1978). Studies carried out on dry tissue by neutron activation gave higher numerical values but indicate relationships in the zinc concentrations of different tissues similar to those found in the older studies. Relatively high values are found in the kidney, hair, nails, and especially teeth, as well as in the liver, bone, and muscle (Tipton and Cook, 1963; Liebscher and Smith, 1968). It is interesting that in some carnivores the concentration of zinc in the tapetum lucidum is in the range of 61,000 to 146,000 ppm dry weight (Vallee, 1959). People in the Far East tend to contain a little more zinc (Tipton et al., 1965).

Apparently, concentrations in the tissues and excreta of heavily exposed people have been reported only rarely. Trevisan et al. (1982) reported that workers exposed to air concentrations above 1.4 mg Zn/m^3 had mean plasma values of 1.4 mg/liter and a urinary excretion of 0.8 mg Zn/gm creatinine, compared to corresponding values in controls of 0.9 mg/liter plasma and 0.5 mg Zn/gm creatinine.

12.4.2 ZINC PHOSPHIDE

12.4.2.1 Identity, Properties, and Uses

Chemical Name Zinc phosphide.

Structure Zn_3P_2.

Synonyms As a rodenticide, zinc phosphide has been manufactured under the tradenames Fasco Field rat powder®, Kilrat®, Mouse-Con®, and Rumetan®. The CAS registry no. is 1314-84-7.

Physical and Chemical Properties Zinc phosphide has the empirical formula P_2Zn_3 and a molecular weight of 258.09. It forms a gray-black crystalline powder with a faint garlic odor and taste. It has a density of 4.55, a melting point above 420°C, and a boiling point of 1100°C. It is insoluble in water and alcohol. Zinc phosphide is stable when dry but spontaneously flammable on contact with acids. It is decomposed by acids into phosphine and is slightly corrosive to metals.

Formulations and Uses Technical zinc phosphide is 80–90% pure. Rodenticidal baits contain 0.5 or 1.0% of the compound; pastes contain 5–10%. As reviewed by von Oettingen (1947), zinc phosphide has been used not only as a rodenticide but also as an insecticide for control of mole crickets.

12.4.2.2 Toxicity to Laboratory Animals

Basic Findings The oral LD 50 of zinc phosphide for rats is 40.5 mg/kg (Dieke and Richter, 1946). Because the complete reaction of 40.5 mg of zinc phosphide produces 10.6 mg of phosphine and because the fatal dosage of phosphine for rats exposed to vapor concentrations ranging from 564 to 7.5 mg/m^3 varies from only 13.5 to 8.9 mg/kg (see Section 14.6.2.2), the toxicity of zinc phosphide is fully accounted for by the toxicity of the phosphine it produces when hydrolyzed by the acid of the stomach. The symptoms produced by the two compounds are similar except that respiratory exposure to the gas may have a slightly greater tendency to produce pulmonary edema and associated symptoms. However, the emetic action of its zinc moiety reduces the toxicity of zinc phosphide to humans and other animals that can vomit. The usual emetic doses of hydrated zinc sulfate in humans (1000–2000 mg) are equivalent to zinc intakes of 3.2–6.4 mg/kg, while the oral LD 50 of zinc phosphide for rats is equivalent to a zinc uptake of 30.8 mg/kg. Thus, a dangerous dose has a powerful emetic action in humans. At the same time, little injury from a dangerous dose of zinc phosphide can be attributed to the zinc moiety.

Absorption, Distribution, Metabolism, and Excretion According to Curry et al. (1959), both phosphide and phosphine were demonstrated in the liver of rats poisoned by zinc phosphide, but was only demonstrable in those that had survived long enough to excrete most of the poison. Although this conclusion probably is correct, the data do not support the authors' assumption that phosphide is absorbed in particulate form.

It is reported that the main urinary excretion product of zinc phosphide in rats and guinea pigs is hypophosphite (Curry et al., 1959).

12.4.2.3 Toxicity to Humans

Accidental and Intentional Poisoning One of the best-described cases of poisoning by zinc phosphide involved a 37-year-old woman who, with suicidal intent, drank a mixture of 180 gm of the rodenticide with water. Vomiting began 1 hr after ingestion and was frequent and violent. She was discovered in a state of shock after about 5 hr. On admission to hospital, her skin was cold and blue; the heart was inaudible, no limb pulses were palpable, and blood pressure was unobtainable. The carotid pulse was 80 per minute. The breath smelled of phosphine. Rectal temperature was 33°C. Treatment was entirely appropriate and almost certainly prolonged the patient's life. Besides very thorough gastric lavage and the use of detoxifying antidotes, the important features of treatment included rehydration and efforts to combat severe metabolic acidosis. Within 8 hr, 1200 mEq of sodium bicarbonate was administered. An attempt to induce diuresis was promptly but only briefly successful. Peripheral limb pulses returned, blood pressure reached 90/60 mm Hg, and by 21 hr after ingestion the patient was conscious, rational, and oriented, and she gave a lucid account of the events leading to her condition. However, complications had developed already and others appeared later. By 16 hr after ingestion, serum bilirubin had risen to 2.2 mg/100 ml. Hepatic tenderness appeared, and other tests of liver function became abnormal. Blood pressure and urine output decreased, and blood urea reached 30 mg/100 ml. A thrombotest showed 28% of normal coagulation activity. Variable tetany appeared; although blood calcium was low (3.3 mEq/liter), the condition did not respond to injection of calcium gluconate. Abdominal pain became severe. The extremities again became pulseless and icy cold. Fever and rapid breathing preceded a rapidly developing confusional state. For a brief period, the patient seemed to suffer terrifying hallucinations, and toward the end she screeched repeatedly. Unexpected cardiac arrest occurred 41 hr after ingestion (Stephenson, 1967).

In a drunken state, a 19-year-old woman in her 30th or 31st week of pregnancy ingested an unknown amount of zinc phosphide intended as a rodent bait. She soon lost consciousness and was cyanotic when brought to hospital. However, her pulse was detectable and her blood pressure normal. Treatment included gastric lavage and supportive measures. Recovery was complete by the third day. A baby girl later was born at term by normal labor; she was normal at birth and in subsequent development (Kuptsov and Aslanov, 1970).

Symptoms are basically the same regardless of route of administration whether oral, vaginal (Santini, 1955), respiratory (Elbel and Holsten, 1936), or directly into the subcutaneous and muscular tissues (Blisnakov and Iskrov, 1961).

In a review of cases where there was enough information to reach a conclusion, it was found that there was no mortality following three industrial accidents with zinc phosphide. However, mortality was 66% in three domestic accidents, 69% in 26 suicides, and 38% in eight attempted murders. Ten patients who died did so within 7–58 hr after ingestion, with an average of 24.6 hr. Patients who survived for 3 days were out of danger, although some suffered liver and/or kidney injury for days before full recovery (Stephenson, 1967). Apparently no exception to this rule regarding survival has been observed even though Rimalis and Bochkarnikov (1978) reported a case in which hepatorenal insufficiency was noted 5 days after ingestion, and the patient was not discharged until 36 days after ingestion.

Use Experience Zinc phosphide has given rise only rarely to occupational poisoning, although accidental poisoning of children by the baits is a real possibility. In one case, inhalation of dust from grain coated with the compound was followed several hours later by vomiting, diarrhea, cyanosis, rales, tachycardia, meteorism, restlessness, fever, albuminuria, and eventual recovery (Elbel and Holsten, 1936). In another instance reviewed by von Oettingen (1947) it apparently was not the applicator but workers in a fish-processing plant who were affected by phosphine generated from zinc phosphide after the rodenticide had come in contact with acid brine used for curing fish.

Dosage Response Adults have been killed by doses of 4000 or 5000 mg (Gilli, 1948; Frketić et al., 1957). However, others have survived as much as 25,000 mg (Paszko, 1961), 50,000 mg (Simonović, 1954), or even 100,000 mg (Rimalis and Bochkarnikov, 1978). Early vomiting improves the prognosis. In fact, one of two young women who had ingested similar amounts of zinc phosphide in a suicide pact survived with only transient symptoms because she had been induced to vomit; the other, who would not vomit, died in spite of gastric lavage 1 hr after ingestion (Mannaioni, 1960).

Laboratory Findings Phosphine may be detected most readily by odor. The concentration of zinc in the tissues is increased; in one case the serum level was between 5.9 and 6.1 ppm (Stephenson, 1967). For zinc in normal tissues, see Section 12.4.1.3. Other findings may include metabolic acidosis, reducing agents in the urine, increased serum bilirubin and other abnormal tests of liver function, thrombocytopenia, methemoglobin, and ECG abnormalities. The reducing substances in the urine include glucose but may induce hypophosphite and dissolved phosphine (Stephenson, 1967).

Pathology When death is rapid, abnormal findings may be restricted to pulmonary edema (Frketić et al., 1957; Mannaioni, 1960; Paszko, 1961; Puccini, 1961; Stephenson, 1967) or to this and cerebral edema (Mannaioni, 1960; Puccini, 1961). Other findings that may be present especially in persons who survive longer include: centrilobular necrosis of the liver, tubular necrosis of the kidneys, mucosal hemorrhage of the stomach, and bloody pleural, peritoneal, or pericardial fluid (Stephenson, 1967).

Treatment of Poisoning Treatment is entirely symptomatic (Hayes, 1975).

12.5 CADMIUM

Cadmium is a metal in the same periodic group as zinc and mercury. The toxicity of cadmium is especially evident when there is a deficiency of zinc, and within limits cadmium toxicity may be counteracted by supplementing the diet with zinc.

On the other hand, cadmium and inorganic mercury are toxicologically similar; following systemic absorption, both are especially likely to injure the kidney.

A wide range of cadmium concentrations are in human food—0.005–0.1 mg/kg wet weight. Kidney and oysters may have concentrations exceeding 1 mg/kg. Drinking water usually has concentrations below 5 μg/liter, but higher levels may be found due to cadmium impurities in the zinc of galvanized pipes and cadmium-containing solders in pipe fittings. More details are available in reviews of cadmium toxicity (Friberg *et al.*, 1986; Foulkes, 1974).

Several cadmium salts showed some promise as insecticides, but their use never became extensive. Recently, a number of cadmium salts have been used as fungicides on turf.

12.5.1 Cadmium Chloride

12.5.1.1 Identity, Properties, and Uses

Chemical Name Cadmium chloride.

Structure $CdCl_2$.

Synonyms The CAS registry no. for cadmium chloride is 10108-64-2.

Physical and Chemical Properties The empirical formula for cadmium chloride is $CdCl_2$ and the molecular weight is 183.32. The compound forms colorless, odorless crystals with a density of 4.05, a melting point of 568°C, and a boiling point of 960°C. It is freely soluble in water and acetone, slightly soluble in methanol and ethanol, and practically insoluble in ether.

Use Cadmium chloride is a fungicide for turf.

12.5.1.2 Toxicity to Laboratory Animals

Basic Findings Fifteen to 30 minutes after a single large dose, animals show salivation and diarrhea in response to the severe irritation of the mucosa of the gastrointestinal tract. Those that can vomit do so. Following sufficiently large repeated doses, animals grow poorly, but the nature of their disability is not distinctive (Lehman, 1951, 1952).

The oral LD 50 of cadmium chloride to rats is 88 mg/kg (Lehman, 1951, 1952). In dogs and rabbits, the lethal intravenous dosage is in the order of 2–5 mg/kg, suggesting that the compound is poorly absorbed from the gastrointestinal tract. The lowest oral emetic dose of cadmium in cats varies from 4.1 to 6.0 mg/kg (Schwartze and Alsberg, 1923).

Rats fed cadmium chloride at a dietary level of 135 ppm (about 6.7 mg/kg/day) showed marked anemia, stunted growth, and increased mortality. Forty to 50% of the red cells of survivors were reticulocytes. Some animals at 45 ppm showed anemia after a year of dosing. Some rats fed a dietary level of 15 ppm of cadmium chloride (about 0.75 mg/kg/day) for a year showed bleaching of the incisor teeth and, in rare instances, anemia. Toxicity was increased by a low-protein diet (Fitzhugh and Meiller, 1941).

Lehman (1951, 1952) reported that rats fed cadmium chloride for long periods show hyperplasia of the bone marrow and spleen and centrolobular degenerative changes in the liver.

Absorption, Distribution, Metabolism, and Excretion Absorption from the gastrointestinal tract usually is limited by rapid and violent vomiting. Absorption may occur from the respiratory tract following exposure to dusts and aerosols. Dermal absorption is not significant.

Once absorbed, cadmium is tenaciously stored and only slowly excreted. Cadmium is believed to be carried to the liver attached to serum albumin. In the liver, it induces metallothionein, a protein of molecular weight 6000 that avidly binds cadmium. It is lost from the liver as a cadmium–metallothionein complex, filtered at the glomerulus, and taken up by the proximal tubular cells of the kidney. Once inside the kidney cell, the metallothionein-cadmium complex is broken down by lysosomes to release free cadmium. The latter can induce metallothionein synthesis in the kidney cells. However, if the rate of release of cadmium exceeds the ability of the cell to produce metallothionein, the cadmium will attach to other "sensitive sites" and damage the cell. The ability of cadmium to induce metallothionein and to bind avidly to this protein is believed to account for its long-term storage in the body (Friberg *et al.*, 1986). Storage is mainly in the pancreas, liver, and kidney (Friberg, 1956) and, following respiratory exposure, in the lung.

Biochemical Effects Nonfatal doses of cadmium induce the synthesis of metallothionein, as discussed above, and may cause an increased tolerance for the ion. When groups of mice were given four-tenths of the LD 50 dosage of cadmium chloride previously determined for the strain and then challenged 48 hr later, the intraperitoneal LD 50 was increased from 5.2 mg/kg in controls to 6.7 mg/kg. The difference was statistically significant. A significant increase was obtained with cadmium acetate also (Jones *et al.*, 1979).

Effects on Organs and Tissues Cadmium chloride and some other cadmium compounds have produced sarcomas at the site of injection. Efforts to produce neoplasia at sites other than the point of injection have been unsuccessful, except that some rats developed interstitial cell tumors of the testes following testicular atrophy and castration changes in the pituitary caused by cadmium (WHO, 1973, 1976b; Friberg *et al.*, 1974).

Cadmium is teratogenic in the rat, and the dosage is unusually critical. Severe anomalies were produced in rat pups when the dams received a single intravenous injection of Cd^{2+} at the rate of 1.25 mg/kg on any of several days (9–15) of gestation. However, a dosage of 1.1 mg/kg was not terato-genic, and 1.35 mg/kg was fatal to all embryos (Samarawickrama and Webb, 1979).

At least a portion of the injury caused by cadmium is secondary to injury to blood vessels. This is notably true of the testis and proximal end of the caput epididymis in rats given a single remote subcutaneous injection of cadmium chloride at a rate of 5.5 mg/kg. That the injury is vascular is shown by a blanching of the affected parts as early as 5 hr after injection and their deep red-violet color about 48 hr after dosing. Injury restricted to the internal spermatic artery and associated pampiniform venous plexus serving the affected parts is inflammatory, as shown histologically. The injury may be prevented by zinc acetate injected subcutaneously at 100 times the molar rate of the cadmium chloride. Other blood vessels, including those to the main body of the epididymis and the vas deferens and all vessels to the female reproductive tract, are uninjured by cadmium. Whatever it is in the susceptible blood vessels that makes them react differently from other vessels is under hormonal control. The testes of most mice preconditioned for 7 or more weeks by either of two estrogens were not injured by cadmium chloride (Gunn et al., 1961, 1963).

In calves, intravenous dosages as low as 0.05 mg/kg produced tubular disorganization in the testis and impaired spermatogenesis (Pate et al., 1970).

Death is due to shock if it occurs after a single large dose. The cause of death is difficult to determine after repeated dosing. Kidney damage may be outstanding, but signs of poisoning involving the central nervous system, liver, and hematopoietic system may be observed in addition to direct irritative effects on the respiratory and gastrointestinal systems.

Treatment of Poisoning in Animals The use of calcium disodium EDTA 4 hr after a single intravenous dose of cadmium can cause as much as a 50-fold increase in the renal excretion of cadmium in rabbits. Under these conditions, the drug may be life saving, and there is no detectable injury to the kidney. However, the possibility of kidney damage when the drug was given for a week after cadmium was given for 3 weeks has been raised (Friberg, 1956). The contribution of the drug to the injury is difficult to decide because cadmium itself is nephrotoxic. It is possible that damage could be avoided by using a small dose of drug so that excretion of cadmium is only moderate at any one time.

The possible danger of chelating agents for treating cadmium poisoning may be related to the effects of thionein, an endogenous chelating agent. Cadmium bound to thionein was seven to eight times more toxic than ionic cadmium. However, not only was zinc-thionein (2.4 mg of Zn/kg) not toxic, but it protected against an otherwise fatal dosage of cadmium (Webb and Etienne, 1977).

An intraperitoneal dosage of cadmium acetate was fatal to all untreated mice. Some survived this dosage when treated orally with N-acetyl, d,l-penicillamine (NAPA), more survived with 2,3-dimercaptosuccinic acid (DMSA); and most survived with sodium, 2,3-dimercaptopropanesulfonate (DMPS). DMPS was most effective at mole ratios to cadmium of 20 to 60 and was less effective at either higher or lower values (Jones et al., 1978).

12.5.1.3 Toxicity to Humans

Accidental and Intentional Poisoning Apparently, the limited use of cadmium chloride as a pesticide has not led to poisoning of anyone. However, the evidence that has accumulated about the high toxicity of cadmium and its very tenacious storage leave no doubt that cadmium in any form should not be used as a pesticide.

Dramatic but not fatal poisoning used to occur fairly frequently when fruit juices or other acid foods were held for a time in cadmium-plated vessels. The citric or other organic salts formed on standing were fully ionized in the presence of hydrochloric acid in the stomach. Signs and symptoms included salivation, nausea, persistent vomiting, mild diarrhea, abdominal pain, and tenesmus. Illness often began suddenly 0.25–5 hr after ingestion; the interval was usually less than 2 hr unless food was eaten at the same time. Recovery usually was well advanced in 1–2 hr (Cangelosi, 1941; Frant and Kleeman, 1941). The amount of cadmium necessary to produce these effects was not great. Schwartz and Alsberg (1923) cited a case of voluntary ingestion of cadmium sulfate, equivalent to about 18 mg of metallic cadmium, which produced vomiting. Mild illness is produced by concentrations as low as 15 ppm.

Use Experience and Environmental Exposure The few episodes of acute occupational poisoning by cadmium have all been associated with inhalation of dust or fumes. The cases were characterized by severe pulmonary irritation, and persons who died showed marked hyperplasia of the lung epithelium and thickening and edema of the alveolar septa. Signs of severe gastrointestinal irritation were present in a high proportion of cases.

Less severe but more prolonged occupational exposure to cadmium may produce a distinctive form of emphysema leading to dyspnea and often accompanied by a low-grade anemia. The most typical feature of chronic cadmium poisoning is kidney damage. The first sign is the excretion of low-molecular-weight proteins. This condition is known as tubular proteinuria because these proteins are normally reabsorbed by the tubular cells in the kidney (Friberg, 1950; Piscator, 1966). At high exposure, more severe effects in kidney function occur, such as aminoaciduria (Clarkson and Kench, 1956), glucosuria, and phosphaturia (Piscator, 1966).

By far the largest number of cases of cadmium poisoning have occurred in Japan as a result of environmental exposure. These cases differed greatly from those caused by cadmium under other circumstances, being characterized by osteomalacia, skeletal deformity, and very severe pain. In fact, the condition took its name "itai-itai disease" from the predominance of pain. The entire matter has been reviewed critically by Friberg et al. (1974), who concluded that there was no doubt that cadmium was the cause but that there was reason to believe that high intake of cadmium and deficient consumption of certain essential food items, especially calcium and vitamin D, had been contributing factors. In spite of the very different clinical manifestations seen in itai-itai disease, it is thought that the basic injury is to the kidney as in other forms of chronic poisoning by cadmium and that the osteomalacia is secondary.

As reviewed by Friberg *et al.* (1974), great interest was aroused by a series of studies on rats during the 1960s indicating that moderate intake of cadmium (5 ppm in drinking water) produced hypertension. The level of cadmium that the controls received in food and drinking water was so low that it was difficult to achieve in the laboratory and impossible to realize in an ordinary environment. Some other studies on dietary cadmium failed to produce hypertension, but it is not clear whether the difference depended on strain of animals or other variables in the experimental situations. The possibility that cadmium predisposes to hypertension led to epidemiological studies focused on people with hypertension or on the population of cities where the levels of cadmium in the air were higher than in control areas. The results were ambiguous. However, epidemiological studies focused on people with really high exposure to cadmium (workers with years of exposure to cadmium or patients with itai-itai disease) have been uniformly negative. The results do not exclude the possibility that cadmium influences blood pressure, but if such an effect exists, it must involve some complex interaction (for example, with sodium). It is difficult to see how cadmium can be an important variable influencing hypertension in the general population if it does not produce hypertension in heavily exposed persons.

Dosage Response Apparently, no information is available on the minimal dosage of a cadmium salt that has been fatal in humans. According to reports cited by Schwartze and Alsberg (1923) doses of 250–1000 mg of cadmium bromide produced illness, and a 33-mg dose of cadmium sulfate produced vomiting. These doses correspond to dosages of cadmium ion of about 1.5–6.0 and 0.25 mg/kg, respectively. The permissible respiratory occupational intake (as Cd) is 0.07 mg/kg/day.

Laboratory Findings Friberg *et al.* (1974) have given reasons for thinking that some of the early reports of concentrations of cadmium in environmental samples and human tissues were incorrectly high because the chemical methods used formerly were not entirely specific. This is an unusual situation because improvement in chemical methods often leads to more complete recovery and recognition of the material analyzed and thus to higher values. Considering only results based on dependable chemical methods, it now seems likely that blood levels in normal adults usually are <0.01 ppm. The renal cortex usually contains cadmium at concentrations of 20–50 ppm, higher than the concentrations in any other tissue. The highest concentration is reached at about 50 years of age, and levels then decline gradually. The kidneys contain about one-third of the total body burden, and the kidneys and liver together contain about half the body burden. Normal urinary

excretion is about 0.002 mg/person/day or less, but levels increase with age.

Intake is about 0.05 mg/person/day from food, with much less from water, air, and even cigarette smoking. The amount of cadmium in ordinary food is one-seventh to one-fifth of the intake thought to be required to produce the storage of 200 ppm in the kidney and consequent kidney damage. Absorption of cadmium ingested in food and water ranges form 4.7 to 7.0% but may be higher if calcium and protein are deficient. Retention of cadmium from smoke or fumes may be 25–50%.

The placenta is an efficient barrier to small concentrations of cadmium; the newborn contains less than 0.001 mg. The biological half-life for cadmium in the whole body lies between 20 and 30 years. Thus cadmium has an unusually great tendency to accumulate in the body (Friberg *et al.*, 1974). In workers, cadmium in the blood is mainly in the cells; the concentration in whole blood usually is between 0.01 and 0.1 ppm. Concentrations in the kidney cortex may be around 300 ppm. The liver may contain proportionately more than would be expected in persons without special exposure. Cadmium is transported in the circulation at least in part bound to metallothionin. When workers begin to excrete protein in their urine, their excretion of cadmium increases, sometimes dramatically, and their blood levels fall correspondingly. Based on results in animals and on autopsy findings in workers, a concentration of 200 ppm in the kidney is the threshold for kidney injury as reflected by kidney function tests and the urinary excretion of protein. More recent data are available based on direct *in vivo* measurement of the kidney content of cadmium in occupationally exposed workers using a neutron activation technique (Ellis *et al.*, 1984). This has allowed the development of more sophisticated dosage–response models (Kjellström, 1985) that estimate, for example, that a daily intake of about 200 μg Cd via food for 45 years will give a 10% chance of mild kidney effects. The equivalent occupational exposure would be 10 years at about 50 μg Cd/m^3.

Besides the proteinuria, other laboratory findings may include mild hypochronic anemia, mild jaundice, and the presence of microscopic blood in the urine.

Persons mildly poisoned by cadmium may show blood levels as high as 6.2 ppm and urinary levels as high as 2.2 ppm (Cotter, 1958).

Treatment of Poisoning Cotter (1958) treated three patients whose major exposure was to cadmium, including at least one without any other exposure. The patients suffered one or more of the following: mental disturbance, cough and other respiratory disturbance, mild jaundice, mild anemia, and abnormal urinary findings. Treatment consisted of 500 mg of calcium disodium EDTA by mouth every 2 hr while the patient was awake and for a period of 1 week. All the patients showed marked clinical improvement. There was no evidence of kidney damage from the treatment, and in fact the proteinuria present before treatment gradually cleared completely. Icterus disappeared, and the red cell count and hemoglobin level improved. Before treatment, blood cadmium levels in the three patients were 0.022–6.2 ppm, and urinary cadmium was 0.036–2.2 ppm. The concentrations fell to undetectable levels following treatment.

A patient who had marked irregularity of the heartbeat and other ECG abnormalities 3 hr after ingesting cadmium showed marked improvement following intravenous injection of calcium gluconate and magnesium sulfate, and she was almost normal within 48 hr after ingestion (Lydtin *et al.*, 1965). However, evidence from animals indicates that some chelating agents such as EDTA can cause renal accumulation by redistribution from other tissues, and therefore application of chelating agents to cases of human poisoning should be viewed with great caution.

12.6 MERCURY

There is no evidence that any quantity of mercury is beneficial to any form of life. However, the element is widely distributed in the environment, and traces of it occur in food, water, and tissues even in the absence of occupational exposure.

Mercury is toxic no matter what its chemical combination. However, different forms of mercury have different absorption, distribution, and excretion characteristics; at the same rate of intake, they reach and maintain different concentrations in different tissues. For this and perhaps other reasons they have distinguishable toxic effects.

In recent years the only mercury pesticides used in significant amounts were organic compounds; some of them constitute a real hazard. It is said that mercury vapor formerly was used in India for the disinfection of stored grain. Several inorganic mercury salts are still listed as fungicides. There is no evidence that the use of mercury vapor or inorganic mercury compounds as pesticides constitutes a significant hazard at this time, largely because such use is limited. Even so, some information on the toxicity of these forms of mercury is necessary for understanding the toxicology of the organic mercury fungicides. Finally, among the organic mercurials, the short-chain alkyl compounds are far more toxic than the phenyl or alkoxyalkyl compounds as discussed in Section 12.6.3.

Valuable reviews (Bidstrup, 1964; Berlin *et al.*, 1969c; Clarkson, 1972; WHO, 1976a; Berlin, 1986) of the toxicology of mercury and its compounds are available.

12.6.1 ELEMENTAL MERCURY

12.6.1.1 Identity, Properties, and Uses

Synonyms Synonyms for elemental mercury (Hg) include mercure (French), mercurio (Italian), kwik (Dutch), quecksilber (German), quicksilver, and RTEC (Polish). The CAS registry no. is 7439-97-6.

Physical and Chemical Properties Elemental mercury is a heavy, silver-white metal which is liquid at room temperature. Its atomic number is 80, and its atomic weight is 200.59.

Mercury has a melting point of $-38.9°C$, a boiling point of 356.9°C, and a density at 0°C of 13.5955. The vapor pressure is 2×10^{-3} mm at 25°C; air saturated at this temperature contains 19.5 mg of mercury (Giese, 1940). Mercury is insoluble in water, alkalies, and most common solvents. Mercury is not attacked by dilute hydrochloride and sulfuric acids but will dissolve in dilute nitric acid and hot, concentrated sulfuric acid. It oxidizes slowly.

Use See Section 12.6.

12.6.1.2 Toxicity to Laboratory Animals

Basic Findings The toxicity of elemental mercury is essentially limited to the vapor, and, therefore, it is not convenient to determine dosage in a milligram per kilogram basis.

Inhalation of a concentration of 28.8 mg/m³ for only 1 hr produced microscopic evidence of mild damage to the brain, kidney, heart, and lung of rabbits. Inhalation of this atmosphere for 4 hr produced severe damage, and exposure for 6 hr/day for 5 days was fatal to some rabbits. A concentration of 6 mg/m³ for 6 weeks or more produced severe but nonfatal injury of the same organs and of the colon also. The kidneys and brains were injured within 6 weeks by exposure to 0.86 mg/m³, but this injury was reversible. Both rabbits and dogs tolerated daily exposure to 0.1 mg/m³ for 86 weeks without functional or microscopic injury (Ashe *et al.*, 1953).

Rats apparently are less susceptible. When they were exposed for only 2 hr each day for 30 days at a concentration of 17 mg/m³, they developed only a delay in escape response plus an increase in the duration and severity of reflexive fighting behavior and of actual fighting (Beliles *et al.*, 1968).

Absorption, Distribution, Metabolism, and Excretion Inhaled mercury vapor diffuses across the alveolar regions of the lung into the bloodstream (Berlin *et al.*, 1969a). Mercury vapor is a monatomic gas which is highly diffusible and lipid soluble (Hursh, 1985). Once in the bloodstream, mercury vapor enters the red blood cells, where it is oxidized to divalent inorganic mercury under the influence of catalase (Magos *et al.*, 1978b; Halbach and Clarkson, 1978). The oxidation can be inhibited by alcohol, thereby decreasing the retention of inhaled vapor (Nielsen-Kudsk, 1965, 1969). Despite oxidation in the red blood cells, dissolved mercury vapor persists in the plasma for sufficient time for it to be transported to other tissues. This explains why 10 times more mercury is retained in the brain after exposure to mercury vapor than after an equivalent intravenous dose of mercuric mercury in both mice (Berlin and Johansson, 1964) and in primates (Berlin *et al.*, 1969b). Placental transport of mercury is also greater after exposure to the vapor (Clarkson *et al.*, 1972). Oxidation by catalase also takes place in fetal tissues (Dencker *et al.*, 1983).

When mice and rats were exposed to ²⁰³Hg for 6 hr daily for 10 days, whole-body autoradiography showed that the highest concentrations of radioactivity were in the kidney, brain, and heart. The brain stem and cerebellar nuclei, the cerebral cortex, and the spinal cord contained a greater concentration of radioactivity than did the cerebral cortex, basal ganglia, and the septum. The walls of the brain ventricles, the choroid plexus, and some other areas in close contact with the cerebrospinal fluid showed high activity. Microautoradiograms confirmed these findings and revealed selective localization in the Purkinje cells and in the neurons of the nucleus dentatus (Cassano *et al.*, 1969). Except for these differences, the pattern of organ distribution of mercury after exposure to vapor or mercuric salts is generally similar, with the highest concentrations always found in the kidney cortex. Excretion is mainly by urine and feces at roughly similar rates but there is a small loss of mercury in expired breath (Rothstein and Hayes, 1960, 1964; Clarkson and Rothstein, 1964).

12.6.1.3 Toxicity to Humans

Experimental Exposure   Using a group of four volunteers in each experiment, the concentrations of radioactive mercury vapor in the inspired and expired air were compared. The inspired air contained from 0.050 to 0.350 mg/m^3. The dead space for the vapor corresponded to the physiological dead space, indicating that all mercury vapor that reached the alveoli was absorbed (Nielsen-Kudsk, 1965, 1969; Teisinger and Fiserova-Bergerova, 1965). A later study in five volunteers confirmed that retention occurs almost entirely in the alveoli. Overall retention was 74%. Examination of the subjects in a whole-body counter yielded average half-lives for mercury as follows: lung, 1.7 days; head, 21 days; kidney region, 64 days; and standard chair position, 58 days (Hursh *et al.*, 1976).

Accidental and Intentional Poisoning   Occupational poisoning by mercury vapor has been almost exclusively chronic and the result of prolonged exposure to only slightly excessive levels. However, truly acute poisoning is possible as a result of occupational or other exposure to unmeasured but certainly very high levels of vapor.

Use Experience   Acute poisoning by metallic mercury is rare. Inhalation of vapor by laboratory workers in a closed space led to bronchial irritation, violent coughing, and severe headache, followed in a few hours by fever, dyspnea, and nausea. Stomatitis appeared in 3 days. Dyspnea and fatigue lasted several months (Christensen *et al.*, 1937). Both renal and nervous involvement are unusual in acute poisoning (Browning, 1969).

Neal *et al.* (1937, 1941a) gave a very thorough account of chronic mercurialism in the fur-cutting and felt-hat industries. Although mercuric nitrate was the material used to treat fur from which felt was made, the mercury was gradually released from the fur and felt in the form of metallic mercury vapor. Thus the workers had a mixed exposure to dust of mercury compounds (especially the nitrate) and to vapor of the element. The clinical picture of poisoning was similar to that observed among smaller groups whose occupational exposure involved metallic mercury only (West and Lim, 1968; Browning, 1969).

The incidence of chronic mercurialism is roughly proportional to the concentration of mercury in the air at concentrations of 0.1 mg/m^3 and upward, and within each range of concentration the incidence increases with duration of employment (Neal *et al.*, 1941a). Patients often gave a history of gastrointestinal disturbances and sore mouth. Salivation, gingivitis, and the loss of teeth were common. However, the major signs included fine tremors and psychic disturbances often called erethism. The tremor usually was noticed first in the hands and later in the tongue, eyelids, face, and legs. It became worse during intentional movement or after the slightest emotional strain. The psychic disturbance took the form of irritability, excitability, timidity, irascibility, and difficulty in getting along with people. These signs were noted more frequently by an examiner than they were reported by the patient. They tended to be replaced by depression or despondency. Headache, drowsiness, insomnia, weakness, slurred speech, excessive sweating, dermographia, and vasomotor disorders all pointed to disorder of some part of the nervous system. Ataxia was seen occasionally and hemiplegia more rarely. In advanced cases there might be hallucinations, loss of memory, and intellectual deterioration. Death might follow symptoms resembling cerebral pachymeningitis (Neal *et al.*, 1941a).

More recent studies have indicated that a number of nonspecific symptoms, such as insomnia, introversion, and anxiety, may be produced at concentrations somewhat below 0.1 mg/m^3 (for review, see USEPA, 1984).

Laboratory Findings   Laboratory tests often reveal albumin and red cells in the urine, generally in the absence of illness related to kidney dysfunction. Occasionally a typical nephrosis is seen (Friberg *et al.*, 1953). Kazantzis *et al.* (1962) reported the nephrotic syndrome in workers exposed to mercury vapor and certain mercury compounds. Buchet *et al.* (1980) noted an increase in urinary excretion of high molecular weight proteins suggestive of a glomerular disturbance in workers exposed to mercury vapor in the range of 0.05 to 0.1 mg/m^3. The glomerular effect may have an immunological basis (Druet *et al.*, 1982).

Treatment of Poisoning   Conflicting reports have been published about the value of both BAL and calcium disodium EDTA for treating chronic poisoning by mercury vapor (Browning, 1969). Sunderman (1978) found that BAL (2,3-dimercapto-1-propanol) was more effective in alleviating the signs and symptoms of mercury vapor poisoning than D-penicillamine or sodium diethyldithiocarbamate. However, treatment with complexing agents may not be necessary as the prognosis is good with virtually complete regression if exposure ceases (Berlin, 1986).

12.6.2 MERCURIC CHLORIDE

12.6.2.1 Identity, Properties, and Uses

Chemical Name   Mercuric chloride.

Structure $HgCl_2$.

Synonyms Mercuric chloride also is known as corrosive sublimate, mercury biochloride, and mercury perchloride. The CAS registry no. is 7487-94-7.

Physical and Chemical Properties Mercuric chloride has the empirical formula Cl_2Hg and a molecular weight of 271.52. It is an odorless, white, crystalline powder with a metallic taste. At 25°C, it has a density of 5.4. It melts at 277°C, and sublimes unchanged at about 300°C. Its vapor pressure is 1.4×10^{-4} torr at 35°C. Mercuric chloride is soluble in ethanol, methanol, acetone, ethyl acetate, and diethyl ester. It is slightly soluble in acetic acid, pyridine, and carbon disulfide. Its solubility in water at 20°C is 69 gm/liter. Mercuric chloride is unstable in the presence of alkalies and is decomposed to metallic mercury by sunlight in the presence of organic matter. It is readily reduced to mercurous chloride and elemental mercury.

History, Formulations, and Uses Mercuric chloride first was used for crop protection in 1891. It formerly was used as a fungicide in soil application to control potato scab and clubroot of brassicas and as an insecticide against root maggots of crucifers. It now is used in seed treatment of potatoes and as a wood preservative. Formulations include wettable powders, dusts, and solutions for injection into tree trunks.

12.6.2.2 Toxicity to Laboratory Animals

Basic Findings The oral LD 50 of mercuric chloride is 37 mg/kg in the rat (Lehman, 1951, 1952) and 10 mg/kg in the mouse (Goldberg *et al.*, 1950). In rabbits the intramuscular LD 50 is 7.3 mg/kg (Braun *et al.*, 1946).

In dogs, a single intravenous dose at the rate of 2 mg/kg produced effects ranging from slight to fatal. Under these conditions, death was the result of progressive azotemia, oliguria, and uremia. Moderate poisoning was characterized by transient azotemia with mild uremic symptoms followed by recovery (Balint, 1968).

Absorption, Distribution, Metabolism, and Excretion Mercuric chloride can be absorbed by any portal. However, injury by it is generally accidental and involves ingestion. The mercuric ion is distributed to all tissues, but it reaches distinctly higher concentrations in the kidney as tabulated in Section 12.6.3.3. Excretion is mainly in the urine. Small concentrations may be found in the feces also. Following a single nonfatal dose, excretion declines rapidly, reaching low levels within a week but continuing as traces for long periods.

Biochemical Effects There is evidence that inorganic mercury is bound mainly by metallothionein in the kidney of rats (Wisniewska *et al.*, 1970), although binding to proteins of greater molecular weight and also to small, dialyzable organic molecules has been observed. The two heavier classes were found mainly in the serum and in liver and kidney homogenates but to only a slight degree in the urine. The dialyzable compounds were mainly in the urine with traces in the kidney (Jakubowski *et al.*, 1970).

As might be expected, regeneration of the renal tubular epithelium after poisoning by mercuric chloride is accompanied by increased DNA synthesis and related changes (Cuppage *et al.*, 1969).

When a high dosage of 2,4-dinitrophenol (but not other metabolic inhibitors) was administered to rats just before they received mercuric chloride, accumulation of mercury in the kidney was prevented. It was concluded that the selective accumulation of mercury in the kidney is energy-dependent and that transport of the ion is mainly directly into the renal tissue from the peritubular capillaries and not by way of glomerular filtration (Clarkson and Magos, 1970).

Effect on Organs and Tissues Mercuric ion in sufficient concentration causes a reversible precipitation of protein. Concentrations of the ion high enough to cause this effect may be reached as a result of direct contact with the skin, the mucous membranes of the eye, or the mucosa of the gastrointestinal tract. However, the mercuric ion produces systemic toxicity at much lower concentrations through inhibition of many enzymes, especially those containing the SH group. After a large dose, death is due to shock and circulatory collapse; arrhythmias may be present, and ventricular fibrillation may be the terminal event. After a somewhat smaller dose, death is due to renal damage leading to anuria.

Dilatation and hyperemia of the glomeruli was detected within 3 hr, earliest necrosis of the proximal tubules was seen within 6 hr, and tubular regeneration began by the fourth day in dogs that received a single intravenous injection of mercuric chloride at the rate of 2 mg/kg. Renal failure could not be accounted for by the slight decrease in renal blood flow but appeared to be due to a definite decrease in glomerular filtration rate and possibly the leakage of tubular fluid (Balint, 1968; Balint *et al.*, 1969).

In another study, an increase in the smooth endoplasmic reticulum of cells of the pars recta of the proximal tubules of rats was detected within 30 min after an intraperitoneal injection at the rate of 5 mg/kg. Discrete mitochondrial changes began half an hour later (Holgersen *et al.*, 1969).

The necrosis of the kidney tubule cells of rats following subcutaneous injection of mercuric chloride at dosage of 0.1–4.0 mg/kg/day for several days was reflected not only by characteristic histology but by the shedding of cells in the urine and by an increase of urinary glutamic-oxaloacetic transaminase activity in the intact animal. The urinary output of cells reached a peak in a few days and then declined in spite of continued administration of the compound. The peak came earlier at higher dosage levels. A transient increase in transaminase corresponded with the peak of renal cell exfoliation, but the enzyme activity was a less sensitive test. Histological examination showed that the decline in cellular exfoliation was associated with tubular regeneration. The new cells were relatively immune to the effects of mercuric ion, but the basis of the tolerance is unknown (Prescott and Ansari, 1969).

Mercuric chloride at a concentration of $3.5 \times 10^{-5} M$ acted as a mitogen in cultures of lymphoid cells from rats, guinea pigs, and rabbits (Pauly *et al.*, 1969).

12.6.2.3 Toxicity to Humans

Experimental Exposure Mercuric chloride or the mercury ion from it is absorbed transepidermally. Details of this process have been studied by electron microscopy in biopsies of skin from volunteers to whom the compound had been applied (Silberberg *et al.*, 1969).

Accidental and Intentional Poisoning Ingestion of mercuric chloride leads immediately to a burning metallic taste, thirst, and soreness of the throat followed soon by salivation, severe gastric pain, bloody diarrhea, and often vomiting.

If the patient does not die promptly in shock following a dose of about 1 gm, the onset is delayed for a few hours. Damage to the capillaries leads to stomatitis, loosening of the teeth, progressive renal damage, and continuing diarrhea. If the blood pressure is maintained, there may be an initial diuresis resulting from suppression of the renal tubular resorption. Progressive injury leads to a diminished flow of urine and eventually to anuria.

Inorganic mercury is excreted so efficiently that persons who survive one or a few doses usually recover completely.

Laboratory Findings See Section 12.6.3.4.

Pathology Local corrosive effects may be the only indication of injury of persons who die rapidly of shock following a large dose of mercuric chloride. In case of longer survival, renal tubular necrosis is the major finding.

Treatment of Poisoning Both BAL and penicillamine are effective in treating poisoning by inorganic mercury compounds (Hayes, 1975).

12.6.3 ORGANIC MERCURY COMPOUNDS: SIMILARITIES AND DISTINCTIONS

12.6.3.1 Uses

The organic mercury compounds are used as seed dressings for the prevention of seed-borne disease of grains, vegetables, cotton, peanuts, soybeans, sugar beets, and ornamentals. They may be used for the control of fungus diseases of turf, fruits, cereals, and vegetables but not under conditions that will leave any measurable residue in the food of humans or animals. At least in other countries, organic mercury compounds have been used for the preservation of wood (Ahlmark, 1948) and in the paper, plastics, and fabric industries (Lundgren and Swensson, 1960).

About 1915, phenylmercury fungicides began to replace

mercuric chloride, which had been in use for seed treatment before the turn of the century. Alkyloxyalkylmercury compounds were introduced next, and ethylmercury was tested as early as 1929. Alyklmercury fungicides were used extensively in the 1940s and thereafter.

The following discussion is necessarily incomplete. Additional information may be found in a book by Bidstrup (1964) and in a health criteria document issued by the World Health Organization (1976a). The first of these references is notable for a tabulated description of cases caused by different forms of mercury.

12.6.3.2 Compounds and Their Characteristics

Mercury is bivalent in the organic compounds used as fungicides. Most of these compounds fall into three major classes depending on whether the organomercury cation involves an (*a*) alkyl (*e.g.*, methyl or ethyl), (*b*) phenyl, or (*c*) alkoxyalkyl (*e.g.*, methoxyethyl) group. Compounds of each group may involve a wide range of inorganic or organic anions, including chloride, bromide, iodide, nitrate, hydroxide, acetate, dicyandiamide, toluene-sulfonate, benzoate, methanedinaphthyldisulfonate, and others. There are other bivalent organomercury compounds not used as fungicides, for example, dialkyl mercury compounds, certain local antiseptics, and the mercurial diuretics, but they are not discussed further here.

Vapor pressure is an important factor determining the availability of organic mercury compounds for absorption. Table 12.1, derived in part from a detailed review by Swensson and Ulfvarson (1963), shows the concentrations of mercury and some of its compounds in saturated atmospheres. This helps to explain the observed extreme hazard of methyl mercury compounds in workplaces. Only a lack of use limits the hazards of the very highly volatile dialkyl compounds. The high reported range of volatility of some alkoxyalkyl compounds depends at least in part on the fact that they often contain metallic mercury as a contaminant (Lindström, 1961). In fact, commercial formulations of all organic mercury compounds are likely to contain related compounds and metallic mercury resulting from the manufacturing process or from slow decompensation catalyzed by light.

Table 12.1

Saturated Vapor Concentration of Mercury and Certain Groups of Its Compounds at 20°C

Group	Concentrations (mg/m³)
Metallic mercury	14
Dialkyl compounds	10,000
Methyl compounds	0.3–94
Ethyl compounds	0.05–9.0
Phenyl compounds	0.001–0.017
Methoxyethyl compounds	0.002–2.6

12.6.3.3 Absorption, Distribution, Metabolism, and Excretion

Absorption These compounds are absorbed slowly by the skin and more efficiently by the respiratory and gastrointestinal tracts. Some of the alkyl compounds are highly volatile thus increasing the hazard of their inhalation. There is no indication of any significant difference in the rate of absorption of different compounds at the same rate of dosage.

Distribution and Storage Alkyl and aryl mercury compounds, like metallic mercury vapor, are transported mainly in association with the erythrocytes. This is in contrast to the inorganic mercury ion, which is bound mainly to plasma protein. Methoxyethyl compounds are evenly distributed between red cells and plasma.

There are striking differences in the distribution and storage of different classes of organic mercury compounds, and this appears to be the basis for the differences in their toxic effects when given in repeated doses. The mercury content of different organs of rats following repeated doses of typical compounds is shown in Table 12.2. It may be seen that mercury from methoxyethyl mercuric hydroxide reaches about the same concentrations in the blood and vital organs as those from mercuric nitrate. However, the distribution of mercury derived from methylmercuric hydroxide is entirely different, being about 15 times as high in the brain, 100 times as high in the blood, but only one-tenth as high in the kidney. The behavior of mercury derived from phenylmercuric hydroxide is intermediate between that of alkyl mercury and inorganic mercury but much more nearly like the latter (Ulfvarson, 1962). Similar results were obtained in chickens (Swensson and Ulfvarson, 1968a).

Metabolism Differences in distribution and storage of organic mercury pesticides are generally assumed to be due to differences in mobility across cell membranes, affinities for tissue ligands, and rates of metabolism to inorganic mercury. The latter is illustrated by the greater stability of alkyl compounds as compared to the more rapid degradation of methoxyethyl and phenol compounds (Gage, 1964; Daniel et al., 1971; Norseth and Clarkson, 1970).

Methyl mercury is readily transported across the placenta in rodents (Childs, 1973). In humans, cord blood levels closely parallel and are about 20% higher than the corresponding levels in maternal blood (Skerfving, 1974; Bakir et al., 1973).

Species vary considerably in the relative distribution of alkyl mercury between brain and blood (Berlin et al., 1969b).

Table 12.2 shows that somewhat more mercury was stored in the liver and kidney when a phenyl compound was injected for 2 weeks than when inorganic mercury was injected at an equivalent rate. The same thing was seen in much exaggerated form when phenylmercuric acetate and mercuric acetate were fed at equivalent doses for a year or more; there was 10 to 20 or more times greater storage of the phenyl compound depending on dosage. The difference was attributed at least in part to greater absorption of the phenyl compound (Fitzhugh et al., 1950).

Excretion Following injection of equivalent amounts of mercury, urinary excretion of phenyl compounds is almost twice that of inorganic mercury and more than 10 times greater than that of methyl mercury (Friberg, 1959; Swensson et al., 1959). That is, the same level of excretion is achieved only at high blood and tissue levels of alkyl compounds.

In rats, following a single dose, the excretion of various forms of mercury was more rapid at first and then slower. For both mercuric nitrate and phenylmercuric hydroxide the "half-lives" were 5 days during the first 9 days and 10 days during the subsequent 30 days. The half-lives were 16 and 26 days for methylmercuric hydroxide during the same intervals (Swensson and Ulfvarson, 1968b).

Half-lives may be different in different species. The half-life of methyl mercury in the mouse is about 7 days as compared to an average 70 days in humans and may be as high as 700 days in certain marine mammals (for review, see Clarkson, 1972).

The half-time of methyl mercury in blood in humans averages about 50 days, whereas that of inorganic mercury is about 30 days (for review, see Clarkson et al., 1988). Information on phenyl mercury compounds is not available.

Although dimethylmercury apparently has not been used as a pesticide, it is of interest because of its formation in aquatic environments. Most of the dimethylmercury injected into mice was rapidly exhaled. The remaining part was metabolized to methyl mercury, on which the entire toxic effect depended (Oestlund, 1969).

12.6.3.4 Laboratory Findings in Humans

The record of mercury levels in human tissues and excreta is complicated by the fact that early analytical methods lacked the necessary sensitivity and made no distinction between inorganic and organic mercury. In fact, this distinction has not yet been made for many different occupational situations or for a reasonably complete spectrum of dietary patterns. As a result, the mercury concentrations in human tissues discussed below are expressed in terms of total mercury.

Blood Goldwater and Hoover (1967) have reported blood levels of mercury in 812 people from 15 countries with no known special exposure to mercury. Approximately 75% of the sam-

Table 12.2
Average Mercury Content of Fresh Tissue of Rats[a,b]

Compound	Blood (ppm)	Liver (ppm)	Kidney (ppm)	Brain (ppm)
$Hg(NO_3)_2$	0.028	0.372	20.1	0.024
Methyl Hg OH	3.04	0.676	2.9	0.155
Phenyl Hg OH	0.313	0.566	26.2	0.008
Methoxyethyl Hg OH	0.033	0.248	26.9	0.009

[a] From data of Ulfvarson (1962).
[b] Treatment of rats is 0.1 mg Hg/day every other day for 2 weeks.

ples were less than 0.5 μg/liter and about 90% were less than 20 μg/liter. Mercury in blood is greatly influenced by dietary fish consumption in otherwise nonexposed people. Methyl mercury in fish can make a substantial and dominant contribution to blood levels. Certain populations that depend on fish for their main source of protein can develop levels in excess of 299 μg/liter (for review, see WHO, 1976a).

In groups occupationally exposed to mercury vapor, blood levels are proportional to time-weighted average air concentrations for long-term exposures (1 year or more) and on a group basis (Smith *et al.*, 1970). In general, time-weighted air concentrations in the range of 50 to 100 μg Hg/m³—values corresponding to maximum allowable limits—correspond to blood levels in the range of 35 to 70 μg/liter. Values of 500 to 1000 or 1300 μg/liter have been reported in patients (Berlin *et al.*, 1969c; Birke *et al.*, 1967).

Urine A study of urine samples from 1107 people in 15 different countries (Goldwater and Hoover 1967) revealed that approximately 80% of the samples had mercury concentrations below 0.5 μg/liter (the detection limit of the analytical method), 90% were below 10 μg/liter, and 95% were below 20 μg/liter. Studies in other populations are consistent with these figures (Buchet *et al.*, 1980; Gotelli *et al.*, 1985).

Smith *et al.* (1970) have reported that urine concentrations of mercury are proportional to the time-weighted average air concentrations of mercury vapor in groups of exposed workers. In general, average air concentrations in the range of 50 to 100 μg Hg/m³ (the maximum values expected in industrial atmosphere) would correspond to urine concentrations in the range of 100 to 200 μg/liter (WHO, 1980).

Exposure to alkyl mercury compounds results in elevated urinary concentrations of mercury (Bakir *et al.*, 1973) but the increase is small and urinary concentrations are not a viable biological indicator (for discussion, see Clarkson *et al.*, 1988). Urinary concentrations may be markedly increased after occupational (Goldwater, 1973) or accidental (Gotelli *et al.*, 1985) exposure to aryl mercury compounds. However, the quantitative relations between exposure and urinary excretion have not been described.

Hair In a study of 559 samples in 13 countries, Airey (1983) noted a correlation between hair concentrations and average fish consumption. Thus he found the mean hair concentration to be 1.4 ppm in individuals consuming fish once or less per month, 1.9 ppm for consumption once every 2 weeks, 2.5 ppm for consumption once a week, and 11.6 ppm for consumption once or more per day.

This correlation is probably due to intake of methyl mercury in fish. A close correlation has been noted in both population (Birke *et al.*, 1972; Amin-Zaki *et al.*, 1976; Phelps *et al.*, 1980) and experimental studies (Hislop *et al.*, 1983; Kershaw *et al.*, 1980) between mercury concentration in hair next to the scalp and the simultaneous blood concentration after exposure to methyl mercury. The average ratio of hair to blood concentrations is about 250 : 1. Studies in volunteers who received

measured amounts of methyl mercury in fish indicate that there is a 20-day delay between the blood concentration and the appearance of mercury in hair next to the scalp (Hislop *et al.*, 1983). Methyl mercury appears to be incorporated into the hair during its formation and remains stable. Because there is little variation in the rate of growth of head hair (1.15 cm/month) it is possible to determine the sequence of past exposures of persons to methyl mercury (Amin-Zaki *et al.*, 1976; Al-Shahristani and Shihab, 1976).

Hair concentrations after exposure to other forms of mercury (mercury vapor, inorganic and aryl compounds) have not been reported in any detail. In the case of occupational exposure, the probability of external contamination should be considered. Factors affecting hair concentration and the use of washing procedures have been reviewed by Airey (1983).

Tissues Information on tissue levels of mercury are generally restricted to the chief target tissues such as brain, kidney, and liver. Measurements have also been reported on placental tissues from the viewpoint of biological monitoring. Determinations on tissue in the early part of this century are not included because of the possibility of contamination with mercury added to tissue fixatives.

Studies of the outbreak of methyl mercury poisoning in Minamata, Japan, in the 1950s provided data on control (nonexposed) groups. Brain levels were reported to be less than 0.1 ppm (for review, see Takeuchi and Eto, 1977). Five autopsy cases in Yugoslavia (Kosta *et al.*, 1975) revealed values in the brain in the range of 0.001–0.007 ppm. Mottet and Brody (1974) reported levels in 60 hospital autopsy cases in the United States with no known exposure to mercury in the range 0.006–0.965 for the cerebellum and 0.008–0.470 for the cerebrum. A recent report (Nylander *et al.*, 1987) suggests that brain levels in otherwise nonexposed individuals increased according to the number of mercury amalgam tooth fillings. Measurements in the occipital lobe cortex in 34 individuals yielded an average value of 0.011 ppm with a range of 0.002 to 0.029 ppm. Linear regression analysis indicated that the mercury concentrations increased with the number of amalgam surfaces in the teeth.

Kidney values for nonexposed people are reported to be in the range of 0.18–2.6 ppm in Japan (Takeuchi and Eto, 1977), 0.01–0.37 ppm in Yugoslavia (Kosta *et al.*, 1975), 0.006–0.4 ppm in the United States (Mottet and Brody (1974), and average values of 0.433 ppm in seven people with mercury amalgams and 0.049 ppm in five people with no mercury amalgams in Sweden (Nylander *et al.*, 1987).

Liver levels in nonexposed people are reported to be 0.16–1.3 ppm in Japan (Tsubaki and Irukayama, 1977), 0.01–0.05 ppm in Yugoslavia (Kosta *et al.*, 1975), and 0.008–1.43 ppm in the United States (Mottet and Brody, 1974).

Fatal cases of methyl mercury poisoning in Minamata had brain levels in the range 2.6–25 ppm, liver levels in the range 22–70 ppm, and kidney levels in the range 21–144 ppm. These individuals had died about 3 months after the end of exposure. Liver levels in the autopsy cases after an outbreak of methyl mercury in Iraq (Magos *et al.*, 1976) were reported to be in the range 1.4–76 ppm (Takeuchi and Eto, 1977).

Little information is available on human tissue levels after exposure to other forms of mercury. Kosta *et al.* (1975) noted elevated levels (sometimes a thousandfold higher than in controls) in thyroid, pituitary, kidney, and liver in mercury miners who had died many years after retirement.

The average level of mercury in 38 placentas from residents in Iowa (United States) was 2.3 ppm. In another study in Ohio, 29 placentas yielded an average of 6.7 ppm, of which 5.3 ppm was in the inorganic form.

Other Findings A close correlation between selenium and mercury concentrations in a variety of autopsy tissues from retired miners and other residents of the mining village of Idria, Yugoslavia, was reported by Kosta *et al.* (1975). The atomic ratio of selenium to mercury was almost exactly 1:1 over a wide range of concentrations. These observations, along with experimental data on animals (for a recent report, see Magos *et al.*, 1984), suggest that inorganic mercury forms a complex with selenium that may persist for long periods in human tissues.

12.6.3.5 Treatment of Poisoning in Animals and Humans

Treatment in Animals The literature on the treatment of poisoning by mercury in animals and people was already very extensive in 1967 when Swensson and Ulfvarson reviewed it and added their own thorough studies in animals. On the basis of information on both animals and humans, they emphasized that therapeutic effect depends on the form of mercury causing poisoning and also on whether treatment begins early in the course of acute poisoning or after chronic poisoning already is established. Of compounds that they tested and that have ever been put to clinical use, BAL and D-penicillamine had a therapeutic effect in acute poisoning by inorganic mercury salts. BAL was also useful in acute poisoning by phenyl mercury. No useful treatment was found for acute poisoning by methyl mercury. Whereas penicillamine may have conferred some benefit in acute poisoning by methoxyethyl mercury, BAL did great harm: all animals died in convulsions following the second dose. All of the chelating agents had some influence on the distribution of mercury in different organs and on its excretion. However, there was no definite connection between the lifesaving effect of an antidote and its effect on distribution or excretion of mercury. An increase in excretion of mercury was not a precondition for lifesaving effect. On the other hand, each chelating agent not only has its own toxicity but also may increase the toxicity of one or more forms of mercury, whether by increasing its concentration in the brain or kidney or in some other way.

Zimmer and Carter (1979) confirmed that BAL is useless in methyl mercury poisoning but, contrary to some earlier results, found that D-penicillamine enhanced weight gain and prevented further development of neurotoxic signs in rats poisoned by methyl mercury chloride.

In some instances, studies concerned directly with therapy have been confirmed by studies on distribution. For example Berlin and Ullberg (1963) showed that BAL greatly increased the uptake of phenyl mercury or methyl mercury by the brain. Zimmer and Carter (1979) reported a similar result with methyl mercury.

More recent work has served to confirm most of the findings, but further progress has been limited. To be sure, an almost endless array of new chelating agents have been synthesized and tested for ability to increase the excretion of mercury, to cause a redistribution of it, and/or to increase the survival of experimental animals. There has been progress in understanding the complications of using systemically acting chelating agents. Following intravenous injection of mercuric chloride, Gabard (1976) tabulated not only the urinary and fecal excretion of ^{203}Hg but also its distribution in red cells, plasma, liver, kidneys, brain, femur, muscle, spleen, and intestine of different groups of rats following treatment with one of 15 chelating agents. It was concluded that the only agent that had a truly favorable effect was sodium 2,3-dimercaptopropane-1-sulfonate (DMPS). Whether this would be true in humans as well as the rat is, of course, unproved. It seems certain, however, that the general problem of complex effects on distribution of metals following systemic chelation applies to all species.

There also has been some progress in the treatment of acute poisoning. What has been lacking is study of possible ways of hastening the reversal of toxic effects or at least halting their progression once they have become established following some weeks or months of intake of alkyl mercury. Unfortunately, almost all recent human cases of mercury poisoning have been the result of such exposure. That the situation is not entirely hopeless was shown by the work of Magos *et al.* (1978a).

When rats were given six oral doses of ^{203}Hg at a rate of 8 mg/kg/day in the form of methyl mercury chloride, there was a progressive loss of weight after five or six doses, and this was followed by necrosis of granule cells of the cerebellum and by functional disturbances of the central nervous system. In rats that received dimercaptosuccinic acid for 3 days as an additive to drinking water (75 mg/30 ml) beginning 1–5 days after the last dose of methyl mercury, body weight was regained, progression of cerebellar damage stopped, and CNS dysfunction improved somewhat. Both the body burden and brain content of mercury were decreased by 60%.

The possible danger that a systemic chelating agent will increase the toxicity of mercury may be avoided completely by using a nonabsorbable chelating agent that serves to reduce the absorption or reabsorption of mercury from the intestine and thus to promote fecal excretion. One of these mercury-binding polymers (MBP) decreased the half-life of intraperitoneally administered methyl mercury in mice from 10.0 to 4.5 days and increased the LD 50 from 10.0 to 12.7 or 13.4 mg/kg, depending on the exact method of administration of the antidote (Harbison *et al.*, 1977).

A possible new approach to the treatment of poisoning by mercury, especially methyl mercury, was suggested by Kostyniak *et al.* (1975). In an *in vitro* study, they used a soluble and dialyzable chelating agent to free methyl mercury from protein binding and then removed the complex by passing the blood through a semipermeable dialysis tube. Using cysteine at a concentration of 10 m*M* in whole blood, up to 44% of methyl mercury and up to 94% of the cysteine were removed by one pass through the dialyzer.

Treatment in Humans   It must be emphasized that removal of poison before absorption occurs and complete care of the patient is nowhere more important than in connection with poisoning by mercury (see Section 8.2).

Unfortunately, specific therapy is complex and (with the exception of the generally recognized value of BAL in acute poisoning by inorganic mercury compounds) is unsatisfactory.

As reviewed by Swensson and Ulfvarson (1967), there was little agreement about the value of chelation treatment in chronic poisoning by alkyl compounds, and there has been no greater agreement since the review. Unithiol has been recommended for treatment of poisoning by ethylmercuric compounds and full recovery has been reported in some instances (Shustov and Tsyganova, 1970; Nizov and Shestakov, 1971; Alekseyeva and Mishin, 1971). Other investigators [Engleson and Herner, 1952; American Medical Association (AMA), 1955; Lundgren and Swensson, 1960; Pierce *et al.,* 1972; Bakir *et al.,* 1973, 1976; Nagi and Yassin, 1974; Al-Damluji, 1976b], who held that conventional chelation therapy with penicillamine, *N*-acetyl-D,L-penicillamine, or dimercaprol sulfonate was of very questionable clinical value (although it might increase urinary excretion and reduce blood levels), referred mainly or entirely to methylmercuric compounds. The difference may be real and may depend on the distinction between ethyl and methyl or on the particular drugs used for therapy, but neither possibility is certain.

There may be some merit in treating sequelae of alkyl mercury poisoning, perhaps because inorganic mercury may be left in the tissues (Ahlborg and Ahlmark, 1949; Lundgren and Swensson, 1960). EDTA has also been used as an antidote, but its value is not established (Glomme and Gustavson, 1959).

On the basis of chemical studies, Canty and Kishimoto (1975) advised caution in the use of BAL for treating poisoning by phenyl mercury. Animal studies indicate that BAL would be very dangerous if used for alkoxyalkyl mercury poisoning. To be sure, there have not been enough cases of poisoning by alkoxy or phenyl mercury compounds to reach any conclusion regarding the relative effectiveness of chelation therapy in these conditions in people.

In addition to conventional chelation therapy, one should consider the most recent developments in orally administered, unabsorbable resin chelators that trap mercury that enters the intestine in the bile or in other ways and ensures its excretion. One such resin was put to use during the latter part of the 1972 outbreak of methyl mercury poisoning in Iraq and was found to reduce blood levels of mercury (Bakir *et al.,* 1973; Clarkson *et al.,* 1981a). However, as suggested by Dr. Mark M. Jones, there has been no proof that the various synthetic resins now

available are superior—or even equal—to activated charcoal. Because charcoal is available, it ought to be used at least until a resin can be obtained.

A neuromuscular disorder similar to myasthenia gravis and responsive to neostigmine was uncovered in the course of electrophysiological testing of Iraqi patients poisoned by methyl mercury. Subsequently, neostigmine therapy (gradually increased to 15–22.5 mg plus 2–3 mg of atropine sulfate intramuscularly daily in split doses) produced a remarkable clinical improvement. Substitution of a placebo resulted in substantial loss of strength that was restored when therapy was resumed (Rustam *et al.,* 1975). The success of this particular therapy would seem to have little bearing on the view expressed earlier by Rustam and others (LeQuesne *et al.,* 1974; Rustam and Hamdi, 1974; von Burg and Rustam, 1974a,b) that *sensory* changes (including paresthesias of the hands, feet, and sometimes the buccal cavity and tongue; defective appreciation of pin prick or light touch; recognition of objects by touch; and position of the fingers associated with fine movements) are exclusively or almost exclusively central in origin.

12.6.4 ALKYL MERCURY COMPOUNDS

12.6.4.1 Identity, Properties, and Uses

Compounds and Synonyms   Of the entire range of alkyl mercury compounds, ethyl and methyl compounds have been used as pesticides. Methyl mercury was available in the form of several salts—each sold under one or more propietary names including the bis-methylmercuric sulfate (Cerewet®), the cyanoguanidine or dicyandiamide (Agrosol®, Morsodren®, Panogen®, Panospray®), the nitrile (Chipcote®), and the propionate (Metasol MP®). Ethyl mercury also was available in the form of several salts including the chloride (Ceresan®, Granosan®), the phosphate (Lignasan®, New Improved Ceresan®, New Improved Granosan®), the *p*-toluenesulfonanilide (Ceresan M®, Granosan M®), the 1,2,3,6-tetrahydro-3,6-endomethano-3,4,5,6,7,7-hexachlorophthalimide (50-CS-46, Emmi®, PX-332), and the thiosalicylate (Elcide®, Merfamin®, Mertorgan®, Merzonin®). Ethylmercuricthiosalicylate also was known by the nonproprietary names mercurothiolate, thimerosal, and thiomersalate.

Properties   See Section 12.6.3.2.

Uses   Most of the individual compounds are used as fungicides in treating seeds, especially those of cereals, sorghum, sugar beets, cotton, and flax. Used in this way, they control diseases caused by seed-borne infection and protect germinating seedlings from soil-borne pathogens (WHO, 1974).

12.6.4.2 Toxicity to Laboratory Animals

Basic Findings   The acute oral LD 50 value for representative compounds in rats is approximately 30 mg/kg (Lehman, 1951, 1952). The total dose of an alkyl mercury compound necessary to produce chronic poisoning in cats is about the same, that is, 6–24 mg/kg expressed as mercury (Kurland *et al.*, 1960).

Rats tolerated 0.5 mg (about 2.8 mg/kg/day) of ethyl mercury chloride daily for 150 days without sign of poisoning, but twice that dosage produced typical signs in 34 to 84 days (Akitake, 1968).

Methyl mercury affects mainly the central nervous system. However, the effects differ markedly for adult versus prenatal exposures, so the two situations will be discussed separately.

Effects on the Mature Nervous System Methyl mercury produces focal damage to specific areas of the brain—the neuronal cells of the visual cortex, particularly neurons situated in the deep sulci, appear to be most susceptible to damage (for a review, see Berlin, 1986). Effects most similar to those observed in humans are seen in nonhuman primates and rats.

Inhibition of protein synthesis is one of the earliest biochemical effects that precede the appearance of overt signs of intoxication in animals.

Effects on the Developing Nervous System Spyker *et al.* (1972) treated mice on day 7 and day 9 of pregnancy with a single (8 mg/kg) dose of methyl mercury. The young did not differ from the controls in size, weight, and appearance. However, when tested at 30 days of age, their behavior was abnormal in an open field test and in swimming. The brain showed abnormalities in the Purinje and granule cells of the cerebellum (Chang *et al.*, 1977). More recently, Sager *et al.* (1984) reported that after a single (8 or 4 mg/kg) dose of methyl mercury to neonatal mice, the cell division of cerebellar granule cells was drastically reduced. The lower dose produced effects in male mice but not in females. It is thought that methyl mercury produces these effects by damaging microtubules, essential for cell division. For further discussion, see Sager and Matheson (1988).

12.6.4.3 Toxicity to Humans

Alkyl mercury fungicides commonly have been the cause of occupational poisoning even in developed countries, especially when anything but the best equipment was used for applying them to seed. Furthermore, their application to seed created the possibility that they would be eaten in quantity, especially by peasants who were hungry and did not know about either the delayed onset of symptoms or the impossibility of adequately decontaminating the seed (see Section 7.1.2.4, Hayes, 1975). Finally, outbreak of poisoning clinically similar to that caused by eating treated seed resulted from eating animals that had consumed contaminated feed or from eating fish that had absorbed alkyl mercury from industrial wastes.

Symptomatology Acute poisoning by organic mercury has been reported infrequently in humans, although cases of such poisoning by methyl (Swensson, 1952) and other alkyl compounds (Lundgren and Swensson, 1949; Veichenblau, 1932) have occurred. There have been many cases of chronic poisoning involving organic mercury.

The classical description of poisoning by an alkyl mercury compound is that of Edwards (1865). The patient may complain of headache; paresthesia of the tongue, lips, fingers, and toes; and other nonspecific dysfunction. In mild cases, the symptoms do not develop beyond this point, and in such instances they usually disappear gradually.

Some but not all workers equally exposed to alkyl mercury compounds complain of a metallic taste in the mouth and slight gastrointestinal disturbances, such as excessive flatus and diarrhea (Bloom *et al.*, 1955; Ritter and Nussbaum, 1945). However, the acute symptoms associated with irritation of the gastrointestinal system and renal failure caused by inorganic mercury compounds are seldom observed in poisoning by alkyl mercury compounds and then almost exclusively in acute poisoning. Even the mild digestive disturbances and sore mouth seen in moderate, chronic, occupational poisoning by inorganic mercury are relatively rare. Instead, the nervous symptoms appear first, sometimes after relatively slight exposure and after weeks or months of latency. Diagnosis is complicated not only by the latency but also by the insidiousness of the onset. The patient may be unable to state with any certainty when he or she first noticed important symptoms.

Early signs of more severe poisoning include fine tremors of the extended hands, loss of side vision, and slight loss of coordination, especially with the eyes closed as in the finger-to-nose test. Incoordination is especially noticeable in speech, writing, and gait. Incoordination may progress to the point of inability to stand or to carry out other voluntary movements. Occasionally there is muscle atrophy and flexure contractures. In other cases, there are generalized myoclonic movements. There may be difficulty in understanding ordinary speech, although hearing and the understanding of slow deliberate speech often remain unaffected. Irritability and bad temper are frequently present and may progress to mania. Occasionally the mental picture deteriorates to stupor or coma (Herner, 1945; Ahlmark, 1948; Ahlborg and Ahlmark, 1949; Hunter *et al.*, 1940). Especially in children, mental retardation may be added to the symptoms of poisoning already mentioned (Engleson and Herner, 1952; Kurland *et al.*, 1960).

Patients frequently become gradually much worse after their illness is recognized and exposure is stopped.

The alkyl mercury compounds are strong irritants of the skin and may cause blisters or other dermatitis with or without associated systemic illness (Hunter *et al.*, 1940; Vintinner, 1940).

Study of 43 cases in the 1972 outbreak in Iraq showed that a few entered hospital with complaints that suggested psychiatric disturbances, and over half of them were consistently depressed. Blood mercury levels were consistently higher in depressed than in nondepressed patients (Maghazaji, 1974).

Signs and symptoms of poisoning in children are similar to those in adults (Nagi and Yassin, 1974).

Duration of Illness The duration of illness in fatal cases ranged from about a month to 15 years (Hunter *et al.,* 1940). Intercurrent infection, aspiration pneumonia, and inanition are the immediate causes of death in protracted cases (Kurland *et al.,* 1960). Ten years after poisoning, neurological disorders persisted with little or no improvement among 26 victims of Minamata disease (Tokutomi *et al.,* 1961). Symptoms often persist for years even in mild poisoning (Tsubaki, 1968).

Recovery from poisoning by alkyl mercury is so slow and the effects of chelation therapy are so unimpressive that it was thought some years ago that no recovery is possible. Observations repeated at long intervals have indicated that some improvement does occur except perhaps in very severe cases.

Twelve patients who were poisoned by ethyl mercury during the 1960 outbreak in Iraq were reexamined in 1973 and showed considerable improvement (Al-Damluji, 1976a). The most severely poisoned patients who survived the 1971–1972 outbreak caused by methyl mercury improved slowly, although ataxia, diminution of visual fields and visual acuity, and paresthesias were still present 2 years later. During the same period, most patients originally graded mild or moderate lost their symptoms completely (Al-Damluji, 1976b). Some children who had suffered mild or moderate poisoning by methyl mercury recovered completely in the course of 2 years. Over half of the children who had suffered severe poisoning remained physically and mentally incapacitated. The degree of clinical progress shown by the children in Iraq was better than that of some other groups, but the difference may have depended on the prompt termination of exposure rather than on the age of the patients (Amin-Zaki *et al.,* 1978).

Perinatal Poisoning Infants exposed to methyl mercury *in utero* may be severely and permanently injured even though their mothers remain asymptomatic. On the other hand, infants who received no mercury *in utero* but received it in their mother's milk may escape without clinical signs. Such cases were observed in association with the outbreak of methyl mercury poisoning in Iraq during the winter and spring of 1971 to 1972. Four infants had blood levels above 1.0 ppm, and one had levels above 1.5 ppm without sign of injury, even though 0.2 ppm is the minimal toxic level for adults (Amin-Zaki *et al.,* 1974a).

In the Minamata area during the period 1955–1959, 22 infants of a total of about 400 were born defective. Most of the mothers of these defective children did not have typical Minamata disease, but most of them experienced numbness during pregnancy. All ate fish frequently (Kutsuna, 1966). Experience in Iraq was quite different: in only one of 15 infant–mother pairs exposed to methyl mercury was the infant affected and the mother free of clinical signs (Amin-Zaki *et al.,* 1974b). The cause of the difference is uncertain, but it might be associated with the stages of gestation at which exposure occurred. Whether teratogenesis occurs, as distinct from fetal intoxication, has been discussed (Berlin *et al.,* 1969b) but is not yet clear.

Follow-up studies of prenatally exposed infants in Iraq have revealed a milder form of affliction characterized by delayed achievement of developmental milestones, abnormal reflexes, and a history of seizures (Marsh *et al.,* 1980, 1981).

Possible Distinctions between Poisoning by Methyl Mercury and Ethyl Mercury There is some indication that, compared to methyl compounds, the illness produced by ethylmercuric compounds involves relatively greater injury to the gastrointestinal system (aphthous stomatitis, catarrhal gingivitis, nausea, liquid stool, pain, and laboratory evidence of liver disorder) and the cardiovascular and hematopoietic systems and less disorder of sensation and coordination (deafness, ataxia) (WHO, 1962; Bogomaz, 1969; Shustov and Tsyganova, 1970; D'yachuk, 1972; Alekseyeva and Mishin, 1971). The contrast between the two has been pointed out on the basis of outbreaks in Iraq, the one in 1960 caused by ethyl mercury and the one in 1972 caused by methyl mercury (Al-Damluji, 1976b). However, poisoning by ethyl mercury may be fatal (Ljubetskii *et al.,* 1961; Gis' and Pozner, 1970; Mal'tsev, 1972), and those who survive may have residual nervous symptoms (Gis' and Pozner, 1970; Mal'tsev, 1972). A description of poisoning by ethyl mercury in children (Mal'tsev, 1972) makes it appear impossible to distinguish poisoning by ethyl and methyl mercury. At present it is unclear whether an important, clinical distinction is justified between poisoning by ethyl and methyl mercury either in adults or in children.

Outbreaks from Eating Treated Grain Several outbreaks caused by eating seeds dressed with methyl or ethyl mercury are listed in Table 7.14 and discussed briefly in the associated text. Findings reached in study of these and some other outbreaks have been used as appropriate throughout this section and Section 12.6.3. However, no attempt is made here to describe the epidemics themselves. The largest one, in which 6148 patients were admitted to hospital and 452 died there, was described at length in the proceedings of a Conference on Intoxication Due to Alkylmercury-Treated Seed (WHO, 1976a) and was summarized by Skerfving and Copplestone (1976).

Outbreaks from Eating Poisoned Animals On December, 1969, an 8-year-old girl developed ataxia, decreased vision, and depression of consciousness progressing to coma over a period of 3 weeks. Two weeks after she became sick, her 13-year-old brother developed a similar illness, which also progressed to coma in 2–3 weeks. At the end of December, their 20-year-old sister developed similar symptoms and became semicomatose. All were hospitalized and given supportive therapy. The use of chelating drugs was of very doubtful value. In May, two patients remained comatose, the other semicomatose (Storrs *et al.,* 1970a,b; Likosky *et al.,* 1970). The 40-year-old mother in the family was pregnant at the time. She did not become ill, and she ate no more pork after the sixth month of gestation. However, her urinary mercury levels were elevated during the 7th and 8th months. A 3062-g male infant was delivered at term. He became dusky at 1 minute of life, and intermittent gross tremulous movements of the extremities persisted for several days. The cry was weak and high pitched, but otherwise the child seemed clinically normal. Urinary mercury values were markedly elevated. The EEG and EMG were normal 3 days after birth and remained so at 6 weeks. However, at 3 months of age the EEG was abnormal, and remained so. Clinical abnormality progressed even more rapidly with increased tone of the extremities at 6 weeks, generalized myoclonic jerks by 6 months, and hypertonicity, irritability, and nystagmoid eye movements without fixation of the eyes at 8 months. These effects were the result of mercury via the placenta, for the child was never breast-fed (Snyder, 1971, 1972).

During the investigation it was learned that in October 1969, 14 of 17 hogs owned by the family became ill with blindness and a gait disturbance; 12 of these 14 died, and two became blind. In September, one hog had been butchered for family food and the meat was eaten by seven of nine family members from September through December. Further investigation revealed that in August 1969, the father had obtained floor sweepings from a plant for treating seed grain with methyl mercury dicyandiamide and had included this grain in food for the hogs. It was never revealed how the waste grain escaped safe disposal even though its danger was recognized and, during many years of treating seed, similar material from the same factory had never been permitted to reach the public.

High levels of mercury were found in the urine of the patients (0.16–0.21 ppm) and of other members of the family who remained well (0.06–0.20 ppm). The seed grain and pork contained almost equal concentrations of mercury (32.8 and 27.5 ppm, respectively) (Storrs et al., 1970a,b; Curley et al., 1971). Mass spectral analysis demonstrated the presence of methyl, ethyl, and probably methoxyethyl mercury in what was left of the waste grain that had been fed to the hogs (Curley et al., 1971). Thus, poisoning had been caused by a mixture of alkyl compounds. Although the concentrations of mercury in the urine was not above that occasionally reported for normal people, it was diagnostic in view of the known exposure to methyl mercury.

A similar tragedy might have occurred when another family acquired improperly discarded, treated seed grain, fed it to chickens, and ate the eggs. However, the matter came to the attention of the police and the agricultural authorities after feeding had progressed only about 2 months. Exposure was stopped promptly before there was illness of chickens or people. The levels of organic and inorganic mercury in egg yolks were 0.596 and 1.902 ppm, respectively; the corresponding values in albumin were 2.719 and 0.098 ppm, mere fractions of what had been found in the pork. Total mercury in blood of family members ranged from 0.009 to 0.020 and corresponded to the number of eggs eaten per day (Atwood et al., 1976).

At least two epidemics were associated with the ingestion of seafood contaminated by industrial waste (Kurland et al., 1960; Tsubaki and Irukayama, 1977).

The first of these outbreaks, which occurred at Minamata, Japan, alerted the medical community to the great danger, and Minamata disease became a synonym for chronic poisoning by organic mercury compounds. There is now considerable evidence that the compound in seafood responsible for poisoning is dimethyl mercuric sulfide (CH_3—Hg—S—CH_3) (Tokutomi et al., 1961).

It was clear from the epidemiology of Minamata disease that mercury could reach dangerous concentrations in fish and shellfish. However, there was some doubt where the conversion took place, especially since spent catalyst from the factory was found to contain about 1% methyl mercury. Later, it was shown that microorganisms are capable of methylating inorganic mercury (Jensen and Jernelöv, 1969). The methylation of mercury can occur both enzymatically and nonenzymatically, but both reactions depend ultimately on bacteria either to form the enzymes or to produce methyl cobalamine, which permits the nonenzymatic reaction. At any given concentration of inorganic mercury, alkylation will tend to be increased if the number of bacteria is increased whether by sewage or other nutrients (Wood et al., 1968). A full discussion of the interconversion of mercury and its compounds, including especially the formation of methyl mercury from industrial wastes or from mercury ores, is beyond the scope of this book, but information may be found in the report of an Expert Committee (1971).

It must be mentioned, however, that methyl mercury was produced when normal human fecal matter was incubated anaerobically with $^{203}HgCl_2$. On the other hand, the organic compound tended to disappear, and the concentration of $^{14}CH_3Hg^+$ decreased at a constant rate when incubated with feces. It was concluded that the intestinal flora can contribute substantially to the methyl mercury burden in humans (Edwards and McBride, 1975). Although methylation of mercury in the human intestine seems to be a fact, evaluation of its toxicological importance must be based on measurements in vivo.

Dosage Response Apparently no useful information on dosage response to alkyl mercury compounds has come from accidents resulting from occupational exposure. Epidemiological studies of populations exposed to unusually high concentrations of methyl mercury in food have defined three categories differing in intensity and duration of exposure. People were poisoned in Iraq when they consumed contaminated grain for an average of 1–2 months at an average mercury intake of 0.08 mg/kg/day and a maximum of about 0.2 mg/kg/day. People were poisoned in Japan when they ate contaminated fish for months or a few years at average and maximal mercury intakes of about 0.03 and 0.10 mg/kg/day. People in Sweden and various other parts of the world where fish have relatively high levels of methyl mercury were not affected by a maximal mercury intake of 0.005 mg/kg/day lasting many years or for life (WHO, 1976a). A dosage–response analysis of both adult and prenatal exposures in Iraq revealed that the developing nervous system is more susceptible than the mature nervous system, probably by a factor of three (Clarkson et al., 1981b).

Laboratory Findings Three men each swallowed 0.01 mg of ^{203}Hg in the form of methylmercuric nitrate. Whole-body counting indicated that mercury accumulated mainly in the liver (50% of dose) and the head (10%). The main excretion route was the feces but urinary excretion (as a fraction of total excretion) increased with time up to 30 days after intake. The whole-body retention curves followed a single exponential curve with half-lives between 70 and 74 days. Pharmacokinetic calculation indicated a plateau after 10 weeks of constant intake, the steady-state concentration being 15.2 times greater than the weekly dosage when both were expressed on a milligram per kilogram basis (Aberg *et al.*, 1969). See also Section 12.6.3.4.

Treatment   See Sections 8.2 and 12.6.3.6.

Pathology   Extensive and relatively characteristic pathology has been reported in humans and experimental animals killed by alkyl mercury compounds. The most common findings are (*a*) bilateral cortical atrophy around the anterior end of the calcarine fissure with disappearances of the striation of Gennari (associated with constriction of the visual fields) and (*b*) gross atrophy of the folia in the depths of the sulci of the lateral lobes and the declive of the cerebellum involving the granule cell layer (associated with ataxia). The hypothalamus, midbrain, and basal ganglia may be involved. The changes in the brain involve gliosis as well as abnormality and loss of specific neurons. The bodies of the Purkinje cells are spared, although the axons are affected. The classical description of the pathology is that of Hunter and Russell (1954) based on a patient who had had industrial exposure to methyl mercury for only 4 months and who had been followed medically from the time of onset until his death from pneumonia and complications a little over 15 years later. The disease had progressed slowly at first, but by the end of the 1st year the patient was quite helpless although still alert and intelligent, and he remained so until his death. Reference to poisoning by alkyl mercury as the "Hunter-Russel syndrome" may be traced to this paper, which pointed out, among other things, the marked difference of pathology associated with alkyl mercury in humans and in experimental animals. Changes in peripheral nerves and the posterior columns have been reported in animals (Hunter *et al.*, 1940; Swensson, 1952), but Hunter was unable to find such changes in humans.

12.6.5 ALKOXYALKYL MERCURY COMPOUNDS

12.6.5.1 Identity, Properties, and Uses

Methoxyethyl mercury silicate frequently was formulated with other fungicides or insecticides for protection of cereal grain against both fungi and insects. Examples of proprietary names, which designate each total formulation and must not be confused with formulations of ethyl mercury involving the word "Ceresan®" include Ceresan-Aldrin® (with aldrin and HCB), Ceresan Gamma M® (with anthraquinone, hexachlorobenzene, and lindane), Ceresan-Morkit® (with anthraquinone and hexachlorobenzene), and Ceresan Universal Trockenbeize® (meth-

oxyethyl mercuric silicate with hexachlorobenzene). Methoxyethylmercuric chloride was known by several proprietary names including Agallol®, Aretan®, and Ceresan Universal Nassbeize®. For a comparison of the vapor pressures of alkoxyalkyl compounds with those of other organic mercury compounds, see Section 12.6.3.2.

12.6.5.2 Toxicity to Laboratory Animals

No information on the toxicity of alkoxyalkyl mercury compounds has been found.

12.6.5.3 Toxicity to Humans

Poisoning by alkoxyalkyl mercury compounds usually begins with loss of appetite, flatulence, and diarrhea. The patient may complain of loss of weight, exhaustion, and headache. Albuminuria is a common finding and may be accompanied by generalized edema. Signs of injury of the central nervous system are less prominent than in poisoning by alkyl mercury compounds, but numbness of the fingers and toes and some degree of ataxia and weakness may occur (Bonnin, 1951; Dérobert and Marcus, 1956; Wilkening and Litzner, 1952; Zeyer, 1952).

A 60-year-old man who had worked during the autumn and winter for 5 years treating grain with methoxyethyl mercury silicate was hospitalized with a nephrotic syndrome. Because no infectious etiology was found and because the attack was brief and without recurrence, it was suspected that methoxyethyl mercury may have been the cause. However, there were no signs of chronic mercurialism and no real proof of the suspected relationship (Strunge, 1970).

Acrodynia was recognized in a 5-year-old boy exposed on a farm to a methyloxyethyl mercury seed disinfectant. The symptoms, which were typical, included an exanthem with scaling of the skin of the hands and feet, extreme apathy, anorexia, photophobia, sleeping during the day and inability to sleep at night, muscular weakness with tremor of the extremities, heavy sweating, hypertension, and tachycardia. The concentrations of mercury in the blood and urine were 0.04 and 0.055 ppm, respectively. The clinical picture improved within 4 weeks; the skin cleared in 2 months, and the patient gained weight; hypertension and tachycardia disappeared slowly (Prediger, 1976). It is unclear whether treatment with cortisone was helpful.

A disease of children eventually named acrodynia because of the severe pain it caused in the extremities or "pink disease" because of the dusky pink color of these parts was described at least as early as 1828. There was no constructive clue to its cause until Warkany and Hubbard (1948) reported that mercury was present in the urine in 18 of 20 suspected cases, and the concentration exceeded 0.05 ppm in 15 of them. The two cases without mercury already had been recognized as atypical, but they indicated that an acrodynia-like condition may occur without demonstrable mercury. The paper also pointed out that the concentration of mercury in the urine of children treated with calomel often exceeds 0.05 ppm, and, therefore, some special susceptibility must be involved in the relatively few instances in which exposure to mercury is followed by acrodynia. A great many more cases confirmed the relationship (Warkany and Hubbard, 1951, 1953). When measures were taken by physicians, pharmaceutical companies, and regulatory agencies to stop the mercurial medication of infants and children, acrodynia became extremely rare (Warkany, 1966).

Following communications with Warkany, Bivings and Lewis (1948) first used BAL to treat acrodynia. The value of such treatment remains unclear.

The alkoxyalkyl mercury compounds, like the alkyl ones, can cause toxic dermatitis ranging from mild irritation to the production of slowly healing ulcers.

Treatment is symptomatic. See Sections 8.2 and 12.6.3.6.

12.6.6 ARYL MERCURY COMPOUNDS

12.6.6.1 Identity, Properties, and Uses

Compounds and Synonyms   Phenyl mercury was available in the form of several salts each sold under one or more proprietary names including the acetate (Gallotox®, Liquiphene®, Mersolite ®, Nylmerate®, Phix®, Riogen®, Scutl®, Tag Fungicide®, Tag HL-331®, also known by the acronyms PMA, PMAC, PMAS), the nitrate (Merphenyl®, Phenmerzyl nitrate®, Phermerite®), the cyanamide (also known as barbak), the methylenebis (2-naphthyl-3-sulfonic acid (Conotrane®, phenyl mercuric Fixtan®, Fibrotan®, Hydraphen®, Penotrane®, Septotan®, Versotrane®, also known as P.M.F. and as hydraga-phen), the borate (Famosept®, Imerfen®, Merfen®), the dimethyldithiocarbamate (Merbam®), the monoethanolammonium lactate (Puratized Agricultural Spray®, Puratized N5E®, the *N*-urea (Puratized Apple Spray®), the propionate (Metasol P-6®), the quinolinate (Metasol DPO®), the triethanolamine lactate (Dowicide 1a®, Dowicide 1®, Leytosan®, Natriphene®), and the hyrdoxychlorophenol (Semesan®, Uspulun®).

Properties   For a comparison of the vapor pressure of phenyl mercury with that of other organic mercury compounds see Section 12.6.3.2.

Uses   The individual compounds are used as fungicides for apples, pears, and other fruits, potatoes, tree wounds, bulbs, textiles, timber, leather, and wood pulp. A few are used as topical antiseptics and bactericides. The acetate is used as an herbicide for crabgrass as well as a fungicide.

12.6.6.2 Toxicity to Laboratory Animals

Basic Findings   The oral LD 50 of phenyl mercury acetate in rats was found to be 60 mg/kg (Piechocka, 1968). The same parameter for another phenyl mercury compound was 30 mg/kg (Lehman, 1951, 1952). In mice, oral LD 50 values for phenylmercuric acetate and another phenylmercuric salt were both 70 mg/kg (Goldberg *et al.*, 1950).

Dietary mercury levels of 40 ppm (about 2 mg/kg/day) or lower in the form of either mercuric acetate or phenylmercuric acetate were tolerated by rats for 2 years without any change in rate of growth, mortality, or organ weights. A dietary level of 160 ppm (about 8 mg/kg/day) of mercuric acetate produced slight reduction in growth of male rats only, while the same rate of ingestion of phenylmercuric acetate interfered to a marked degree with the growth of both sexes and shortened their survival. The action of both compounds in the rat appeared to be on the kidney. A dietary level of 0.5 ppm of the phenyl compound produced detectable histological change in the kidney, but 10–20 times as much mercuric acetate was required to produce the same effect (Fitzhugh *et al.*, 1950).

12.6.6.3 Toxicity to Humans

Accidental and Intentional Poisoning   Poisoning by aryl mercury compounds usually involves the blood with symptoms of weakness secondary to anemia and infection secondary to leukopenia (Cotter, 1947). In some instances, a nonspecific neurasthenia occurs even though anemia is mild (Massmann, 1957) or absent (Swensson and Ulfvarson, 1963). In reporting an unsuccessful suicide with phenyl mercury, Ishida (1970) noted that the patient displayed no significant neurological manifestations.

Apparently the only serious illnesses ascribed to a phenyl mercury compound were a case resembling amyotrophic sclerosis and several cases of "combined motor system involvement" (Brown, 1954), but the relationship of cause and effect is difficult to evaluate in the absence of other similar cases. Although significant injury to the kidney apparently has not been reported in persons exposed to phenyl mercury compounds, the results of animal studies suggest such injury might occur. One case of mild kidney damage in a heavily exposed person has been reported, but the renal injury may have resulted from an acid burn of the skin and not from mercury (Goldwater *et al.*, 1964).

Use Experience   In many instances phenyl mercury fungicides have been used extensively without untoward effect even though workers may have increased levels of mercury in their hair (Kinoshita and Ogima, 1968; Tokutomi, 1968).

Three cases of acrodynia were reported in several thousand infants exposed to a phenyl mercury acetate added to a diaper wash as a fungicide (Gotelli *et al.*, 1985). A follow-up investigation of several hundred of these infants revealed urinary levels of mercury up to 500 μg/liter. No clinical effects were found. Some infants had a mild enzymuria that subsequently disappeared.

Laboratory Findings   See Section 12.6.3.4.

Pathology   Decrease in anterior horn cells with demyelination of the lateral columns of the spinal cord (associated with a case said to resemble amyotrophic sclerosis) has been reported;

the difference may be related to the fact that a phenyl mercury compound was involved (Brown, 1954).

Treatment of Poisoning   See Sections 8.2 and 12.6.3.6.

12.7 THALLIUM

Thallium stands between mercury and lead in the periodic table, and the compounds of these metals show marked similarities. All of them may produce immediate local irritation followed by delayed effects in various organs, notably the nervous system.

Thallium compounds cause little difficulty in industry in spite of their high toxicity. Most cases of poisoning by compounds of thallium, including even the small number that are truly occupational, involve compounds intended for use as pesticides. Most of the cases involve accidental ingestion, suicide, or murder. Moeschlin (1965) stated that in Europe thallium had replaced arsenic as a homicidal poison.

Thallium sulfate has been more widely used as a pesticide than any other compound of thallium. It has produced many cases of poisoning and serves as a good example of the toxicity of thallium generally.

A very thorough review of the toxicology of thallium is that of Heyroth (1947).

12.7.1 THALLIUM SULFATE

12.7.1.1 Identity, Properties, and Uses

Chemical Name   Thallous sulfate.

Structure Tl_2SO_4.

Synonyms   Proprietary names for thallium sulfate include Bonide Antzix ant killer®, GTA ant bane®, GTA bait®, Magikil Jelly ant bait®, Martin's Rat-Stop®, Liquid Mission Brank ant-roach killer®, and Rex ant bait®. The CAS registry no. is 7446-18-6.

Physical and Chemical Properties   Thallium sulfate has the empirical formula O_4STl_2 and a molecular weight of 504.85. It forms a colorless, odorless, dense powder of rhomboid prisms, with a density of 6.77 and a melting point of 632°C. Its vapor pressure is inappreciable. Its solubility in water at 20°C is 4.87%; at 100°C, 18.45%.

History, Formulations, and Uses   Thallium sulfate was introduced as a rodenticide in the United States during the 1930s. Syrups and jellies for sweet-eating ants and grain baits for ground squirrels and prairie dogs formerly were available with concentrations as high as 3%.

12.7.1.2 Toxicity to Laboratory Animals

The oral LD 50 of thallium sulfate to rats is 15.8 ± 9.0 mg/kg. (Dieke and Richter, 1946). Other investigators have found similar values for rats (Munch and Silver, 1931; Lehman, 1951, 1952) and dogs (Gettler and Weiss, 1943).

Poisoned animals show restlessness, ataxia, and convulsive movements followed by paresis, tremor, dyspnea, loss of weight, hemorrhagic diarrhea, and death from respiratory failure.

Thallium is a cumulative poison. The oral administration of thallium acetate to rats at a rate of about 0.45 mg/kg/day caused depilation in 6 weeks and death within 4 months. It was noteworthy that the rats had lost little weight and, except for depilation, looked rather well shortly before they died (Hanzlik *et al.*, 1928).

Although the chronicity index has not been measured specifically, it appears to be greater than 35.

Absorption, Distribution, Metabolism, and Excretion
Thallium is easily absorbed by the skin as well as by the respiratory and the gastrointestinal tracts. In industry, absorption is mainly respiratory, while nearly all accidental and intentional poisoning involves ingestion.

Following acute poisoning, thallium accumulates in the skin mainly in active hair follicles and much less in those in a resting phase. It seems likely that thallium produces alopecia by disturbing the formation of keratin and that an excess of cystine may counteract this effect (Thyresson, 1951).

Excretion of thallium is slow, amounting to about 3.2% of the body burden per day in humans and 7.5% in the rat. Excretion is almost entirely by the urine in humans (Barclay *et al.*, 1953), but is about 60% by the feces in rats (Thyresson, 1951; Barclay *et al.*, 1953; Lund, 1956a).

In the rabbit, thallium is secreted by glomerular filtration, but about half is resorbed by the tubules. Renal clearance is doubled when potassium sulfate is used as a diuretic. There is some evidence that both the storage and excretion of thallium are related to those of potassium (Lund, 1956a).

In the rat, thallium accompanies both gastric and intestinal secretions at concentrations corresponding to that of the plasma (Lund, 1956a). Somewhat more detailed observations are available for rabbits. In that species, thallium appears in the gastric juice a few minutes after subcutaneous injection of the toxin. The concentration here depends on that in the blood but never becomes quite equal to it. The concentration of thallium is high in the cystic bile and consequently in the upper portion of the small intestine. The concentration of thallium gradually decreases in the colon and in the terminal portion again reaches the concentration of the blood. The fact that the concentration of thallium in the portal vein is higher than that in the peripheral blood indicates the presence of an enterohepatic circulation (Frey and Schlechter, 1939).

Thallium crosses the placental barrier in rats and mice (Gibson *et al.*, 1967), in rabbits (Frey and Schlechter, 1939), and in humans. Characteristic hair loss and nail bands were seen in a baby born 60 days after the mother ingested 750 mg of thallium sulfate (von Martius, 1953).

Mode of Action Thallium sulfate affects almost every tissue in the body, as may be seen from the description of accidental poisoning in Section 12.7.1.3. The most serious effect is on the nervous system, but there are notable effects on the cardiovascular system, the kidney, the gastrointestinal system, and the hair and nails.

It is presumed that thallium inhibits enzymes, but nothing is really known of a biochemical lesion. In fatal cases, there usually is extensive peripheral paralysis and cardiovascular involvement. The immediate cause of death may be peripheral respiratory failure or cardiac arrest.

Pharmacological Effects In anesthetized rats, intravenous dosages of thallium sulfate ranging from 3 to 100 mg/kg produced a dosage-related decrease in blood pressure and heart rate. The hypotension was secondary to decreased contractile force and slower rate of the heart and to a reduction of peripheral vascular tone (Lameijer and Van Zweiten, 1975). It may be that these results were conditioned by anesthesia. Poisoned people often show hypertension and tachycardia.

Pathology By far the most thorough study of tissue changes in rats poisoned by thallium is that of Herman and Bensch (1967), which must be consulted for details. Briefly, renal eosinophilic casts, enteritis, and severe colitis were present consistently in acute poisoning. In subacute poisoning, the brain contained frequent foci of perivascular cuffing and rare foci of recent necrosis. In chronic poisoning, no abnormality was visible by light microscopy, but degenerative changes frequently were present in the mitochondria of the kidney, liver, and intestines, and sometimes in those of the brain, seminal vesicles, and pancreas. Other changes included autophagic vacuoles and lipid droplets. The changes were not specific for thallium. These findings were similar to but more detailed than those of Cortella (1928).

Treatment of Poisoning in Animals BAL has not been found effective in treating animals poisoned by thallium (Braun et al., 1946; Moeschlin, 1965; Lund, 1956b; Thyresson, 1951). A wide range of other drugs including EDTA and several other chelating agents have been tried without success.

Moeschlin (1965) found that cysteamine (mercaptoethylamine, Becapton®) at a rate of 30 mg/kg caused increased survival of both mice and guinea pigs poisoned by thallium sulfate.

Lund (1956b) found dithizone (diphenylthiocarbazone) effective in rats at an oral rate of 20 mg/kg/day for 5 days. A similar result was found in dogs (Mathew and Low, 1960; Doak et al., 1965) and mice (Stavinoha et al., 1959). Kurnatowski and Polakowski (1966) confirmed the lifesaving effect of dithizone in rats but found that it did not protect the collecting tubules of the kidney. However, a distinct regeneration of the tubular epithelium was seen by day 6 after the

poison was administered. Later, Polakowski (1974) measured the oral and parenteral toxicity of dithizone in rats, mice, and rabbits and showed that even nonfatal doses may injure the liver and heart. Excretion of some elements was increased but that of others was decreased. The total excretion of thallium was increased by 41% or more, both fecal and especially urinary excretion being greater (Schwetz et al., 1967). Therapy with dithizone was unsatisfactory in cats (Zook et al., 1968), but the dosage (70 mg/kg, 3 times a day) may have been excessive. It must be recalled that dithizone given in large intravenous doses may produce diabetes and other serious, permanent effects (Hayes, 1975). However, only a transient effect was produced in the rabbits by 500 mg/kg orally. Diabetes has not been encountered in animals or people given therapeutic doses.

When animals poisoned by thallium are treated with dithiocarb, the chelate produces the same kinds of injury and is just as toxic as a soluble salt of thallium. When given to thallium-poisoned animals, dithiocarb causes convulsions because it doubles the concentration of thallium in the brain (Rauws et al., 1969; Kamerbeek et al., 1971a). Dithiocarb is relatively ineffective as an antidote (Stavinoha et al., 1959).

Thyresson (1951) found that cystine (2% in the diet) moderately increased the urinary excretion of thallium in rats but not its fecal excretion. The protection given by cystine in chronic poisoning appeared greater than could be accounted for by the increase in excretion. Lund (1956b) confirmed that cystine increased thallium secretion moderately but failed to demonstrate any antidotal effect.

Potassium chloride (0.75% as drinking water) caused a 50–80% increase in the urinary excretion of thallium in rats, and activated charcoal (500 mg/kg twice daily) did the same for fecal excretion. Furthermore, both reduced mortality as compared to controls (Lund, 1956b).

A suspension of ferric ferrocyanide administered to rats at the rate of 50 mg/rat (about 200 mg/kg) twice daily for 9 days prevented death and weight loss of rats, even though treatment was withheld until the fourth day after thallium sulfate was injected intravenously at a dosage that produced 80% mortality of control rats, mainly within 6–7 days. Studies showed that absorption of [204]thallium was decreased and excretion of [204]thallium was increased by even a single dose of ferric ferrocyanide at the same rate (Heydlauf, 1969). Dvořák (1969) reported similar results and emphasized the importance of using a colloidal suspension. Guenther (1971) found that use of a 2% suspension as the drinking water of rats increased the loss of intravenously injected [204]thallium from their organs by a factor of 2.8 and increased the LD 50 by a factor of 2.3. Contrary to other results, it was found that the treatment had to be started during the first 24 hr.

Ferric ferrocyanide was more effective than rhyolytic pumice in rats (Dvořák, 1974).

12.7.1.3 Toxicity to Humans

The most complete review of human thallotoxicosis is that of Munch (1934).

Therapeutic Use Apparently thallium sulfate has not been used as a drug. Thallium acetate was used as a dipilatory agent in treating fungal infections of the hair. Single oral doses at the rate of 4–10 mg/kg were employed. An interval of 2–6 months (usually 3 months) was recommended before readministration. Use of thallium was discontinued because it was found impossible to adjust the dosage so that the toxic effects were restricted to the loss of hair. However, children who survived treatment were reported to grow normally.

A review (Munch, 1934) showed there was serious poisoning in 5.5% of 8006 cases treated with a single oral dose of thallium acetate at different recommended dosage rates, mostly 8 mg/kg. There were 8 deaths in the series. No deaths were reported at dosages lower than 8 mg/kg, but such dosages were unreliable in causing hair loss, and one case of poisoning occurred at a dosage of 4 mg/kg. In addition to the illnesses already mentioned, there were 11 nonfatal and 22 fatal cases associated with overdosage or with the administration of ordinary doses to undernourished children.

Adults were more susceptible to poisoning than children, so the drug was given orally only to children under 10 or 12 years of age (Felden, 1928). However, thallium acetate ointments were used for treating hypertrichosis in adults. Munch (1934) tabulated 59 intoxications, some involving severe polyneuropathy, muscular atrophy, marked cerebral involvement, and blindness following use of 3–8% ointments for 1 week to several months. There were no deaths in this series.

In all, Munch (1934) recorded 692 cases, including 31 deaths, associated with the medicinal use of thallium. The numbers do not include an indeterminate number of cancer cases treated with thallium.

Accidental and Intentional Poisoning Signs and symptoms are referable mainly to the gastrointestinal tract, nervous system, and the hair and nails; the heart and kidneys may also be involved. After large doses, gastroenteritis is evident in about 12–14 hours, while neurological symptoms may be delayed 2–5 days. Following smaller doses, onset may be delayed as much as 3 weeks (Reed *et al.*, 1963).

Gastrointestinal manifestations include severe paroxysmal abdominal pain, vomiting, diarrhea, anorexia, stomatitis, salivation, and weight loss. Neurological manifestations during the first days of illness may include paresthesias, headache, cranial nerve damage (ptosis, strabismus, optic atrophy), myoclonic or choreiform movements, convulsions, delirium, and coma. The occurrence of high fever is probably the result of brain injury; it indicates a bad prognosis. Vascular collapse and death may occur in 24–48 hours, but the course is usually more prolonged. Death may be caused by respiratory paralysis, pneumonia, or circulatory disturbances. Peripheral neuropathy, particularly in the legs, is common with severe pain, paresthesias, muscle weakness, tremor, ataxia, and atrophy (Sollmann, 1957). Obstinate constipation may interfere with treatment. Loss of hair begins after 1 to 2 weeks have elapsed. Several days before spontaneous shedding, impending alopecia is indicated by the ease with which the hair may be pulled out.

In the more protracted cases, ataxia, choreiform movements, dementia, depression, and psychosis may be prominent. The neurological changes must be characterized as diverse (Steinberg, 1961) and sometimes as bizarre. Neurologic damage may be permanent. In fact, chronic neurological defects were found in 54% of 48 patients who survived and were followed up. A blue gingival line and dermatological abnormalities, including white bands in the nails, may appear. Liver damage occurs but is not prominent clinically. Kidney damage may occur (Munch *et al.*, 1933; Chamberlain *et al.*, 1958; Reed *et al.*, 1963).

Death may occur promptly from shock, or it may be delayed as much as 19 days after onset (Cavanagh *et al.*, 1974). In a series of 72 children who ingested thallium, 9 died and 26 (36%) were left with persistent neurological damage. Prognostically unfavorable signs were gastrointestinal disturbances, cardiovascular abnormalities, coma, convulsions, and mental abberation (Reed *et al.*, 1963).

The clinical course and pathology of thallium poisoning tend to be chronic in those who survive the acute effects of a single dose. Most of those left with sequelae reach a stable state and are not subject to recrudescences. However, in at least one case there were intermittent attacks over a period of 5 years. Thallium was found on two occasions 2 years apart, but the concentrations found at autopsy were lower than those usually found in acute fatal cases. Although the source was never found, it was concluded that ingestion had been repeated either as the result of a psychotic self-medication or through the criminal intent of someone else (Gefel *et al.*, 1970; Dr. M. Liron, personal communication, July 8, 1979).

There was at least one small outbreak of thallium poisoning of people who ate a thallium-poisoned goat. A Bedouin family had seven goats. All of the goats ate treated grain intended as rodent poison. Six goats that died were thrown into a gorge, where they were eaten by four dogs, which died within 2 weeks. When the last goat became sick, it was killed and roasted even though the poison grain was present in its stomach. All eight members of the family ate some of the meat; those who ate only one meal remained well, but two girls who ate two meals became mildly sick a week later. In one, who was 18 weeks pregnant, the illness included loss of hair, but the child born 5 months later was healthy with no sign of falling hair (Ben-Assa, 1962).

An outbreak of poisoning resulting from the use of thallium-treated grain as food is listed in Table 7.14.

In chronic poisoning, symptoms can be nonspecific, and thallium intoxication may not be suspected unless depilation occurs. Although characteristic of thallium toxicity, hair loss also can result from poisoning with other metals and certain drugs. The same is true of the white bands on the nails.

The findings already summarized are confirmed in many other reports of accidents, murders, and especially suicides (Grulee and Clark, 1951; Bental *et al.*, 1961; Goulon, 1963; Taber, 1964; Gerdts, 1964; Hausman and Wilson, 1964; Sørensen, 1965; Potes-Gutierrez and Del Real, 1966; Reibscheid *et al.*, 1966; Marten, 1969; Koblenzer and Weiner, 1969; Curry *et al.*, 1969; Gharib, 1970; Gefel *et al.*, 1970;

Bank *et al.*, 1972; Freund *et al.*, 1971; Ossa *et al.*, 1975; Chinen *et al.*, 1977; Gastel *et al.*, 1978; Vasil'eva *et al.*, 1978).

Atypical Cases of Various Origins   Mild to moderate loss of hair lasting months or years and in some instances associated with fatigue, loss of memory, mild aching of the arms and legs, or neuroses were attributed to thallotoxicosis by Hubler (1966), and the relationship was substantiated by the occasional finding of thallium in the patients' urine. No direct contact with thallium formulations was recognized, and it was concluded that no specific exposure is required to produce the effect. No control study was carried out to examine the analytical methods used or to learn whether completely unaffected people have equally high urinary levels of thallium.

Dosage Response   Even in children, who are less susceptible than adults, serious poisoning has followed a single dose of thallium acetate at a rate of 4 mg/kg. Twice that dosage poisoned 5.5% of treated patients. Moeschlin (1965) reported that death of an adult had followed a dosage of only 8 mg/kg, but that most fatalities involved dosages in the range of 10 to 15 mg/kg or higher.

A patient who survived attempted suicide excreted 494.5 mg of thallium in the course of 15 weeks of treatment (Jindrichova and Rockova, 1969). This measured excretion was almost as great as the minimal fatal dose.

On the other hand, treated patients have survived a dose as high as 2000 mg (about 28.6 mg/kg) (Kamerbeek *et al.*, 1971b).

Treatment with Prussian blue proved difficult because of gastrointestinal symptoms in a patient who had ingested 7400 mg of thallium sulfate, and she died 51 hr after ingestion (Tauris, 1975).

The occupational intake of thallium considered safe is 0.014 mg/kg/day.

Laboratory Findings   In a study in which some 30 samples were analyzed from each of two persons killed by thallium, the following concentrations were found in important tissues: brain, 2.8 and 12.0 ppm; liver, 14.6 and 38.0 ppm; kidney, 8 and 28 ppm; and blood, 3 and 6 ppm. An extensive review of the literature revealed that earlier reports showed wider ranges. For example, most liver values lay between 3.8 and 90.1 ppm, but one value regarded as exceptional was reported as 560 ppm (Weinig and Schmidt, 1966). Other reports including more recent ones (Munch *et al.*, 1933; Domnitz, 1960; Grunfeld and Hinostroza, 1964; Arena *et al.*, 1965; Henke and Bohn, 1969; Nielsen, 1974) have shown a similar wide range of values but no trend to consistently higher or lower values. Values for the thallium content of various bones tend to be about the same as those for the liver of the same fatally poisoned person and not much higher, as in the case of lead. The concentration of thallium may be high in the intestinal contents, and often is higher in the large than in the small intestine. This may be true even in cases where the patient survives several weeks follow-

ing ingestion. Weinig and Schmidt (1966) recorded values as high as 333 ppm in the cecum in one case and values of 84 and 29 ppm, respectively, in the large and small intestine of a person who had survived 30 days and whose liver contained only 3.5 ppm.

Over a period of 12 days, a total of 225 mg of radioactive thallium was administered to a woman known to be dying of osteogenic sarcoma. This amount of thallium was tolerated without any effect on the clinical course. An average of 3.2% of the amount remaining in the body was excreted in each 24 hr period. The level of thallium in the blood rose to 3% of the administered dose 2 hr after each dosing and then fell to a level of 1.6% for as much as 48 hr. Excretion was chiefly in the urine (15.3% of the total dose in 5.5 days), but there was some in the feces (0.4% in 3 days). At death from sarcoma 24 days after the first dose, thallium was found in all tissues, but chiefly in the scalp hair, kidney, heart, and spleen. In general, nerve tissues and fatty tissues were quite low in activity, while the endocrine glands were of intermediate activity. The complete range of concentration was 0.88–9.5 ppm (Barclay *et al.*, 1953).

Diagnosis of poisoning often can be confirmed by analysis for thallium in urine, blood, or hair. The concentration of thallium in normal tissue is low. The concentration in serum does not exceed 0.03 ppm (Gofman *et al.*, 1964). Urinary levels as high as 10–50 ppm have been found in a patient who survived (Mathews and Anzarut, 1968). In a group of poisoned children 1–6 years of age, the excretion of thallium soon after hospitalization was usually 1–3 mg/24 hr, but in one patient it reached a level of 15.4 mg/24 hr (Chamberlain *et al.*, 1958). Similar concentrations (2–4 ppm) were found in a poisoned adult (Gettler and Weiss, 1943). In a case of subacute, nonfatal poisoning, the concentration of thallium in the urine varied from 0.2 to 0.3 ppm when first measured a month after ingestion and then declined more and more slowly to values of 0.05 to 0.06 ppm 20 days later (Rodermund *et al.*, 1968).

Proteinuria, cylindruria, and sometimes hematuria and oliguria may be present as indications of renal damage. Liver function tests may be abnormal. The blood picture and bone marrow are usually normal. However, there may be increased coproporphyrin and/or, more rarely, uroporphyrin in the urine. The serum iron may be slightly increased, suggesting a disturbance in the uptake of iron by the reticuloendothelial system. According to Moeschlin (1965), the spinal fluid shows a marked increase in protein, sometimes involving the globulin, but no increase in cells; a slight gold-sol and mastix reaction of the parenchymatous type may be present also. In other cases, the spinal fluid may be entirely normal (Chamberlain *et al.*, 1958). Examination of the spinal fluid is not useful in prognosis (Reed *et al.*, 1963).

One or more bands of dark pigment may be demonstrated in hair near the root in as little as 4 days after ingestion. The bands do not contain increased thallium (Moeschlin, 1965).

In many patients there is flattening or inversion of the T-waves in some leads of the electrocardiogram.

In the few patients who have epileptic seizures, the electroencephalogram shows long stretches of low-voltage theta waves and low-voltage fast activity interrupted at intervals by slow high-amplitude waves that may be single or in groups, including regular runs of waves at the rate of 6 or 7/second (Moeschlin, 1965). Other investigators have emphasized the slow, high-amplitude waves. Patients with abnormal electroencephalographic findings frequently die or fail to recover completely, while those with normal records usually survive without sequelae (Reed *et al.*, 1963).

Pathology Only visceral congestion and hyperemia and punctate hemorrhages of the gastrointestinal tract may be found if death occurs soon after exposure. In cases with longer survival, alopecia may be present. The skin is dry, and microscopic examination reveals marked lesions of the epithelium, follicles, and glands. Damage to the intestinal mucosa is common. There may be fatty degeneration of the heart and liver, degeneration of kidney tubules and the adrenal medulla, and edema and congestion of the lungs. At least a part of the varied tissue damage is explained by histological damage in the capillaries. Degeneration and demyelination occur in peripheral nerves. Similar changes have been found in one or more cases in the paravertebral sympathetic chain, the fasciculus gracilis, and in various other tracts or nerves, including the optic nerve. There may be retrograde injury to neurons in ganglia and nerve nuclei (Gettler and Weiss, 1943; Heyroth, 1947; Moeschlin, 1965; Karkos, 1971; Bank *et al.*, 1972). The dying back may affect both motor and sensory nerves (Cavanagh *et al.*, 1974). Finally, severe damage to a wide range of brain nuclei may be found (Kennedy and Cavanagh, 1976).

Differential Diagnosis In the absence of alopecia, neurological signs may be so confusing that differential diagnosis must include infection and degenerative, traumatic, and neoplastic disease as well as intoxication by other compounds (Chamberlain *et al.*, 1958). Compared to poisoning by arsenic, thallium produces less prompt and usually less severe gastrointestinal disorder, little or no depression of the blood cells, and a prompter, more varied effect on the nervous system. Although it occurs late and is not completely diagnostic, alopecia is especially helpful in suggesting poisoning by thallium.

Treatment of Poisoning The treatment of choice (following efforts to remove as much ingested poison as possible) would appear to include ferric ferrocyanide (Prussian blue) or activated charcoal, forced diuresis (with a moderate supplementation of total potassium chloride), and supportive measures as required. Among the latter, trihexyphenidyl (Artane) may be of value in selected cases. This compound, which is ordinarily used to treat Parkinsonism, caused a striking reduction in tremors in one series of cases of thallium poisoning (Stein and Perlstein, 1959).

Ferric ferrocyanide in divided oral doses at a total rate of 250 mg/kg/day or even greater should be administered to minimize absorption of thallium from the intestine. Daily doses should be given to reduce reabsorption of the poison from the intestine. Although fecal excretion of thallium is ordinarily small in humans, the material is excreted into the gastrointestinal tract as in animals. Frey and Schlechter (1939) reported a case in which moderate quantities of thallium were found in the vomitus as late as the 35th day after onset.

Rauws and van Heyst (1979) found that different preparations of Prussian blue differed in their ability to adsorb thallium. In general, colloidally soluble preparations are effective, but ideally every batch intended for antidotal use should be tested for thallium-binding capacity.

No side effects were seen from ferric ferrocyanide even at a dosage of 416 mg/kg/day. Duodenal intubation is not required for administering this material. Its effects are dramatic when administered soon after ingestion and rewarding even when given in long-standing intoxication. It may promote substantial fecal excretion, even though the concentration of thallium in the urine has decreased to less than 0.5 mg/24 hr (Barbier, 1974). On the contrary, when hemodialysis, forced diuresis, and Prussian blue were used in combined treatment, slightly more thallium was recovered in the urine than in the dialysate and only very little was found in the feces (Drasch and Hauck, 1977). It is not yet clear how the different forms of removal of thallium compete with one another, just which method is best, or whether combined treatment is necessarily better than the best single treatment.

If ferric ferrocyanide is not available at once, the patient should be treated with repeated doses of activated charcoal (500 mg/kg twice daily) until Prussian blue can be obtained.

Hemodialysis for 5.5 hr reduced the concentration of thallium in the serum of a patient from 0.885 to 0.170 ppm; 16.26 mg was in the dialysate, and forced diuresis later led to the excretion of 8.96 mg in the urine (Piazolo *et al.*, 1971). Although used by others, hemodialysis has been considered of doubtful value (Paulson *et al.*, 1972).

According to Koch *et al.* (1972) it is possible by forced diuresis of 12 liters/day to increase the urinary excretion of thallium to 3.5 times what it would be otherwise. They reported that in this way they recovered (in 10.6 days) 62% of 507 mg of thallium a patient was thought to have ingested.

In another case in which the ingested dosage was much larger (1300–1800 mg) and the symptoms severe, forced diuresis was combined with hemodialysis, ferric ferrocyanide, and laxatives and enemas (Loew *et al.*, 1972). A similar multiple approach was used by Jax *et al.* (1973), Stevens *et al.* (1974), Van Hees *et al.* (1975), Drasch and Hauck (1977), and Graben *et al.* (1978).

Hypertension and tachycardia associated with thallium poisoning are reported to respond to 150 mg of propranolol per day (Merguet *et al.*, 1969) or to propranolol and phentolamine combined (Hantschmann, 1970), but whether a clinical benefit is achieved is obscure.

Potassium chloride (2000 mg every 4 hr) greatly increased confusion in a patient poisoned by thallium; however, excretion of thallium was increased, and the confusion gradually lessened as treatment was continued for 6 days (Papp *et al.*, 1969). Another patient treated at a slightly lower rate showed no increase in excretion but did show progression of peripheral neurological injury during treatment (Innis and Moses, 1978).

The following paragraphs are concerned with different systemic chelating agents and one nonabsorbable chelating agent. This review justifies recommending the nonabsorbable agent, Prussian blue, and avoidance of most if not all of the available systemic chelating agents.

No controlled study of antidotes for treating thallium poisoning in humans has been reported. An attempt to evaluate dithizone, BAL, and CaEDTA retrospectively indicated that none of them, including dithizone, offered any definite advantage (in terms of survival without sequelae) over supportive treatment only (Reed et al., 1963). Thus, at best, the systemic chelating agents make the results in the severe cases in which they tend to be used similar to the unsatisfactory results in the less severe cases in which no antidote is employed.

Although potassium iodide and sodium thiosulfate formerly were recommended for treatment of poisoning by thallium, there is no objective evidence that they are effective in humans and animal studies show them worthless.

A number of systemic chelating agents have been tried. There are reports of improvement after the administration of BAL (Mazzei and Schaposnik, 1949; Welty and Berrey, 1950; Stein and Perlstein, 1959; Grunfeld, 1963). However, it now is generally felt both on the basis of clinical experience and animal experiments that EDTA or BAL are not useful in the treatment of thallium intoxication (Foreman, 1961).

Sodium diethyldithiocarbamate (dithiocarb) was used in treating one case (Bass, 1963). Although the patient survived, he became worse following each treatment. Both survival and exacerbation of symptoms were attributed to the mobilization and excretion of thallium, but no quantitative information was given. Kamerbeek et al. (1970) found that dithiocarb did increase excretion of thallium, but the level of consciousness fell in patients treated with it; animal experiments showed this was caused by a redistribution of thallium to the brain. The very severe illness in another patient who was thought to have ingested only 500 mg of thallium sulfate (Keller et al., 1971) may have been conditioned by treatment with dithiocarb.

In one study, dithizone, another chelating agent, was considered effective in five of six severely ill children in an oral dosage of 10 mg/kg twice a day for 4 to 21 days (Chamberlain et al., 1958). Dithizone was considered successful in other cases (Mathews and Anzarut, 1968; Parra et al., 1973), including one in which BAL had failed (Bendl, 1969). However, the treatment certainly failed in some instances (Arena et al., 1965). The mechanism of action was unknown because the apparent clinical improvement in certain cases was not accompanied by increased excretion. Similar findings were reported by Smith and Doherty (1964). However, the fact that dithizone is clinically effective in more than one species of animal indicates that a thorough study of its mode of action might be rewarding. For further discussion of dithizone see Sections 4.2.7.3 and 4.2.8.1.

After demonstrating that ferric ferrocyanide is much more adsorptive than activated charcoal for thallium ion, Kamerbeek

et al. (1971b) administered ferric ferrocyanide to patients poisoned by thallium. The dosage was 10,000 mg/person/day for 10 to 14 days. All the patients recovered, although one who had ingested what was considered a fatal dose was left with a slight ataxia and paresis of the legs. The treatment caused no side effects.

Van Der Merwe (1972) reported the treatment of two patients with ferric ferrocyanide at a dosage of 250 mg/kg/day (3.75 g in 50 ml of 15% mannitol administered by duodenal tube and repeated four times a day) for about 2 weeks. Although each patient was thought to have ingested about 700 mg of thallium sulfate and although each was hospitalized too late for gastric lavage (which was done) to be effective, both patients recovered. The symptoms were limited to hyperthesia and pain beginning in 3 or 4 days and then gradually clearing and to some loss of hair 10–14 days after ingestion of the poison. Mannitol was used to prevent or delay the onset of paralytic ileus, which would render the Prussian blue useless.

12.8 LEAD

Traces of lead occur in many rocks in addition to those that qualify as ores. Lead thus finds its way into soil and water and hence into food and into human and animal tissues even in remote places where there is no use of the metal or its compounds (see Table 12.3). In spite of its widespread distribution in tissues, there is no indication that lead has any beneficial effect. The concentrations found in the general population are tolerated, and similar concentrations must have been tolerated since time immemorial. People with regulated occupational exposure show no ill effect in spite of slightly higher tissue

Table 12.3

Concentration of Lead in Soil, Water, Beverages, Food, and Air

Material	Range of concentrations (ppm)
Rocks (means)[a]	8–20
Virgin soils[a]	0.03–108
Agricultural soils[a]	0.5–>1000
Urban soils[b]	28–360
Seawater[a]	0.001–0.008
Fresh water[a]	0.001–0.055
Drinking water (U.S. cities)[c]	<0.004–>0.055
Beverages including wine[a]	0.004–1.51
Food of vegetable origin[a]	0.003–6
Food of animal origin[a]	0.003–10
City air[a,d]	0.0005–0.020[e]

[a] deTreville (1964).
[b] Kehoe (1961).
[c] Taylor (1962).
[d] WHO (1977).
[e] mg/m^3.

levels. However, studies in volunteers show that the safety factor of lead is less than 10. The daily intake of lead by the general population is about 0.4 mg/person/day. A volunteer who was given lead (in the form of a soluble salt) at the rate of 3 mg/day began to show signs of mild poisoning in less than 4 months. Other volunteers tolerated dosing at the rate of 0.3, 1, and 2 mg/person/day for periods as great as 21 months (Kehoe, 1961).

Stable isotopes of lead (^{204}Pb and ^{207}Pb) were used to study lead kinetics and metabolism in a volunteer without ever increasing the total intake of lead above the person's normal level (0.367 mg/day). It was concluded that approximately two-thirds of his intake was dietary and the remainder was respiratory as judged by absorbed lead measured in the blood (Rabinowitz and Wetherill, 1973). A similar experiment on another subject, who received the same food and similar atmospheric exposure, revealed a distinctly lower blood lead level. This was explained by lesser absorption from the gut and to a smaller extent by other factors. In the course of the second experiment, the concentration of lead in the air was greatly reduced by a filter. The response of the blood lead was prompt, and its slope indicated that, prior to the reduction, about 0.015 mg/day had been absorbed from the unfiltered atmosphere. This was the same value as that measured less directly for the first subject. Because of the difference in gastrointestinal absorption, the contributions of food and air to blood lead were more nearly equal in the second subject (Rabinowitz *et al.*, 1974).

The present minor importance of lead compounds as pesticides justifies very little attention to them in this book. Although almost all accidental deaths caused by arsenic compounds are caused by pesticides, not one of many recent deaths caused by lead were caused by compounds intended for use as pesticides (Hayes and Pirkle, 1966). However, the great importance of other lead compounds as causes of accidental poisoning and the long persistence of lead arsenate following its earlier heavy use as a pesticide require some discussion of lead here. Those requiring additional information may find it in several reviews (Aub *et al.*, 1926; Cantarow and Trumpeter, 1944; Kehoe 1964; U.S. Public Health Service, 1966; Browning, 1969; Goldwater, 1972a; Goyer, 1974; WHO, 1977).

12.8.1 LEAD ARSENATE

12.8.1.1 Identity, Properties, and Uses

Chemical Name Lead arsenate.

Structure PbHAsO$_4$.

Synonyms Other names for lead arsenate include acid lead arsenate, dibasic lead arsenate, dilead arsenate, dilead orthoarsenate, diplumbic hydrogen arsenate, lead hydrogen arsenate, and standard lead arsenate. Trade names include Arsinette®,

Gypsine®, Ortho L10 Dust®, and Ortho L40 Dust®. The CAS registry no. is 10102-48-4.

Physical and Chemical Properties Lead arsenate has the empirical formula AsHO$_4$Pb and a molecular weight of 347.13. It is a white, odorless powder with a density of 5.79. It decomposes above 280°C. It is soluble in dilute nitric acid and alkali but insoluble in water. It is stable to light, air, and water. It is not stable in acid, alkali, or sulfides.

History, Formulations, and Uses Lead arsenate first was used as an insecticide in 1894. It is used for the control of moths, leaf rollers, and other chewing insects and in soil treatments for Japanese and Asiatic beetles in lawns. It is formulated as pastes or powders. Pastes contain at least 28.4% PbO, 14% As$_2$O$_5$; powder contains at least 62% PbO, 32% As$_2$O$_5$; neither contains more than 0.25% As$_2$O$_5$ in water-soluble form. Lead arsenate may be used with summer oil emulsions, spray lime, wettable sulfur, and certain hydrocarbons and nicotine sulfate. An indefinite lead arsenate mixture called basic lead arsenate (see Table 12.10) also is used in the form of dusts with sulfur or clay, and in water suspensions. Production of lead arsenate and of calcium arsenate is illustrated in Fig. 1.8.

12.8.1.2 Toxicity to Laboratory Animals

Symptomatology The signs of acute poisoning by lead arsenate in rats are similar to those of other arsenic compounds (see Section 12.12.1). The animals show violent gastroenteritis and diarrhea and die from exhaustion and dehydration. Convulsions and general paralysis may occur before the onset of gastroenteritis. Death may occur within a few hours to several days.

Following repeated doses, dogs may develop convulsions and paralysis not unlike the signs of encephalopathy seen in subacute poisoning in humans. Rats show nephropathy at least histologically and thus reproduce another injury seen in humans. Anemia is commonly present. Many of the subtle effects of chronic lead poisoning observed in humans are poorly reproduced in animals, although Aub *et al.* (1926) produced a convincing "wristdrop" in cats by weighing the paw.

Dosage Response Voight *et al.* (1948) reported a marked difference between the oral LD 50 values of lead arsenate in the rabbit (125 mg/kg) and rat (825 mg/kg). However, Lehman (1951, 1952) reported a value for the rat (100 mg/kg) not very different from that reported earlier for the rabbit.

Dogs fed lead at rates of 0.33–1.10 mg/kg developed signs of poisoning in 120–215 days, and only some of them survived 229 days until the end of the experiment. Young animals were more susceptible than old ones. Dogs fed lead at rates of 1.8–2.6 mg/kg/day developed the first signs of poisoning in 14–44 days, and most of them died following convulsions and paralysis in 51–84 days after the beginning of feeding. Within the dosage range used, there was an approximately straight-line inverse relationship between rate of intake and the time at which signs of poisoning began. Dogs fed arsenic trioxide at arsenic rates corresponding to those obtained from lead arsenate remained well (Calvery *et al.*, 1938). A no-effect level for lead was not demonstrated.

Male rats, but not females, were said to show decreased growth rate when fed lead arsenate at an average lead rate of about 0.21 mg/ kg/day (Laug and Morris, 1938), but the difference was of questionable statistical significance. There was a slight increase in the dry weight of the kidney relative to body weight, but this may have been the result of a nutritional disturbance caused by pair feedings. It is possible that 0.21 mg/kg/day is a threshold level for toxicity in the rat. This result is very similar to that reported earlier by Smyth and Smyth (1932), who found a dosage of 0.265 mg/kg/day for 16 weeks harmless, 1.03 mg/kg/day questionably harmful, and a dosage of 3.93 mg/kg/day definitely harmful.

Fairhall and Miller (1941) found that a dosage of 24 mg/kg/day caused some failure of growth in the course of a 2-year experiment. Horwitt and Cowgill (1937) found that an intake of about 5 mg/kg/day produced no effect on growth, but an intake of about 10 mg/kg/day did produce anemia and growth retardation. Slight but reproducible growth retardation was reported by Laug and Morris (1938) in an experiment in which rats on a special low-lead diet received a supplement that added only 0.213 mg/kg/day to their lead intake.

Since lead arsenate contains two toxic elements, it might be predicted that its toxicity would show an influence of both kinds of poisoning. Fairhall and Miller (1941) reported evidence that this is true; for example, it was clear that increased hemosiderin of the spleen was an effect of arsenic, while certain inclusion bodies in the kidney were an effect of lead. Furthermore, as described below, this study suggests that rats are more susceptible to mortality caused by prolonged exposure to the arsenic moiety of lead arsenate, while the work of Calvery *et al.* (1938) cited above suggests that dogs are more susceptible to the lead moiety.

One group of rats was fed lead arsenate at an approximate rate of 10 mg/rat/day, which would be about 40 mg/kg/day when they reached adulthood. Other groups were fed lead carbonate and calcium arsenate at such a rate that they received an equivalent dosage of lead and arsenic, respectively. A control group received the same diet but none of the chemicals. During the 2-year course of the experiment, lead carbonate did not increase the mortality significantly over that of the controls (42%). However, both arsenic compounds caused an approximately equal increase in mortality (56% or more after 2 years). At the end of 1 year, half of the living animals were killed and their tissues analyzed. Similar analyses were made on the rats that survived for 2 years. Animals fed lead arsenate stored more arsenic than lead in their soft tissues, even though the rate of arsenic intake was less (21.6% of molecule as compared to 60.7%). The storage of lead in bone was very great, as expected. More interesting was the fact that (with the possible exception of arsenic in the liver) all organs stored less arsenic and less lead when they were fed simultaneously as lead arsenate than when fed separately at the same rates. The

difference (at least for lead) was attributed to decreased absorption or increased excretion, but the possibility that solubility might be involved could not be excluded (Fairhall and Miller, 1941).

Absorption, Distribution, Metabolism, and Excretion
Absorption of lead arsenate is generally gastrointestinal. This is likely to be true following respiratory exposure to coarse dusts as well as after ingestion. Dermal absorption is extremely small.

Lead and arsenic derived from lead arsenate are distributed separately in the body. Lead is stored in highest concentration in the bone with much lower concentrations in soft tissues. Arsenic, although constituting a smaller proportion of the molecule, is stored in the liver and in some instances in the kidney at higher concentrations than those for lead (Fairhall and Miller, 1941).

Lead is transferred to the fetus of animals and humans (Legge and Goadby, 1912; Calvery 1938; Morris *et al.*, 1938; Horiuchi *et al.*, 1959).

Dogs and rats fed lead at a constant rate store less lead when fed a normal or high-calcium diet than when fed a low-calcium diet (Calvery *et al.*, 1938; Grant *et al.*, 1938). In fact, the metabolism of lead is very similar to that of calcium. The same factors act on both, and each tends to displace the other.

Rats store lead at the lowest measurable dietary intake, and storage is proportional to intake (Laug and Morris, 1938).

When rats ingest lead at ordinary dietary levels, it is stored in highest concentration in bone, but when feeding is at a high level for a few weeks, the highest concentration is in the kidney (Laug and Morris, 1938).

Mode of Action   Lead is a protoplasmic poison leading to changes in many organs. It is reported that the bacterial decomposition of organic matter in water is inhibited by lead at a concentration of 0.1 ppm, a concentration sometimes reached in the blood and often exceeded in the tissues of people in the general population.

It is thought that the action of lead is particularly marked in the blood vessels and that some effects are secondary to this injury. However, there is little doubt that the nervous system and kidneys, especially the tubules, are affected directly. It is thought by some that the cramps, diarrhea, and constipation characteristic of lead poisoning represent a direct action on smooth muscle rather than the nerves and that wristdrop and footdrop represent a similar action on striated muscle (Aub *et al.*, 1926).

Lead is stored to a very marked degree. It is perhaps the classic example of a cumulative poison.

The cause of death in acute poisoning is usually shock. In subacute poisoning, death usually follows severe injury to the brain evidenced by convulsions and coma. Persons or animals with severe chronic poisoning become cachectic and exhibit such diffuse injury that it is difficult to assign a single cause of death.

Although many enzymes are inhibited by lead, no specific inhibition has been identified as the biochemical lesion.

Although not related to lead arsenate specifically, it is interesting to note that much lead poisoning in children is related to pica, which causes them to consume other lead compounds of very low solubility. Studies in rats showed that calcium deficiency is one component of lead pica in that species. Weanling rats were offered a choice of distilled water and either 0.08, 0.16, 0.32, or 0.64% lead acetate solution. Those eating a low-calcium diet ingested lead acetate solutions in much greater proportions than did controls on a normal diet or those receiving a diet deficient in iron. Increased ingestion occurred even at the high concentrations of lead acetate, which normal weanlings avoided. Repeated injections of lead acetate did not cause weanlings to change their ingestion of lead, but, at least in females, did produce a significant increase in the ingestion of calcium (Snowdon and Sanderson, 1974).

Effects on Organs and Tissues Leukocyte cultures from mice poisoned rapidly by a dietary level of 10,000 ppm of lead acetate showed a great increase of gaps usually in single chromatids; some acentric chromatin fragments were found also (Muro and Goyer, 1969).

The feeding of very high doses of lead phosphate, lead acetate, or basic lead acetate has led to cancer of the kidney in rats (Zollinger, 1953; Boyland et al., 1962; Van Esch et al., 1962). No increase in tumors was found in male rats that received 25 ppm lead in their drinking water from weaning until natural death, although the animals showed weight loss from the 24th month onward (Schroeder et al., 1970).

A thorough review of the tumorigenicity of lead salts in general (WHO, 1972) revealed that lead acetate, lead subacetate, and lead phosphate are carcinogenic in rats and/or mice. The kidney is the most important and perhaps only target organ. There is no evidence that lead salts cause cancer of any site in humans. The dosages necessary to cause the condition in animals far exceed the maximal tolerated dosage in humans.

Treatment of Poisoning in Animals CaNa$_2$-EDTA was more effective than unithiol in promoting excretion of lead (Soroka and Sorokina, 1969).

12.8.1.3 Toxicity to Humans

Experimental Exposure One man was given lead arsenate at the rate of 40 mg/day or about 0.57 mg/kg/day for 50 days without ill effect (Cardiff, 1940). In a separate study, two men ingested lead arsenate at a rate of 100 mg/man/day for 10 days without injury (Fairhall and Neal, 1938). These levels are far above the level of lead in soluble form found to produce mild poisoning in a somewhat longer period. The difference in effect presumably is due to the insolubility of lead arsenate, although duration of exposure may play a part also.

Accidental and Intentional Poisoning There have been astonishingly few reports of poisoning by lead arsenate. Tobaldin

et al. (1966) did report cases of nonfatal poisoning in two girls, ages 8 and 10 years. The initial symptoms of gastrointestinal irritation were what one would expect in acute poisoning by a metal salt. The authors concluded that the effects were the result of both elements.

Use Experience In an apple-raising area, many people, including children, ate apples sprayed with lead arsenate so that the average intake of the compound was about 5 mg/person/day. They suffered no ill effect, and the only change was a marginal increase in the levels of lead in the blood and of lead and arsenic in the urine as compared with samples from an urban community (Neal et al., 1941b).

In a 14-month study of 542 formulators and applicators of lead arsenate sprays for apple orchards, Neal et al. (1941b) found only seven who had a combination of clinical and laboratory findings directly referable to the absorption of the compound. Whether the very mild observed conditions represented poisoning was left moot, but it was noted that not a single case met the criteria established by the Committee on Lead Poisoning of the American Public Health Association. Dermatitis was infrequent and not related to exposure to lead arsenate. The fertility of married orchardists was normal. The degree of exposure of these orchardists was indicated by average lead concentrations of 5.74 mg/m^3 during mixing and 0.45 mg/m^3 during spraying. Arsenic values were proportionally smaller.

These orchardists, who had had many years of heavy exposure to lead arsenate as applicators and the arsenic content of whose urine in 1938 averaged 0.141 ppm (men) and 0.098 ppm (women), were studied again in 1968 and 1969. The standard total mortality ratio (SMR) for the orchardists compared to the general population of the same state was only 0.65. The corresponding SMRs for heart disease, cancer, and stroke were 0.60, 0.66, and 0.76, respectively, indicating that this cohort experienced less total mortality and less mortality from heart disease, cancer, and stroke (Nelson et al., 1973).

During 1945, when, because of World War II, much agricultural work was done by Mexican laborers, a study in the same agricultural community found similar concentrations of lead in air for the same kind of work but found that during October 60% of the laborers had urinary lead levels in excess of 0.15 ppm, and 40 of them were hospitalized for lead intoxication (Farner et al., 1949). It is difficult to determine what bearing the latter paper had on the usual pattern of spraying tree fruit with lead arsenate. It contained no medical information. It discussed respiratory exposure at length but attributed the hospitalization to lead intoxication by mouth. The possibility was not excluded that the exposure of the Mexican workers was not directly occupational.

Character of Poisoning by Lead Since the insecticide lead arsenate has not been a notable source of intoxication, it seems desirable to add a description of poisoning caused by lead encountered in other ways.

In recent years, lead poisoning has occurred most frequently and severely in children who live in slums. They ingest lead paint applied many years earlier to their homes and now flaking and peeling from many surfaces. Another common source of poisoning has been lead dissolved from old automobile radiators used in the distillation of illicit whiskey. Under present conditions, lead is not a common source of poisoning in industry.

The signs and symptoms of lead poisoning differ with the dosage rate. In acute poisoning, which is rarely seen nowadays, the symptoms are principally gastrointestinal with colic (which may be so severe that it can be confused with appendicitis), vomiting, and diarrhea followed later by constipation. With lesser degrees of exposure, there are subacute symptoms, including not only mild abdominal pain and constipation, but also irritability, headache, drowsiness, confusion, incoordination, muscular weakness, toxic psychosis, vomiting, convulsions, and coma. The more dramatic neurological signs go to make up what is called encephalopathy. This may come on progressively over a period of 3–6 weeks or it may appear suddenly in a child who has shown no particular illness but may present with convulsions. It is the subacute disease which is most likely to be encountered in children. Usually nothing this severe is found now in industrial workers.

Chronic lead poisoning presents a very diverse picture involving constipation, some pain (particularly in the abdomen and also in the arms and legs), some headache, fatigue, occasionally tremor (but even this is unusual now), and some weakness of extensor muscles (but usually not fully developed paralysis involving wristdrop or footdrop). Weakness of muscles tends to occur in those that are used most; for example, it begins earliest and is most severe in the right hand of right-handed people. There may be a lead line about a millimeter back from the edge of the gums, particularly in persons who have poor dental hygiene and presumably produced by sulfides in the mouth. It has been shown by Japanese investigators that exposure to lead produces a rather high rate of sterility among both males and females. Finally, there is considerable evidence that sufficient exposure to lead may eventually produce nephropathy. In a study of the renal function of 102 Romanian patients with lead poisoning, dysfunction was more frequent in those with episodes of lead colic and long occupational exposure. Decreased urea clearance was the earliest sign and was followed by deteriorating creatinine clearance. Continued exposure to lead produced persistent urea retention and creatinemia frequently accompanied within several years by arterial hypertension. Undercompensated and decompensated renal failure was found in 17 of the 102 patients. Impairment of renal function was considered the result of impairment of intrarenal circulation (Lilis et al., 1968).

In addition, lead produces a number of subtle injuries that may contribute to the patient's debility and may persist after the anemia, ataxia, and other visible signs have been alleviated. The failure of plasma renin activity and aldosterone secretion rate to increase normally in response to sharp restriction of dietary sodium has been interpreted as evidence of injury to the juxtaglomerular apparatus (Sandstead et al., 1969b). Injury to the iodine-concentrating mechanism of the thyroid has also been demonstrated (Sandstead et al., 1969a).

Rakow and Lieben (1968) emphasized the chronicity of even the mild gastrointestinal and renal effects of controlled occupational exposure. They studied 24 men who 10 years earlier had experienced lead poisoning sufficiently severe that all of them had been separated from contact. Six of the men had returned to and remained in jobs involving relatively high exposure to lead and two others also were still employed by the same lead plant but at jobs involving somewhat lower exposure. Three men had returned to their jobs but remained only a short time, and 13 never returned to the plant. All 24 men were still actively employed. Urine lead levels in the nonexposed group ranged from 0.006 to 0.112 ppm with a mean of 0.047 ppm. In the group of eight who were still in the same plant, the urinary lead ranged from 0.035 to 0.81 ppm with a mean of 0.249 ppm. The man with the highest urinary level had a blood lead level of 1.72 ppm. Albuminuria was evident in 21.7% of the cases compared to 3 to 6% in the general population. Of the eight men still in the plant, 75% complained of symptoms referable to the neuromuscular and gastrointestinal systems; however, 44% of the unexposed men also complained of similar symptoms.

Storage and Excretion of Lead The concentrations of lead in the blood and excreta of the general population, in healthy workers, and in persons poisoned by lead are shown in Tables 12.4 to 12.6. Blood and especially urine values tend to reflect recent intake rather than body burden. On the other hand, urinary excretion following a test dose of a chelating agent gives a good indication of the body burden (see *Use of Chelating Agents to Mobilize Lead* in Section 8.1.4.1.

The greatest amount of information on the relationship between lead poisoning and storage involves blood lead. Some biochemical changes can be demonstrated dependably at blood levels at which there is no clinical disturbance. Because of individual variation and other factors, there is no way to be

Table 12.4
Concentration of Lead in Human Blood

Exposure	Concentration (ppm)	Reference
General population	0.20–0.59	Kehoe (1961)
	0.27[a]	
	0.000–1.00	Goldwater and Hoover (1967)
	0.18[a]	
	0.07–0.53[b]	Gofman et al. (1964)
	<0.01–1.093	Kubota et al. (1968)
	0.13[a]	
	0.30[a]	Zurlo et al. (1970)
Workers	0.20–0.79	Zurlo et al. (1970)
	0.51[a]	
	0.1–0.7[c]	Fleming (1964)
	0.6[a,c]	
Cases	0.7–2.0[c]	Fleming (1964)
	0.9[a,c]	

[a] Mean or median values.
[b] Plasma values.
[c] Values for workers exposed to tetraethyl lead.

Table 12.5
Concentration of Lead in Human Urine

Exposure	Concentration (ppm)	Reference
General population	0.000–0.118	Goldwater and Hoover (1967)
	0.033[a]	
	0.000–0.160[b]	Whitaker et al. (1962)
	0.015[a,b]	
	0.038[a]	Zurlo et al. (1970)
Workers	0.01–0.15[c]	Fleming (1964)
	0.08[a,c]	
Cases	0.08–0.40[c]	Fleming (1964)
	>0.19[a,c]	
	0.000–0.500[b]	Whitaker et al. (1962)
	0.146[a,b]	

[a] Mean or median values.

[b] Values for children. A range of 0.000–0.120 ppm with a mean of 0.024 ppm was found in children suspected of poisoning but without clear clinical signs.

[c] Values for workers exposed to tetraethyl lead.

certain at what level a particular ill effect will occur in an individual or in some members of a small group. However, a useful and conservative guide consists of a series of levels below which specific effects have not been demonstrated. An expert group (WHO, 1977) has compiled such a list that may be summarized as follows: slight decrease of hemoglobin, 0.5 ppm; subclinical peripheral electrophysiological changes, 0.4–0.5 ppm; brain dysfunction, 0.5–0.6 ppm in children and 0.6–0.7 ppm in adults; acute or chronic encephalopathy, 0.6–0.7 ppm in children and 0.8 ppm in adults; nephropathy, 0.7 ppm for a prolonged period.

Among children in Chicago, there was a seasonal variation in blood lead levels regardless of whether those levels remained in the normal range or indicated excessive absorption. The levels were highest in June and lowest during November to January (Blanksma et al., 1969). The reason for the cycle is unknown. Other factors may influence the level. For example, black children deficient in glucose-6-phosphate dehydrogenase had significantly higher whole-blood lead levels after correction for anemia and higher levels in the red cells than nondeficient children with similar exposure (McIntire and Angle, 1972).

Table 12.6
Concentration of Lead in Human Feces

Exposure	Concentration (ppm)	Reference
General population	0.18–0.34[a]	Fleming (1964)
	0.25[a,b]	
Workers	0.6–1.0[a]	Fleming (1964)
	<1.5[a,b]	
Cases	1.1 or more[a]	Fleming (1964)
	>1.5[a,b]	

[a] Values for workers exposed to tetraethyl lead.

[b] Mean or median values.

About 90% of inorganic lead in the blood is found in the red cells (Kehoe, 1961). Organic lead is transported mainly in the plasma.

Neal et al. (1941b) found that regular consumption of commercially washed apples bearing a maximal lead residue of 0.018 grains/lb (2.5 ppm) did not produce a measurable increment in blood lead values over those of persons who did not live in an apple-growing region and who ate few apples, even washed ones. However, consumption of unwashed apples bearing residues in the order of 0.285 to 0.331 grains/lb (40–47 ppm) at an average rate of about a quarter-pound apple per day and, therefore, about 5 mg of lead/person/day produced an increment in the blood lead level of 0.07 ppm (0.000194 ppm per single apple).

The average blood and urinary values for the entire year for persons who had no special exposure to lead arsenate, those who consistently ate sprayed apples, and those who formulated and applied the compound are shown in Table 12.7. The values for consumers are essentially the same as those found in large samples of the general population (see Tables 12.4 and 12.5).

Not shown in Table 12.7 is the fact that the blood and urinary lead values of the orchardists varied significantly during the year, being higher during July and August (when exposure was maximal) and for some time thereafter, and least during the spring when the orchardists had been longest removed from exposure. There was a similar pattern for urinary arsenic, but the difference was not statistically significant because of greater variability of the data.

Based on values for orchardists during winter and spring and on all values for former orchardists whose occupational exposure was completely interrupted, lead storage and excretion fell rapidly at first and then more slowly so that both blood and urine values approached those for consumers in about 5 years. The excretion of arsenic was more rapid, approaching the level of consumers in about 2 years. Although the average values for orchardists followed the described trend closely, the individual values showed marked variation (Neal et al., 1941b).

Table 12.7
Range and Average of Concentrations of Lead and Arsenic in Persons Relative to Exposure to Lead Arsenate[a]

	General population[b] (ppm)	Consumers[c] (ppm)	Orchardists[c] (ppm)
Blood lead		0.04–0.59	0.04–1.09
		0.268[d]	0.439[d]
Urine lead	0.008–0.051	0.009–0.119	0.009–0.419
	0.0297[d]	0.0353[d]	0.0883[d]
Urine arsenic	0.000–0.60	0.019–0.699	0.019–2.039
	0.0145[d]	0.0620[d]	0.1405[d]

[a] From data of Neal et al. (1941b).

[b] Bethesda, Maryland. General population had no special exposure.

[c] Wenatchee, Washington. Consumers regularly ate sprayed apples. Orchardists formulated and applied the compound.

[d] Mean or median values.

The concentrations of lead in certain vital organs and in bones are shown in Table 12.8. Different authors have found essentially similar ranges of values for the lead content of the general population. The wider ranges are based on larger population samples. Schroeder and Tipton (1968) reported that the average storage of lead in adults living in the United States was greater than that of persons living in most other countries. However, the average values varied by a factor of less than three from those in remote, nonindustrialized areas of Africa. Furthermore, the values for all areas were subject to "tremendous variation." Reports indicate that different organs differ from one country to another in their relative avidity for lead even though the total storage is essentially similar (Schroeder and Tipton, 1968), but the finding is completely unexplained and open to some question on physiological grounds.

Kehoe (1961) presented limited data indicating there was no increase of lead storage with increasing age. Schroeder and Tipton (1968) reached the same conclusion regarding most samples from persons living in Europe, Africa, and Asia. However, they found that the concentrations of lead in the kidney, liver, lung, pancreas, and spleen of Americans increased up through the fifth or sixth decade and decreased thereafter. The concentration of lead in the aorta increased with age in Europeans, Africans, and Asians as well as in Americans. The data are difficult to interpret. The values for American infants were very low, but there were no corresponding values available for infants from other continents. The values for adults of different continents differed by a factor of two or less (aorta, pancreas, liver, kidney) or not at all (spleen, heart, lung, brain). Slightly later studies in England confirmed that concentrations of lead were low in the tissues of infants but differed in showing no further increase in concentration after the second decade of life except in bone, spleen, lung, and aorta, in which accumulation continued indefinitely. Because about 95% of the lead in adults was in bone, it followed that the increase in total body burden during the course of a lifetime was considerable. However, the greater body burden in those who died at an advanced age did not exclude the possibility that their lead intake had been higher when they were young and when the other subjects were yet unborn (Barry and Mossman, 1970).

Other Laboratory Findings Lead poisoning is characterized by anemia and evidence of immaturity of the red cells. The anemia is seldom severe, and it is hypochronic. There are usually 4–4.5 million cells per mm^3, and the hemoglobin is usually 70–80% of normal. Reticulocytes frequently constitute more than 3% of the red cells, the upper limit of normal. Basophilic stippling, also considered an evidence of immaturity, is one of the most common indications of lead poisoning. Cells showing this stippling occur in other conditions and may be found in as many as 0.01% of red cells of normal people. In lead poisoning, 1% of the red cells may be stippled. The stippled cells may be counted most easily and accurately in a dark field; done in this way the count tends to be about twice as high as that obtained by the ordinary method. The counting of stippled cells is a sensitive, satisfactory, and in some situations cheap way of monitoring workers potentially exposed to lead (Cressal, 1968).

Lead inhibits δ-aminolevulinic acid (δALA) dehydrogenase, leading to an increase of aminolevulinic acid and coproporphyrin III in the urine (see Section 2.4.17.2). The red cells also contain increased coproporphyrin, which renders them more fluorescent than normal erythrocytes under ultraviolet light. The concentration of δ-ALA in the urine is proportional to the concentration of lead in the blood only at blood levels above 0.5 ppm (Hernberg et al., 1970) and proportional to lead in the urine only at levels above about 0.146 ppm (Barnes et al., 1972). However, the logarithm of erythrocyte δ-ALA-dehydrase is indirectly proportional to blood lead over at least the range of 0.03 to 0.95 ppm, and measurement of this enzyme has been proposed as a screening procedure to detect absorption of lead above any selected level (Hernberg and Nikkanen, 1970; Hernberg et al., 1970). Measurement of activity of δ-ALA-dehydrase is undoubtedly the most sensitive test of the action of lead on heme synthesis and probably the most sensitive test of any biochemical effect of lead. However, the reason for proposing it as a screening test is the relative ease and speed of measuring the enzyme compared with measuring blood lead (Hernberg et al., 1970).

Under occupational conditions that led to an increase of

Table 12.8
Concentration of Lead in Certain Vital Organs and Bones[a]

Sample	General population (ppm)		Persons killed by lead (ppm)
Brain	0.1–6.9[b]		2.0–5.8[b]
	0–6.1	(0.10)[c]	
	0.08–0.31	(0.15)[d]	
	0.01–0.8	(0.12)[e]	
Kidney	0.15–1.6[b]		6.1–25.9[b]
	0.97–6.5	(1.1)[c]	
	0.58–3.2	(1.2)[d]	
	0.01–1.7	(0.7)[e]	
Liver	0.4–2.8[b]		5–80[b]
	0.4–7.5	(1.7)[c]	
	0.74–4.6	(1.7)[d]	
	0.03–3.1	(1.0)[e]	
Flat bone	2.1–11.1[b]		107–268[b]
	2.2–12.5[d]	(1.1)[c,f]	
	0.75–19.5	(8.7)[e]	
	0.01–28.5		
Long bone	6.7–35.9[b]		131[b]
	3.1–29.8[d]		
	0.2–49.5	(21.0)[e]	

[a] Mean or median values are given in parentheses.
[b] Kehoe (1961).
[c] Schroeder and Tipton (1968).
[d] Horiuchi et al. (1959).
[e] Barry and Mossman (1970) (males only).
[f] Value for skeleton without distinguishing flat and long bones.

blood lead from an average of 0.34 to an average of 0.45 ppm within 1 month after starting work, δ-ALA-dehydrase activity decreased from an average of 14.55 to 8.25 mU/ml of red cells. The same exposure approximately doubled the rate of abnormal metaphases involving mainly chromatid and one-break chromosome aberrations (Forni *et al.*, 1976).

Damage to the kidney may be indicated by glycosuria, proteinuria, and aminoaciduria.

Children with excessive exposure to lead show increased x-ray density at the metaphysical ends of long bones, and this may be a key to diagnosis (Rennert *et al.*, 1970).

Pathology　Renal biopsies in human cases with proteinuria were completely normal by light microscopy but by electron microscopy showed definite and constant alterations of fine structure, which have been described in detail and confirmed by experiments with rabbits (Macadam, 1969).

Treatment of Poisoning　Acute lead poisoning is unusual. If it occurs, every effort should be made to remove unabsorbed lead (see Section 8.2).

In chronic poisoning, which is far more common, much lead already has been absorbed, and the problem is to relieve illness preferably by a means that also promotes excretion. The specific antidote of choice is calcium disodium edetate. Calcium trisodium penetate (CaNa$_3$-DTPA) (see Table 8.10) has essentially identical characteristics but is not available in the United States. Both compounds substantially increase urinary excretion of lead without increasing fecal excretion (Iampol'skaia and Dashash, 1968).

Although BAL alone is not recommended for treatment of lead poisoning, combined treatment with BAL and CaNa$_2$-EDTA caused more rapid excretion of lead and more rapid and complete relief of illness than did CaNa$_2$-EDTA alone in lead encephalopathy (Chisolm, 1968).

In lead poisoning in childhood, prolonged oral treatment with penicillamine was found beneficial (Chisolm, 1968). It is the only agent effective for oral treatment of lead poisoning, and some investigators (Cramer and Selander, 1968) have preferred it to calcium disodium edetate.

For many years treatment of lead poisoning was attempted through manipulation of the lead stores. The poison would be mobilized for excretion by administering citrate, but the mobilization was often accompanied by increased symptoms. Deposit of lead in the bones could be promoted by administration of calcium, but this tended to prolong the problem. When BAL became available, it was tried as a treatment of lead poisoning but with limited success.

The introduction of calcium disodium EDTA met with immediate success. It is still an excellent drug. Whether penicillamine now offers an overall advantage will have to be determined by further experience (see Section 8.2.3.4). Ohlsson (1962) pointed out that calcium disodium EDTA may have undesirable side effects, some of which may be associated with its tendency to cause an initial increase in the concentration of lead in the blood and presumably the soft tissues. Whether penicillamine is inherently safer or less safe, as Hammond (1973) concluded from animal studies, is not clear.

More rapid excretion of lead may be produced by a combination of calcium disodium EDTA and penicillamine than by either drug alone (Ohlsson, 1962), but there is no real evidence that the combination offers a clinical advantage.

When a patient with a high blood level (2.6 ppm) and unexpectedly mild symptoms of lead poisoning was treated with calcium disodium edetate, urinary excretion of zinc increased and was 3.5 times greater than that of lead; acid dehydrase activity fell and was lowest when the blood lead to serum zinc ratio was greatest (1.47). Oral administration of zinc sulfate (100 mg, three times a day for 5 days) resulted in a significant increase in dehydrase activity. *In vitro* addition of zinc chloride to the patient's erythrocytes resulted in reactivation of the enzyme. It was suggested that zinc plays a protective role in lead toxicity, and zinc supplementation may be a useful adjunct to chelation therapy for lead poisoning (Thomasino *et al.*, 1977).

Although chelating agents are the key to treating poisoning by lead, symptomatic care of the patient must not be neglected. A person who has cramps or colic may be helped by atropine, hot water bottles, and the injection of calcium.

12.9 TIN

Tin is in the same periodic group as lead. Under conditions of use, inorganic tin compounds have proved essentially harmless, although inhalation of stannic oxide commonly leads to a benign pneumoconiosis. Organic tin compounds have produced gastrointestinal disturbances, tremor, convulsions, paralysis, and death in animals. Triethyltin compounds, which readily cross the blood–brain barrier, produce severe neurological disturbances in both animals and humans (see Section 12.9.2). Thus, lead and tin may injure the same organs, and some alkyl compounds of both are especially dangerous. However, the situation is far from simple. Alkyl derivatives of lead, like those of antimony, bismuth, and mercury, damage nerve cells, whereas triethyltin produces an interstitial edema of the white matter without damage to the cells. Some tin compounds that are closely related chemically have very different toxic effects. Triethyltin causes edema of the central nervous system; diethyltin causes hypertrophy of the bile ducts in some species. The same compound may be highly toxic to one species and essentially harmless to another. An example is dibutyltin, which is highly toxic to rats but not to guinea pigs. In addition to these differences observed in the same laboratory, there are unusually large quantitative differences in the toxicity of certain compounds (e.g., triphenyltin) as observed in different laboratories. Unexplored possibilities to explain the quantitative differences include the strain of rat and the supply of essential trace elements such as zinc.

Traces of inorganic tin are widely distributed in nature. In addition to the amount naturally present in food, tin may be added from foil and plated cans used as containers. Organic tin does not occur naturally. No conclusion about its safety can be drawn from experience with inorganic compounds. Organic tin compounds have some importance as fungicides and they have been proposed as insecticides or antifeeding compounds for insects. So far, these uses have led to no serious difficulty. However, the fact that related compounds have produced serious injury and death in humans serves as a warning that any tin compound proposed for use as a pesticide should be studied with particular care.

The following sections are confined to recognized pesticides and to an extremely brief summary of ethyltin compounds. Although the latter compounds have only been proposed as pesticides, it is necessary to keep them in mind in any consideration of pest control based on tin. Comprehensive reviews of the toxicology of tin are those of Barnes and Stoner (1959) and LeBreton (1962).

12.9.1 FENTIN ACETATE

12.9.1.1 Identity, Properties, and Uses

Chemical Name   Triphenyltin acetate.

Structure $(C_6H_5)_3$ Sn—OC(O)—CH$_3$.

Synonyms   Fentin acetate (BSI, ISO) is the common name in use. A trade name for the compound is Brestan. Code designations include ENT-25,208, GC-6,936, Hoe-2,824, and VP-1, 940. The CAS registry no. is 900-95-8.

Physical and Chemical Properties   Fentin acetate has the empirical formula $C_{20}H_{18}O_2Sn$ and a molecular weight of 409.06. It forms white odorless crystals that melt at 122–124°C. The vapor pressure at 30°C is 1.33×10^{-6} torr. Its solubility in water at 20°C is 28 mg/liter. It is poorly soluble in organic solvents. Fentin acetate is stable when dry but rapidly hydrolyzed by water to the hydroxide, a white solid that melts at 118 to 120°C. The hydroxide practically is insoluble in water but is soluble in most organic solvents.

History, Formulations, and Uses   Fentin acetate was introduced in 1954. It is used as a fungicide on turnips, potatoes, celery, beans, and other crops. The technical product is 90–95% pure. It is formulated as wettable powders of 20 and 60% concentration and applied at a rate of approximately 160–260 gm of active ingredient per hectare. Fentin acetate also is used as an antifeeding compound for insect control.

12.9.1.2 Toxicity to Laboratory Animals

Basic Findings   Rats poisoned by a single dose of fentin acetate show sluggishness, unsteadiness, moderate diarrhea, anorexia, bloody stain around the nose and eyes, and wheezing.

The acute toxicity of fentin acetate is shown in Table 12.9. It is clear that absorption from the gastrointestinal tract is poor compared with that from the peritoneum.

Table 12.9
Acute Toxicity of Fentin Acetate

Species	Route	LD 50 (mg/kg)	Reference
Rat	oral	136[a]	Klimmer (1964)
Rat, F	oral	491[b]	Stoner (1966)
Rat	dermal	450	Klimmer (1964)
Rat	ip	13.2	Klimmer (1964)
Rat, M	ip	8.5	Stoner (1966)
Rat, F	ip	11.9	Stoner (1966)
Mouse, M	oral	81.3	Stoner (1966)
Mouse, M	ip	7.9	Stoner (1966)
Guinea pig	oral	21	Klimmer (1964)
Guinea pig, M	oral	10	Stoner et al. (1955)
Guinea pig	ip	5.3	Klimmer (1964)
Guinea pig, M	ip	3.74	Stoner (1966)
Rabbit	oral	30–50	Klimmer (1964)
Rabbit	ip	10	Klimmer (1964)

[a] In methylcellulose.
[b] In arachis oil.

Klimmer (1964) found that 70% of rats dosed by stomach tube at a daily rate considered equivalent to 50 ppm in the diet died of secondary infection in an average of 26.6 days. Stoner (1966) found that rats survived a dietary level of 200 ppm for 10 weeks, but most died when the concentration was raised to 300 ppm. The difference in response almost certainly depended on the dosage schedule. Even a level of 25 ppm may reduce food intake, growth, and the number of leukocytes in the blood (Verschuuren et al., 1966).

Guinea pigs are more susceptible than rats to triphenyltin acetate, on both an acute and a long-term basis. Dietary levels of 50 ppm are fatal in a few weeks. Levels as low as 5 ppm cause growth inhibition and reduction in hemoglobin and white cells in the blood (Stoner, 1966; Verschuuren et al., 1966). Even at 1 ppm, food intake was reduced (Stoner, 1966). The injury is not merely one of starvation; treated guinea pigs grow more slowly than pair-fed controls (Stoner and Heath, 1967).

The effect of fentin acetate is highly cumulative in the guinea pig. The logarithmic mean survival time on 25 ppm was twice that on 50 ppm (Stoner, 1966). However, the log mean survival time (>190 days) on 12 ppm was greater than would be predicted on the basis of a completely cumulative effect (Stoner and Heath, 1967).

Histologically, only a few animals fed triphenyltin acetate displayed interstitial edema of the brain. Dietary levels of 20 ppm and higher significantly increased the water content of the brain and spinal cord in guinea pigs. A dietary level of 500 ppm significantly increased the water content of the spinal cord of rats, but only in the females (Verschuuren et al., 1966). In spite of these morphological and chemical changes in the brain and spinal cord at high levels of intake, the symptomatology does not suggest that injury to the central nervous system is critical in poisoning by triphenyltin acetate.

Triphenyltin acetate (and chloride) produced marked testicular atrophy in rats when fed for 20 days at a concentration giving an intake of 20 mg/kg/day (Pate and Hayes, 1968). The effect was more striking than that reported for triphenyltin hydroxide but the difference probably was explained by the higher dosage involved.

The second segment of the logtime–logdosage curve for fatal dosages of triphenyltin acetate in guinea pigs was presented by Scholz (1965). As expected (see Section 2.2.3.2), it closely fits a straight line.

Fentin acetate was not tumorigenic when administered to mice for about 18 months at the maximal tolerated level (Innes *et al.,* 1969).

Absorption, Distribution, Metabolism, and Excretion
Absorption from the skin is poor (Stoner, 1966). During oral dosing of sheep for 20 days with fentin acetate at the rate of 10 mg/day, ^{113}Sn was found in the milk at an average concentration of 0.0017 ppm. Tin was present as fentin acetate and in two unidentified forms. Seventeen days after dosing was stopped, the concentration had fallen to the limits of detectability. During treatment, the concentration of ^{113}Sn was 0.0029 ppm in the blood and 0.0075 ppm in the urine. Eight days after dosing was stopped, the liver, kidney, lung, pancreas, gallbladder, and brain contained higher concentrations of ^{113}Sn than did other organs, and the level was still increased in the liver after 218 days (Herok and Götte, 1964). In cows and sheep, triphenyltin is excreted chiefly in the feces (Brügemman *et al.,* 1964; Herok and Götte, 1964).

Triphenyltin is rapidly distributed to all tissues, including the brain of rats. It can still be detected in the brains of rats and guinea pigs more than 30 days after a single dose (Heath, 1966).

Mode of Action A single dose in the fatal range produces irritation of mucous membranes and death due to respiratory failure. Repeated doses produce no injury unless they are large enough to interfere with food intake. However, the cause of death following repeated doses is not clear. Starvation undoubtedly contributes. In some but not all laboratories, secondary infection has been an important cause of death of animals receiving this compound (Klimmer, 1964; Verschuuren *et al.,* 1966). A basis for susceptibility to infection was found in guinea pigs, which showed reduced lymphopoiesis, including atrophy of the white pulp of the spleen (Verschuuren *et al.,* 1966). It may be that increased susceptibility to infection explains the morbidity and mortality caused by fentin acetate to a far greater extent than has been proved. Infection is difficult to recognize in the absence of inflammation.

Other lesions that have been reported in rats included reduced size of the ovary, decreased number of mature follicles, increased atresia of early follicle growth, and a pronounced decrease in the number of corpora lutea. Females receiving fentin acetate at a rate of 20 mg/kg/day showed these effects within 5 days. These changes implied decreased fertility, but fertility was not tested directly (Newton and Hays, 1968). With

the closely related compound fentin hydroxide, Gaines and Kimbrough (1968) found that the fertility of male rats decreased after 64 days on a dietary level of 100 or 200 ppm. However, fertility improved later as the animals adapted and began to eat more food. The infertility as well as testicular atrophy seen at 500 ppm were attributed to starvation.

12.9.1.3 Toxicity to Humans

Poisoning of two pilots and three mechanics followed the aerial application to field crops of a mixture of fentin acetate and manganese ethylenedithiocarbamate without stringent observation of safety regulations. The pilots were severely ill. Gastrointestinal irritation was the main problem, but the liver was affected in one. Illness in the mechanics was mainly subjective (Horacek and Demcik, 1970).

Laboratory Findings Apparently there is no report of tissue levels of tin following poisoning by fentin acetate. The occurrence of tin in normal people is discussed in Section 12.9.2.3.

12.9.2 ETHYLTIN AND RELATED COMPOUNDS

12.9.2.1 Identity, Properties, and Uses

Compounds and Their Characteristics Alkyltin compounds occur in the following forms: $RSnX_3$, R_2SnX_2, R_3SnX, and R_4Sn, where R is an alkyl group linked directly to tin and X is a simple or complex ion. It has been found that the toxicity of these compounds and of certain phenyltin compounds to mammals and fungi depends mostly on the R constituent and to only a minor degree on the nature of X. Tributylin salts have the greatest fungicidal activity, and the effectiveness decreases with changes in the R component in the following order: tributyl > tri-*n*-propyl = tri-*iso* propyl > triethyl = diethylphenyl > triphenyl > trihexyl > trimethyl > trioctyl = diethyl. The monoethyl- and tetraethyl-tin compounds were ineffective as fungicides (Van der Kerk and Luijten, 1954). Triethyltin salts have the greatest toxicity for mammals.

12.9.2.2 Toxicity to Laboratory Animals

Basic Findings The toxicity of ethyltin trichloride is low. An intravenous dose at the rate of 70–150 mg/kg quickly produced hyperpnea, vasodilatation, prostration, and muscular tremors in rabbits, but they recovered in about an hour. Rats showed no distinctive signs after an intraperitoneal dose of 200 mg/kg (Stoner *et al.,* 1955).

Diethyltin compounds do not produce clearly neurological effects. They produce a more generalized illness similar to that caused by the triphenyltin. They also produce in the rat and mouse but not the rabbit, guinea pig, cat, or hen a characteristic injury of the bile ducts (Barnes and Stoner, 1959). The lesion was first described in great detail in connection with dibutyltin dichloride (Barnes and Magee, 1958). The injury starts within 60 min of an intravenous dose or 4 hr of an oral dose as a localized lesion of the lower part of the bile duct. The initial lesion, accompanied by an apparently minor extravasation of bile into the surrounding pancreatic tissue, sets up a chain of events leading to: (*a*) partial blockage of the bile duct and its great dilatation, (*b*) inflammation of the walls of the main vessels of the portal tracts, (*c*) thrombosis in some of these vessels, and (*d*) sharply localized areas of necrosis resembling infarcts within the liver parenchyma. The bile duct may rupture, leading to peritonitis and fat necrosis. It is of interest that this unusual injury apparently occurs only in species in which the pancreatic ducts enter the lower part of the common bile duct rather than entering the duodenum directly. It is also of interest that the general toxic effects of dibutyltin are prevented by BAL, but the local action on the biliary tract is not prevented.

It is difficult to evaluate relatively minor changes reported by Calley *et al.* (1967a,b) in the liver parenchyma of rats and mice dosed with dibutyltin compounds, since their studies apparently were done under conditions that failed to produce the typical lesions of the biliary system.

Triethyltin produces significant swelling of the brain and spinal cord and a striking noninflammatory interstitial edema of their white matter without detectable damage to the nerve cells. Chemical study indicates that the fluid between the fibers is an ultrafiltrate of plasma. Even among compounds that produce brain edema, triethyltin tin was considered unique in not affecting the gray matter (Magee *et al.*, 1957). Later it was found that hexachloraphene produces a similar lesion (Kimbrough and Gaines, 1971). Poisoning by triethyltin is manifested by progressive weakness, paralysis, and convulsions. In rats, the sulfate is about equally toxic orally, intravenously, or intraperitoneally. The intraperitoneal LD 50 is 5.7 mg/kg (Stoner *et al.*, 1955). Rats fed triethyltin hydroxide at a dietary level of 20 ppm lost weight, but only a little more rapidly than pair-fed controls. Unlike the controls, they showed ataxia of the hind legs in 7–9 days when they had consumed a total of about 10 mg/kg. Weakness progressed until the hind legs lay motionless while the rats dragged themselves about using their front legs. The hind legs were not completely paralyzed and could be withdrawn if pinched. If feeding were continued, the front legs, too, became weak, and the rats lay helplessly on their sides, although they would still attempt to eat. About two-thirds of them died during the third week, but the remainder appeared to become resistant. Their food intake increased and they showed partial recovery. Recovery was more certain if they were transferred to a dietary level of 10 ppm when they first reached a state of prostration. Such rats appeared almost normal after 6 weeks on the lower concentration, although there was some wasting of the muscles of the hind legs and some difficulty in balancing on the edge of a cage. No further improvement occurred even if the rats were returned to a normal diet, but the histological lesion cleared. If, on the other hand, the rats were continued on diets containing triethyltin hydroxide, they gradually became irritable, tremorous, and unwell. The tremor was made worse by intentional movement. Some of these rats suffered intermittent or almost continuous convulsions (Stoner *et al.*, 1955; Magee *et al.*, 1957).

Tetraethyltin has the same effect as triethyltin but acts more slowly because its toxic action really depends on its metabolism to triethyltin (Cremer, 1958).

In general, methyltin compounds are less toxic than corresponding ethyltin compounds. For trialkyl compounds, the toxicity decreases gradually as the length of the side chains is increased beyond two. In the dialkyl series, the propyl and butyl compounds are more toxic than either ethyl or methyl, and toxicity remains high through octyl (Barnes and Stoner, 1958).

Absorption, Distribution, Metabolism, and Excretion There is considerable variation in the absorption of alkyl tin compounds. For example, in the rat triethyltin is equally toxic by mouth and by intraperitoneal injection; but in the hen it is not toxic orally. In the rat, diethyltin is toxic when given by stomach tube, but it apparently reacts with some constituent in the food so that even high dietary concentrations are without effect.

Ethyltin trichloride injected intraperitoneally is almost all excreted unmetabolized in the urine, with only trace amounts in the bile; when the compound is given by mouth it is excreted in the feces, indicating very limited absorption from the gastrointestinal tract (Bridges *et al.*, 1967).

Diethyltin dichloride injected intraperitoneally is partially metabolized to ethyltin, much of which is excreted in the urine; a portion of the unmetabolized compound is excreted in the bile and eventually appears in the feces. The conversion of diethyltin to ethyltin apparently occurs in the tissues and in the gut, although the conversion has been demonstrated *in vitro* only in cecal contents and not in liver homogenate (Bridges *et al.*, 1967).

When the triethyltin chloride is injected intravenously into rats, guinea pigs, or hamsters, it reaches a higher concentration in the liver than in other tissues, including the brain. In the rat, this relative distribution is maintained from 10 min to 5 days after injection. In 4 days, rats excrete about 50% of an intravenous dose, mostly in the feces. The compound is probably excreted in the bile of rats, and it certainly reaches high concentrations in the bile of guinea pigs and hamsters (Rose and Aldridge, 1968).

Mode of Action Dialkyltin compounds inhibit α-keto oxidase activity leading to the accumulation of pyruvate. This is considered important in the toxic action. BAL blocks this inhibition and the acute toxicity (Aldridge and Cremer, 1955; Barnes and Stoner, 1959).

Triethyltin is the most effective known inhibitor of oxidative phosphorylation, being active at 1×10^{-7} M *in vitro*. This inhibition is not blocked by BAL (Aldridge and Cremer, 1955).

Inhibition of phosphorylation must interfere with energy exchange everywhere in the body. It does not explain why the visible lesion is confined to the white matter of the central nervous system (Barnes and Stoner, 1959).

A single intravenous dose of triethyltin sulfate at the rate of 7.5 mg/kg reduces the body temperature of rats about 6°C at a room temperature of 20°C and thus reduces incorporation of ^{32}P from orthophosphate into the brain phospholipids. There is no fall in body temperature and no abnormality of ^{32}P metabolism if the rats are kept at 33°C, even though this temperature does not interfere with toxicity and the development of edema (Rose and Aldridge, 1966).

12.9.2.3 Toxicity to Humans

Therapeutic Use Tin and various inorganic compounds of it were promoted during the early part of this century for treating staphylococcal infection or helminthic infestation. These treatments were usually harmless to patients and pathogens alike, although Bar (1956) reported a case of poisoning by stannous oxide. However, in 1953, a large outbreak of poisoning followed the introduction in France of an organic tin preparation called "Stalinon" for treating staphylococcal infection of the skin, osteomyelitis, anthrax, and acne. The preparation was supposed to be diethyltin diiodide, but it contained about 10% of triethyltin iodide and a little less ethyltin triiodide. One report tabulated 224 cases, including 103 deaths (LeBreton, 1962). There were a few additional cases and deaths reported by others. It was estimated that about 1000 people took the medicine.

Symptoms began in 1–30 days after dosage was started. The total dose varied from 81 to 1094 mg or about 1–16 mg/kg in fatal cases. Signs and symptoms included headache, vomiting, photophobia, dizziness, abdominal pain, marked weight loss, hypothermia, bradycardia, retention of urine, alteration of consciousness, psychic changes, convulsions, coma, and paralysis. In spite of this array of abnormalities and the high mortality rate, many patients presented without any diagnostic signs. Some patients had abnormalities of the fundus of the eye, the spinal fluid, or the electroencephalogram, but these changes were often absent in patients who went on to die. The level of consciousness was the best prognostic sign; only one patient who became comatose survived. A few patients recovered rapidly, but most who lived required several months to recover, and one required 18 months. Still others were left with permanent sequelae, including blindness and severe, flaccid paraplegia. Death occurred as early as the day of onset; in most instances it came 1–3 weeks after onset but was delayed 36 days in one case.

The symptomatology and the autopsy findings indicated edema of the white matter of the brain as the cause of death. Consistent with this view was the finding that surgical decompression of the brain constituted the only useful treatment; six of eight patients treated in this way survived (Alajouanine et al., 1958; LeBreton, 1962). Thus, the action was characteristic of triethyltin, not of diethyltin, which constituted a little more than 80% of the preparation. It appears that humans react the same as other animals to triethyltin but are far more sensitive.

Laboratory Findings In the victims of "Stalinon," the concentration of tin was similar in the heart, lung, liver, and kidney, although it tended to be slightly lower in the heart and higher in the liver. The range for pooled viscera was 1.5–16 ppm with a mean of 5.6 ppm. The concentration in the brain was consistently higher, with a range of 5.1–39 ppm and a mean of 17.3 ppm (LeBreton, 1962).

In the United States and France, tin may be found in most samples of all organs except the brain, which rarely contains a detectable quantity in normal people. The median concentration in most organs is no more than 1 ppm (Kehoe et al., 1940a; LeBreton, 1962; Tipton and Cook, 1963).

The concentration of tin in the blood of normal Americans averages 0.14 ppm and that in urine 0.018 ppm (Kehoe et al., 1940a). The concentration in normal plasma does not exceed 0.47 ppm (Gofman et al., 1964).

The distribution of tin in the organs of the French patients was entirely different from that found in experimental animals injected intravenously with triethyltin chloride, where more tin is retained by the liver than by the brain. Whether the difference depends on species or on the fact that "Stalinon" was a mixture is not clear.

12.10 BISMUTH

Bismuth is a heavy metal immediately following lead in the periodic table. It is in the same group as arsenic and antimony.

Bismuth compounds used as pesticides are highly insoluble. They have proved safe when used as drugs in doses far larger than any likely to arise from their use as pesticides.

In persons without special exposure, the concentration of bismuth in the plasma does not exceed 0.20 ppm (Gofman et al., 1964).

12.10.1 BISMUTH SUBCARBONATE

12.10.1.1 Identity, Properties, and Uses

Chemical Name Bismuth subcarbonate.

Structure $(BiO)_2CO_3$.

Synonyms Synonyms include bismuth oxycarbonate and basic bismuth carbonate. The CAS registry no. is 5892-10-4.

Physical and Chemical Properties Bismuth subcarbonate has the empirical formula CBi_2O_5 and a molecular weight of 510.01. It is an odorless, tasteless powder that is practically insoluble in water or alcohol but soluble in mineral acids and concentrated acetic acid.

Use When added to arsenical and fluoride formulations, bismuth subcarbonate tended to increase the feeding of insects on poisoned foliage.

12.10.1.2 Toxicity to Laboratory Animals

Basic Findings Apparently the toxicology of the specific bismuth compounds used or proposed as pesticides has not been studied in animals. It seems reasonable to suppose, however, that sufficient dosages of relatively insoluble pesticides would produce changes similar to all but the most acute injuries produced by soluble bismuth compounds.

Using compounds (sodium bismuth citrate and sodium bismuth glycolate) that were soluble initially but formed flocks over a period of hours, Sollmann and Seifter (1942) found that bismuth dosages of 2.5–3.5 mg/kg killed 66% of rabbits following intravenous injection during 10 min but slightly larger dosages (2.8–5.0 mg/kg as bismuth) were required when each injection was protracted over a period of 10–14 hr. The fatal dosage after intramuscular injection was 5–10 times higher than that by slow intravenous injection. A few of the deaths were the result of shock associated with the colloidal suspension. Acute deaths were more common following repeated injections and in this instance were the result of thrombosis secondary to vascular inflammation. Under the conditions used, death from typical bismuth nephritis in rabbits occurred within several hours to 24 days after injection. Poisoning in dogs also involved nephritis. Excretion of bismuth was slower and storage more prolonged in dogs than in rats.

Pathology The tissue changes in rabbits caused by several bismuth compounds used in the treatment of syphilis were found to be characteristic of bismuth and not dependent on specific compounds or any particular route of administration. The major lesion involved the epithelium of the convoluted tubules of the kidney. These cells showed all types of degeneration from cloudy swelling to calcification. The glomeruli did not appear primarily damaged, but the glomerular capillaries frequently contained coagulated masses of erythrocytes. The lesions of the liver were much less conspicuous than those of the kidney, but cloudy swelling and small areas of necrosis flooded by erythrocytes did occur. Other organs showed no dependable or characteristic pathology. The picture produced by bismuth was similar to that seen in mercury poisoning and opposite to that associated with arsenic, where liver lesions predominated (Lucke and Klauder, 1923).

12.10.1.3 Toxicity to Humans

Therapeutic Use Bismuth subcarbonate is used to furnish mechanical protection and to exclude irritants from external ulcers, fistulas, or inflamed mucous membranes or from gastrointestinal inflammations or ulcers. It helps to allay diarrhea. Formerly it was used as an adjuvant to more active amoebacides against intestinal amoebae and as an opaque medium in roentgenoscopy. The usual oral dose in treating peptic ulcer is 1000–2000 mg suspended in fluid before each meal. The material is harmless unless applied to extensive burns or ulcers or left in fistulas for long periods. Formerly the compound was given as an x-ray contrast medium at a dose of about 50,000 mg. The disadvantage compared to barium sulfate was not toxicity but a delay in emptying of the stomach (Sollmann, 1957).

Treatment of Poisoning BAL has been used for treating poisoning by any bismuth compound. Other treatment is symptomatic.

12.10.2 BISMUTH SUBSALICYLATE

12.10.2.1 Identity, Properties, and Uses

Chemical Name Bismuth subsalicylate.

Structure See Fig. 12.1.

Synonyms Other names for bismuth subsalicylate include basic bismuth salicylate and salicylic acid basic bismuth salt. The CAS registry no. is 14882-18-9.

Physical and Chemical Properties Bismuth subsalicylate has the empirical formula $C_7H_5BiO_4$ and a molecular weight of 362.11. It forms microscopic prisms that are decomposed by boiling water and by alkalies into a more basic salt. It is almost insoluble in water or alcohol.

Use Bismuth subsalicylate is a fungicide, especially for the control of bluemold disease of tobacco seedlings.

12.10.2.2 Toxicity to Laboratory Animals

See Section 12.10.1.2.

12.10.2.3 Toxicity to Humans

Therapeutic Use The compound is sometime used orally to allay diarrhea or to soothe gastritis or peptic ulcer. The dose

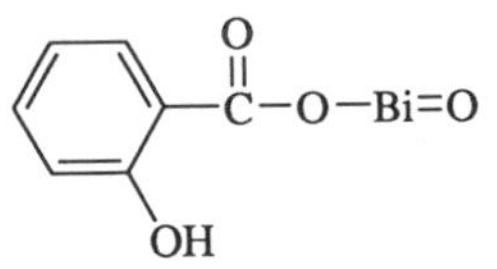

Bismuth subsalicylate

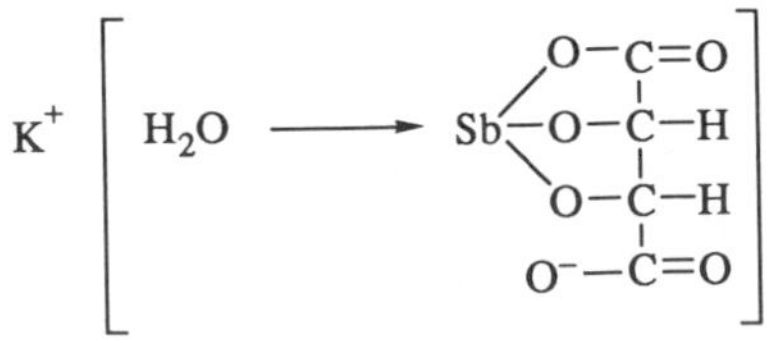

Antimony potassium tartrate

Figure 12.1 Two organometallic pesticides.

varies from 500 to 2000 mg and may be given three times a day. Before the advent of penicillin, bismuth subsalicylate was much used in the treatment of syphilis, and it may still be used in patients who are intolerant to penicillin. It is given by intramuscular injection as a 10% suspension in oil at the rate of 130 mg/week, usually for 8–10 weeks. This treatment results within about 3 weeks in a urinary excretion of about 1 mg/day. By using a dose of 260 mg, a urinary level of 2 mg/day can be achieved in 1 week.

Even when its use was extensive, the gradual intramuscular injection used against syphilis rarely led to serious poisoning. It was customary to stop treatment if gingivitis, albuminuria, cutaneous eruptions, or marked diarrhea appeared. If one of these signs was ignored and dosing continued, serious ulcerative stomatitis with salivation was likely to appear and soon be followed by one or more of the following: malaise, headache, insomnia, depression, asthenia, join pains, nausea, loss of appetite, diarrhea, loss of weight, albuminuria, and skin reactions (such as puritis, herpes zoster, purpura, and sometimes serious exfoliative dermatitis). Jaundice and conjunctival hemorrhage were rare complications of treatment. A line of bismuth sulfide often appeared at the gingival margin along with similar blotches on the mucosae of the mouth, tongue, throat, colon, rectum, cecum, and appendix. The bismuth line was not a contraindication to treatment. Even when illness occurred, it was usually less severe than that associated with other heavy metals. Specifically, the stomatitis and albuminuria were less severe than those caused by mercury and the cutaneous eruptions less severe than those caused by arsphenamine (Sollmann, 1957).

Six examples of poisoning by bismuth subsalicylate were reported by Peters (1942). These cases, arising from treatment of syphilis, involved the simultaneous occurrence of stomatitis and albuminuria. Peters noted that bismuth, like lead, tended to be mobilized during acidosis, and he advised caution in administering bismuth to patients subject to acidosis. Although different side effects have been described in connection with different bismuth compounds, many of the effects probably are common to bismuth regardless of its form. Browning (1969) cited numerous reports of poisoning by other compounds.

After treatment, the highest concentration of bismuth was found in the kidneys and the lowest in the brain and blood. Bismuth freely crosses the placental barrier (Sollmann, 1957).

Pathology   Two patients who died following bismuth therapy but not as a result of it both showed refractile globules in the nuclei and cytoplasm of the epithelium of the convoluted tubules. Similar globules were found in the renal epithelial cells of rats following injection with one of the same compounds (Pappenheimer and Maechling, 1934).

Treatment of Poisoning   BAL has been used for treatment of poisoning by any bismuth compound. Other treatment is symptomatic.

12.11 ANTIMONY

Antimony is a metal. It follows tin in the periodic table, and it belongs to the same group as arsenic. The trivalent compounds of antimony, like those of arsenic, are more toxic than the pentavalent ones. The toxic effects of antimony compounds closely resemble those of arsenic compounds, but antimony causes greater vomiting and is excreted more rapidly.

Traces of antimony are widely distributed in the environment.

Eight or more compounds of antimony had some use as insecticides before DDT became available. However, antimony potassium tartrate was the only one of much commercial importance. The toxicity of this compound is typical of the group.

A useful review of the toxicology of antimony, which emphasizes the industrial aspects, is that of Fairhall and Hyslop (1947).

12.11.1 ANTIMONY POTASSIUM TARTRATE

12.11.1.1 Identity, Properties, and Uses

Chemical Name   Antimony potassium tartrate.

Structure   See Fig. 12.1.

Synonyms   Other names include antimony tartrate, potassium antimonyl tartrate, tartar emetic, tartarized antimony, and tartrated antimony. A code designation is ENT-50,434. The CAS registry no. is 28300-74-5.

Physical and Chemical Properties   Antimony potassium tartrate has the empirical formula $C_4H_4KO_7Sb$ and a molecular weight of 324.92. It forms transparent crystals or powder with a sweetish, metallic taste. The density is 2.6. It is soluble in water and glycerol, insoluble in alcohol. Crystals effloresce upon exposure to air.

Formulations and Uses   The compound serves as a poison in baits to control insects, especially thrips, and as an emetic (for people or pets) in baits to control rodents. The insect baits usually are applied as sprays containing 0.36–0.48% of the compound in the liquid formulation. The rodent baits are pastes or solids containing 0.3–3% of the compound, specifically 0.30% with thallium sulfate and zinc phosphide, 1.12% with arsenic trioxide, and 3.00% with ANTU.

12.11.1.2 Toxicity to Laboratory Animals

Basic Findings   The intraperitoneal LD 50 for mice is 46–50 mg/kg for the different isomers of antimony potassium tartrate (Haskins and Luttermoser, 1950). The subcutaneous and intravenous LD 50 values in mice are 55 and 65 mg/kg, respectively (Ercoli, 1968). The oral LD 50 for the same species is 600 mg/kg. The marked difference between these values is an indication of poor gastrointestinal absorption even in an animal that does not vomit. Other species are somewhat more susceptible, with an intraperitoneal LD 50 of 30 mg/kg (11 mg/kg as antimony) in rats and 25 mg/kg in guinea pigs (Bradley and Fredrick, 1941). (The metal itself is about one-tenth as toxic, and various industrial compounds are 1/100 to 1/400 as toxic in terms of antimony content (Bradley and Fredrick, 1941).

Animals poisoned by antimony compounds showed dyspnea, loss of weight, weakness, loss of hair, and evidence of cardiac insufficiency. Those that survived began to regain weight within 5–10 days (Bradley and Fredrick, 1941).

Absorption, Distribution, Metabolism, and Storage Ingestion of the compound usually leads to repeated vomiting. Thus, removal of the material from the gastrointestinal tract and inherently poor absorption combine to limit the amount of the compound reaching the tissues. Excretion is mainly urinary. It is much faster than that of arsenic and is almost complete in 72 hr (Osol *et al.*, 1967). The rate of excretion varies considerably in different species, being slower in mice and monkeys and more rapid in rats. The synergistic action of salts of tris(*p*-aminophenyl)carbonium on the toxicity of tartar emetic to *Schistosoma mansoni* was not accompanied by any significant effect on the distribution or rate of excretion of tartar emetic and must, therefore, have involved the parasite only (Waitz *et al.*, 1965).

Although the acute toxicity of soluble antimony is greater than that of soluble lead, the excretion of antimony is sufficiently rapid that no significant storage occurs (Bradley and Fredrick, 1941).

Following single or repeated doses of tartar emetic, there was no really marked accumulation of antimony in any organ, but the concentration was always greatest in the liver, and it reached an average of 65 ppm in hamsters killed by repeated intraperitoneal injection (Gellhorn *et al.*, 1946). A similar relationship was found in dogs, where the concentration of antimony decreased in the following order: liver > thyroid > parasites > kidney cortex > other organs (Brady *et al.*, 1945).

Mode of Action Antimony combines with sulfydryl groups including those in several enzymes important for tissue respiration. The antidotal action of BAL depends on its ability to prevent or break the union between antimony and vital enzymes (Sollmann, 1957).

The most characteristic toxic effect is vomiting, which is largely reflex in origin. Although vomiting may occur after intravenous injection, a larger dose is required and the action is more delayed than when the drug is given by mouth (Sollmann, 1957). Furthermore, the action is largely reflex even after injection, for the compound is excreted through the walls of the stomach (Osol *et al.*, 1967).

The cause of death is essentially the same as that in acute arsenic poisoning. Serious injury almost always involves the gastrointestinal system and may involve the cardiovascular system, the kidneys, or other organs leading in any event to a condition of shock. The rapid excretion of antimony makes important sequelae or delayed death unusual.

Pathology Rats killed by an intraperitoneal injection of tartar emetic showed degenerative changes of the myocardium, congestion of the glomeruli and degeneration of the tubules of the kidney, and extensive centrolobular hepatic necrosis. Injury to the heart was detected histologically in rats receiving daily doses of antimony too small to reduce the rate of growth. On the contrary, antimony produced no serious blood changes following either single or repeated doses (Bradley and Fredrick, 1941).

12.11.1.3 Toxicity to Humans

Therapeutic Use When antimony potassium tartrate is rubbed on the skin in the form of an ointment, it produces little irritation at first but produces a pustular eruption if applied for long periods. This is due to decomposition of the double salt by the acid secretions of the follicles leading to formation of the more irritant antimonous oxide and other compounds (Sollmann, 1957).

Antimony potassium tartrate was once used as an emetic for treating patients poisoned by a wide variety of compounds. The drug still has some use as a diaphoretic or expectorant in certain cough syrups. It has been used for treating a number of tropical diseases, and it still is the drug of choice for treating infection by *Schistosoma japonicum*. It is not used to treat *S. mansoni* or *S. haematobium* infections because less toxic agents are effective (AMA, 1977).

The dose of tartar emetic varies greatly according to these different uses. As an emetic, the dose was usually 30–60 mg. The small safety factor is indicated by the fact that in one case a dose of 130 mg proved fatal (Osol *et al.*, 1967). The dose in cough remedies or expectorants varies from 1 to 8 mg repeated two or three times daily. As an intravenous injection for treating *S. japonicum* infection in adults, a freshly prepared 0.5% solution should be injected extremely slowly on alternate days according to the following schedule: 8 ml initially increased by 4 ml with each subsequent dose until the 11th day (when 28 ml is given) and then 28 ml on alternate days until a total of 500 ml (2500 mg) has been given or until side effects become severe. Each dose should be given 2 hr after a light meal and the patient should remain recumbent for 1 hr after treatment (AMA, 1977). These therapeutic doses may be compared with 5 mg/person/day, the rate of respiratory intake of antimony considered safe for workers exposed to various antimony compounds.

Use of antimony potassium tartrate has been abandoned as an emetic to give patients, but it is still used as an emetic to combine with certain rodenticides to make them less harmful if they are accidentally consumed by people or pets. Presumably the compound is more stable in rodenticide formulations than ipecac, which now is considered a faster and safer emetic for patients.

The doses of antimony potassium tartrate received from cough medicines generally cause no side effects. Excessive doses either by mouth or intravenously produce symptoms resembling those of acute or subacute arsenic poisoning. In fact, the resemblance is so close that a distinction may be impossible unless the cause is known as the result of history or chemical analysis. There is, however, a tendency for antimony to produce earlier more profuse vomiting, less systemic absorption, more rapid excretion, and thus a shorter course without severe neurological sequelae. Symptoms include a metallic taste, extreme nausea, copious vomiting, frequent hiccough, burning pain in the stomach, colic, frequent stools and tenesmus, fainting, bradycardia often with ECG irregularities, hypotension, difficult and irregular breathing, cutaneous anesthesia, convulsive movements, painful cramps in the legs or joints, jaundice, anuria, prostration, and death (Osol *et al.*, 1967; AMA, 1977).

Laboratory Findings Antimony is found in essentially all organs of all normal people. The range of concentration in hair is 0.08 to 6.58 ppm; that in bone is 0.03 to 1.98 ppm. Of the soft tissues, lung, liver, prostrate, and uterus contain the highest concentration of antimony. A concentration as high as 0.52 ppm has been observed in the lung, but the average concentration in that organ is only 0.06 ppm and the averages in other tissues are less (Liebscher and Smith, 1968). The concentration in normal plasma does not exceed 0.31 ppm (Gofman *et al.*, 1964).

Following intravenous injection of tartar emetic, only about 2.5% of the dose was recovered from the urine during the first 24 hr. The rate of recovery fell only very slowly in subsequent days (Boyd and Roy, 1929).

Analysis of 315 electrocardiograms taken on 100 patients during various stages of treatment with tartar emetic and Fuadin for schistosomiasis revealed one or another abnormality in 11–99% of the patients. Abnormalities in one or more leads included increased amplitude of P waves, a fusion of ST segment and T wave, decreased amplitude of T wave, and prolongation of the Q-T interval. The duration of these changes was variable but was noted up to 2 months after treatment stopped (Schroeder *et al.*, 1946).

Pathology At autopsy of persons who have died following ingestion of a large dose, ulcerations usually are found in the esophagus and stomach but not in the intestine. In subacute cases, fatty degeneration of the liver, kidney, and heart may be present; degenerative changes in the nervous system are less common. Persons who died, perhaps as a result of individual susceptibility, following the usual, intravenous, therapeutic dose of tartar emetic showed marked degeneration of the liver, some necrosis of the renal tubular epithelium, and varying degrees of hemorrhage (McKenzie, 1932).

Treatment of Poisoning BAL is effective in treating poisoning by antimony potassium tartrate, but this is not true of all organic antimony compounds.

12.12 ARSENIC

Arsenic is a metalloid. It belongs to the same group as phosphorus. Each of these elements combines with hydrogen to form a highly toxic gas, arsine and phosphine, respectively. Arsenic is followed in the periodic table by selenium, an element of somewhat similar toxicity.

Arsenic compounds occur in many rocks and thus find their way into soil, water, and food, being especially high (3 to 170 ppm) in some seafood (Monier-Williams, 1949). Arsenic is a normal constituent of the human body, a fact recognized since the work of Gautier (1899). Two laboratories have independently reported that arsenic, at least in the inorganic form, is an essential nutrient in minipigs and goats (Anke *et al.*, 1976, 1978) and in rats and chicks (Nielsen *et al.*, 1975; Uthus and Nielsen, 1985). If an element is found to be essential in animals, it is highly probable it is essential in humans. However, we lack knowledge of a biochemical mechanism and physiologic role of arsenic.

For recent reviews of arsenic, see WHO (1981), USEPA (1983), and Ishinishi *et al.* (1986).

12.12.1 ARSENICAL PESTICIDES

12.12.1.1 Identity, Properties, and Uses

Compounds and Their Characteristics Elementary arsenic forms two oxides: the trioxide, As_2O_3, and the pentoxide, As_2O_5. Arsenic trioxide (trivalent) reacts with water to form arsenous acid, H_3AsO_3, which is known only in solution and forms three series of salts: orthoarsenites (e.g., Na_3AsO_3), metaarsenites (e.g., $NaAsO_2$), and pyroarsenites (e.g., $Na_4As_2O_5$). Arsenic pentoxide (pentavalent) reacts with water to form three acids that may be isolated: orthoarsenic acid, H_3AsO_4; metaarsenic acid, $HAsO_3$, and pyroarsenic acid, $H_4As_2O_7$. These acids form the corresponding salts: orthoarsenates, metaarsenates, and pyroarsenates. A few organic arsenic compounds also are used as pesticides. Although a great many arsenicals have had some use as pesticides, the ones shown in Table 12.10 are of the greatest importance.

Table 12.10
Some Arsenical Pesticides

Name	Synonym	Formula
Arsenic trioxide	white arsenic	As_2O_3
Sodium arsenite		Na_3AsO_3, $NaAsO_2$, $Na_4As_2O_5$
Paris green	copper aceto-meta-arsenite	$Cu(CH_3COO)_2\ 3Cu(AsO_2)_2$
Lead arsenate	acid lead arsenate standard lead arsenate dilead arsenate	$PbHAsO_4$
Basic lead arsenate	lead hydroxyarsenate	$Pb_4(PbOH)(AsO_4)_3 \cdot H_2O$
Calcium arsenate		a complex mixture
Dimethylarsinic acid	Arsan® cacodylic acid Phytar® Silvisar®	$(CH_3)_2AsO(OH)$
Disodium methyl arsenate		$Na_2CH_3AsO_3 \cdot 6H_2O$

It is beyond the scope of this book to discuss the highly toxic compounds of arsenic (arsine and certain war gases) or those of low toxicity employed therapeutically in medicine and agriculture (drugs and feed additives).

Formulations, Uses, and Production   Arsenites are more soluble and more rapidly toxic than corresponding arsenates; therefore, arsenites are used as rodenticides and herbicides and in insecticidal baits. Paris green, although an arsenite, may be applied to foliage, but inorganic arsenates are less phytotoxic and, therefore, preferred for application to crops as insecticides. Some organic arsenates (dimethylarsinic acid and disodium methyl arsenate) are herbicides. The use of arsenical insecticides in agriculture decreased greatly following the introduction of DDT and later poisons, but the use of arsenical herbicides has increased.

12.12.1.2   Toxicity to Laboratory Animals

Symptomatology   The acute effects of arsenic in animals are similar to those observed in humans (see Section 12.12.1.3). The degree of irritation of the gastrointestinal tract involved in poisoning by arsenic trioxide depends on its purity. A commercial preparation that was 97.8% pure was much more irritant yet slightly less toxic than a sample of greater than 99.999% purity (Harrisson et al., 1958).

Dogs fed sodium arsenite at a rate of about 2.7 mg/kg/day showed anorexia, listlessness, and weight loss leading to cachexia and eventually death. Mild to moderate anemia was present prior to death. Neither skin lesions nor polyneuropathy apparently has been observed in experimental animals. Thus, except for weight loss and anemia in some species, arsenic poisoning as it occurs in humans is poorly reproduced in animals.

Dosage Response   The literature indicates a tremendous variation in the oral toxicity of arsenic compounds. Table 12.11, prepared from a careful study of arsenic trioxide by Harrisson et al. (1958), shows that the variation is real but can be accounted for largely by whether the compound is administered dry or in solution and to a lesser extent by the purity of the sample and by the species, strain, and weight of the experimental animals. Harrisson and his colleagues found no significant difference in the response of males and females. They acknowledged that arsenic of coarse grind might be less easily dissolved and hence less toxic than fine powder. However, in the particular samples they studied, the coarser preparation was actually more toxic because of its greater purity. Thus a combination of variables must be taken into account.

The LD 50 values of suspensions of calcium arsenate (298 mg/kg) and of Paris green (100 mg/kg) in rats are similar to that of powdered arsenic trioxide. The LD 50 value of lead arsenate is distinctly higher (1050 mg/kg) (Gaines, 1969).

Chronic effects in animals as a result of long-term (2 years) feeding included reduced growth rates with greater effects in the female (Byron et al., 1967). A marked enlargement of the

Table 12.11

Effect of Purity and Dosage Form of Arsenic Trioxide on Its Oral Toxicity in Male Animals of Different Species, Strains, and Weights[a]

Experimental animal	Weight (gm)	Dosage form	LD 50 value (mg As/kg) 97.8% As_2O_3	99.999% As_2O_3
Swiss mouse	20–25	solution	42.9 ± 2.1	39.4 ± 4.7
Swiss mouse	35–40	solution		47.6 ± 3.3
C57H16 mouse		solution		25.8 ± 1.8
Dba2 mouse		solution		32.4 ± 2.3
C3H mouse		solution		25.8 ± 1.8
Sprague–Dawley rat	125–200	solution	23.6 ± 1.4	15.1 ± 1.8
Sprague–Dawley rat	125–200	dry	214.0 ± 8.4	145.2 ± 8.7

[a]From data of Harrisson et al. (1958).

common bile duct is a characteristic feature. A no-adverse-effect level in rats is about 1.6 mg As/kg/day as arsenite and about twice as high for sodium arsenate. Dogs appear to be somewhat more susceptible than rats. Neither skin lesions nor polyneuropathy has been observed in experimental animals. Thus, except for weight and anemia observed in dogs (Kiyono et al., 1974), arsenic poisoning as it occurs in humans is poorly reproduced in animals.

Absorption, Distribution, Metabolism, and Excretion   Arsenic is absorbed chiefly by the gastrointestinal and respiratory tracts. However, some is absorbed by the intact skin, and systemic illness may follow application of arsenical ointment to eczematous skin.

Gastrointestinal absorption of the soluble trivalent compounds of arsenic appears to be high (Coulson et al., 1935; Crecelius, 1977; Mappes, 1977; Buchet et al., 1981a,b) in both animals and humans. The organic form of arsenic present in shellfish and other marine foods is also well absorbed from the gastrointestinal tract. Soluble arsenates are also well absorbed.

Arsenic is rapidly cleared from the bloodstream except in the case of rats, where its methylated derivatives bind to hemoglobin. In fact, both tri- and pentavalent forms of arsenic are rapidly methylated, so their distributions are somewhat similar. Initial accumulation is in liver, kidneys, and lung, from which arsenic is cleared rapidly; long-term accumulation is in skin, squamous epithelium of the upper gastrointestinal tract, thyroid, the lens of the eye, and the skeleton. It is also accumulated in hair. Human autopsies have also confirmed accumulation in karatinized tissues and the skeleton.

Both tri- and pentavalent forms of arsenic readily cross the placenta (for review, see Clarkson et al., 1983). The pentavalent form accumulated in the skeleton of the fetus in late gestation. Little arsenic crossed the blood–brain barrier.

Most arsenic in tissues is found to be protein bound. Trivalent arsenic is well known to bind to tissue —SH groups (Webb, 1966).

Both tri- and pentavalent arsenic can be interconverted by oxidation–reduction reactions in mammalian tissues. The biochemical mechanisms are not known. Monomethyl and dimethyl derivatives are produced in experimental animals and humans presumably by methylation of the trivalent form. Substantial species differences exist in methylation rates and in the relative proportions of the monomethyl and dimethyl forms. Arsenobetaine, the organic form of arsenic in marine organisms, is not further metabolized in the body.

Methylation of arsenic may be regarded as a detoxication process, as the methylated derivative is less toxic than the inorganic form. Factors affecting the methylation rate are therefore important. There is evidence that the efficiency of methylation decreases at higher doses. Populations having certain dietary deficiencies (e.g., in methionine) may be more susceptible to arsenic poisoning.

After absorption of either the tri- or pentavalent form, urinary excretion is the dominant pathway. In chronic exposure, this route accounts for 60–70% of total excretion. Methylation rate is important, as the methylated species is more rapidly excreted than the inorganic form. For example, urinary excretion is lowest in the marmoset monkey, which is unable to methylate arsenic (Vahter *et al.,* 1982). Excretion also takes place by feces, skin, hair, and milk. Fecal excretion may be preceded by extensive enterohepatic recirculation according to data for experimental animals (Klaassen, 1974).

Tolerance   It was reported during the last century that the mountaineers of Styria and certain other regions ate arsenic once or twice a week as a tonic and thus accustomed themselves to doses of 400 mg or more per day. Their blood and urinary arsenic levels and even the absorbability of the material they ate are apparently unknown. However, the reality of tolerance to inorganic arsenic has been demonstrated by tests in dogs (Cloetta, 1906), rabbits (Cloetta, 1906), and rats (Norris and Elliott, 1945; Joachimoglu, 1916). Tolerance does not depend on decreased absorption from the gastrointestinal tract, for it may be induced by intraperitoneal injection (Norris and Elliott, 1945).

Biochemical Effects   Arsenic inhibits pyruvate oxidase and the phosphatases. The blood level of pyruvate increases in poisoned animals or people. There is a reduction of tissue respiration leading to a wide range of functional and some morphological changes. Many other sulfhydryl-containing enzymes are involved also, and it is impossible to assign relative importance to them. However, studies on antidotes have made it clear that chemical reaction of trivalent arsenic with sulfhydryl groups, including those in susceptible enzymes, is the biochemical lesion (Peters, 1952). Further studies by Peters' group (for review, see Clarkson, 1983) revealed that the inhibition of pyruvate oxidase was due to the binding of trivalent arsenic, as the oxyanion, to neighboring —SH groups of α-

lipoic acid. Pentavalent arsenic, also as the oxyanion, is able to substitute for phosphate anions in the cell's transport and enzymic processes. The result is replacement of phosphates by arsenate in high-energy phosphorylated substrates, leading to uncoupling of oxidative phosphorylation reactions (for a review, see Jennette, 1981).

Altered biochemical functions in the liver mitochondria of rats fed arsenic are associated with considerable physical distortion of the mitochondrial membrane components. The same degree of biochemical change is associated with less electron microscopic change in the mouse (Fowler and Woods, 1979).

Although arsenic inhibits many enzymes, it increases the activity of liver microsomal enzymes. Arsenic trioxide at a dietary level of 1000 ppm for 15 days induced several enzymes, and even at 100 ppm hexobarbital sleeping time was decreased. Rats develop some tolerance to arsenic, and its toxicity is decreased by phenobarbital (Wagstaff, 1972; Kourounakis *et al.,* 1973).

Effects on Organs and Tissues   The chief pharmacodynamic action is dilatation and increased permeability of the capillaries. This action is strongest in the intestines, regardless of route of absorption. Local action on capillaries causes congestion, stasis, thrombosis, ischemia, and necrosis. Such necrosis extends into the bone in some instances. Injury to the kidneys is due primarily to capillary injury, but there is always some injury to the epithelium. Initial injury to the nervous system is also based on circulatory disturbance, but later there is direct injury to the nerve cells. Injury to the liver by arsenic is usually minor. A few single cases or clusters of cases involving cirrhosis have been described. In many of these cases, alcohol was a complicating and perhaps critical factor in the etiology.

The cause of death depends on the size of the dose and, therefore, on the speed of action. If death occurs within a day or two, it is caused by shock characterized by a severe fall in blood pressure. Vasodilatation is most marked in the splanchnic area, but death occurs in experimental animals even if the intestines are tied off early. The action on capillaries is direct, for it follows perfusion of excised organs with solutions of arsenic. The dilatation is not due to a loss of contractility; the vessels continue to react to splanchnic stimulation until very late, and they react to epinephrine even later (Loeb, 1912).

If death is delayed 3–14 days, it is caused by dehydration, electrolyte imbalance, and a more gradual fall in blood pressure.

Most animal studies testing for carcinogenicity of arsenic have been negative (for review, see USEPA, 1984). Studies on rats should be viewed with caution in view of the unusual metabolism of arsenic in this species.

Effects on Reproduction and Development   Few studies have been made on the effect of arsenic on reproduction and development. Treatment of pregnant animals with high doses of inorganic arsenic results in fetal resorptions and, in surviving offspring, defects in the genitourinary tract (for review, see Clarkson *et al.,* 1983).

Pathology The injury produced by arsenic compounds in most species is not characteristic although the enlargement of the rat's common bile duct by sodium arsenite and sodium arsenate is indeed striking. Using a strain of rat that occasionally showed spontaneous enlargement of the duct, Byron *et al.* (1967) found that the duct enlarged in 45 of 49 rats fed sodium arsenite at a dietary As level of 250 ppm and in 42 of 48 rats fed sodium arsenate at a dietary As level of 400 ppm. Lower dietary levels produced a lower incidence of enlargement. Some of the ducts measured more than 7 mm in diameter, and their walls were as much as 10 times thicker than normal. The condition was reminiscent of that produced in rats by dibutyltin dichloride and a few nonmetal compounds. No parallel condition in humans has been recognized.

Treatment of Poisoning in Animals Dimercaptosuccinic acid increased the rate of excretion of radioactive arsenic by poisoned rats and increased their survival compared with controls (Okonishnikova, 1965).

12.12.1.3 Toxicity to Humans

Experimental Exposure See Laboratory Findings.

Therapeutic Use Arsenic in the form of arsenic trioxide, potassium arsenite solution (Fowler's solution), or arsenious acid solution formerly was used extensively as a tonic in treating nutritional disturbances, neuralgia, rheumatism, arthritis, asthma, chorea, malaria, syphilis, tuberculosis, diabetes, skin disease, and every kind of blood disturbance. Some skin conditions were treated locally, and arsenic was used to destroy some superficial epitheliomas. In fact, both Hippocrates and Galen recommended a naturally occurring arsenic disulfide for treating ulcers, and cautery of tumors by arsenic salts was practiced by Avicenna in the tenth century and by Guy de Chauliac in the fourteenth. Fowler's solution was used in some treatment of leukemia until rather recently (Sollmann, 1957).

Experience in the systemic use of inorganic arsenicals showed that their prolonged administration at the usual rate of 0.04–0.09 mg/kg/day frequently produced mild poisoning. The various systemic and cutaneous effects described below under Use Experience have been produced by arsenical therapy also.

Accidental and Intentional Poisoning For many years, arsenic has been the most important single cause of accidental deaths associated with pesticides in the United States. It caused 36, 26, 29, 31, and 17% of such cases in 1956, 1961, 1969, 1973, and 1974, respectively (Hayes and Vaughn, 1977). Accidental poisoning by arsenic pesticides is almost always acute and often involves children. Experience in many other countries, for example, Poland (Brodniewicz and Szuber, 1960), Australia (Southby, 1965), and New Zealand (Kennedy, 1961; Bailey, 1964), has indicated the disproportionate importance of arsenical pesticides as a cause of pesticide poisoning. Contamination of well-water by arsenical pesticides has

been a cause of outbreaks of poisoning in Russia (Planques *et al.*, 1960; Khasanov, 1971) and possibly in Hungary (Nagy *et al.*, 1975a,b).

The first symptom is often a feeling of constriction of the throat, followed by difficulty in swallowing and epigastric discomfort. Abdominal pain and vomiting often start within an hour of ingestion, although the onset may be delayed until the next day, particularly if foul play is involved and the dosage is controlled. Death may result from a severe fall in blood pressure and collapse as in "dry" cholera. Generally, death is delayed for 1.5–3 days after onset and sometimes as much as 14 days. In this event, death follows vomiting and profuse, watery, painful diarrhea; the clinical picture is similar to cholera because of the "rice water" character of the stools and the great dehydration of the patient. Although arsenic is not truly corrosive, the extreme distention of the capillaries may lead to their rupture and thus to ecchymoses or even bleeding into the stomach or intestine and eventually, but infrequently, bloody vomiting and diarrhea. The patient has great thirst and difficulty in swallowing and articulation. Although the abdomen is painful, it is not tender. Descriptions of cases of this kind can be found in great profusion in the older literature, for example, Orfila (1814–1815) and Christison (1845).

If the patient survives the acute phase, skin eruptions, a moderate depression of blood cells, and polyneuropathy may appear.

The pseudoinflammatory reaction may extend to the conjunctiva, gums, mouth, pharynx, and bronchi, and it may persist in the gastrointestinal tract. Thus, conjunctivitis, rhinitis, cough, or bronchopneumonia may be present. Dermatitis is especially prominent in the palms and soles and other areas subject to pressure. White transverse bands in the nails frequently appear in about 6 weeks and may accompany polyneuropathy, which often appears 1–3 weeks after ingestion. The bands migrate to the free edge of the nails at approximately the normal rate of about 5 months from matrix to edge. Although these lines, first described by Mees (1919), may have other causes, their occurrence in conjunction with polyneuropathy is almost pathognomonic of arsenic poisoning. Skin eruptions may progress to exfoliative dermatitis, especially following exposure to organic arsenicals. Peripheral circulatory difficulty characterized by blanching or flushing of the skin may be present, especially in the fingers.

Some authors (Leng-Levy *et al.*, 1969) have emphasized the importance of cardiac involvement in the total syndrome, and the frequency of ECG changes would support this view. Among various forms of cardiac involvement, Wang and Mazzia (1969) emphasized the unusual susceptibility of persons severely poisoned by arsenic to ventribular fibrillation and cardiac arrest during anesthesia.

Arsenical polyneuropathy involves paresthesia, pain, burning, and tenderness of the affected limbs (Heyman *et al.*, 1956). Trouble in walking or in grasping objects may at first be secondary to pain. Later the pain may disappear with astonishing suddenness, but the patient may be left with loss of (*a*) proprioception, (*b*) other sensory functions, and (*c*) motor function. The relative importance of different changes varies from case to case. The legs and arms are affected about equally, although difficulty usually is first noticed in the feet. Muscle atrophy may be pronounced (McCutchen and Utterback, 1966). Tendon reflexes are, of course, weak or absent. Mental confusion may be present and may be evident as an apparent inability of the patient to grasp the seriousness of the condition or the possible implications of foul play.

Tsuchiya (1977) reviewed an outbreak of arsenic poisoning that differed from others in two ways: most of the victims were less than 12 months of age, and the compound involved was found to be pentavalent. The arsenic was a contaminant of sodium phosphate intentionally added to milk as a stabilizer. Different lots of the powdered milk product contained 0–34 ppm of arsenic. Symptoms began early in the summer of 1955; following investigation, sale of this milk powder was banned on August 24, 1955. Many of the signs and symptoms (diarrhea, vomiting, anorexia, and others) were typical of acute poisoning by trivalent arsenic but the prominence of many other difficulties (dermatitis, loss of hair, melanosis, leukoderma, and irritation of the eyes and upper respiratory system) was typical of subchronic or chronic poisoning, as one might expect with exposure lasting several months. However, neuritis was not observed, and electrical measurements indicated no dysfunction of the peripheral nervous system. In view of the fact that there were a total of 12,131 cases and 130 deaths, one would have expected hundreds if not thousands of cases of polyneuropathy if trivalent arsenic had been involved. Other differences from ordinary arsenic poisoning were the presence of fever and of liver swelling in the majority of cases. The contrast is especially remarkable in view of the demonstrated interconversion of the two valence forms. The poisoned infants were treated with BAL; rapid weight gain was considered the most striking benefit. Survivors were examined in June 1956, and it was concluded that most were normal—another contrast in view of the severity of the initial illness.

It seems clear that the majority of cases of arsenic poisoning have been associated with trivalent compounds, but in some instances the identity—and thus the valence—of the offending compound has not been reported. The large outbreak just mentioned suggests that there are two distinctly different forms of arsenic poisoning, depending on valence.

Arsine (AsH_3) is not used as a pesticide and ordinarily plays no part in the danger of arsenical pesticides. However, arsine was the cause of the illness of eight children and one adult who 48 hr earlier had helped to clean a dip vat that had been charged with chlordimeform and monobasic calcium phosphate. All of the patients showed albuminuria, and some showed hematuria, abdominal pain, dysuria, and headache. A diagnosis of arsine poisoning was made in the absence of any known source of arsenic. However, the next day, the farmer recalled that an arsenical dip had been used in the vat 2 years earlier, and arsenic later was measured in the acid mud (pH 6.5) of the vat and in the urine of the patients. Fortunately (and consistently with the delayed onset), all the cases were mild and the recoveries complete (Rathus *et al.*, 1979).

Use Experience Poisoning has not been a significant problem in pesticide applicators; cases reported in vineyard workers in Germany may have involved the drinking of contaminated wine. Poisoning is well known from other occupational sources, including the manufacture of pesticides. However, according to Buchanan (1962), who reviewed the industrial toxicology of arsenic in detail, even the use of arsenic compounds in industry has not proved an important cause of occupational morbidity and mortality.

Poisoning that is caused by repeated occupational exposure usually involves the frequently insidious onset of loss of appetite, weight loss, weakness, nausea, alternating diarrhea and constipation, colic, peripheral neuropathy, dermatitis, some loss of hair, giddiness, and headache. In general, gastrointestinal involvement is less and dermal involvement is greater than in poisoning caused by one or a few doses. Prolonged exposure may lead to gradual mental and physical deterioration and a state of cachexia suggestive of a malignant or endocrine disorder. Cyanosis of the face may be present as a result of statis in the injured capillaries rather than systemic anoxia. The dermatitis may be erythrematous, pustular, or even ulcerative. Burning and itching may be present and there may be serous discharge. With most arsenic compounds, the skin lesions tend to be most marked in the area of greatest contact. They are considered mainly the result of direct toxic action. The eruption may involve the face, eyelids, conjunctivae, or even cornea. There may be irritation of the nose, pharynx, and trachea leading to hoarseness and chronic cough. Perforation of the nasal septum has occurred.

A highly characteristic dermatitis confined to the scrotum, inguinal area, and nasolabial folds may follow moderate occupational exposure to Paris green. The lesions begin with erythema, frequently become eczematous and weeping, and may start to heal with the formation of a black scab. A sensitization reaction may be involved because the distribution does not correspond to the distribution of insecticide on the skin, and the dermatitis generally occurs in the absence of typical systemic poisoning.

In less acute cases, hyperkeratosis, hyperhidrosis, or melanosis may occur. These changes are considered evidence of chronic systemic action. The hyperpigmentation is most marked on surfaces exposed to light; it does not extend to mucous membranes. There may be a speckled depigmentation of pigmented areas giving the so-called raindrop appearance.

In persons exposed to sufficient arsenical dust, the onset of illness is characterized by dyspnea and oppression and pain in the chest. These symptoms may be followed by nausea, diarrhea, and other usual signs of poisoning but generally of a mild degree.

The polyneuropathy that may follow repeated exposure to arsenic resembles that seen in persons who survive one or a few doses. Disturbance of sight, taste, and smell may occur. There may be disturbance of bladder function. It is said that arsenical polyneuropathy is particularly severe and unremitting in chronic alcoholics.

There is no doubt that compounds similar or identical to

those used as pesticides have caused skin cancer in humans. The earliest evidence comes from patients treated with potassium arsenite (Fowler's solution) (Hutchinson, 1887; Neubauer, 1947; Sommers and McManus, 1953; Sanderson, 1963; Minkowitz, 1964; Fierz, 1966) and from people who consumed water with a naturally high arsenic content (Neubauer, 1947; Tseng et al., 1968). In these instances, intake of arsenic was oral. The situation was somewhat less clear in connection with certain winegrowers in Germany and France (Roth, 1957a; Liebegott, 1952; Galy et al., 1963a,b; Latarjet et al., 1964; Denk et al., 1969; L'Epee et al., 1973). Whereas the initial impression was that exposure to lead arsenate was dermal and respiratory—as, indeed, it was—the critical intake of arsenic may have been oral and associated with contamination of wine by arsenic, making the exposure of the winegrowers entirely similar to that of people who drank arsenic in Fowler's solution or in water.

Two histopathological types of skin cancer have been associated with arsenic—squamous carcinomas in the keratin areas and basal cell carcinomas. Skin cancers caused by arsenic differ from those resulting from ultraviolet light by occurring in areas of the body not exposed to sunlight, e.g., soles of the feet. The appearance of skin cancer is preceded by a characteristic sequence of changes in skin epithelium.

Hyperpigmentation is followed by hyperkeratosis, which, histologically, has been described as keratin proliferation of a verrucose nature with derangement of the squamous portions of the epithelium. The latent period for initiation of exposure to appearance of skin cancer ranges from 6 to 50 years when arsenic was used medicinally, e.g., Fowler's solution. When exposure was from contaminated drinking water, the shortest latency was about 24 hours.

A considerable body of evidence now associates lung cancer with occupational exposure to arsenic. Perry et al. (1948) in the United Kingdom and Ott et al. (1974), Baetjer et al. (1975), and Mabuchi et al. (1979) in the United States found an excess risk of lung cancer associated with exposure to arsenic in industries manufacturing arsenic pesticides. A number of studies of copper smelters in the United States, Sweden, and Japan (for review, see USEPA, 1984) have also implicated arsenic as a cause of lung cancer.

Arsenic has been mentioned in connection with the carcinogenicity of cigarettes (Satterlee, 1956), and it is true that residues of arsenic in tobacco increased from an average of 16.2 ppm in 1932–1934 to an average of 42 ppm in 1950–1951 (Satterlee, 1956). However, the concentration of arsenic in tobacco decreased later, so that in 1958 the average concentration in 17 brands was only 6.2 ppm (Guthrie et al., 1959).

In a few instances, people with arsenical keratoses or other late effects of arsenic ingestion have presented with a wide variety of internal cancers, and the possibility that the internal cancers were caused by arsenic has been raised (Roth, 1957b; Atkinson, 1969; Brady et al., 1977). However, recent reviews (USEPA, 1984) regard the evidence as equivocal.

Dosage Response   A dose of 5–50 mg of arsenic trioxide is toxic. A dose of 128 mg (about 1.8 mg/kg) is said to have proved fatal to an unhabituated adult, but recovery has occurred after much larger doses. In fact, recovery occurred in one case after what was thought to be 20,000 mg (Cosic and Kusik, 1966). Very young children may be more susceptible. Study of 291 exposure incidents involving a single kind of ant bait in the form of a bottle containing one-half ounce (15 ml) of sweetened 0.61% sodium arsenite solution permitted a poison control center to conclude that a dosage of less than 1 mg/kg can cause serious illness in a child and 2 mg/kg can cause death (Peoples et al., 1977).

The effectiveness of arsenical rat poisons varies greatly with the grind of the powder; very fine powders approach the toxicity of solutions containing an equivalent amount of arsenic. Thus, the ease of absorption influences the toxicity to a marked degree.

The repeated dose necessary to produce poisoning is less well known. The "therapeutic" dose of arsenic trioxide (1–2 mg three times daily) that used to be employed as a tonic frequently led to mild poisoning. Two milligrams three times a day for an adult is a rate of only about 0.06 mg/kg/day expressed as As.

Cancer associated with arsenic has not been reported in persons exposed to air concentrations of 0.1 mg/m³ or less even for long periods. It has been estimated that exposure to air concentrations of 50 μg As/m³ occupationally for 24 years would result in a 200% excess risk of lung cancer (WHO, 1981). Data from a population in Taiwan (Tseng, 1977) led a WHO Task Group on Environmental Health Criteria for Arsenic (WHO, 1981) to conclude that the lifetime risk for skin cancer due to arsenic in drinking water is about 5% for a total dose of 10 gm in an assumed life span of 70 years.

Arsenic has been measured in human tissue and body fluids in both "nonexposed" and exposed individuals. In people exposed to normal environmental levels, hair and nails have the highest concentration with skin and lung next in order (Liebscher and Smith, 1968). Unfortunately, only total arsenic is reported, and we do not know the levels of specific forms of arsenic.

Tissue levels change rapidly after a single dose of arsenic. In six human subjects who ingested a tracer dose of arsenate labeled with the ^{74}As isotope, more than 5% of the dose was excreted in urine within 5 days (Tam et al., 1979). In three people who ingested 500 μg of arsenic as arsenate in drinking water, 45% of the dose was excreted in urine within 45 days. Ingestion of the same amount of arsenic as the mono- or dimethyl derivative resulted in about 75% of the dose being excreted in urine within 4 days (Buchet et al., 1981a).

Arsenic is rapidly cleared from blood in humans (for review, see USEPA, 1984). If exposure is continuous, blood levels should quickly attain a steady state and should be proportional to average daily intake. However, it was not possible to detect any increase in blood levels in individuals exposed to arsenic in drinking water until the level in drinking water rose to 100–300 µg As/liter (Valentine *et al.*, 1979). Most drinking water samples are below 10 µg As/liter (WHO, 1981).

Normal concentrations in blood of nonexposed adults are in the range 1–4 µg As/liter. Individuals exposed to elevated arsenic in drinking water may have blood levels up to 50–60 µg As/liter (for review, see Vahter, 1988). When considering blood levels in nonexposed people, the possibility of intake of organic arsenic in seafood should be taken into account. Ingestion of shrimp with a high natural arsenic content causes blood levels to rise to 50 µg As/liter within 2 hr (Vahter, 1988).

Levels of total arsenic in urine in nonexposed people are in the range 5–50 µg As/liter. However, ingestion of seafood can increase urinary levels up to 1000 µg As/liter. Urinary arsenic in occupational exposure is usually in the range of hundreds of micrograms per liter—values that can easily be confounded by ingestion of seafood. Vahter (1988) has reviewed published studies indicating that long-term daily ingestion of drinking water at 100 µg As/liter results in an average urinary concentration of 60 µg As/liter. Vahter (1988) goes on to suggest that a better index of exposure to inorganic arsenic may be obtained by measuring the urinary concentrations of inorganic arsenic and the two metabolites mono- and dimethyl arsenic.

Hair concentrations of total arsenic in nonexposed individuals are usually less than 2 µg As/gm. In subjects occupationally exposed or ingesting arsenic in contaminated drinking water, hair concentrations can rise to 50 µg As/gm.

The methylated derivatives of arsenic and the organic arsenic in seafood are not accumulated in the hair (Vahter, 1988), so total arsenic in hair should reflect the body levels of inorganic arsenic. Inorganic arsenic is accumulated into hair at the time of formation of the hair strand. Once incorporated into the strand, its concentration remains unchanged. Thus the "segmental" analysis of hair section by section measured from the scalp should quantitatively reveal the sequence of part absorption (Smith, 1964).

The use of hair as a monitor of absorbed inorganic arsenic is limited by the possibilities of external contamination from water, soaps, and shampoos. No satisfactory washing procedure has been developed for removing external arsenic from the hair sample (Atalla *et al.*, 1965). Since trivalent arsenic is known to bind selectively to the —SH groups of keratin in hair, it is likely that accumulation in hair may depend not only on inorganic versus organic forms of arsenic but also on the oxidation state of inorganic arsenic.

Concentrations of arsenic in nails in nonexposed persons are in the range of 0.01–3 µg As/gm with an average of about 0.3 µg As/gm. Values over 100 µg As/gm have been reported in cases of chronic arsenic poisoning (see Vahter, 1988). Arsenic is probably incorporated into the growing tissue of nails, so its concentration may vary along the growth direction of the nail.

The concentrations of arsenic in the organs of people in the general population and in persons killed by arsenic are shown in Table 12.12. There should be no difficulty in confirming a diagnosis of poisoning by analysis of organs if the deceased person had no occupational exposure to arsenic and if arsenical embalming fluid does not complicate the picture. Apparently no

Table 12.12
Concentration of Arsenic in Human Organs

Sample	General population (ppm)	Persons killed by arsenic (ppm)
Brain	0.001–0.036[a,b]	0.5–20[c]
Kidney	0.002–0.363[a,b]	5–150[c]
Liver	0.005–0.246[a,b]	10–500[c]
		7–127[d]
		110–132[a,e]
		3[f]
		1.2–73[g]
Spleen	0.001–0.132[a,b]	5–250[c]
Lung		1.6[f]

[a] Concentration in dry tissue.
[b] Liebscher and Smith (1968).
[c] Sollmann (1957).
[d] Gonzales *et al.* (1954).
[e] Boylen and Hardy (1967).
[f] Buchanan (1962).
[g] Hayes and Vaughn (1977).

information is available on the concentration of arsenic in the organs of occupationally exposed persons who died of unrelated causes. Thus, it is not certain whether the analysis of organs always offers clear evidence about whether the death of a person with occupational or other special exposure to arsenic was or was not caused by the material. In any event, levels less than 0.2 ppm (dry weight) should be ignored; levels higher than 0.2 ppm should be evaluated carefully, although they occasionally occur in normal persons.

Pathology In acute poisoning, erosion and inflammation of the stomach and upper intestinal tract may be marked. The liver may show degenerative lesions. Unless death is very rapid, the severe dehydration produced by acute poisoning gives the body an emaciated appearance, even though a normal amount of fat may remain. The alimentary canal shows a large amount of fluid, shreds of mucus, and false membrane in the absence of marked corrosion—a picture similar to that in cholera. Central necrosis may be found in the follicles of the spleen and the tonsils. The body may decay more slowly than would be expected in the same amount of time at the same temperature.

When death follows long repeated exposure, there is usually fatty degeneration of the myocardium, kidney, and liver, and the liver is often enlarged. Cachexia may be marked, and severe edema may be present. The nerves may show demyelinization and disintegration of axons.

Treatment of Poisoning If ingestion is suspected, the stomach should be emptied by vomiting or lavage with warm water and activated charcoal followed by a saline cathartic. BAL (dimercaprol) is a specific antidote. Dehydration should be combated with saline infusions, guided, where possible, by laboratory studies. If available, an artificial kidney may be used. According to Lasch (1961), much arsenic can be removed by hemodialysis. The diet should be liquid and supplemented with vitamins. D-Penicillamine has been found at least as effective as BAL for treating human cases, and it has been recommended in all situations in which oral administration is appropriate (Peterson and Rumack, 1977). Soviet authors generally prefer unithiol to BAL for treating poisoning by arsenic compounds other than arsine (Mizyukova and Petrun'kin, 1974), and they are almost certainly correct on the basis of both effectiveness and safety. The relative value of unithiol and D-penicillamine is uncertain.

12.13 PHOSPHORUS

Compounds of phosphorus are a major constituent of protoplasm and essential to life. However, the element itself in its reactive white or yellow form is highly toxic. Red phosphorus and the less common black phosphorus are much less reactive and, therefore, relatively harmless.

12.13.1 PHOSPHORUS

12.13.1.1 Identity, Properties, and Uses

Chemical Name White phosphorus.

Synonyms Because of discoloring impurities, white phosphorus is sometimes known as yellow phosphorus. Trade names for the rodenticide include Bonide Blue Death rat killer®, Common Sense cockroach and rat preparations®, and Rat-Nip®. The CAS registry no. is 7723-14-0.

Physical and Chemical Properties Phosphorus has an atomic weight of 30.97376. It has three main allotropic forms: white, black, and red, all of which melt to form the same liquid. White phosphorus is the most highly reactive solid form, and it is the only one used as a pesticide. Red phosphorus is used for the manufacture of some fertilizers and pesticides. Under ordinary conditions, phosphorus is present as the molecule P_4. White phosphorus is a colorless or pale yellow crystalline solid with a waxy appearance and garlic-like order. When stored in water, it increases the water's acidity and corrodes the container at the liquid–air interface. The density of white phosphorus at 20°C is 1.83. It has a melting point of 44.1°C and a boiling point of 280°C. It is practically insoluble in water but soluble in absolute alcohol (1 gm/400 ml); in benzene (1 gm/31.5 ml); in chloroform (1 gm/40 ml); in oil of turpentine (1 gm/60 ml); and in almond oil (1 gm/100 ml). White phosphorus ignites spontaneously in moist air at about 30°C and in dry air at a higher temperature.

Formulations and Uses Pastes in collapsible tubes and jars containing 1.5–2% or even as much as 5% phosphorus were formerly used for rat, mouse, and cockroach control.

12.13.1.2 Toxicity to Experimental Animals

Oral and subcutaneous lethal doses of 2–12 mg/kg for rabbits and dogs are quoted from the literature around 1900 (Spector, 1955). It appears that no measurement of the acute or chronic toxicity of phosphorus has been made in a way that would permit proper quantitation. Rabbits and guinea pigs were not killed by a dosage of 0.66 mg/kg/day but they developed a cirrhosis-like condition (Mallory, 1933).

Absorption, Distribution, Metabolism, and Excretion Phosphorus is absorbed from the respiratory and gastrointestinal tracts. It can cause severe burns to the skin, but it is said that not enough is absorbed from the burned areas to cause systemic poisoning. The dead tissue may be protective by permitting time for complete oxidation to phosphoric acid. Whether dilute formulations such as may occur in the gastrointestinal tract would be absorbed from the skin in harmful amounts has not been tested.

Unreacted elementary phosphorus may be demonstrated in the tissues of people who die several days after ingesting phosphorus but not in those who die after longer periods.

No quantitative study of the excretion of phosphorus seems to have been made.

Mode of Action The mode of action is unknown. It has not been possible to associate the main clinical or pathological features of intoxication with inhibition of any particular enzyme or class of enzymes, although some are inhibited. It is common to speak of phosphorus as a protoplasmic poison, but it is difficult to distinguish its possible direct effects on the liver, kidney, brain, and heart from the effects of anoxia on those organs. The peripheral vascular dilatation, which is the first and most pervasive systemic effect of phosphorus, contributes to all the disorders that may be seen in various organs. However, the mechanism of this dilatation is not clear.

Phosphorus not only leads to structural damage of vital organs but also produces serious disruption of their metabolic function, as evidenced by hypoglycemia, azotemia, inhibition of glycogen formation in the liver, and many other disorders. Apparently there has been no recent review of the metabolic effects of phosphorus. Early reviews (Rubitsky and Myerson, 1949; Sollmann, 1957) list a great variety of biochemical effects, but nothing that could be termed a biochemical lesion.

It is interesting that the signs and symptoms of poisoning by phosphorus are similar to those of poisoning by phosphine. This is especially true if one considers poisoning by zinc phosphide or aluminum phosphide, in which phosphine is released in the stomach and symptoms involving direct irritation of the lungs are minimal. Poisoning by phosphorus apparently has not been studied quantitatively in rats. Therefore, it is not possible to compare in this species the toxicity of preformed phosphine and of phosphine equivalent from phosphorus. It can be stated that in the rat the LD 50 for phosphine gas is 8.9 mg/kg (Section 14.6.2) and that for phosphine derived from zinc phosphide is 10.6 mg/kg (Section 12.4.2.2), whereas that for white phosphorus (expressed as phosphine equivalent) in humans may be estimated at roughly 16 mg/kg. The values are certainly of the same order of magnitude. The difference is in the direction one would expect if the conversion of phosphorus to phosphine is incomplete. Such differences as exist in the kind of injury caused by ingested phosphorus and ingested phosphine (in the form of a phosphide) might be due to differences in distribution of phosphine in the tissue related to the place of its formation.

These qualitative and quantitative relationships could be explained if phosphorus were converted to phosphine in the intestine before absorption or in the liver after absorption. Such conversion probably has not been looked for and certainly has not been demonstrated, although it commonly is stated that small quantities of phosphine are formed in the putrefraction of organic matter containing phosphorus.

Treatment of Poisoning in Animals Mineral oil (50 to 100 ml) prolonged the life of some 10- to 12-kg dogs and saved others from a 500-mg dose of phosphorus, which was uniformly fatal to controls that received saline cathartics or no treatment (Atkinson, 1921).

12.13.1.3 Toxicity to Humans

Therapeutic Use It was observed about 100 years ago that continued small doses of phosphorus to growing animals result in a layer of dense bone under the proliferating epiphyseal cartilage. In adults, the haversian and marrow canals are gradually filled with dense bone. These observations led to the ill-advised use of phosphorus in treating rickets, osteoporosis, and fractures (Sollmann, 1957). It was claimed that children up to 8 years old suffered no dangerous effects from 0.5 mg/day, although some vomited at first. The smallest dosage that exceptionally produced dangerous effects was 1 mg/day. The effects included gastrointestinal disturbance, necrosis of the jaw, and rarely typical phosphorus poisoning.

Accidental and Intentional Poisoning Apparently the most thorough clinical study of poisoning by phosphorus is that of Diaz-Rivera et al. (1950, 1961) based on a series of 56 cases involving suicide. Practically all poisoning by phosphorus has been caused by accidental or suicidal ingestion or occasionally by murder. The mortality was high.

It has been conventional to describe phosphorus poisoning in three stages: initial, latent, and systemic. This convention was recognized by the turn of the century (Hann and Veale, 1910) and was followed in a review by Rubitsky and Myerson (1949). It is universally agreed that persons who ingest large doses die quickly in profound shock. Thus, the three stages are possibly applicable only in cases in which the dose is small enough to permit survival for a week or more. Even in regard to such cases, there is apparent disagreement concerning the distinctness of the three stages.

The initial symptoms include nausea, severe epigastric pain, headache, dizziness, and weakness. Diarrhea is uncom-mon. Vomiting is frequent but does not occur in all cases. Hematemesis may be present. The patient may be very nervous. These symptoms are commonly attributed directly or indirectly to irritation of the gastric mucosa (Diaz-Rivera et al., 1950). However, absorption of phosphorus must begin at once, for the very first symptoms are similar regardless of the severity of poisoning, and in severe cases the absorption of a fatal dose requires only a few hours.

The initial symptoms are usually very distressing so that victims of accidental poisoning and many suicides seek medical attention promptly. However, LaDue et al. (1944) reported the death of a 15-month-old girl on the fifth day of illness, although the symptoms (abdominal pain and intermittent vomiting) during the first 4 days were so mild they did not interfere with the child's play; diagnosis was on the basis of autopsy findings and not confirmed by chemical analysis or a history of ingestion.

The onset of poisoning may be delayed as much as 5 hr but is often within half an hour or less.

The latent stage is characterized by a temporary and misleading improvement in the patient's condition and sense of well being. However, according to Diaz-Rivera et al. (1950), the so-called asymptomatic period is seldom as pleasant as may appear in the literature. In spite of some apparent improvement, their patients were seldom free of nausea, anorexia, a disagreeable taste in the mouth, eructations, or epigastric or generalized abdominal pain; some had constipation, and a few vomited. This period of relative relief starts within the first 48 hr, and the severe symptoms observed in those not destined to survive begin within the first 4–5 days. In some cases the latent stage may last until 10 days after ingestion (Rubitsky and Myerson, 1949).

In some cases, the improvement leading to what might otherwise constitute a latent phase is retained, and the patient goes on to complete recovery (LaDue et al., 1944).

The third stage is ushered in by the reappearance of severe vomiting, abdominal pain, and sometimes hematemesis. Severe damage to several organs becomes apparent. The liver is usually enlarged and very tender; jaundice, hypoprothrombinemia, and a bleeding tendency appear. Hypoglycemia is severe in some cases. Bleeding may be from the gums, stomach, intestine, or kidney, or in rare cases there may be extensive superficial ecchymoses (Hann and Veale, 1910). Injury to the kidney is evident by oliguria and azotemia. Injury to the brain results in severe restlessness, toxic delirium, and toxic insanity. These have been attributed to cerebral anoxia, but it seems impossible to exclude the possibility of direct toxic effect. The early appearance and rapid progression of hepatic, renal, or cerebral signs portend a bad prognosis, and death frequently occurs by the eighth day or earlier. Severe agitation, coma, shock, early azotemia, and severe hypoglycemia are the most certain signs of impending death. However, the actual occurrence of death is often sudden. Occasionally death is due to massive hematemesis but more often has been attributed to cardiac arrest.

In cases destined to survive, the third or systemic stage of poisoning begins relatively late, and the signs and symptoms are relatively mild compared to those in fatal cases. Recovery is usually established by the 14th day, although asymptomatic hepatomegaly may persist as long as 30 days after intoxication, and abnormalities of the electrocardiogram have been found as much as 27 days after ingestion.

Although cirrhosis of the liver may be a sequela of poisoning (LaDue et al., 1944; Moeschlin, 1965), recovery in other cases is complete.

Following a sufficiently large dose of phosphorus, the initial symptoms, including gastric irritation, headache, dizziness, weakness, and severe thirst, are rapidly replaced by signs of shock. The blood pressure falls rapidly; cyanosis, pallor, and coma appear. The clinical picture is one of irreversible peripheral vascular collapse, accompanied by a tremendous decrease in cardiac output. Death frequently occurs in the first 12 hr. The great majority of cases of phosphorus poisoning die before the appearance of a clear-cut picture of hepatic damage. Patients who survive 13–24 hr often develop a toxic psychosis with maniacal manifestations before death.

The majority of patients who die during the second day of illness have a fairly normal blood pressure at the time of hospital admission. Hepatomegaly appears in them within an average of 18 hr. Azotemia, but not jaundice, is usually present at the time of death, which may be due to vascular collapse or to sudden cardiac complication.

Patients who die during the third or fourth day develop hepatomegaly within the first 36 hr and live to develop jaundice as well as azotemia, oliguria, and other signs of kidney failure. Toxic psychosis may appear. Electrocardiographic changes are definite. Death is probably due in many instances to myocardial damage. Thus, patients who die within the second through the fourth day develop a picture of systemic poisoning often with little or no indication of a latent stage.

Although cases in which death occurs 5 days or more after ingestion may be considered examples of the hepatorenal syndrome, the final event is often preceded by a profound drop in blood pressure entirely similar to that found in more rapid poisoning.

A 30-year-old man who had swallowed a substantial dose of phosphorus presumably with suicidal intent developed in addition to the usual symptoms and signs of poisoning also symptoms, signs, and ECG changes indicating myocardial infarction. The patient recovered. On the ninth day, the acute S-T segment changes began to resolve, and 2 days later the Q wave changes diagnostic of infarct were no longer visible. Following more specialized ECG studies, it was concluded that ischemic myocardial necrosis had not occurred, and the ECG changes had been the result of metabolic derangement secondary to poisoning (Pietras et al., 1968).

A positive Chvostek sign and increased neuromuscular irritability were observed on the 15th day of acute, typical phosphorus poisoning from which the patient had already recovered to a considerable degree. Blood levels of calcium and phosphate were low, and urinary excretion of calcium exceeded intake. Both the clinical and laboratory findings spontaneously reverted to normal in 3 days. The lesion was considered to have been in the proximal renal tubules. Three other cases of hypocalcemia in phosphorus poisoning were reviewed and it was concluded that this complication may be more frequent than formerly supposed (Cushman and Alexander, 1966).

Phosphorus may be effective as an abortifacient, although it may kill the mother also (Piribauer and Wallenko, 1961).

Use Experience   Formerly, chronic poisoning, characterized by necrosis of the mandible and maxillary bone, was caused by prolonged inhalation of phosphorus in industry. This kind of phosphorus poisoning might be accompanied by signs of mild liver and kidney damage, but in some cases necrosis of the jaw was the only evidence of injury (Heimann, 1946). The history of the condition commonly called "phossy jaw" has been reviewed in detail by Hughes et al. (1962) who also described the much milder condition that still occasionally occurs in industry. In spite of continuing clinical observation and modern biochemical studies, the cause of the condition remains obscure. However, it appears to be an osteomyelitis that progresses because of a local, probiotic effect of elemental phosphorus. Although the condition is an osteomyelitis, it differs clinically and radiologically from other osteomyelitis. The organisms involved vary from case to case and may not even be recognized pathogens.

Under present conditions, phosphorus is not an important problem in industry. In a similar way, phosphorus used as a rodenticide is rarely a source of occupational poisoning, but it is highly dangerous to children who find and ingest it.

Dosage Response   A daily dose of 1 mg given with therapeutic intent sometimes produced gastrointestinal disturbance, necrosis of the jaw, and rarely typical phosphorus poisoning.

A dose of 15 mg may be severely toxic, and as little as 50 mg (about 0.7 mg/kg) has proved fatal to an adult (Sollmann, 1957). As little as 2 mg is reported to have killed an infant (Rabinowitch, 1943). On the contrary, patients have recovered after doses thought to range from 350 to 715 (Caley and Kellock, 1955; Fletcher and Galambos, 1963).

Phosphorus is better absorbed and more toxic if ingested in a finely divided state rather than in lumps. Diaz-Rivera et al. (1950) gave evidence that even a uniform, finely ground paste of phosphorus was more quickly and completely absorbed when suspended in water, or especially when dissolved in an alcoholic beverage. Study of a series of 56 cases, in which a single formulation of phosphorus was ingested with suicidal intent, revealed a clear relationship between the amount ingested and the severity and outcome of intoxication. In this particular series, the smallest fatal dose was estimated as 190 mg (about 3 mg/kg). In 33 cases in which the dose ingested was 780 mg or less (up to about 13 mg/kg), the mortality was 18% and the time from ingestion to death was 4 days or more. In 21 individuals who ingested 1570 mg (about 26 mg/kg), the mortality was 90% and death occurred in a few hours to 3 days. Higher doses were uniformly, rapidly fatal.

Laboratory Findings Urinalysis may show albuminuria, cylindruria, hematuria, and grossly abnormal concentrations of several amino acids. Liver function tests, including prothrombin time, become abnormal but usually not before hepatomegaly and jaundice are evident. Hypoglycemia may be severe; blood urea nitrogen, creatinine, and ammonia may be elevated. Any changes in the peripheral blood are small in degree and in no way characteristic. The phosphorus content of the blood is usually normal. EKG changes have been described in detail by Diaz-Rivera *et al.* (1961).

In the absence of a history of exposure, the garlic-like odor of the patient's breath often gives the first indication that phosphorus is involved. In addition, phosphorus may be detected in vomitus and feces—and according to Rubitsky and Myerson (1949), in the breath—by the light it emits in a dark room. Elementary phosphorus may be detected in excreta, gastric contents, and tissues in smaller concentration but with no greater certainty by chemical analysis. It is claimed that phosphorus and phosphine in tissue can be separately demonstrated (Curry *et al.*, 1958).

Pathology If death is sufficiently prompt, there is no pathology except irritation of the esophagus and stomach. Perforation may occur. Following survival for several days, fatty degeneration is striking in the liver, heart, and kidney but may be found in all organs, including the brain. Hepatic necrosis may be extensive, with changes occurring first in the periphery of lobules. The earliest signs of definite morphological change of the liver were found in a patient who died 6 hr after ingesting phosphorus.

Periportal necrosis with degenerative changes extending toward the center of the lobules have been observed in biopsies from patients who survived. Later biopsies showed that fibrosis occurred in some but not all cases. When present, the fibrosis was periportal, sometimes forming septa between portal areas. The degree of fibrosis could not be explained by dosage or by the degree of injury evident during the acute phase and must have depended in part on one or more unidentified factors (LaDue *et al.*, 1944; Fletcher and Galambos, 1963; Greenberger *et al.*, 1964).

Differential Diagnosis If history of phosphorus exposure is unavailable, the initial symptoms may be confused with the gastroenteritis caused by agents such as arsenic. There is a characteristic odor of garlic to the breath and vomitus in phosphorus poisoning. Luminescence of the gastric contents or feces in a darkened room is pathognomonic. Diagnosis in the absence of a history of exposure is much easier if the patient survives long enough to develop signs of hepatic, renal, and central nervous system dysfunction.

Treatment of Poisoning Since there is no specific therapy, the removal of phosphorus by vomiting or gastric lavage with large volumes of fluid is of utmost importance. According to Diaz-Rivera *et al.* (1950), early vomiting or gastric lavage may be of benefit, and at times lifesaving among patients ingesting doses of 780 mg or less, but for larger doses the outcome is almost always death, regardless of treatment. Potassium permanganate, 0.1% solution, or 2% hydrogen peroxide is used in preference to water since they may oxidize phosphorus to harmless phosphates. Mineral oil (200–250 ml), which helps to prevent phosphorus absorption, should be administered by gastric tube. Additional doses of 30–40 ml should be given by mouth every 3 hr for the first 24 hr. Absorption can be increased by digestible fats and oils, and for that reason they are contraindicated. The treatment of shock and acute hepatic or renal failure is instituted when necessary. According to some authors, shock caused by phosphorus responds to vasopressor agents, but in connection with poisoning associated with suicide Diaz-Rivera *et al.* (1950) found these agents generally ineffective.

A high carbohydrate, high protein, low fat diet supplemented with heavy doses of vitamin B and crude liver extract is generally advised. It has been reported but not confirmed that a combination of methionine and cystine can prevent necrosis of the liver (Rubitsky and Myerson, 1949).

The use of cortisone acetate resulted in dramatic improvement in one case of severe poisoning after the ingestion of 825 mg of phosphorus, which is ordinarily a fatal dose. The drug was given in an initial intramuscular dose of 200 mg followed by 50 mg ever 6 hr. Oral administration was used after 48 hr. Doses were decreased on the 8th day and again later, and eventually stopped on the 65th day. The drug was given in the hope that it would improve both glycogen deposition and detoxification in the liver (Bayne *et al.*, 1952).

It should be mentioned that although BAL has been tried in the treatment of phosphorus poisoning, there is neither clinical nor theoretical justification for it. If signs of calcium deficiency appear, calcium gluconate should be given.

If phosphorus contacts the skin, it should be removed with water and later with a 1% solution of copper sulfate. Additional details about the treatment of phosphorus burns were given by Rabinowitch (1943).

12.14 SULFUR

Sulfur follows phosphorus in the periodic table. It is in the same group as oxygen and selenium. Sulfur is an important constituent of protoplasm.

12.14.1 ELEMENTAL SULFUR

12.14.1.1 Identity, Properties, and Uses

Chemical Name Sulfur.

Synonyms Synonyms for sulfur include brimstone, colsul, flour sulfur, and flowers of sulfur. Trade names include Corosul D and S®, Kolofog®, Kolospray®, Magnetic 70, 90 and 95®, Spersul®, Sulforon®, and Thiovit®. The CAS registry no. is 7704-34-9.

Physical and Chemical Properties The atomic weight of sulfur is 32.064. The element exists in several allotropic forms of which the orthorhombic, cyclooctasulfur (also called α-sulfur) is stable at ordinary temperatures and pressures. The stable form consists of amber-colored crystals with a density of 2.06. When this is heated to 94.5°C, it forms monoclinic, cyclooctasulfur (β-sulfur), which melts at 115°C and boils at about 444.6°C. The vapor pressure of sulfur is 3.96×10^{-6} torr at 30.4°C. Sulfur is soluble in carbon disulfide, slightly soluble in petroleum ether and alcohols, and insoluble in water.

Formulations and Uses Sulfur is used as an acaricide and fungicide in the form of dusts, wettable powders, and pastes.

12.14.1.2 Toxicity to Laboratory Animals

In the intestine, sulfur is converted to hydrogen sulfide; the reaction is more rapid and complete if the sulfur is in colloidal rather than crystalline or powdered form. With the colloid, an oral dosage of 175 mg/kg was rapidly fatal to some rabbits; prior to death they showed convulsions, unconsciousness, a hydrogen sulfide odor of the breath, a fall in blood pressure, bradycardia, and stimulation of respiration followed by respiratory arrest (Greengard and Wolley, 1940a). Part of the absorbed sulfur is excreted and part enters into the general metabolic pool. When radioactive sulfur was fed to sheep, activity appeared in their wool within 2 weeks, and continued feeding of sulfur changed the physical properties of the fibers by changing the number of disulfide linages (Clark and Buhrke, 1954).

12.14.1.3 Toxicity to Humans

Experimental Exposure Volunteers who ingested daily doses of 500 or 750 mg of colloidal sulfur absorbed it completely and excreted most of it, mainly as the sulfate, within 24 hr. Fecal excretion of sulfur was not measurably increased. After ingestion of a single dose, excretion rose to a peak within the first 2–4 hr and then declined gradually to normal in 14–20 hr. Absorption of powdered (100 mesh) sulfur was far less complete and was delayed until 8–16 hr after ingestion (Greengard and Woolley, 1940b).

Therapeutic Use Binz (1897) cited an earlier reference on the medicinal use of sulfur by the followers of Hippocrates. In relatively recent times elemental sulfur has been used as a laxative and as an ointment for treatment of scabies and fungal infections. These uses were effective. In addition, sulfur ointments were used for various other skin diseases, and colloidal sulfur was injected either intravenously or intramuscularly for treatment of tuberculosis, syphilis, and especially arthritis (Sollmann, 1957). The injections especially for arthritis were probably an extension of the traditional treatment of rheumatism and various other conditions by baths in water from sulfur springs.

The oral, purgative dose of noncolloidal sulfur was 2000–4000 mg. Sulfur in combination with molasses constituted a favorite "spring tonic" of earlier times. Its purgative action was due to hydrogen sulfide, which was formed by gradual reduction of a part of the sulfur. If the dose were retained, a dangerous amount of hydrogen sulfide might be formed, but this was rare and is unlikely in the absence of mechanical obstruction. It has long been recognized that hydrogen sulfide was formed and was exhaled in the breath and apparently secreted by the skin. Silver ornaments worn by patients treated with sulfur were turned black (Binz, 1897).

Accidental and Intentional Poisoning Poisoning by lime sulfur (calcium polysulfides) probably should be attributed to sulfur because it decomposes to form sulfur in the presence of acid, including that in the stomach. Wakasugi and Fukui (1974) reported the suicide of a 22-year-old student who was found dead beside a 400-ml bottle labeled calcium polysulfide. The yellowish material with a sulfide odor was found on the face and hands as well in the stomach. Findings at autopsy were numerous but nonspecific.

12.15 SELENIUM

Selenium is a metalloid. It follows arsenic in the periodic table and falls in the same group as sulfur, which it resembles in many of its chemical reactions.

The toxic properties of plants grown on certain soils and eventually shown to depend on selenium have been known for a long time. In fact, the loss of hooves by horses and cows that eat these poisonous plants is so characteristic, one can be confident this was the disease observed by Marco Polo (1254–1327) in western China and described by him. The disease has been carefully studied and its quantitative relationship to selenium established.

It is only recently that selenium has been shown to be an essential trace element. Thus, selenium is one of those elements known first as a poison but later found necessary for life. The difference is one of dosage. Deficient diets contain less than 0.1 ppm of selenium; normal diets contain 0.1 ppm or somewhat more; toxic diets may contain as little as 5 ppm, but toxicity is more likely at concentrations of about 25 ppm.

Selenium is widely, but unevenly, distributed in nature. Traces of it ranging from 0.0000 to 0.01 ppm are found in community drinking water (Taylor, 1962). Food also contains selenium. For example, commercial wheat contains from 0.1 to 1.9 ppm. Selenium often is found in relatively high concentrations in acid soils of semiarid areas. Soils containing more than 0.5 ppm may lead to concentrations greater than 5 ppm in plants sometimes eaten by livestock and thus constitute a potential hazard. Much higher concentrations may occur in plants either because the soil in which they grow contains up to 30 ppm or because certain ones, namely some species of *Astragalus* and all species of *Stanleya, Oonopsis,* and *Xylorrhizia* (Kingsbury, 1964), are especially adapted to high concentrations of selenium and, in fact, dependent on the element.

The highest concentration of selenium reported in field-grown wheat is 63 ppm (Moxon, 1958). Most vegetables contain far less but onions may contain up to 17.8 ppm (Underwood, 1956). (Indicator plants of the genera just mentioned may contain concentrations approaching 15,000 ppm (Trelease and Beath, 1949). Livestock do not eat these plants unless driven by starvation, but their presence indicates the possibility of a problem in the soil, and if they are eaten, only a small amount of such plants may cause poisoning.

At least a portion of the selenium in plant tissues is in the form of analogs of ordinary sulfur compounds. Thus Se-methyl-selenocysteine has been identified in plant tissue but is difficult to separate from its sulfur analog (Trelease *et al.*, 1960).

If a high proportion of their diet contains high residues of selenium, livestock, especially cattle, at first become depressed and unaware of their surroundings. Gastrointestinal stasis leads to pain indicated by grunting, grinding of the teeth, and excessive salivation. A period of excitement may follow in which the animals wander aimlessly. There may be partial blindness and usually is some degree of paralysis. The aimless, stumbling wandering is recalled by the term "blind staggers," which is the common name for this form of poisoning.

Autopsy usually reveals multiple small hemorrhages in the heart, kidney, and spleen. Gastroenteritis may be present and the kidney may be soft and friable (Radeleff, 1964).

If the intake of selenium is smaller but more prolonged, livestock develop a more chronic condition called "alkali disease." It may even be intermittent if the animals receive excessive residues only part of the time. The disease is characterized by emaciation, lack of vitality, loss of long hair from the tails of horses and cattle and from the manes of horses, and deformity of the hooves leading to pain and lameness. In severe cases, the hooves may be lost. The animals are often anemic. Congestive heart failure is common, and on autopsy atrophy and fibrosis of the heart are prominent. Cirrhosis of the liver and scarring of the kidney and erosion of the joints of the long bones may also be found at death (Radeleff, 1964).

Rats fed grain grown in affected areas show many of the signs seen in poisoned livestock, including reduced food intake, weight loss, paralysis of the hind legs, hemorrhage into the gastrointestinal tract and the subcutaneous tissues and muscle fascia near the joints, and atrophy of the thymus and reproductive organs. Pathology is not marked in rats that die early because it requires some time to develop. Animals receiving smaller doses develop anemia and characteristic liver changes involving necrosis and atrophy accompanied by regeneration and leading to a grossly nodular appearance and to edema and other secondary changes (Franke, 1934).

Adult sheep are not very susceptible to selenium poisoning. However, lambs born to ewes fed high levels of this element may have abnormal eyes and deformed feet.

Dietary levels above 5 ppm are teratogenic to poultry (Franke and Tully, 1935).

It was shown by Schwarz *et al.* (1957) and by Schwarz and Foltz (1958) that rats maintained on a diet containing an undetectable amount of selenium (less than 0.1 ppm) develop liver necrosis, and chicks on the same diet develop an exudative diathesis. The selenium normally present in the diet of animals is in organic form. However, the rats and chicks remained healthy and developed normally when their deficient diet was supplemented by selenium at a dietary level of 0.04 ppm (rats) or 0.1 ppm (chicks). Selenium was equally effective whether in the form of sodium selenite or some organic selenium compounds. However, selenium is an integral part of Factor 3, a normally occurring dietary agent that prevents liver necrosis in the rat (Schwarz and Foltz, 1957), and, on a molar basis, the selenium in Factor 3 is some three to four times more effective than the other forms of selenium studied (Schwarz and Foltz, 1958). Even elementary selenium was effective if fed at a substantially higher level. This result was confirmed and extended by many authors. Although the actions of selenium and vitamin E are similar in many respects, it has been shown that selenium is an essential nutrient in both rats (McCoy and Weswig, 1969) and chicks (Thompson and Scott, 1970) even when their diet is fully supplemented by the vitamin.

More recent progress in showing that selenium is a necessary constituent of certain enzymes and other critical molecules was reviewed by Stadtman (1974) and by Underwood (1977). Although most details cannot be given here, the essentiality of selenium is emphasized by the finding that at least in *Escherichia coli,* selenium in the form of 4-selenouridine is an integral part of RNA (Hoffman and McConnell, 1974).

It was later found that muscular dystrophy (white muscle disease), a spontaneous myopathy of lambs raised in certain areas, could be prevented to a large extent by supplementing the deficient diet of their mothers with selenium at the rate of 0.1 ppm using sodium selenite (Muth *et al.,* 1958). The disease can be prevented (or, if not too advanced, it can be cured) by subcutaneous injection of 1 mg of sodium selenate per lamb (Lagacé, 1961). Radeleff (1964) mentions that traces of selenium will prevent certain myodystrophic conditions of horses as well as those of cattle and sheep. In addition to muscular dystrophy in several species and exudative diathesis in chickens, other diseases of domestic animals that occur spontaneously in selenium-deficient areas and may be corrected by selenium supplements include pancreatic fibrosis in chickens, hepatosis dietetica in pigs, unthriftiness in sheep and cattle, and reproductive disorders in various species (Underwood, 1977).

The beneficial effects of selenium may be due in part to interaction with other metals. For example, micromolar concentrations of selenium partially prevented the *in vitro* inhibition of colony formation by mouse bone marrow cells and by certain tumor cells caused by low concentrations of organic and inorganic mercury (Strom *et al.,* 1979).

Even dietary levels that permit reproduction and lead to no recognizable disease may be inadequate for maximal growth. On the other hand, the optimal level of dietary selenium is astonishly close to the toxic level, as was discussed in connection with the logprobit model and quantitative study of the effects of small dosages (Section 2.2.7.4).

Although illness of people has been attributed to excessive industrial environmental exposure to selenium (Dudley, 1938; Lemley, 1940; Lemley and Merryman, 1941), there is no agreement about the nature of the disease, and its existence has been questioned (Smith, 1941). The fact that people remain healthy in areas where livestock are subject to alkali disease has been explained by the facts that human diet is more varied and that much human food is brought in from other areas so that the dosage received by people is less than that received by livestock. This argument was less applicable in pioneer times, when both food and feed were raised locally. It remains true, of course, that people eat only plants that are relatively inefficient in accumulating selenium. Animals may be driven by starvation to eat plants of high selenium content. Thus people tend to receive a lower dosage than livestock living in the same areas and the people probably have a higher protein intake. However, the urinary excretion of selenium by healthy people living on seleniferous soil varies from 0.02 to 1.33 ppm (Smith and Westfall, 1936), and the daily output of some workers may reach 5 mg (Vesce, 1947). There is, therefore, some evidence that humans are less susceptible than livestock to poisoning by selenium.

Nearly all injury caused by a wide variety of selenium compounds in industry arises not from their systemic toxicity but from their irritation of the skin, eyes, and respiratory tract (Browning, 1969).

Apparently no form of uncomplicated selenium deficiency has been reported in people. However, increased growth in children suffering from kwashiorkor (Schwarz, 1961) and other malnutrition (Majaj and Hopkins, 1966) has been reported following administration of selenium.

Additional information on the toxic and nutritional effects of selenium may be found in reviews by Frost and Lish (1975) and by Underwood (1977).

12.15.1 SODIUM SELENATE

12.15.1.1 Identity, Properties, and Uses

Chemical Name Sodium selenate.

Structure $Na_2SeO_4 \cdot 10H_2O$.

Synonyms Trade names include Sel-Kaps®, Sel-Tox®, SS02®, and SS-20®. Code designations for the compound include P-40. The CAS registry no. is 10112-94-4.

Physical and Chemical Properties Sodium selenate has the empirical formula Na_2O_4Se. The anhydrous salt and the hydrate have molecular weights of 188.94 and 369.11, respectively. The compound forms white, nonflammable crystals which have a density of 3.098 and are very water-soluble.

Use Sodium selenate is an insecticide used in horticulture for the control of mites, aphids, and mealybugs.

12.15.1.2 Toxicity to Laboratory Animals

Basic Findings Animals given enough of a selenium compound to produce poisoning in 15 min show spasmotic contractions of the flanks, dyspnea, tetanic spasms, and death from respiratory failure (Franke and Moxon, 1936). Pathological changes include congestion of the liver with areas of focal necrosis; congestion of the kidney; endocarditis; myocarditis; and atony of smooth muscle of the gastrointestinal tract, gallbladder, and bladder.

The intraperitoneal dosage of selenium (as sodium selenate) that kills 75% of rats in 48 hr is 5.25–5.75 mg/kg. The lowest dosage causing death is 3.75 mg/kg. Sodium selenate is only slightly less toxic than sodium selenite (Franke and Moxon, 1936). Lehman (1951, 1952) reported the oral LD 50 values of both compounds as 2.5 mg/kg. The intravenous dosage of selenium (as sodium selenate) fatal to 50% of rats lies between 3 and 4 mg/kg. Rabbits are more susceptible; an intravenous dosage of 2.5 mg/kg killed all those tested, as was true of an oral dosage of 4.0 mg/kg (Smith et al., 1937).

Animals showing signs of poisoning have urinary concentrations of selenium ranging from 0.6 to 3.0 ppm (Smith, 1941).

Rats receiving selenium compounds (generally sodium selenite) in their diets show acute, subacute, and chronic pathologic pictures entirely similar to those seen in rats fed poisonous field-grown grain (Franke and Potter, 1935). Rats that received selenium (as sodium selenate) at a dietary level of 100 ppm ate little food and all died in 8–16 days; those receiving 50 ppm all died in 10–97 days. A dietary level of 15 ppm was tolerated for 72 days or more, but food intake was about half of normal. All rats survived a dietary level of 7.5 ppm (about 0.37 mg/kg/day) for 6 months, and their growth was normal (Smith et al., 1937).

Rats maintained on a diet deficient in protein (10%) were severely poisoned by a wheat selenium at a dietary level of 10 ppm, but the same concentration of selenium had virtually no effect on rats maintained on an isocaloric diet containing adequate protein, whether obtained from casein, wheat protein, lactalbumin, ovalbumin, yeast protein, liver protein, or even gelatin. Several individual amino acids were not protective (Smith, 1939, 1941; Smith and Stohlman, 1940; Lewis et al., 1940; Gortner, 1940).

Oral intake of selenium compounds leads to restricted food intake and marked loss of weight. Weight loss also occurred in an experiment involving subcutaneous administration, even though food intake was increased above the control level (Cameron, 1947). In spite of this difference, the rats showed many changes found in the other studies, including both atrophy and hypertrophy of liver lobes. Curiously enough, there was no cirrhosis (the injured liver was smooth), and the lobular distribution of hypertrophy and atrophy were reported to be opposite to that described and clearly illustrated by Franke (1934).

Absorption, Distribution, Metabolism, and Excretion Various compounds of selenium are freely absorbed from the respiratory and gastrointestinal tracts. Dermal absorption is less important.

Experimental animals store more selenium in the liver, kidney, spleen, pancreas, heart, and lung than in other organs. Values as high as 30 ppm were found in the liver and 18 ppm in the kidneys of rabbits fed selenium-bearing oats for 8–9 months. At dosage rates intended to be equal, organic selenium produced higher storage and more prolonged retention (Smith *et al.*, 1938).

Selenium is excreted chiefly in the urine but about 3–10% is metabolized and excreted by the lungs, and there is some fecal excretion even when sodium selenate is administered subcutaneously (McConnell, 1942). When sodium selenite is administered in the same way, 17–52% is exhaled within 8 hr (Schultz and Lewis, 1940).

Selenium crosses the placental barrier in both animals and humans (Westfall *et al.*, 1938; Hadjimarkos *et al.*, 1959). The concentration varied from 0.13 to 0.24 ppm in the placenta and from 0.07 to 0.18 ppm in cord blood.

Mode of Action Excessive amounts of selenium decrease the activity of succinic hydrogenases (Klug *et al.*, 1950). It is not clear whether this represents the biochemical lesion. It is of interest, however, that arsenic maintains this enzyme (Klug *et al.*, 1950) and also counteracts the toxicity of selenium in the intact animal (Moxon *et al.*, 1945). Losses of livestock from selenium poisoning are reduced by using salt containing about 40 ppm of arsenic or by the addition of 50–100 ppm of arsanilic acid to the rations of calves and pigs (Radeleff, 1964).

Although selenite inhibits a variety of sulfhydral enzymes *in vitro*, the action is so weak it cannot explain the toxicity of selenium. It is more likely that the toxicity may be explained by the selenium-catalyzed oxidation of such cofactors as glutathione, coenzyme A, and dihydrolipoic acid, and by the resulting disturbance of intermediary metabolism (Tsen and Collier, 1959).

Rats that received repeated, gradually increasing, subcutaneous doses of inorganic selenium developed resistance so that they tolerated (although not without weight loss and signs of chronic intoxication) many doses each more than three times the LD 50. When dosing was stopped, the rats recovered their health and body weight (Cameron, 1947).

Effects on Organs and Tissues When the possible carcinogenicity of selenium and its compounds was reviewed by an IARC Working Group, it was concluded that the available data were insufficient to allow an evaluation of the carcinogenicity of large dosages of selenium compounds in animals. The group concluded that the data provided no suggestion that selenium is carcinogenic in humans. They found evidence for a negative correlation between regional cancer death rates and selenium not convincing, even though they cited considerable evidence along this line as well as evidence that small dosages of selenium tend to protect animals from naturally occurring cancer or cancer induced by classical carcinogens (WHO, 1975). Other more objective reviews (Scott,

1973; Underwood, 1977) have concluded that selenium has not been shown to be carcinogenic and has been shown to be protective.

12.15.1.3 Toxicity to Humans

Accidental and Intentional Poisoning Apparently there is no record of human poisoning by sodium selenate. Ingestion of about 1000 mg of sodium selenite caused a condition similar to arsenic poisoning with death in 5 hr (Moeschlin, 1965).

Laboratory Findings In normal persons without unusual exposure, the concentration of selenium in the liver ranges from 0.55 to 1.34 ppm; in the heart it ranges from 0.14 to 0.67 ppm (Liebscher and Smith, 1968). The concentration in normal urine is 0.01–0.16 ppm (Sterner and Lidfeldt, 1941). The concentration in the urine of most people living in a seleniferous area varies from 0.02 to 1.33 ppm (Smith and Westfall, 1936). The latter range overlaps that for animals poisoned by selenium, but the people are unaffected by their exposure. Heavily exposed industrial workers excreted selenium at levels as high as 6.9 ppm.

The concentrations of selenium in 210 samples of blood from people in 16 cities of the United States ranged from 0.10 to 0.34 and averaged 0.206 ppm. There was some tendency for the blood values for selenium to be higher in geographic areas where the concentrations of selenium are higher in the soil and in plants. However, the variation in the selenium content of blood was much less pronounced than the variation in selenium in locally produced foods (Allaway *et al.*, 1968). The concentration in normal plasma does not exceed 0.15 ppm (Gofman *et al.*, 1964).

Treatment of Poisoning The treatment of selenium poisoning is essentially unknown. A high-protein diet may be helpful. Arsenical feed supplements are beneficial in animals. BAL is not indicated. Some evidence from animal studies suggests that BAL decreases injury to the liver, increases injury to the kidneys, and has no effect on survival.

12.16 FLUORINE

Fluorine is the halogen of lightest atomic weight. Its salts are widely distributed in soil and water and occur in all tissues. The toxic effects of excessive doses of various fluorides have been known for many years. Since about 1940 it has been known that children develop a high level of dental caries if they live where the drinking water contains much less than 1 ppm of the fluoride ion. Children who live where there is naturally a good supply of fluoride in the local water or children whose supply of fluoride is supplemented develop teeth that are more resistant to rotting. Thus fluoride is essential to human health if not to human life.

It was not until the 1970s that evidence began to accumulate that fluoride is essential for optimal growth in rats and for reproduction and prevention of anemia in mice. Not all inorganic fluorine compounds are equally effective when added to a basic diet containing <0.04 ppm F to give an equal concentration of fluorine (2.5 ppm). Furthermore, the relative contributions of fluoride, monofluorophosphate, hexafluorosilicate, and monofluoropyruvate are different in regard to growth as compared to normal development of the teeth or to the deposition of fluorine in bones (Milne and Schwarz, 1974).

Sodium fluoride is the prototype of inorganic fluorides used as pesticides. It has received some study in this connection and a great deal more in connection with industrial air pollution on the one hand and the prevention of dental caries on the other. The remaining inorganic fluoride pesticides, cryotite, sodium fluorosilicate, and even zinc hexafluorosilicate, owe their toxicity to fluoride ion, which they release slowly on contact with water. Through their often careless use, the inorganic fluoride pesticides have been an important cause of accidental acute poisoning. There is no indication that they have been a source of any chronic condition. The fluorine compounds that have given rise to chronic effects (mainly fluorosis of teeth and bone) in both humans and animals are in all instances not pesticides.

For those several reasons, it seems best to confine the sections on fluoride pesticides to information on the compounds themselves, emphasizing acute effects, and to outline what is known of the long-term environmental and occupational effects of fluorine compounds in this section. These long-term effects offer the best available indication of what continuing rate of intake of fluoride pesticides would be required to produce chronic injury.

The only moderately common effect of continued excessive intake of fluoride in humans is mottling of the enamel of the teeth. This effect involves chalky patches alternating with areas of staining. No mottling has been reported where the concentration of fluoride in drinking water is less than 0.3 ppm and practically none at levels below 0.6 ppm. Mottling is exceptional and slight when the concentration in drinking water is 1 ppm. The incidence and degree of mottling increase in proportion to the fluoride concentration in water within the range of 2 to 10 ppm.

Chronic fluorosis was first described as occurring among animals that obtained excessive fluorides from their pastures. The residues deposited on vegetation consist of dust from indigenous soil (certain phosphate deposits or volcanic ash) or from the stack of gases of factories making phosphate fertilizer, some other phosphorus chemicals, steel, and aluminum. The compounds include native minerals, silicon tetrafluoride, and hydrofluorosilicic acid. Affected animals have stiff-legged gait, swollen hock joints, palpable lumps on their bones, and severely and irregularly worn teeth (Heyroth, 1963).

The pain the animals show is a direct result of the deformity of their bones and the erosion of their articular surfaces. Lameness may lead to inability to feed; this contributes to weight loss, rough coat, reduced milk production, and infertility often seen in poisoned animals (Radeleff, 1964).

Under field conditions, cattle are most susceptible, and other species are less so in the following order: cattle>sheep >swine>horses>turkeys>chickens (Radeleff, 1964). An extensive review of the literature (Schmidt and Rand, 1952) revealed that the highest dosages that did not produce fluorosis were 1–3 mg/kg/day in cattle, 5–12 mg/kg/day in swine, 10–20 mg/kg/day in rats and guinea pigs, and 35–70 mg/kg/day in chickens.

Mottling of the enamel in humans does not occur if excessive exposure to fluorides begins after the permanent teeth are formed. Although the bones may be affected at any time of life, even mild effects of this kind generally occur only after prolonged, poorly regulated, generally industrial exposure and, therefore, only in adults. It is probably because of this age distribution that essentially all reports of fluorosis in people involve osteosclerotic changes in bone marked by greater opacity to x-ray, thickening of the lamina, exostoses, and calcification of the ligamentous attachments.

Table 12.13 shows various indices of excessive repeated fluoride intake that have been associated with detectable effects in humans. In most instances, even workers who exhibit radiological evidence of skeletal fluorosis suffer no disabling symptoms. However, about half of a group with an average urinary concentration of 16.1 ppm and with urinary levels up to 43.4 ppm complained of lack of appetite, nausea, and shortness of breath and showed some degree of anemia. A smaller proportion of the men had other complaints (Brun *et al.*, 1941, or Roholm, 1937).

The beneficial effect of fluoride in reducing the prevalence of dental caries was discovered much more recently than the toxic effects of higher doses. The beginning of this discovery, which has permitted our children's teeth to be so much better than our own, has been traced back to (*a*) the observation of Eager (1901) connecting "Chiaie teeth" (now called mottled teeth) with drinking water and air charged with volcanic vapors now known to be fluorides and (*b*) the subsequent demonstration by Dean (1942a,b) of a quantitative relationship between caries in 7257 children and the concentrations of fluoride in their drinking waters. The decrease in caries is a linear function of the logarithm of fluoride concentration (Hodge, 1950). The use of fluoridation has been reviewed in detail (Shaw, 1954; Campbell, 1963). Briefly, when the concentration of fluoride is optimum, no ill effects will result and caries rates will be only 35–40% of those in communities using water supplies with little or no fluoride. The optimal concentration is about 1 ppm. However, the dosage obtained from drinking water depends on the average amount of water consumed, and this depends on temperature. Therefore, the official recommendation for a particular community depends on its annual average maximal daily air temperatures as shown in Table 12.14. The recommendations take into account the usual range of fluoride intake from food.

Of 165 community water supplies analyzed for fluorine in 1961, 81 fell below the lowest optimal average of 0.7 ppm, while only 21 were above the highest optimal average of 1.2

Table 12.13
Effect of Prolonged Intake of Fluoride in Humans

Water (ppm)	Air (mg/m³)	Approximate intake (mg/kg/day)	Urinary output	Effect	Reference
<0.6		<0.01	<0.6 ppm	rotting of teeth	
1		0.03	~1 ppm	optimal tooth development; no injury	
6		0.17	7.8 ppm	mottled dental enamel	
		0.2–0.35		fluorosis in many	Møller and Gudjonnson (1932)
	12–26[a]	0.2–1.0	16.1	fluorosis[b]	Roholm (1937)
			2.4–43.4 ppm	fluorosis progressive with duration of employment	Brun et al. (1941)
	0.14–3.43		<9.03 mg/24 hr	fluorosis by X ray in some	Agate et al. (1949)
			≥10	fluorosis by X ray	Largent et al. (1951)
			6 ppm	slight fluorosis in a few	Heyroth (1952)

[a] Fluoride content calculated from gravimetric measurement of cryolite dust, slightly over half of which was of respirable size.
[b] First detectable by X ray after an average of 8.0 years of exposure, the shortest time observed being 2.8 years.

ppm, and only six supplies had an average concentration above 1.29 ppm. The highest observed value was 10 ppm (Taylor, 1962).

Effects on Reproduction Female mice maintained on a low-fluoride diet (0.1–0.3 ppm) for two generations showed a progressive decline in litter production. Mice receiving the same diet supplemented with fluoride reproduced normally (Messer et al., 1972). On the other hand, high levels (100 ppm and especially 200 ppm) of fluoride also reduced litter production (Messer et al., 1972, 1973).

More information on the value of fluoride and on the injuries produced by both deficient and excessive intake of it may be found in a WHO monograph entitled Fluorides and Human Health (WHO, 1970). Another valuable source of information that emphasizes effects on domestic animals is a chapter by Underwood (1977). More general works on the pharmacology and toxicology of fluorides are those by Roholm (1937), Largent (1961), Hodge and Smith (1965), and Smith (1966, 1970).

12.16.1 SODIUM FLUORIDE

12.16.1.1 Identity, Properties, and Uses

Chemical Name Sodium fluoride.

Structure NaF.

Synonyms Trade names for sodium fluoride include Floridine®, Florocid®, Flura-Drops®, Karidium®, Pergantine®, T-Fluoride®, and Villiaumite®. Code designations include FDA-101. The CAS registry no. is 7681-49-4.

Physical and Chemical Properties Sodium fluoride has the empirical formula FNa and a molecular weight of 41.99. It forms an odorless, noninflammable, white crystalline powder with a salty taste. It has a density of 2.78, a melting point of 993°C, and a boiling point of 1704°C. It is soluble in water and slightly soluble in alcohol.

Formulations and Uses Sodium fluoride is toxic to all forms of life. It has been used as an insecticide, rodenticide, and herbicide and as a fungicide for preservation of timber. Its toxicity to plants generally has restricted its use as an insecticide to bait formulations. The commercial product varies in purity from 93 to 99%. It should be colored to help distinguish it from table salt or flour.

Table 12.14
Recommended Limits for Fluoride in Drinking Water[a]

Annual average of maximum daily air temperatures[b] (°F)	(°C)	Lower level (ppm)	Optimum level (ppm)	Upper level (ppm)
50.0–53.7	10.0–12.0	0.9	1.2	1.7
53.8–58.3	12.1–14.6	0.8	1.1	1.5
58.4–63.8	14.7–17.6	0.8	1.0	1.3
63.9–70.6	17.7–21.4	0.7	0.9	1.2
70.7–79.2	21.5–26.2	0.7	0.8	1.0
79.3–90.5	26.3–32.5	0.6	0.7	0.8

[a] Modified from U.S. Public Health Service (1962).
[b] Based on temperature data obtained for a minimum of 5 years.

12.16.1.2 Toxicity to Laboratory Animals

Oral LD 50 values of 200 and 180 mg/kg have been reported for sodium fluoride in rats (Lehman, 1951, 1952; Smyth *et al.,* 1969) and 200 mg/kg was reported for rabbits (Muehlberger, 1930). An intraperitoneal LD 50 of 49 mg/kg was found in mice (Nofre *et al.,* 1963).

Rats fed a diet containing sodium fluoride at fluoride levels of 7–14 ppm for 6 weeks developed dental fluorosis detectable only by the aid of a lens as fine lines of impaired calcification. When the dietary concentration of fluoride was 226 ppm, the incisors became chalky and pitted. Dietary levels from 225 to 452 ppm inhibited body growth, and levels of 904 ppm or more produced marked weight loss and death in a few weeks. Fluorine interfered with reproduction only at levels of feeding that stunted the growth of the female, and there was no evidence of specific damage to the reproductive organs (Smith and Leverton, 1934).

Absorption, Distribution, Metabolism, and Excretion
Following oral administration of sodium fluoride to rabbits, the fluoride concentration of plasma rose rapidly from a range of 0.01 to 0.07 ppm to a maximal level usually within 1 hr and then usually declined with a half-life of 4 or 5 hr. Doses of 100 to 140 mg/kg gave 1-hr concentrations of 12–14 ppm. Plasma concentrations of 28 ppm at 1 hr led to death within 12 hr, but levels somewhat less than 24 ppm usually were associated with survival for at least 24 hr, although not permanently (Hall *et al.,* 1972).

Biochemical Effects A 2% solution of sodium fluoride kills the cells of mucous membranes and produces corrosion. Lower concentrations also have local action if applied for long periods. Thus, the compound at concentrations of 10 to 25 ppm has been used as an antiseptic or food preservative (Sollmann, 1957).

Enzymes strongly inhibited by fluoride *in vitro* include lipases, esterases, and phosphatases. Although many enzymes are known to be affected, the biochemical lesion has not been identified.

According to Kochmann (1934), parathyroid hormone is so effective in combating fluoride poisoning in mice that the relationship could be used as an assay method for the hormone. A further indication of involvement of the parathyroid glands is the report (Pavlovic and Tihomirov, 1932) that these glands show marked degeneration in acute poisoning and less severe effects following smaller repeated doses. However, the changes in blood calcium level during poisoning are not sufficient to explain toxicity even in acute poisoning. The antagonistic effect of injected calcium is considered due to precipitation of fluoride, not primarily correction of calcium deficiency.

In fluorosis uncomplicated by systemic illness, fluoride ion appears to be deposited in place of hydroxyl ion in the hydroxyapatite of bone (Neuman *et al.,* 1950; McCann, 1953). There is little or no change in the calcium (McClure and Mitchell, 1931; Lantz and Smith, 1934) or phosphate (Phillips, 1932; Smith and Lantz, 1935) content of the bone. A part of the fluorine deposited in bone is readily excreted after fluoride feeding is stopped, but another part is more firmly held (Savchuck and Armstrong, 1951; Miller and Phillips, 1953).

12.16.1.3 Toxicity to Humans

Therapeutic Use In areas where there is a deficiency of fluoride in the drinking water, the incidence of dental caries can be reduced by administering sodium fluoride at a rate of 2.2 mg/day (Arnold *et al.,* 1960). However, to be of value the drug must be taken consistently during the years when the permanent teeth are being formed. Since few children or their parents can remember to carry out this preventive procedure, it is much more efficient to treat municipal water supplies so that the concentration of fluoride ion is in the range of 0.7 to 1.3 ppm. This may be done by adding sodium fluoride at a rate of 1.5 to 3.0 ppm.

Larger doses given therapeutically are discussed under Dosage Response.

Accidental and Intentional Poisoning Acute, nonfatal poisoning is characterized by gastroenteritis (sudden nausea and vomiting, abdominal cramps, burning pain, and diarrhea) lasting for 3–6 hr and followed by collapse involving stupor and weakness lasting for about 36 hr (Vallee, 1920; Sharkey and Simpson, 1933). Tetany may occur as a result of calcium depletion. In fatal poisoning, muscular weakness appears early and is accompanied by a marked fall in blood pressure; tremor may be followed by clonic convulsions; dyspnea may be accompanied by a grayish-blue cyanosis. Death from respiratory and cardiac arrest may occur a few minutes to 10 hr or more after ingestion but usually in 3 or 4 hr.

Table 7.14 lists a large outbreak of poisoning caused by the eating of sodium fluoride. In a much smaller outbreak, two people were killed by the compound when it was sold and used as flour (Fazekas, 1968).

Dosage Response Death has followed ingestion of as little as 4000 mg of sodium fluoride (about 57 mg/kg) (Sollmann, 1957; Peters, 1948). Baldwin (1899) calculated the doses of four people who survived severe poisoning as 9000, 6000, 5000, and 1000 mg. Prolonged, heroic treatment saved one patient who had intentionally ingested 120,000 mg (Abukurah *et al.,* 1973), but good treatment may fail following a much smaller dose (Whelton *et al.,* 1973).

Two adults were able to withstand a dose of 250 mg with minimal illness. One volunteer experienced slight nausea and epigastric distress lasting about 5 hr and salivation, which was intense for 15–30 min and stopped in half an hour; an itching sensation on his hands and feet lasted for about a week (Rabuteau, 1867). Another volunteer, who took 250 mg of sodium fluoride on an empty stomach, experienced nausea, which appeared in 2 min and in 20 min increased to a maximum accompanied by greatly increased salivation and some retching but no vomiting. Two hours after the dose, lunch was eaten but was immediately vomited. Slight nausea continued throughout the following day but disappeared on the second day (Baldwin, 1899).

Sodium fluoride produced no injury when given to children at the rate of 2.2 mg/child/day.

Sodium fluoride was explored many years ago as a disinfectant and as a systemic treatment for malaria, epilepsy, and headache in children. In the course of these studies, it was found that a dose greater than a quarter of a grain (16.25 mg) produced nausea and vomiting in children; doses, therefore, were limited to 8–11 mg three times a day. The urine passed by each of three men 1–2 hr after each received 8 mg of sodium fluoride resisted bacterial decomposition, showing that the material was excreted rapidly with this property intact. Urine passed later became turbid at the usual rate (Kolpinski, 1886).

Sodium fluoride was administered to more than 70 patients in an exploration of its therapeutic effects in cancer and hypertension. The average dose for adults was 80 mg four times a day; for children the dose varied from 20 to 50 mg four times a day. In most instances the period of therapy was several months. To avoid irritation of the stomach from the formation of hydrofluoric acid, the medication was given as enteric coated tablets or with an amphoteric antacid. Sodium fluoride also was given intravenously at a maximal dosage of 30 mg/kg. In one case a total dose of 5600 mg was administered in this way during a period of 9 days. No evidence of acute or chronic systemic toxicity or parenchymatous damage from these treatments was observed. Certain neoplasms were controlled temporarily, and there was some tendency for hypertension to be reduced (Black *et al.*, 1949).

The threshold limit value (2.5 mg/m^3) permits a safe occupational intake of 0.36 mg/kg/day. This rate is higher than that found necessary to provide lifetime protection of the teeth, namely 0.029 mg/kg/day.

Laboratory Findings   In a fatal case, the concentrations of fluoride in the blood and liver were 6.63 and 6.86 ppm, respectively (Dodinval-Versie *et al.*, 1966). A patient who was saved only by heroic measures had a serum level of 2 ppm (Abukurah *et al.*, 1973). The mean fluoride content of plasma is in the range of 0.14 to 0.19 ppm, even when the fluoride content of drinking water varies from 0.15 to 2.5 ppm. This indicates the existence of a homeostatic mechanism. However, when the fluoride content of drinking water is as high as 5.4 ppm, this regulatory mechanism is overwhelmed to some extent, and mean plasma concentrations of 0.26 ppm have been observed (WHO, 1970).

The normal concentration of fluoride in most soft tissues is in the range of 0.5 to 1.0 ppm, and this is maintained by a homeostatic mechanism.

Bones and teeth normally contain much higher concentrations, usually in the range of 100 to 300 ppm. When fluoride intake is excessive the concentration of fluoride in the bones increases, but bone structure is not altered unless the concentration in the bones exceeds 2500 ppm (Hodge and Smith, 1965).

The homeostasis of fluoride depends, at least in part, on its ready excretion in the urine. In fact, the concentration of fluoride in urine corresponds numerically with the concentration in drinking water as shown in Table 12.15, adapted from Heyroth (1963). When the concentration of fluoride in water was reduced from 8 to 1 ppm, the concentrations in the urine of those who drank the water decreased from 6 to 8 to about 2 ppm in the course of 27 months (Likins *et al.*, 1956).

In case of poisoning, blood calcium may be decreased, and there is usually a general disruption of fluid balance as a result of vomiting. Albuminuria is common.

Pathology   In acute fatal poisoning there is corrosion of the stomach and sometimes other parts of the gastrointestinal tract. Frequently there is edema of the brain and lungs and petechial hemorrhages of the lungs and heart.

Treatment of Poisoning   Vomiting should be promoted or gastric lavage carried out if the poison itself has not already produced copious vomiting. Liquid given between bouts of vomiting or used for gastric lavage should contain calcium (lime water, 1% calcium chloride solution, calcium gluconate, or even milk) to form the highly insoluble calcium fluoride. After the stomach has been cleared, a cathartic should be given. Milk of magnesia is best because it precipitates fluoride as well as clearing the intestine. Vomitus and excreta should be washed away quickly to prevent burns (Peters, 1948).

Calcium gluconate (20 ml of a 10 or 20% solution) should be given intravenously at once. It should be repeated as required by the blood calcium level. It not only may alleviate carpopedal spasm but may raise the blood pressure to normal from a shock level (Rao *et al.*, 1969).

The marked success of treating animals with parathyroid hormone (see Section 12.16.1.2) suggests that it should be used in human cases and, in fact, success has been reported by Müller and Bock (1958).

Additional treatment should be symptomatic depending on the progress of the case but should emphasize restoration of fluid balance. In one very severe case, an intravenous atrial pacemaker was necessary to control ventricular fibrillation;

Table 12.15

Concentration of Fluoride in Drinking Water and in the Urine of Persons Who Drink This Water[a]

Fluoride in water (ppm)	Mean urinary output (ppm)
2	2.09
5.5	5.46
6	7.80
8	8.71

[a] Modified from Heyroth (1963), by permission of John Wiley and Sons, Inc.

feeding through a gastrostomy was necessary for 30 days (Abukurah *et al.*, 1973).

12.16.2 SULFURYL FLUORIDE

12.16.2.1 Identity, Properties, and Uses

Chemical Name   Sulfuryl fluoride.

Structure SO_2F_2.

Synonyms   Sulfuryl fluoride is manufactured under the trade name Vikane®. The CAS registry no. is 2699-79-8.

Physical and Chemical Properties   Sulfuryl fluoride has the empirical formula F_2O_2S and a molecular weight of 102.07. It is an odorless, colorless gas with a melting point of $-135.82°C$ and a boiling point of $-55.38°C$. The vapor pressure is 13×10^3 torr at 25°C. The solubility in water at 25°C is 0.75 g/kg. Sulfuryl fluoride is of low solubility in most organic solvents but is miscible with methyl bromide. It is stable and noncorrosive. It is not hydrolyzed by water, but by NaOH solution.

History, Formulations, and Uses   Sulfuryl fluoride was first introduced in 1957. It is used for the fumigation of structures against drywood termites. Technical sulfuryl fluoride is 95% pure.

12.16.2.2 Toxicity to Laboratory Animals

Both sexes of rats, guinea pigs, and rabbits and female rhesus monkeys tolerated air concentrations of 100 ppm (417 mg/m^3) without apparent adverse effect when exposed 7 hr a day, 5 days a week, for 6 months. Observations included survival, general appearance, behavior, and the appearance of internal organs of animals killed at the end of the experiment (Stewart, 1957). Later it was reported that a concentration of 20 ppm produced detectable effects in rats, mice, and guinea pigs exposed 7 hr a day for 6 months, but the injury present after 12 months was reversible when exposure was discontinued. Some evidence of fluorosis was observed in the incisors of mice but not in those of rats or guinea pigs (ACGIH, 1971).

Although the long-term effects of sulfuryl fluoride are those of excess fluoride, it seems possible that some or all of the acute effects are those of the intact molecule.

Biochemical Effects   In the absence of studies on mammals, it is necessary to refer to an excellent study on termites. First it was shown that termites fumigated with a nonlethal concentration of [^{35}S]sulfuryl fluoride excreted inorganic sulfate, indicating that fluoride had been released. Then, using the labeled metabolic pool technique (see Section 3.3.3 in Hayes, 1975), separate studies of termites prefed sodium [^{14}C]acetate or on [^{32}P]phosphate showed that fumigated termites exhibited a spectrum of metabolic changes characteristic of fluoride toxicity (Meikle *et al.*, 1963).

12.16.2.3 Toxicity to Humans

Accidental and Intentional Poisoning   A case attributed to sulfuryl fluoride involved a 30-year-old man who was exposed for about 4 hr to unknown concentrations of a 99:1 mixture of it with chloropicrin. While still at work, he experienced nausea, vomiting, crampy abdominal pain, and itching. When admitted to hospital soon afterward, vital signs were normal; the only abnormalities observed were reddening of the conjunctival, pharyngeal, and nasal mucosae; diffuse rhonchi; and paresthesia of the lateral surface of the right leg. The serum was positive for fluoride. The signs and symptoms resolved quickly; the patient was discharged on the fourth hospital day. He returned three times as an outpatient, complaining of persistent scratching of the throat, flatulence, and difficulty in reading. Ophthalmological examination revealed no abnormality, and the patient was discharged with a strong suspicion that emotional factors played a significant role in his disorder (Taxay, 1966). In his discussion of the case, Taxay reviewed unpublished reports of animal experiments apparently indicating that dosages sufficient to produce illness from a single exposure produce respiratory irritation, central nervous system depression, and possible liver and kidney injury. Certainly the patient's major objective findings involved irritation of the eyes and respiratory tract. Only a series of cases would reveal whether the patient's signs and symptoms were typical or even whether they were due primarily to sulfuryl fluoride.

A totally different sort of case listed by Hayes (1976) involved a 25-year-old man with a postmortem blood alcohol level of 0.156% who was found lifeless in a residence that had been fumigated with sulfuryl fluoride under canvas. He was unknown to the rightful occupants of the house, and it was unclear how he had gotten in undetected.

Dosage Response   The threshold limit value (20 mgm^3) would permit occupational exposure at the rate of 2.86 mg/kg/day, equivalent to a fluoride exposure of 0.42 mg/kg/day.

Treatment of Poisoning   Treatment is symptomatic (see Sections 8.2 and 12.16.1.3).

12.16.3 ZINC HEXAFLUOROSILICATE

12.16.3.1 Identity, Properties, and Uses

Chemical Name   Zinc hexafluorosilicate.

Structure $ZnSiF_6 \cdot 6H_2O$).

Synonyms   Other names for zinc hexafluorosilicate include zinc fluosilicate, zinc fluorosilicate, and zinc silicofluoride. The CAS registry no. is 16871-71-9.

Physical and Chemical Properties   The anhydride of zinc hexafluorosilicate has the empirical formula F_6SiZn and a molecular weight of 207.46. The hexahydrate forms white crystals which are soluble in water.

Use   Mothproofing agent.

12.16.3.2 Toxicity to Laboratory Animals

The oral lethal dose for the guinea pig was reported as 100 mg/kg (Simonin and Pierron, 1937).

12.16.3.3 Toxicity to Humans

Accidental and Intentional Poisoning   A suicide served to show that poisoning by zinc hexafluorosilicate is typical of poisoning by the fluoride ion. A 35-year-old man drank half a glassful of a 5–10% solution of a commercial formulation. Following ingestion, emesis and tetanic convulsions occurred in 3.4 hr and death in 4.5 hr. Pathology was typical of fluoride poisoning (von Kraemer and Giebelmann, 1975).

Laboratory Findings   In two cases, including the suicide just mentioned, analysis showed that the concentration of zinc was increased over normal values more dependably in the blood than in the liver or kidneys. In fact, in the suicide, the concentration of zinc in these organs was within the range of normal (Giebelmann and Peplow, 1974). Even in cases in which analysis of stomach contents for zinc hexafluorosilicate is definitive, it would seem best to analyze the tissues for fluoride.

Treatment of Poisoning   See Sections 1.8 and 12.16.1.3.

12.17 CHLORINE

Chlorine is a halogen that can occur as the highly toxic gas Cl_2. However, the chloride ion is essential to life. Its concentration as NaCl in normal human blood is 4500–5000 ppm.

Unlike compounds of lead or mercury, which have toxic properties common to the element, compounds of chlorine, whether inorganic or organic, have little in common, although certain groups of them may exhibit similarities. Thus there seems to be no characteristic chlorine toxicity as there is a mercury toxicity. This does not deny that the toxicity of many organic compounds can be modified and often substantially increased by chlorine substitution in the molecule. Such substitutions have been developed by living organisms and much more recently by chemists. Examples of naturally occurring organic chlorine compounds include ochratoxin A (Van der Merwe *et al.*, 1965), the compound now called penitrem A (Wilson *et al*, 1968), and cyclochlorotine (Ishikawa *et al.*, 1970).

12.17.1 SODIUM CHLORATE

12.17.1.1 Identity, Properties, and Uses

Chemical Name   Sodium chlorate.

Structure $NaClO_3$.

Synonyms   Trade names for sodium chlorate include Altacide®, Chlorax®, De-Fol-Ate®, Drop Leaf®, Klorex®, Ortho-C-1-Defoliant®, Rasikal®, Shed-A-Leaf®, Val-Drop®, and Weed Killer®. The CAS registry no. is 775-09-9.

Physical and Chemical Properties   Sodium chlorate has the empirical formula $ClNaO_3$ and a molecular weight of 106.45. It forms an odorless white powder with a density of 2.5 and a melting point of 248°C. It liberates oxygen at about 300°C and decomposes upon heating. The solubility of sodium chlorate in water at 0°C is 790 gm/liter. It is soluble in ethanol and glycerol. A strong oxidizing agent, sodium chlorate reacts with organic materials in the presence of sunlight.

History, Formulations, and Uses   Sodium chlorate has been in use as a weed killer since 1910. The commercial product is about 99% pure and is applied at rates of about 100 to 200 kg/ha. In some formulations, sodium chloride or other salts are included as fire retardants. Sodium borate may be formulated with sodium chlorate for both its fire retardant and herbicidal action.

12.17.1.2 Toxicity to Laboratory Animals

The oral LD 50 of sodium chlorate in the rat is 1200 mg/kg (Edson, 1960). The intraperitoneal LD 50 in the mouse is 596 mg/kg (Nofre *et al.*, 1963).

Sodium chlorate is a strong oxidizing agent. In the body it produces methemoglobin, a process involving the conversion of iron from the normal ferrous state to the ferric state. In addition, chlorate destroys red blood corpuscles, liberating hemoglobin and other proteins. The intact red cell has considerable power to reduce methemoglobin, but the mechanism apparently cannot operate after hemolysis. Thus, a high percentage of hemoglobin in the plasma may be in the form of methemoglobin while the percentage of metaglobin in the intact cells is low (Knight *et al.*, 1967).

Repeated doses of chlorate, large enough to produce illness and weight loss but too small to be harmful if given only once, injure the kidney tubules severely without producing detectable methemoglobinemia (Richardson, 1937). This situation apparently has no parallel in human clinical experience but could be involved with livestock.

12.17.1.3 Toxicity to Humans

Accidental and Intentional Poisoning   The majority of deaths caused by sodium chlorate have been the result of suicide (Timperman and Maes, 1966; Mengele *et al.*, 1969; Motin *et al.*, 1970; Oliver *et al.*, 1972). The chance of ingesting a fatal dose accidentally is small unless the compounds is mistaken for a drug and taken purposely, as occurred when the potassium salt mistakenly was substituted for potassium chloride (Cochrane and Smith, 1940). However, completely typical, near-fatal poisoning occurred when a 13-year-old boy "tasted" crystals of this weed killer which he found in his father's shed. In spite of intensive treatment, recovery did not begin until about the 15th day and required a little over 40 days (Starvou *et al.*, 1978).

Poisoning is characterized by gastritis (nausea, vomiting, and pain), anoxia (cyanosis, collapse, and terminal convulsions) secondary to methemoglobinemia, possible liver injury, and nephritis (lumbar pain and oliguria). Nephritis presumably is the direct result of chlorate ion as well as secondary to the destruction of corpuscles. The blood pressure tends to fall and the heartbeat becomes irregular. The liver and spleen may be enlarged and tender. The urine, if any, is brown or black in color and contains casts, red cells, free hemoglobin, and methemoglobin. The blood is brownish in color, and the plasma contains free hemoglobin and free methemoglobin. The red cell count is very low and the white cell count high (Sollmann, 1957; Knight *et al.*, 1967).

Onset may be delayed as much as 12 hr (Mengele *et al.*, 1969).

Death from sodium chlorate poisoning has occurred from 4 hr to 34 days after ingestion with an average of just over 4 days (Knight *et al.*, 1967; Mengele *et al.*, 1969; Motin *et al.*, 1970).

An entirely different kind of danger also arises from the strong oxidizing action of sodium chlorate. Its storage constitutes a special fire hazard.

Sodium chlorate can explode if subjected to intense heat with or without sudden pressure. If mixed with sulfur, sugar, or some other oxidizable materials, it forms an explosive mixture that may be more powerful than gunpowder (in which the oxidant is KNO_3). McGregor and Jackson (1969) described the pattern of hand injuries resulting from the accidental explosion of homemade sodium chlorate mixture bombs in 11 teenage patients and discussed the management of the injury.

Use Experience When used as a pesticide, sodium chlorate may cause irritation of the skin, eyes, or upper respiratory tract.

Dosage Response Dermal absorption associated with agricultural use of sodium chlorate is not sufficient to cause systemic poisoning. Even by mouth, a large dose is required to produce illness. A 6.35% solution of potassium chlorate was long used as a gargle, or a 300-mg tablet was allowed to dissolve slowly in the mouth to treat pharyngitis before modern antibiotics became available. The toxicities of the sodium and potassium salts are similar. It was considered that a dose of 10,000 mg was toxic and 15,000–20,000 mg was fatal (Cochrane and Smith, 1940; Sollmann, 1957). The smallest recorded fatal dose was 7500 mg (Bernstein, 1930). However, vigorous treatment saved one person who had ingested about 40,000 mg (Knight *et al.*, 1967).

Laboratory Findings In a fatal case in which chlorate could not be demonstrated in the blood or organs, it was found at a concentration of 6000 ppm in the urine (Oliver *et al.*, 1972).

Methemoglobin levels of workers exposed to sodium chlo-

rate were greater than those of a control group but always less than 10% (Maki, 1972).

In acute poisoning, blood potassium and urea may be increased. Even in a patient who eventually survives, the plasma may have a dark, opaque, muddy brown appearance, and spectroscopy may show hemoglobin, oxyhemoglobin, methemoglobin, and methemalbumin. The red cells may appear black and shiny like coal dust. During recovery, kidney function may return to normal very slowly and not always completely (Knight *et al.*, 1967).

Treatment of Poisoning In case of irritation of the skin or mucous membranes, the area should be thoroughly flushed with water. Every effort should be made to remove the material if ingestion has occurred. There is no specific antidote, but oxygen, peritoneal dialysis, and exchange transfusions may be lifesaving even after a dose as high as 40 gm. Dialysis is important because 95% of small doses of chlorate are excreted by the kidney, but larger doses so injure that organ that the body is almost powerless to remove the poison unaided (Knight *et al.*, 1967).

12.18 MISCELLANEOUS ELEMENTS

Boron, the only element discussed under this heading, has atomic number 5 and an atomic weight of 10.81. It precedes carbon in the periodic table and is in the same group as aluminum.

Although boron has long been recognized as essential to the growth of higher plants, there is no evidence so far that it is essential for animals. The lowest dietary level yet attained was 0.15 ppm (Underwood, 1977). On the other hand, the addition of 5 ppm boron (as sodium metaborate) to the drinking water of mice during their entire lifetime was without effect on their body weight, tumor incidence, or longevity (Schroeder and Mitchener, 1975).

As might be expected of an element essential to plants, boron is found in all animal tissues. As reviewed by Underwood (1977), measurements of daily intake of boron have varied from 0.4 to 20 mg/person/day, depending largely if not entirely on the quantity of fruits and vegetables in the diet. The concentrations in normal human soft tissues, including brain, range from 0.06 to 0.6 ppm; concentrations in bone and teeth are somewhat higher, especially in hard-water areas.

Boron has been used as an insecticide in the form of boric acid and borax, both mainly for the control of cockroaches. The acid is slightly more toxic, but the kind of illness produced by the two compounds is the same.

12.18.1 BORIC ACID

12.18.1.1 Identity, Properties, and Uses

Chemical Name Boric acid.

Structure H_3BO_3.

Synonyms Boric acid also is known as boracic acid and as orthoboric acid. The CAS registry no. is 10043-35-3.

Physical and Chemical Properties Boric acid has the empirical formula BH_3O_3 and a molecular weight of 61.84. It forms odorless, white crystals with a pearly lustre and faintly bitter taste. It is slightly corrosive at room temperature. The density of boric acid is 1.435 at 15°C. It has a melting point of about 171°C but also may decompose upon heating. Its solubility in water at 20°C is 4.88 gm/100 ml; in cold alcohol, 1 gm/18 ml; in boiling alcohol, 1 gm/6 ml; and in glycerine, 1 gm/4 ml. It is stable up to 100°C.

Formulations and Uses Boric acid has slight fungicidal properties. Its main use as a pesticide is in the form of tablets for the control of roaches.

12.18.1.2 Toxicity to Laboratory Animals

Basic Findings The oral LD 50 values of boric acid are 2660 and 3450 mg/kg in rats and mice, respectively. The corresponding intravenous values are 1330 and 1780 mg/kg (Pfeiffer *et al.*, 1945), indicating relatively rapid and complete absorption from the gastrointestinal tract. Animals poisoned by boric acid showed depression, ataxia (occasionally convulsions), a fall in body temperature, a violet-red color of the skin and mucous membranes, and, in dogs, persistent vomiting and meningismus (Pfeiffer *et al.*, 1945).

Growth of rats was inhibited when their drinking water contained boric acid at a concentration of 2500 ppm, resulting in a dosage of about 325 mg/kg/day; growth was unaffected at a concentration of 1000 ppm (about 130 mg/kg/day).

The mechanism of the toxic action of boron is not known. However, it is clear that no injury is done unless one or a few doses overpower the body's rather considerable ability to excrete the ion so that its concentration in the tissues and especially in the brain increases to >10 ppm from the normal level of <1 ppm.

Absorption, Distribution, Metabolism, and Excretion The similarity of the oral and intravenous LD 50 values indicates that absorption from the gastrointestinal tract is rapid and virtually complete.

Following intraperitoneal injection, a peak concentration was reached in about 1.0–1.5 hr in brain and in about 0.5 hr in other tissues. The concentrations of borate in the tissues were directly proportional to dosage over the range of 18 to 700 mg/kg (Locksley and Sweet, 1954).

In acute poisoning, the concentration of boric acid reaches high levels in all tissues, the high concentration in the brain being especially noteworthy. In a typical experiment, the concentrations were about 1110, 910, and 260 ppm in brain, liver, and body fat, respectively (Pfeiffer *et al.*, 1945).

Boric acid is excreted unchanged in the urine. Following intravenous injection in dogs, this excretion became maximal in 1–2 hr and then declined gradually; at the same time, there was an initial, brief depression of phosphorus excretion followed by a gradual rise, which at 6 hr exceeded the control value for phosphorus by five times (Pfeiffer *et al.*, 1945). The significance of this increase in excretion of phosphorus is unknown.

The half-life of boric acid in the blood of mice is about 65 min (Locksley and Sweet, 1954).

12.18.1.3 Toxicity to Humans

Experimental Exposure Pfeiffer *et al.* (1945) demonstrated by animal studies and by a review of human case histories that boric acid is absorbed easily from injured skin. By studies in adult volunteers who were heavily exposed to 5% solution or to 10% boric acid ointment, they showed by analysis of the urine that no detectable boron was absorbed from the intact skin. Goldbloom and Goldbloom (1953) confirmed this negative result in 10 volunteers.

Accidental and Intentional Exposure Most poisoning by boric acid has occurred in connection with its former use as a local antiseptic applied to irritated skin, burns, or wounds or from its mistaken inclusion in the feeding formula for babies. However, children also have ingested the compressed tablets made to combat roaches.

Illness usually begins about 8 hr after ingestion. Signs include vomiting, diarrhea, rapidly progressing prostration, tremors, meningismus, and convulsions. An erythematous eruption of the skin that may progress to exfoliative dermatitis is characteristic. The eruption tends to be prominent on the palms, soles, and buttocks. Death may occur in less than a day or after as much as a week (Pfeiffer *et al.*, 1945; Young *et al.*, 1949; Goldbloom and Goldbloom, 1953; Wong *et al.*, 1964). In very severe cases, onset may be within an hour and death within 4 hr (McNally and Rukstinat, 1947).

Goldbloom and Goldbloom (1953) raised the possibility that Ritter's disease was, in fact, acute boric acid poisoning.

Dosage Response The fatal dose is thought to be 2000–3000 mg for infants, 5000–6000 mg for children, and 15,000–20,000 mg for adults (Young *et al.*, 1949).

When through error a 42-year-old patient received an intravenous infusion of about 15,000 mg of boric acid as a 2.5% solution with 10% dextrose, she showed slight flushing, slight nausea, one episode of vomiting, and no further trouble. A total of 14,650 mg of boric acid was recovered from the urine (McIntyre and Burke, 1937). It is not clear whether this case is to be viewed as an example of individual variation—and good luck—or whether it reflects the relative protective effect of very gradual administration.

In newborns, who may be more susceptible than older infants, active treatment was successful in saving all those thought to have ingested 4000 mg and one thought to have ingested 4500 mg, but was not successful against higher doses (Wong *et al.*, 1964).

Laboratory Findings Fisher and Freimuth (1958) reported the cases of two children who failed to show any illness after drinking a solution of boric acid; their blood boron levels when first examined were 13.0 and 13.8 ppm, respectively, The authors questioned an earlier report that 8.7 ppm is a fatal level and stated that, in their experience, levels of 87–175 ppm or higher (500–1000 ppm or more expressed as boric acid) are found in cases of fatal poisoning. These results are consistent with those of Boggs and Anrode (1955), who reported the recovery of a mildly ill infant whose initial blood boron level of 48 ppm was soon reduced to 31 ppm by an exchange transfusion. The report by others of low blood boron values associated with serious or fatal poisoning may have been the result of faulty analytical techniques. One baby whose initial blood boron level was 94 ppm died in spite of vigorous treatment, but two with initial levels of 49 and 34 ppm survived (Segar, 1960).

In fatal cases the concentration of boric acid in the brain has ranged from 250 to 2555 ppm (McNally and Rust, 1928; Fellows *et al.*, 1948; Young *et al.*, 1949); that is, boron levels of 44–447 ppm. In many cases, the highest concentration was found in the brain, but in some instances the highest concentration was in the lung or liver.

Metabolic acidosis, jaundice, and increased blood urea may be present (Wong *et al.*, 1964).

Pathology In fatal cases, pathological changes may be minimal but may include degeneration of the kidney tubules; slight degeneration of liver cells; engorgement, focal hemorrhage, and leukocytic infiltration of the skin; and edema and congestion of the brain and spinal cord (Goldbloom and Goldbloom, 1953; Wong *et al.*, 1964).

Treatment of Poisoning Treatment of poisoning by boron is symptomatic. There is no pharmacological or specific antidote. Therefore removal of the poison is of particular importance.

Boggs and Anrode (1955) demonstrated the effectiveness of exchange transfusion in removing boric acid from the body. Later, Segar (1960) showed that 4 hr of peritoneal dialysis removed about the same amount of boric acid as one exchange transfusion and concluded that continuous dialysis for 24–28 hr is, therefore, much more efficient than exchange transfusion for this purpose. Peritoneal dialysis was also used and recommended by Wong *et al.* (1964).

Animal experiments showing that the compound is excreted readily in the urine (Pfeiffer *et al.*, 1945) would justify the use of forced diuresis.

REFERENCES

Aamodt, R. L., Ramble, W. F., O'Reilly, S., Johnston, E., and Henkin, R. I. (1975). Studies on the metabolism of Zn-65 in man. *Fed. Proc., Fed. Am. Soc. Exp. Biol.* **34**, 922 (Abstr. 3981).

Aamodt, R. L., Ramble, W. F., Johnston, G. S., Foster, D., and Henkin, R. I. (1979). Zinc metabolism in humans after oral and intravenous administration of Zn-69m. *Am. J. Clin. Nutr.* **32**, 559–569.

Aberg, B., Ekman, L., Falk, R., Greitz, U., Presson, G., and Snihs, J.-O. (1969). Metabolism of methyl mercury (203-Hg) compounds in man. *Arch. Environ. Health* **19**, 478–484.

Abukurah, A. R., Moser, A. M., Baird, C. L., Randall, R. E., Jr., Setter, J. G., and Blanke, R. V. (1973). Acute sodium fluoride poisoning. *Fluoride* **6**, 68–69.

Agate, J. N., Bell, G. H., Boddie, C. F., Bowler, R. G., Bucknell, M., Cheeseman, E. A., Douglas, T. H. J., Druett, H. A., Garrad, J., Hunter, D., Perry, K. M. A., Richardson, J. D., and Weir, J. B. V. (1949). "Industrial Fluorosis," Memo. No. 22. Med. Res. Counc. Br., London.

Ahlborg, G., and Ahlmark, A. (1949). Alkly mercury compound poisoning: Clinical aspect and risks of exposure. *Nord. Med.* **41**, 503–504.

Ahlmark, A. (1948). Poisoning by methyl mercury compounds. *Br. J. Ind. Med.* **5**, 117–119.

Airey, D. (1983). Total mercury concentrations in human hair from 13 countries in relation to fish consumption and location. *Sci. Total Environ.* **31**, 157–180.

Akitake, T. (1968). Experimental study on poisoning by organic mercury compounds. *Igaku Kenkyu* **38**, 357–378 (in Japanese).

Alajouanine, T., Derobert, L., and Thieffry, S. (1958). Clinical study of a group of 210 cases of intoxication by organic salts of tin. *Rev. Neurol.* **98**, 85–96 (in French).

Al-Damluji, S. F. (1976a). Organomercury poisoning in Iraq: History prior to the 1971–72 outbreak. *Bull. W.H.O.* **53**, Suppl., 11–13.

Al-Damluji, S. F. (1976b). Intoxication due to alkylmercury-treated seed—1971–72 outbreak in Iraq: Clinical aspects. *Bull. W.H.O.* **53**, Suppl., 65–81.

Aldridge, W. N., and Cremer, J. E. (1955). The biochemistry of organotin compounds diethyltin dichloride and triethyltin sulphate. *Biochem. J.* **61**, 406–418.

Alekseyeva, T. I., and Mishin, G. P. (1971). Treatment of cases of Granosan poisoning. *Sov. Med.* **5**, 137–138 (in Russian).

Allaway, W. H., Kubota, J., Losee, F., and Roth, M. (1968). Selenium as an integral part of factor 3 against dietary necrotic liver degeneration. *J. Am. Chem. Soc.* **79**, 3292–3293.

Al-Shahristani, H., and Shihab, K. (1976). Mercury in hair as an indicator of total body burden. *Bull. W.H.O.* **53**, Suppl., 105–112.

American Conference of Governmental Industrial Hygienists (ACGIH) (1971). "Documentation of the Threshold Limit Value for Substances in Workroom Air." Am. Conf. Govt. Ind. Hyg., Cincinnati, Ohio.

American Conference of Governmental Industrial Hygienists (ACGIH) (1981). "Documentation of the Threshold Limit Values," pp. 283–285. Am. Conf. Govt. Ind. Hyg., Cincinnati, Ohio.

American Medical Association (AMA) (1955). Council on Pharmacy and Chemistry. Report of the Committee on Pesticides. *J. Am. Med. Assoc.* **157**, 237–241.

American Medical Association (AMA) (1977). "AMA Drug Evaluations." Publishing Sciences Group, Littleton, Massachusetts.

Amin-Zaki, L., Elhassani, S., Majeed, M. A., Clarkson, T. W., Doherty, R. A., and Greenwood, M. R. (1974a). Studies of infants postnatally exposed to methylmercury. *J. Pediatr.* **85**, 81–84.

Amin-Zaki, L., Elhassani, S., Majeed, M. A., Clarkson, T. W., Doherty, R. A., and Greenwood, M. (1974b). Intra-uterine methylmercury poisoning in Iraq. *Pediatrics* **54**, 587–595.

Amin-Zaki, L., Elhassani, S., Majeed, M. A., Clarkson, T. W., Doherty, R. A., Greenwood, M. R., and Giovanoli-Jakubczak, T. (1976). Perinatal methylmercury poisoning in Iraq. *Am. J. Dis. Child.* **130**, 1070–1076.

Amin-Zaki, L., Majeed, M. A., Clarkson, T. W., and Greenwood, M. R. (1978). Methylmercury poisoning in Iraqi children: Clinical observations over two years. *Br. Med. J.* **1**, 613–616.

Andersen, R. A. (1981). Nutritional role of chromium. *Sci. Total Environ.* **17**, 13–19.

Anke, M., Gran, M., and Parschefeld, M. (1976). The essentiality of arsenic for animals. *Trace Subst. Environ. Health* **10**, 403–409.

Anke, M., Gran, M., Parschefeld, M., Groppel, B., and Hennig, A. (1978). Essentiality and function of arsenic. *Trace Elem. Metab. Man Anim., Proc. Int. Symp., 3rd, 1977*, pp. 248–252.

Ansari, M. S., Miller, W. J., Lassiter, J. W., Neathery, M. W., and Gentry, R. P. (1975). Effects of high but nontoxic dietary zinc on zinc metabolism and adaptations in rats. *Proc. Soc. Exp. Biol. Med.* **150**, 534–536.

Arena, J. M., Watson, G. A., and Sakhadeo, S. S. (1965). Fatal thallium poisoning: A plea for a safer pesticide. *Clin. Pediatr. (Philadelphia)* **4**, 267–270.

Arnold, F. A., Jr., McClure, F. J., and White, C. L. (1960). Sodium fluoride tablets for children. *Dent. Prog.* **1**, 8–12.

Ashe, W. F., Largent, E. J., Dutra, F. R., Hubbard, D. M., and Blackstone, M. (1953). Behavior of mercury in the animal organism following inhalation. *Arch. Ind. Hyg. Occup. Med.* **7**, 19–43.

Atalla, L. T., Silva, C. M., and Lima, F. W. (1965). Activation analysis of arsenic in human hair—some observations on the problem of external contamination. *An. Acad. Bras. Cienc.* **37**, 433–441.

Atkinson, H. V. (1921). The treatment of acute phosphorus poisoning. *J. Lab. Clin. Med.* **7**, 148–150.

Atkinson, S. C. (1969). Arsenical keratoses and internal cancer (urinary bladder and nasopharynx). *Arch. Dermatol.* **99**, 237–238.

Atwood, R. G., Gates, P., Patnode, M., LacQuaye, R., Clarkson, T., Greenwood, M., and Smith, J. C. (1976). Organic mercury exposure—Washington. *Morbid. Mortal. Wkly. Rep.* **25**, 133.

Aub, J. C., Fairhall, L. T., Minot, A. S., Reznikoff, P., and Hamilton, A. (1926). Lead poisoning. *In* "Medicine Monograph," Vol. 7, pp. i–x and 1–265. Williams & Wilkins, Baltimore, Maryland.

Aughey, E., Grant, L., Furman, B. L., and Dryden, W. F. (1977). The effects of oral zinc supplementation in the mouse. *J. Comp. Pathol.* **87**, 1–14.

Baetjer, A. M., (1950a). Pulmonary carcinoma in chromate workers. I. Review of the literature and report of cases. *AMA Arch. Ind. Hyg. Occup. Health* **2**, 123–125.

Baetjer, A. M., (1950b). Pulmonary carcinoma in chromate workers. II. Incidence on basis of hospital records. *AMA Arch. Ind. Hyg. Occup. Health* **2**, 505–516.

Baetjer, A. M., Damron, C., and Budacz, V. (1959). The distribution and retention of chromium in men and animals. *Arch. Ind. Health* **20**, 136–150.

Baetjer, A. M., Lilienfeld, A. M., and Levin, M. L. (1975). Cancer and occupational exposure to inorganic arsenic. *Proc. Int. Congr. Occup. Health, 18th, 1975*, Abstr., p. 393.

Bailey, R. R. (1964). The farmer and his poisons. *N.Z. Med. J.* **63**, 655–659.

Bakir, F., Damluji, S. F., Amin-Zaki, L., Murtadha, M., Khalidi, A., Al-Rawi, N. Y., Tikriti, S., Dhahir, H. I., Clarkson, T. W., Smith, J. C., and Doherty, R. A. (1973). Methylmercury poisoning in Iraq. *Science* **181**, 230–241.

Bakir, F., Al-Khalidi, A., Clarkson, T. W., and Greenwood, R. (1976). Clinical observations on treatment of alkylmercury poisoning in hospital patients. *Bull. W.H.O.* **53**, Suppl., 87–92.

Baldwin, H. (1899). The toxic action of sodium fluoride. *J. Am. Chem. Soc.* **21**, 517–521.

Balint, P. (1968). Pathogenesis of mercuric chloride-induced renal failure in the dog. *Acta Med. Acad. Sci. Hung.* **25**, 287–297 (in Hungarian).

Balint, P., Fekete, A., and Harza, T. (1969). Intrarenal circulation in mercuric chloride-induced renal failure. *Experientia* **25**, 722–723.

Bank, W. J., Pleasure, D. E., Suzuki, K., Nigro, M., and Katz, R. (1972). Thallium poisoning. *Arch. Neurol. (Chicago)* **26**, 456–464.

Bar, M. J. (1956). Concerning an accident due to tin. *Arch. Mal. Prof., Med. Trav. Secur. Soc.* **17**, 506–508 (in French).

Barbier, F. (1974). Treatment of thallium poisoning. *Lancet* **2**, 1528.

Barclay, R. K., Peacock, W. C., and Karnofsky, G. A. (1953). Distribution and excretion of radioactive thallium in the chick embryo, rat and man. *J. Pharmacol. Exp. Ther.* **107**, 178–187.

Barnes, J. M., and Magee, P. N. (1958). The biliary and hepatic lesion produced experimentally by dibutyltin salts. *J. Pathol.* **75**, 267–279.

Barnes, J. M., and Stoner, H. B. (1958). Toxic properties of some dialkyl and trialkyl tin salts. *Br. J. Ind. Med.* **15**, 15–22.

Barnes, J. M., and Stoner, H. B. (1959). The toxicology of tin compounds. *Pharmacol. Rev.* **11**, 211–231.

Barnes, J. R., Smith, P. E., and Drummond, C. M. (1972). Urine osmolality and δ-aminolevulinic acid excretion. *Arch. Environ. Health* **25**, 450–455.

Barrowman, J. A., Bonnett, R., and Bray, P. J. (1973). Biliary excretion of zinc in rats. *Biochem. Soc. Trans.* **1**, 985–989.

Barry, P. S. I., and Mossman, D. B. (1970). Lead concentrations in human tissues. *Br. J. Ind. Med.* **27**, 339–351.

Bass, M. (1963). Thallium poisoning: A preliminary report. *J. Am. Osteopath. Assoc.* **63**, 229–235.

Bauer, G. C. H., Carlsson, A., and Lindquist, B. (1956). A comparative study of metabolism of 140Ba and 45Ca in rats. *Biochem. J.* **63**, 535–542.

Bauer, G. C. H., Carlsson, A., and Lindquist, B. (1957). Metabolism of Ba140 in man. *Acta Orthop. Scand.* **26**, 241–254.

Bayne, J. R. D., Beck, J. C., Lowenstein, L., and Browne, J. S. L. (1952). Cortisone acetate in the treatment of acute phosphorus poisoning. *Can. Med. Assoc. J.* **67**, 465–467.

Becker, W. M., and Hoekstra, W. G. (1971). Ion transport in plant cells. *In* "Intestinal Absorption of Metal Ions, Trace Elements and Radionuclides" (S. C. Skovya and D. Waldron-Edward, eds.), pp. 229–256. Pergamon, New York.

Behrbohm, P. (1957). Allergic contact eczema from chromate wood preservatives. *Berfus-dermatosen* **5**, 271–282 (in German).

Beliles, R. P., Clark, R. S., and Yuile, C. L. (1968). The effects of exposure to mercury vapor on behavior of rats. *Toxicol. Appl. Pharmacol.* **12**, 15–21.

Ben-Assa, B. (1962). Indirect thallium poisoning in a Bedouin family. *Harefuah* **62**, 378–380 (in Hebrew).

Bendl, B. J. (1969). Thallium poisoning: Report of a case successfully treated with dithizone. *Arch. Dermatol.* **100**, 443–446.

Bental, E., Lavy, S., and Amir, N. (1961). Electroencephalographic changes due to arsenic, thallium and strychnine poisoning. *Confin. Neurol.* **21**, 233–240.

Berlin, M. H. (1986). Mercury. *In* "Handbook on the Toxicology of Metals" (L. Friberg, G. F. Nordberg, and V. B. Vouk, eds.), 2nd ed., Vol. 2, pp. 387–445. Elsevier, Amsterdam.

Berlin, M. H., and Johansson, L. G. (1964). Mercury in mouse brain after inhalation of mercury vapor and after intravenous injection of mercury salt. *Nature (London)* **204**, 85–86.

Berlin, M. H., and Ullberg, S. (1963). Increased uptake of mercury in mouse brain caused by 2,3-dimercaptopropanol. *Nature (London)* **197**, 84–85.

Berlin, M. H., Nordberg, G. F., and Serenius, F. (1969a). On the site and mechanism of mercury vapor resorption in the lung. A study in the guinea pig using mercuric nitrate Hg-203. *Arch. Environ. Health* **18**, 42–50.

Berlin, M. H., Fazackerley, J., and Nordberg, G. (1969b). The uptake of mercury in the brain of mammals exposed to mercury vapor and to mercuric salts. *Arch. Environ. Health* **18**, 719–729.

Berlin, M. H., Clarkson, T. W., Friberg, L. T., Gage, J. C., Goldwater, L. J., Jernelov, A., Kazantzis, G., Magos, L., Nordberg, G. F., Radford, E. P., Ramel, C., Skerfving, S., Smith, R. G., Suzuki, T., Swensson, A., Tejning, S., Truhart, R., and Vostal, J. (1969c). Maximal allowable concentrations of mercury compounds. *Arch. Environ. Health* **19**, 891–905.

Bernstein, R. (1930). Potassium chlorate poisoning (suicide by means of Pebeco toothpaste). *Sommerkersamml. Vergiftungsfallen* **1**(A7), 15–16.

Berry, J. P., Hourdig, J., Galle, P., and Laquie, G. (1978). Chromium concentration by proximal renal tubule cells: An ultrastructural microanalytical and cytochemical study. *J. Histochem. Cytochem.* **26**, 651–657.

Bidstrup, P. L. (1964). "Toxicity of Mercury and Its Compounds." Elsevier, Amsterdam.

Bidstrup, P. L., and Case, R. A. M. (1956). Carcinoma of the lung in workmen in the bichromates-producing industry in Great Britain. *Br. J. Ind. Med.* **13**, 260–264.

Binz, C. (1897). "Lectures on Pharmacology for Practitioners and Students," (P. W. Latham, ed.), Vol. II. New Sydenham Society, London.

Birke, G., Johnels, A. G., Plantin, L. O., Sjöstrand, B., and Westermark, T. (1967). Mercury poisoning through eating fish? *Sven. Laekaritidn.* **64**, 3628–3637.

Birke, G., Johnels, A. G., Plantin, L. O., Sjöstrand, B., Skerfving, S., and

Westermark, T. (1972). Studies on humans exposed to methyl mercury through fish consumption. *Arch. Environ. Health* **25**, 77–91.

Bivings, L., and Lewis, G. (1948). Acrodynia: A new treatment with BAL. *J. Pediatr.* **32**, 63–65.

Black, M. M., Kleiner, I. S., and Bloker, H. (1949). The toxicity of sodium fluoride in man. *N.Y. State J. Med.* **49**, 1187–1188.

Blanksma, L. A., Sachs, H. K., Murray, E. F., and O'Connell, M. J. (1969). Incidence of high blood levels in Chicago children. *Pediatrics* **44**, 661–667.

Bligh, P. H., and Taylor, D. M. (1963). Comparative studies of the metabolism of strontium and barium in the rat. *Biochem. J.* **87**, 612–618.

Blisnakov, C., and Iskrov, G. (1961). Fatal poisoning by parenteral injection of zinc phosphide. *Folia Med.* **3**, 73–76 (in German).

Bloom, G., Lundgren, K.-D., and Swensson, A. (1955). Exposure and hazards from organic mercury compounds in connection with seed dressing on small farms. *Nord. Hyg. Tidskr.* **36**, 110–117.

Boggs, T. R., and Anrode, H. G. (1955). Boric acid poisoning treated by exchange transfusion. *Pediatrics* **16**, 109–114.

Bogomaz, M. S. (1969). Food poisoning with Granosan. *Vrach. Delo* **1**, 142–143.

Bonnin, M. (1951). Organic mercury dust poisoning. *Rep. Adelaide Hosp.* **31**, 11–13.

Boyd, T. C., and Roy, A. C. (1929). Observations on the excretion of Sb in urine. *Indian J. Med. Res.* **17**, 94–108.

Boyden, R., Potter, V. R., and Elvehjen, C. A. (1938). Effect of feeding high levels of copper to albino rats. *J. Nutr.* **15**, 397–402.

Boyland, E., Dukes, C. E., Grover, P. L., and Mitchley, B. C. V. (1962). The induction of renal tumors by feeding lead acetate to rats. *Br. J. Cancer* **16**, 283–288.

Boylen, G. W., Jr., and Hardy, H. L. (1967). Distribution of arsenic in nonexposed persons (hair, liver, and urine). *Am. Ind. Hyg. Assoc. J.* **28**, 148–150.

Bradley, W. R., and Fredrick, W. G. (1941). Toxicity of antimony—animal studies. *Ind. Med. (Ind. Hyg. Sect.)* **2**, 15–22.

Brady, F. J., Lawton, A. H., Cowie, D. B., Andrews, H. L., Ness, A. T., and Ogden, G. E. (1945). Localization of trivalent radio-active Sb following intravenous administration to dogs infected with *Diofilaria immitis*. *Am. J. Trop. Med.* **25**, 103–107.

Brady, J., Liberatore, F., Harper, P., Greenwald, P., Burnett, W., Davies, J. N. P., Polan, A., Vianna, N., and Bishop, M. (1977). Angiosarcoma of the liver: An epidemiologic survey. *J. Natl. Cancer Inst. (U.S.)* **59**, 1383–1385.

Braun, H. A., Lusky, L. M., and Calvery, H. O. (1946). The efficacy of 2,3-dimercaptopropanol (BAL) in the therapy of poisoning by compounds of antimony, bismuth, chromium, mercury and nickel. *J. Pharmacol. Exp. Ther.* **87**, Suppl., 119–125.

Brenniman, G. R., Namekata, T., Kojola, W. H., Carnow, B. W., and Levy, P. S. (1979). Cardiovascular disease death rates in communities with elevated levels of barium in drinking water. *Environ. Res.* **20**, 318–324.

Bridges, J. W., Davis, D. S., and Williams, R. T. (1967). The fate of ethyltin and diethyltin derivatives in the rat. *Biochem. J.* **105**, 1261–1267.

Brinton, H. P., Frasier, E. S., and Koven, A. L. (1952). Morbidity and mortality experience among chromate workers. *Public Health Rep.* **67**, 835–847.

Brodniewicz, A., and Szuber, T. (1960). Poisoning of the population with rodenticides in Poland. *Zdrowie* **75**, 159–167 (in Polish).

Brown, I. A. (1954). Chronic mercurialism. *Arch. Neurol. Psychiatry* **72**, 674–681.

Browning, E. (1969). "Toxicity of Industrial Metals," 2nd ed. Appleton-Century-Crofts, New York.

Brügemann, J., Barth, K., and Niesar, K. H. (1964). Part II. Experimental studies on the occurrence of triphenylacetate residues in beet leaves and silage, in animals fed them, and in their excretions. *Zentralbl. Veterinaermed., Reihe A* **11**, 4–19 (in German).

Brun, G. C., Buchwald, H., and Roholm, K. (1941). Excretion of fluoride in urine in chronic fluoride poisoning of cryolite workers. *Acta Med. Scand.* **106**, 261–273 (in German).

Bruner, H. D. (1950). Effect of BAL on distribution of intravenously administered zinc using Zn^{65}. *Fed. Proc., Fed. Am. Soc. Exp. Biol.* **9**, 260.

Buchanan, W. D. (1962). "Toxicity of Arsenic Compounds." Am. Elsevier, New York.

Buchet, J. P.,. Roels, H., Bernard, A., and Lauwerys, R. (1980). Assessment of renal function of workers exposed to inorganic lead, cadmium and mercurcy vapor. *J. Occup. Med.* **22**, 241–750.

Buchet, J. P., Lauwerys, R., and Roels, H. (1981a). Comparison of the urinary excretion of arsenic metabolites after a single oral dose of sodium arsenite, monomethyl arsonate and dimethyl arsenate in man. *Int. Arch. Occup. Environ. Health* **48**, 71–79.

Buchet, J. P., Lauwerys, R., and Roels, H. (1981b). Urinary excretion of inorganic arsenic and its metabolites after repeated ingestion of sodium meta arsenite by volunteers. *Int. Arch. Occup. Environ. Health* **48**, 111–118.

Byron, W. R., Bierbower, G. W., Brouwer, J. B., and Hansen, W. H. (1967). Pathologic changes in rats and dogs from two-year feeding of sodium arsenite or sodium arsenate. *Toxicol. Appl. Pharmacol.* **10**, 132–147.

Caley, J. P., and Kellock, I. A. (1955). Acute yellow phosphorus poisoning with recovery. *Lancet* **1**, 539–541.

Calley, D. J., Guess, W. L., and Autian, J. (1967a). Hepatotoxicity of a series of organotin esters. *J. Pharm. Sci.* **56**, 240–247.

Calley, D. J., Guess, W. L., and Autian, J. (1967b). Ultrastructural hepatotoxicity induced by an organotin ester. *J. Pharm. Sci.* **56**, 1267–1272.

Calvery, H. O. (1938). Chronic effects of ingested lead and arsenic. A review and correlation. *JAMA, J. Am. Med. Assoc.* **111**, 1723–1729.

Calvery, H. O., Laug, E. P., and Morris, H. J. (1938). The chronic effects on dogs of feeding diets containing lead acetate, lead arsenate, and arsenic trioxide in varying concentrations. *J. Pharmacol. Exp. Ther.* **64**, 364–387.

Cameron, G. R. (1947). Liver atrophy produced by chronic selenium intoxication. *J. Pathol. Bacteriol.* **59**, 539–545.

Campbell, I. R. (1963). "The Role of Fluoride in Public Health—The Soundness of Fluoridation of Communal Water Supplies." Kettering Laboratory, University of Cincinnati, Cincinnati, Ohio.

Campbell, J. K., and Mills, C. F. (1979). The toxicity of zinc to pregnant sheep. *Environ. Res.* **20**, 1–13.

Cangelosi, J. T. (1941). Acute cadmium metal poisoning. *U.S. Nav. Med. Bull.* **39**, 408–410.

Cantarow, A., and Trumpeter, M. (1944). "Lead Poisoning." Williams & Wilkins, Baltimore, Maryland.

Canty, A. J., and Kishimoto, R. (1975). British anti-Lewisite and organomercury poisoning. *Nature (London)* **253**, 123–125.

Cardiff, I. D. (1940). How toxic is arsenate of lead? *J. Ind. Hyg.* **22**, 333–346.

Cassano, G. B., Viola, P. L., Ghetti, B., and Amaducci, L. (1969). The distribution of inhaled mercury (Hg-203) vapors in the brain of rats and mice. *J. Neuropathol. Exp. Neurol.* **28**, 308–320.

Castagnou, R., Paoletti, C., and Larcebeau, S. (1957). Absorption and distribution of barium administered intravenously or orally to rats. *C. R. Hebd. Seanes Ser. Acad. Sci. D* **244**, 2994–2996. (in French).

Cavanagh, J. B., Fuller, N. H., Johnson, H. R. M., and Rudge, P. (1974). The effects of thallium salts, with particular reference to the nervous system changes. *Q. J. Med.* **43**, 293–319.

Chamberlain, P. H., Stavinoh, W. B., Davies, H., Kniker, W. T., and Panos, T. C. (1958). Thallium poisoning. *Pediatrics* **22**, 1170–1182.

Chang, L. W., Reuhl, K. R., and Spyker, J. M. (1977). Ultrastructural study of the latent effects of methyl mercury on the nervous system after prenatal exposure. *Environ. Res.* **13**, 171–185.

Chawla, S. C., and Mehta, S. P. (1973). A study of host and environmental factors in cases of accidental poisoning admitted in Irwin Hospital. *Indian J. Med. Res.* **61**, 724–731.

Childs, E. A. (1973). Kinetics of transplacental movement of mercury fed in a tuna matrix to mice. *Arch. Environ. Health* **27**, 50–52.

Chinen, M., Mori, T., Anjirei, K., Nakamura, Y., Tamanaha, E., Kiyamu, M., Nakamoto, F. (1977). Six cases of intoxication due to thallium in a single district. *Acta Paediatr. Jpn., Overseas Ed.* **81**, 1125–1126. (in Japanese).

Chisolm, J. J., Jr. (1968). The use of chelating agents in the treatment of acute and chronic lead intoxication in childhood. *J. Pediatr.* **73**, 1–38.

Christensen, H., Krogh, M., and Nielsen, M. (1937). Acute mercury poisoning in a respiration chamber. *Nature (London)* **139**, 626–627.

Christison, R. (1845). "A Treatise on Poisons in Relation to Medical Jurisprudence, Physiology, and the Practice of Physic." E. Barrington and G. D. Haswell, Philadelphia, Pennsylvania.

Chugh, K. S., Singhal, P. C., and Sharma, B. K. (1975). Methemoglobinemia in acute copper sulfate poisoning. *Ann. Intern. Med.* **82**, 226–227.

Chugh, K. S., Singhal, P. C., Sharma, B. K., Das, K. C., and Datta, B. N. (1977). Acute renal failure following copper sulphate intoxication. *Postgrad. Med. J.* **53**, 18–23.

Clark, G. L., and Buhrke, V. E. (1954). Effect of elemental sulfur in the diet on load-extension hysteresis in single wood fibers. *Science* **120**, 40.

Clarkson, T. W. (1972). Recent advances in the toxicology of mercury with emphasis on the alkylmercurials. *CRC Crit. Rev. Toxicol.* **1**, 203–234.

Clarkson, T. W. (1983). Molecular targets of metal toxicity. *In* "Chemical Toxicity and Clinical Chemistry of Metals" (S. S. Brown and J. Savory, eds.), pp. 211–226. Academic Press, New York.

Clarkson, T. W., and Kench, J. E. (1956). Urinary excretion of amino acids by men absorbing heavy metals. *Biochem. J.* **62**, 361–372.

Clarkson, T. W., and Magos, L. (1970). Effect of 2,4-dinitrophenol and other metabolic inhibitors on the renal disposition and excretion of mercury. *Biochem. Pharmacol.* **19**, 3029–3037.

Clarkson, T. W., and Rothstein, A. (1964). Excretion of volatile mercury rats injected with mercuric salts. *Health Phys.* **10**, 1115–1121.

Clarkson, T. W., Magos, L., and Greenwood, M. R. (1972). The transport of elemental mercury into fetal tissue. *Biol. Neonate* **21**, 239–244.

Clarkson, T. W., Magos, L., Cox, C., Greenwood, M. R., Amin-Zaki, L., Majeed, M. A., and Damluji, S. F. (1981a). Tests of efficacy of antidotes for removal of methylmercury in human poisonings during the Iraq outbreak. *J. Pharmacol. Exp. Ther.* **218**, 74–83.

Clarkson, T. W., Cox, C., Marsh, D. O., Myers, G. J., Al-Tikriti, S., Amin-Zaki, L., and Dabbagh, A. R. (1981b). Dose–response relationships for adult and prenatal exposures to methylmercury. *In* "Measurement of Risk" (G. G. Berg and H. D. Maillie, eds.), pp. 111–130. Plenum, New York.

Clarkson, T. W., Nordberg, G. F., Sager, P. R., *et al.* (1983). An overview of the reproductive and developmental toxicity of metals. *In* "Reproductive and Developmental Toxicity of Metals" (T. W. Clarkson, G. F. Nordberg, and P. R. Sager, eds.), pp. 1–26. Plenum, New York.

Clarkson, T. W., Hursh, J. B., Sager, P. R., and Syversen, T. L. M. (1988). Mercury. *In* "Biological Monitoring of Toxic Metals" (T. W. Clarkson, L. Friberg, G. F. Nordberg, and P. R. Sager, eds.), pp. 199–246. Plenum, New York.

Cloetta, M. (1906). On the cause of tolerance to arsenic. *Arch. Exp. Pathol. Pharmakol.* **54**, 196–205 (in German).

Cochrane, W. J., and Smith, R. P. (1940). A fatal case of accidental poisoning by chlorate of potassium: With a review of the literature. *Can. Med. Assoc. J.* **42**, 23–26.

Cortella, E. (1928). Research on changes in the central nervous system in intoxication by thallium acetate. *G. Ital. Dermatol. Sifilol.* **69**, 1167–1176.

Cosic, V., and Kusic, R. (1966). Acute poisoning with arsenic trioxide. *Vojnosanit. Pregl.* **23**, 601–603 (in Serbo-Croatian).

Cotter, L. H. (1947). Hazard of phenylmercuric salts. *Occup. Med.* **4**, 305–309.

Cotter, L. H. (1958). Treatment of cadmium poisoning with EDTA. *JAMA, J. Am. Med. Assoc.* **166**, 735–736.

Coulson, E. J., Remington, R. E., and Lynch, K. M. (1935). Metabolism in the rat of the naturally occurring arsenic of shrimp as compared with arsenic trioxide. *J. Nutr.* **10**, 255–270.

Cox, C. J. (1954). Acute fluoride poisoning and crippling chronic fluorosis. *In* "Fluorides as a Public Health Measure" (J. H. Shaw, ed.). Am. Assoc. Adv. Sci., Washington, D.C.

Cramer, K., and Selander, S. (1968). Penicillamine in lead poisoning. *Postgrad. Med. J.* **44**, October Suppl., 45–48.

Crecelius, E. A. (1977). Changes in the chemical speciation of arsenic following ingestion by man. *Environ. Health Perspect.* **19**, 147–150.

Cremer, J. E. (1958). The biochemistry of organotin compounds. The conversion of tetraethyltin into triethyltin in mammals. *Biochem. J.* **68**, 685–692.

Cressal, S. F. M. (1968). Punctate basophilia and lead absorption. *Singapore Med. J.* **9**, 170–173.

Cuppage, F. E., Cunningham, N., and Tate, A. (1969). Nucleic acid synthesis in the regenerating nephron following injury with mercuric chloride. *Lab. Invest.* **21**, 449–457.

Curley, A., Sedlak, V. A., Girling, E. F., Hawk, R. E., Barthel, W. F., Pierce, P. E., and Likosky, W. H. (1971). Organic mercury identified as the cause of poisoning in humans and hogs. *Science* **172**, 65–67.

Curry, A. S., Rutter, E. R., and Lim, C. H. (1958). The detection of yellow phosphorus and phosphides in biological material. *J. Pharm. Pharmacol.* **10**, 635–637.

Curry, A. S., Price, D. E., and Tryhorn, F. G. (1959). Absorption of zinc phosphide particles. *Nature (London)* **184**, 642–643.

Curry, A. S., Grech, J. L., Spiteri, L., and Vassallo, L. (1969). Death from thallium poisoning: A case report. *Eur. J. Toxicol.* **2**, 260–269.

Cushman, P., Jr., and Alexander, B. H. (1966). Renal phosphate and calcium excretory defects in a case of acute phosphorus poisoning. *Nephron* **3**, 123–128.

Daniel, J. W., Gage, J. C., and Lefevre, P. A. (1971). Metabolism of methoxyethylmercury salts. *Biochem. J.* **121**, 411–415.

Davies, D. J. A., and Bennett, B. G. (1983). Summary exposure assessment—copper. *In* "Exposure Commitment Assessments of Environmental Pollutants," Vol. 3, p. 15, MARC, Global Environ. Monit. Syst. University of London, London.

Dean, G. (1950). Seven cases of barium carbonate poisoning. *Br. Med. J.* **2**, 817–818.

Dean, H. T. (1942a). Geographical distribution of endemic dental fluorosis (mottled enamel). *In* "Fluorine and Dental Health" (F. R. Mouton, ed.), pp. 6–11. Am. Assoc. Adv. Sci., Washington, D.C.

Dean, H. T. (1942b). The investigation of physiological effects by the epidemiological method. *In* "Fluorine and Dental Health" (F. R. Moulton, ed.), pp. 23–31. Am. Assoc. Adv. Sci., Washington, D.C.

Dencker, L., Nillson, A., Ronnback, C., and Walinder, G. (1976). Uptake and retention of ^{133}Ba and ^{140}Ba—^{140}La in mouse tissue. *Acta Radiol.: Ther., Phys., Biol.* [N.S.] **15**, 273–287.

Dencker, L., Danielsson, B., Khayat, A., and Lindren, A. (1983). Deposition of metals in the embryo and fetus. *In* "Reproductive and Developmental Toxicity of Metals" (T. W. Clarkson, G. F. Nordberg, and P. R. Sager, eds.), pp. 607–631. Plenum, New York.

Denk, R., Holzmann, H., Lange, H. J., and Greve, D. (1969). Chronic arsenic injuries in autopsied Moselle winegrowers. *Med. Welt* **20**, 557–567 (in German).

Dérobert, L., and Marcus, O. (1956). Occupational poisoning by inhalation of organic mercury compounds. *Ann. Med. Lég.* **36**, 294–296 (in French).

deTreville, R. T. P. (1964). Natural occurrence of lead. *Arch. Environ. Health* **8**, 212–221.

Díaz-Rivera, R. S., Collazo, P. J., Pons, E. R., and Torregrosa, M. V. (1950). Acute phosphorus poisoning in man: A study of 56 cases. *Medicine (Baltimore)* **29**, 269–298.

Díaz-Rivera, R. S., Ramos-Morales, F., Garcia-Palmieri, M. R., and Ramirez, E. A. (1961). The electrocardiographic changes in acute phosphorus poisoning in man. *Am. J. Med. Sci.* **241**, 758–765.

Dieke, S. H., and Richter, C. P. (1946). Comparative assays of rodenticides on wild Norway rats. *Public Health Rep.* **61**, 672–679.

Diengott, D., Rozsa, O., Levy, N., and Muammar, S. (1964). Hypokalaemia in barium poisoning. *Lancet* **2**, 343–344.

Doak, R. L., Schmidtke, R. P., Wallach, J. D., Davies, L. E., and Niemeyer, K. H. (1965). Thallium intoxications: A specific antidote, supportive therapy and clinical evaluation. *VM/SAC, Vet. Med. Small Anim. Clin.* **60**, 1227–1231.

Dodinval-Versie, J., Dodinval, P., and Andre, A. (1966). Fatal poisoning by sodium fluoride in an insecticide. Difficulties of the toxicological study. *Ann. Méd. Lég.* **46**, 155–162 (in French).

Domnitz, J. (1960). Thallium poisoning. A report of six cases. *South. Med. J.* **53**, 590–593.

Drasch, G., and Hauck, G. (1977). Monitoring the progress of intensive treatment of thallium poisoning. *Arch. Toxicol.* **38**, 209–215 (in German).

Drinker, K. R., Thompson, P. K., and Marsh, M. (1927a). An investigation of the effect of long-continued ingestion of zinc in the form of zinc oxide, by cats and dogs, together with observations upon the excretion and storage of zinc. *Am. J. Physiol.* **80**, 31–64.

Drinker, K. R., Thompson, P. K., and Marsh, M. (1927b). An investivation of the effect upon rats of long-continued ingestion of zinc compounds, with special reference to the relation of zinc excretion to zinc intake. *Am. J. Physiol.* **81**, 284–306.

Druet, P., Bellon, B., Sapin, C., Druet, E., Hirsch, F., and Fournie, G. (1982). Nephrotoxin induced changes in kidney immunobiology with special reference to mercury induced glomerulonephritis. *In* "Nephrotoxicity Assessment and Pathogenesis" (P. H. Bach, F. W. Bonner, J. W. Bridges, and E. A. Lock, eds.), pp. 206–221, Wiley, New York.

Dudley, H. C. (1938). Toxicology of selenium. Toxic and vesicant properties of Se oxychloride. *Public Health Rep.* **53**, 94.

Dvořák, P. (1969). Colloidal hexacyanoferrate(II) as an antidote in thallium poisoning. *Z. Gesamte Exp. Med. Einschl. Exp. Chir.* **151**, 89–92 (in German).

Dvořák, P. (1974). Removal of thallium in rats by rhyolitic pumice. *Res. Exp. Med.* **162**, 63–66 (in German).

D'yachuk, I. A. (1972). Hygienic assessment of the working conditions in seed treatment facilities. *Gig. Tr. Prof. Zabol.* **16**, 45–47 (in Russian).

Eager, J. M. (1901). Denti di Chiaie (Chiaie teeth). *Public Health Rep.* **16**, 2576–2577.

Eckert, H., and Jerochin, S. (1982). Copper sulfate mediated changes of the lung: An experimental contribution to pathogenesis of vineyard sprayer's lung. *Z. Erkr. Atmungsorgane* **148**, 270–276.

Edson, E. F. (1960). Applied toxicology of pestides. *Pharm. J.* **185**, 361–367.

Edwards, G. N. (1865). Two cases of poisoning by mercuric methide. *St. Bart's Hosp. Rep.* **1**, 141.

Edwards, T., and McBride, B. C. (1975). Biosynthesis and degradation of methylmercury in human faeces. *Nature (London)* **253**, 462–464.

Elbel, H., and Holsten, K. (1936). On the hazard of the mouse poison "Delicia." *Dtsch. Z. Gesamte Gerichtl. Med.* **26**, 178–180 (in German).

Elinder, C.-F., Kjellström, T., Linnman, L., and Pershagen, G. (1978). Urinary excretion of cadmium and zinc among persons from Sweden. *Environ. Res.* **15**, 473–484.

Ellis, K. J., Yuen, K., Yasumura, S., and Cohen, S. H. (1984). Dose–response analysis of cadmium in man: Body burden vs kidney dysfunction. *Environ. Res.* **33**, 216–226.

Engleson, G., and Herner, T. (1952). Alkyl mercury poisoning. *Acta Paediatr.* **41**, 289–294.

Ercoli, N. (1968). Chemotherapeutic and toxicological properties of antimonyl tartrate–dimethylcysteine chelates. *Proc. Soc. Exp. Biol. Med.* **129**, 284–290.

Evan, A. P., and Dail, W. G. (1974). The effects of sodium chromate on the proximal tubules of the kidney. *Lab. Invest.* **30**, 704–715.

Evans, E. H. (1945). Casualties following exposure to zinc chloride smoke. *Lancet* **249**, 368–370.

Evans, G. W. (1973). Copper homeostasis in the mammalian system. *Physiol. Rev.* **53**, 535–570.

Evans, G. W., and Johnson, P. E. (1978). Copper and zinc binding ligands in the intestinal mucosa. *Trace Elem. Metab. Man Anim., Proc. Int. Symp., 3rd, 1977*, pp. 98–105.

Expert Committee (1971). "Methyl Mercury in Fish. A Toxicologic–Epidemiologic Evaluation of Risks." Report from an Expert Group, *Nord. Hyg. Tidskr., Suppl. 4.* Uno S. Andersons Tryckeri, Stockholm.

Fairhall, L. T., and Hyslop, F. (1947). The toxicology of antimony. *Public Health Rep., Suppl.* **195**.

Fairhall, L. T., and Miller, J. W. (1941). A study of the relative toxicity of the molecular components of lead arsenate. *Public Health Rep.* **56**, 1610–1625.

Fairhall, L. T., and Neal, P. A. (1938). The absorption and excretion of lead arsenate in man. *Public Health Rep.* **53**, 1231–1245.

Farner, L. M., Yaffe, C. D., Scott, N., and Adley, F. E. (1949). The hazards associated with the use of lead arsenate in apple orchards. *J. Ind. Hyg. Toxicol.* **31**, 162–168.

Fazekas, I. G. (1964). Lethal copper sulfate poisoning following eating of sprayed grapes. *Acta Med. Leg. Soc.* **17**, 129–138 (in German).

Fazekas, I. G. (1968). Two fatal cases of sodium fluoride poisoning. *Orv. Hetil.* **109**, 2493–2496 (in Hungarian).

Fazekas, I. G., Felkai, B., and Melegh, B. (1953). The central nervous system in barium chloride poisonisng. *Virchows Arch. Pathol. Anat. Physiol.* **324**, 110–115 (in German).

Felden, B. F. (1928). Epilation with thallium acetate in the treatment of ringworm of the scalp in children. *Arch. Dermatol.* **17**, 182–193.

Fellows, A. W., Campbell, J. S., and Wadsworth, R. C. (1948). Boric acid—poison. *J. Maine Med. Assoc.* **39**, 339–350.

Fierz, U. (1966). Studies on the side-effects of therapy of skin diseases with arsenic based on patients' histories. *Arch. Klin. Exp. Dermatol.* **227**, 286–290 (in German).

Fisher, R. S., and Freimuth, H. C. (1958). Blood boron levels in human infants. *J. Invest. Dermatol.* **30**, 85–86.

Fitzhugh, O. G., and Meiller, F. H. (1941). The chronic toxicity of cadmium. *J. Pharmacol. Exp. Ther.* **72**, 15.

Fitzhugh, O. G., Nelson, A. A., Laug, E. P., and Kunze, F. M. (1950). Chronic oral toxicities of mercuriphenyl- and mercuric salts. *Arch. Ind. Hyg.* **2**, 433–442.

Fleming, A. J. (1964). Industrial hygiene and medical control procedures. *Arch. Environ. Health* **8**, 266–270.

Fletcher, G. F., and Galambos, J. T. (1963). Phosphorus poisoning in humans. *Arch. Intern. Med.* **112**, 846–852.

Foreman, H. (1961). Use of chelating agents in treatment of metal poisoning (with special emphasis on lead). *Fed. Proc., Fed. Am. Soc. Exp. Biol.* **20**, 191–196.

Forni, A., Cambiaghi, G., and Secchi, G. C. (1976). Initial occupational exposure to lead. *Arch. Environ. Health* **31**, 73–78.

Foulkes, E. C. (1974). Excretion and retention of cadmium, zinc, and mercury by rabbit kidney. *Am. J. Physiol.* **227**, 1356–1360.

Fowler, B. A., and Woods, J. S. (1979). The effects of prolonged oral arsenate exposure on liver mitochondria of mice: Morphometric and biochemical studies. *Toxicol. Appl. Pharmacol.* **50**, 177–187.

Franke, K. W. (1934). A new toxicant occurring naturally in certain samples of plant foodstuffs. I. Results obtained in preliminary feeding trials. *J. Nutr.* **8**, 597–608.

Franke, K. W., and Moxon, A. L. (1936). A comparison of the minimum fatal doses of selenium, tellurium, arsenic, and vanadium. *J. Pharmacol. Exp. Ther.* **58**, 454–459.

Franke, K. W., and Potter, V. R. (1935). A new toxicant occurring naturally in certain samples of plant foodstuffs. IV. Toxic effects of orally ingested selenium. *J. Nutr.* **10**, 213–221.

Franke, K. W., and Tully, W. C. (1935). Low hatachability due to deformities in chicks. *Poult. Sci.* **14**, 273–277.

Frant, S., and Kleeman, I. (1941). Cadmium food poisoning. *JAMA, J. Am. Med. Assoc.* **117**, 86–89.

Franz, R.-D. (1962). Toxicity of a trace metal. *Naunyn-Schmiedebergs Arch. Exp. Pathol. Pharmakol.* **244**, 17–20 (in German).

Freund, M., Leffkowitz, M., and Elian, M. (1971). Clinical manifestations of thallium poisoning. *Harefuah* **81**, 140–141 (in Hebrew).

Frey, J., and Schlechter, M. (1939). Experimental investigation of the quantitative excretion of thallium in various body fluids. *Naunyn Schmiedebergs Arch. Exp. Pathol. Pharmakol.* **193**, 530–538 (in German).

Friberg, L. (1950). Health hazards in the manufacture of alkaline accumulators with special reference to chronic cadmium poisoning. *Acta Med. Scand., Suppl.* **240**, 1–124.

Friberg, L. (1956). Edathamil calcium disodium in cadmium poisoning. *Arch. Ind. Health* **13**, 18–23.

Friberg, L. (1959). Studies on the metabolism of mercuric chloride and methyl mercuric dicyandiamide. *Arch. Ind. Health* **20**, 42–49.

Friberg, L., Hammarström, S., and Nyström, A. (1953). Kidney injury after chronic exposure to inorganic mercury. *Arch. Ind. Hyg. Occup. Health* **8**, 149–153.

Friberg, L., Piscator, M., Nordberg, G. F., and Kjellström, T. (1974). "Cadmium in the Environment." CRC Press, Cleveland, Ohio.

Friberg, L., Kjellström, T., and Nordberg, G. F. (1986). Cadmium. *In* "Handbook on the Toxicology of Metals" (L. Friberg, G. F. Nordberg, and V. B. Vouk, eds.), 2nd ed., Vol. 2, pp. 130–184. Elsevier, Amsterdam.

Frketić, J., Magdić, A., and Štajduhar-Djurić, Z. (1957). Zn phosphide poisoning. *Arh. Hig. Rada Toksikol.* **8**, 15–24.

Frost, D. V., and Lish, P. M. (1975). Selenium in biology. *Annu. Rev. Pharmacol.* **15**, 259–284.

Gabard, B. (1976). The excretion and distribution of inorganic mercury in the rat as influenced by several chelating agents. *Arch. Toxicol.* **35**, 15–24.

Gage, J. C. (1964). Distribution and excretion of methyl and phenyl mercury salts. *Br. J. Ind. Med.* **21**, 197–201.

Gaines, T. B. (1969). Acute toxicity of pesticides. *Toxicol. Appl. Pharmacol.* **14**, 515–534.

Gaines, T. B., and Kimbrough, R. D. (1968). Toxicity of fentin hydroxide to rats. *Toxicol. Appl. Pharmacol.* **12**, 397–403.

Galy, P., Touraine, R., Brune, J., Gallois, P., Roudier, R., Loire, R., L'heureux, P., and Wiesendanger, T. (1963a). Bronchopulmonary cancers in chronic arsenic poisoning of winegrowers of Beaujolais. *Lyon Med.* **210**, 735–744 (in French).

Galy, P., Touraine, R., Brune, J., Roudier, P., and Gallois, P. (1963b). Pulmonary cancer from arsenic in winegrowers of Beaujolais. *J. Fr. Med. Chir. Thorac.* **17**, 303–311 (in French).

Gastel, B., Innis, R., and Moses, H., III (1978). Thallium poisoning. *Johns Hopkins Med. J.* **142**, 27–31.

Gautier, A. (1899). On the normal occurrence of arsenic in animals and its localization in certains organs. *C. R. Hebd. Seances Acad. Sci., Ser. D* **129**, 929–936 (in French).

Gefel, A., Liron, M., and Hirsche, W. (1970). Chronic thallium poisoning. *Isr. J. Med. Sci.* **6**, 380–382.

Gellhorn, A., Tupikova, N. A., and van Dyke, H. B. (1946). Tissue distribution and excretion of 4 organic antimonials after single or repeated administration to normal hamsters. *J. Pharmacol. Exp. Ther.* **87**, 169–180.

Gerdts, E. (1964). Thallium poisoning. *Tidsskr. Nor. Laegeforen.* **84**, 1556–1558.

Gettler, A. O., and Weiss, L. (1943). Thallium poisoning. III. Clinical toxicology of thallium. *Am. J. Clin. Pathol.* **13**, 422–429.

Gharib, M. (1970). Enigmatic alopecia. *Clin. Pediatr.* **9**, 622.

Gibson, J. E., Sigdestad, C. P., and Becker, B. A. (1967). Placental transport and distribution of thallium-204 sulfate in newborn rats and mice. *Toxicol. Appl. Pharmacol.* **10**, 408.

Giebelmann, V. R., and Peplow, E. (1974). Concentration of zinc in man following poisoning by zinc hexafluorosilicate. *Dtsch. Gesundheitswes.*, **29**, 1378–1379 (in German).

Giese, A. C. (1940). Mercury poisoning. *Science* **91**, 476–477.

Gili, R. (1948). On a case of acute fatal poisoning by zinc phosphide. *Zacchia* **23**, 144–152.

Gis', Yu. F., and Pozner, A. Z. (1970). The clinical picture of Granosan intoxication in children. *Pediatriya (Moscow)* **49**, 80–81 (in Russian).

Glomme, J., and Gustavson, K. H. (1959). Treatment of experimental acute mercury poisoning by chelating agents BAL and EDTA. *Acta Med. Scand.* **164**, 175.

Gofman, J. W., deLalla, O. F., Kovich, E. L., Lowe, O., Martin, W., Piluso, D. L., Tandy, R. K., and Upham, F. (1964). Chemical elements of the blood of man. *Arch. Environ. Health* **8**, 105–109.

Goldberg, A. A., Shapiero, M., and Wilder, E. (1950). Antibacterial colloidal electrolytes: The potentiation of the activities of mercuric-, phenylmercuric-, and silver ions by colloidal sulphonic anion. *J. Pharm. Pharmacol.* **2**, 20–26.

Goldbloom, R. B., and Goldbloom, A. (1953). Boric acid poisoning. Report of four cases and a review of 109 cases from the world literature. *J. Pediatr.* **43**, 631–643.

Goldwater, L. J. (1972a). An assessment of the scientific justification for establishing 2 μg/m³ as the maximum safe level for airborne lead. *Ind. Med. Surg.* **41**(7), 13–18.

Goldwater, L. J. (1972b). Normal mercury in man. *In* "Mercury: A History of Quicksilver" (L. J. Goldwater, ed.), pp. 135, 177. York Press, Baltimore, Maryland.

Goldwater, L. J. (1973). Aryl and alkoxyalkylmercurials. *In* "Mercury, Mercurials and Mercaptans" (M. W. Miller and T. W. Clarkson, eds.), pp. 56–67. Thomas, Springfield, Illinois.

Goldwater, L. J., and Hoover, A. W. (1967). An international study of "normal" levels in lead in blood and urine. *Arch. Environ. Health* **15**, 60–63.

Goldwater, L. J., Ladd, A. C., Berkhout, P. G., and Jacobs, M. B. (1964). Acute exposure to phenylmercuric acetate. *J. Occup. Med.* **6**, 227–228.

Gonzales, T. A., Vance, M., Helpern, M., and Umberger, C. (1954). "Legal Medicine Pathology and Toxicology," 2nd ed. Appleton-Century-Crofts, New York.

Gortner, R. A., Jr. (1940). Chronic selenium poisoning of rats as influenced by dietary protein. *J. Nutr.* **19**, 105.

Gotelli, C. A., Astolfi, E., Cox, C., Cernichiari, E., and Clarkson, T. W. (1985). Early biochemical effects of an organic mercury fungicide on infants: "Dose makes the poison." *Science* **227**, 638–640.

Goulon, M. (1963). Intoxications by thallium. *Rev. Prat.* **13**, 1321–1324.

Goyer, R. A., ed. (1974). Perspective on low level lead toxicity. *Environ. Health Perspect.* **7**, 1–252.

Graben, N., Doss, M., and Kloppel, H. A. (1978). Disturbance of porphyrin metabolism in thallium poisoning. *Med. Klin. (Munich)* **73**, 1114–1116 (in German).

Grant, R. L., Calvery, H. O., Laug, E. P., and Morris, H. J. (1938). The influence of calcium and phosphorus on the storage and toxicity of lead and arsenic. *J. Pharmacol. Exp. Ther.* **64**, 446–457.

Great Britain Ministry of Agriculture, Fisheries and Food. (1981). "Survey of Copper and Zinc in Food," Food Surveillance Paper No. 5. Stationery Office, London.

Greenberger, N. J., Robinson, W. L., and Isselbacher, K. J. (1964). Toxic hepatitis after ingestion of phosphorus with subsequent recovery. *Gastroenterology* **47**, 179–183.

Greengard, H., and Woolley, J. R. (1940a). Studies on colloidal sulfur-polysulphide mixture. I. Toxicity. *J. Am. Pharm. Assoc., Sci. Ed.* **29**, 289–292.

Greengard, H., and Woolley, J. R. (1940b). Studies on colloidal sulfur-polysulfide mixture. Absorption and oxidation after oral administration. *J. Biol. Chem.* **132**, 83–89.

Gross, W. G., and Heller, V. G. (1946). Chromates in animal nutrition. *J. Ind. Hyg.* **28**, 52–56.

Grulee, C. G., Jr., and Clark, E. H. (1951). Thallotoxicosis in a preschool nursery. *Am. J. Dis. Child.* **81**, 47–51.

Grunfeld, O. (1963). Hazards to health: Thallium poisoning treated with BAL. *N. Engl. J. Med.* **269**, 1138–1140.

Grunfeld, O., and Hinostroza, G. (1964). Thallium poisoning. *Arch. Intern. Med.* **114**, 132–138.

Guenther, M. (1971). The effect of colloidal ferrihexacyanoferrate(II) on the distribution and toxicity of thallium. *Arch. Toxicol.* **28**, 39–45 (in German).

Gunn, S. A., Gould, T. C., and Anderson, W. A. (1961). Zinc protection against cadmium injury to rat testes. *Arch. Pathol.* **71**, 272–281.

Gunn, S. A., Gould, T. C., and Anderson, W. A. (1963). The selective injurious response of testicular and epididymal blood vessels to cadmium and its prevention by zinc. *Am. J. Pathol.* **42**, 685–702.

Guthrie, B. E., Wolf, W. R., and Veillen, C. (1978). Background correction and related problems in the determination of chromium in urine by graphite furnace atomic absorption spectrophotometry. *Anal. Chem.* **50**, 1900–1902.

Guthrie, F. E., McCants, C. B., and Small, H. G., Jr. (1959). Arsenic content of commercial tobacco, 1917–1958. *Tob. Sci.* **3**, 62–64.

Hadjimarkos, D. M., Bonhorst, C. W., and Mattice, J. J. (1959). The selenium concentration in placental tissue and foetal cord blood. *J. Pediatr.* **54**, 296–298.

Halbach, S., and Clarkson, T. W. (1978). Enzymic oxidation of mercury vapor by erythrocytes. *Biochim. Biophys. Acta* **523**, 522–531.

Hall, L. L., Smith, F. A., and Hodge, H. C. (1972). Plasma fluoride levels in rabbits acutely poisoned with sodium fluoride. *Proc. Soc. Exp. Biol. Med.* **139**, 1007–1009.

Halsted, J. A., Smith, J. C., and Irwin, M. I. (1974). A conspectus of research on zinc requirements of man. *J. Nutr.* **104**, 345–378.

Hambridge, K. M. (1971). Use of static argon atmosphere in emission spectrochemical determination of chromium in biological materials. *Anal. Chem.* **43**, 103–107.

Hambridge, K. M., and Droegnueller, W. (1974). Changes in plasma and hair concentrations of zinc, copper, chromium and manganese during pregnancy. *Obstet. Gynecol.* **44**, 666–670.

Hambridge, K. M., Franklin, M. C., and Jacobs, M. A. (1972). Changes in hair chromium concentrations with increasing distances from hair roots. *Am. J. Clin. Nutr.* **25**, 380–383.

Hammond, P. B. (1973). The effect of D-penicillamine on the tissue distribution and excretion of lead. *Toxicol. Appl. Pharmacol.* **26**, 241–246.

Hann, R. G., and Veale, R. A. (1910). A fatal case of poisoning by phosphorus with unusual subcutaneous haemorrhages. *Lancet* **1**, 163–164.

Hantschmann, L. (1970). The development of high blood pressure in thallium poisonings. *Hippokrates* **41**, 150–151.

Hanzlik, P. J., Talbot, E. P., and Gibson, E. E. (1928). Continued administration of iodide and other salts. *Arch. Intern. Med.* **42**, 579–589.

Harbison, R. D., Jones, M. M., MacDonald, J. S., Pratt, T. H., and Coates, R. L. (1977). Synthesis and pharmacological study of a polymer which selectively binds mercury. *Toxicol. Appl. Pharmacol.* **42**, 445–454.

Harrisson, J. W. E., Packman, E. W., and Abbott, D. D. (1958). Acute oral toxicity and chemical and physical properties of arsenic trioxides. *Arch. Ind. Health* **17**, 118–123.

Haskins, W. T., and Luttermoser, G. W. (1950). The comparative toxicities of the antimonyl derivatives of the four isomeric potassium acid tartrates. *Am. J. Trop. Med.* **30**, 591–592.

Hausman, R., and Wilson, W. J., Jr. (1964). Thallotoxicosis: A social menace. *J. Forensic Sci.* **9**, 71–88.

Hayes, R. B., Lilienfeld, A. M., and Snell, L. M. (1979). Mortality in chromium chemical production workers: A prospective study. *Int. J. Epidemiol.* **8**, 363–374.

Hayes, W. J., Jr. (1975). "Toxicology of Pesticides." Williams and Wilkins, Baltimore, Maryland.

Hayes, W. J., Jr. (1976). Mortality in 1969 from pesticides including aerosols. *Arch. Environ. Health* **31**, 61–72.

Hayes, W. J., Jr., and Pirkle, C. I. (1966). Mortality from pesticides in 1961. *Arch. Environ. Health* **12**, 43–55.

Hayes, W. J., Jr., and Vaughn, W. K. (1977). Mortality from pesticides in the United States in 1973 and 1974. *Toxicol. Appl. Pharmacol.* **42**, 235–252.

Heath, D. F. (1966). The retention of triphenyltin and dieldrin and its relevance to the toxic effects of multiple dosing. In "Radioisotopes in the Detection of Pesticide Residues," Int. At. Energy Agency, Vienna.

Hegsted, D. M., McKirbbin, J. M., and Drinker, C. K. (1945). The biological, hygienic, and medical properties of zinc and zinc compounds. *Public Health Rep., Suppl.* **179**.

Heimann, H. (1946). Chronic phosphorus poisoning. *J. Ind. Hyg. Toxicol.* **28**, 142–150.

Henke, G., and Bohn, G. (1969). Detection of a repeated thallium poisoning by activation analysis of hair and nails. *Arch. Toxikol.* **25**, 48–56. (in German).

Herman, M. M., and Bensch, K. G. (1967). Light and electron microscopic studies of acute and chronic thallium intoxication in rats. *Toxicol. Appl. Pharmacol.* **10**, 199–222.

Hernberg, S., and Nikkanen, J. (1970). Enzyme inhibition by lead under normal urban conditions. *Lancet* **1**, 63–64.

Hernberg, S., Nikkanen, J., Mellin, G., and Lilius, H. (1970). Delta-aminolevulinic acid dehydrase as a measure of lead exposure. *Arch. Environ. Health* **21**, 140–145.

Herner, T. (1945). Intoxication with organic compounds of mercury. *Nord. Med., NM* **26**, 833–836.

Herok, J., and Götte, H. (1964). Part III. Radioactive metabolic balance studies with tin triphenylacetate in the lactating sheep. *Zentralbl. Veterinaermed., Reihe A* **11**, 20–28 (in German).

Heydlauf, H. (1969). Ferric-cyanoferrate(II): An effective antidote in thallium poisoning. *Eur. J. Pharmacol.* **6**, 340–344.

Heyman, A., Pfeiffer, J. B., Willett, R. W., and Taylor, H. M. (1956). Peripheral neuropathy caused by arsenical intoxication. *N. Engl. J. Med.* **254**, 401–409.

Heyroth, F. F. (1947). Thallium—a review and summary of medical literature. *Public Health Rep., Suppl.* **197**, 1–23.

Heyroth, F. F. (1952). Toxicological evidence for the safety of the fluoridation of public water supplies. *Am. J. Public Health* **42**, 1568–1575.

Heyroth, F. F. (1963). Halogens, In "Industrial Hygiene and Toxicology" (F. A. Patty, ed.), 2nd rev. ed., pp. 831–856. Wiley (Interscience), New York.

Hislop, J. S., Collier, T. R., White, G. F., Khathing, D. T., and French, E. (1983). The use of keratinised tissues to monitor the detailed exposure of man to methylmercury from fish. In "Chemical Toxicology and Clinical Chemistry of Metals" (S. S. Brown and J. Savory, eds.), pp. 145–148. Academic Press, New York.

Hodge, H. C. (1950). The concentration of fluorides in drinking water to give the point of minimum caries with maximum safety. *J. Am. Dent. Assoc.* **40**, 436–439.

Hodge, H. C., and Smith, F. A. (1965). "Biological Effects of Inorganic Fluorides," Fluorine Chem., Vol. 4. Academic Press, New York.

Hoffman, J., and McConnell, K. (1974). The presence of 4-selenouridine in *Escherichia coli* tRNA. *Biochim. Biophys. Acta* **366**, 109–113.

Holgersen, O. E., Gloor, F., Rohr, H. P., and Torhorst, J. (1969). Early changes in the proximal tubular cell of the rat kidney after sublimate poisoning. Degenerative and adaptive phenomena in the proximal tubular cell. *Virchows Arch. B* **3**, 324–338 (in German).

Honstead, J. F., and Brady, D. N. (1967). The uptake and retention of ^{32}P and ^{65}Zn from the consumption of Columbia River fish. *Health Phys.* **13**, 455–463.

Horacek, V., and Demcik, K. (1970). Group poisoning in the spraying of field crops with Brestan-60 (triphenyltin acetate). *Prac. Lek.* **22**, 61–66 (in Czech).

Horiuchi, K., Horiguchi, S., and Suekane, M. (1959). Studies on the industrial lead poisoning. I. Absorption, transportation, deposition and excretion of lead. 6. The lead contents in organ tissues of the normal Japanese. *Osaka City Med. J.* **5**, 41–70.

Horwitt, M. K., and Cowgil, G. R. (1937). The effects of ingested lead on the organism. I. Studies on the rat. *J. Pharmacol. Exp. Ther.* **61**, 300–310.

Hubler, W. R. (1966). Hair loss as a symptom of chronic thallotoxicosis. *South. Med. J.* **59**, 436–441.

Hughes, J. P. W., Baron, R., Buckland, D. H., Cooke, M. A., Craig, J. D., Duffield, D. P., Grosart, A. W., Parkes, P. W. J., and Porter, A. (1962). Phosphorus necrosis of the jaw: A present-day study. *Br. J. Ind. Med.* **19**, 83–99.

Hunter, D., and Russell, D. S. (1954). Focal cerebral and cerebellar atrophy in a human subject due to organic mercury compounds. *J. Neurol., Neurosurg. Psychiatry* **17**, 235–241.

Hunter, D., Bomford, R. R., and Russels, D. S. (1940). Poisoning by methyl mercury compounds. *Q. J. Med.* **33**, 192–213.

Hursh, J. B. (1985). Partition coefficients of mercury (^{203}Hg) vapor between air and biological fluids. *J. Appl. Toxicol.* **5**, 327–332.

Hursh, J. B., Clarkson, T. W., Cherian, M. G., Vostad, J. J., and Vander Mallie, R. (1976). Clearance of mercury (mercury-197, mercury-203) vapor inhaled by human subjects. *Arch. Environ. Health* **31**, 302–309.

Hutchinson, J. (1887). Arsenic cancer. *Br. Med. J.* **2**, 1280–1281.

Iampol'skaia, B. A., and Dashash, A. (1968). Paths of lead removal in patients with chronic lead intoxication under the influence of complexon therapy with pentacin (CaNa$_3$-DTPA). *Gig. Tr. Prof. Zabol.* **12**, 54–56 (in Russian).

Innes, J. R. M., Ulland, B. M., Valerio, M. G., Petrucelli, L., Fishbein, L., Hart, E. R., Pallotta, A. J., Bates, R. R., Falk, H. L., Gart, J. J., Klein, M., Mitchell, I., and Peters, J. (1969). Bioassay of pesticides and industrial chemicals for tumorigenicity in mice: A preliminary note. *J. Natl. Cancer Inst. (U.S.)* **42**, 1101–1114.

Innis, R., and Moses, H., III (1978). Thallium poisoning. *Johns Hopkins Med. J.* **142**, 27–31.

International Agency for Research on Cancer (IARC) (1980). IARC monographs on the evaluation of the carcinogenic risk of chemicals to humans: Some metals and metallic compounds. *IARC Sci. Publ.* **23**, 205–323.

Ishida, F. (1970). Studies on organic mercury poisoning. *Kumamoto Med. J.* **44**, 638–652. (in Japanese).

Ishikawa, I., Ueno, Y., and Tsunoda, H. (1970). Chemical determinations of the chlorine-containing peptide, a hepatotoxic mycotoxin of *Penicillium islandicum* Sopp. *J. Biochem. (Tokyo)* **67**, 753.

Ishinishi, N., Tsuchiya, K., Vahter, M., and Fowler, B. A. (1986). Arsenic. *In* "Handbook on the Toxicology of Metals" (L. Firberg, G. F. Nordberg, and V. B. Vouk, eds.), 2nd ed., Vol. 2, pp. 43–83. Am. Elsevier, New York.

Jakubowski, M., Piotrowski, J., and Trojanowska, B. (1970). Binding of mercury in the rat: Studies using 203-HgCl$_2$ and gel filtration. *Toxicol. Appl. Pharmacol.* **16**, 743–753.

Jax, W., Grabensee, B., and Schroeder, E. (1973). Therapy of thallium poisoning. *Med. Welt* **24**, 691–693 (in German).

Jennette, K. W. (1981). The role of metals in carcinogenesis: Biochemistry and metabolism. *Environ. Health Perspect.* **40**, 233–252.

Jensen, S., and Jernelöv, A. (1969). Biological methylation in aquatic organisms. *Nature (London)* **223**, 753–754.

Jindrichova, J., and Rockova, I. (1969). Orientational proof of thallium poisoning in the hair. *Vnitr. Lek.* **15**, 471–475.

Joachimoglu, G. (1916). On the question of tolerance to arsenic. *Arch. Exp. Pathol. Pharmakol.* **79**, 419–442 (in German).

Johansson, A. T., Curstedt, T., Robertson, B., and Camner, P. (1984). Lung morphology and phospholipids after experimental inhalation of soluble cadmium, copper and cobalt. *Environ. Res.* **34**, 295–309.

Jones, M. J., Weaver, A. D., and Weler, W. L. (1978). The relative effectiveness of some chelating agents as antidotes in acute cadmium poisoning. *Res. Commun. Chem. Pathol. Pharmacol.* **22**, 581–588.

Jones, M. J., Schoenheit, J. E., and Weaver, A. D. (1979). Pretreatment and heavy metal LD50 values. *Toxicol. Appl. Pharmacol.* **49**, 41–44.

Jones, M. M., Basinger, M. A., and Tarka, M. P. (1980). The relative effectiveness of some chelating agents in acute copper intoxication in the mouse. *Res. Commun. Chem. Pathol. Pharmacol.* **27**, 571–577.

Kamerbeek, H. H., van Heijst, A. N. P., Rauws, A. G., and ten Ham, M. (1970). Therapeutic problems in thallium poisoning: A clinical trial with diethyldithiocarbamate. *Ned. Tijdschr. Geneeskd.* **114**, 457–460 (in Dutch).

Kamerbeek, H. H., Rauws, A. G., ten Ham, M., and van Heijst, A. N. P. (1971a). Dangerous redistribution of thallium by treatment with sodium diethyldithiocarbamate. *Acta Med. Scand.* **189**, 149–154.

Kamerbeek, H. H., Rauws, Λ. G., ten Ham, M., and van Heijst, A. N. P. (1971b). Prussian blue in therapy of thallotoxicosis: An experimental and clinical investigation. *Acta Med. Scand.* **189**, 321–324.

Karkos, J. (1971). Neuropathological findings in thallium encephalopathy. *Neurol. Neurochir. Pol.* **21**, 911–915 (in Polish).

Katoh, Y., Torikai, S., Ohkubo, Y., and Kigawada, R. (1977). A case of acute renal insufficiency due to copper sulfate. *J. Kanagawa Med. Assoc.* **4**, 39 (in Japanese).

Kayne, K. J., Komar, G., Laboda, H., and Vanderlinde, R. E. (1978). Atomic absorption spectrophotometry of chromium in serum and urine with a modified Perkin-Elmer 603 atomic absorption spectrophotometer. *Clin. Chem. (Winston-Salem, N.C.)* **24**, 2151–2154.

Kazantzis, G., Schiller, K. F. R., Asscher, A. W., and Drew, R. G. (1962). Albuminuria and the nephrotic syndrome following exposure to mercury and its compounds. *Q. J. Exp. Med.* **31**, 403–418.

Kehoe, R. A. (1961). The metabolism of lead in man in health and disease (The Harben Lectures, 1960). *J. R. Inst. Public Health* **24**, 81–97, 101–120, 129–143.

Kehoe, R. A., Cholak, J., and Storey, R. V. (1940a). A spectrochemical study

of the normal ranges of concentration of certain trace metals in biological materials. *J. Nutr.* **19**, 579–592.

Kehoe, R. A., Cholak, J., and Storey, R. V. (1940b). Manganese, lead, tin, aluminum, copper, and silver in normal biological material. *J. Nutr.* **20**, 85–98.

Kehoe, R. A. (1964). Normal metabolism of lead. *Arch. Environ. Health* **8**, 232–235.

Keller, R., Thimme, W., Dissmann, W., Buschmann, H. J., Dross, K., and Daugs, J. (1971). Thallium poisoning with consumptive coagulopathy. *Schweiz. Med. Wochenschr.* **101**, 511–515 (in German).

Kennedy, D. (1961). Notes on the casualties with poisons in New Zealand. *WHO Inf. Circ. Toxic. Pestic. Man*, No. 7, p. 5.

Kennedy, P., and Cavanagh, J. B. (1976). Spinal changes in the neuropathy of thallium poisoning. *J. Neurol. Sci.* **29**, 295–301.

Kershaw, T. G., Dhahir, P. J., and Clarkson, T. W. (1980). The relationship between blood levels and dose of methylmercury in man. *Arch. Environ. Health* **35**, 8–35.

Khasanov, Y. Kh. (1971). A rare case of poisoning with pesticide-contaminated water. *Gig. Sanit.* **36**, 96 (in Russian).

Kimbrough, R. D., and Gaines, T. B. (1971). Hexachlorophene effects on the rat brain: Study of high doses by light and electron microscopy. *Arch. Environ. Health* **23**, 114–118.

Kingsbury, J. M. (1964). "Poisonous Plants of the United States and Canada." Prentice-Hall, Edgewood Cliffs, New Jersey.

Kinoshita, Y., and Ogima, I. (1968). Symposium on clinical observations on public nuisances and agricultural pesticide poisonings. 4. Pesticide pneumonitis. *Nippon Naika Gakkai Zasshi* **57**, 1219–1221 (in Japanese).

Kirchgessner, M., Weser, U., and Muller, H. L. (1967). Dynamics of copper absorption. 7. Copper absorption with supplements of gluconic, citric, salicylic, and oxaic acids. *Z. Tierphysiol., Tierenaehr. Futtermittelkd.* **23**, 28–30 (in German).

Kirschbaum, B. B., Sprinkel, F. M., and Oken, D. E. (1981). Proximal tubule brush border alterations during the course of chromate nephropathy. *Toxicol. Appl. Pharmacol.* **58**, 19–30.

Kiyono, S., Hasui, K., Takasu, K., and Seo, M. (1974). Toxic effect of arsenic trioxide in infant rats. *J. Physiol. Soc. Jpn.* **36**, 253–254.

Kjellström, T. (1985). Critical organs, critical concentrations and whole-body dose-response relationships. *In* "Cadmium and Health: A Toxicological and Epidemiological Appraisal" (L. Friberg, C.-G. Elinder, T. Kjellström, and G. F. Nordberg, eds.), pp. 231–246. CRC Press, Boca Raton, Florida.

Klaassen, C. D. (1974). Biliary excretion of arsenic in rats, rabbits, and dogs. *Toxicol. Appl. Pharmacol.* **29**, 447–457.

Klimmer, O. R. (1964). Part IV. Toxicological studies on triphenylacetate of tin (TPZA). *Zentralbl. Veterinaermed., Reihe A* **11**, 29–39.

Kline, R. D., Hayes, V. W., and Cromwell, G. L. (1971). Effects of copper, molybdenum and sulfate on performance, hematology and copper stores of pigs and lambs. *J. Anim. Sci.* **33**, 771.

Klug, H. L., Moxon, A. L. Petersen, D. F., and Potter, V. R. (1950). Inhibition of succinic dehydrogenase by selenium and its release by arsenic. *Arch. Biochem.* **28**, 253–259.

Knight, R. K., Trounce, J. R., and Cameron, J. S. (1967). Suicidal chlorate poisoning treated with peritoneal dialysis. *Br. Med. J.* **3**, 601–62.

Koblenzer, P. J., and Weiner, L. B. (1969). Alopecia secondary to thallium intoxication. *Arch. Dermatol.* **99**, 777.

Koch, R., Winter, R., Tillmann, P., and Wiessmann, B. (1972). Forced diurasis in thallium poisoning. *Med. Welt* **23**, 649–651 (in German).

Kochmann, M. (1934). Evaluation of parathyroid hormone by means of sodium fluoride. *Dtsch. Med. Wochenschr.* **60**, 1062–1063 (in German).

Kolpinski, L. (1886). Preliminary notes on some of the properties of sodium fluoride. *Med. News* **49**, 202–205.

Kosta, L., Byrne, A. R., and Zelenko, V. (1975). Correlation between selenium and mercury in man following exposure to inorganic mercury. *Nature (London)* **254**, 238–239.

Kostyniak, P. J., Clarkson, T. W., Cestero, R. V., Freeman, R. B., and Abbasi, A. H. (1975). An extracorporeal complexing hemodialysis system for the treatment of methylmercury poisoning. I. In vitro studies of the effects of four complexing agents on the distribution and dialyzability of methylmercury in human blood. *J. Pharmacol. Exp. Ther.* **192**, 260–269.

Kourounakis, P., Szabo, S., Villeneuve, C., and Gagnon, M. (1973). Effect of pharmacologic or surgical conditioning upon intoxication with arsenicals. *J. Eur. Toxicol.* **6**, 232–236.

Koven, A. L., Buhrow, C. J., Walters, F. J., Brinton, H. P., Bales, R. E., Yaffe, C. D., Byers, D. H., and Hook, M. E., (1953). Health of workers in the chromate industry. *U.S., Public Health Service Publ.*, **192**, pp. i–xii and 1–131.

Kubota, J., Lazar, V. A., and Losee, F. (1968). Copper, zinc, cadmium, and lead in human blood from 19 locations in the United States. *Arch. Environ. Health* **16**, 788–793.

Kuptsov, V. V., and Aslanov, M. O. (1970). A case of a favorable course of pregnancy and birth after severe poisoning with zinc phosphide. *Pediatr., Akush. Ginekol.* **32**, 61 (in Ukrainian).

Kurland, L. T., Faro, S. N., and Siedler, H. (1960). Minamata disease. *World Neurol.* **1**, 370–394.

Kurnatowski, A., and Polakowski, P. (1966). Morphological investigation of kidneys in experimental thallium intoxication treated with dithizone. *Acta Physiol. Pol.* **17**, 293 (in Polish).

Kutsuna, M., ed. (1966). "Minamata Disease: An Investigation of Intoxication by Organic Mercury." Kumamoto University Medical School, Kumamoto, Japan (see Berlin *et al.*, 1969c).

LaDue, J. S., Schenken, J. R., and Kuker, L. H. (1944). Phosphorus poisoning: A report of sixteen cases with repeated liver biopsies in a recovered case. *Am. J. Med. Sci.* **208**, 223–234.

Lagacé, A. (1961). White muscle disease in lambs. *J. Am. Vet. Med. Assoc.* **138**, 188.

Lameijer, W., and Van Zweiten, P. A. (1975). Acute cardiovascular toxicity of thallium (I) ions. *Arch. Toxicol.* **35**, 49–61.

Langard, S., and Norseth, T. (1975). A cohort study of bronchial carcinomas in workers producing chromate pigments. *Br. J. Ind. Med.* **32**, 335–342.

Lantz, E. M., and Smith, M. C. (1934). The effect of fluorine on calcium and phosphorus metabolism in albino rats. *Am. J. Physiol.* **109**, 645–654.

Largent, E. J. (1961). "Fluorosis, the Health Aspects of Fluorine Compounds." Ohio State Univ. Press, Columbus.

Largent, E. J., Bovard, P. G., and Heyroth, F. F. (1951). Roentgenographic changes and urinary fluoride excretion among workmen engaged in the manufacture of inorganic fluorides. *Am. J. Roentgenol. Radium Ther.* **65**, 42–48.

Lasch, F. (1961). Successful treatment of an acute severe arsenic poisoning. *Med. Klin. (Munich)* **56**, 62–63 (in German).

Laskin, S., Kuschner, M., and Drew, R. T. (1970). Studies in pulmonary carcinogenesis. *In* "Inhalation Carcinogenesis" (M. H. Hanna, Jr., P. Nettesheim, and J. R. Gilbert, eds.), Symp. Ser. No. 18. U.S. At. Energy Comm., Oak Ridge, Tennessee.

Latarjet, R., Galy, P., Maret, G., and Gallois, P. (1964). Bronchopulmonary cancers and arsenic poisoning in winegrowers of Beaujolais. *Mem. Acad. Chir.* **90**, 384–390 (in French).

Laug, E. P., and Morris, H. P. (1938). The effect of lead on rats fed diets containing lead arsenate and lead acetate. *J. Pharmacol. Exp. Ther.* **64**, 388–410.

LeBreton, R. (1962). "Toxicological Study of Tin and Its Derivatives." Tours Imp. Mame., France (in French).

Legge, T. M., and Goadby, K. W. (1912). "Lead Poisoning and Lead Absorption." Longmans, Green, New York.

Lehman, A. J. (1951). Chemicals in foods: A report to the Association of Food and Drug Officials on current developments. II. Pesticides. Section I. Introduction. *Q. Bull.—Assoc. Food Drug Off.* **15**(I), 122–133.

Lehman, A. J. (1952). Chemicals in foods: A report to the Association of Food and Drug Officials on current developments. II. Pesticides. Section II. Dermal toxicity. Section III. Subacute and chronic toxicity. Section IV. Biochemistry. Section V. Pathology. *Q. Bull.—Assoc. Food Drug Off.* **16** (II), 3–9; (III), 47–53; (IV), 85–91; (v), 126–132.

Lemley, R. E. (1940). Selenium poisoning in the human. *Lancet* **60**, 528–536.

Lemley, R. E., and Merryman, M. P. (1941). Selenium poisoning in the human subject. *Lancet* **61**, 435–438.

Leng-Levy, J., Aubertin, J., Leng, B., Magendie, P., Marion, J., and Mauriac, M. (1969). Myocardiac attacks in the course of occupational arsenic poisoning. *Arch. Mal. Prof. Med. Trav. Secur. Soc.* **30**, 434–436 (in French).

L'Epee, P., Texier, L., Lazarini, H. J., Ducombs, G., Doignon, J., Larcebau, S., and Miegeville, M. J. (1973). Late-developing cutaneous arsenicalism. Arsenical cancers. *Arch. Mal. Prof. Med. Trav. Secur. Soc.* **34**, 457–461 (in French).

LeQuesne, P., Damluji, S. F., and Rustam, H. (1974). Electrophysiological studies of peripheral nerves in patients with organic mercury poisoning. *J. Neurol., Neurosurg. Psychiatry* **37**, 333–339.

Lewi, Z., and Bar-Khayim, Y. (1964). Food poisoning from barium carbonate. *Lancet* **2**, 342–343.

Lewis, H. B., Schulz, J., and Gortner, R. A., Jr. (1940). Dietary protein and the toxicity of sodium selenite in the white rat. *J. Pharmacol. Exp. Ther.* **68**, 292–299.

Liebegott, G. (1952). On the relations between chronic arsenic poisoning and malignant neoplasms. *Zentralbl. Arbeitsmed. Arbeitsschutz* **2**, 15 (in German).

Liebscher, K., and Smith, H. (1968). Essential and nonessential trace elements. A method of determining whether an element is essential or nonessential in human tissue. *Arch. Environ. Health* **17**, 881–890.

Likins, R. C., McClure, F. J., and Steere, A. C. (1956). Urinary excretion of fluoride following defluoridation of a water supply. *Public Health Rep.* **71**, 217–220.

Likosky, W. H., Hinman, A. R., and Barthel, W. F. (1970). Organic mercury poisoning, New Mexico. *Neurology* **20**, 401.

Lilis, R., Gavrilescu, N., Nestorescu, B., Dumitriu, C., and Roventa, A. (1968). Nephropathy in chronic lead poisoning. *Br. J. Ind. Med.* **25**, 196–202.

Lindstrom, O. (1961). Liquid seed treatment studies. *Trans. R. Inst. Technol., Stockholm*, No. 185.

Ljubetskii, K. Z., Krazil'shchikov, D. G., and Reshetova, T. E. (1961). On the problem of food poisoning with Granosan. *Gig. Sanit.* **26**, 68–71.

Locksley, H. B., and Sweet, W. H. (1954). Tissue distribution of boron compounds in relation to neutron-capture therapy of cancer. *Proc. Soc. Exp. Biol. Med.* **86**, 56–63.

Loeb, A. (1912). On the vascular action of arsenic. *Verh. Ges. Dtch. Naturforsch. Aerzte* **2**, 489–491 (in German).

Loew, H., Tillmann, P., Winter, R., Wiessmann, B., Koch, R., and Schiller, M. (1972). Thallium removal by hemodialysis as compared to copious diuresis in a severe thallium intoxication. *Med. Welt* **23**, 1411–1412 (in German).

Lucke, B., and Klauder, J. V. (1923). Histological changes produced experimentally in rabbits. *J. Pharmacol. Exp. Ther.* **21**, 313–321.

Lund, A. (1956a). Distribution of thallium in the organism and its elimination. *Acta Pharmacol. Toxicol.* **12**, 251–259.

Lund, A. (1956b). The effect of various substances on the excretion and the toxicity of thallium in the rat. *Acta Pharmacol. Toxicol.* **12**, 260–268.

Lundborg, M., and Camner, P. (1984). Lysozyme levels in rabbit lung after inhalation of nickel, cadmium, cobalt and copper chlorides. *Environ. Res.* **34**, 335–342.

Lundgren, K.-D., and Swensson, A. (1949). Occupational poisoning by alkyl mercury compounds. *J. Ind. Hyg. Toxicol.* **31**, 190–200.

Lundgren, K.-D., and Swensson, A. (1960). A survey of results of investigations on some organic mercury compounds used as fungicides. *Am. Ind. Hyg. Assoc. J.* **21**, 308–311.

Lydtin, H., Korfmacher, I., Frank, U., and Zollner, N. (1965). Barium poisoning. *Muench. Med. Wochenschr.* **107**, 1045–1048 (in German).

Mabuchi, K. A., Lilienfeld, A. M., and Snell, L. (1979). Lung cancer among pesticide workers exposed to inorganic arsenicals. *Arch. Environ. Health* **34**, 312–319.

Macadam, R. F. (1969). The early glomerular lesion in human and rabbit lead poisoning. *Br. J. Exp. Pathol.* **50**, 239–240.

Machle, W., and Gregorius, F. (1948). Cancer of the respiratory system in the United States chromate-producing industry. *Public Health Rep.* **63**, 1114–1117.

MacKenzie, R. D., Brerrum, R. U., Decker, G. F., Hoppert, C. A., and Laugham, R. F. (1958). Chronic toxicity studies. II. Hexavalent and trivalent chromium administered in drinking water to rats. *AMA Arch. Ind. Health* **18**, 232–234.

MacKenzie, R. D., Anwar, R. A., Byerrum, R. U., and Hoppert, C. A. (1959). Absorption and distribution of ^{51}Cr in the albino rat. *Arch. Biochem. Biophys.* **79**, 200–205.

Magee, P. N., Stoner, H. B., and Barnes, J. M. (1957). The experimental production of oedema in the central nervous system of the rat by triethyltin compounds. *J. Pathol. Bacteriol.* **73**, 107–124.

Maghazaji, H. I. (1974). Psychiatric aspects of methylmercury poisoning. *J. Neurol., Neurosurg. Psychiatry* **37**, 954–958.

Magos, L., Bakin, F., Clarkson, T. W., Al-Jawad, A. M., and Al-Soffi, M. H. (1976). Tissues levels of mercury in autopsy specimens of liver and kidney. *Bull. W.H.O.* **53**, Suppl., 93–97.

Magos, L., Peristianis, G. C., and Snowden, R. T. (1978a). Postexposure preventive treatment of methylmercury intoxication in rats with dimercaptosuccinic acid. *Toxicol. Appl. Pharmacol.* **45**, 463–475.

Magos, L., Halbach, S., and Clarkson, T. W. (1978b). Role of catalase in the oxidation of mercury vapor. *Biochem. Pharmacol.* **27**, 1373–1377.

Magos, L., Clarkson, T. W., and Hudson, A. R. (1984). Differences in the effects of selenite and biological selenium on the chemical form and distribution of mercury after the simultaneous administration of $HgCl_2$ and selenium to rats. *J. Pharmacol. Exp. Ther.* **228**, 478–483.

Majaj, A. S., and Hopkins, L. L., Jr. (1966). Selenium and kwashiorkor. *Lancet* **2**, 592–593.

Maki, S. (1972). Agricultural chemicals and their toxicity. *Ringyo to Yakuzai* **39**, 15–20 (in Japanese).

Mallory, F. B. (1933). Phosphorus and alcoholic cirrhosis. *Am. J. Pathol.* **9**, 557–567.

Maloof, C. C. (1955). Use of edathamil calcium in treatment of chrome ulcers of the skin. *AMA Arch. Ind. Health* **11**, 123–125.

Mal'tsev, P. V. (1972). Granosan poisoning in children. *Fel'dsher Akush* **37**, 14–16 (in Russian).

Mancuso, T. F., and Hueper, W. C. (1951). Occupational cancer and other health hazards in a chromate plant: A medical appraisal. I. Lung cancer in chromate workers. *Ind. Med. Surg.* **20**, 358–363.

Mannaioni, P. F. (1960). Clinical–toxicological considerations in some cases of acute poisoning by zinc phosphide. *Minerva Med.* **51**, 3721–3724.

Mappes, R. (1977). Experiments on the excretion of arsenic in urine. *Int. Arch. Occup. Environ. Health* **40**, 267–272.

Marsh, D. O., Myers, G. J., Clarkson, T. W., Amin-Zaki, L., Tikriti, S., and Mjeed, M. A. (1980). Fetal methylmercury poisoning: Clinical and toxicological data in 29 cases. *Ann. Neurol.* **7**, 348–355.

Marsh, D. O., Myers, G. J., Clarkson, T. W., Amin-Zaki, L., Tikriti, S., and Majeed, M. A. (1981). Dose–response relationship for human fetal exposure to methylmercury. *Clin. Toxicol.* **18**, 1311–1318.

Marten, J. (1969). Acute thallium poisoning in an eleven-year-old boy. *Cesk. Pediatr.* **24**, 233–237.

Massmann, W. (1957). Observations on the circulation with phenylmercury pyrocatechol. *Zentralbl. Arbeitsmed. Arbeitsschutz* **7**, 9–13 (in German).

Mathew, G. W., and Low, D. G. (1960). Thallium intoxication in dogs. *J. Am. Vet. Med. Assoc.* **137**, 544–549.

Mathews, J., and Anzarut, A. (1968). Thallium poisoning. *Can. Med. Assoc. J.* **99**, 72–75.

Mathur, A. K., Chandra, S. V., and Tandon, S. K. (1977). Comparative toxicity of trivalent and hexavalent chromium in rabbits. III. Morphological changes in some organs. *Toxicology* **8**, 53–61.

Mazzei, E. S., and Schaposnik, F. (1949). Subacute poisoning by thallium treated with BAL. *Br. Med. J.* **2**, 791–792.

McCann, H. G. (1953). Reactions of fluoride ion with hydroxapatite. *J. Biol. Chem.* **201**, 247–259.

McClure, F. J., and Mitchell, H. H. (1931). The effect of fluorine on the calcium metabolism of albino rats and the composition of the bones. *J. Biol. Chem.* **90**, 297–320.

McConnell, K. P. (1942). Respiratory excretion of selenium studied with the radioactive isotope. *J. Biol. Chem.* **145**, 55–60.

McCoy, K. E. M., and Weswig, P. H. (1969). Some selenium responses in the rat not related to vitamin E. *J. Nutr.* **98**, 383–389.

McCutchen, J. J., and Utterback, R. A. (1966). Chronic arsenic poisoning resembling muscular dystrophy. *South. Med. J.* **59**, 1139–1145.

McGregor, I. A., and Jackson, I. T. (1969). Sodium chlorate bomb injuries of the hand. *Br. J. Plast. Surg.* **22**, 16–29.

McIntire, M. S., and Angle, C. R. (1972). Air lead: Relation to lead in blood of black school children deficient in glucose-6-phosphate dehydrogenase. *Science* **177**, 520–522.

McIntyre, A. R., and Burke, J. C. (1937). Intravenous boric acid poisoning in man. *J. Pharmacol. Exp. Ther.* **60**, 112–113.

McKenzie, A. (1932). Fatalities following administration of intravenous tartar emetic. *Trans. R. Soc. Trop. Med. Hyg.* **25**, 407–410.

McNally, W. D., and Rukstinat, G. (1947). Two deaths due to boric acid. *Med. Rec.* **160**, 284–288.

McNally, W. D., and Rust, C. A. (1928). The distribution of boric acid in human organs in six deaths due to boric acid poisoning. *JAMA, J. Am. Med. Assoc.* **90**, 382–383.

Mees, R. A. (1919). Nails with arsenical polyneuritis. *JAMA, J. Am. Med. Assoc.* **72**, 1337.

Meikle, R. W., Stewart, D., and Globus, O. A. (1963). Drywood termite metabolism of Vikane fumigant as shown by labeled pool technique. *J. Agric. Food Chem.* **11**, 226–230.

Mengele, K., Schwarzmeier, J., Schmidt, P., and Moser, K. (1969). Clinical aspects and studies of erythrocyte metabolism in poisoning by sodium chlorate. *Int. Z. Klin. Pharmakol., Ther. Toxikol.* **2**, 120–125 (in German).

Merguet, P., Schuemann, H. J., Murata, T., Rausch-Stroomann, J.-G., Schroeder, E., Paar, D., and Bock, K. D. (1969). Studies on the pathogenesis of hypertonia and sinus tachycardia in human thallium poisoning. *Arch. Klin. Med.* **216**, 1–20 (in German).

Mertz, W. (1967). Biological role of chromium. *Fed. Proc., Fed. Am. Soc. Exp. Biol.* **26**, 186–193.

Messer, H. H., Armstrong, W. D., and Singer, L. (1972). Fertility impairment in mice on a low fluoride intake. *Science* **177**, 893–894.

Messer, H. H., Armstrong, W. D., and Singer, L. (1973). Influence of fluoride intake on reproduction in mice. *J. Nutr.* **103**, 1319–1326.

Miller, R. F., and Phillips, P. H. (1953). The metabolism of fluorine in the bones of the fluorine-poisoned rat. *J. Nutr.* **51**, 273–281.

Milne, D. B., and Schwarz, K. (1974). Effect of different fluorine compounds on growth and bone fluoride levels in rats. *In* "Trace Elements in Metabolism" (W. G. Hoekstra, J. W. Suttie, H. E. Ganther, and W. Mertz, eds.), University Park Press, Baltimore, Maryland.

Minkowitz, S. (1964). Multiple carcinomata following ingestion of medicinal arsenic. *Ann. Intern. Med.* **61**, 296–299.

Mizyukova, I. G., and Petrun'kin, V. Y. (1974). Unithiol and mecaptide as antidotes in poisonings with arsenic-containing substances. *Vrach. Delo* **2**, 126–129 (in German).

Moeschlin, S. (1965). "Poisoning Diagnosis and Treatment," 1st Am. ed. Grune & Stratton, New York.

Møller, F., and Gudjonsson, S. V. (1932). Cases of massive fluorosis of the bones and tendons (fluorosis in workmen handling cryolite). *Acta Radiol.* **13**, 269–294.

Monier-Williams, G. W. (1949). "Trace Elements in Food." Chapman & Hall, London.

Morris, H. P., Laug, E. P., Morris, H. J., and Grant, R. L. (1938). The growth and reproduction of rats fed diets containing lead acetate and arsenic trioxide and the lead and arsenic content of newborn and suckling rats. *J. Pharmacol. Exp. Ther.* **64**, 420–445.

Morton, W. (1945). Poisoning by barium carbonate. *Lancet* **2**, 738–739.

Motin, J., Maret, G., Traeger, J., Fries, D., and Guibaud, P., (1970). Attempted suicide with sodium chlorate. *Bull. Med. Leg. Toxicol. Med.* **13**, 177–179 (in French).

Mottet, N. K., and Brody, R. L. (1974). Mercury burden in human autopsy organs and tissues. *Arch. Environ. Health* **29**, 18–24.

Moxon, A. L. (1958). Selenium. *In* "Trace Elements" (C. A. Lamb, O. G. Bentley, and J. M. Beattie, eds.). Academic Press, New York.

Moxon, A. L., Paynter, C. R., and Halverson, A. W. (1945). Effect of route of administration on detoxication of selenium by arsenic. *J. Pharmacol. Exp. Ther.* **84**, 115–119.

Moynahan, E. J. (1974). Acrodermatitis enteropathica: A lethal inherited human zinc-deficiency disorder. *Lancet* **2**, 399–400.

Muehlberger, C. W. (1930). Toxicity studies of fluorine insecticides. *J. Pharmacol. Exp. Ther.* **39**, 246–248.

Müller, W., and Bock, K. D. (1958). On an acute poisoning with fluorosilicic acid. *Med. Klin. (Munich)* **53**, 502–503 (in German).

Munch, J. C. (1934). Human thallotoxicosis. *JAMA, J. Med. Assoc.* **102**, 1929–1934.

Munch, J. C., and Silver, J. (1931). "The Pharmacology of Thallium and Its Use in Rodent Control," Tech. Bull. No. 238, pp. 1–28. U.S. Dept. Agric., Washington, D.C.

Munch, J. C., Ginsburg, H. M., and Nixon, C. E. (1933). The 1932 thallotoxicosis outbreak in California. *JAMA, J. Med. Assoc.* **100**, 1315–1319.

Muro, L. A., and Goyer, R. A. (1969). Chromosome damage in experimental lead poisoning. *Arch. Pathol.* **87**, 660–663.

Muth, O. H., Oldfield, J. E., Remmert, L. F., and Schubert, J. R. (1958). Effects of selenium and vitamin E on white muscle disease. *Science* **128**, 1090.

Nagi, N. A., and Yassin, A. K. (1974). Organic mercury poisoning in children. *J. Trop. Med. Hyg.* **77**, 128–132.

Nagy, G., Varga, G., Thurzo, A., and Szilagyi, M. (1975a). Endemic chronic arsenic poisoning caused by water. *Borgyogy. Venerol. Sz.* **51**, 19–26 (in Hungarian).

Nagy, G., Varga, G., and Thurzo, T. (1975b). Clinical and hygienic aspects of chronic endemic poisonings due to contaminated drinking-water. *Orv. Hetil.* **116**, 497–500 (in Hungarian).

National Research Council (NRC) (1979). "Zinc." University Park Press, Baltimore, Maryland.

Neal, P. A., Jones, R. R., Bloomfield, J. J., Dalla Valle, J. M., and Edwards, T. I. (1937). A study of chronic mercurialism in the hatters' fur-cutting industry. *Public Health Bull.* **234**, 1–70.

Neal, P. A., Flinn, R. H., Edwards, T. I., Reinhart, W. H., Hough, J. W., Dalla Valle, J. M., Goldman, F. H., Armstrong, D. W., Gray, A. S., Coleman, A. L., and Postman, B. F. (1941a). Mercurialism and its control in the felt hat industry. *Public Health Bull.* **263**, 1–134.

Neal, P. A., Dreessen, W. C., Edwards, T. I., Reinhart, W. H., Webster, S. H., Castberg, H. T., and Firhall, L. T. (1941b). A study of the effect of lead arsenate exposure on orchardists and consumers of sprayed fruit. *Public Health Bull.* **267**, 1–181.

Nelson, W. C., Lykins, M. H., Mackey, J., Newill, V. A., Finklea, J. F., and Hammer, D. I. (1973). Mortality among orchard workers exposed to lead arsenate spray: A cohort study. *J. Chronic Dis.* **26**, 105–118.

Nettesheim, P., Hanna, M. G., Jr., Dorethy, D. G., Newell, R. F., and Hellman, A. (1971). Effect of calcium chromate dust, influenza virus, and 100 R whole-body X radiation on lung tumor incidence in mice. *J. Natl. Cancer Inst. (U.S.)* **47**, 1129–1144.

Neubauer, O. (1947). Arsenical cancer. A review. *Br. J. Cancer* **1**, 192–251.

Neuman, W. F., Neuman, M. W., Main, E. R., O'Leary, J., and Smith, F. A. (1950). The surface chemistry of bone. II. Fluoride deposition. *J. Biol. Chem.* **187**, 655–661.

Newton, D. W., and Hays, R. L. (1968). Histological studies of ovaries in rats treated with hydroxyurea, triphenyltin acetate, and triphenyltin chloride. *J. Econ. Entomol.* **61**, 1668–1669.

Nielsen, F. H., Givand, S. H., and Myron, D. R. (1975). Evidence of a possible requirement for arsenic in the rat. *Fed. Proc., Fed. Am. Soc. Exp. Biol.* **34**, 923.

Nielsen, J. S. (1974). Acute thallium poisoning treated with Prussian blue. *Ugeskr. Laeg.* **136**, 2930–2931.

Nielsen-Kudsk, F. N. (1965). Absorption of mercury vapor from the respiratory tract in man. *Acta Pharmacol. Toxicol.* **23**, 250–262 (in Danish).

Nielsen-Kudsk, F. N. (1969). Uptake of mercury vapor in blood *in vivo* and *in vitro* from Hg-container air. *Acta Pharmacol. Toxicol.* **27**, 149–160.

Nikitina, Y. I. (1974). Course of labor and puerperium in the vineyard workers and milkmaids in Crimea. *Gig. Tr. Prof. Zabol.* **18**, 17–20.

Nizov, A. A., and Shestakov, H. M. (1971). Contribution to the clinical aspects of Granosan poisoning. *Sov. Med.* **11**, 150–152. (in Russian).

Nofre, C., Dufour, H., and Cier, A. (1963). Comparative general toxicity of mineral anions in the mouse. *C. R. Hebd. Seances Acad. Sci., Ser. D* **257**, 791–794 (in French).

Norris, E. R., and Elliott, N. W. (1945). Tolerance to arsenic trioxide in the albino rat. *Am. J. Physiol.* **143**, 635–638.

Norseth, T., and Clarkson, T. W. (1970). Studies on the biotransformation of 203-Hg-labeled methyl mercury chloride in rats. *Arch. Environ. Health* **21**, 717–727.

Nylander, M., Friberg, L., and Lind, B. (1987). Mercury concentrations in the human brain and kidneys in relation to exposure from dental amalgam fillings. *Swed. Dent. J.* **11**, 179–187.

Occupational Safety and Health Administration (OSHA) (1978). "Air Contaminants," 29 CFR 2910.1000, pp. 99–102. Occup. Saf. Health Admin., Washington, D.C.

Oestlund, K. (1969). Studies on the metabolism of methyl mercury and dimethyl mercury in mice. *Acta Pharmacol. Toxicol.* **27**, Suppl. 1, 1–132.

Ogawa, E. (1976). Experimental study on absorption, distribution and excretion of trivalent and hexavalent chromes. *Jpn. J. Pharmacol.* **26**, 92.

Ohlsson, W. T. L. (1962). Penicillamine as lead-chelating substance in man. *Br. Med. J.* **1**, 1454–1456.

Okonishnikova, I. E. (1965). Experimental therapy and prophylaxis of acute poisoning with arsenic compounds. *Gig. Tr. Prof. Zabol.* **9**, 38–43.

Okubo, T., and Tsuchiya, K. (1979). Epidemiological study of chromium platers in Japan. *Biol. Trace Elem. Res.* **1**, 35–44.

Oliver, J. S., Smith, H., and Watson, A. A. (1972). Sodium chlorate poisoning. *J. Forensic Sci. Soc.* **12**, 445–448.

Orfila, M. J. B. (1814–1815). "Traité des Poisons Tirés des Règnes Minéral, Végétal et Animal ou Toxicologie Générale Considérée sous les Rapports de la Pathologie et de la Médecine Légale." Crochard, Paris.

Osol, A., Pratt, R., and Altschule, M. D. (1967). "The United States Dispensatory and Physicians' Pharmacology," 26th ed. Lippincott, Philadelphia, Pennsylvania.

Ossa, A. P., Soto, H. R., Wolff, F. C., and Armas, M. R. (1975). Acute thallium poisoning. *Rev. Med. Chile* **103**, 256–259.

Ott, G. O., Holder, B. B., and Gordon, H. L. (1974). Respiratory cancer and occupational exposure to arsenicals. *Arch. Environ. Health* **29**, 250–255.

Papp, J. P., Gay, P. C., Dodson, V. N., and Pollard, H. M. (1969). Potassium chloride treatment in thallotoxicosis. *Ann. Intern. Med.* **71**, 119–123.

Pappenheimer, A. M., and Maechling, E. H. (1934). Inclusions in renal epithelial cells following the use of certain bismuth preparations. *Am. J. Pathol.* **10**, 577–588.

Parra, M. A. A., Albornoz, A. L., and Lopez, J. R. (1973). Thallium—urinary excretion with dithizone. *Bull. Med. Leg. Toxicol. Med.* **16**, 155–159.

Pascale, L. R., Waldstein, S. S., Engbring, G., Dubin, A., and Szanto, P. B. (1952). Chromium intoxication with special reference to the liver. *JAMA, J. Med. Assoc.* **149**, 1385–1389.

Paszko, W. (1961). A case of zinc phosphide poisoning. *Pol. Tyg. Lek.* **16**, 1618–1619 (in Polish).

Pate, B. D., and Hays, R. L. (1968). Histological studies of testes in rats treated with certain insect chemosterilants. *J. Econ. Entomol.* **61**, 32–34.

Pate, F. M., Johnson, A. D., and Miller, W. J. (1970). Testicular changes in calves following injection with cadmium chloride. *J. Anim. Sci.* **31**, 559–564.

Paulson, G., Vergara, G., Young, J., and Bird, M. (1972). Thallium intoxication treated with dithizone and hemodialysis. *Arch. Intern. Med.* **129**, 100–103.

Pauly, J. L., Caron, G. A., and Suskind, R. R. (1969). Blast transformation of lymphocytes from guinea pigs, rats and rabbits induced by mercuric chloride *in vitro*. *J. Cell biol.* **41**, 847–850.

Pavlovic, R. A., and Tihomirov, D. M. (1932). Morphological changes in the parathyroid gland of rabbits in experimental poisoning by sodium fluoride. *C. R. Seance Soc. Biol. (Paris)* **110**, 497–499 (in French).

Pekarek, R. S., Hauer, E. C., Wannemacher, R. W., and Biesel, W. R. (1974). The direct determination of serum chromium by an atomic absorption spectrophotometer with a heated graphite atomizer. *Anal. Biochem.* **59**, 283–292.

Pennypacker, E., Shrair, H. R., Lane, W. T., and Schrack, W. D., Jr. (1975). Acute copper poisoning—Pennsylvania. *Morbid. Mortal. Wkly. Rep.* **24**, 99.

Peoples, S. A., Maddy, K. T., Johnston, L., Ray, C., and Weindler, F. (1977). Poison exposures of children in California due to ingestion of liquid-formation pesticides containing sodium arsenite. *Clin. Toxicol.* **10**, 477.

Perry, K., Bowler, R. G., Buckell, H. M., Druett, H. A., and Schilling, R. S. F. (1948). Studies in the incidence of cancer in a factory handling inorganic compounds of arsenic. II. Clinical and environmental investigations. *Br. J. Ind. Med.* **5**, 6.

Petering, H. O., Johnsson, M. A., and Temmer, K. L. (1971). Studies of zinc metabolism in the rat. 1. Dose–response effects of cadmium. *Arch. Environ. Health* **23**, 93–101.

Peters, E. E. (1942). Bismuth stomatitis and albuminuria. *Am. J. Syph.* **26**, 84–95.

Peters, J. H. (1948). Therapy of acute fluoride poisoning. *Am. J. Med. Sci.* **216**, 278–285.

Peters, R. A. (1952). British anti-Lewisite. I. The biochemistry of arsenic. *R. Inst. Public Health Hyg. J.* **15**, 89–103.

Peterson, R. G., and Rumack, B. H. (1977). D-Penicillamine therapy of acute arsenic poisoning, *J. Pediatr.* **91**, 661–666.

Pfeiffer, C. C., Hallman, L. F., and Gersh, I. (1945). Boric acid ointment. A study of possible intoxication in the treatment of burns. *JAMA, J. Am. Med. Assoc.* **128**, 266–274.

Pfeil, E. (1935). Lung tumors as occupational illness in chromate factories. *Dtsch. Med. Wochenschr.* **61**, 1197–1200 (in German).

Phelps, R. W., Clarkson, T. W., Kershaw, T. G., and Wheatley, B. (1980). Interrelationships of blood and hair mercury concentrations in a North American population exposed to methylmercury. *Arch. Environ. Health* **35**, 161–168.

Phillips, P. H. (1932). Plasma phosphatase in dairy cows suffering from fluorosis. *Science* **76**, 239–240.

Piazolo, P., Franz, H. E., Brech, W., Walb, D., and Wilk, G. (1971). Management of thallium poisoning by hemodialysis. *Dtsch. Med. Wochenschr.* **96**, 1217–1218, 1221–1222 (in German).

Piechocka, J. (1968). Chemical and toxicological studies of the fungicide phenylmercury acetate. 2. Studies of mercury absorption by some organs in the rat and mercury excretion following poisoning with phenylmercury acetate as compared to mercury chloride. *Rocz. Panstw. Zakl. Hig.* **19**, 389–393.

Pierce, P. E., Thompson, J. F., Likosky, W. H., Nickey, L. N., Barthel, W. F., and Hinman, A. R. (1972). Alkyl mercury poisoning in humans. Report of an outbreak. *JAMA, J. Am. Med. Assoc.* **220**, 1439–1442.

Pietras, R. J., Stavrakos, C., Gunnar, R. M., and Tobin, J. R., Jr. (1968). Phosphorus poisoning simulating acute myocardial infarction. *Arch. Intern. Med.* **22**, 430–434.

Pimentel, J. C., and Marques, F. (1969). Vineyard sprayer's lung: A new occupational disease. *Thorax* **24**, 678–688.

Pimentel, J. C., and Menezes, A. P. (1975). Liver granulomas containing copper in vineyard sprayer's lung. A new etiology of hepatic granulomatosis. *Am. Rev. Respir. Dis.* **111**, 189–195.

Pimentel, J. C., and Menezes, A. P. (1976). Liver damage in vineyard fungicide applicators. *J. Med. (Lisbon)* **90**, 409–415.

Piribauer, J., and Wallenko, H. (1961). Fatal phosphorus poisoning. *Med. Klin. (Munich)* **56**, 1043–1046. (in German).

Piscator, M. (1966). "Proteinuria in Chronic Cadmium Poisoning." Beckman's, Stockholm.

Piscator, M. (1979). Copper. *In* "Handbook on the Toxicology of Metals" (L. Friberg, G. Nordberg, and V. Vouk, eds.), pp. 411–420. Elsevier/North-Holland Biomedical Press, Amsterdam.

Planques, J., Brustier, V., Bourbon, P., Pitet, G., and Broussy, G. (1960). Distribution of arsenic in the human organism in an outbreak of chronic poisoning. *Ann. Med. Leg.* **40**, 509–515.

Polakowski, P. (1974). Pharmacological properties of dithizone and its influence on excretion and distribution of various metals in tissues after experimental poisoning. *Pol. Tyg. Lek.* **29**, 199–200 (in Polish).

Potes-Gutierrez, J., and Del Real, E. (1966). Acute thallium intoxication. *Ind. Med. Surg.* **35**, 618–619.

Prasad, A. S. (1966). Metabolism of zinc and its deficiency in human subjects. *In* "Zinc Metabolism" (A. S. Prasad, ed.). pp. 250–303. Thomas, Springfield, Illinois.

Prediger, V. (1976). Seed disinfectants as a cause of acrodynia. *Monatsschr. Kinderheilkd.* **124**, 36–37 (in German).

Prescott, L. F., and Ansari, S. (1969). The effects of repeated administration of mercuric chloride on exfoliation of renal tubular cells and urinary glutamicoxaloacetic transaminase activity in the rat. *Toxicol. Appl. Pharamcol.* **14**, 97–107.

Puccini, C. (1961). On poisoning by zinc phosphide. *Minerva Med.* **81**, 216–223.

Pundit, A. N., and Bhave, S. A. (1983). Copper and Indian childhood cirrhosis. *Indian Pediatr.* **20**, 893–899.

Rabinowitch, I. M. (1943). Treatment of phosphorus burns. *Can. Med. Assoc. J.* **48**, 291–296.

Rabinowitz, M. B., and Wetherill, G. W. (1973). Lead metabolism in the normal human: Stable isotope studies. *Science* **182**, 725–727.

Rabinowitz, M. B., Wetherill, G. W., and Kopple, J. D. (1974). Studies of human lead metabolism by use of stable isotope tracers. *Environ. Health Perspect.* **7**, 145–153.

Rabuteau, A. P. A. (1867). Experimental study of the physiological effects of fluorides and of metal compounds in general (in French). Thesis, Paris (cited by Cox, 1954).

Radeleff, R. D. (1964). "Veterinary Toxicology." Lea & Febiger, Philadelphia, Pennsylvania.

Rahill, W. J., and Walser, M. (1965). Renal tubular resorption of trace alkaline earths compared with calcium. *Am. J. Physiol.* **208**, 1165–1170.

Rakow, A. B., and Lieben, J. (1968). Twenty-four cases of lead poisoning, ten years later. *Arch. Environ. Health* **16**, 785–787.

Rao, S. H., Gopal, E. R., and Raj, R. (1969). A case of acute sodium fluoride intoxication. *J. Assoc. Physicians India* **17**, 373–374.

Rathus, E., Stinton, R. G., and Putnam, J. L. (1979). Arsine poisoning, country style. *Med. J. Aust.* **1**, 163–166.

Rauws, A. G., and van Heyst, A. N. (1979). Check of Prussian blue for antidotal efficacy in thallium intoxication. *Arch. Toxicol.* **43**, 153–154.

Rauws, A. G., ten Ham, M., and Kamerbeek, H. H. (1969). Influence of the antidote dithiocarb on distribution and toxicity of thallium in the rat. *Arch. Int. Pharmacodyn. Ther.* **182**, 425–426.

Reed, D., Crawley, J., Faro, S. N., Pieper, S. J., and Kurland, L. T. (1963). Thallotoxicosis. *JAMA, J. Am. Med. Assoc.* **183**, 516–522.

Reibscheid, S., Stella, S., and de Padua Vilcla, M. (1966). Poisoning with thallium. Report of two cases. *Hospital (Rio de Janeiro)* **70**, 715–724 (in Portuguese).

Rennert, O. M., Weiner, P., and Madden, J. (1970). Asymptomatic lead poisoning in 85 Chicago children. *Clin. Pediatr.* **9**, 9–13.

Richards, M. P., and Cousins, R. J. (1976). Metallothionein and its relationship to the metabolism of dietary zinc in rats. *J. Nutr.* **106**, 1591–1599.

Richardson, A. P. (1937). Toxic potentialities of continued administration of chlorate for blood and tissues. *J. Pharmacol. Exp. Ther.* **59**, 101–113.

Rimalis, B. T., and Bochkarnikov, V. V. (1978). Acute hepatorenal insufficiency in some rare acute exogenous poisoning. *Klin. Med. (Moscow)* **56**, 125–128 (in Russian).

Ritter, W. L., and Nussbaum, M. A. (1945). Occupational illnesses in cotton industries. III. The mercury hazard in seed treating. *Miss. Doct.* **22**, 262–264.

Rodermund, O. E., Goenechea, S., and Sellier, K. (1968). Poisoning with thallium. Report of two cases. *Hospital (Rio de Janeiro)* **70**, 715–724.

Roholm, K. (1937). "Fluorine Intoxication." H. K. Lewis and Co., London.

Rose, M. S., and Aldridge, W. N. (1966). Triethyltin and the incorporation of (^{32}P) phosphate into rat brain phospholipids. *J. Neurochem.* **13**, 103–108.

Rose, M. S., and Aldridge, W. N. (1968). The interaction of triethyltin with components of animal tissues. *Biochem. J.* **106**, 821–828.

Roth, F. (1957a). On the late effects of chronic arsenicism of Mosel wine-growers. *Dtsch. Med. Wochenschr.* **82**, 468 (in German).

Roth, F. (1957b). Arsenic liver tumors (hemangioendotheliomas). *Z. Krebsforsch.* **61**, 468–503.

Rothstein, A., and Hayes, A. L. (1960). Metabolism of mercury in the rat studied by isotope techniques. *J. Pharmacol. Exp. Ther.* **130**, 166–176.

Rothstein, A., and Hayes, A. L. (1964). The turnover of mercury in rats exposed repeatedly to mercury vapor. *Health Phys.* **10**, 1099–1113.

Royle, H. (1975). Toxicity of chromic acid in the chromium plating industry. *Environ. Res.* **10**, 141–163.

Rubitsky, H. J., and Myerson, R. M. (1949). Acute phosphorus poisoning. *Arch. Intern. Med.* **83**, 164–178.

Rustam, H., and Hamdi, T. (1974). Methyl mercury poisoning in Iraq: A neurological study. *Brain* **97**, 499–510.

Rustam, H., von Burg, R., Amin-Zaki, L., and El Hassani, S. (1975). Evidence for a neuromuscular disorder in methylmercury poisoning. *Arch. Environ. Health* **30**, 190–195.

Sager, P. R., and Matheson, D. W. (1988). Mechanisms of neurotoxicity related to selective disruption of microtubules and intermediate filaments. *Toxicology* **49**, 479–492.

Sager, P. R., Aschner, M., and Rodier, P. M. (1984). Persistent, differential alterations in developing cerebellar cortex of male and female mice after methylmercury exposure. *Dev. Brain Res.* **12**, 1–11.

Samarawickrama, G. P., and Webb, M. (1979). Acute effects of cadmium during pregnancy and embryo-fetal development in the rat. *Environ. Health Perspect.* **28**, 245–249.

Sanderson, K. V. (1963). Arsenic and skin cancer. *Trans. St. Johns Hosp. Dermatol. Soc.* **49**, 115–122.

Sandstead, H. H., Stant, E. G., Brill, A. B., Arias, L. I., and Terry, R. T. (1969a). Lead intoxication and the thyroid. *Arch. Intern. Med.* **123**, 632–635.

Sandstead, H. H., Michelakis, A. M., and Temple, T. E. (1969b). chronic lead intoxication, its effect on the reninaldosterone response to sodium deprivation. *Arch. Environ. Health* **20**, 356–363.

Santini, M. (1955). Poisoning by zinc phosphide introduced per vagina. *G. Med. Leg. Infortunistica Tossicol.* **1**, 104–110.

Satterlee, H. S. (1956). The problem of arsenic in American cigarette tobacco. *N. Engl. J. Med.* **254**, 1150–1154.

Savchuck, W. B., and Armstrong, W. D. (1951). Metabolic turnover of fluoride by the skeleton of the rat. *J. Biol. Chem.* **193**, 575–585.

Schaidt, G., Geldmacher-von Mallinckrodt, M., and Opitz, O. (1979). On the distribution of zinc in the body fluids and organs following fatal zinc poisoning. *Beitr. Gerich. Med.* **37**, 351–355.

Schmidt, H. J., and Rand, W. E. (1952). A critical study of the literature on fluoride toxicology with respect to cattle damage. *Am. J. Vet. Res.* **13**, 38–49.

Scholz, J. (1965). Chronic toxicity testing. *Nature (London)* **207**, 870–871.

Schroeder, E. G., Rose, F. A., and Most, H. (1946). Effect of antimony on the electrocardiogram. *Am. J. Med. Sci.* **212**, 697–706.

Schroeder, H. A. (1973). Recondite toxicity of trace elements. *Essays Toxicol.* **4**, 108–199.

Schroeder, H. A., and Mitchener, M. (1975). Life-term effects of mercury, methyl mercury, and nine other trace metals on mice. *J. Nutr.* **105**, 452–458.

Schroeder, H. A., and Tipton, I. H. (1968). The human body burden of lead. *Arch. Environ. Health* **17**, 965–978.

Schroeder, H. A., Mitchener, M., and Nason, A. P. (1970). Zirconium, niobium, antimony, vanadium and lead in rats: Life term studies. *J. Nutr.* **100**, 59–68.

Schryver, H. F., Hintz, H. F., and Lowe, J. W. (1980). Absorption, excretion and tissue distribution of stable zinc and ^{65}zinc in ponies. *J. Anim. Sci.* **51**, 896–902.

Schultz, J., and Lewis, H. B. (1940). The excretion of volatile selenium compounds after the administration of sodium selenite to white rats. *J. Biol. Chem.* **133**, 199–207.

Schwartze, E. W., and Alsberg, C. L. (1923). Studies on the pharmacology of cadmium and zinc with particular reference to emesis. *J. Pharmacol. Exp. Ther.* **21**, 1–22.

Schwarz, K. (1961). Developmenet and status of experimental work on Factor 3–selenium. *Fed. Proc., Fed. Am. Soc. Exp. Biol.* **20** (Pt. I), 666–673.

Schwarz, K., and Foltz, C. M. (1957). Selenium as an integral part of Factor 3 against dietary necrotic liver degeneration. *J. Am. Chem. Soc.* **79**, 3292–3293.

Schwarz, K., and Foltz, C. M. (1958). Factor 3 activity of selenium compounds. *J. Biol. Chem.* **233**, 245–251.

Schwarz, K., Bieri, J. G., Briggs, G. M., and Scott, M. L. (1957). Prevention of exudative diathesis in chicks by Factor 3 and Se. *Proc. Soc. Exp. Biol. Med.* **95**, 621–625.

Schwetz, B. A., O'Neil, P. V., Voekler, F. A., and Jacobs, D. W. (1967). Effects of diphenylthiocarbazone and diethyldithiocarbamate on the excretion of thallium by rats. *Toxicol. Appl. Pharmacol.* **10**, 79–88.

Scott, M. L. (1973). The selenium dilemma. *J. Nutr.* **103**, 803–810.

Segar, W. E. (1960). Peritoneal dialysis in the treatment of boric acid poisoning. *N. Engl. J. Med.* **262**, 798–800.

Sharda, B. (1984). Indian childhood cirrhosis: Dietary copper. *Indian Pediatr.* **21**, 182.

Sharkey, T. P., and Simpson, W. M. (1933). Accidental sodium fluoride poisoning. *JAMA, J. Am. Med. Assoc.* **100**, 97–100.

Sharrett, A. R., Carter, A. P., Orheim, R. M., and Feinleib, M. (1982). Daily intake of lead, cadmium, copper and zinc from drinking water: The Seattle study of trace metal exposure. *Environ. Res.* **28**, 456–475.

Shaw, J. J., ed. (1954). "Fluoridation as a Public Health Measure." Am. Assoc. Adv. Sci. Washington, D.C.

Shustov, V. IA., and Tsyganova, S. I. (1970). Clinical aspects of subacute intoxication with Granosan. *Kazan. Med. Zh.* **2**, 78–79.

Silberberg, I., Prutkin, L., and Leider, M. (1969). Electron microscopic studies of transepidermal absorption of mercury: Histochemical methods for demonstration of electron densities in mercury-treated skin. *Arch. Environ. Health* **19**, 7–14.

Simonin, P., and Pierron, A. (1937). Acute toxicity of fluorine compounds. *C. R. Seance Soc. Biol. Ses. Fil.* **124**, 133–134 (in German).

Simonović, I. (1954). Zinc phosphide poisoning. *Arh. Hig. Rada* **5**, 355–358.

Skerfving, S. (1974). Methylmercury exposure, mercury levels in blood and hair, and health status in Swedes consuming contaminated fish. *Toxicology* **2**, 3–23.

Skerfving, S. B., and Copplestone, J. F. (1976). Poisoning caused by the consumption of organomercury-dressed seed in Iraq. *Bull. W.H.O.* **54**, 111–112.

Smith, D. H., and Doherty, R. A. (1964). Thallitoxicosis: Report of three cases in Massachusetts. *Pediatrics* **34**, 480–490.

Smith, F. A., ed. (1966) "Handbuch der Experimentelten Pharmakologie," Vol. 20, Part 1. Springer-Verlag, Berlin.

Smith, F. A., ed. (1970). "Handbuch der Experimentelten Pharmakologie," Vol. 20, Part 2. Springer-Verlag, Berlin.

Smith, H. (1964). The interpretation of the arsenic content of hair. *J. Forensic Sci. Soc.* **4**, 192–199.

Smith, M. C., and Lantz, E. M. (1935). The effect of fluorine upon the phosphatase content of plasma, bones, and teeth of albino rats. *J. Biol. Chem.* **112**, 303–311.

Smith, M. C., and Leverton, R. M. (1934). Comparative toxicity of fluorine compounds. *Ind. Eng. Chem., Ind. Ed.* **26**, 791–797.

Smith, M. I. (1939). The influence of diet on the chronic toxicity of selenium. *Public Health Rep.* **54**, 1441–1453.

Smith, M. I. (1941). Chronic endemic selenium poisoning. A review of the more recent field and laboratory studies. *JAMA, J. Am. Med. Assoc.* **116**, 562–567.

Smith, M. I., and Stohlman, E. F. (1940). Further observations on the influence of dietary protein on the toxicity of selenium. *J. Pharmacol. Exp. Ther.* **70**, 270–278.

Smith, M. I., and Westfall, B. B. (1936). The selenium problem in relation to public health. *Public Health Rep.* **51**, 1496.

Smith, M. I., Westfall, B. B., and Stohlman, E. F. (1937). Elimination of Se and its distribution in tissues. *Public Health Rep.* **52,** 1171.

Smith, M. I., Westfall, B. B., and Stohlman, E. F. (1938). Studies on the fate of Se in the organism. *Public Health Rep.* **53,** 1199.

Smith, R. G., Vorwald, A. J., Patil, L. S., and Mooney, T. F. (1970). Effects of exposure to mercury in the manufacture of chlorine. *Am. Ind. Hyg. Assoc. J.* **31,** 687–700.

Smith, S. E., and Larson, E. J. (1946). Zinc toxicity in rats: Antagonistic effects of copper and liver. *J. Biol. Chem.* **163,** 29–38.

Smyth, H. F., and Smyth, H. F., Jr. (1932). Relative toxicity of some fluoride and arsenical insecticides. *Ind. Eng. Chem.* **24,** 229–232.

Smyth, H. F., Jr., Carpenter, C. P., Weil, C. S., Pozzani, U. C., Striegel, J. A., and Nycum, J. S. (1969). Range-finding toxicity data: List VII. *Am. Ind. Hyg. Assoc. J.* **30,** 470–476.

Snowden, E. M. (1958). Trace elements in human tissue. 3. Strontium and barium in non-skeletal tissue. *Biochem. J.* **70,** 712–715.

Snowden, E. M., and Stitch, S. R. (1957). Trace elements in human tissue. 2. Estimation of the concentrations of stable strontium and barium in human bone. *Biochem. J.* **67,** 104–109.

Snowdon, C. T., and Sanderson, B. A. (1974). Lead pica produced in rats. *Science* **183,** 92–94.

Snyder, R. D. (1971). Congenital mercury poisoning. *N. Engl. J. Med.* **284,** 1014–1016.

Snyder, R. D. (1972). The involuntary movements of chronic mercury poisoning. *Arch. Neurol. (Chicago)* **26,** 379–381.

Sollmann, T. (1957). "A Manual of Pharmacology and Its Applications to Toxicology and Therapeutics," 8th ed. Saunders, Philadelphia, Pennsylvania.

Sollmann, T., and Seifter, J. (1942). Intravenous injection of soluble bismuth compounds. *J. Pharmacol. Exp. Ther.* **74,** 134–154.

Sommers, S. C., and McManus, R. G. (1953). Multiple arsenical cancers of skin and internal organs. *Cancer (Philadelphia)* **6,** 347.

Sørensen, O. H. (1965). Thallium poisoning. *Ugeskr. Laeg.* **127,** 804–807.

Soroka, V. P., and Sorokina, A. A. (1969). The effect of unithiol and CaNa$_2$-EDTA on urinary trace element excretion in dogs. *Gig. Tr. Prof. Zabol.* **13,** 40–41.

Southby, R. (1965). Fatal poisoning in children under five years of age: A survey in Victoria for the years 1955 to 1963. *Med. J. Aust.* **1,** 533–538.

Spector, W. S. (1955). "Handbook of Toxicology." Carpenter Litho and Printing Co., Springfield, Illinois.

Spyker, J. M., Sparber, S. B., and Goldberg, A. M. (1972). Subtle consequences of methylmercury exposure: Behavioral deviations in offspring of treated mothers. *Science* **177,** 621–623.

Stadtman, T. C. (1974). Selenium biochemistry. *Science* **183,** 915–922.

Starvou, A., Butcher, R., and Sakula, A. (1978). Accidental self-poisoning by sodium chlorate weedkiller. *Practitioner* **221,** 397–399.

Stavinoha, W. B., Emerson, G. A., and Nash, J. B. (1959). The effects of some sulfur compounds on thallotoxicosis in mice. *Toxicol. Appl. Pharmacol.* **1,** 638–646.

Steffee, C. H., and Baetjer, A. M. (1965). Histopathologic effects of chromate chemicals. *Arch. Environ. Health* **11,** 66–75.

Stein, M. D., and Perlstein, M. A. (1959). Thallium poisoning: Report of two cases. *Am. J. Dis. Child.* **98.** 80–85.

Steinberg, H. J. (1961). Accidental thallium poisoning in adults. *South. Med. J.* **54,** 6–9.

Stephenson, J. B. P. (1967). Zinc phosphide poisoning. *Arch. Environ. Health* **15,** 83–88.

Sterner, J. H., and Lidfeldt, V. (1941). The selenium content of "normal" urine. *J. Pharmacol. Exp. Ther.* **73,** 205–211.

Stevens, W., Van Peteghem, C., Heyndrickx, A., and Barbier, F. (1974). Eleven cases of thallium intoxication treated with Prussian blue. *Int. J. Clin. Pharmacol., Ther. Toxicol.* **10,** 1–22.

Stewart, D. (1957). Sulfuryl fluoride: A new fumigant for control of the drywood termite *Kalotermes minor* Hagen. *J. Econ. Entomol.* **50,** 7–11.

Stokinger, H. H. (1963). The metals (excluding lead). *In* "Industrial Hygiene and Toxicology" (F. A. Patty, ed.), Vol. 2, pp. 987–1194, Wiley (Interscience), New York.

Stokinger, H. E. (1981). Copper. *In* "Patty's Industrial Hygiene and Toxicology" (G. D. Clayton and F. E. Clayton, eds.), 3rd rev. ed., Vol. 2A, pp. 1620–1630. Wiley, New York.

Stoner, H. B. (1966). Toxicity of triphenyltin. *Br. J. Ind. Med.* **23,** 222–229.

Stoner, H. B., and Heath, D. F. (1967). The cumulative action of triphenyltin. *Food Cosmet. Toxicol.* **5,** 285–286.

Stoner, H. B., Barnes, J. M., and Duff, J. I. (1955). Studies on the toxicity of alkyl tin compounds. *Br. J. Pharmacol. Chemother.* **10,** 16–25.

Storrs, B., Thomson, J. Fair, G., Dickerson, M. S., Nickey, L., Barthel, W., and Spaulding, J. E. (1970a). Organic mercury poisoning. Alamogordo, New Mexico. *Morbid. Mortal. Wkly. Rep.* **19,** 25–26.

Storrs, B., Thompson, J., Nickey, L., Barthel, W., and Spaulding, J. E. (1970b). Follow-up organic mercury poisoning—New Mexico. (1970b). *Morbid. Mortal. Wkly. Rep.* **19,** 169–170.

Strom, S., Johnson, R. L., and Uyeki, E. M. (1979). Mercury toxicity to hemopoietic and tumor colony-forming cells and its reversal by selenium *in vitro. Toxicol. Appl. Pharmacol.* **49,** 431–436.

Strunge, P. (1970). Nephrotic syndrome caused by a seed disinfectant. *J. Occup. Med.* **12,** 178–179.

Sunderman, F. W., Sr. (1978). Clinical response to therapeutic agents in poisoning from mercury vapor. *Ann. Chem. Lab. Sci.* **8,** 259–269.

Suttle, N. F., and Mills, C. F. (1966a). Studies on the toxicity of copper to pigs. 1. Effects of oral supplements of zinc and iron salts on the development of copper toxicosis. *Br. J. Nutr.* **20,** 135–145.

Suttle, N. F., and Mills, C. F. (1966b). Studies on the toxicity of copper to pigs. 2. Effects of protein source and other dietary components on the response to high and moderate intakes of copper. *Br. J. Nutr.* **20,** 149.

Swensson, A. (1952). Investigations on the toxicity of some organic mercury compounds which are used as seed disinfectants. *Acta Med. Scand.* **143,** 365–384.

Swensson, A., and Ulfvarson, U. (1963). Toxicology of organic mercury compounds used as fungicides. *Occup. Health Rev.* **15,** 5–11.

Swensson, A., and Ulfvarson, U. (1967). Experiments with different antidotes in acute poisoning by different mercury compounds: Effects on survival and on distribution and excretion of mercury. *Int. Arch. Gewerbepathol. Gewerbehyg.* **24,** 12–50.

Swensson, A., and Ulfvarson, U. (1968a). Distribution and excretion of various mercury compounds after single injections in poultry. *Acta Pharmacol. Toxicol.* **26,** 259–272.

Swensson, A., and Ulfvarson, U. (1968b). Distribution and excretion of mercury compounds after single injection. *Arch. Ind. Health* **20,** 432–443.

Syed, I. B., and Hosain, F. (1972). Determination of LD50 of barium chloride and allied agents. *Toxicol. Appl. Pharmacol.* **22,** 150–152.

Taber, P. (1964). Chronic thallium poisoning: Rapid diagnosis and treatment. *J. Pediatr.* **65,** 461–463.

Takeuchi, T., and Eto, K. (1977). Pathology and pathogenesis of Minamata disease. *In* "Minamata Disease" (T. Tsubaki and K. Irukayama, eds.), pp. 103–142. Am. Elsevier, New York.

Tam, G. K. H., Charbonneau, S. M., Bryce, F., Pomroy, C., and Sandi, E. (1979). Metabolism of inorganic arsenic (^{74}As) in humans following oral ingestion. *Toxicol. Appl. Pharmacol.* **50,** 319–322.

Tandon, S. K., Mathur, A. K., and Gaur, J. S. (1977). Urinary excretion of chromium and nickel among electroplaters and pigment industry workers. *Int. Arch. Occup. Environ. Health* **40,** 71–76.

Tauris, P. (1975). Acute thalium poisoning. *Ugeskr. Laeg.* **137,** 473–474 (in Danish).

Taxay, E. (966). Vikane inhalation. *J. Occup. Med.* **8,** 425–426.

Taylor, D. M., Bligh, P. H., and Duggan, M. H. (1962). The absorption of calcium, strontium, barium and radium from the gastrointestinal tract of the rat. *Biochem. J.* **83,** 25–29.

Taylor, F. B. (1962). Effectiveness of water utility quality control practices. *J. Am. Water Works Assoc.* **54,** 1257–1264.

Taylor, F. H. (1966). The relationship of mortality and duration of employment as reflected by a cohort of chromate workers. *Am. J. Public Health* **56,** 218–229.

Teisinger, J., and Fiserova-Bergerova, V. (1965). Pulmonary retention and excretion of mercury vapors in man. *Ind. Med. Surg.* **34,** 580–584.

Thomasino, J. A., Zuroweste, E., Brooks, S. M., Petering, H. G., Lerner, S. I., and Finelli, V. N. (1977). Lead, zinc, and erythrocyte δ-aminolevulinic acid dehydratase: Relationships in lead toxicity. *Arch. Environ. Health* **32,** 244–247.

Thompson, J. N., and Scott, M. L. (1970). Impaired lipid and vitamin E absorption related to atrophy of the pancreas in selenium-deficient chicks. *J. Nutr.* **100,** 797–809.

Thyresson, N. (1951). Experimental investigation on thallium poisoning in the rat. *Acta Derm.-Venereol.* **31,** 3–27.

Timperman, J., and Maes, R. (1966). Suicidal poisoning by sodium chlorate. A report of three cases. *J. Forensic Med.* **13,** 123–129.

Tipton, I. H., and Cook, M. J. (1963). Trace elements in human tissue. Part II. Adult subjects from the United States. *Health Phys.* **9,** 103–145.

Tipton, I. H., Schroeder, H. A., Perry, H. M., Jr., and Cook, M. J. (1965). Trace elements in human tissue. Part III. Subjects from Africa, the Near and Far East and Europe. *Health Phys.* **11,** 403–451.

Tobaldin, G., Castellani, E., Ferrari, B., and Montanari, M. G. (1966). Acute intoxication by lead arsenate. *Arcisp. S. Anna Ferrara* **19,** 177–1006.

Tokutomi, H. (1968). Symposium on clinical observations on public nuisances and agricultural pesticide poisonings. 3. Organic mercury poisoning. *Nippon Naika Gakkai Zasshi* **57,** 1212–1216.

Tokutomi, H., Okajima, T., Kanai, J., Tsunoda, M., Ichiyasu, Y., Misumi, H., Shimomura, K., and Takaba, M. (1961). Minamata disease: An unusual neurological disorder occuring in Minamata, Japan. *Kumamoto Med. J.* **14,** 47–64.

Trelease, S. F., and Beath, O. A. (1949). "Selenium." Published by the authors, New York.

Trelease, S. F., DiSomma, A. A., and Jacobs, A. L. (1960). Seleno-amino acid found in *Astragalus bisulcatus*. *Science* **132,** 618.

Trevisan, A., Buzzo, A., and Gori, E. P. (1982). Biological indices of occupational exposure to low concentrations of zinc. *Med. Lav.* **73,** 614–618 (in Italian).

Tsen, C. C., and Collier, H. B. (1959). Selenite as a relatively weak inhibitor of some sulfhydryl enzymes. *Nature (London)* **183,** 1327–1328.

Tseng, W. P. (1977). Effects and dose–response relationships of skin cancer and blackfoot disease with arsenic. *Environ. Health Perspect.* **19,** 109–119.

Tseng, W. P., Chu, H. M., How, S. W., Fong, J. M., Lin, C. S., and Yeh, S. (1968). Prevalence of skin cancer in an endemic area of chronic arsenicism in Taiwan. *J. Natl. Cancer Inst. (U.S.)* **40,** 453.

Tsubaki, T. (1968). Symposium on clinical observations on public nuisances and agricultural pesticide poisonings. 3. Organic mercury poisoning. 3a. Clinical features of organic mercury intoxication. *J. Jpn. Soc. Intern. Med.* **57,** 1217–1218 (in Japanese).

Tsubaki, T., and Irukayama, K., eds. (1977). "Minamata Disease: Methylmercury Poisoning in Minamata and Nigata, Japan." Am. Elsevier, New York.

Tsuchiya, K. (1977). Various effects of arsenic in Japan depending on type of exposure. *Environ. Health Perspect.* **19,** 35–42.

Ulfvarson, U. (1962). Distribution and excretion of some mercury compounds after long term exposure. *Int. Arch. Gewerbepathol. Gewerbehyg.* **19,** 412–422.

Underwood, E. J. (1956). "Trace Elements in Human and Animal Nutrition." Academic Press, New York.

Underwood, E. J. (1977). "Trace Elements in Human and Animal Nutrition." 4th ed. Academic Press, New York.

U.S. Department of Health and Human Services (1982). "The Health Consequences of Smoking—Cancer," A report of the Surgeon General, U.S. Govt. Printing Office, Washington, D.C.

U.S. Environmental Protection Agency (USEPA) (1983). "Health Assessment Document for Inorganic Arsenic," Rep. No. EPA-600/8-83-021F. U.S. Environ. Prot. Agency, Washington, D.C.

U.S. Environmental Protection Agency (USEPA) (1984). "Mercury Health Effects Update. Health Issue Assessment," Rep. No. EPA-600/8-84-019F. U.S. Environ. Prot. Agency, Washington, D.C.

U.S. Environmental Protection Agency (USEPA) (1987). "Summary Review of the Health Effects Associated with Copper," Rep. No. EPA 600/8-87-001. U.S. Environ. Prot. Agency, Washington, D.C.

U.S. Public Health Service (1962). "Public Health Service Drinking Water Standards," Publ. No. 956. U.S. Public Health Serv., Washington, D.C.

U.S. Public Health Service (1966). "Symposium on Environmental Lead Contamination," Publ. No. 1440. U.S. Public Health Serv., Washington.

Uthus, E. O., and Nielsen, F. H. (1985). Consequence of arsenic deprivation in laboratory animals. In "Arsenic, Industrial, Biomedical and Environmental Perspectives" (W. H. Lederer, ed.), pp. 173–189. Van Nostrand-Reinhold, New York.

Vahter, M. E. (1988). Arsenic. In "Biological Monitoring of Toxic Metals" (T. W. Clarkson, L. Friberg, G. F. Nordberg, and P. R. Sager, eds.), pp. 303–321. Plenum, New York.

Vahter, M. E., Marafante, E., Lindgren, A., and Dencker, L. (1982). Tissue distribution and subcellular binding of arsenic to marmoset monkeys after injection of ^{74}As-arsenite. *Arch. Toxicol.* **51,** 65–77.

Valentine, J. L., Kang, H. K., and Spivey, G. (1979). Arsenic levels in human blood, urine and hair in response to exposure via drinking water. *Environ. Res.* **20,** 24–32.

Vallee, B. L. (1959). Biochemistry, physiology, and pathology of zinc. *Physiol. Rev.* **39,** 443–490.

Vallee, B. L. (1962). Zinc. In "Mineral Metabolism: An Advanced Treatise: (C. L. Comar and F. Bronner, eds.), Vol. 2B, pp. 443–482. Academic Press, New York.

Vallee, C. (1920). Nonfatal poisoning by sodium fluoride. *J. Pharm. Chim.* **21,** 5–8.

Van der Kerk, G. J. M., and Luijten, J. G. A. (1954). Investigations on organo-tin compounds. III. The biocidal properties of organo-tin compounds. *J. Appl. Chem.* **4,** 314–319.

Van Der Merwe, C. F. (1972). The treatment of thallium poisoning: A report of 2 cases. *S. Afr. Med. J.* **46,** 960–961.

Van der Merwe, K. J., Steyn, P. S., and Fourie, L. (1965). Mycotoxins. Part II. The constitution of ochratoxins A, B, and C. Metabolites of *Aspergillus ochraceus* Wilh. *J. Chem. Soc., London,* pp. 7083–7088.

Van Esch, G. J., Van Genderen, H., and Vink, H. H. (1962). The induction of renal tumors by feeding of basic lead acetate to rats. *Br. J. Cancer* **16,** 289–297.

Van Hees, P. A. M., Jansen, A. P., Fennis, J. F. M., and Van 'T Laar, A. (1975). Forced diuresis in thallium intoxication. *Neth. J. Med.* **18,** 125–128.

Van Reen, R., and Pearson, P. B. (1953). Effect of excessive dietary zinc on growth and liver enzymes of rat. *Fed. Proc., Fed. Am. Soc. Exp. Biol.* **12,** 283.

Vasil'eva, S. N., Aleksandrova, T. G., Rybakova, M. G., Bryukhanov, V. A., Bulavintseva, O. A., and Bulavintsev, A. G. (1978). Domestic poisoning with thallium. *Klin. Med. (Moscow)* **56,** 130–132 (in Russian).

Veichenblau, L. (1932). New occupational illnesses in agriculture. *Muench. Med. Wochenschr.* **79,** 432–433 (in German).

Veillen, C., Wolf, W. R., and Guthrie, B. E. (1979). Determination of chromiun in biological materials by stable isotope dilution. *Anal. Chem.* **51,** 1022–1024.

Verschuuren, H. G., Kroes, R., Vink, H. H., and Van Esch, G. J. (1966). Short-term toxicity studies with triphenyltin compounds in rats and guinea pig. *Food Cosmet. Toxicol.* **4,** 35–45.

Versieck, J., Hoste, J., Barbier, F., Steyaert, H., DeRudder, J., and Michels, H. (1968). Determination of chromium and cobalt in human serum by neutron activation analysis. *Clin. Chem. (Winston-Salem, N.C.)* **24,** 303–308.

Vesce, C. A. (1947). Experimental intoxication by selenium: Morphological changes of the endocrine glands. *Folia Med. (Naples)* **30,** 209–217.

Vintinner, F. J. (1940). Dermatitis venenata resulting from contact with an aqueous solution of ethyl mercury phosphate. *J. Ind. Hyg.* **22,** 297–299.

Voight, J. L., Edwards, L. D., and Johnson, C. H. (1948). Acute toxicity of arsenate of lead to animals. *J. Am. Pharm. Assoc., Sci. Ed.* **37**, 122–123.

von Burg, R., and Rustam, H. (1974a). Conduction velocities in methylmercury poisoned patients. *Bull. Environ. Contam. Toxicol.* **12**, 81–85.

von Burg, R., and Rustam, H. (1974b). Electrophysiological investigations of methylmercury intoxication in humans. Evaluation of peripheral nerve by conduction velocity and electromyography. *Electroencephalogr. Clin. Neurophysiol.* **37**, 381–392.

von Kraemer, M., and Giebelmann, R. (1975). Fatal poisoning by zinc hexafluorosilikate. *Dtsch. Gesundheitswes.* **29**, 1378–1379 (in German).

von Martius, C. O. (1953). Clinical and spectroanalytic observations on acute poisoning by thallium sulphate. *Dtsch. Arch. Klin. Med.* **200**, 596–602 (in German).

von Oettingen, E. W. (1947). The toxicity and potential dangers of zinc phosphide and of hydrogen phosphide (phosphine). *Public Health Rep., Suppl.* **203**, 1–17.

Wagstaff, D. J. (1972). Arsenic trioxide: Stimulation of liver enzyme detoxication activity. *Toxicol. Appl. Pharmacol.* **22**, 310.

Wahlberg, J. E. (1965). Percutaneous absorption of trivalent and hexavalent chromium. *Arch. Dermatol.* **92**, 315–318.

Waitz, A., Ober, R. E., Meisenhelder, J. E., and Thompson, P. E. (1965). Physiological distribution of Sb after administration of ^{124}Sb-labeled tartar emetic to rats, mice, and monkeys, and the effects of tris (*p*-aminophenyl)carbonium pamoate on this distribution. *Bull. W.H.O.* **33**, 537–546.

Wakasugi, C., and Fukui, M. (1974). A case report of fatal intoxication by ingestion of calcium polysulfide. *Nippon Hoigaku Zasshi* **28**, 102–103 (in Japanese).

Walsh, F. M., Crosson, F. J., Bayley, M., McReynolds, J., and Pearson, B. J. (1977). Acute copper intoxication. Pathophysiology and therapy with a case report. *Am. J. Dis. Child.* **131**, 149–151.

Wang, B. C., and Mazzia, V. D. B. (1969). Arsenic poisoning as anesthetic risk. *N.Y. State J. Med.* **69**, 2911–2912.

Ware, R. A., Chang, L. W., and Burkholder, P. M. (1974). Ultrastructural evidence for fetal liver injury induced by in utero exposure to small doses of methylmercury. *Nature,* **251**, 236–237.

Warkany, J. (1966). Postmortem of a disease. *Am. J. Dis. Child.* **112**, 147–156.

Warkany, J., and Hubbard, D. M. (1948). Mercury in the urine of children with acrodynia. *Lancet* **204**, 829–830.

Warkany, J., and Hubbard, D. M. (1951). Adverse mercurial reactions in the form of acrodynia and related conditions. *Am. J. Dis. Child.* **81**, 335–373.

Warkany, J., and Hubbard, D. M. (1953). Acrodynia and mercury. *J. Pediatr.* **42**, 365–386.

Wastrous, R. M., and McCaughey, M. B. (1945). Occupational exposure to arsenic in manufacture of arsphenamine and related compounds. *Ind. Med. Surg.,* **14**, 639–646.

Webb, J. L. (1966). Arsenicals. *In* "Enzyme and Metabolic Inhibitors" (J. L. Webb, ed.), Vol. 3, pp. 595–793. Academic Press, New York.

Webb, M., and Etienne, A. T. (1977). Studies on the toxicity and metabolism of cadmium-thionein. *Biochem. Pharmacol.* **26**, 25–30.

Webster, S. H. (1941). Lead and arsenic content of urines from 46 persons with no known exposure to lead or arsenic. *Public Health Rep.* **56**, 1953–1961.

Weinig, E., and Schmidt, G. (1966). Distribution of thallium in the organism in fatal thallium poisonings. *Arch. Toxicol.* **21**, 199–215 (in German).

Welty, J. A., and Berrey, B. H. (1950). Acute thallotoxicosis: Report of two cases treated with BAL. *J. Pediatr.* **37**, 756–758.

West, I., and Lim, J. (1968). Mercury poisoning among workers in California's mercury mills. *J. Occup. Med.* **10**, 697–701.

Westfall, B. B., Stohlman, E. F., and Smith, M. I. (1938). The placental transmission of selenium. *J. Pharmacol. Exp. Ther.* **64**, 55–57.

Whelton, A., Snyder, D. S., and Walker, W. G. (1973). Acute toxic drug ingestions at the Johns Hopkins Hospital 1963 through 1970. *Johns Hopkins Med. J.* **132**, 157–167.

Whitaker, J. A., Austin, W., and Nelson, J. D. (1962). Edathamil calcium disodium (Versenate) diagnostic test for lead poisoning. *Pediatrics* **29**, 384–388.

Wilkening, H., and Litzner, St. (1952). Injuries especially to the kidney from alkylmercury compounds. *Dtsch. Med. Wochenschr.* **77**, 432–434. (in German).

Wilson, B. J., Wilson, C. H., and Hayes, A. W. (1968). Tremorgenic toxin from *Penicillium cyclopium* grown on food materials. *Nature (London)* **220**, 77–78.

Wisniewska, J. M., Trojanowska, B., Piotrowski, J., and Jakubowski, M. (1970). Binding of mercury in the rat kidney by metallothionein. *Toxicol. Appl. Pharmacol.* **16**, 754–763.

Wong, L. C., Heimbach, M. D., Truscott, D. R., and Duncan, B. D. (1964). Boric acid poisoning. Report of 11 cases. *Can. Med. Assoc. J.* **90**, 1018–1023.

Wood, J. M., Kennedy, F. S., and Rosen, C. G. (1968). Synthesis of methylmercury compounds by extracts of a methanogenic bacterium. *Nature (London)* **220**, 173–174.

World Health Organization (WHO) (1962). Accidental food poisoning with Agrosan. Communication to World Health Organization from S. A. Raza Ali. *WHO Inf. Circ. Toxic. Pestic. Man* No. 9, p. 23.

World Health Organization (WHO) (1970). "Fluorides and Human Health." World Health Organ., Geneva.

World Health Organization (WHO) (1972). "IARC Monographs on the Evaluation of Carcinogenic Risk of Chemicals to Man," Vol. 1, Int. Agency Res. Cancer, Lyon, France.

World Health Organization (WHO) (1973). Some inorganic and organometallic compounds. *IARC Monogr. Eval. Carcinog. Risk Chem. Man* **2**, 1–181.

World Health Organization (WHO) (1974). "The use of mercury and alternative compounds as seed dressings. Report of a Joint FAO/WHO Meeting." *W.H.O. Tech. Rep. Ser.* **555**.

World Health Organization (WHO) (1975). Some aziridines, N-, S-, and O-mustards and selenium. *IARC Monogr. Eval. Carcinog. Risk Chem. Man* **9**, 1–268.

World Health Organization (WHO) (1976a). "Environmental Health Criteria. I. Mercury." World Health Organ., Geneva.

World Health Organization (WHO) (1976b). "Cadmium, nickel, some epoxides, miscellaneous industrial chemicals and general considerations on volatile anaesthetics. *IARC Mongr. Eval. Carcinog. Risk Chem. Man* **11**, 1–306.

World Health Organization (WHO) (1977). "Environmental Health Criteria. 3 Lead." World Health Organ., Geneva.

World Health Organization (WHO) (1980). Recommended health-based limits in occupational exposure to heavy metals. *W.H.O. Tech. Rep. Ser.* **647**.

World Health Organization (WHO) (1981). "Environmental Health Criteria 18. Arsenic." World Health Organ., Geneva.

Young, E. G., Smith, R. P., and MacIntosh, O. C. (1949). Boric acid as a poison. *Can. Med. Assoc. J.* **61**, 447–450.

Zeyer, H. G. (1952). Methoxyethylmercury oxalate poisoning. *Zentralbl. Arbeitsmed. Arbeitsschutz* **2**, 68–72 (in German).

Zimmer, L., and Carter, D. E. (1979). Effects of complexing treatment administered with the onset of methyl mercury neurotoxic signs. *Toxicol. Appl. Pharmacol.* **51**, 29–38.

Zimnoch, L., Rudzki, Z., and Kurlowicz-Sidun, B. (1975). Histochemical studies on the rat kidney in acute poisoning with phenylmercuric acetate. *Patol. Pol.* **26**, 247–256.

Zollinger, H. U. (1953). Renal adenoma and carcinoma produced in rats by chronic lead poisoning and their relations to the corresponding human tumors. *Virchows Arch. Pathol. Anat. Physiol.* **323**, 694–712 (in German).

Zook, B. C., Holzworth, J., and Thornton, G. W. (1968). Thallium poisoning in cats. *J. Am. Vet. Med. Assoc.* **153**, 285–299.

Zurlo, N., Griffni, A. M., and Vigliani, E. C. (1970). The content of lead in blood and urine of adults living in Milan, not occupationally exposed to lead. *Am. Ind. Hyg. Assoc. J.* **31**, 92–95.

Pesticides Derived from Plants and Other Organisms

David E. Ray
MRC Laboratories, United Kingdom

13.1 INTRODUCTION

Different groups of pesticides derived from living organisms are entirely unrelated chemically and pharmacologically. They range from relatively simple alkaloids such as nicotine, with a molecular weight of only 162.23, through proteinaceous poisons to virulent living organisms. They range in toxicity from harmless and fragile pheromones, which are used as attractants, to ricin, which has been considered as a chemical warfare agent.

The distinction between synthetic compounds and those derived from living organisms is somewhat artificial. In practice, related compounds are assigned to one category or the other, depending on whether the particular compound of the group that was first known and used was of synthetic or of natural origin. For example, pyrethrum and later the naturally occurring pyrethrins were well known for years before the first synthetic pyrethroid was made; as a result, pyrethroids are thought of as variants of natural compounds, even though they have not been found in nature and are unlikely to occur. By contrast, synthetic sodium fluoroacetate acquired a reputation as a rodenticide and was explored as a systemic insecticide before it was realized that the potassium salt is the active principal of a poisonous plant. Thus pyrethroids are discussed in this chapter as derivatives of living organisms (see Section 13.2), but the organic fluorides are discussed as synthetic organic rodenticides (see Section 19.2).

Perhaps the only unifying feature of the diverse array of poisons derived from living organisms is the popular view that "natural" substances are harmless. On this matter of safety, an Expert Committee of the World Health Organization (WHO) (1967) pointed out that "all the most poisonous materials so far known are, in fact, of natural origin." The committee went on to state:

> Therefore, any material—living or dead—which it is proposed to introduce as a pest control agent should be subjected to the same searching examination for potential toxicity to man as is applied to the synthetic pesticides. Furthermore, it may be very difficult to lay down satisfactory criteria for testing the safety of such agents as novel viruses or bacteria. Microbial toxins could be submitted to a conventional pharmacological and toxicological examination, but a precise assessment of hazard could only follow a detailed study of the mode of action, which might take a very long time. Such considerations apply only to non-viable biological control materials that come into intimate contact with man.

The Committee recommends that WHO take steps to ensure that the safety of any biological agent proposed for use in pest control should be assessed in a laboratory with the specialized knowledge appropriate to the study of the particular agent under investigation.

13.2 PYRETHRUM AND RELATED COMPOUNDS

History and Development The insecticidal properties of pyrethrum flowers (genus *Chrysanthemum*, most commonly *C. cineraraefolum*) have been recognized since at least the middle of the last century, when commercial sale of "insect powder" from Dalmatian pyrethrum flower heads began. Commercial production of the flowers subsequently started in Japan and, most importantly, in East Africa (McLaughlin, 1973). In addition to their insect-killing activity, an attractive feature of the natural pyrethrins (pyrethrum) as insecticides was their lack of persistence in the environment and their rapid "knock down" activity whereby flying insects very quickly become incoordinated and unable to fly. Prior to the development of DDT, pyrethrum was a major insecticide for both domestic and agricultural use, despite its poor light stability. Its usefulness was extended in the 1950s by the introduction of piperonyl butoxide and other compounds as synergists, which greatly reduced the unit cost of crop treatment. Poor light stability and high cost continued to be a problem until the

Table 13.1

Pyrethrins of the Form

Compound	R	R'
Pyrethrin I	$(CH_3)_2-C=CH-$	$-CH_2-CH=CH-CH=CH_2$
Pyrethrin II	$CH_3-O-C(O)-C(CH_3)=CH-$	$-CH_2-CH=CH-CH=CH_2$
Cinerin I	$(CH_3)_2-C=CH-$	$-CH_2-CH=CH-CH_3$
Cinerin II	$CH_3-O-C(O)-C(CH_3)=CH-$	$-CH_2-CH=CH-CH_3$
Jasmolin I	$(CH_3)_2-C=CH-$	$-CH_2-CH=CH-CH_2-CH_3$
Jasmolin II	$CH_3-O-C(O)-C(CH_3)=CH-$	$-CH_2-CH=CH-CH_2-CH_3$

development of synthetic pyrethroids with increased stability and insecticidal activity (Elliott, 1977). For example, deltamethrin (see Section 13.2.4), which was developed by Dr. Elliott, is light stable and rapidly biodegradable and is, gram for gram, 2680–5560 times more toxic to houseflies than rats. This compares with ratios of 58–90 for pyrethrum or 11.3 for DDT (Glomot, 1982). The natural pyrethrins are now used mainly as domestic insecticides, while the synthetic pyrethroids represented 20–25% of the world foliar insecticide market in 1983 (Hervé, 1985) and the proportion is increasing steadily. As various researchers have approached the problem of producing new synthetic pyrethroids, over a thousand structures have been synthesized. Some of these show considerable divergence from the original pyrethrins (Casida *et al.*, 1983), a few even lacking the cyclopropane ring of chrysanthemic acid. Major differences between the naturally occurring pyrethrins and the pyrethroids discussed in this chapter may be seen by comparing Tables 13.1 and 13.2.

Mode of Action Pyrethrum and the synthetic pyrethroids are sodium channel toxins which, because of their remarkable potency and selectivity, have found application in general pharmacology as well as in toxicology (Lazdunski *et al.*, 1985). Their actions on the nerve membrane sodium channel are now well understood at the receptor level (Chinn and Narahashi, 1989; Lombet *et al.*, 1988; Vijverberg and de Weille, 1985). Pyrethroids have a very high affinity for membrane sodium channels, with dissociation constants of the order of 4×10^{-8} M (Soderlund, 1985), and produce subtle changes in their function. Inexcitable cells, by contrast, are little affected by pyrethroids; Baeza-Squiban *et al.* (1987) found no cytotoxicity at 10^{-4} M and cell growth inhibition only at 10^{-5} M for a number of pyrethroids. After modification by pyrethroids, sodium channels continue in many of their normal functions, retaining their selectivity for sodium ions and link with membrane potential (Narahashi, 1986). The kinetics of the sodium channel are drastically changed, however. Although the activation of sodium current by membrane depolarization is little

affected by pyrethroids, the rate of inactivation of this current (which terminates the action potential) is greatly slowed in modified channels. Thus, in neuroblastoma cells, although the sodium current amplitude was unaffected by the pyrethroid tetramethrin, the mean channel open time was greatly extended (Narahashi, 1985). A major consequence of this is that while the amplitude and duration of action potentials are little affected by pyrethroids, they are followed by a slowly inactivating abnormal "tail" current. At high concentrations of pyrethroid this may become sufficiently large to depolarize the nerve membrane completely and block excitability. This is usually a high-dose effect, but at lower concentrations the tail current is still sufficient to cause repetitive activity. Thus one (normal) action potential leads to a train of abnormal action potentials which follow it, since the tail current continues to act as a stimulus to the nerve membrane. Such an effect can be produced by modification of as few as 0.1% of the sodium channels (Narahashi, 1985) because most excitable membranes have a large excess of channels over that required to propagate an action potential. The effect of this small but significant subpopulation of modified channels is thus that at low doses pyrethroids cause stable repetitive firing, and at high doses (such as may rarely be reached *in vivo*) depolarization and conduction block (Vijverberg and de Weille, 1985). A further characteristic of the pyrethroids is that, although they have a very high affinity for active sodium channels, they have little effect on inactive or closed channels, which have therefore to be activated for *in vitro* studies Jacques *et al.*, 1980). The pyrethroids are thus known as *open channel blockers*.

A complicating factor is introduced by the existence of at least four isomeric forms of the pyrethroids, as indicated in Fig. 13.1. The interaction with the sodium channel complex is highly stereospecific (Soderlund, 1985), with the 1R and 1S cis isomers binding competitively to one site and the 1R and 1S trans isomers binding noncompetitively to another (Narahashi, 1986). The 1S forms do not modify the channel function but do block the effect of the 1R isomers. In whole mammals the 1R isomers are thus active and the 1S isomers inactive and essen-

Table 13.2
Pyrethroids of the Form

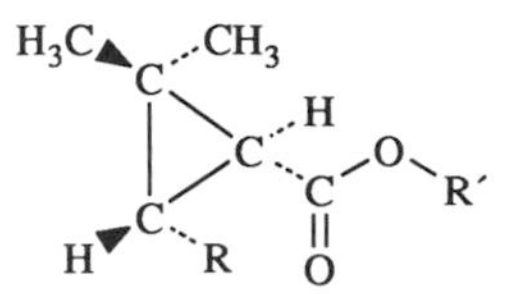

Compound	R	R′
Barthrin	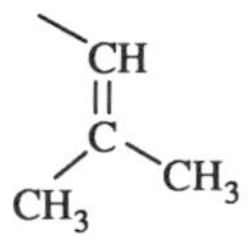	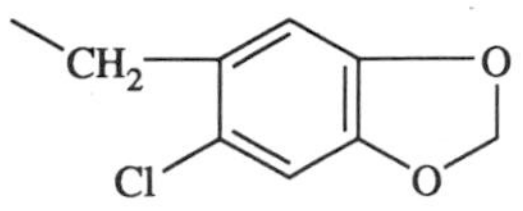
Cypermethrin	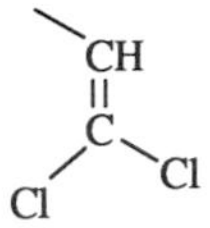	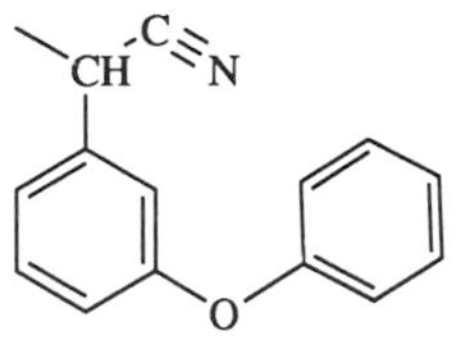
Deltamethrin	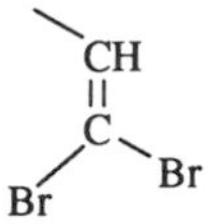	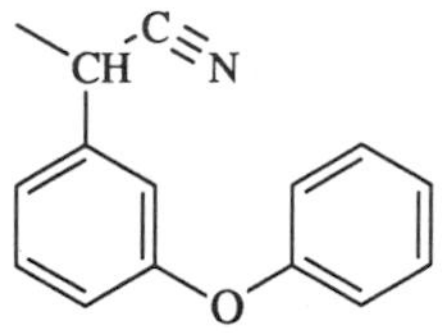
Permethrin	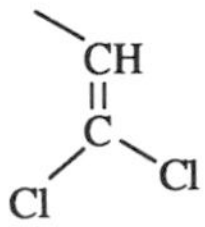	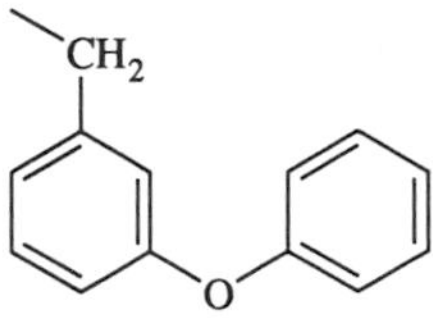
Phenothrin	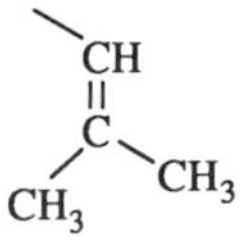	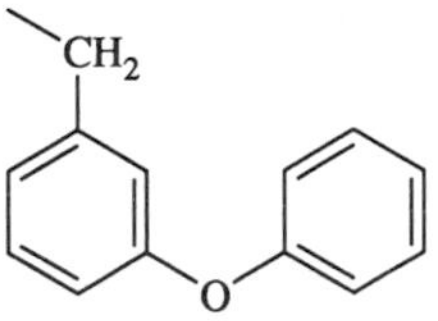

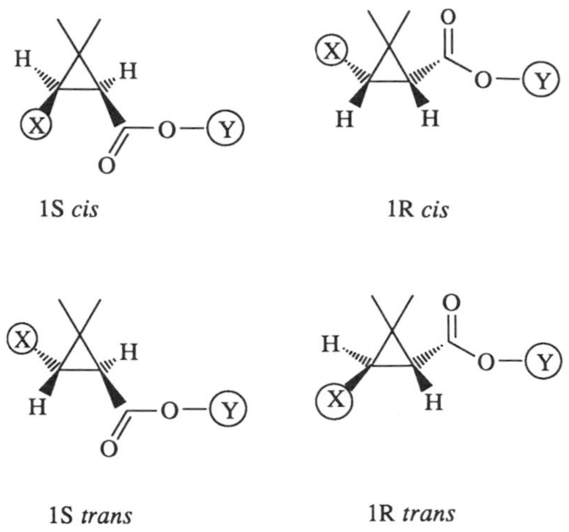

Figure 13.1 Isomerism about the cyclopropane ring. The ring is drawn in the plane of the page.

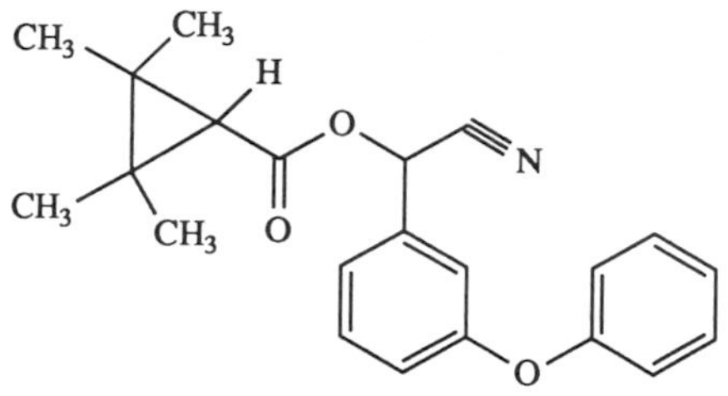

1S cis   1R cis

1S trans   1R trans

Fenproponate

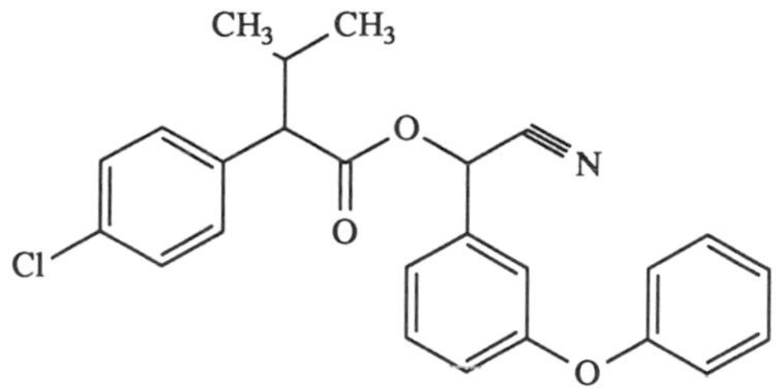

Fenvalerate

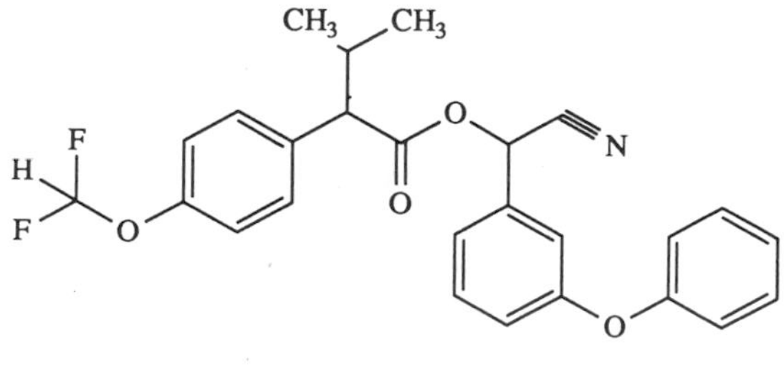

Flucythrinate

Figure 13.2 Other pyrethroids.

tially nontoxic. This is the explanation for much of the wide variation in reported toxicity of racemic mixtures of pyrethroids as detailed for pyrethrum (Section 13.2.1) and permethrin (Section 13.2.8). Isomerism at the third carbon of the cyclopropane ring gives cis and trans isomers which show insecticidal activity (Elliott *et al.*, 1978) but differential mammalian toxicity, with the cis isomers being about ten times more potent than the trans ones (Gray, 1985). A final isomeric center is generated if a cyano substituent is added to the alcohol (see Table 13.2 and Fig. 13.2), giving eight possible isomers. Again this affects potency, with only the α-*S* and not the α-*R* forms being toxic to both insects and mammals. This stereospecificity has been exploited in the synthesis of pure isomers such as deltamethrin (Section 13.2.4) to produce a remarkable degree of selective toxicity (Glomot, 1982).

Interaction with sodium channels is not the only mechanism of action proposed for the pyrethroids. Their effects on the central nervous system have led various workers to suggest actions via antagonism of γ-aminobutyric acid (GABA)-mediated inhibition, modulation of nicotinic cholinergic transmission, enhancement of noradrenaline release, or actions on calcium ions. Since neurotransmitter-specific pharmacological agents offer only poor or partial protection against poisoning (see Therapeutic Agents), it is unlikely that one of these effects represents the primary mechanism of action of the pyrethroids, and most neurotransmitter release is secondary to increased sodium entry [e.g., Eells and Dubocovich, (1988)]. Deltamethrin inhibits binding of ligand to the mammalian GABA complex by 50% at $1.7 \times 10^{-7} M$ (Lawrence et al., 1985) and GABA-stimulated chloride flux is reduced to 28% by $1 \times 10^{-6} M$ cis-cypermethrin (Abalis et al., 1986). These effects are specific for type II pyrethroids but in vivo GABA action is prolonged (Joy et al., 1990) and in vitro inhibition is seen only at 200 times the concentration needed to enhance sodium flux (Soderlund, 1985). An even more marked differential is seen in invertebrates, with sodium effects at $10^{-12} M$ and GABA effects at $10^{-6} M$ (Chalmers et al., 1987). Pyrethroids, however, potentiate pentylenetetrazole convulsions by interaction with benzodiazepine binding sites (Devaud et al., 1986) at more reasonable doses, and this may indicate a potential for an action via GABA. Pyrethroids have no anticholinesterase activity (Ray and Cremer, 1979) and have little effect on acetylcholine sensitivity of muscle (Sherby et al., 1986) but do inhibit acetylcholine-activated calcium flux at $10^{-7} M$ and slow the desensitization of the nicotinic receptor (Sherby et al., 1986). This may lead to some degree of potentiation of nicotinic transmission in the central nervous system (CNS). A more sensitive effect is the stimulation of noradrenaline release from brain synaptosomes, which has an ED 50 of only $2.9 \times 10^{-9} M$ for deltamethrin, although noncyano pyrethroids were ineffective (Brooks and Clark, 1987). This noradrenaline release parallels increased calcium entry and may indicate an action via voltage-sensitive calcium or sodium channels. Related effects are seen in whole animals, where deltamethrin markedly increases plasma noradrenaline (Cremer and Seville, 1982) and enhances the noradrenaline-mediated contraction of mesenteric blood vessels and cardiac contractility (Forshaw and Bradbury, 1983). It has been suggested that the calcium effects may be mediated by an action on calmodulin, but calmodulin-stimulated phosphodiesterase activity is inhibited by pyrethroids only at 10^{-6} to $10^{-4} M$ (Rashatwar and Matsumara, 1985). Narahashi (1986) has also described a *decrease* in fast calcium current in neuroblastoma cells at concentrations similar to those prolonging sodium current. The significance of this is not yet clear, but it may be related to the *depression* of neurosecretion measured *in vitro* after *in vivo* dosing of pyrethroids (Dyball, 1982).

Other biochemical changes are the marked increases in cerebellar cyclic GMP seen during type II intoxication (Aldridge et al., 1978). This would appear to be entirely secondary to the increased motor activity, however (Brodie, 1983), and could not be reproduced in cerebellar slices (Lock and Berry, 1981). Similarly, there are changes in the concentration of several neurotransmitters in the brain which parallel the motor symptoms (Aldridge et al., 1978; Hudson et al., 1986) but which are probably only of secondary importance. Pyrethroids have been shown to inhibit mitochondrial Mg^{2+}-ATPase activity, but only at $2 \times 10^{-5} M$ (Prasada Rao et al., 1984).

Metabolism The relative resistance of mammals to the pyrethroids is almost wholly attributable to their ability to hydrolyze the pyrethroids rapidly to their inactive acid and alcohol components, since direct injection into the mammalian CNS leads to a susceptibility similar to that seen in insects (Lawrence and Casida, 1982). Some additional resistance of homeothermic organisms can also be attributed to the negative temperature coefficient of action of the pyrethroids (van den Bercken et al., 1973), which are thus less toxic at mammalian body temperatures, but the major effect is metabolic. Metabolic disposal of the pyrethroids is very rapid (Gray et al., 1980), which means that toxicity is high by the intravenous route, moderate by slower oral absorption, and often unmeasurably low by dermal absorption. This is illustrated by the intravenous and oral toxicities of a range of pyrethroids shown in Table 13.3 Indirect measurements using the magnitude of biological effect on muscle indicate half-lives of 6–195 min for a range of pyrethroids in the rat (Wright et al., 1987), and the initial half-time for loss of deltamethrin from the brain of rats is 10–30 min (Gray and Rickard, 1982b). This early rapid fall is followed by a much slower loss with a time constant of 1 or 5 days from brain and body fat, where pyrethroids are sequestered in lipid which has a very low pyrethroid esterase capacity (Marei et al., 1982).

The metabolic pathways for the breakdown of the pyrethroids vary little between mammalian species but vary somewhat with structure. This literature has been ably summarized by Leahey (1985), and further references to the metabolism of specific pyrethroids are given in the sections on individual compounds (13.2.1 to 13.2.9). Essentially, pyrethrum and allethrin are broken down mainly by oxidation of the isobutenyl side chain of the acid moiety and of the unsaturated side chain of the alcohol moiety with ester hydrolysis playing an unimportant part, whereas for the other pyrethroids ester hydrolysis predominates. These reactions can take place in both liver and plasma and are followed by hydroxylation and conjugation to glucuronides or sulfates, which are then excreted in the urine. A number of factors modify the rate of breakdown, notably stereospecificity, with trans isomer hydrolysis being catalyzed by esterases but cis isomer hydrolysis being catalyzed at a rather lower rate by oxidases. This slower breakdown of cis isomers may contribute to their greater mammalian toxicity, but their higher inherent affinity for the sodium channel complex is thought to be the predominant factor (Gray, 1985). An additional influence on the rate of metabolism is the presence of an α-cyano group, which slows both hydrolysis and oxidation.

Since metabolic disposal largely determines toxicity, inhibi-

Table 13.3
Acute Toxicity of Pyrethroids

Type I	LD 50[a]	Intermediate	LD 50	Type II	LD 50
Allethrin[b,c]	3.5 (200)	Cyphenothrin[d]	5 (—)	Cyfluthrin[d]	5 (—)
Barthrin[e]	— (23,600)	Fenproponate[b–d]	2.5 (28)	Cyhalothrin[f]	— (144)
Bioallethrin[g]	4 (1030)	Flucythrinate[h]	— (67)	Cypermethrin[b,c]	55 (900)
Bioresmethrin[g,i]	340 (>8000)			Deltamethrin[b,d,i]	2.3 (52)
Cismethrin[g,i]	6.5 (63)			Fenvalerate[b,f,i]	75 (450)
Fenfluthrin[c,d]	1 (120)			cis-Fluorocyphenothrin[d,i]	0.6 (—)
trans-Fluorocyphenothrin[i]	6 (—)				
Kadethrin[b,c]	0.5 (—)				
Permethrin[b,c,i]	>250 (1500)				
Phenothrin[b,f]	472 (>5000)				
Pyrethrin I[b,g]	5 (340)				
Pyrethrin II[b,g]	1 (>600)				
Resmethrin[b,g]	165 (1347)				
Tetramethrin[b,c]	2.3 (>4000)				

[a] Approximate LD 50 in rats via the intravenous or (oral) route in milligrams per kilogram. Female data given where available.
[b] Lawrence and Casida (1982).
[c] R. D. Verschoyle (personal communication).
[d] Wright et al. (1988).
[e] Ambrose (1963).
[f] FAO/WHO (1985).
[g] Verschoyle and Barnes (1972).
[h] FAO/WHO (1986).
[i] Verschoyle and Aldridge (1980).

tion of oxidative and hydrolytic activity with synergists such as piperonyl butoxide or DEF (an organophosphate used as an agricultural defoliant) greatly increases toxicity (Lawrence and Casida, 1982; Casida et al., 1983). This may be of importance in cases of mixed exposures.

Poisoning Syndromes The pyrethroids are essentially functional toxins, producing their harmful effects largely secondarily, as a consequence of neuronal hyperexcitability. This is shown by the lack of pathological effects in the central nervous system even after repeated severe intoxication (A. W. Brown, personal communication) and the production of only reversible, relatively nonspecific lesions in the peripheral nerves of animals showing protracted and severely abnormal motor symptoms (Parker et al., 1985). Despite this dependence on a relatively well-defined mode of action, the pyrethroids are capable of generating a bewildering variety of effects in mammals and insects, which, although showing some analogies with those produced by other sodium channel toxins (Gray, 1985; Lazdunski et al., 1985) and with DDT (Narahashi, 1986), have many unique characteristics (Ray, 1982b). Fortunately, a degree of simplification can be achieved by considering the effects produced by topical application and by systemic intoxication separately and also by dividing the systemic effects into two major classes. Such a division has been made by a number of authors for systemic effects in insects (Clements and May, 1977; Gammon et al., 1981; Salgado et al., 1983), in amphibians (Ruigt and van den Bercken, 1986),

and in mammals (Barnes and Verschoyle, 1974; Verschoyle and Aldridge, 1980; Wright et al., 1988). Generally speaking, there is fairly good agreement between species (Wright et al., 1988), with most noncyano substitute pyrethroids falling into group I and most of the cyano pyrethroids into group II (Table 13.3). Some authors have objected to such a division on the grounds that qualitatively similar electrophysiological changes are produced by all active pyrethroids in both invertebrates (Leake et al., 1985) and mammals (Staatz-Benson and Hosko, 1986) or because some pyrethroids show intermediate characteristics (Verschoyle and Aldridge, 1980; Gammon et al., 1981). There is good evidence, however, that the intermediate compounds represent a true overlap between the classes (Wright et al., 1988). Such a division will be used in this chapter, although the chemical basis for the division is far from clear, with fluorocyphenothrin, for example, falling into type I or type II depending on its isomeric form (Table 13.3).

The type I pyrethroids produce the simplest poisoning syndrome and produce sodium tail currents with relatively short time constants (Wright et al., 1988). Poisoning closely resembles that produced by DDT and was first clearly distinguished by Verschoyle and Aldridge (1980). It involves a progressive development of fine whole-body tremor, exaggerated startle response, incoordinated twitching of the dorsal muscles, hyperexcitability, and death (Ray, 1982b). The tremor is associated with a large increase in metabolic rate and leads to hyperthermia, which, with metabolic exhaustion, is the usual cause of death. Respiration and blood pressure are well sustained

(Ray, 1982b) but plasma noradrenaline, lactate, and to a lesser extent adrenaline are greatly increased (Cremer and Seville, 1982). Type I effects are generated largely by action on the central nervous system, as shown by the good correlation between brain levels of cismethrin and tremor (White *et al.*, 1976) and the induction of tremor by small quantities of cismethrin directly injected into the CNS (Gray and Rickard, 1982a; Staatz *et al.*, 1982). Poisoning is associated with marked increases in both spinal (Carlton, 1977; Staatz-Benson and Hosko, 1986) and brain stem excitability (Forshaw and Ray, 1986), although not with marked effects on the higher centers. Thus lethal doses of cismethrin do not induce cortical electroencephalogram (EEG) spiking (Ray, 1982a) although supralethal doses in paralyzed, ventilated animals do (Staatz and Hosko, 1985). Also, when cismethrin is injected into the lateral ventricles tremor is seen only when enough is given to reach the brain stem (Gray and Rickard, 1982a) and, although primary increases in reflex excitability are seen in the brain stem and spinal cord, only secondary effects are seen at the cerebellar, thalamic, and cerebral cortical levels (Ray, 1982a). In addition to these central effects, there is evidence for repetitive firing in sensory nerves, which although a small effect in one study (Staatz-Benson and Hosko, 1986) was more pronounced in others (Forshaw and Ray, 1986; Wright *et al.*, 1988). Such repetitive firing is analogous to that seen in amphibians (Vijverberg *et al.*, 1982) and probably contributes to the hyperexcitable state produced by the central actions of the type I pyrethroids.

The type II pyrethroids produce a more complex poisoning syndrome and act on a wider range of tissues. They give sodium tail currents with relatively long time constants (Wright, *et al.*, 1988), which may be the reason for their ability to act on the whole range of excitable tissues. First noted by Barnes and Verschoyle (1974), type II poisoning in rats involves progressive development of nosing and exaggerated jaw opening similar to that seen in response to an irritant placed on the tongue, salivation which may be profuse, increasing extensor tone in the hind limbs causing a rolling gait, incoordination progressing to a very coarse tremor, choreoform movements of the limbs and tail often precipitated by sensory stimuli, generalized choreoathetosis (writhing spasms), tonic seizures, apnea, and death (Ray, 1982b). At lower doses more subtle repetitive behavior is seen (Brodie and Aldridge, 1982). In dogs, similar symptoms are seen but salivation and upper airway hypersecretion and gastrointestinal symptoms are more prominent (Thiebault *et al.*, 1985). Unlike the type I syndrome, type II pyrethroids generally decrease rather than increase the startle response to sound (Crofton and Reiter, 1984), although this is a complex response and at low doses some type II pyrethroids give an increased startle (Hijzen and Slangen, 1988). The cerebral cortical response to sound is also depressed (Ray, 1980) and the latency of the visual response increased (Dyer, 1985). As in type I poisoning, plasma noradrenaline is increased by type II pyrethroids, but there is also a large increase in adrenaline and in blood glucose (Ray and Cremer, 1979; Cremer and Seville, 1982) which is not seen in type I poisoning. Type II

but not type I pyrethroids also increase cardiac contractility both directly by action on cardiac muscle and via circulating and locally released catecholamines (Forshaw and Bradbury, 1983). They also cause repetitive firing and potentiate contraction in skeletal muscle (Forshaw *et al.*, 1986). These effects are limited to a large degree by physiological compensation, which maintains blood pressure at normal levels in intact rats despite some arrhythmias, and by the inability of skeletal muscle to sustain repetitive firing for more than a few seconds at normal discharge frequencies. Both effects are therefore of secondary importance in the normal animal. As with type I pyrethroids, the primary action is on the central nervous system, since symptoms correlate well with brain concentrations (Rickard and Brodie, 1985) and can be reproduced in part by microinjection into the CNS (Brodie, 1985; Staatz *et al.*, 1982). The former injection studies showed, however, that actions at all levels of the neuroaxis are needed to reproduce the full range of effects. Thus, although choreoathetosis can be reproduced in spinal rats (Bradbury *et al.*, 1983), other symptoms are generated at higher levels and are associated with EEG spiking at cortical and subcortical sites which ultimately progresses to slow-wave activity and loss of consciousness not seen for type I pyrethroids (Ray, 1980). Although there is evidence for increased neuronal activity in both the spinal cord (Staatz-Genson and Hosko, 1986) and brain (Ray, 1980; Staatz and Hosko, 1985), the type II pyrethroids do not produce the repetitive activity in sensory nerves seen after type I pyrethroids (Wright *et al.*, 1988). This again is analogous to the effects seen in amphibians (Vijverberg *et al.*, 1982). As might be expected, both classes of pyrethroid produce large increases in brain glucose utilization, this being most marked in motor areas (Cremer *et al.*, 1983; Cremer and Seville, 1985). Such increases seem to be secondary to increased neuronal activity and are paralleled by increased brain blood flow except in the cerebral cortex, where the flow increase is disproportionally large. This component of the blood flow increase is cholinergically mediated and can be blocked by atropine without affecting the motor actions (Lister and Ray, 1988) as the motor actions can be blocked without preventing the blood flow increase (Bradbury *et al.*, 1983). A final factor distinguishing type II pyrethroids is their ability to depress resting chloride conductance, thereby amplifying any sodium or calcium effects (Forshaw and Ray, 1990).

Intermediate signs representing a combination of types I and II are produced by some pyrethroids (Table 13.3). These appear to represent a true combination of the I and II classes (Wright *et al.*, 1988) and thus represent a transitional group. Evidence in support of this is given by measurement of the time constants of the sodium afterpotential produced by the pyrethroids. These are short for the type I and long for the type II pyrethroids. For the whole range of pyrethroids, time constants range from 5 to 1772 msec in amphibians (Vijverberg and de Weille, 1985) and 2.3 to 33 msec in mammals (Wright, *et al.*, 1988), and the intermediate structures fit in the middle of these ranges.

Topical application of pyrethrins and pyrethroids to skin

produces additional effects unrelated to their systemic actions. The plant products associated with impure pyrethrum extracts can give rise to contact dermatitis, described in Section 13.2.1.3, and in addition the pure synthetic pyrethroids have a separate irritant effect if they reach sufficient concentration in the skin. This irritation is not associated with inflammation (Flannigan and Tucker, 1985a) and appears to be unique to the pyrethroids. It lasts for up to 24 hr and, when intense, is associated with numbness (paresthesia) and is produced by all classes of pyrethroid although most readily by the type II pyrethroids. The effect is annoying but not disabling and does not appear to be associated with any lasting ill effects (Le-Quesne et al., 1980). An animal model has been developed (Cagen et al., 1984) and also a clinical test, which, in animals, can detect nerve hyperexcitability up to 24 hr after exposure (Parkin and LeQuesne, 1982). Since veratrine produces a similar response to the pyrethroids in a guinea pig model of paresthesia (McKillop et al., 1987), it appears likely that repetitive firing in sensory nerves is involved in the irritation. The peripheral nerve damage produced by repeated systemic dosage (see cypermethrin, fenvalerate, permethrin) is a different effect, since it appears only when severe motor symptoms are produced (Rose and Dewar, 1983).

Therapeutic Agents   Since the pyrethroids appear to be essentially functional toxins, they produce few if any specific neuropathological effects. Therapy can thus be directed at limiting hyperexcitability and its consequences—hyperthermia, choreoathetosis, hypersecretion, seizures, etc.—until the pyrethroids are removed from the body by metabolism. As already stated, the pyrethroids have little selectivity for specific neurotransmitter systems and so general membrane-stabilizing agents are usually the most effective. An exception to this rule is the remarkable efficacy of diazepam against intraventricularly administered type II pyrethroids (Gammon et al., 1982). This route produces atypical effects, however, probably due to high local concentrations in the hippocampus, and diazepam is only poorly effective against systemic pyrethroids in rats (Staatz et al., 1982), effective only against the terminal seizures of the type II syndrome in another study (Cremer et al., 1980), and only moderately effective in the dog (Thiebault et al., 1985). Atropine is effective against the profuse salivation of the type II syndrome (Ray and Cremer, 1979) but prevents the other actions only at very high nonspecific doses.

The anesthetics phenobarbital and pentobarbital are effective especially against type I pyrethroids [Food and Agriculture Organization/World Health Organization (FAO/WHO), 1980], although only at anesthetic concentrations, as is urethane (LeClercq et al., 1986; Wright et al., 1988). The muscle relaxant mephenesin has a degree of selectivity, preventing choreoathetosis at moderate doses but giving full protection against both classes of pyrethroid only at doses producing a marked loss in muscle tone (Bradbury et al., 1983). Similar effects are also produced by other spinally acting muscle relaxants such as methocarbamol, chlorphenesin, chloroxazone, and metaxalone (Gray and Gray, 1990) but not by peripherally acting agents

such as dantrolene. The sedative clomethiazole is also effective against the type II pyrethroid deltamethrin (Thiebault et al., 1985), blocking the major signs with greater specificity than diazepam. Combined diazepam–clomethiazole therapy was found to be effective (with atropine to prevent dyspnea due to excess saliva, etc.) but did not decrease toxicity to the same extent as full anesthesia (LeClercq et al., 1986).

The skin irritation and paresthesia produced by topical application of pyrethroids are alleviated by application of vitamin E cream (Flannigan and Tucker, 1985b). Similar effects can be shown in guinea pigs, where pre- or posttreatment of skin with vitamin E cream markedly reduced the licking, biting, and scratching responses elicited by dermal application of fenvalerate (Malley et al., 1985). The vitamin E was effective if applied from 29 hr before to 15 min after the pyrethroid and protection lasted for more than 5 hr, but the concentration required to give greater protection than that of the corn oil solvent alone was very high (50%) and the specificity and mechanism of action of vitamin E protection are unclear. Similarly, in humans considerable relief can be obtained by use of presumably inert preparations such as corn oil or Vaseline as well as vitamin E (Tucker et al., 1983). Clearly, any lipophilic agent which removes absorbed pyrethroid from the skin should be effective against this distressing if not harmful action of the pyrethroids since they are only very slowly absorbed through the skin (Scott and Ramsey, 1987). Topical treatment with local anesthetic has been described in humans and in animals (FAO/WHO, 1982; Malley et al., 1985), but the effects of such treatment may be more inconvenient than the paresthesia itself. Indeed, it may even be considered that *preventive* therapy against paresthesia is undesirable, as the paresthesia serves as an indicator of poor work and handling practices, and that it would be better to improve these even though there is no evidence to suggest that such low-level dermal exposures are harmful in themselves.

13.2.1 PYRETHRUM

13.2.1.1 Identity, Properties, and Uses

Chemical Name   The six known insecticidally active compounds in pyrethrum are esters of two acids and three alcohols. Specifically, pyrethrin I is the pyrethrolone ester of chrysanthemic acid, pyrethrin II is the pyrethrolone ester of pyrethric acid, cinerin I is the cinerolone ester of chrysanthemic acid, cinerin II is the cinerolone ester of pyrethric acid, jasmolin I is the jasmolone ester of chrysanthemic acid, and jasmolin II is the jasmolone ester of pyrethric acid. There is much evidence indicating that the biological activity of these molecules depends on their configuration (Elliott, 1969, 1971). Actually, free rotation is possible about all the acyclic single bonds, permitting a wide range of molecular shapes. However, preferred conformations can be deduced, and spectral methods such as nuclear magnetic resonance (NMR) can indicate average conformation. The present consensus about conformation of the molecules is indicated in Table 13.1.

Structure   See Table 13.1

Synonyms   "Insect powder" made from "Dalmatian insect flowers" (*Chrysanthemum cinerariaefolium*) is called pyrethrum powder or simply pyrethrum. The powder itself was formerly used as an insecticide, but now it is usually extracted. The primary extract yields, after concentration, a dark viscous material containing approximately 30–35% pyrethrins and about 50% impurities (oleoresin concentrate), which may be diluted and standardized to contain 25% pyrethrins (oleoresin extract). The oleoresin may be processed further to form a refined extract containing 50–55% total pyrethrins and about 23% impurities. The six active ingredients are known collectively as pyrethrins; those based on chrysanthemic acid are called pyrethrins I, and those based on pyrethric acid are called pyrethrins II. Purified separate isomers or mixtures of isomers are available only in the laboratory; they are too expensive for practical use.

Physical and Chemical Properties   The empirical formulas and molecular weights are:

Pyrethrin I	$C_{21}H_{28}O_3$	328.4
Pyrethrin II	$C_{22}H_{28}O_5$	372.4
Cinerin I	$C_{20}H_{28}O_3$	316.4
Cinerin II	$C_{21}H_{28}O_5$	360.4
Jasmolin I	$C_{21}H_{30}O_3$	330.4
Jasmolin II	$C_{22}H_{30}O_5$	374.4

Stability   Pyrethrins are decomposed by exposure to light with loss of insecticidal activity. They also are rapidly oxidized and inactivated by air. Antioxidants used to help protect insecticidal residues of pyrethrins include minute concentrations of pyrocatechol, pyrogallol, and hydroquinone; 1-benzene-azo-2-naphthol is used to protect against the effects of sunlight. As the pyrethrins approach 100% purity, their stability decreases; pyrethrins I and II are less stable than the other compounds. They must be stored in glass wrapped in metal foil, sealed in polythene, at a temperature of about −25°C.

Formulations, Uses, and Production   Pyrethrins, generally combined with a synergist, are used in sprays and aerosols against a wide range of flying insects. The usual household formulation contains about 0.5% active pyrethrum principles. They are also extensively used in veterinary flea powders for cats and dogs.

13.2.1.2 Toxicity to Laboratory Animals

Pyrethrum and the pyrethrins produce typical type I motor symptoms in mammals. The acute oral LD 50's for pyrethrins I and II are given in Table 13.3 as 340 and >600 mg/kg, respectively (Verschoyle and Barnes, 1972), and Casida *et al.* (1971)

found values of 450–2000 and over 2900 mg/kg for the two pyrethrins when given as divided doses over 12–54 hr. There is, however, a great divergence in the published literature with regard to the acute toxicity of unpurified pyrethrum extract, with oral LD 50 values in rats ranging from 200 to 1870 mg/kg (Hayes, 1982). This would appear to be largely attributable to variations in the constituents of the pyrethrum extracts used, and toxicity was also highly dependent on the concentration of the dosing solutions. This conflicting older literature is well reviewed by Barthel (1973). In a study using a range of pyrethrin extracts, rat oral LD 50 values ranged from 273 to 796 mg/kg (Malone and Brown, 1968).

When pyrethrins were fed at a dietary level of 1000 or 5000 ppm for 2 years, the liver lesions included bile duct proliferation and focal necrosis of the liver cells (Lehman, 1965). Pyrethrins, especially synergized pyrethrins, produced enlargement, margination, and cytoplasmic inclusions in the liver cells of rats. At a dietary level of 1000 ppm pyrethrins and 10,000 ppm piperonyl butoxide, the changes were well developed in only 8 days but of course were not maximal. The changes were proportional to dosage and similar to those produced by DDT. The effects of the two materials were additive (Kimbrough *et al.*, 1968). No relevant pathology was detected in rats fed pyrethrins at a dietary level of 8000 ppm for 5 weeks (Griffin, 1973). The resulting dosage (911 mg/kg/day) was more than double what we would expect for the dietary concentration, indicating a very unusual diet or careless arithmetic. Furthermore, one would expect liver changes in such rats. In fact, the presence of liver enlargement has been confirmed, and its expected correspondence with the induction of a number of microsomal enzymes has been demonstrated (Springfield *et al.*, 1973). Pregnant rats fed 150 mg/kg on days 6–15 showed only a small increase in the number of resorptions and no malformations (Khera *et al.*, 1982). Pyrethrum is not mutagenic in bacterial reversion tests (Moriya *et al.*, 1983).

Metabolism is rapid and involves oxidation at several sites. Hydrolysis of the ester bond is only a minor pathway (Casida, 1973).

With regard to the dermal effects of pyrethrum, Rickett *et al.* (1972) were able to demonstrate both immediate and delayed hypersensitivity in guinea pigs sensitized by a single subcutaneous injection of ground flowers suspended in Freund's complete adjuvant. A hexane extract, similar to pyrethrum oleoresin, produced a moderate reaction, and various aqueous extracts elicited strong reactions. A commercially refined extract proved negative. The allergens in the aqueous extracts could not be dialyzed. Methylene chloride extracts of flowers previously extracted by hexane were irritating to the skin. Further study (Rickett and Tyskiewicz, 1973) revealed that two types of allergens were present in crude pyrethrum oleoresin. The more potent were compounds similar to those extracted from pyrethrum flowers by saline. They were thought to be glycoproteins or glycopeptides ranging in molecular weight from about 60,000 to 200,000. The second class of allergens were sesquiterpene lactones, principally pyrethrosin, but they were of minor importance due to their low concentrations in the oleoresin. The allergenicity of sesquiterpene lactones has been confirmed (Hausen and Schulz, 1973).

13.2.1.3 Toxicity to Humans

Experimental Exposure   When 200 people (177 women and 23 men) were patch tested with a 1% water dispersion of pyrethrins, no evidence of primary irritancy or of sensitization was found (unpublished report, cited by FAO/WHO, 1971). Mitchell *et al.* (1972) found all the active ingredients of pyrethrum, except pyrethrin II, to be inactive on patch test in a patient who had a history of allergenic dermatitis to pyrethrum and who reacted positively to pyrethrum flower heads and powder, extracts of the plant, and pyrethrosin. It would appear that the contact dermatitis produced by crude pyrethrum extracts is due to impurities. This is borne out by the lack of any such reaction to the pure synthetic pyrethroids (Flannigan and Tucker, 1985a).

Therapeutic Use   Sensitivity was produced in 10–26% of unselected test populations by repeated application of pyrethrum ointment (Lord and Johnson, 1947). On the other hand, the insecticide has been considered so innocuous that an ointment containing 0.75% pyrethrin was recommended for treatment of scabies, and such use led to only a few cases of dermatitis, some of doubtful relation to the treatment (Sweitzer and Tedder, 1935; Sweitzer, 1936). Pyrethrins have been used extensively for the control of human body lice. The formulation employed during the early part of World War II was called MYL powder; its use was discontinued only after the more effective and long-lasting DDT louse powder became available (Simmons, 1959). Pyrethrins are still effective for control of head lice (Gerberg, 1973).

Pyrethrum was used orally as an anthelmintic in some areas for many years with no apparent ill effects (Gnadinger, 1936).

Accidental and Intentional Poisoning   Very little injury by pyrethrum has been the result of recognized accidents. There is one report of a 2-year-old girl in Montreal who died after eating about half an ounce of insect powder (Anonymous, 1889). An 11-month-old infant was playing with a box of pyrethrum powder when the top came off and the child's mouth, nostrils, and entire face were covered with the powder. Within moments, the baby suffered pallor, intermittent convulsions, and then vomiting. As soon as a physician arrived, he found the child collapsed, reddened by pain when pulled up by the hands, and refusing to nurse. The heart sounds were feeble and slow and the respiration was labored. The face and mucous membranes were washed carefully. Two doses of syrup of ipecac (10 g each at an interval of 5 min) produced abundant vomiting. Except for a slight inflammation of the conjuctivae and extreme reddening of the lips and tongue, the child was essentially recovered in 1.5 hr and resumed nursing (Bosredon, 1897).

Use Experience   Injury to humans from pyrethrum has most frequently resulted from the allergenic properties of the mate-

rial rather than its direct toxicity. Although the allergy usually has been associated with occupational or therapeutic contact, it is impossible to exclude the possibility of injury associated with other kinds of exposure.

Many reports of pyrethrum dermatitis involved contact with flowers in connection with harvesting, weighing, or grinding (McCord *et al.*, 1921; Tonking, 1936). However, dermatitis (Kesten and Laszlo, 1931; Schwartz, 1934) and especially allergy of the respiratory tract (Feinberg, 1934; Ramirez, 1930) may result from exposure to pyrethrum formulations intended for use in the home or workplace.

Superficial corneal abrasions have been reported after use of a 0.17% synergized pyrethrin shampoo to control head lice in children (Clarke, 1986), although this may have been the result of ingredients other than pyrethrins.

Dosage Response   Under practical conditions, pyrethrum and its derivatives are probably the least toxic to mammals of all the insecticides currently in use. The death of a 2-year-old child following the eating of $\frac{1}{2}$ ounce (14,000 mg) of powder was attributed to pyrethrum poisoning (Anonymous, 1889). No information is available on the dosage necessary to elicit an allergic reaction in susceptible persons. When pyrethrins were used as an anthelmintic, the dosage suggested was 20 mg for adults and 10 mg for children given daily for 3 days in the form of an emulsion formed by adding an alcoholic solution to water (Chevalier, 1930).

The concentration of 5 mg/m^3, considered safe for occupational exposure, would determine a respiratory intake of 0.7 mg/kg/day.

Laboratory Findings   Positive patch tests with pyrethrum are helpful in diagnosis. Eosinophilia may accompany the acute allergic reaction. Examination of mucous nasal smears from individuals with vasomotor rhinitis reveals numerous eosinophils following exposure.

13.2.2 BARTHRIN

13.2.2.1 Identity, Properties, and Uses

Chemical Name   2,2-Dimethyl-3-(2-methyl-1-propenyl)cyclopropanecarboxylic acid (6-chloro-1,3-benzodioxol-5-yl) methyl ester, or 2,2-dimethyl-3-(2-methylpropenyl)cyclopropanecarboxylic acid 6-chloropiperonyl ester.

Structure   See Table 13.2.

Synonyms   Barthrin is the common name in use. Other names for the compound are 6-chloropiperonyl chrysanthemumate and chrysanthemummonocarboxylic acid 6-chloropiperonyl ester. A code designation is ENT-21,557. The CAS registry number is 70-43-9.

Physical and Chemical Properties   Barthrin has the empirical formula $C_{18}H_{21}ClO_4$ and a molecular weight of 336.83.

It is a pale yellow oily liquid that boils at 155–171°C at 0.2 mm Hg and at 184–206°C at 0.7 mm Hg. It is soluble in kerosene.

History and Use Patented in 1959, barthrin is a synthetic pyrethroid insecticide, now no longer in production.

13.2.2.2 Toxicity to Laboratory Animals

Barthrin is a typical type I pyrethroid and has a low mammalian toxicity; the oral LD 50 in male rats is 23,600 mg/kg. Daily oral doses of 11,800 mg/kg for 15 days had no adverse effect (Ambrose, 1963).

13.2.2.3 Toxicity to Humans

No primary irritation, sensitization, or allergic response was observed among seven volunteers who received ten daily applications of 0.5 ml of undiluted technical barthrin on gauze covered by a plastic adhesive compress. The pads were attached to the left antecubital fossa for about 8 hr/day, 5 days/week. Ten days after the last 0.5-ml application, each subject was challenged with 0.1 ml of undiluted barthrin (Ambrose, 1963).

Treatment would be symptomatic if ever required.

13.2.3 CYPERMETHRIN

13.2.3.1 Identity, Properties, and Uses

Chemical Name (R,S)-α-Cyano-3-phenoxybenzyl-2,2-dimethyl $(1R,1S)$-cis,trans-3-(2,2-dichlorovinyl)cyclopropane-carboxylate. There are eight isomeric forms.

Structure See Table 13.2.

Synonyms Cypermethrin (ANSI, BSI, ISO) is the common name in use. Trade names are Polytrin®, Stockade®, Folcord®, Ripcord®, and Cymbush®. Code designations for the compound include NRDC149, WL43467, PP383, CCN52, and OMS2002. The CAS registry number is 52315-07-8.

Physical and Chemical Properties Cypermethrin has the empirical formula $C_{22}H_{19}O_3NCl_2$ and a molecular weight of 416.31. The racemic mixture is a viscous yellow liquid and the pure isomers are colorless crystals with melting points between 60 and 80°C. The density is 1.12 gm/ml at 22°C and the vapor pressure 4×10^{-8} mm Hg at 70°C. Its water solubility is 9 μg/liter, but it is freely soluble in most organic solvents. It is light stable.

History, Formulations, and Uses Cypermethrin was first described by Dr. M. Elliott in 1974 and was introduced commercially in 1977 as an emulsifiable concentrate to be used against a wide range of insect pests.

13.2.3.2 Toxicity to Laboratory Animals

Cypermethrin produces typical type II motor symptoms in mammals (Lawrence and Casida, 1982). The acute oral LD 50 in female rats is given in Table 13.3 as 900 mg/kg, but this varies with the cis/trans ratio and the vehicle used from 367 to 2000 mg/kg (FAO/WHO, 1980). Values ranging from 82 to 779 mg/kg were obtained for mice. The intravenous LD 50 in rats is approximately 55 mg/kg (R. D. Verschoyle, personal communication) but dermal toxicity is very low, the acute LD 50 being in excess of 4800 mg/kg and five consecutive daily doses of 5000 mg/kg/day producing 20–30% mortality (FAO/WHO, 1980). Rats receiving 750 ppm of the potent cis isomer of cypermethrin in their diet for 5 weeks showed gross motor symptoms but no fatalities, whereas 1500 ppm caused deaths from 4 to 17 days. Fatalities were associated with axonal swelling and demyelination in the sciatic nerve. This peripheral nerve damage was not seen in the 750-ppm group, in survivors from the higher-dose group, or in rats fed a racemic mixture of 1000 ppm for 2 years (FAO/WHO, 1980). Dogs were rather less susceptible to cypermethrin, dietary levels of 1500 ppm for 13 weeks producing motor symptoms but no fatalities. Cypermethrin has been reported to have no teratogenic or mutagenic activity (FAO/WHO, 1980), but Amer and Aboul-ela (1985) have reported that cypermethrin increased the incidence of polychromatic erythrocytes with micronuclei in mouse bone marrow. This increase was significant after feeding cypermethrin at 900 but not 300 ppm in the diet for 7 days and disappeared after a 14-day recovery period. No deaths were seen at this dosage. Intraperitoneal injections of cypermethrin at 180 mg/kg (LD 60), three doses of 60 mg/kg over 10 days (LD 20), or two dermal doses at 360 mg/kg over 7 days (LD 20) produced similar transient effects. The authors concluded that this indicated that cypermethrin showed mutagenic potential. Another report (L'vova, 1984) found negative effects in mouse bone marrow and in cultured human lymphocytes but an increase in chromosome aberrations in yeasts, while Pluijmen et al. (1984) found no mutagenic effects in *Salmonella* or hamster cells and Waters et al. (1982) also failed to see any effect on mouse bone marrow.

Metabolism of cypermethrin in rats closely resembles that of other α-cyano-3-phenoxybenzyl pyrethroids, with rapid hydroxylation and cleavage at the ester bond (Crawford et al., 1981). This occurs over hours, but there is a much slower elimination of cypermethrin sequestered in body fat with a half-life of 18 days for the cis isomer or 3.4 days for the trans isomer (Rhodes et al., 1984).

13.2.3.3 Toxicity to Humans

Dermal exposure to cypermethrin during spray application at up to 46 mg/hr led to an estimation that approximately 3% was absorbed (FAO/WHO, 1980). A further study in which workers were monitored over seven fortnightly spraying sessions under tropical conditions showed absorption to be less than that expected from an oral dose of 1 mg per session (FAO/WHO,

1982). These exposures gave rise to no adverse effects, but LeQuesne *et al.* (1980) reported that pesticide workers exposed to cypermethrin and other pyrethroids developed a transient abnormal facial sensation similar to that described for fenvalerate after accidental direct contact with solutions or after use of fine powder formulations. The facial sensation was not associated with any abnormal neurological or electrophysiological changes. Similar sensations were produced by experimental dermal application of cypermethrin to the ear lobe of human volunteers at 130 $\mu g/cm^2$ (Flannigan and Tucker, 1985b). Cypermethrin was the first pyrethroid to be reported as having caused a human fatality. In Greece a man died 3 hr after eating a meal cooked in a 10% cypermethrin concentrate used in error instead of oil. Nausea, prolonged vomiting with colicky pain, tenesmus, and diarrhea began within a few minutes after eating the meal and progressed to convulsions, unconsciousness, and coma. Death due to respiratory failure occurred despite intensive emergency treatment. Other family members developed less severe symptoms and survived after intensive hospital treatment. Tissue residues of cypermethrin were below detection levels, but 0.7 gm remained in the stomach (Poulos *et al.*, 1982). Unfortunately, the quantity of cypermethrin ingested by any of those poisoned is unknown. He *et al.* (1989) have described 45 cases of moderate intoxication including oral ingestion of up to 140 mg/kg, all of which survived after gastric lavage. Signs of intoxication were typical of those described for deltamethrin. Urinary excretion of cypermethrin metabolites was complete 48 hr after the last of 5 daily tracer doses of 1.5 mg (Eadsforth *et al.*, 1988).

13.2.4 DELTAMETHRIN

13.2.4.1 Identity, Properties, and Uses

Chemical Name *S*-α-Cyano-3-phenoxybenzyl-(1*R*)-*cis*-3-(2,2-dibromovinyl)-2,2-dimethylcyclopropanecarboxylate. It is a single isomer.

Structure See Table 13.3.

Synonyms Deltamethrin (BSI, ISO) (formerly decamethrin) is the common name in use. Trade names are K-Othrine®, Butox®, and Decis®. Code designations include NRDC 161, OMS 1998 and RU 22974. The CAS registry number is 52918-63-5.

Physical and Chemical Properties Deltamethrin has the empirical formula $C_{22}H_{19}Br_2NO_3$ and a molecular weight of 505.24. It is a white or slightly beige powder that melts between 98 and 101°C. The vapor pressure is 1.5×10^{-8} mm Hg at 25°C. Its water solubility is less than 2 μg/liter, but it is readily soluble in most organic solvents. It is stable to light.

History, Formulations, and Uses Deltamethrin was first described by Dr. M. Elliott in 1974 and was introduced com-

mercially in 1978 to be used against a wide range of insect pests.

13.2.4.2 Toxicity to Laboratory Animals

Deltamethrin produces typical type II motor symptoms in mammals (Barnes and Verschoyle, 1974; Verschoyle and Aldridge, 1980). The acute oral LD 50 in female rats is given in Table 13.3 as 52 mg/kg and published values for rats range from 31 to 139 mg/kg (Kavlock *et al.*, 1979; FAO/WHO, 1981). Values ranging from 21 to 34 mg/kg were obtained for mice but of 300 mg/kg for dogs (Thiebault *et al.*, 1985). The intravenous LD 50 in rats and dogs was between 2 and 2.6 mg/kg (Verschoyle and Aldridge, 1980; Thiebault *et al.*, 1985) and the dermal toxicity in excess of 2940 mg/kg (FAO/WHO, 1981). Rats and dogs given oral doses of 10 mg/kg/day for 13 weeks showed some motor symptoms but no fatalities and showed no pathological changes (FAO/WHO, 1981). The dogs showed diarrhea, vomiting, and depression of the gag and patellar reflexes and hind limb placing reaction in addition to the typical type II motor symptoms. In another study, rats given 15 daily oral doses of 10 mg/kg (LD 50) showed severe motor symptoms, but a full neuropathological examination of the central nervous system showed no pathological changes (A. W. Brown, personal communication). Deltamethrin has no teratogenic or mutagenic activity (Kavlock *et al.*, 1979; Pluijmen *et al.*, 1984).

Metabolism of deltamethrin in rats involves rapid ester cleavage and hydroxylation (Ruzo *et al.*, 1978; Shono *et al.*, 1979). Deltamethrin has a half-life in rat brain of 1–2 days, but it is rather more persistent in body fat, with a half-life of 5 days (Marei *et al.*, 1982).

13.2.4.3 Toxicity to Humans

He *et al.* (1989) have reported 158 cases of dermal deltamethrin poisoning after agricultural use with inadequate handling precautions, and a further 167 cases of accidental or suicidal poisoning mostly by the oral route at doses estimated at 2–250 mg/kg. Oral ingestion caused epigastric pain, nausea (60%), vomiting (57%) and coarse muscular fasciculations, with higher doses of 100–250 mg/kg causing coma within 15–20 min. Two cases were fatal. Repeated motor seizures with upper limb flexion and lower limb extension, opisthotonos, and unconsciousness were also seen as frequently as 10–30 per day and only resolving after 2–3 weeks. Recovery was then rapid with no persisting ill effects. As in animals the "seizures" were poorly controlled by anesthetics, phenytoin, diazepam or chlorpromazine whilst atropine was effective against the hypersalivation and pulmonary edema. Less severe systemic poisoning caused sharp EEG waves without motor signs. No inhibition of blood cholinesterase was seen in unmixed exposures. Perhaps the most interesting feature of these cases is the long duration of intoxication, which followed a time course more like that expected for loss of pyrethroid from body fat than from blood or brain. This may be a particular feature of high-level exposures by the dermal route.

Workers exposed to deltamethrin during its manufacture over 7–8 years experienced transient cutaneous and mucous membrane irritation which could be prevented by use of gloves and face masks, but no other ill effects were seen. Similar findings were obtained for agricultural use in Yugoslavia (FAO/WHO, 1983), and Chinese workers exposed to deltamethrin dusts experienced facial burning, itching, and numbness, i.e., paresthesia (He *et al.*, 1989). Workers handling deltamethrin concentrates, especially in aromatic solvents, without adequate protection of the facial skin experienced more severe irritation. This involved an initial painful pruritis and a blotchy erythema and burning sensation, which persisted for several days (FAO/WHO, 1982). This irritant effect of deltamethrin has not been studied in greater detail in humans, but there is no reason to suppose that it differs in principle from that produced by other pyrethroids such as fenvalerate.

13.2.5 FENPROPONATE

13.2.5.1 Identity, Properties, and Uses

Chemical Name α-Cyano-3-phenoxybenzyl-2,2,3,3-tetramethylcyclopropanecarboxylate. There are eight isomeric forms.

Structure See Table 13.2.

Synonyms Fenproponate and fenpropathrin are the common names in use. Trade names are Danitol® and Meothrin®. Code designations for the compound include S3206, SD41706, WL41706, and OMS1999. The CAS registry number is 39515-41-8.

Physical and Chemical Properties Fenproponate has the empirical formula $C_{22}H_{23}NO_3$ and a molecular weight of 349.43. The racemic mixture is a yellow viscous liquid and the pure isomers are colorless crystals with melting points between 45 and 50°C. Its water solubility is 330 μg/liter at 25°C, and it is freely soluble in most organic solvents. It is light stable.

History, Formulations, and Uses Fenproponate was first developed by Sumitomo in 1971 and introduced commercially in 1980 as an emulsifiable concentrate to be used against a wide range of insect pests.

13.2.5.2 Toxicity to Laboratory Animals

Fenproponate produces intermediate or mixed motor symptoms in mammals (Lawrence and Casida, 1982; Wright *et al.*, 1987). This means that a fine tremor characteristic of the type I syndrome is superimposed on the facial movements, salivation, and abnormal gait characteristic of the type II syndrome and that the higher-dosage symptoms become complex, involving both hyperexcitability and seizures. The oral LD 50

in female rats is 17–46 mg/kg and the intravenous LD 50 2.5 mg/kg for a 50 : 50 *R* : *S* mixture (R. D. Verschoyle, personal communication). When synergized with piperonyl butoxide the intraperitoneal LD 50 in rats was 3.7 mg/kg (Lawrence and Casida, 1982).

Metabolism of fenproponate in rats involves rapid oxidase-catalyzed ester cleavage followed by hydroxylation (Crawford and Hutson, 1977).

13.2.5.3 Toxicity to Humans

In a study of transient abnormal facial sensation produced by the pyrethroids (LeQuesne *et al.*, 1980), fenproponate was the compound most frequently associated with symptoms. This was after direct application of concentrates to the facial skin or after exposure to dusts. Symptoms involved a tingling sensation, not associated with loss of normal sensation, distributed over the face, especially under the eyes and around the nose. These symptoms appeared within 0.5–3 hr, persisted for 0.5–8 hr, were not associated with any abnormal neurological or electrophysiological changes, and would appear to represent a milder form of the paresthesia reported for other pyrethroids (Flannigan *et al.*, 1985).

13.2.6 FENVALERATE

13.2.6.1 Identity, Properties, and Uses

Chemical Name (*R,S*)-α-Cyano-3-phenoxybenzyl (1*R*,1*S*)-2-(4-chlorophenyl)-3-methyl-1-butyrate. There are four isomeric forms.

Structure See Fig. 13.2. It should be noted that fenvalerate is not based on a cyclopropane ring structure.

Synonyms Fenvalerate (BSI, ISO) is the common name in use. Trade names are Sumicidin®, Belmark®, and Pydrin®. Code designations for the compound include S5602, WL43775, SD43775, and OMS2000. The CAS registry number is 51630-58-1.

Physical and Chemical Properties Fenvalerate has the empirical formula $C_{25}H_{22}ClNO_3$ and a molecular weight of 419.91. The racemic mixture is a yellow viscous liquid. The density is 1.17 gm/ml at 23°C and the vapor pressure 2.8×10^{-7} mm Hg at 25°C. Its water solubility is approximately 2 μg/liter, but it is freely soluble in most organic solvents. It is light stable.

History, Formulations, and Uses Fenvalerate was first developed by Sumitomo in 1973 and was introduced commercially in 1976 as an emulsifiable concentrate to be used against a wide range of insect pests.

13.2.6.2 Toxicity to Laboratory Animals

Fenvalerate produces typical type II motor symptoms in mammals (Verschoyle and Aldridge, 1980; Lawrence and Casida,

1982; Wright *et al.*, 1987). The acute oral LD 50 in rats is given in Table 13.3 as 450 mg/kg but can be as high as 3000 depending on solvent (FAO/ WHO, 1980). In common with other pyrethroids, the intravenous route is far more effective, with an LD 50 of 50–100 mg/kg (Verschoyle and Aldridge, 1980), and dermal application is far less effective, with an LD 50 of 5000 mg/kg (FAO/WHO, 1980). Rats receiving 2000 ppm in their diet for 90 days died, but others receiving 1500 ppm for 15 months showed typical motor symptoms but did not die. Rats showing severe motor symptoms developed axonal swelling and demyelination in the sciatic nerve (Parker *et al.*, 1985). These changes appeared to be reversible (FAO/WHO, 1980). Fenvalerate has no teratogenic or mutagenic activity (Zhu *et al.*, 1986; Pluijmen *et al.*, 1984). In both rats and dogs fed 500–1000 ppm fenvalerate, granulomatous changes and giant cell infiltration were seen in the liver (Parker *et al.*, 1984; Okuno *et al.*, 1986). These were, however, a foreign-body response to deposition of crystals of the cholesterol 2-(4-chlorophenyl)-isovalerate ester in the liver (Miyamoto *et al.*, 1986). The esters are formed by microsomal carbaryl esterases and are highly specific for fenvalerate (Kaneko *et al.*, 1988).

Despite its lack of a cyclopropane ring in the acid, fenvalerate is rapidly metabolized in rats by ester cleavage and hydroxylation, as are the more traditional pyrethroids (Ohkawa *et al.*, 1979). Elimination from body fat is slow, with a half-life of 7–10 days; elimination from brain is less slow, with a half-life of 2 days (Marei *et al.*, 1982), presumably due to the more effective perfusion of brain and the presence of esterases in brain tissue.

13.2.6.3 Toxicity to Humans

Despite early reports of negative findings (FAO/WHO, 1980), fenvalerate produced local irritant symptoms in 73% of plant nursery workers handling treated seedlings (Kolmodin-Hedman *et al.*, 1982). Tingling or burning sensations were also described by LeQuesne *et al.* (1980) after accidental splashing of the facial skin with fenvalerate. A study of human volunteers who were exposed to fenvalerate applied to the ear lobe (Flannigan and Tucker, 1985b) confirmed this and reported that paresthesia (i.e., numbness combined with irritating abnormal sensation) could be experienced in severe cases. The threshold application appeared to be less than 10 $\mu g/cm^2$. All reports agree that the sensation appears after a latent period of about 30 min and persists for 0.5–24 hr, depending on severity. He *et al.* (1989) reported 196 cases of poisoning, three of which, involving ingestion of up to 2000 mg/kg, were fatal despite gastric lavage. Intoxication was as described for deltamethrin. A 20% emulsion rapidly produced skin irritation.

13.2.7 FLUCYTHRINATE

13.2.7.1 Identity, Properties, and Uses

Chemical Name α-Cyano-3-phenoxybenzyl-(*S*)-2-[4-(difluoromethoxy)phenyl]-3-methylbutyrate. There are four isomeric forms.

Structure See Fig. 13.2. Like fenvalerate, flucythrinate is not based on a cyclopropane ring structure.

Synonyms Flucythrinate (ANSI, BSI, ISO) is the common name in use. Trade names include Pay-off® and Cybolt®. Code designations for the compound include AC222750, CL222705 and OMS2007. The CAS registry number is 70124-77-5.

Physical and Chemical Properties Flucythrinate has the empirical formula $C_{26}H_{23}F_2NO_4$ and a molecular weight of 451.47. The technical material is a viscous brown liquid with a density of 1.19 gm/ml at 22°C. Its vapor pressure is 8.7×10^{-9} mm Hg at 25°C. Its water solubility is less than 0.5 mg/liter, but it is freely soluble in most organic solvents. It is light stable.

History, Formulations, and Uses Flucythrinate was described by the American Cyanamid Corporation in 1979 and is marketed as an emulsifiable concentrate to be used against a wide variety of insect pests.

13.2.7.2 Toxicity to Laboratory Animals

Flucythrinate appears to produce intermediate or mixed motor symptoms in mammals, although this cannot be considered certain as the only published description is imprecise (FAO/WHO, 1986). The acute oral LD 50 in female rats is 67 mg/kg and in mice 76 mg/kg. Rats fed 300 ppm for 28 days showed severe motor symptoms, and rats fed 150 ppm showed moderate motor symptoms. In both cases these disappeared within 48 hr of reverting to normal diet. Flucythrinate has no teratogenic or mutagenic activity (FAO/WHO, 1986).

Flucythrinate is rapidly metabolized by ester cleavage and oxidation (FAO/WHO, 1986).

13.2.7.3 Toxicity to Humans

Experimental application of flucythrinate to the ear lobe of human volunteers at 130 $\mu g/cm^2$ caused a marked paresthesia which began 30 min after application and persisted for 24 hr. Flucythrinate produced the most severe paresthesia of the four pyrethroids tested (Flannigan and Tucker, 1985b). A second study using forearm skin and application at 13.8 mg/cm² produced paresthesia after a delay of 4–5 hr lasting for 3 days (Flannigan and Tucker, 1985b), indicating that the thinner facial skin is more sensitive than other areas.

13.2.8 PERMETHRIN

13.2.8.1 Identity, Properties, and Uses

Chemical Name 3-Phenoxybenzyl-(1*R*, 1*S*)-*cis*,*trans*-3-(2,2-dichloro vinyl)-2,2-dimethylcyclopropanecarboxylate. There are four isomeric forms.

Structure See Table 13.2.

Synonyms   Permethrin (ANSI, BSI, ISO) is the common name in use. Trade names include Ambush®, Kafil®, Eksmin®, and Pounce®. Code designations for the compound include FMC33297, OMS1821, PP557, WL43479, and NRDC143. The CAS registry number is 52645-53-1. The *cis* isomer is also known as cispermethrin (NRDC148) and the *trans* isomer as biopermethrin (NRDC147).

Physical and Chemical Properties   Permethrin has the empirical formula $C_{21}H_{20}Cl_2O_3$ and a molecular weight of 391.30. When pure, it is a white crystalline powder melting between 34 and 39°C. Cispermethrin melts between 63 and 65°C and biopermethrin between 44 and 47°C. Its water solubility is less than 1 mg/liter but it is freely soluble in most organic solvents. It is not light stable but is 10–100 times more stable than the pyrethrins.

History, Formulations, and Uses   Permethrin was first described by Dr. M. Elliott in 1973. It is used as a broad-spectrum insecticide in a variety of formulations. The *cis/trans* ratio varies depending on conditions of manufacture and can also vary with time due to differential rates of hydrolysis and photolysis. A common ratio is 40:60 for agricultural use, with veterinary preparations having lower ratios.

13.2.8.2 Toxicity to Laboratory Animals

Permethrin produces typical type I motor symptoms in mammals (Verschoyle and Aldridge, 1980; Lawrence and Casida, 1982). The acute oral LD 50 in female rats is given in Table 13.3 as 1500 mg/kg but varies greatly with *cis/trans* ratio, as the mammalian toxicity is almost entirely attributable to the *cis* isomer with LD 50 values for racemates ranging from 430 to 8900 mg/kg (FAO/WHO, 1980). Rats fed 3000 ppm permethrin in their diet for 6 months showed typical motor symptoms in the early stages of the study but no other changes except for a slight increase in liver weight associated with an increase in smooth endoplasmic reticulum. Rats fed 5000 ppm or more for 14 days developed acute poisoning and deaths occurred. Animals showing severe symptoms showed axonal swelling and myelin degeneration in the sciatic nerve (FAO/WHO, 1980). Permethrin has no teratogenic or mutagenic activity (FAO/WHO, 1982; Waters *et al.*, 1982; Pluijmen *et al.*, 1984). Very low levels of permethrin in the diet of chickens (0.1 ppm for 3–6 weeks after hatching) have been reported to reduce immune responsiveness (McCorkle *et al.*, 1980), and permethrin suppresses the response of mouse lymphocytes to mitogens *in vitro* at $2 \times 10^{-5} M$ (Stelzer and Gordon, 1984). This *in vitro* suppression showed little stereospecificity and was shown by both type I and type II pyrethroids, and the authors suggested that it might result from a nonspecific interaction with membrane lipids. The possibility of immune suppression by pyrethroids has been little investigated as yet, but many investigators have fed high levels of pyrethroids in long-term studies without reporting increases in infections.

Permethrin is rapidly metabolized in rats and other species by ester cleavage and hydroxylation (Gaughan *et al.*, 1977a). It is rather more persistent in body lipid, however, with half-lives of 4–5 days in brain and body fat (Marei *et al.*, 1982).

13.2.8.3 Toxicity to Humans

In spraying trials in Kenya it was estimated that permethrin absorption did not exceed 2 mg per 12-hr period. After oral dosage of 2 or 4 mg permethrin, urinary excretion accounted for 18 or 35% of the dose, with most being excreted over the first 12 hr (FAO/WHO, 1982). No systemic symptoms have been reported, but skin irritation has been described by several workers. Flannigan *et al.* (1985) found that the threshold application to the ear lobe was approximately 130 μg/cm². Kolmodin-Hedman *et al.* (1982) found that 63 or 33% of workers in a plant nursery developed symptoms, depending on the *cis/trans* ratio, although LeQuesne *et al.* (1980) found no permethrin-related symptoms after moderate exposure to concentrates in three subjects. The symptoms were similar to those described for fenvalerate.

A man developed a fatal motor neuron disease shortly following acute exposure to an aerosol spray of 454 mg permethrin with 9 gm chlordane in a confined space (Pall *et al.*, 1987). The only initial symptom was loss of consciousness for a half-hour followed by development of muscle wasting and fasciculation from 2 weeks, and it would appear unlikely that this typical case of motor neuron disease was directly related to the permethrin exposure.

13.2.9 PHENOTHRIN

13.2.9.1 Identity, Properties, and Uses

Chemical Name   3-Phenoxybenzyl-(1R,1S)-*cis,trans*-3(2-methylprop-1-enyl)-2,2-dimethylcyclopropanecarboxylate.   There are four isomeric forms.

Structure   See Table 13.2

Synonyms   Phenothrin (BSI, ISO) is the common name in use. Trade names include Sumithrin® and Wellcide®. Code designations for the compound include S2539 and OMS1809. The CAS registry number is 26002-80-2.

Physical and Chemical Properties   Phenothrin has the empirical formula $C_{23}H_{26}O_3$ and a molecular weight of 350.46. The racemic mixture is a viscous liquid. The density is 1.058 gm/ml at 25°C and the vapor pressure 1.2×10^{-6} mm Hg at 25°C. Its water solubility is 1.4 mg/liter and it is freely soluble in most organic solvents. Is is not light stable.

History, Formulations, and Uses   Phenothrin was first developed in 1973. It is used as a domestic insecticide in a partially resolved mixture rich in the 1R isomers (Sumithrin) and for grain protection.

13.2.9.2 Toxicity to Laboratory Animals

Phenothrin produces typical type I motor symptoms in mammals (Lawrence and Casida, 1982). The acute oral LD 50 in rats is in excess of 5000 mg/kg and the intravenous LD 50 between 452 and 492 mg/kg (FAO/WHO, 1981). Rats fed 6000 ppm for 2 years showed only a small reduction in weight gain (FAO/WHO, 1981). Phenothrin has been stated to have no teratogenic or mutagenic activity (FAO/WHO, 1985), but Nishi *et al.* (1985) reported it to be mutagenic in *Salmonella* together with a number of other pyrethroids.

Metabolism of phenothrin in the rat is rapid and proceeds by ester cleavage followed by oxidation (Miyamoto *et al.*, 1974).

13.2.9.3 Toxicity to Humans

In an experimental study (FAO/WHO, 1981), human volunteers were given dermal applications of 0.44–0.67 mg/kg/day. As might be expected from animal studies, this produced no systemic toxic effects. Also, no abnormal skin sensation was reported.

13.3 ROTENONE AND RELATED MATERIALS

According to Shepard (1951), rotenone-bearing plants were recorded as fish poisons as early as 1747 in Malaya and 1725 in South America. Actually, their use as a fish poison by many different indigenous peoples probably is ancient, but their use as an insecticide probably is little more than a century old.

Plants known to produce rotenone and other rotenoids belong to at least 68 species of the family Leguminosae, the same as that for peas and beans. The genera most exploited so far are *Derris* and *Lonchocarpus* of the tribe Dahlbergieae. Of possible importance in the future are *Tephrosia, Millettia,* and *Mundulea* of the tribe Galegeae and to a lesser extent *Spatholobus* and *Pachyrhizus* of the tribe Phaseolae. Most commercial rotenone preparations come from *D. elliptica, D. mallaccensis, L. utilis,* and *L. urucu;* preparations from *Derris* are called derris or tuba; those from *Lonchocarpus* are called cubé or timbo. *Derris* is native to Southeast Asia, *Lonchocarpus* to South America.

Rotenone and other active principles often occur chiefly in the roots of rotenone-bearing plants but may be in the leaves (as in *Tephrosia vogeli*), seeds (as in *Millettia pachycarpa*), or bark (as in *Mundulea sericea*).

Regardless of the genus or the particular part of the plant involved, the active constituents of rotenone-bearing plants may be extracted with ether or acetone as a resin. Rotenone constitutes anywhere from 2 to 40% of these resins. The remainder consist of rotenoids and noninsecticidal materials, including oils containing sesquiterpenes, two unidentified crystalline compounds, and lonchocarpic acid. Roots of *L. utilis* may contain as much as 25% total extractives and roots of *D. elliptica* may contain up to 31%. The concentrations in differ-

ent lots of cubé imported by the United States from Peru during one entire year ranged from 2.5 to 11.5% and averaged 6.07%.

More detail on the toxicity of rotenone than can be covered in this book was reviewed by Haley (1978).

13.3.1 ROTENONE

13.3.1.1 Identity, Properties, and Uses

Chemical Name and Structure Rotenone is (2R,6aS,12aS)-1,2,6,6a,12,12a-hexahydro-2-isopropenyl-8,9-dimethoxychromeno[3,4-b]furo[2,3-h]chromen-6-one. Its structure is depicted in Fig. 13.3. Rotenone is only one of the compounds extracted from derris root and cubé. Five other naturally occurring, closely related rotenoids are known. They include sumatrol (which differs from rotenone only by having a hydroxide group on carbon 15), elliptone (which differs from rotenone by having a double bond between carbons 20 and 21 and no side chain on carbon 20), malaccol (which is elliptone hydroxylated at the 15 position), deguelin (which is similar to rotenone but has three carbons and a double bond in the E ring and has the side chain saturated), and l-α-toxicarol (which is identical to deguelin, except that is hydroxylated on carbon 15). Although rotenone generally is considered to be the active ingredient in these resins, the other constituents show considerable insecticidal activity and may deserve further study (Metcalf, 1955).

Synonyms Synonyms for rotenone (BSI, ISO) include derris (JMAF), nicouline, and tubatoxin. The CAS registry number is 83-79-4.

Physical and Chemical Properties The empirical formula is $C_{23}H_{22}O_6$, and the molecular weight is 394.43. Rotenone forms colorless crystals which melt between 162 and 163°C but a dimorphic form melts between 185 and 186°C.

Rotenone is sparingly soluble in water (15 mg/liter at 100°C) but is readily soluble in many organic solvents and oils.

Rotenone is readily oxidized and racemized in the presence of light and the process is accelerated in alkaline solution. Cheng *et al.* (1972) reported at least 20 decomposition products including 6aβ,12αβ-rotenolone and rotenonone.

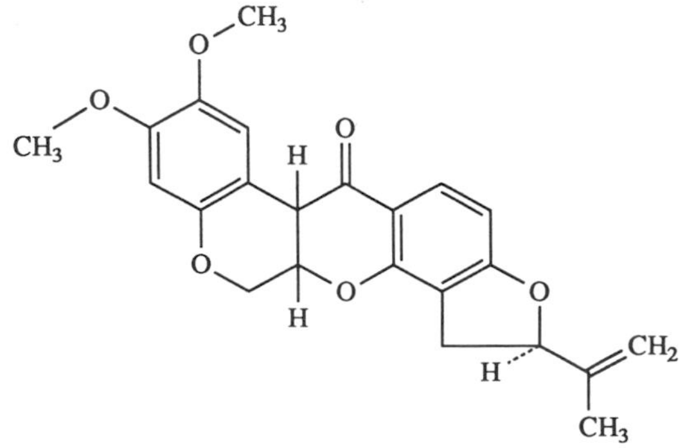

Figure 13.3 Structure of rotenone.

Hydrolysis is associated with development of a red color and with a reduction in toxicity, although the 6aβ,12αβ-rotenolone has an ip LD 50 to mice of 4.1 mg/kg, only slightly higher than that of rotenone (Cheng *et al.*, 1972).

History, Formulations, Uses, and Production The insecticidal properties of derris root were known to the Chinese many years ago and have long been used by island natives to poison fish. Rotenone was first isolated from derris root in 1895 by E. Geoffrey. The use of the extract as a pesticide was first patented in Britain in 1912. The structure of rotenone was established in 1932 by E. B. LaForge.

Rotenone is a fish poison used primarily to control fish stocks in conserved waters. It has some selectivity of action when pure, killing marine fish but not invertebrates (Gilmore *et al.*, 1981). It is also active as a nonsystemic pesticide against a wide variety of insects, arachnids, and mollusks. Its rapid photodecomposition means that it is active only for about 1 week on plants or 2–6 days in water, and this limits its commercial use, although rotenone still finds use as a domestic garden insecticide. Total estimated consumption in the United States in 1978 was estimated at 15,000,000 pounds (Gosalvez and Diaz-Gil, 1978). It has been used in veterinary medicine but has a poor therapeutic index (Fox and DeLeon, 1982).

Formulations include dusts of 0.75–5% concentration, crystalline preparations of 97% purity, and emulsified solutions of up to 50% and resins of 42–45% concentration intended for manufacture. The dusts are stabilized with phosphoric acid to reduce oxidation.

13.3.1.2 Toxicity to Laboratory Animals

Rotenone is a highly potent mitochondrial poison, blocking NADH oxidation, and this property dominates its actions in animals. It has been used extensively as a model mitochondrial toxin (e.g., Heikkila *et al.*, 1985). The toxicology of rotenone was extensively reviewed by Haley in 1978.

Symptomatology Small parenteral doses cause a transient stimulation of respiration in all species and may cause emesis in dogs (Haag, 1931).

Signs of serious poisoning in animals include initial respiratory stimulation followed by respiratory depression, incoordination, clonic or tonic convulsions, muscle tremors, and death from respiratory failure (Haag, 1931; Ambrose and Haag, 1936; Shimkin and Anderson, 1936; Lehman, 1951, 1952). The heart continues to beat and the blood pressure is maintained for a relatively long time after respiration has stopped.

Death occurs within 30 min or less in about half of the animals that receive rotenone intraperitoneally, but others die after a delay of as much as 14 days. Death is slower following an oral dose; about half the animals die in less than 2 days, while the remainder live for 3–10 days or more (Shimkin and Anderson, 1936; Lehman, 1951, 1952).

Irritation and Sensitization Derris powder or ointment produces only a mild rash or no irritation of human or animal skin. The dust produces intense irritation of the rabbit eye, accompanied by the formation of pus. No anesthetic effect, such as is seen in the human mouth following application of either rotenone or derris, can be observed in the eye. Complete recovery can be expected in several days (Ambrose and Haag, 1936).

Dosage Response The acute toxicity of rotenone is shown in Table 13.4 and can be seen to vary greatly, as does the toxicity of many poorly water-soluble toxins, depending on particle size, dispersion, and degree of solution. Ground material administered as a suspension in vegetable gums may have oral LD 50 values of 200 mg/kg (rats) or more than 3000 mg/kg (rabbits). On the contrary, the LD 50 of rotenone dissolved in olive oil is 25 mg/kg (rats) or less (guinea pigs) (Lightbody and Matthews, 1936; Ambrose and Haag, 1937). Birds have about the same range of susceptibility as mammals (Cutkomp, 1943). Samples of the natural product varied considerably in oral toxicity, even when tested under the same conditions, and the same sample varied considerably in toxicity in different species. However, the kind of poisoning produced by derris is apparently indistinguishable from that caused by crystalline rotenone (Ambrose and Haag, 1936; Matthews and Lightbody, 1936), and the same is true of the analogs and derivatives (Ambrose and Haag, 1937).

The acute oral toxicity of cubé is similar to that of derris. One sample of cubé was found to have oral LD 50 values of

Table 13.4
Acute Toxicity of Rotenone

Species	Route	LD 50 (mg/kg)	Reference
Rat	oral	64[a]	Shimkin and Anderson (1936)
Rat	oral	25[a,b]	Lightbody and Matthews (1936)
Rat	oral	132	Lehman (1951)
Rat	oral	60	Santi and Tóth (1965)
Rat	ip	2.2[a]	Shimkin and Anderson (1936)
Rat	ip	1.6	Santi and Tóth (1965)
Rat	iv	0.3	Lehman (1954)
Rat	iv	0.2	Santi and Tóth (1965)
Mouse	ip	5.4[a]	Shimkin and Anderson (1936)
Mouse	ip	2.8	Cheng et al. (1972)
Guinea pig	oral	13[a,b]	Lightbody and Matthews (1936)
Guinea pig	oral	130[a]	Shimkin and Anderson (1936)
Guinea pig	oral	75[b,c]	Haag (1931)
Guinea pig	ip	13[a]	Shimkin and Anderson (1936)
Guinea pig	ip	2[c]	Haag (1931)
Rabbit	oral	1500[c]	Haag (1931)
Rabbit	dermal	100–200	Lehman (1954)
Rabbit	iv	0.35[c]	Haag (1931)
Rabbit	iv	0.65[c]	Haag (1931)
Cat	iv	0.65[b]	Haag (1931)

[a] Calculated from original mortality fractions.
[b] Oil solution.
[c] Minimal lethal dose.

160 mg/kg in rats, 190 mg/kg in guinea pigs, 860 mg/kg in rabbits, and 320 mg/kg in dogs (Ambrose and Haag, 1936).

When rats and dogs were exposed in a chamber to a cloud of derris dust in such a way that the onset of poisoning began in only a few minutes, it was found by measuring the total amount of dust used and the amount recovered from the chamber after exposure that the uniformly fatal dose (which was largely respiratory) was smaller than the fatal oral dose (Ambrose and Haag, 1936).

Dogs fed rotenone at the rate of 5 mg/kg/day for a month appeared well but showed fatty changes of the liver and kidneys. A dosage of 10 mg/kg/day killed three of five dogs, and one that was killed showed severe toxic injury of the liver, with possibly one-third of the bulk occupied by fat. Rabbits were more tolerant (Haag, 1931).

Adult dogs tolerated derris at dietary levels as high as 400 ppm (8.0 mg/kg/day) without weight loss. However, the same diet leading to only slightly greater dosage (8.8 mg/kg/day) lessens the growth of pups (Ambrose and Haag, 1938).

Some workers (Ambrose et al., 1943) found that their rats tolerated a dietary level of 80 ppm with only a moderate retardation of growth during the first 35 days of feeding, regardless of the fat content of the diet. On the contrary, when rotenone and sulfoxide were given to rats in their drinking water, with both at a level of 2.5 ppm, there was marked retardation of growth (Brooks and Price, 1961). Thus, the synergist may enhance the toxicity of rotenone for mammals as well as insects.

Absorption, Distribution, Metabolism, and Excretion Rotenone is metabolized rather effectively by the liver. In order to produce the same clinical effect, the compound must be injected into a mesenteric vein at about 10 times the dose required for injection into a femoral vein (Haag, 1931).

Rat and mouse liver enzymes and intact mice hydroxylate rotenone at carbons 7 and 24. *In vitro*, the change is produced by microsomes in the presence of nicotinamide-adenine dinucleotide phosphate. The products include rotenolone I, rotenolone II, 8'-hydroxyrotenone, 6',7'-dihydro-6',7'-dihydroxyrotenone, two rotenolones of each of the latter compounds, and uncharacterized polar materials. The toxicity of certain of these rotenoids to mice is similar to that of rotenone (Fukami et al., 1967). However, metabolism of at least a part of the rotenone molecule eventually is complete. One mechanism of detoxication of natural rotenone (5'β-rotenone) or one of its metabolites was found to be 3-O-demethylation, as indicated by recovery of 27 and 13% of the administered radiocarbon as ^{14}C-labeled carbon dioxide within 50 hr after administration to mice and rats, respectively. Within the same period, the animals excreted 7–17% of the radioactivity in their urine (Unai et al., 1973). In another study, 19.5 and 20.0% of the dose were recovered in the urine of mice and rats, respectively, within 24 hr after oral administration (Fukami et al., 1969).

Biochemical Effects In isolated rat liver mitochondria, the aerobic oxidation of pyruvate is almost completely inhibited by $6.0 \times 10^{-7} M$ rotenone, but the same concentration has no effect on the oxidation of succinate. The inhibition of pyruvate oxidation is decreased by methylene blue but not by uncoupling of phosphorylation through $10^{-4} M$ dinitrophenol. In the presence of rotenone, the flavoprotein, NADH dehydrogenase, and cytochromes b, c, a, and a_3 are found to be in the oxidized state. It therefore was thought that rotenone blocks the electron transport system between NADH and the flavoprotein (Lindahl and Öberg, 1961). Later, extensive evidence indicated that the block was at the next step, that is, between the flavoprotein and ubiquinone (coenzyme Q) (Gutman et al., 1970a,b, 1971, 1972). Rotenone is one of the most potent known inhibitors of the NADH dehydrogenase system. Ernster et al. (1963) showed that 20 pmol/mg protein produces 50% inhibition of mitochondrial pyruvate oxidation. Radiolabel studies showed this to be equivalent to 2 moles rotenone per "mole" of NADH dehydrogenase. The site at which rotenone acts involves Fe-S proteins and is the same as the site at which amytal produces its inhibition, although rotenone is more selective and shows less affinity for other proteins (Storey, 1981).

The block of NADH oxidation can lead to increased incorporation of acetate into long-chain fatty acids by isolated mitochondria (Hull and Whereat, 1967). This may be a link with the fatty changes seen in the liver after long-term feeding.

Effects on Reproduction Dietary levels of 75 and 150 ppm of rotenone were tolerated by pregnant guinea pigs but injured the young, which were either born dead or failed to thrive after birth, suggesting that rotenone or a toxic metabolite is excreted in the milk (Haag, 1931). Khera et al. (1982) found that daily oral administration of rotenone to female rats at 5 mg/kg on days 6–15 of pregnancy resulted in reduced maternal weight gain and that 10 mg/kg/day killed 60% of the dams. As might be expected from the maternal toxicity, the high dose increased the number of resorptions, but without producing significant fetal abnormalities. Some skeletal malformations such as extra ribs were seen at 5 mg/kg/day although this dose rate did not increase resorptions. Dosing at 2.5 mg/kg/day had no effects.

Effects on Organs and Tissues There is some disagreement in the literature regarding the carcinogenic potential of rotenone. Gosalvez and Merchan (1973) reported an increased incidence of mammary tumors in rats given 1.7 mg/kg/day intraperitoneally in oil for 42 days, but this finding was not reproduced by Freudental et al. (1981). Although the latter authors also found dietary administration at 125–1000 ppm in hamsters or 500–1000 ppm in rats not to be tumorigenic, Gosalvez and Merchan (1973) reported that oral administration of 13.5 mg/kg rotenone over 45 days produces tumors and quoted an unpublished report of E. L. Long that, although tumors were not seen above 10 ppm rotenone in the diet, tumor incidence was maximal in rats fed 5 ppm (Gosalvez, 1983). Innes et al. (1969), however, found no tumors in mice fed 3 ppm for 18 months, the time of peak tumor incidence in rats. Gosalvez (1983), in reviewing these findings, suggested that rotenone may cause tumors only in vitamin-deficient animals. Rotenone suppresses weight gain at or above 50 ppm in the diet of rats (Gosalvez, 1983) or hamsters (Freudenthal et al., 1981) and so suppression of cell division may limit carcinogenic potential, but Gosalvez suggested that increased serum growth hormone, progesterone, and estrogen levels may be involved in rotenone carcinogenesis and showed a parallel between tumor incidence and low-level rotenone-induced obesity in rats. The tumors produced were encapsulated mammary adenomas with numerous mitochondrial lesions (Merchan et al., 1978). Waters et al. (1982) reported no mutagenic effects of rotenone in mouse bone marrow. The high cytotoxicity of rotenone at 2×10^{-8} M (Murakami and Fukami, 1983) or 10^{-7} M (Garry and Moore, 1974) makes in vitro studies difficult, and there are no reports of cell transformation by rotenone. Rotenone is nonmutagenic in bacterial reversion tests (Moriya et al., 1983).

Rotenone is a potential spindle poison. At concentrations ranging from 1×10^{-7} to $1 \times 10^{-5} M$, the compound causes an increase in the mitotic index of cultured hamster cells within 15 min. The index reaches a peak, the height of which is proportional to the concentration of the compound. This effect can be demonstrated since the cell line used is unusually resistant to the metabolic action of rotenone (Barham and Brinkley, 1976a). The action of rotenone is similar to that of colchicine, except that the latter is delayed at low concentrations. It is thought that rotenone acts on the spindle by preferential binding at sulfhydryl and disulfide bonds in its protein structure (Meisner and Sorensen, 1966). Detailed study of cultured mammalian cells by both light and electron microscopy confirmed that rotenone reversibly inhibits spindle microtubule assembly (Barham and Brinkley, 1975, 1976b). However, rotenone delayed cell progression in all phases of the cell cycle. This was thought to be a direct result of respiratory inhibition, even though amytal, which blocks electron transport at the same site as that blocked by rotenone, does not arrest cell progression at mitosis. Thus, the total effect of rotenone was thought to depend on inhibition of respiration and, separately and more importantly, on inhibition of microtubule assembly (Barham and Brinkley, 1975, 1976a), although the relevance of the microtubule effect in cells not unusually resistant to metabolic inhibition is unclear.

Fukami et al. (1959) studied the relation between chemical structure and the toxicity of rotenone and 34 of its derivatives. Without exception, those with strong insecticidal activity blocked nerve conduction and also inhibited oxidation, as discussed in the preceding section. Some blocked conduction and inhibited respiration but lacked strong insecticidal activity. The apparent discrepancy may be due to rapid degradation of the less toxic compounds by insects (Narahashi, 1971).

Pathology Some animals show pulmonary congestion on autopsy but the findings are not diagnostic or sufficient to explain death (Shimkin and Anderson, 1936; Ambrose and Haag, 1936). Guinea pigs killed by an oral dose show rather severe irritation of the entire gastrointestinal tract, especially the stomach. Rabbits show much less gastrointestinal irritation (Haag, 1931).

Derris at dietary levels of 79 ppm in rats and 130 ppm in dogs produces liver injury. Both species show periportal irritation. Rats also show midzonal necrosis, while dogs exhibit constriction of the hepatic veins and passive congestion (Ambrose and Haag, 1938).

13.3.1.3 Toxicity to Humans

Experimental Exposure When derris powder was applied to the armpits of four persons twice daily for 30 days, one developed a mild rash at the site of application; the rash disappeared within 24 hr. The others experienced no inconvenience, except that one person noted a very mild smarting. When applied to the forearms as a 10% ointment in anhydrous lanolin, no local irritation or anesthesia was observed. About 10 min after derris or a water extract of it was taken into the mouth of volunteers, all experienced a slight sensation of numbness, as well as a metallic taste; these effects lasted 3 or 4 hr (Haag, 1931; Ambrose and Haag, 1936).

Accidental and Intentional Poisoning There is only one report of accidental poisoning by rotenone in the published literature. A previously healthy 3.5-year-old girl died after drinking about 10 ml of an insecticidal preparation of rotenone (DeWilde et al., 1986). Symptoms were initial vomiting and drowsiness leading rapidly to coma, depressed respiration, and apnea. Despite artificial ventilation begun within 2–2.5 hr of ingestion, the girl died at 8–8.5 hr. Postmortem showed anoxic damage in the cerebrum, lungs, and heart and serohemorrhagic pleural effusion. There was also evidence of an acute renal tubular necrosis, but the authors suggested that this could have been due to various etherial oils present in the insecticide. HPLC analysis of postmortem tissues showed rotenone concentrations of 6×10^{-6} to 1×10^{-5} mol/kg and the estimated oral dose was 40 mg/kg. Given that tissue concentrations 10 times lower than those found in this case completely inhibit mitochondrial respiration (see previous section), there can be no doubt that death was due to rotenone poisoning. The authors remark that the etherial herb extracts also present in the preparation may have facilitated gastrointestinal absorption of the water-insoluble rotenone, although 40 mg/kg is well within the oral LD 50 values quoted in Table 13.4. It is particularly noteworthy that the insecticide was labeled as "Natural product—Non toxic."

Ingestion of rotenone was a common means of suicide by natives of New Ireland but not other parts of the Mandated Territory of New Guinea. When such persons were brought to medical attention while still alive, they were found to be in a state of collapse with feeble pulse and dilated pupils. Some, especially those suspected of having taken a very small dose, recovered following gastric lavage and stimulants. The only finding in numerous autopsies was that of acute congestive heart failure. The root was not generally found in the stomach, as vomiting before death was the rule. However, the deceased often had been seen eating the root, and sometimes a nibbled piece was found beside the body (Holland, 1938).

Use Experience LeCointe (1936) mentioned the primitive industrial conditions for processing rotenone-bearing plants in the Amazon valley. Physicians observed some cases of severe irritation of the throat with partial destruction of the soft palate as well as of the anterior pillars and, very frequently, an irritation of the conjunctiva followed by ulcerative keratitis. Inflammation of the skin was notable in skin folds or where perspiration led to accumulation of the powder. The author held high hopes that improved industrial hygiene would correct the situation.

Difficulties have not been confined to those working with raw products in the tropics but have affected factory workers in temperate climates. All workers in Lyon who encountered the fine powder developed in 2 or 3 days a violent dermatitis of the genital region. It was characterized by a red-violet color, slight edema, and some itching. In 24 hr, if exposure was stopped, the irritated skin underwent desquamation in plaques of different sizes. If contact persisted, the dermatitis became worse; itching, erythema, and the leatherlike texture increased. The skin became covered with large, flat, excoriated, oozing papules in patches 0.5 cm in diameter. The dermatitis recurred with each new exposure. Workers also experienced ulcerative rhinitis and temporary but complete loss of the sense of smell. In some instances there was irritation of the lips and tongue. The situation was corrected by modern ventilation and by issuing a dust mask to each worker (Racouchot, 1939). Gosalvez and Diaz-Gil (1978) estimated that there was a residue of 14–58 μg/kg on raw green beans treated with rotenone as an insecticide and concluded that this may represent a carcinogenic risk. Little of this rotenone would survive cooking, however.

Treatment of Poisoning Treatment is symptomatic.

13.4 NICOTINE AND RELATED COMPOUNDS

Three closely related compounds (nicotine, nornicotine, and anabasine, shown in Fig. 13.4) were commonly used as insecticides, although only the most potent, nicotine, is now used to any extent. In the past, nicotine and nornicotine have sometimes both been present in a single formulation marketed as nicotine. Nicotine is usually obtained from *Nicotiana tabacum* but it also occurs in *N. rustica* and in *Duboisia,* another genus of the Solanaceae, and in three other taxonomically diverse genera, namely *Asclepias* (Asclepidaceae), *Equisetum* (Equisetaceae), and *Lycopodium* (Lycopodiaceae). Nornicotine predominates in *N. sylvestris* and *D. hopwoodii.* Anabasine may be extracted from *Nicotiana glauca* but usually is obtained from *A. aphylla,* a member of the Chemopodiaceae. Thus these chemically closely related compounds are derived from plants of five families, six genera, and many species.

13.4.1 NICOTINE

13.4.1.1 Identity, Properties, and Uses

Chemical Name *S*-3-(1-Methylpyrrolidin-2-yl)pyridine.

Structure See Fig. 13.4.

Synonyms Nicotine (BSI, ISO) has been sold as Destruxol® and Black Leaf®. The CAS registry number is 54-11-5.

Physical and Chemical Properties The empirical formula for nicotine is $C_{10}H_{14}N_2$ and the molecular weight 162.23. It is a colorless liquid melting at $-80°C$ and boiling at 247°C and has a density of·1.009 gm/cm³ at 20°C. Its vapor pressure is 4.25×10^{-2} mm Hg at 25°C, and it has a burning acrid taste and characteristic odor. It is hygroscopic and miscible with water below 60°C and readily forms basic salts, the nicotine ion having pK values of 6.16 and 10.96. It is readily soluble in organic solvents. It is easily oxidized and turns brown after exposure to air. Nicotine exists in two isomeric forms, the natural *S* isomer or the *R* isomer. The *S* form is 1–8 times less toxic than the synthetic *R* form (Martin, 1986).

Formulations, Uses, and Production Nicotine is obtained from the dried leaves of *N. tabacum* and *N. rustica,* in which it occurs to the extent of 2–8% combined with citric and malic acids. Solutions of the free base are used for fumigation. Nicotine sulfate is used as a stomach poison for leaf-eating insects. Formulations include sprays and dusts (0.05–4.0%) and a concentrated solution of the sulfate (40% nicotine).

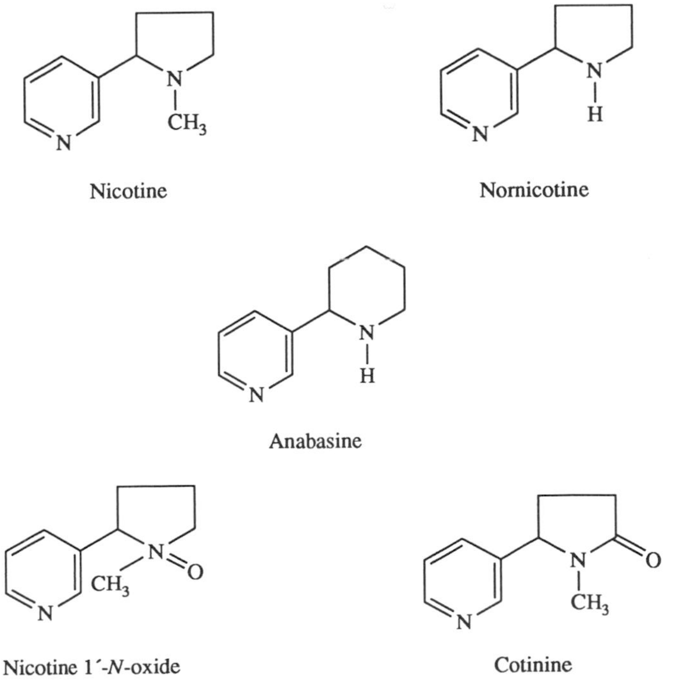

Nicotine   Nornicotine

Anabasine

Nicotine 1′-*N*-oxide   Cotinine

Figure 13.4 Nicotine, nornicotine, and anabasine with two important metabolites of nicotine.

In 1970 imports of nicotine in the United States amounted to a little over 21,000 kg, although its importance as an insecticide is declining as more effective modern substitutes are developed. A little-known use of nicotine permits the capture of dangerous, unmanageable, feral or wild animals. A syringe containing a proper dose constitutes a projectile fired from a gun, using carbon dioxide as the propellant. The syringe is so designed that it injects its contents only after it is embedded in the animal's muscle (Hayes *et al.*, 1959; Jenkins *et al.*, 1961). The therapeutic index (minimal effective dosage divided by approximate lethal dosage) varied from 1.5 to 4.3 in a series of 14 species that were tested (Feurt *et al.*, 1958). The very high concentrations of nicotine used in such darts (285 mg/ml) represent a potential hazard to users (Haigh and Haigh, 1980).

An excellent recent review covering the occupational and medicinal usage and toxicity of nicotine and related alkaloids is that of Holmstedt (1988).

13.4.1.2 Toxicity to Laboratory Animals

Symptomatology With the decline in the importance of nicotine as an insecticide, most modern studies have been directed toward chronic low-level exposure related to tobacco smoking. The acute toxicity of nicotine results from its stimulation of nicotinic acetylcholine receptors in both the peripheral and central nervous systems. Since nicotine both stimulates and at higher doses inhibits both sympathetic and parasympathetic ganglia as well as acting centrally, its actions in the whole mammal are complex and highly dependent on dose and rate of absorption (Gilman *et al.*, 1985).

The most sensitive indicator of nicotine action is an increase in motor activity, which is seen at dosages as low as 0.05 mg/kg (subcutaneous) in the rat and is followed by tremor at intravenous doses ranging from 0.35 to 0.6 mg/kg. Seizures are seen at intravenous doses of 0.23–0.84 mg/kg in rats, mice, and dogs and vomiting at 1.5 mg/kg iv in dogs (Schievelbein, 1982). Dogs poisoned by nicotine become restless and then manifest a brief period of apnea, followed by hyperpnea, followed in turn by a rapid decrease in the strength of respiration terminating in apnea. The blood pressure falls during the first period of apnea but returns to about the normal level as the final respiratory failure begins; as this failure is established, convulsions occur, the blood pressure rises to a peak, and the heart beats very fast. Moments later, the convulsions subside, and the blood pressure rapidly falls as the animal dies. The entire process requires less than 5 min. If respiration is resumed after the convulsions stop, the animal usually survives. The convulsions can be avoided, and the dogs can be made slightly less susceptible to nicotine either by ether anesthesia or by giving them an initial nonfatal dose of nicotine (Franke and Thomas, 1933).

Dosage Response The acute toxicity of nicotine and a few of its salts is shown in Table 13.5. Only LD 50 values have been included; much of the information on toxicity in the literature reviewed by Larson *et al.* (1961) is expressed as "lethal dose"

Table 13.5
Acute Toxicity of Nicotine and Some of Its Salts

Species	Route	LD 50 (mg/kg)	Reference
Rat	oral	188	Ambrose and DeEds (1946)
Rat	oral	52.5[a]	Lazutka *et al.* (1969)
Rat	oral	56.7[b]	Lazutka *et al.* (1969)
Rat, F	oral	83[b]	Gaines (1969)
Rat, F	dermal	285[b]	Gaines (1969)
Rat, M	sc	47[c]	Holck *et al.* (1937)
Rat, F	sc	37[c]	Holck *et al.* (1937)
Rat	ip	30	Ambrose and DeEds (1946)
Rat, M	ip	14.6	Blum and Zacks (1958)
Rat, M	iv	2.8	Larson *et al.* (1949)
Rat, M	iv	27.5[d]	Larson *et al.* (1949)
Mouse	oral	24	Heubner and Papierkowski (1938)
Mouse	oral	3.34[a]	Lazutka *et al.* (1969)
Mouse	oral	8.55[b]	Lazutka *et al.* (1969)
Mouse	sc	16	Heubner and Papierkowski (1938)
Mouse	sc	55[e]	Bogdanski and Dattoli (1952)
Mouse	ip	10.3	Larson *et al.* (1945)
Mouse	ip	11.0	Haag (1937)
Mouse	ip	11.8	Haag (1940)
Mouse, M	iv	0.55	Larson *et al.* (1949)
Mouse, M	iv	7.1[d]	Larson *et al.* (1949)
Guinea pig[f]	sc	40[b]	Hatcher (1904)
Guinea pig[g]	sc	15[b]	Hatcher (1904)
Guinea pig	sc	25[c]	Haag (1933)
Rabbit	sc	20[b]	Hatcher (1904)
Rabbit	iv	6[c]	Haag (1933)
Rabbit	iv	6.25	Haag (1940)
Rabbit, M	iv	5.9	Larson *et al.* (1949)
Rabbit, M	iv	9.4	Larson *et al.* (1949)

[a] Nicotine base.
[b] Nicotine sulfate.
[c] Calculated from original data.
[d] Anesthetized.
[e] Nicotine salicylate.
[f] Adult.
[g] Young.

or in other nonstatistical terms that are difficult to interpret. As already mentioned, the complex and sometimes antagonistic consequences of nicotinic stimulation, coupled with differing rates of absorption, result in considerable variation in the LD 50 values between different species and routes of administration. This is shown in Table 13.5. One further factor causing variation is the desensitization of the nicotinic receptor seen after prolonged exposure to nicotine or related agents (Volle, 1980) and the corresponding development of increasing tolerance to repeated doses (tachyphylaxis). This was first shown by Ruppert (1942). Tachyphylaxis begins in less than 10 min and disappears by 150 min after administration of the initial, sublethal dose (Ruppert, 1942; Hazard and Savini, 1953). Tachyphylaxis explains the lesser effect of doses absorbed over a period of minutes (as in smoking) rather than in a period of seconds (as in rapid intravenous injection). It even accounts for an observation of Bogdanski and Dattoli (1952), namely that a given subcutaneous dose of nicotine is less toxic in dilute solution than in concentrated solution. Due to this long time course of nicotine tachyphylaxis, factors other than receptor desensitization are probably involved (Banerjee *et al.,* 1982).

Anesthesia is another variable in the acute toxicity of nicotine. Unanesthetized dogs were susceptible to smaller dosages, and those that died did so more quickly than anesthetized animals (Franke and Thomas, 1932).

In feeding tests, some of which lasted over a year, rats were unable to survive on diets containing more than 500 ppm nicotine as the sulfate. Diets containing more than 60 ppm inhibited growth, and the degree of inhibition increased with increasing concentration. Paired feeding studies showed that most of the inhibition of growth was due to reduced food intake but that an additional small part of the effect was attributable to the nicotine *per se* (Wilson and DeEds, 1936).

Absorption, Distribution, Metabolism, and Excretion

Nicotine is rapidly absorbed from all mucosal surfaces, including those of the mouth, gastrointestinal tract, and lung. Since nicotine readily forms salts in acid solution, its penetration through biological membranes is strongly pH dependent. Thus it is not rapidly absorbed from the stomach, or reabsorbed from the bladder if the urine is acidic (Borzelleca, 1963). It is also more slowly absorbed from acidic than alkaline smoke. When it is present as the free alkaloid it is capable of rapid penetration, however (Schievelbein, 1982), and readily passes the blood–brain barrier, establishing a brain/blood ratio of 5.6:1 within 1 min of injection into mice.

The metabolism of nicotine is highly complex and is reviewed by Gorrod and Jenner (1975) and Schievelbein (1982). Metabolism is mainly by cytochrome P-450 linked microsomal oxidative pathways in the liver. Cotinine (Fig. 13.4) is a major metabolite, which then undergoes further oxidation. Following small doses, about 4–12% is excreted unchanged in the urine (Haag and Larson, 1942; Larson and Haag, 1942). Following larger doses, a higher proportion is excreted, and the rate of increase is linear; 30% of the dose was recovered unmetabolized from the urine of a dog dosed intravenously at the rate of 48 mg/kg (Finnegan *et al.,* 1947). Urinary excretion of nicotine is virtually complete in the rat in 16 hr (Ganz *et al.,* 1951) and in the dog in 16–36 hr (Finnegan *et al.,* 1947; Bennett *et al.,* 1954).

Following a single very small (0.04 mg) intravenous dose of $2'$-^{14}C-labeled nicotine in cats, 90% of the activity in the brain 15 min after injection still was in unmetabolized form. However, metabolism was more rapid in other tissues; ^{14}C-labeled cotinine could be detected in the blood within 2.5 min. Within 24 hr, 55% of the total activity has been excreted but only 1% as unchanged nicotine (Turner, 1969). The half-life of nicotine in the blood is 50–60 min (Rotenberg, 1982).

Biochemical Effects

According to Ruddon and Cohen (1970), induction of hepatic microsomal enzymes could be produced in the rat by acute doses of nicotine but only when convulsive doses were given several times a day. Administration in drinking water at a rate of 5.9 mg/kg/day did increase the production of microsomal protein and induce some but not all enzymes; how-

ever, activity was not maintained when dosage was reduced to 4.4 mg/kg/day.

Based on the concentrations of nicotine alkaloid in the drinking water and on the measured ingestion of the water, the average dosages of two groups of rats were calculated as 1.14 and 4.56 mg/kg/day, respectively. When administered for 34 weeks, the higher but not the lower dosage increased activities of isocitric dehydrogenase linked to NADP, particulate acid phosphatase, and both soluble and particulate β-glucuronidase and increased mortality, compared to that in controls, from 20.5 to 37.5% during hypoxia, lasting 12 hr in 6% oxygen (Wenzel and Richards, 1970).

Rabbits that had received cholesterol and corn oil in their diets and also had received intramuscular injections of nicotine at a rate of 2.28 mg/kg 5 days a week for 6 weeks showed greater atherosclerosis, more serum lecithin and cephalin, and less free cholesterol than controls on the same diet. *In vitro,* nicotine formed a fairly stable complex with heparin in a ratio of about 20:1. It was concluded that some of the effects of nicotine may depend on its formation of a complex with heparin (Stefanovich *et al.,* 1969).

Pharmacological Action

The pharmacology of nicotine is well described in standard works such as Gilman *et al.* (1985) and has been the subject of a number of comprehensive reviews such as those of Silvette *et al.* (1962), Volle (1980), Martin (1986), and Benowitz (1986) and so will only be briefly summarized here.

Nicotine simulates the action of acetylcholine at nicotinic receptors in the central nervous system, autonomic ganglia, and some peripheral nerves. Its K_d for brain receptors is 5×10^{-10} to 2×10^{-8} M (Martin, 1986) and there appear to be multiple binding sites. Its central actions result in tremor and convulsions, stimulation and then depression of ventilation, and induction of vomiting by a direct action on the medulla. Ventilation is stimulated by peripheral actions on the aortic and carotid chemoreceptors, and adrenal catecholamine secretion is increased at low doses and suppressed at high doses by a sympathomimetic action. Autonomic ganglia are also stimulated or inhibited at higher doses. Heart rate and blood pressure are largely dominated by sympathetic effects and show increases compounded by adrenal catecholamines. The gastrointestinal tract is dominated by parasympathetic effects and shows hypersecretion followed by block as well as increased tone and peristalsis. Death is usually a result of block of neuromuscular transmission in the respiratory muscles or a consequence of seizures. In addition to its action on cholinergic transmission, nicotine can act at noncholinergic sites (Martin, 1986) and also activate receptors on sensory nerve endings and vagal C fibers.

Effects on Organs and Tissues

Mice given nicotine subcutaneously at 2.7 mg/kg/day during their second or third trimester showed a shortened gestation period (Nasrat *et al.,* 1986), and rats given 6 mg/kg/day as a divided subcutaneous dose from days 4 to 20 of gestation did not gain weight normally and produced pups of reduced body weight and brain development (Slotkin *et al.*, 1986). The growth reduction was made up by rebound growth during the last week of gestation and first two postgestational weeks. Fetal brain ornithine decarboxylase activity was elevated while maturation was delayed, which may indicate a specific action of nicotine on brain as there was none of the normal sparing of brain development seen after generalized insult. That nicotine is also capable of producing generalized effects is shown by its potentiation of the teratogenic effects of a carbonic anhydrase inhibitor via uterine vasoconstriction (Ugen and Scott, 1985).

The carcinogenic potential of tobacco is well established, but there is debate about the role of nicotine, which, although probably not carcinogenic itself, can be converted to carcinogens such as N'-nitrosonornicotine and 4-(methylnitrosamino)-1-(3-pyridyl)-1-butanone. The metabolites cotinine and nicotine $1'$-N-oxide are not carcinogenic or cocarcinogenic, although they do produce hyperplasia of the bladder epithelium (Hoffmann *et al.*, 1985).

Treatment of Poisoning in Animals   Artificial respiration is almost always lifesaving in dogs poisoned by nicotine, provided it is begun before there is a severe fall in blood pressure (Franke and Thomas, 1933, 1936).

13.4.1.3 Toxicity to Humans

Experimental Exposure   An intravenous dose of 2.0 mg of nicotine bitartrate (about 0.6 mg of nicotine) produced a small to moderate increase in respiration, heart rate, and blood pressure in almost all of 46 volunteers. Some subjects showed electrocardiographic (ECG) changes. Individual variation was marked, but each person showed only limited variation in response to successive exposures. Smokers and nonsmokers did not differ significantly in their reactions. Symptoms occurred in about three-fourths of the subjects; dizziness was most common, but tingling and faintness also were common; nausea occurred three times and anginal pain twice (both in association with ECG changes). One of the nonsmokers given the same dose perspired profusely and became pale and cold. In a few minutes he became nauseated and vomited. The pulse was thready and, for a short time, the blood pressure was unobtainable. He then retched for 5 min, felt nauseated for an hour, and was weak for several hours. It was concluded that the effect of nicotine in coronary heart disease probably involves both constriction of the coronary arteries and increased work of the heart (Boyle *et al.*, 1947).

Similar conclusions were reached in a recent study in which volunteers were given 4 mg nicotine in chewing gum (Kaijser and Berglund, 1985). This produced an increase in myocardial oxygen consumption not paralleled by an equivalent increase in blood flow, presumably due to vasoconstriction. Intravenous nicotine at up to 3 mg produced increases in blood pressure and heart rate in eight volunteers but an initial slowing of the heart in four. Other symptoms included nausea and euphoria (Henningfield *et al.*, 1985).

In humans, the excretion of nicotine is highly variable unless the pH of the urine is controlled. During a period when the urine is made alkaline by repeated doses of a mixture of alkaline citrate and carbonate, the excretion of nicotine is only about 25% of that when the urine is made acid by repeated doses of ammonium chloride. The difference is thought not to involve the primary excretion but rather reabsorption from alkaline urine (Haag and Larson, 1942).

Accidental and Intentional Poisoning   Beeman and Hunter (1937) described 24 fatal cases of nicotine poisoning resulting from the drinking of insecticides. They reported that at the time nicotine ranked fourth among different poisons, including carbon monoxide and alcohol (first and second), as a cause of death. During the years 1930 through 1934, there were 106 accidental deaths and 182 fatal suicides caused by nicotine in the United States. Additional cases were reviewed by Franke and Thomas (1936).

Among deaths in New Zealand during 1957 to 1960, 24 of 49 suicides and 4 of 14 accidents associated with pesticides involved nicotine (Kennedy, 1962). In Israel between 1953 and 1958, 3 of 46 cases of pesticide poisoning admitted to only one hospital were caused by nicotine (Eschar, 1961). In England and Wales, where there were nine deaths from pesticides during 1952 to 1971, one involved nicotine swallowed by a 21-month-old boy (Hearn, 1973).

Nicotine poisoning in humans resembles that in animals in its rapidity and in the importance of respiratory failure and circulatory collapse. The conditions differ in the rarity of convulsions in humans. Following ingestion, many patients die in 5 min or less; those who live more than 30 min usually survive (Beeman and Hunter, 1937).

Dermal exposure to nicotine alkaloid produces the same range of signs and symptoms as that produced by ingestion. Onset may be as little as 15 or 20 min after exposure (Lockhart, 1933; Faulkner, 1933). However, unlike cases involving ingestion, onset of poisoning after contamination of the skin may be delayed 2–4 hr (Wilson, 1930; Gindhart, 1939). Regardless of the time of onset, signs and symptoms of poisoning may be more prolonged following dermal absorption as compared to ingestion. Three weeks after a man sat on a chair on which 40% free alkaloid had been spilled, he still experienced weakness, sweating, vertigo on change of position, insomnia, nervousness, and a mild, constant substernal pressure not aggravated by exertion. All of these symptoms gradually cleared over a period of an additional 3 weeks (Faulkner, 1933). Persistence of symptoms for a week or more is not unusual (Wilson, 1930; Knack, 1932; Wehrlin, 1938).

Benowitz *et al.* (1987) reported a case of dermal intoxication after an attempted therapeutic application of 40% nicotine sulfate, which illustrates that tolerance can develop rapidly at toxic doses in humans. Thus, nausea and vomiting developed within 15 min and lethargy with periodic apnea within 2 hr, at which point the skin was washed, but plasma nicotine remained elevated at 200–300 ng/ml over 8 hr. The nausea and apnea persisted for only 4 hr, however, indicating marked tachyphylaxis in the face of a sustained plasma level of nicotine. Chronic ingestion of nicotine vie chewing gum at an estimated daily dose of 60 mg/day for 2 months caused a man to develop atrial fibrillation (Stewart and Catterall, 1985). It was noted that blood nicotine remained detectable for 14 hr after chewing as opposed to less than 8 hr after smoking, suggesting a greater potential for accumulation of dose by this route.

Use Experience Nicotine was applied to nearly 30,000 pear trees late in the dormant season of 1946–1947 for control of the pear psylla. A product containing 97–99% nicotine was applied with blower equipment as a concentrated mist spray, using kerosene or water containing 16 oz of alkaloid per gallon (125 ml/liter). No symptoms were experienced by workers who made preliminary tests, but many operators who applied the material on a large scale soon showed signs of poisoning. Those most seriously affected had weird dreams, a heavy feeling in the chest, difficulty in breathing, and violent nausea, which continued in some cases for as long as 10 hr. Susceptible individuals could not work more than 1 or 2 days without becoming sick. After recovering, they could not work with the alkaloid again without recurrent illness. Most of the workers had no warning symptoms. Those who had dreams as a first symptom were replaced immediately. All workers complained of a burning sensation of exposed skin when they first encountered the spray. Absorption through the skin seemed to be more detrimental than inhalation of fumes, although the fumes tended to aggravate nausea once nicotine had been absorbed.

Dust-type respirators were useless, but gas masks with special cannisters to absorb the fumes were effective. Rubber gloves and aprons were used in certain operations. All workers kept their collars buttoned and their sleeves rolled down, and they changed clothes frequently. They chewed and swallowed one charcoal tablet per hour. A lanolin-type skin cream protective against lime–sulfur sprays proved useless, but a cream that did not dissolve nicotine was used later. Using all these precautionary measures, all individuals were able to work without discomfort (Haines and Davis, 1948). The fact that oral charcoal was considered useful in association with dermal and respiratory exposure is interesting in view of the demonstrated secretion of nicotine into the stomach of various species of animals.

Nicotine is the probable cause of "green tobacco sickness" (Gehlbach et al., 1974, 1975, 1979) and can act as a hapten causing dermatitis (Sudan et al., 1984).

Dosage Response Many accidents and suicides have involved ingestion of the entire contents of a 1-ounce (29.6 ml) bottle of a 40% nicotine formulation. The resulting dose of about 12,000 mg has caused death in 1–10 min (Beeman and Hunter, 1937). In one case, 3176 mg of nicotine was recovered from the stomach contents and viscera (Smith, 1951). In another case just over 10,000 mg was recovered (Møller and Simesen, 1939).

A number of authors cited by Larson et al. (1961, 1968, 1971, 1975) have estimated that a dose of nicotine between 50 and 60 mg may be fatal. Although this estimate may be accurate, I have been unable to locate the report of any case on which it was based. Some evidence that 60 mg of nicotine might be fatal is offered by cases in which serious illness followed this or a somewhat smaller dose. Thus, Axtrup (1945) described an illness involving marked derangement of the EEG, as well as the more commonly observed signs of poisoning, in a 3-year-old boy who merely had licked the cork from a bottle of concentrated nicotine solution.

On the other hand, much larger doses have sometimes been ingested without a fatal outcome. In one instance a 33-year-old man survived at attempt at suicide in which he swallowed 4 ml of pure nicotine. Of course, much of the dose was lost by vomiting (Schmidt, 1931).

Maddock and Collier (1933) showed that the intravenous injection of 1.0 mg of nicotine alkaloid caused approximately the same increase in blood pressure and heart rate and decrease in skin temperature of the fingers and toes as was produced by smoking a cigarette. They quoted the work of others indicating that the smoke from two-thirds of a cigarette contains about 3.78 mg of nicotine, of which about 2.5 or 3.3 mg is retained, depending on whether the smoke is puffed or inhaled. The objective results were essentially similar in another series of studies in which the intravenous dose was 2 mg of nicotine bitartrate, equivalent to 0.6 mg of alkaloid, but some of the subjects experienced transient symptoms, some severe (Boyle et al., 1947).

A surprisingly small amount of nicotine base may produce serious illness through dermal absorption. Severe poisoning occurred in a girl employed in the manufacture of nicotine insecticide when she accidently spilled about 7.5 ml of a 95% solution on her coveralls. The coveralls were changed and some of the remaining poison was quickly removed by wiping the sleeve of her shirt and washing her arm. However, she collapsed in 20 min, and her life was saved only by prompt artificial respiration after she stopped breathing (Lockhart, 1933). Although it is impossible to determine how much nicotine reached the skin in this case, it must have been much less than the approximately 7120 mg spilled. In another instance a 35-year-old man happened to sit on a chair, on the seat of which a little 40% solution of free nicotine had been spilled. The clothing was wet in an area about the size of the palm of his hand. He became ill within 15 min and was unconscious for 3 hr (Faulkner, 1933).

Although not directly related to the question of dosage, it is important to recall that dilute solutions may cause poisoning. In one accident, two men were poisoned by a 0.23% solution of nicotine used to treat peach trees (Wilson, 1930).

The threshold limit value is 0.5 mg/m^3, indicating that occupational intake at the rate of 0.07 mg/kg/day is considered safe.

Laboratory Findings The laboratory findings are not

characteristic, except that nicotine may be found in the urine and in the tissues.

In a case of suicide, the following concentrations of nicotine were found: heart blood, 100 ppm; heart, 290 ppm; brain, 11 ppm; kidneys, 45 ppm; liver, 62 ppm; and spleen, 910 ppm; only a trace was found in the urine. Essentially identical values were obtained when the formalin-preserved tissues were re-analyzed after 1 year of storage under cool dark conditions (Tiess and Nagel, 1966).

The concentration of nicotine in the blood of smokers may be as great as 2 ppm but is generally less than 0.4 ppm. The nicotine is bound to the red cells (Larson *et al.*, 1961). The concentration in the blood in a fatal case was 28 ppm. In the same case, other concentrations were urine, 104 ppm; spleen, 124 ppm; liver, 52 ppm; kidney, 19 ppm; and brain, 9 ppm; the blood alcohol was 0.18% (Møller and Simesen, 1939). In another case, a concentration of 793 ppm in the brain was reported (Orsós, 1936).

Nicotine is excreted in human milk in concentrations up to 0.5 ppm (Perlman and Dannenberg, 1942).

Chronic exposure to nicotine and other constituents of tobacco smoke are clearly implicated in the pathogenesis of coronary heart disease, although because of the nature of exposure it is difficult to define causative agents. Some possibilities are reviewed by Benowitz (1986) and include increased plasma free fatty acids, platelet aggregation, coronary vasoconstriction, and circulating catecholamines.

In addition to smoking, cigarettes also provide a readily available source of nicotine and have been responsible for poisoning after ingestion by children (Saxena and Scheman, 1985) and in an adult following use of a homemade tobacco enema (Garcia-Estrada and Fischman, 1977).

Treatment of Poisoning   Artificial respiration is the most important measure. If the patient does not need it at once, preparation for it should be made while the patient is given activated charcoal or permanganate. The poison itself usually will have produced vomiting, but if the stomach has not been cleared thoroughly this should be done.

One of the earliest medical accounts of poisoning by tobacco (Bleasdale, 1906) tells of a 2-year-old boy who survived even though he was completely dependent on artificial respiration for about 40 min and partially dependent for another 20 min. At least one other case of successful resuscitation has been reported (Lockhart, 1933).

Because of the pH dependence of absorption, alkaline solutions are to be avoided in therapy.

13.4.2 ANABASINE

13.4.2.1 Identity, Properties, and Uses

Chemical Name   (*S*)-3-(2-Piperidinyl)pyridine or 2-(3-pyridyl)piperidine.

Structure   See Fig. 13.4.

Synonyms   Anabasine (JMAF) is the common name in use, but the compound in racemic form was once known as neonicotine. The CAS registry number is 494-52-0.

Physical and Chemical Properties   The empirical formula for anabasine is $C_{10}H_{14}N_2$ and the molecular weight 162.24. Anabasine is a liquid that freezes at 9°C and boils at 270–272°C. It is miscible with water and most organic solvents and forms salts with acids.

History, Formulations, Uses, and Production   The compound now called anabasine was made by Smith (1931), who described the synthesis and proposed the name neonicotine in a paper presented at a meeting of the American Chemical Society on April 8, 1930 and published on January 12, 1931. Later, the same compound was isolated by Orechoff and Menschikoff (1931) from *Anabasis aphylla,* a member of the Chenopodiaceae, native to parts of Russia. Anabasine is no longer produced as an insecticide in the United States or the United Kingdom. It is not clear if it is produced in other parts of the world, but, as with nicotine, its usefulness as an insecticide is now very limited indeed.

13.4.2.2 Toxicity to Laboratory Animals

Guinea pigs poisoned by anabasine show hyperexcitability, incoordination, tremor, clonic and tonic seizures, depression, and finally death, apparently from respiratory failure. Compared to nicotine, the acute toxicity of anabasine is slightly greater in guinea pigs and substantially greater in rabbits. Data given by Haag (1933) permit calculation of subcutaneous LD 50 values of 16 and 26 mg/kg for anabasine and nicotine, respectively, in guinea pigs and corresponding intravenous LD 50 values of 1.6 and 7.0 mg/kg in rabbits.

Anabasine is readily absorbed from the skin and from mucous membranes.

Pregnant pigs given 2.6 mg/kg anabasine twice daily in their food on days 30–37 or 43–53 of gestation showed tremor, protrusion of the nictitating membrane, and ataxia that persisted 2–3 days after dosage ended. This resulted in a large proportion of limb defects and cleft palates in the offspring (Keeler *et al.,* 1984). This teratogenicity may well be the consequence of a nicotinic pharmacological action on the uterus, as in the case of nicotine itself.

13.4.2.3 Toxicity to Humans

Accidental and Intentional Poisoning   According to Danilin and Shabaeva (1969), only six cases of poisoning by anabasine or its derivatives had been reported in the Soviet literature before they reported the details of a seventh case. A 29-year-old man was rushed to a clinic only 30 min after he had used a "tar" containing the compound as part of an enema to treat his rectal prolapse. He defecated promptly and experienced sharp generalized weakness, vertigo, and nausea. When examined, he was in critical condition. Although conscious, he was suffering cardiovascular disturbances, cyanosis of the hands and feet, and reduced body temperature. Thirty-five minutes after first aid, his respiration became severely depressed and he became markedly cyanotic and lost consciousness. Artificial respiration with enriched oxygen was administered. It was almost 8 hr until the patient breathed again spontaneously. He was discharged in 2 weeks. Anabasine was found in the patient's urine but not in the stomach washings collected on admission. Anabasine sulfate was present in the clyster flask. No sequelae were found when the patient was reexamined 1.5 years later.

Whereas this episode may seem strange, the use of nicotine as an enema has been reported for many years and from widely distant places. For example, Eberle (1830), while recommending the treatment "in cases of obstinate constipation," warned against its danger and cited the death of a charming little boy in less than 20 min. See also Garcia-Estrada and Fischman (1977) for a more recent case.

Treatment of Poisoning Treatment is the same as that for nicotine. See Section 13.4.1.3.

13.5 SABADILLA AND RELATED INSECTICIDES

Sabadilla (veratrin) is derived from *Schoenocaulon officinale,* a member of the lily family. However, one of its main alkaloids, veratridine, is present in veratrum derived from *Veratrum album* and to a lesser extent *Veratrum viride,* belonging to a closely related family, Melanthaceae. This phenomenon of having identical or similar toxicants produced by distinctly different plants is not unusual. Nowhere is it exhibited better than in connection with the digitalis-like glycocides, which are produced not only by botanically diverse plants but also by certain toads. Another example involves nicotine and related compounds (see Section 13.4).

One is warned against confusing veratrin and veratrum because they have different sources and different uses. However, they do have in common that both have been used in medicine and as insecticides, and, as already mentioned, they involve one important alkaloid, veratridine, in common. Most of their active constituents, including this one, are amine bases of steroid structure.

13.5.1 SABADILLA AND RELATED COMPOUNDS

13.5.1.1 Identity, Properties, and Uses

Scientific Name, Synonyms, and Structure Sabadilla is the dried ripe seeds of *S. officinale,* a plant of the lily family. When used as an insecticide, the ground seeds or formulations of them also are known as cevadilla, caustic barley, sabane dust, sabacide, and Shirlan®. A code designation for one com-

mercial formulation is ENT-123. The CAS registry number is 802-85-77.

The seeds contain about 0.3% alkaloids, of which cevadine (crystalline veratrine; CAS registry number 62-59-9) and veratridine (amorphous veratrine; CAS registry number 71-62-5) are the most important (Shanes, 1952). Other alkaloids present include sabadinine, sabadilline, and sabadine. The seeds also contain sabadillic and veratric acids, fatty oil, and resin. The structure of cevadine is shown in Fig. 13.5.

Physical and Chemical Properties Cevadine has the empirical formula $C_{32}H_{49}NO_9$ and a molecular weight of 591.72. It forms flat needles that decompose at 213–214.5°C. One gram of cevadine dissolves in about 15 ml alcohol or ether. The compound is slightly soluble in water.

History, Formulations, Uses, and Production It was recorded in the latter part of the sixteenth century that the Indians of New Spain were using sabadilla to combat vermin breeding in wounds and sores, as they no doubt had done much earlier. The Spaniards probably used it at about this time as a louse powder (Allen *et al.,* 1944). Sabadilla is no longer produced as an insecticide in the United States or the United Kingdom due largely to its poor selectivity of action and poor persistence on crops. It was used for control of insects infesting farm animals and as a domestic insecticide. Before the advent of modern insecticides, the import of sabadilla in the United States was as much as 42,628 kg/year.

Veratrin-containing plant extracts appear to be used to some extent in Eastern Europe, where "natural" pesticides are still popular, and veratrin has been found effective at suppressing weevil damage to stored grain (Nawrot, 1983).

13.5.1.2 Toxicity in Laboratory Animals

Basic Findings Since the veratrum alkaloids have a potent and highly specific effect on membrane sodium channels, their effects in mammals are largely on excitable tissues. Animals poisoned by sabadilla show retching, muscular spasms, ataxia, and coma. Illness begins rapidly, and death from respiratory or

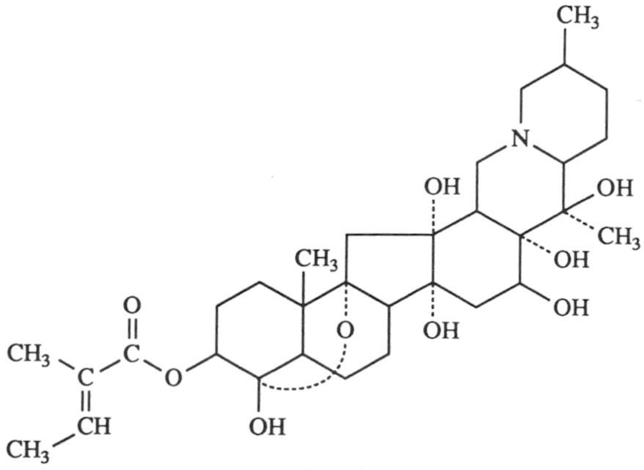

Figure 13.5 Structure of cevadine.

cardiac arrest may occur as early as 3–10 min or as late as 24 hr (Lehman, 1951, 1952).

Reports on the acute toxicity of sabadilla and its constituents (see Table 13.6) are not consistent. The ground powder was found to have far less toxicity than that of its constituent alkaloids and their concentration in the powder would lead one to expect. It may be that the alkaloids in the sample of powder tested had been been liberated fully either by aging, heat, or alkali.

In a study of 25 samples of sabadilla, it was found that no freshly powdered sabadilla seed was insecticidally active. However, the powder gradually becomes active merely by aging, or the constituents could be activated immediately by extraction with kerosene at 150°C, by heating the seed to 150°C for 1 hr and then extracting with cool kerosene, or by treating the seed with soda ash and then extracting with kerosene at 60°C. The extracts lost activity rapidly on exposure to light but were stable for at least 2 years when stored in brown bottles (Allen *et al.*, 1944).

The veratrum alkaloids are known to be teratogenic in sheep and cattle feeding on alkaloid-producing plants. Sabadilla itself does not appear to be teratogenic, but the related cyclopamine is teratogenic after a single oral dose of 120 mg/kg in hamsters (Keeler, 1978) and may be a significant impurity.

Pharmacological Actions   The veratrum alkaloids are very widely used as pharmacological tools, a review being that by Catterall (1980). Like the pyrethroids (Section 13.2), the veratrum alkaloids act on the membrane sodium channel and increase sodium flux. They act, however, at a separate site from the pyrethroids and produce two distinct effects: first, an activation of the sodium current at more negative membrane potentials so that there is an appreciable depolarizing current even at the normal resting potential, and second, a block of the time-dependent inactivation of the sodium current that normally follows the action potential. This block of inactivation is distinct from the slowing of inactivation produced by the pyrethroids and is also associated with a marked slowing of the rate of *activation* of the sodium current. Thus, in muscle, the

resting potential shows a gradual decline, hastened by stimulation, and nerves pass through a brief phase of hyperexcitability followed by depolarization and blockage (Dankó *et al.*, 1981). In neuroblastoma cells the half-maximal effect on sodium current is reached at 4.4×10^{-5} M cevadine, but calcium currents are reduced at 2.9×10^{-5} M (Romey and Lazdunski, 1982), which suggests that the primary effect of cevadine may be via increased sodium current in muscle but via decreased calcium current in other tissues.

As might be expected from its action on sodium channels, in addition to being a strong irritant, cevadine produces systemic actions including a characteristic prolonged contracture of skeletal muscle, slowing of the heart at least partially due to vagal stimulation, convulsions probably of medullary origin, and a rapid fall of blood pressure. The action on muscle is direct, for it occurs even after curare.

Intravenous dosages of cevadine as low as 0.025–0.050 mg/kg produced sudden slowing of the heart accompanied by a fall in blood pressure followed by marked cardiac arrhythmia or temporary arrest. This was due to stimulation of the vagus center, for it did not occur when the vagi were divided (Pilcher and Sollmann, 1915).

13.5.1.3 Toxicity to Humans

Therapeutic Use   The alkaloids of sabadilla are easily absorbed. Dermal absorption following use of salves or decoctions as "counterirritants" has produced not only severe irritation but also serious systemic symptoms (Sollmann, 1957).

Use Experience   As early as 1901, Sollmann noted that poisoning was rare, but he failed to record the conditions under which it did occur. He stated without documentation that in humans veratrine poisoning was characterized by burning of the mouth and later of the stomach, increased salivation, vomiting, diarrhea, abdominal pain, headache, dizziness, dilatation of the pupils, muscular twitching, and a slow, weak, irregular pulse. The patient remained oriented and therefore anxious. Death was caused by respiratory and circulatory collapse. In nonfatal cases, the symptoms were slow to disappear. Two patients who received repeated small doses became weak and thin and suffered bloody diarrhea, insomnia, disturbance of the intellect, and delirium. Thus, the possibility of cumulative action appears real.

In the course of their studies, Allen *et al.* (1944) noted the "sternutatory action produced during inhalation of the suspended toxicant" and speculated that this property might limit acceptance of the product.

Treatment of Poisoning   Treatment is entirely symptomatic.

13.6 OTHER BOTANICAL INSECTICIDES

In addition to those already described, there are many other insecticidal compounds derived from plants. Some such as the

Table 13.6
Acute Toxicity of Sabadilla and Some Constituent Alkaloids

Compound and species	Route	LD 50 (mg/kg)	Reference
Sabadilla			
rat	oral	4000	Lehman (1951, 1952)
Veratrine			
mouse	ip	7.5	Swiss and Bauer (1951)
blackbird	oral	18	Schafer *et al.* (1983)
Cevadine			
mouse	ip	3.5	Ikawa (1945)
mouse	ip	3.5	Swiss and Bauer (1951)
Veratridine			
mouse	ip	1.35	Swiss and Bauer (1951)
mouse	iv	0.42	Krayer *et al.* (1944)
rat	ip	3.5	Mendez and Montes (1943)

isobutylamides and azadirachtin are still in the developmental stage, but many more have been little exploited save for purely local use. For example, *Datura metal* has been used in the Gold Coast to combat vermin. The seeds of *Delphinium staphisagria*, of which the common name is lousewort, have been used for centuries against head lice in Europe. *Haplphyton cimicidum* was used in Mexico and other parts of Central America to combat head lice, cockroaches, and other insects. *Sophora flavescens* was used as an insecticide in China and Japan. These and many other botanical materials were explored by entomologists before the era of modern synthetic insecticides began. It would probably be an oversimplification to conclude that this screening operation sorted out the really effective materials, which then were exploited commercially. There is no way to predict what value may eventually be found in the products that were passed over. Certainly, there was nothing about pyrethrum powder *per se* to suggest that it would one day be possible and economical to synthesize pyrethroids that are stable to light and have other marked advantages over naturally occurring pyrethrins.

The lipid amides are a recently developed class of insecticides derived from black peppers and related plants (Miyakado *et al.*, 1985; Adesina, 1986). They are derived from long-chain aliphatic isobutylamides such as pellitorine, *N*-(2-methylpropyl)-2,4-decadienamide (CAS registry number 18836-52-7) and appear to owe their insecticidal activity to a pyrethroid-like interaction with membrane sodium channels. No mammalian studies are as yet reported for these potentially very important agents or for azadirachtin, an insect growth-inhibiting limonoid from the Indian neem tree (Yamasaki and Klocke, 1987).

13.7 PESTICIDES OF ANIMAL ORIGIN

Although not themselves of biological origin, a number of pesticides are structurally related to the annelid toxin nereistoxin, which is indeed a minor metabolite of several of them. These insecticides—cartap, bensultap, sha chong shuang (a Chinese pesticide), and thiocyclam (Fig. 13.6) were developed as nereistoxin analogs and share a common mechanism of action.

Nereistoxin itself is *N,N*-dimethyl 1,2-dithiolan-4-amine (CAS 1631-58-9) and was first isolated from the marine annelid *Lumbriconereis heteropoda* in 1934 by Nitta, who noted that flies feeding on the dead worms became paralyzed. Sattelle *et al.* (1985) found that nereistoxin produced an incomplete (<60%) curare-like block of cholinergic ganglionic transmission in cockroaches at 2×10^{-8} to $1 \times 10^{-6} M$ and an additional postsynaptic depolarization at 1×10^{-5} to $1 \times 10^{-3} M$. In mammals, death is by respiratory paralysis following blockade of neuromuscular transmission. High doses produce seizures by a central action, while lower doses produce increased intestinal motility, lacrimation, and salivation (Schopp and DeClue, 1980). The mechanism of action in vertebrates appears to involve inhibition of the nicotinic acetylcholine re-

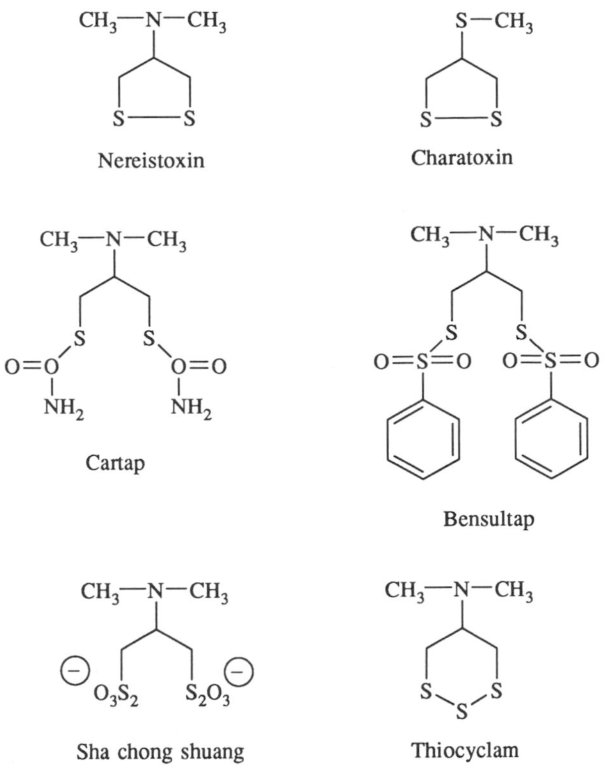

Figure 13.6 Nereistoxin, charatoxin, and insecticides related to nereistoxin.

ceptor ion channel, frog motor end-plate current being inhibited by 68% at $1 \times 10^{-4} M$ and binding of acetylcholine to isolated *Torpedo* electric organ membrane by 24% (Eldefrawi *et al.*, 1980), although this is complicated by nereistoxin also acting as a partial cholinergic agonist at lower concentrations (0.5×10^{-5} and $1 \times 10^{-4} M$). There are some analogies with charatoxin, a toxin isolated from the alga *Chara globularis* (see Fig. 13.6), which is itself also the basis for a number of experimental pesticides (Nielsen and Pedersen, 1984) although charatoxin acts on the low-affinity noncompetitive blocker site (Sherby *et al.*, 1986).

Nereistoxin has an intravenous LD 50 in mice of 30 mg/kg and an oral LD 50 of 118 mg/kg (Konishi, 1972), and in dogs intravenous administration of 1 mg/kg gives a lethal 50% block of neuromuscular transmission (Schopp and DeClue, 1980). Most of the insecticidal analogs of nereistoxin are of lower potency but share the same mechanism of action, and one of them, cartap, is described in greater detail in the next section. Of the others, thiocyclam (CAS 31895-21-3) has a rat oral LD 50 of 310 mg/kg, and bensultap (CAS 17606-31-4) of 1105 mg/kg (Sakai, 1984). Both are used against lepidopteran and coleopteran pests.

13.7.1 CARTAP

13.7.1.1 Identity, Properties, and Uses

Chemical Name Cartap is *S,S'*-[2-(dimethylamino)-1,3-propanediyl] dicarbamothioate. It is normally used as the hydrochloride.

Structure See Fig. 13.6

Synonyms Cartap is the common name in use. Trade names include Padan®, Thiobel®, and Vegetox®. The CAS registry number is 15263-53-3 for cartap or 15263-52-2 for cartap hydrochloride.

Physical and Chemical Properties Cartap hydrochloride has the empirical formula $C_7H_{15}N_3O_2S_2HCl$ and a molecular weight of 273.81. It forms colorless crystals which melt between 179 and 181°C with decomposition. Its water solubility is 178 gm/liter and it is only slightly soluble in methanol and insoluble in many other organic solvents. It is hydrolyzed to an inactive nereistoxin polymer in neutral or alkaline solutions (Obayashi and Asaka, 1983).

History, Formulations, and Uses Cartap was introduced in Japan in 1967 and is used as 25 and 50% water-soluble powders, 2% dusts, or 4–10% granules against a range of insects, especially weevils and caterpillars

13.7.1.2 Toxicity to Laboratory Animals

Cartap produces its acute toxicity by neuromuscular blockade leading to respiratory failure. In rats the acute oral LD 50 is 325–390 mg/kg, in mice 150–225 mg/kg, and in monkeys 100–200 mg/kg. Cartap is more toxic by the subcutaneous and intravenous routes, with rat LD 50 values of 41 and 40 mg/kg, respectively, but in rabbits the dermal LD 50 was 820 mg/kg (FAO/WHO, 1977). Rats and mice fed cartap in their diet for 3 months showed reductions in weight gain at 40 or 135 mg/kg/day, respectively, but no other effects, and rabbits given daily dermal doses of 60 mg/kg for 3 weeks also showed weight loss and slight dermal irritation.

Cartap is rapidly absorbed, metabolized, and excreted in the urine of both rats and mice, 94 and 89% of the total dose being excreted within 24 hr in these two species (FAO/WHO, 1979). The half-life in the blood of rabbits is 13.9 hr, and blood levels peak 2 hr after oral administration (Jin *et al.*, 1984). Cartap is readily hydrolyzed to nereistoxin and dihydronereistoxin, which are then methylated and oxidized. Nereistoxin represents 1–2% of the urinary metabolites (FAO/WHO, 1979).

Daily oral dosage of pregnant female rats at 50 mg/kg/day from days 6 to 15 (maternal LD 5) produced a small reduction in fetal weight but no malformations. Cartap had no mutagenic effects in microbial or mouse bone marrow assays (FAO/WHO, 1979; Maryanska-Nadachowska and Rudek, 1983). Significant protection from the effects of an oral dose of 50 mg/kg cartap was seen in rabbits given intravenous cystine, the ED 50 being 40 mg/kg (FAO/WHO, 1977).

13.7.1.3 Toxicity to Humans

No specific studies in humans have been reported, but detailed medical examinations of workers involved in the manufacture of cartap showed no adverse effects, although there was no quantification of the degree of exposure (FAO/WHO, 1977).

13.8 INSECT GROWTH REGULATORS

A number of recently developed insecticides act not on the nervous system, which shares many common features with that of vertebrates, but on the highly species-specific insect hormonal systems controlling metamorphosis and molting. These insecticides have the advantage of very low mammalian toxicity, but their extreme species specificity, lack of rapid kill, and poor stability have limited usage until suitable formulations and control strategies are developed. Their applications in insect control and public health are reviewed by Mian and Mulla (1982).

Juvenile hormone, discovered by Wigglesworth (1935, 1936), was extracted and characterized by Williams (1956), who proposed its use in insect control. Juvenile hormones are one of the three types of internal secretions used by insects to regulate growth and metamorphosis. The juvenile hormones are synthesized and released to the hemolymph in a regulated way by the corpora allata in the head of each insect. Each immature larva has an absolute requirement for these hormones if it is to progress through the usual larval stages. Then, in order for the mature larva to metamorphose into a sexually mature adult, the concentration of the hormone must become very low. The adult must secrete it again if eggs are to be produced, but it must be absent from the egg for normal development to occur. A number of active juvenile hormones have been synthesized (Schwarz *et al.*, 1970; Sláma *et al.*, 1974) and their physiology has been reviewed by Wigglesworth (1970) and Sláma *et al.* (1974).

Although pure juvenile hormones have very low mammalian toxicity, some technical preparations are teratogenic after a single injection of 0.5–1.5 gm/kg (Wright and Smalley, 1977), so impurities may represent an unexpected hazard.

Mice tolerated a single oral dose of one of the natural juvenile hormones (C-17 JH shown as B in Fig. 13.7) or of a close analog at a rate of 5000 mg/kg without any sign of toxicity (Siddall and Slade, 1971). Because terpenes from plants are metabolized readily by mammals, it seems unlikely that repeated absorption of the natural hormones or of analogs that are simple hydrocarbons would be injurious.

It was noticed that paper made from balsam fir wood inhibited insect metamorphosis, and various "paper factors" were identified (Fig. 13.7C) and a large number of synthetic derivatives developed (Sláma, 1971). The most active compounds have an acyclic terpenoid skeleton. However, activity may be retained in spite of some variation in length and in spite of the presence of nitrogen or chlorine in the molecule (Schwarz *et al.*, 1970). Although the natural hormones identified so far are not known to occur in plants, the differences seem minor, and the hormones appear to follow the "isoprene rule," which, according to Simonsen and Owen (1947), has been the most valuable working hypothesis for elucidating the structure of terpenes.

Juvenile hormone I suppresses mitosis in cultured mouse cells at 10 mg/liter (Zielinska *et al.*, 1981), and it has been shown that synthetic C-18 juvenile hormone at concentrations

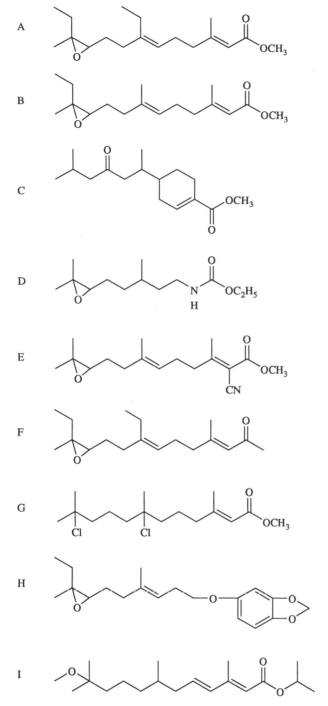

Figure 13.7 Some juvenile hormones and selected analogs. (A and B) Naturally occurring hormones from *Hyalophola cecropia:* A, C-18 JH; B, C-17 JH. (C) Paper factor; (D–I) synthetic analogs, including methoprene (I).

of 2–100 mg/liter *in vitro* is cytocidal and inhibits the synthesis of protein, DNA, and to a lesser degree RNA. Two juvenile hormone analogs were somewhat less active, but all were inactivated by serum (Chmurzynska *et al.,* 1979). There is, however, no evidence that the compounds could survive metabolism and reach effective concentrations in mammals *in vivo* even if serum were not inhibitory.

Synthetic juvenile hormones in use include methoprene (Al-

tosid), which has the CAS registry number 40596-69-8, and altozar, CAS registry number 41096-46-2. Methoprene is in use as a broad-spectrum insect growth inhibitor. It is of extremely low mammalian toxicity, has no teratogenic effects in rats when given orally at 1000 mg/kg despite a transient loss of maternal weight (Hackel, 1983), and is not genotoxic in a fly wing mosaicism test (Szabad and Bennettova, 1986). It is also rapidly metabolized by mammals (Mian and Mulla, 1982). A second class of growth regulators act on chitin synthesis, and some insecticides such as diflubenzuran (Dimilin) act by interfering with these (Mian and Mulla, 1982).

13.9 ATTRACTANTS

It is a common observation that flies are attracted to food and that different species are attracted to different foods—fruit flies to fruit, flesh flies to flesh, etc. The fact that the common names reflect the insects' preferences is an indication of how long the relationship has been known for some species.

Much more recently, but still long ago, it was noticed that females of some species of moths attract males of the same species, sometimes from considerable distances.

Modern study has revealed a vast array of materials that influence the behavior of insects. Actions or processes affected include attraction to food, biting, swallowing, growth, aggregation, defense, courtship, mating, egg laying, and many of the special behavior patterns that characterize social insects, including trailing and alarm reactions. The ability of a single pheromone to subserve multiple functions in different environmental contexts has been noted, especially in social insects. Persons interested in the intricate and varied subject of insect communication by chemicals may find a wealth of information in books restricted to this matter (Beroza, 1970; Wood *et al.,* 1970; Shorey and McKelvey, 1977) or to the even broader subject of chemical communication by a wide range of animals (Shorey, 1976). A more recent review is that by Plimmer *et al.* (1982).

Two approaches have been used in discovering insect attractants. First, compounds have been isolated from natural sources, identified, synthesized, and then proved by laboratory and field tests to be active. Second, a large number of chemicals have been tested against a given insect species to find an attractant, and then related compounds were synthesized in an effort to find a more effective analog.

Of the naturally occurring attractants, the sex pheromones of the Lepidoptera and the attractant pheromones of the Coleoptera have been most thoroughly explored. More of the former are long-chain unsaturated acetates but a few are straight-chain, usually unsaturated alcohols or aldehydes or even saturated hydrocarbons. One of the acetates, propylure, is shown in Fig. 13.8A. Attractant pheromones of Coleoptera are even more varied; they include terpene alcohols (see Fig. 13.8B–D), terpene aldehydes, an unusual bicyclic ketal structure (see Fig. 13.8E, F), acids (see Fig. 13.8G), and esters. Synthetic attractants are highly diverse (see Fig. 13.8H–L). It is not known how

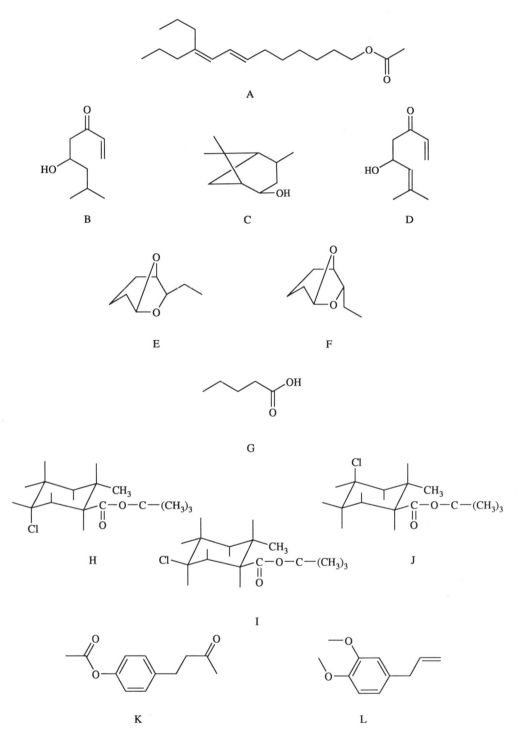

Figure 13.8 Some naturally occurring (A–F) and synthetic (G–K) insect attractants. The compounds are (A) propylure, the natural attractant of the pink bollworm moth; (B–D) principal components of the natural attractant of *Ips confusus*, a wood-boring beetle; (E and F) *exo-* and *endo*-brevicomin, attractant from *Dendroctonus brevicomis*; (G) valeric acid, an attractant produced by *Limonius californicus*; (H–J) isomers A, B₁, and C of trimedlure, which are active as attractants of the Mediterranean fruit fly (the B₂ isomer is not attractive); (K) cue-lure, which attracts the melon fly; and (L) methyl eugenol, which attracts the Oriental fruit fly.

they work. They might resemble some constituent in the insect's food, or those that attract males only might resemble sex phenomones, but this is speculation. The compounds shown in Fig. 13.8H–L are used to detect the Mediterranean fruit fly, the melon fly, and the Oriental fruit fly.

Some of the pheromones are, in fact, mixtures of compounds. In some instances, no single constituent of the mixture is active but a proper ratio of all constituents—four in the case of the boll weevil pheromone—is required for optimal activity (Tumlinson *et al.*, 1970). On the contrary, as little as 15% of the *cis* isomer of propylure is sufficient to nullify the activity of the *trans* isomer (Jacobson, 1969). Some pheromones are most active only in the presence of a compound produced by the host plant. For example, myrcene, a product of pine trees, greatly increases the attractiveness of both *exo-* and *endo-*brevicomin.

In practice, attractants can be used in several ways to control insect populations. They can be used for surveys of pest species, both in the field and in stores, and to help correct the timing and choice of use of conventional pesticides. They can also be used as lures for mass trapping to remove males from the population or to disrupt normal courtship and mating. A particularly efficient application is to lure insects to conventional insecticides, thus reducing cost and environmental exposure. The attractants themselves have the advantage of low toxicity, rapid biodegradability, and remarkable efficiency, since insects are capable of responding to as little as one molecule of certain pheromones (Plimmer *et al.*, 1982). They have the disadvantage that they are often very highly specific and cannot be used to control mixed infestations, and they tend also to be expensive since large-scale synthesis is not required. Much effort is being directed at finding effective slow-release formulations to make usage more economic.

13.10 BOTANICAL RODENTICIDES

In the hope of controlling rodents that rob them of food, health, and property, people have used not only botanical poisons but also inorganic poisons (see Sections 12.1.1, 12.4.2, 12.7.1, 12.11.1, 12.12.1, and 12.13.1) and a variety of synthetic organic compounds (see Chapter 19).

The botanical compounds used for this purpose include strychnine, red squill, and ricin. Of these, strychnine has been used as a drug, and the red squill used to kill rats differs little from the white variety used in human medicine.

The active ingredient of red squill bulbs is scilliroside (CAS registry number 507-60-8), a cardiac glucoside of which the active aglycone is scillirosidin (see Fig. 13.9). Red squill was formerly important as a rodenticide, and it has been suggested (Verbiscar *et al.*, 1986) that it may find increasing usage as rats become resistant to warfarin, although squill is banned as a rodenticide in the United Kingdom on humane grounds. Rats are relatively resistant to the cardiac actions of scilliroside and instead show protracted convulsions and muscular weakness, which develop over 2–10 hr at half of the acutely cardiotoxic dose (Gold *et al.*, 1947). The oral LD 50 in male rats is 5.3 mg/kg and in females is 1.4 mg/kg (Verbiscar *et al.*, 1986); but scilliroside is a potent local emetic, eight times more effective than oubain, and is more effective in continuous feeders such as the rat, which are incapable of vomiting, than in other species.

Strychnine is an alkaloid; red squill contains a number of cardiac glycosides; ricin is a glycoprotein with a molecular weight of approximately 65,000, closely related to other plant toxins such as abrin and modeccin (Stirpe and Barbieri, 1986).

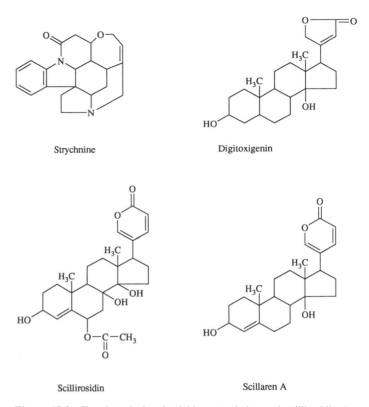

Figure 13.9 Two botanical rodenticides, strychnine and scillirosidin (an aglucone or genin from red squill). Also shown are aglucones from white squill and digitalis, both of which are used as drugs.

13.10.1 STRYCHNINE

13.10.1.1 Identity, Properties, and Uses

Chemical Name   Strychnine or strychnidin-10-one.

Structure   See Fig. 13.9.

Synonyms   Strychnine (BSI, ISO) is manufactured under the trade names Certox®, Kwik-Kil®, Mouse-Red®, Mouse-Tox®, and Ro-Dex®. The CAS registry number is 57-24-9.

Physical and Chemical Properties   The empirical formula for strychnine is $C_{21}H_{22}N_2O_2$ and the molecular weight 334.40. Strychnine forms very bitter orthorhombic, spheroidal prisms from alcohol and appears as white powder. Its melting point is 268–290°C with decomposition. The solubility of strychnine in water at room temperature is 143 mg/liter. It is slightly soluble in benzene and chloroform and very slightly soluble in ether and petroleum ether. Strychnine is a base with pK values of 6.0 and 11.7, and its salts are more soluble in water; for example, the sulfate is soluble in water at 30 gm/liter at 15°C.

Formulations and Uses   Strychnine and its salts are used for destroying birds, rodents, moles, and predatory animals and for acquiring fur-bearing animals. Prepared pelleted baits usually contain 5–10 gm strychnine sulfate/kg. The sulfate is

78.04% strychnine. Both the alkaloid and the sulfate are available as technical powders.

13.10.1.2 Toxicity to Laboratory Animals

Symptomatology The effects of strychnine in animals are so similar to those in humans that there is no need to mention them. Irritation of tissues and sensitization are not associated with strychnine.

Dosage Response The older literature contains many records of lethal doses of strychnine, as summarized by Flury and Zernik (1935). Table 13.7 contains information on its acute toxicity expressed in modern terms. The ED 50 for convulsions is remarkably close to the LD 50. There is no difference in intraperitoneal toxicity between the sulfate, benzoate, salicylate, and orthonitrobenzoate expressed in terms of their alkaloid content. Female rats and mice are slightly more susceptible than males, and young rats are slightly more susceptible than adults (Poe *et al.*, 1936; Lakatos *et al.*, 1964). These results were confirmed and extended by Kato *et al.* (1962, 1963), who found that the sex differential was seen only when the dosage route allowed time for metabolic disposal to become significant, and these authors failed to find a sex difference in susceptibility to strychnine among immature rats or among mice or guinea pigs. The difference in susceptibility among intact adult rats and the lack of difference between other comparable males and females corresponded to the ability of liver homogenates from these animals to metabolize strychnine *in vitro*. SKF 525 A increased the toxicity of strychnine to intact animals and eliminated the sex difference both *in vivo* and *in vitro*.

Reflex enhancement, as measured by the startle response to sound, is seen in rats given strychnine doses of only 0.25 mg/kg (Davis *et al.*, 1986). Individual subcutaneous injection of dogs and guinea pigs at rates of 0.25–0.35 mg/kg every 3–7 days occasionally produced no increase in reflexes but generally produced increased reflexes or convulsions of variable degree. There was no evidence of tolerance. If such injections were repeated for a sufficient length of time, the animal eventually failed to survive a convulsion, but this was hardly evidence for a cumulative effect under these conditions (Hale, 1909).

Bears (*Ursus arctos yesoensis*) are unusually susceptible, 0.5 (but not 0.25) mg/kg being adequate for their control. The meat of bears poisoned by strychnine at a dosage of either 0.5 or 1.0 mg/kg may be eaten safely by people (Inukai, 1969).

Oral LD 50 values of strychnine ranged from 2.9 to 24.7 mg/kg in six species of birds (Tucker and Haegele, 1971).

Absorption, Distribution, Metabolism, and Excretion It is agreed that strychnine is promptly absorbed, mainly from the intestine. With a pK_2 of 11.7, strychnine would not exist as the free alkaloid anywhere in the digestive tract.

Although strychnine acts principally on the spinal cord, it is not concentrated there. In persons killed by the compound, the highest concentrations are found in the blood, liver, and kidney. In dogs killed by the compound, the concentration of strychnine in the liver ranged from 0 to 52 ppm and averaged 6.7 ppm (Hatch and Funnell, 1968).

In rats, strychnine is metabolized by microsomal enzymes of the liver. In one experiment the rates of biotransformation produced by microsomal fractions were 144 and 64 μg/gm of liver/hr in males and females, respectively. Metabolism was reduced to 9–7 μg/gm/hr, respectively, by SKF 525 A (Kato *et al.*, 1962). The rate of metabolism is greater in the guinea pig, reaching 387 μg/gm/hr in microsomal preparations, 649 μg/gm/hr in liver slices, and 1152 μg/gm/hr in liver slices from animals pretreated with phenobarbital. Phenobarbital also induces strychnine-metabolizing enzymes of rats (Kato *et al.*, 1963).

Pharmacological Effects A description of strychnine poisoning in humans is given in Section 13.10.1.3. The picture in animals is similar. The most characteristic feature is the violent response to a sudden, unexpected stimulus, whether of touch, light, or sound. All of the voluntary muscles, including the diaphragm, undergo a sustained contraction or tetanus. Since the extensors, which serve to hold the body erect, are generally stronger than the flexors, the limbs usually are extended and the back is arched in a position of opisthotonos.

Almost all of the actions of strychnine are attributable to its antagonism of the inhibitory neurotransmitter glycine (Barron and Guth, 1987). Glycine is the major inhibitory transmitter in the spinal cord and brain stem, and it is the disturbance of the normal balance between excitation and inhibition produced by

Table 13.7
Acute Toxicity of Strychnine Base

Species	Age (weeks)	Route	ED 50[a] (mg/kg)	LD 50 (mg/kg)	Reference
Rat	adult	oral		16.2	Lehman (1951, 1952)
Rat, M	adult	sc	3.72	4.01	Kato *et al.* (1962)
Rat, F	adult	sc	1.67	1.81	Kato *et al.* (1962)
Rat, M	6	ip		1.4	Poe *et al.* (1936)
Rat, M	10	ip		1.9	Poe *et al.* (1936)
Rat, M	18	ip		2.3	Poe *et al.* (1936)
Rat, M	adult	ip		2.3	Poe *et al.* (1936)
Rat, F	6	ip		0.9	Poe *et al.* (1936)
Rat, F	18	ip		1.1	Poe *et al.* (1936)
Rat, F	adult	ip		1.4	Poe *et al.* (1936)
Rat, M	adult	ip	2.61	2.82	Kato *et al.* (1962)
Rat, F	adult	ip	1.50	1.62	Kato *et al.* (1962)
Rat, M	adult	iv	0.51	0.57	Kato *et al.* (1962)
Rat, F	adult	iv	0.50	0.57	Kato *et al.* (1962)
Mouse, M	8	ip		1.9	Lakatos *et al.* (1964)
Mouse, F	8	ip		1.6	Lakatos *et al.* (1964)
Guinea pig	adult	sc	4.1	4.8	Kato *et al.* (1963)
Guinea pig	adult	ip	9.6	10.9	Kato *et al.* (1963)
Guinea pig	adult	iv	0.34	0.39	Kato *et al.* (1963)
Dog	adult	sc		0.46	Kamel and Afifi (1969)

[a] Dosage producing convulsion.

blockade of glycine receptors in these areas that causes the powerful motor symptoms seen in strychnine poisoning. Glycine is thought to play a role in neurotransmission in higher centers such as the substantia nigra and neostriatum (Pycock and Kerwin, 1981) but the glycine receptors in these areas and in the hippocampus and cerebral cortex are of a subtype insensitive to strychnine (Bristow *et al.*, 1986), which is why strychnine symptoms are largely spinal in origin. Consciousness is retained throughout the most severe strychnine symptoms, a feature which distinguishes them from those produced by agents acting on higher centers. In cats given intravenous strychnine at 0.125–0.5 mg/kg, the enhanced sensory responsiveness of higher centers could be shown to result from a primary action on the brain stem reticular formation which spreads to other areas by recruitment (Faingold *et al.*, 1985).

Strychnine has a high affinity for glycine receptors, with a K_a of 3×10^{-8} M for rat spinal cord synaptosomes, which is 300 times higher than that of glycine itself (Young and Snyder, 1973). Strychnine shows a high degree of specificity for glycine receptors, Curtis *et al.* (1971) showing that in cats intravenous doses of 0.2–0.8 mg/kg antagonized the inhibitory effects of iontophoretically applied glycine on spinal neurons by a factor of five but did not alter the effect of iontophoretically applied GABA at all. At very high doses strychnine has more widespread actions. These are reviewed by Barron and Guth (1987) and include inhibition of sodium, potassium, and chloride conductances and antagonism of GABA and noradrenaline. It is this generalized excitatory action produced at very high (millimolar) doses that enabled topical strychnine to be used to trace neuronal pathways through the CNS by following the spread of strychnine-induced discharges in strychnine neuronography (Wall and Horwitz, 1951).

Pathology   Autopsy findings are entirely nonspecific, reflecting only the presence of violent convulsions and anoxia. Congestion and small hemorrhages may be found in the brain and sometimes in the viscera. In fact, ultrastructural study revealed no difference from controls in the spinal cord synapses of rats killed at the appearance of convulsions following intraperitoneal injection of strychnine chlorhydrate at a rate of 5 mg/kg (Pensa and Ceccarelli, 1968).

Treatment of Poisoning in Animals   It was shown very early (Gies and Meltzer, 1903) that artificial respiration will protect animals from an otherwise fatal dose of strychnine.

Rabbits may be saved from 35 fatal doses of strychnine by small repeated intravenous doses of pentobarbital (Barlow, 1932).

Berger (1949, 1952) showed that the antagonism between strychnine and mephenesin is more complete than that between strychnine and a short-acting barbiturate. Mephenesin, like strychnine, has its major effect on the spinal cord and brain stem.

The oral ED 50 of diazepam used to protect mice from the convulsant action of strychnine (0.63 mg/kg iv) was 16 mg/kg (Randall *et al.*, 1961).

As reported earlier by others, pyrone compounds isolated from the rhizome of *Piper methysticum* were effective antagonists of poisoning when administered 30 min before strychnine. Methysticin (CAS registry number 495-85-2) was the most potent; its maximal effective intraperitoneal dosage was 300 mg/kg, which raised the subcutaneous LD 50 of strychnine from 1.45 to 7.3 mg/kg. This degree of protection was not as great as that offered by phenobarbital, which, at an intraperitoneal dosage of 200 mg/kg, raised the LD 50 of strychnine to 43 mg/kg. What distinguished the pyrenones was that at dosages that did not block polysynaptic reflexes or evoke distinct muscle relaxation (e.g., methysticin at 150 mg/kg ip) they gave complete protection from strychnine at 5 mg/kg, even though 2 mg/kg killed all unprotected mice. The protected mice not only survived but also maintained normal motor activity and food intake (Kretzschmar *et al.*, 1970).

13.10.1.3 Toxicity to Humans

Therapeutic Use   Because it produces increased tone of skeletal muscles, strychnine has been used in the past as a tonic in connection with fatigue, general weakness, incontinence, impotence, collapse of varied origin, paralysis, pneumonia, tuberculosis, and numerous other diseases. When strychnine was used to treat paralysis following a cerebral stoke, the paralyzed muscles were often the first to contract because they lacked cerebral inhibition. Even in this century, it was spoken of as truly representing the specific medicament for all nervous insufficiency. Intensive treatment was recommended with doses increasing to 5 to 6 mg in women and 6 to 7 mg in men. One of the advantages claimed for it was that it was not habit forming (Hartenberg, 1913). The usual dose varied from 1 to 5 mg of the sulfate or 0.6 to 2 ml of the tincture of nux vomica, which contained 0.12% strychnine and the same concentration of related alkaloids. Even as late at 1961 there were five deaths in the United States caused by strychnine intended for use as a drug. Most, if not all, of these fatalities were caused by accidental ingestion rather than therapeutic misadventure. In the same year, there was only one death caused by strychnine intended for killing rats (Hayes and Pirkle, 1966). As many presumably accidental deaths annually caused by strychnine were revealed by special studies of deaths in 1969, 1973, and 1974, but the proportion clearly attributed to strychnine intended as a drug was smaller (Hayes, 1976; Hayes and Vaughn, 1977).

Accidental and Intentional Poisoning   Toxic doses usually produce some tightness and twitching of the muscles, especially those in the face and neck. Movements may be abrupt. Vomiting may occur. Generalized convulsions occur within 15 to 30 min after ingestion. They may be clonic at first but quickly become tonic. The more delayed the onset of the tetanus, the better the prognosis.

The seizure may begin with a cry, more from the expulsion of air than from pain. The patient remains fully conscious and lucid until anoxia supervenes. Therefore, during a seizure, pain is intense because of the violent contraction of the muscles, whose very rigidity prevents an outcry. The chest and diaphragm are fixed, stopping respiration and producing cyanosis. The muscles are hard. The contraction may be violent enough to cause compression fractures of the vertebrae. The seizure is symmetrical. The back is arched so that the victim often rests on the heels and the back of the head. The legs are adducted and extended, the feet curved inward, the arches bowed. The arms may be flexed strongly over the chest or extended rigidly with the fists clenched. The jaws are fixed. Foam gathers at the mouth. The eyes protrude and the pupils dilate. The pulse may be difficult to detect.

The first seizure usually lasts one or a few minutes. In severe, untreated poisoning, each succeeding convulsion tends to last longer than the one before it, and the intervals between convulsions tend to get shorter.

Many convulsions are precipitated by some external stimulus but, because of the patient's great hyperexcitability, the stimulus may be very small. A curious thing about strychnine poisoning is that the victim may tolerate being lifted and moved, provided the action is expected and gentle, but a sudden, unexpected light touch may throw the victim into tonic contraction. Recent cases treated with diazepam emphasize that the complete seizure cycle involves a prodromal period immediately preceding the actual convulsions. The conscious patient can tell the physician about prodromal symptoms, including cramps in the legs and tightness in the chest, and convulsions can be prevented by additional, intravenous drug. The same cases suggest that, no matter how important extraneous stimuli may be in strychnine poisoning, the untreated condition is inherently characterized by the cyclic recurrence of prodromal symptoms, convulsions, remission, prodromal symptoms, etc.

During the remissions, patients are exhausted and understandably anxious. They may sweat. The throat is dry, and they usually are thirsty. Convulsions may recur within a few moments or after several hours. The patient must be watched carefully for about 24 hr.

Death may occur at any time. Rarely, with very large doses, it may follow sudden collapse before convulsions develop but is usually due either to brain damage secondary to apnea from uncontrolled seizures (e.g., Dittrich et al., 1984) or to cardiac arrest (e.g., O'Callaghan et al., 1982). If repeated seizures occur, the contractions eventually become weaker and paralysis is more prominent during intermissions. If recovery occurs, it is remarkably prompt and complete in spite of the violence of the illness. Of course, the patient is very sore from the violent exercise. Some tightness of muscles may persist for a day or two. The intensity of the muscle activity can lead to extreme acidosis due to lactic acid production, but patients have recovered from arterial pH values as low as 6.59 with the aid of artificial ventilation (Loughhead et al., 1978; Lambert et al., 1981; Boyd et al., 1983). In many cases the body temperature remains normal, but it may rise to 38.9°C and remain abnormally high for a day or more, long after convulsions have stopped (Hewlett, 1913), or it may reach 43°C transiently with

survival (Boyd et al., 1983). Hyperthermia was seen in 6 of 25 cases reviewed by Edmunds et al. (1986). Earlier cases are reviewed by Schrader (1937).

The number of fatal accidents caused by strychnine intended for use as a rodenticide decreased from 1939 to 1959 but then leveled off (Hayes, 1975), and cases of accidental poisoning and suicide are still seen. In 1978 and 1981 there were 13 deaths from strychnine poisoning in the United States (Perper, 1985) and in 1983 there were 30 hospital admissions (Dittrich et al., 1984). A disturbing trend is that several recent cases have involved adulteration or replacement of illicit drugs with strychnine, either intravenous heroin (Decker et al., 1982) or inhaled cocaine (O'Callaghan et al., 1982; Boyd et al., 1983).

Dosage Response Patients given doses of 5–7 mg reported a tightness of their muscles, especially those of the neck and jaws, and individual muscles, especially those of the little fingers, may twitch. Apparently, some of the very early therapeutic efforts involved high doses. Eberle (1830) quotes Paris to the effect that doses of 30 mg cause "serious effects" and larger ones cause convulsions and death.

A 20-year-old woman was killed by a dose of strychnine estimated as 135–143 mg (Salm, 1952).

Children may be more susceptible to strychnine than adults. A child died of strychnine poisoning after ingesting an unknown number of cathartic pills, each containing 0.8 mg of strychnine nitrate, an amount only twice the maximal "therapeutic" dose for a child of about the same age (Schwarz, 1954).

On the other hand, larger doses may be survived if treatment is prompt. A patient who swallowed about 15,000 mg of the sulfate, equivalent to about 13,000 mg of strychnine base, vomited an unknown portion of the poison and survived following treatment (Priest, 1938). Others have survived doses at least as great as 250 mg without clearing of the stomach (Bental et al., 1961), or up to 570 or 700 mg when the stomach was cleared (Cotten and Lane, 1966; Sagaragli and Mannaioni, 1974). A 1.5-year-old boy survived a dose of 9.5 mg or greater (Symons and Boyle, 1963).

The threshold limit value of 0.15 mg/m^3 indicates that an occupational intake of 0.02 mg/kg/day is considered safe.

Laboratory Findings A concentration of strychnine in the urine as high as 100 ppm was reported in a patient who survived. Except for the demonstration of the poison itself, laboratory findings are helpful only in control of acidosis. There is little diagnostic value in the electroencephalographic changes reported (Bental et al., 1961).

Strychnine is metabolized by microsomal oxidation in the liver, and the half-life in human plasma is 10 hr, this corresponding to clearance of 7% of the serum strychnine per hour (Edmunds et al., 1986).

From 11 to 20% of a therapeutic dose of 4 mg, whether ingested or injected intramuscularly, is excreted unchanged in the urine. Of the portion excreted by the kidneys, an average of

70% appears in the first 6 hr and nearly 90% in the first 24 hr (Weiss and Hatcher, 1922). Strychnine may be detectable in the urine in 0.5–3 hr in humans (Hewlett, 1913). Following toxic doses, most of the excretion occurs in the first 24 hr, but excretion during the first 6 hr or so may be small, thus accounting for the negligible amounts found in persons killed rapidly by strychnine (Hewlett, 1913). Traces may persist for 4 days (Hewlett, 1913) or even 5 days (Hale, 1909). In animals, excretion of strychnine is increased only slightly by diuresis (Weiss and Hatcher, 1922).

In one case of attempted suicide, myoglobin was found in the plasma on the day of admission and later in the urine. This was correlated with metabolic acidosis; intense muscular weakness; elevation of plasma CPK, LDH, and SGOT; and focal injury of striated muscle revealed by biopsy. These changes occurred even though convulsions were well controlled by diazepam (Bismuth *et al.*, 1977).

Pathology The pathological findings are entirely nonspecific. They usually consist of petechial hemorrhages and congestion of the organs, indicating combined action of severe convulsions and anoxia. Compression fractures and related injury may be found in cases with violent tetanus. In one case, the ventricles of the heart were completely contracted and felt as hard as wood, even though the auricles were dilated. It was believed that death was due to spasm of the ventricles (Lovegrove, 1963).

Treatment of Poisoning There have been many reports of the treatment of poisoning in humans. A recent report and review of the clinical literature is that of Edmunds *et al.* (1986). Because of the very rapid absorption of strychnine and the danger of precipitating convulsions, emptying of the stomach should not be attempted unless it can be done immediately after ingestion or after the patient is completely protected against convulsions. Potassium permanganate or charcoal (see Section 8.2.3.1) may be given to reduce and delay absorption if symptoms are minimal or absent. Charcoal can be very effective at removing strychnine from the stomach, and in mice coadministration of charcoal with strychnine increases the LD 50 by a factor of 400 (Olkkola, 1984). A dramatic early demonstration of the efficacy of oral charcoal was given by a French pharmacist, Touery, who swallowed a lethal dose of strychnine followed by 15 gm of charcoal before the French Academy in 1830 and survived to demonstrate the point (Anderson, 1946).

If symptoms develop, a rapid-acting sedative such as diazepam should be given (Herishanu and Landau, 1972) both to allay fear and to reduce the reflex hyperresponsiveness. The usual adult intravenous dose is 10 mg. Maintenance of the patient with diazepam in a quiet, darkened room controls moderate symptoms (O'Callaghan *et al.*, 1982), although if convulsions develop these need to be controlled by paralysis with succinylcholine or curare and artificial ventilation (Edmunds *et al.*, 1986). Agents other than diazepam have been used successfully to control hyperresponsiveness, such as sodium pen-

tobarbital (Priest, 1938), shorter-acting barbiturates (Symons and Boyle, 1963), and mephenesin. It is possible that strychnine poisoning is counteracted more directly by mephenesin than by barbiturates. A 2-year-old girl in severe opisthotonos relaxed during the slow, intravenous injection of 250 mg of mephenesin (Jacoby and Boyle, 1956). A young adult who suffered tightness of his muscles, reflex hyperirritability, and anxiety responded to the slow, intravenous injection of 500 mg. He was given 1500 mg more in an infusion (Swissman and Jacoby, 1964).

Clearly, it is important to control muscle tone, but it is also important to preserve respiratory reflexes as far as possible to avoid aspirating vomit, and anesthesia is best avoided if possible (Maron *et al.*, 1971).

It has been suggested that peritoneal dialysis and forced diuresis can substantially increase removal of strychnine (Teitelbaum and Ott, 1970), although the small proportion of strychnine excreted in the urine at toxic doses (see earlier) would suggest that diuresis alone would be of little value. Morphine is contraindicated because of respiratory depression. Physostigmine is also contraindicated.

Equipment must be kept ready for mechanical ventilation, and it must be used if spontaneous respiration stops as a result of either excessive anticonvulsant treatment or postconvulsive depression.

13.10.2 RICIN

13.10.2.1 Identity, Properties, and Uses

Chemical Name and Structure Ricin is a toxic glycoprotein of molecular weight 60,000–65,000 isolated from the castor bean (*Ricinus sanquineus*, Euphorbiaceae). The species sometimes is called *R. communis*. The structure of ricin is discussed under Biochemical Effects in Section 13.10.2.2. In one study (Ishiguro *et al.*, 1964) the recovery of crude ricin from defatted castor bean meal was 4.6% by weight, and the recovery of crystalline ricin was 0.21%, a 21.9-fold difference. Ricin is one of a family of related plant toxins including Abrin and Volkensin (Jiménez and Vázquez, 1985).

Synonyms The CAS registry number is 9009-86-3.

Physical and Chemical Properties Commercial ricin is a white powder soluble in 10% sodium chloride solution. It has an isoelectric point of 7.1.

History, Formulations, Uses, and Production Ricin first was isolated from the castor bean in 1889 by Stillmark. The commercial formulation is used as a mole killer. Of course, most castor bean meal is used as fertilizer, being a by-product of the castor oil lubricant industry. Ricin also has been considered as a chemical warfare agent. Recent applications are the use of radiolabeled ricin or ricin–horseradish peroxidase conjugates in histology to trace neuronal pathways (Wiley *et al.*,

1983) and attempts to use targeted ricin conjugates in cancer chemotherapy (Stirpe and Barbieri, 1986).

13.10.2.2 Toxicity to Laboratory Animals

Symptomatology   The appearance of illness is slow, even when large doses of ricin are administered. The animals refuse to eat after a few hours, but the onset of severe symptoms is always rather sudden. Convulsions and opisthotonos are followed by extreme relaxation and again by a return of convulsions. The influence of increasing dosage above the lethal level consists chiefly in shortening the latent period before the appearance of appreciable symptoms and shortening the time to death. Subcutaneous injection of one preparation in rabbits at rates of 1–2 μg/kg produced death in 60–82 hr. Dosages of 20–60 μg/kg produced death in about 48 hr. A dosage of 310 mg/kg produced death in 18 hr (Osborne *et al.*, 1905).

Moderately purified ricin is much less poisonous orally than subcutaneously or intraperitoneally. Osborne *et al.* (1905) presented data suggesting that the factor of difference is about 700 times. This factor is not unlike that for botulinus toxin, which, in spite of its poor absorption, has been demonstrated in the blood following oral administration. Extremely slow digestion of ricin by trypsin was demonstrated by Osborne *et al.* (1905).

It is impossible to discuss the toxicity of ricin except in connection with different preparations of it. In a review of the early literature, Osborne *et al.* (1905) recorded that in 1887 Dixson was first to isolate a highly toxic substance from castor bean seeds. Stillmark in 1889 applied the name ricin to the toxic material he separated from castor beans. The ability of these materials to agglutinate red blood cells was known early, and in 1891 Ehrlich showed that animals were capable of forming protective antibodies against castor bean proteins. The development of immunity was confirmed by Osborne *et al.* (1905). Osborne and his colleagues found their most active preparation to be fatal to rabbits when administered subcutaneously at 0.5 μg/kg.

Ricin purified according to present standards and homogeneous by electrophoresis, ultracentrifugation, chromatography, and crystallization differs greatly from earlier preparations in having neither proteolytic, hemagglutinating, or nonspecific protein-coagulating activity, but it differs little in toxicity from Osborne's best preparation. Thus Ishiguro *et al.* (1964) reported that their best product, which they called ricin D, had a "minimum lethal dose" of 0.001 μg of nitrogen per gram of body weight in mice examined 48 hr after intraperitoneal injection. For the whole molecule, this is equivalent to about 6 μg/kg. Olsnes *et al.* (1974) reported that the intraperitoneal LD 50 values of native and reconstituted ricins in mice were 4 and 8 μg/kg, respectively. A strict comparison of the values given by different authors is impossible. The work of Osborne *et al.* was done before proper methods for measuring toxicity were developed, and even some later investigators have failed to use good statistical procedures. Furthermore, some tests have ignored the very slow action of ricin when given at dosages near the threshold of lethality.

The toxicity and other properties of absolutely pure ricin are of great interest. However, the preparations (ranging from whole beans and bean meal to crude ricin) likely to be encountered by either pests or people contain other toxins—some of them quite potent—that not only inhibit protein synthesis but also have proteolytic, hemagglutinating, and allergenic properties. Thus a wider range of signs and symptoms must be expected in practice than in the laboratory.

Biochemical Effects   Olsnes *et al.* (1974) and more recently Stirpe and Barbieri (1986) have reviewed the now extensive literature on the biochemistry of ricin. Briefly, ricin is a glycoprotein consisting of A and B polypeptide chains joined by S—S bonds. The neutral A chain with a molecular weight of about 32,000 is the active toxicant; the slightly acid B chain with a molecular weight of 34,000 serves to bind the whole molecule to galactose residues on cell surfaces. The A chain inhibits eukaryotic protein synthesis by a highly specific interaction involving hydrolysis of an *N*-glycosidic bond on a specific adenine residue in the ribosomal RNA (Endo *et al.*, 1987; Endo and Tsurugi, 1987). The A chain alone is inactive in intact cells other than macrophages (Stirpe and Barbieri, 1986), and A-chain-like toxins are produced by many plant species. Although binding of the intact toxin to the cell surface is rapid, the reaction could be prevented by antitoxin applied during the first portion of the lag period; later application of antitoxin was without effect. From this it was concluded that the entire molecule is confined to the outside of the cell during the first, relatively brief portion of the lag period, but either it or the A polypeptide chain has entered the cell during the longer, final portion of the lag period. Ricin produces 50% inhibition of protein synthesis in cultured cells at only 1.1×10^{-12} *M* (Stirpe and Barbieri, 1986). From correlations of protein synthesis and plating efficiency of HeLa cells it appears that only one molecule of ricin in the cytosol can produce complete inhibition of protein synthesis (Eiklid *et al.*, 1980). The toxicity of ricin appears to be limited only by its need to bind specifically with galactose residues on the cell surface in order to enter the cell and by its metabolic disposal.

Although the mode of action of ricin in cell-free preparations and in cell cultures is clear, its mode of action in intact animals is less certain. Animals killed by highly purified ricin die before inhibition of protein synthesis is complete.

When injected into peripheral nerves, ricin is transported back to the cell body and causes cell death. This "suicide transport" has been used histologically to identify motor neurons (Helke *et al.*, 1985; Yamamoto *et al.*, 1983), since the ricin is not transported further within the central nervous system either because of differential uptake by nonneuronal cells or because of lack of suitable binding sites on the surface of central neurons (Wiley *et al.*, 1983).

13.10.2.3 Toxicity to Humans

After castor oil has been extracted from the seeds by pressure, solvents, or both, the remaining meal may be used as fertilizer.

The dust is highly irritant. It has caused conjunctivitis with tearing and swelling of the lids, congestion of the nasal passages, dryness and soreness of the throat, swelling of the lips, some bronchial irritation, and a few cases of prolonged asthma of allergic origin. Persons often have been affected, even though their only contact was with dusty, used bags or with dust on the clothing of others who were directly exposed (Zerbest, 1944; Figley and Rawling, 1950; Snell, 1952). The character of the illness, the fact that not all workers are affected, and the ability to sensitize animals indicate an allergic origin (Zerbest, 1944; Figley and Fawling, 1950). However, primary irritation must play some part in the disease, for Snell (1952) recorded that a mill shut down because of the extreme discomfort of its employees only 4 days after it began processing castor beans. All agree that symptoms stop soon after exposure is ended. The chemical nature of the irritant or allergen in castor beans in unknown. Figley and Rawling (1950) spoke of dericinized meal as allergenic but offered no convincing evidence for the absence of ricin.

The systemic illness observed in humans is more diverse than that described in animals. Onset is more prompt. Signs that may represent local irritation are more marked. Tissue changes at autopsy are more striking. It is difficult to determine whether the difference is primarily one of species or due to the fact that the human cases have involved whole beans while animals studies have involved more or less purified preparations. Apparently no cases have been reported involving partially purified material used to kill moles. The probable extreme danger of such a preparation is indicated by the fact that ingestion of only 15–20 castor beans has proved fatal after an illness lasting 12 days (Abdülkadir-Lütfi, 1935). Eating the beans causes nausea, vomiting, colic, and in severe cases hemorrhagic gastritis and enteritis. As poisoning progresses, the patient becomes drowsy, irrational, and comatose. The pulse may become rapid as the blood pressure falls and cyanosis appears. Death may be due to circulatory collapse. In other instances, the kidneys are most critically affected; the patient dies in uremia after suffering oliguria and anuria (Abdülkadir-Lütfi, 1935).

Pathology Ingestion of castor beans produces small hemorrhages, focal necrosis, and especially inflammation and degeneration in the kidneys, liver, heart, and spleen (Abdülkadir-Lütfi, 1935).

Treatment of Poisoning Treatment is entirely symptomatic. Studies in animals suggest that it would be possible to develop an antitoxin.

13.11 ANTIBIOTICS AND FUNGAL TOXINS

It was its antibacterial action that led to the discovery of penicillin. It soon became apparent that penicillin is highly effective against certain bacterial and spirochetal diseases of humans. In due season, a great many other antibiotics were iso-

lated and identified that were effective against different spectra of bacteria, spirochetes, rickettsiae, and fungi. Because these discoveries changed the course of human medicine, it was to be expected that a search would be made for antibiotics useful for attacking pests that are not endoparasitic in humans or in domestic animals. Such searches have been made and with some success.

Some of the antibiotics used for pest control (e.g., griseofulvin, streptomycin, and ivermectin) are the same as those used in medicine. Others (e.g., Antimycin and blasticidin) have been developed separately. As a group, the antibiotics used in pest control combat at least as wide a range of organisms as do those used in medicine. They may control not only bacteria and fungi but also mites and even insects.

13.11.1 BLASTICIDIN-S

13.11.1.1 Identity, Properties, and Uses

Chemical Name (S)-4-[[3-Amino-5-[(aminoiminomethyl)-methylamino]-l-oxopentyl]amino]-1-(4-amino-2-oxo-1-(2H)-pyrimidinyl)-1,2,3,4-tetradeoxy-β-D-erythro-hex-2-enopyranuronic acid.

Structure See Fig. 13.10.

Synonyms Blasticidin-S (JMAF) is the common name in use but the fungicide is also known as BLA-S. The CAS registry number is 2079-00-7.

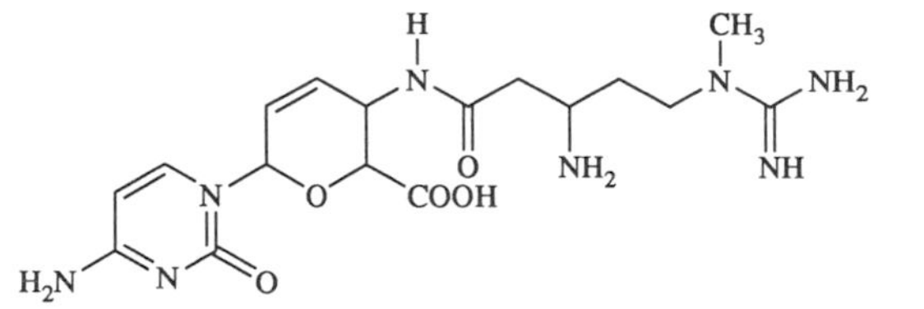

Blasticidin

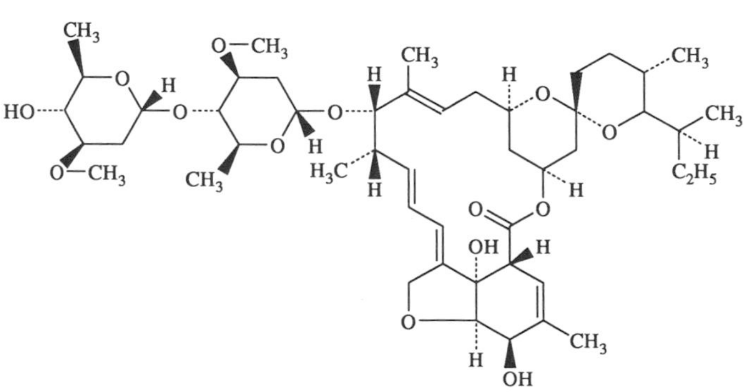

Ivermectin

Figure 13.10 Structure of two fungal toxins, blasticidin-S and ivermectin (22,23-dihydroavermectin B_{1a}).

Physical and Chemical Properties Blasticidin-S has the empirical formula $C_{17}H_{26}N_8O_5$ and a molecular weight of 422.4. It forms white needles with a melting point of 235–236°C with decomposition. It is soluble in water and acetic acid but insoluble in common organic solvents.

History, Formulations, and Uses Blasticidin-S was introduced in Japan in 1969 as a contact fungicide for the control of rice blast (*Picicularia oryzae*) and is still widely used in Japan (Kitagawa *et al.*, 1982). Blasticidin is produced by fermentation using *Streptomyces griseochromogenes*. Because of its phytotoxicity, its benzylaminobenzenesulfonate derivative, which is less injurious to plants, is widely used as the active ingredient in commercial products. Formulations include emulsifiable concentrates (20 gm active ingredient/liter), wettable powders (40 gm active ingredient/kg), and dusts (1.6 gm active ingredient/kg). The compound is used at rates of 10 gm/hectare.

Blasticidin-S is also used in medicine as an antimicrobial.

13.11.1.2 Toxicity to Laboratory Animals

Oral LD 50 values in rats have been given as 40 mg/kg (Martin and Worthing, 1977) or 63 mg/kg (Suzuki, 1977), but dermal toxicity is much lower at 3100 mg/kg for rats or 320 mg/kg in mice (Martin and Worthing, 1977). The intravenous LD 50 in mice is 2.8 mg/kg (Yonehara, 1984). The comparatively low dermal toxicity explains the relative safety of blasticidin under practical conditions of use. Suzuki (1977) found that rats fed 100 ppm blasticidin for 6 months showed some growth suppression but no specific changes.

Effects on Organs and Tissues Serum alkaline phosphatase was reduced over 3–24 hr, recovering in 2 days in rats given oral blasticidin at 3 mg/kg or more, and alkaline phosphatase in the small intestine was reduced similarly at 30 mg/kg (Suzuki, 1977). A similar reduction in blood activity was seen in rats fed 100 ppm blasticidin for 6 months.

An aqueous solution of blasticidin-S injected intratracheally into rabbits produced a pneumonitis characterized by focal destruction of tissues. Three days after injection, nonciliated, presumably undifferentiated, epithelial cells at the terminal portion of the respiratory bronchioles began to proliferate. Within 5–6 days after injection, these proliferations formed glandular structures extending from the bronchiole. Blood capillaries began to surround the glandular structures 7–8 days after treatment. Within 2 more days the glandular cells began to differentiate to form alveoli, so that by 12–14 days after treatment both types of alveolar cells could be distinguished (Ebe, 1969). The proliferation from bronchioles was confirmed by Hirono (1974b), who also showed that when rabbits were injected intratracheally with 1 ml of solution, only those that received >0.1 μg of the fungicide developed any pathological change. Alveoli were destroyed by larger doses, and both the degree of injury and the time required for recovery were increased as the concentration was increased from 0.1 to 10

μg/ml. Blasticidin is not mutagenic in bacterial reversion tests (Moriya *et al.*, 1983).

Factors Influencing Toxicity It was found that the addition of some but not all commercial proteases to blasticidin-S reduced the irritation it produced in the eyes of guinea pigs. However, this reduction was unrelated to enzyme activity and was not destroyed by boiling. The active material, which proved to be calcium acetate, was separated by dialysis and chromatography and identified by infrared spectrophotometry (Sugimoto, 1972a,b, 1978).

13.11.1.3 Toxicity to Humans

Use Experience Blasticidin-S has caused blepharitis, hyperemia of the conjuctiva, and injury to the cornea if splashed in the eye during application (Suga, 1972). Corneal ulcers have been observed (Imaizumi *et al.*, 1972). An extensive survey of ophthalmic disturbances caused by this fungicide revealed that the percentage of applicators who suffered some damage ranged from 4.3 to 34.2% between 1962 and 1968. As many as 7865 users were contacted during a single year. The highest proportion were affected in 1962 and the lowest in 1968. The improvement may have resulted at least in part from the development of a new formulation containing 5% calcium acetate. Calcium acetate and other calcium salts have been shown to alleviate the eye irritation produced by blasticidin in guinea pigs or rabbits and in field tests (Sugimoto, 1972b, 1978). It appears that this involves a direct interaction with the blasticidin, since the calcium salts must be added 30 min before or after its application in order to produce protection.

Not all cases have been confined to the eyes and skin, but the possibility has not been excluded that the injury always involves irritation. Hirono (1974a) reported illness in 22 of 30 persons exposed for 120 min or less. The following signs and symptoms occurred: pain in the pharynx in 15, coughing in 15, dyspnea in 5, headache in 9, nausea in 5, abdominal pains in 10, eye disturbances in 2, dermatitis in 7, and fever in 4. Abnormal spotlike shadows and increased pulmonary markings were found in chest films in 8 of 12 persons examined by x-ray. Three persons were severely ill and were hospitalized. In another series of cases, one of four patients died of pulmonary edema, which may have resulted in part from massive fluid therapy (Suh *et al.*, 1970).

Other reports of injury from blasticidin-S include those of Takano (1972) and Kato *et al.* (1976).

Treatment of Poisoning Treatment is symptomatic.

13.11.2 IVERMECTIN

13.11.2.1 Identity, Properties, and Uses

Chemical Name Ivermectin is a mixture of 80% 22,23-dihydroavermectin B_{1a} and 20%, 22,23-dihydroavermectin B_{1b}.

Structure See Fig. 13.6. Avermectins are complex macrocyclic disaccharides made up of a 16-membered lactone ring with a spiroacetal system of two 6-membered rings and a disaccharide substituent. The avermectins are derived from the soil bacterium *Streptomyces avermitilis* and are divided chemically into two groups, A and B, with the B group having greater biological activity against parasitic nematodes, arthropods, and insects (Wright, 1986). A related avermectin, Abamectin (avermectin B_1), is under development for agricultural use.

Synonyms Ivermectin is the common name in use. The CAS registry number is 70288-86-7.

Physical and Chemical Properties The empirical formula is $C_{48}H_{74}O_{14}$ and the molecular weight is 875.1. Ivermectin forms colorless crystals. Its water solubility is only 4 mg/liter, but it is soluble in polar organic solvents such as butanol at 330 gm/liter.

History, Formulations, Uses, and Production The avermectins were discovered in the 1970s following evaluation of various microbial isolates for antibiotic activity. Ivermectin has little antibiotic activity but was introduced as a potent antiparasitic agent in 1981. Commercial production has been facilitated by isolation of *S. avermitilis* mutants giving 50 times the original yield of avermectins (Campbell *et al.*, 1983). Ivermectin is effective against parasitic nematodes, insects, and arachnids when given subcutaneously, topically, or to a lesser degree orally and is also effective against free-living insects. Formulations include 1% solutions in organic solvents, 2% micellar suspensions, or pastes. Veterinary dosages range from 20 to 300 μg/kg (Campbell and Benz, 1984).

13.11.2.2 Toxicity to Laboratory Animals

Ivermectin acts on insects by potentiation of GABAergic neural and neuromuscular transmission, but since mammals have only central GABAergic synapses which are to a large extent protected by the blood–brain barrier, they are relatively resistent to ivermectin. Some penetration of the blood–brain barrier does occur at relatively high doses, with brain levels peaking between 2 and 12 hr after administration (Campbell *et al.*, 1983), and the primary symptoms seen in a range of mammalian species are CNS depression and consequent ataxia, as might be expected from potentiation of inhibitory GABAergic synapses. Thus, when ivermectin was given to rats intravenously at 4 mg/kg moderate incoordination was seen, while 6 mg/kg produced a state resembling anesthesia which began 1 min after injection and lasted for 4–5 hr. Higher doses cause death due to respiratory depression (D. E. Ray, unpublished observations). Ivermectin also prolongs the action of diazepam and antagonizes photically induced seizures in chickens at an intramuscular dose of 1 or 4 mg/kg (Crichlow *et al.*, 1986). In dogs some excitatory symptoms are seen, oral doses of 2.5 mg/kg producing pupil dilation and 5 mg/kg tremor. Doses of 10 mg/kg produce ataxia with tremor and 40 mg/kg death with respiratory depression (Campbell and Benz, 1984), although some dog strains are unusually susceptible (Campbell, 1985). Lethargy and ataxia are seen in horses at 12 mg/kg intramuscularly and in pigs at 30 mg/kg (Campbell and Benz, 1984). Repeated oral dosage of horses at 2 mg/kg/day for 2 days produced ataxia in half, and 2 mg/kg/day for 14 weeks produced tremor and ataxia in three of four dogs over the fourth to twelfth weeks (Campbell and Benz, 1984).

Ivermectin is well absorbed from subcutaneous or intramuscular injections and moderately well from oral administration. It is little metabolized by mammals; 90% of the administered dose is excreted in the feces and tissue residues are of the parent compound (Campbell, 1985). Plasma half-life varies from 0.5 days in pigs and 1.8 days in dogs to 2.8 days in cattle (Lo *et al.*, 1985), although absorption is usually the limiting factor and antiparasitic activity persists for 1–2 weeks in a range of species.

No adverse effects were reported when pregnant horses were given six intramuscular injections of ivermectin at 0.6 mg/kg over 2 months (Campbell and Benz, 1984).

Pharmacologically, ivermectin acts by potentiation of the release and binding of γ-aminobutyric acid (GABA), and the K_d for binding to the GABA–benzodiazapine receptor complex is $2.5 \times 10^{-9} M$. The binding site is probably separate from those for GABA, benzodiazepines, chloride ions, or the pyrethroids. Similar concentrations potentiate GABAergic actions in mammalian and invertebrate preparations, although at $10^{-6} M$ there are interactions with glycine receptors as well (Wright, 1986). Thus at high concentrations ivermectin can potentiate both of the major mammalian inhibitory neurotransmitters.

13.11.2.3 Toxicity to Humans

Ivermectin has been evaluated as a treatment for microfilarial worm infestations in both the skin and eyes at oral doses of 50–200 μg/kg (Coulaud *et al.*, 1984). It was found effective from 2 weeks and protection lasted for 6–12 months. The only adverse effect was a minor hypersensitivity seen in some patients.

13.12 LIVING ORGANISMS AS PESTICIDES

The idea of biological control of pests, particularly insects, by exploiting their natural enemies in the environment is not new and the early developments are reviewed by Sweetman (1936) and by Laird (1985) in his provocative and wide-ranging review. The use of biological control agents has many potential advantages over chemical control, not least the possibility of high selectivity for the target organisms over their natural predators and other beneficial species. Over 1500 microorganisms or microbial products have been identified as potential insecticides (Miller *et al.*, 1983). Most successful attempts have been directed against insects, as biological control of vertebrates has met with understandably little success (see Section 13.12.2) due to cross-infection problems. The World Health Organisation has investigated viruses, bacteria, fungi, and nematodes as potential insect control agents since all play a part in limiting the growth of natural insect populations.

Viral insecticides are still in the experimental stage, but many are under investigation, as reviewed by Miller *et al.* (1983). The baculoviruses appear to infect only invertebrates and have very narrow host ranges. The viral protein has a molecular weight of 25,000–33,000 and is sufficiently stable to protect the virons until they are solubilized in the alkaline insect gut. Some viruses produce crystalline toxins which may enhance their insect-killing actions. At present the baculoviruses can only be produced *in vivo*, which limits mass production.

Bacterial insecticides represent the largest and widest used group and are reviewed by Burges (1982) and Lysenko (1985). All of those used are spore-formers, since the spores can be readily stored in dried form and applied by conventional means as wettable powders or dusts. Many form a crystalline toxin within the spore, which enhances their pathogenicity to insects. The most widely used is *Bacillus thuringiensis*, which is further described in Section 13.12.1. A closely similar bacterium, *Bacillus papilliae*, was introduced in the United States in the 1940s and has been used against Japanese beetle. It has the advantage that once spores are introduced into the environment the bacterial population is sustained by reinfection of the insect hosts, but the disadvantage that spore production requires expensive *in vivo* production using insect pupae and is now of declining importance. It is highly specific, does not infect vertebrates, and despite production of a crystal toxin is nontoxic to mammals by repeated oral administration (Burges, 1982). Two other bacteria of importance are *Bacillus lentimorbus* and *Bacillus sphaericus*. *Bacillus lentimorbus* is used against Japanese beetle but differs from *B. papilliae* in not producing a crystalline toxin. *Bacillus sphaericus* toxin is also non-crystalline, but the organism is very effective against mosquitoes, is capable of reinfection of insects in the wild, and may supercede *B. thuringiensis* as a mosquito control agent (Burges, 1982).

Fungal insecticides are commercially produced for a variety of specific applications and are again reviewed by Miller *et al.* (1983). More than 500 insect-infecting fungi are known. Their importance in controlling natural insect populations has been recognized since 1834, and *Aschersonia* has been used to control Floridan white fly on citrus since the early 1900s. Fungi have the advantage of forming a stable population in the insects' environment and are capable of infection through the insect cuticle, not just by ingestion as are bacteria. A disadvantage is their susceptibility to widely used fungicides. *Beauveria basiana* is marketed as Boverin and used against Colorado beetle and corn borer in Russia and China. *Metarhizium anisopliae* was first isolated in 1879 and is used against a range of insects as Metaquino. *Hirsutella thompsonii* is used to control citrus rust mite in the United States as Mycar, and *Verticillium lecanii* is used as Vertalec or Mycotal for

aphid control in the United Kingdom. Some fungi such as *Beauveria bassiana* produce toxins (beauvericin) which may be involved in their pathogenicity. *Culicinomyces clavosporus* and *Lagenidium giganteum* are mosquito pathogens.

Nematode insecticides have been investigated by the World Health Organisation for malarial control since 1970. *Romanomermis culicivorax* and *Romanomermis iyengari* are two closely related nematodes isolated from mosquito larvae in the southern United States and India at low natural population densities. Although they must be reared *in vivo*, which is expensive, and there are some resistant mosquito populations, the nematodes are tolerant of many insecticides and insect growth regulators and can be used in combined malaria control programs (Petersen, 1982). They are not infective in rats or mice (Ignoffo *et al.*, 1974) and are rapidly broken down by human gastric juice (Gajana *et al.*, 1978).

Given the enthusiasm of the proponents of biological insect control and its long history, the limited role that these agents play in current pest control may be perhaps surprising. There are, however, a number of difficulties, both practical and fundamental. There are practical difficulties in sustaining a usefully large population of the control agent on crops, or in the case of mosquitoes at the water surface, and in agriculture difficulties associated with the very high host specificity of some agents. More fundamental problems are the potential risk from replicating agents which can increase in the environment and the possibility of transfer of toxin-encoding genes from invertebrate to vertebrate bacteria or viruses (see Section 13.12.1.3). It is clear, however, that current experience with biological control agents is very encouraging and that they can be expected to play an important part in integrated pest control programs in the future (Laird, 1985).

13.12.1 *BACILLUS THURINGIENSIS*

13.12.1.1 Identity, Properties, and Uses

Scientific Name   *Bacillus thuringiensis*, Berliner.

Synonyms   Preparations of *B. thuringiensis* spores include Bactimos®, Bactospeine®, Dipel®, Sporeine®, Technor®, Thuricide®, and Vectobac®.

History, Formulations, and Uses   First isolated by Ishiwata in 1901 from dying silkworm larvae, *B. thuringiensis* was named by Berliner in 1911. It has been extensively studied as a biological control agent and 22 varieties have been described (Whitely and Schnepf, 1986), of which the varieties *israelensis* or serotype H-14, which was discovered in Israel in 1977 and is effective against mosquito and blackfly larvae but not Lepidoptera, and *kurstaki*, which is effective against leaf-eating Lepidoptera larvae, are the most important. Due to intensive selection the insecticidal potency of *B. thuringiensis* strains has increased by two orders of magnitude since the first isolates were studied in the 1920s (Burges, 1982), and the molecular biology of endotoxin production is well understood

(Whitely and Schnepf, 1986). The bacillus is rare in the wild and thrives only in dry conditions where the spores can survive degradation. This means that repeated applications of spores are normally needed during the larval growth season. Production and agricultural usage are reviewed by Krieg and Miltenburger (1984). Formulations include wettable powders, liquid concentrates, and dusts containing about 2.5×10^{10} viable spores/gm, although activity is normally given in international bioassay units (IU). Gamma ray-inactivated spores have been used in some public health applications where human exposure is a particular risk (Krieg and Miltenburger, 1984). It was estimated that over 5000 tons had been used by 1982 (WHO, 1982).

13.12.1.2 Toxicity to Laboratory Animals

In common with a number of other bacteria, *B. thuringiensis* produces a crystal endotoxin during sporulation and also two exotoxins not included in the spore. One exotoxin, an adenine nucleotide known as thuringiensine or β-exotoxin, is thermostable; the other, α-exotoxin, is a thermolabile protein highly toxic to mice. The β-exotoxin is toxic to vertebrates, the parenteral mouse LD 50 being 13–18 mg/kg and 200 mg/kg/day given orally killing mice after 8 days. Birds are even more sensitive, hens dying after 2 weeks of oral administration at 3 mg/kg/day (Burges, 1982). The β-toxin has been used as a broad-spectrum insecticide in the USSR and for fly control in Finland, but because of its high avian toxicity only non-β-endotoxin-producing strains of *B. thuringiensis* are approved elsewhere.

The bacillus does not grow in warm-blooded creatures and six serial passages through mice at 6-hr intervals produced no ill effects. The bacilli disappeared from the blood by 72 hr (Fisher and Rosner, 1959) and other studies have confirmed that the rate of disappearance is similar to that of inert latex particles (Burges, 1982). Shadduck (1980) also found no evidence of growth in mammals but found persistence of some bacilli for 3–4 weeks or longer if applied to the corneal surface. Fisher and Rosner (1959) found no ill effects in rats given 24 gm/kg or 2×10^{12} viable spores/kg orally, and De Barjac *et al.* (1980) found that up to 10^8 bacteria per animal by subcutaneous, oral, ocular, or inhalation dosage had no ill effect in mice, rats, guinea pigs, or rabbits. The only toxic actions of the non-exotoxin-producing bacilli appear to be the convulsions and death seen after injection of more than 5×10^6 bacteria directly into the brain of rats (Shadduck, 1980). The variety *galleriae* used in the Soviet Union, however, produced loss of appetite, fever, and changes in blood chemistry following administration by oral, intravenous, intranasal, and intradermal routes, and bacteria were found in the blood even after oral administration (Pivovarov *et al.*, 1977). These effects may have been related to exotoxin.

No allergenic response to *B. thuringiensis* was elicited in guinea pigs by intracutaneous injection, inhalation, or topical application to the intact or abraded skin (Fisher and Rosner, 1959).

Endotoxin   The parasporal crystals of endotoxin (protoxin) are insoluble in water and have no appreciable toxic effects in mice and other mammalian species (Thomas and Ellar, 1983; Burges, 1982), but when the endotoxin is solubilized by incubation at pH 10–12 or by digestion with proteases it can produce hind-limb paralysis and death in mice. Thomas and Ellar (1983) found the intravenous LD 50 in mice to be about 16 mg/kg, with half of the animals showing a degree of hind-limb paralysis at 6.7 mg/kg. Suckling mice were killed by 2.7 to 6.7 mg/kg given subcutaneously. Oral administration at 17 mg/kg produced no ill effects, however, suggesting inactivation of the polypeptides in the mammalian gut, whereas in the alkaline insect gut the protoxin is in fact activated and produced its major effects on the cells of the gut wall (Burges, 1982). Activation of the endotoxin by autoclaving probably explains the toxic effect of autoclaved spores described by Fisher and Rosner (1959), who found 3×10^8 such spores to kill mice on intraperitoneal injection. Solubilization of the crystal endotoxin liberates at least two toxic proteins which vary between different varieties, *israelensis* giving one of molecular weight 65,000 which accounts for the insect toxicity and represents one-seventh of the total protein, and another of molecular weight 25,000–28,000 which is cytolytic (Hurley *et al.*, 1985), toxic to mammals, and represents less than a fifth of the total protein (Cheung *et al.*, 1987). Two other proteins of molecular weights 98,000 and 93,500 remain insoluble (Thomas and Ellar, 1983). The cytolytic protein appears to be a phosphatidylinositol-specific phospholipase C which releases ectoenzymes such as alkaline phosphatase and acetylcholinesterase from the surface of erythrocytes and cells in culture, increasing osmotic fragility and inhibiting growth (Ikezawa *et al.*, 1985). In insects the whole soluble toxin acts initially on muscle, causing ultrastructural damage, membrane depolarization, and paralysis, but later produces a blockage of ganglionic and neuromuscular transmission by inhibiting calcium uptake (Singh and Gill, 1985). Studies with the purified cytolytic protein showed that this was five times less toxic to insects than the whole solubilized toxin and failed to produce the excitatory symptoms seen after local injection of the whole toxin. This is consistent with the suggestion of Hurley *et al.* (1985) that the protein of molecular weight 65,000 is responsible for most of the insect toxicity, whereas the mammalian toxicity resides in the lower-molecular-weight cytolytic factor. In this context, it is interesting that the solubilized whole endotoxin from the variant *kurstaki* showed high insect but no measurable mammalian toxicity (Thomas and Ellar, 1983).

Effects on Organs and Tissues   No adverse effects have been reported for the approved, non-exotoxin-producing varieties, but the exotoxin appears to have some mutagenic potential. Meretoja *et al.* (1977) found chromosome aberrations in bone marrow cells of rats killed 2 days after administration of what would have been a lethal dose of exotoxin, but not after sublethal doses. In rats that drank culture medium instead of water for 3 months, blood cultures showed an inhibition of mitosis and increased chromosomal aberrations. The exotoxin also inhibits spindles and cytokinesis and induces micronuclei, chromocentric nuclei, and minor deviations in spindle activity in plants (Sharma and Sahu, 1977).

13.12.1.3 Toxicity to Humans

Clearly, the major risk with a biological agent is of infection, and the lack of infectivity of *B. thuringiensis* in animal studies appears to apply also to humans, as only one case has been recorded in over 20 years of usage. This case was that of a farm worker who developed a corneal ulcer 10 days after accidentally splashing one eye with the agricultural preparation Dipel. The ulcer contained active *B. thuringiensis* but resolved 14 days after treatment with topical gentamicin (Samples and Buettner, 1983) without leading to any spread of infection.

There is a potential problem, however, which is related to the close similarities between *B. thuringiensis* and a nonpathogenic bacterium, *Acinetobacter calcoaceticus* var. *anitratus,* which is commonly found on human skin. The only essential difference between the two appears to be the lack of crystalline endotoxin production by *A. calcoaceticus,* and this ability can be transferred by plasmid exchange in actively growing cocultures (Warren *et al.,* 1984; Whiteley and Schnepf, 1986). Such conditions occurred in a contaminated culture used for research, and a laboratory worker sustained an infection after accidental injection of this culture into a finger web space. The infection recovered after 5 days with penicillin therapy and the culture produced only slight inflammation when injected intraperitoneally into mice, guinea pigs, and rabbits. Warren *et al.* found, however, that filtrates of such mixed strains were lethal on intravenous injection to mice, although neither culture alone was toxic. They attributed this to the activation of *B. thuringiensis* protoxin by proteases produced by *A. calcoaceticus* and also suggested that *B. thuringiensis* infection may be missed because of misidentification as *A. calcoaceticus.*

Experimental Exposure   Each of 18 persons ingested 1 gm of a commercial *B. thuringiensis* preparation containing approximately 3×10^9 spores daily for 5 days. In addition to ingestion, five of them inhaled 100 mg of the powder for 5 days. There were no complaints and no positive findings on physical and laboratory examination (Fisher and Rosner, 1959).

The ingestion of foods artificially contaminated with *B. thuringiensis* var. *galleriae* at concentrations of 10^5 to 10^9 cells/gm caused nausea, vomiting, diarrhea, tenesmus, coliclike pains in the abdomen, and fever. Three of four volunteers were affected. The incubation period was 8 hr. It was concluded that bacteria pathogenic to insects can cause food poisoning similar to that caused by other bacteria of the *Bacillus cereus* group (Pivovarov *et al.,* 1977). As in the animal studies, the toxicity of the variant *galleriae* may be due to exotoxin.

Use Experience   Of course, the application of *B. thuringiensis* to crops leads to the formation of an aerosol. When it was

applied by aircraft at a rate of 2 kg of preparation (3×10^9 organisms/gm) per hectare (i.e., 6×10^{12} organisms/hectare), the concentration of viable organisms in the air over the field exceeded background by 42.5 times on the day of application and by 22.5 times 5 days later (Murza *et al.,* 1974).

No complaints were received from eight men exposed for 7 months to fermentation broth, moist bacterial cake, effluent, and the final powder in the course of commercial manufacture of the pesticide (Fisher and Rosner, 1959).

Treatment of Poisoning   Treatment is entirely symptomatic.

13.12.2 *SALMONELLA*

13.12.2.1 Identity, Properties, and Uses

Scientific Name   *Salmonella typimurium* and *Salmonella enteritidis.*

History and Uses   Although it may seem strange that what is now recognized as a human pathogen should be used as a rodent control agent, *S. typhimurium* was used to control wild rodents, mainly field mice, from 1892 to as recently as 1966. This usage was detailed by Hayes (1982), who describes the use of cultures to control plagues of field mice and the difficulties in evaluating their usefulness in the face of rapid fluctuations in population density.

13.12.2.2 Effects in Humans

Danysz (1893) reported self-experimentation on the safety of *Salmonella.*

Evidence appeared as early as 1908 (Handson *et al.,* 1908) that the various cultures were pathogenic for persons not already immune. Usually the illness took the form of acute enteric infections that almost all adults and many infants survived. However, deaths traced to *Salmonella* used for rodent control were recorded by Staub (1920), Wreschner (1921), and Kristensen and Bojlén (1931). Taylor (1956) recorded 23 fatal cases in Britain alone between 1944 and 1955. Mortality usually was low, but in one outbreak death occurred in 6 of 30 recognized cases (Anonymous, 1945). Some fatal cases, as well as numerous outbreaks without mortality, were reviewed by Leslie (1942) and by Wodzicki (1973). The illness sometimes assumed a chronic form, as described by Dathan *et al.* (1947).

Those with a vested interest in the bacterial control of rodents minimized these reports of illness and called attention to the great benefits of rodent control (Bahr, 1947). Annett (1908) replied in this way to the report by Handson *et al.* (1908) before the latter had time to publish.

Faced more or less clearly with the facts, agencies of different governments have taken measures that varied as widely as the effects of *Salmonella* on different people. In some places, all use of *Salmonella* has been banned. In many instances, use has been disapproved but not prohibited. In Poland at one time, use of cultures in food processing plants, food warehouses, restaurants, institutions for child care, and other situations where food might be handled was prohibited, but use for control of field rodents was promoted actively, and people were immunized to withstand infection (Brodniewicz, 1966).

The views of international experts on human and veterinary public health (FAO/WHO, 1967) were summarized as follows: "In connection with salmonellosis in rodents it should be re-emphasized that salmonellas should under no circumstances be used as rodenticides. Rodents rapidly develop resistance to *Salmonella* serotypes; thus, this method has little practical value. Moreover it has been shown in different countries that such practices are a public health hazard because the serotypes used are also dangerous to man."

REFERENCES

Abalis, I. M., Eldefrawi, M. E., and Eldefrawi, A. T. (1986). Effects of insecticides on GABA-induced chloride influx into rat brain microsacs. *J. Toxicol. Environ. Health* **18**, 13–23.

Abdülkadir-Lütfi, N. (1935). Fatal intoxication by castor oil plant seeds. *Dtsch. Med. Wochenschr.* **61**, 416–417 (in German).

Adesina, S. K. (1986). Further novel constituents of *Zanthoxylum zanthoxyloides* root and pericarp. *J. Nat. Prod.* **49**, 715–716.

Aldridge, W. N., Clothier, B., Forshaw, P., Johnson, M. K., Parker, V. H., Price, R. J., Skilleter, D. N., Verschoyle, R. D., and Stevens, C. (1978). The effect of DDT and the pyrethroids cismethrin and decamethrin on acetylcholine and cyclic nucleotide content of rat brain. *Biochem. Pharmacol.* **27**, 1703–1706.

Allen, T. C., Dicke, R. J., and Harris, H. H. (1944). Sabadilla, *Schoenocaulon*, ssp., with reference to its toxicity to houseflies. *J. Econ. Entomol.* **37**, 400–408.

Ambrose, A. M. (1963). Toxicologic studies on pyrethrin-type esters of chrysanthemumic acid. I. Chrysanthemumic acid, 6-chloropiperonyl ester (barthrin). *Toxicol. Appl. Pharmacol.* **5**, 414–426.

Ambrose, A. M., and DeEds, F. (1946). Some comparative observations on *l*-nicotine and myosmine. *Proc. Soc. Exp. Biol. Med.* **63**, 423–424.

Ambrose, A. M., and Haag, H. B. (1936). Toxicological study of derris. *Ind. Eng. Chem., Ind. Ed.* **28**, 815–821.

Ambrose, A. M., and Haag, H. B. (1937). Toxicological studies of derris. Comparative toxicity and elimination of some constituents of derris. *Ind. Eng. Chem.* **29**, 429–431.

Ambrose, A. M., and Haag, H. B. (1938). Toxicological studies of derris. Chronic toxicity of derris. *Ind. Eng. Chem.* **30**, 592–595.

Ambrose, A. M., DeEds, F., and Cox, A. J., Jr. (1943). The effect of high fat diet on chronic toxicity of derris and rotenone. *J. Pharmacol. Exp. Ther.* **78**, 90–92.

Amer, S. M., and Aboul-ela, E. I. (1985). Cytogenic effects of pesticides. III. Induction of micronuclei in mouse bone marrow by the insecticides cypermethrin and rotenone. *Mutat. Res.* **155**, 135–142.

Anderson, A. H. (1946). Experimental studies of the pharmacology of activated charcoal in aqueous solutions. *Acta Pharmacol.* **2**, 69–78.

Annett, H. E. (1908). Virus for the destruction of rats and mice. *Br. Med. J.* **2**, 1524–1525.

Anonymous (1889). Poisoning by insect powder. *Chem. Drug.* **35**, 557.

Anonymous (1945). Food poisoning at Stoke-on-Trent. *Lancet* **2**, 221.

Axtrup, S. (1945). On acute nicotine poisoning. *Acta Paediatr.* **32**, 288–297.

Baeza-Squiban, A., Marano, F., Ronot, X., Adolphe, M., and Puiseux-Dao, S. (1987). Effects of Deltamethrin and its commercial formulation DECIS on different cell types *in vitro*: Cytotoxicity, cellular binding and intracellular localization. *Pestic. Biochem. Physiol.* **28**, 103–113.

Bahr, L. (1947). The ratin bacillus and the "ratin system" through 40 years. *Maanedsskr. Dyrlaeg.* **59**, 161–192.

Banerjee, A., Sharma, A., and Talukder, G. (1982). Action of nicotine on cellular systems. *Life Sci. Adv.* **1**, 327–333.

Barham, S. S., and Brinkley, B. R. (1974). The effect of rotenone on the cell cycle kinetics, the mitotic spindle, and respiratory activity in cultured mammalian cells. *Tex. Rep. Biol. Med.* **33**, 554–557.

Barham, S. S., and Brinkley, B. R. (1976a). Action of rotenone and related respiratory inhibitors on mammalian cell division. 1. Cell kinetics and biochemical aspects. *Cytobios* **15** (58–59), 85–96.

Barham, S. S., and Brinkley, B. R. (1976b). Action of rotenone and related respiratory inhibitors on mammalian cell division. 2. Ultrastructural studies. *Cytobios* **15** (58–59), 97–109.

Barlow, O. W. (1932). The effectiveness of pentobarbital in antidoting strychnine poisoning in the rabbit. *JAMA, J. Am. Med. Assoc.* **98**, 1980–1981.

Barnes, J. M., and Verschoyle, R. D. (1974). Toxicity of new pyrethroid insecticide. *Nature (London)* **248**, 711.

Barron, S. E., and Guth, P. S. (1987). Uses and limitations of strychnine as a probe in neurotransmission. *Trends Pharmacol. Sci.* **8**, 204–206.

Barthel, W. F. (1973). Toxicity of pyrethrum and its constituents to mammals. *In* "Pyrethrum: The Natural Insecticide" (J. E. Casida, ed.), pp. 123–142. Academic Press, New York and London.

Beeman, J. A., and Hunter, W. C. (1937). Fatal nicotine poisoning. A report of twenty-four cases. *Arch. Pathol.* **24**, 481–485.

Bennett, D. R., Tedeschi, R. D., and Larson, P. S. (1954). Studies on the fate of nicotine in the body. VII. Observations on the excretion of nicotine and its metabolites by the dog. *Arch. Int. Pharmacodyn. Ther.* **98**, 221–227.

Benowitz, N. L. (1986). Clinical pharmacology of nicotine. *Annu. Rev. Med.* **37**, 21–32.

Benowitz, N. L., Lake, T., Keller, K. H., and Lee, B. L. (1987). Prolonged absorption with development of tolerance to toxic effects after cutaneous exposure to nicotine. *Clin. Pharmacol. Ther.* **42**, 119–120.

Bental, E., Lavy, S., and Amir, N. (1961). Electroencephalographic changes due to arsenic, thallium, and strychnine poisoning. *Confin. Neurol.* **21**, 233–240.

Berger, F. M. (1949). Spinal cord depressant drugs. *Pharmacol. Rev.* **1**, 243–278.

Berger, F. M. (1952). Central depressant and anticonvulsant properties of glycerol ethers isomeric with mephenesin. *J. Pharmacol. Exp. Ther.* **104**, 450–457.

Beroza, M., ed. (1970). "Chemicals Controlling Insect Behavior." Academic Press, New York.

Bismuth, C., Caramella, J. P., and Rosenberg, N. (1977). Rhabdomyolysis during strychnine intoxication—a description of the two cases. *Nouv. Presse Med.* **6**, 3549–3550 (in French).

Bleasdale, R. (1906). Tobacco poisoning in a child. *Br. Med. J.* **1**, 1155–1156.

Blum, B., and Zacks, S. (1958). Analysis of the relationship between drug-induced convulsions and mortality in rats. *J. Pharmacol. Exp. Ther.* **124**, 350–356.

Bogdanski, D. F., and Dattoli, J. A. (1952). Diparcol in nicotine poisoning. *Fed. Proc., Fed. Am. Soc. Exp. Biol.* **11**, 324.

Borzelleca, J. F. (1963). Drug absorption from the urinary tract of the rat: Nicotine. *Arch. Int. Pharmacodyn. Ther.* **143**, 595–602.

Bosredon (1897). Intoxication by pyrethroid powder. *Bull. Gen. Ther. (Paris)* **132**, 275–276 (in French).

Boyd, R. E., Brennan, P. T., Deng, J.-F., Rochester, D. F., and Spyker, D. A. (1983). Strychnine poisoning: Recovery from profound lactic acidosis, hyperthermia and rhabdomyolysis. *Am. J. Med.* **74**, 507–512.

Boyle, M. N., Wegria, R., Cathcart, R. T., Nickerson, J. L., and Levy, R. L. (1947). Effects of intravenous injection of nicotine on the circulation. *Am. Heart J.* **34**, 65–79.

Bradbury, J. E., Forshaw, P. J., Gray, A. J., and Ray, D. E. (1983). The action of mephenesin and other agents on the effects produced by two neurotoxic pyrethroids in the intact and spinal rat. *Neuropharmacology* **22**, 907–914.

Bristow, D. R., Bowery, N. G., and Woodruff, G. N. (1986). Light microscopic autoradiographic localisation of [3H]glycine and [3H]strychnine binding sites in rat brain. *Eur. J. Pharmacol.* **126**, 303–307.

Brodie, M. E. (1983). Correlations between cerebellar cyclic GMP and motor effects induced by deltamethrin: Independence of olivo-cerebellar tract. *Neurotoxicology* **4**, 1–12.

Brodie, M. E. (1985). Deltamethrin infusion into different sites in the neuraxis of freely-moving rats. *Neurobehav. Toxicol. Teratol.* **7**, 51–55.

Brodie, M. E., and Aldridge, W. N. (1982). Elevated cerebellar cyclic GMP levels during the deltamethrin-induced motor syndrome. *Neurobehav. Toxicol. Teratol.* **4**, 109–113.

Brodniewicz, A. (1966). "Microbial Control of Pest Rodents in Poland During 1926–1950," WHO/EBL/66.82. World Health Organ., Geneva.

Brooks, I. C., and Price, R. W. (1961). Studies on the chronic toxicity of Pro-Noxfish, a proprietary synergized rotenone fish-toxicant. *Toxicol. Appl. Pharmacol.* **3**, 49–56.

Brooks, M. W., and Clark, J. M. (1987). Enhancement of norepinephrine release from rat brain synaptosomes by alpha cyano pyrethroids. *Pestic. Biochem. Physiol.* **28**, 127–139.

Burges, H. D. (1982). Control of insects by bacteria. *Parasitology* **84**, (Symp.), 79–117.

Cagen, S. Z., Malley, L. A., Parker, C. M., Gardiner, T. H., Van Gelder, G. A., and Jud, V. A. (1984). Pyrethroid-mediated skin sensory stimulation characterised by a new behavioural paradigm. *Toxicol. Appl. Pharmacol.* **76**, 270–279.

Campbell, W. C. (1985). Ivermectin: An update. *Parasitol. Today* **1**, 10–11.

Campbell, W. C., and Benz, G. W. (1984). Ivermectin: A review of efficacy and safety. *J. Vet. Pharmacol. Ther.* **7**, 1–16.

Campbell, W. C., Fisher, M. H., Stapley, E. O., Albers-Schöberg, G., and Jacob, T. A. (1983). Ivermectin: A potent new antiparasitic agent. *Science* **221**, 823–828.

Carlton, M. (1977). Some effects of cismethrin on the rabbit nervous system. *Pestic. Sci.* **8**, 700–712.

Casida, J. E. (1973). Biochemistry of the pyrethrins. *In* "Pyrethrum: The Natural Insecticide" (J. E. Casida, ed.), Academic Press, New York and London.

Casida, J. E., Kimmel, E. C., Elliott, M., and Janes, N. F. (1971). Oxidative metabolism of pyrethrins in mammals. *Nature (London)* **230**, 326–327.

Casida, J. E., Ueda, K., Gaughan, L. C., Jao, L. T., and Soderlund, D. M. (1976). Structure–biogradability relationships in pyrethroid insecticides. *Arch. Contam. Toxicol.* **3**, 481–500.

Catterall, W. A. (1980). Neurotoxins that act on voltage-sensitive sodium channels in excitable membranes. *Annu. Rev. Pharmacol. Toxicol.* **20**, 15–43.

Chalmers, A. E., Miller, T. A., and Olsen, R. W. (1987). Deltamethrin: A neurophysiological study of the sites of action. *Pestic. Biochem. Physiol.* **27**, 36–41.

Cheng, H.-M., Yamamoto, I., and Casida, J. E. (1972). Rotenone photodecomposition. *J. Agric. Food Chem.* **20**, 850–856.

Cheung, P. Y., Buster, D., Hammock, B. D., Roe, R. M., and Alford, A. R. (1987). *Bacillus thuringiensis* var. *israelensis* δ-endotoxin: Evidence of neurotoxic action. *Pestic. Biochem. Physiol.* **27**, 42–49.

Chevalier, J. (1930). Pyrethrum (chrysanthemate insecticides), pharmacodynamic and therapeutic studies. *Bull. Sci. Pharmacol.* **37**, 154–165 (in French).

Chinn, K., and Narahashi, T. (1989). Temperature-dependent subconducting states and kinetics of deltamethrin-modified sodium channels of neuroblastoma cells. *Pflugers Arch.* **43**, 571–579.

Chmurzynska, W., Grzelakowska-Sztabert, B., and Zielinska, Z. M. (1979). Interference of a synthetic C_{18} juvenile hormone and related insect growth regulators with macromolecular biosynthesis in mammalian cells. *Toxicol. Appl. Pharmacol.* **49**, 517–523.

Clarke, J. S. (1986). Letter to editor. *Pediatr. Emerg. Care* **2**, 65.

Clements, A. N., and May, T. E. (1977). The actions of pyrethroids upon the peripheral nervous system and associated organs in the locust. *Pestic. Sci.* **8**, 661–680.

Cotten, M. S., and Lane, D. H. (1966). Massive strychnine poisoning. A successful treatment. *J. Miss. State Med. Assoc.* **7**, 466–468.

Couland, J. P., Lariviere, M., Aziz, M. A., Gervais, M. C., Gaxotte, P., Deluol, A. M., and Cenac, J. (1984). Ivermectin in onchoceriasis. *Lancet* **2**, 526–527.

Crawford, M. J., and Hutson, D. H. (1977). The metabolism of the pyrethroid insecticide (±)-α-cyano-3-phenoxybenzyl-2,2,3,3-tetramethyl cyclopropanecarboxylate, WL41706, in the rat. *Pestic. Sci.* **8**, 579–599.

Crawford, M. J., Croucher, A., and Hutson, D. H. (1981). Metabolism of *cis*- and *trans*-cypermethrin in rats. Balance and tissue retention study. *J. Agric. Food Chem.* **29**, 130–135.

Cremer, J. E., and Seville, M. P. (1982). Comparative effects of two pyrethroids, deltamethrin and cismethrin, on plasma catecholamines and on blood glucose and lactate. *Toxicol. Appl. Pharmacol.* **66**, 124–133.

Cremer, J. E., and Seville, M. P. (1985). Changes in regional cerebral blood flow and glucose metabolism associated with symptoms of pyrethroid toxicity. *Neurotoxicology* **6**, 1–12.

Cremer, J. E., Cunningham, V. J., Ray, D. E., and Sarna, G. S. (1980). Regional changes in brain glucose utilization in rats given a pyrethroid insecticide. *Brain Res.* **194**, 278–282.

Cremer, J. E., Cunningham, V. J., and Seville, M. P. (1983). Relationships between extraction and metabolism of glucose, blood flow, and tissue blood volume in regions of rat brain. *J. Cereb. Blood Flow Metab.* **3**, 291–302.

Crichlow, E. C., Mishra, P. R., and Crawford, R. D. (1986). Anticonvulsant effects of ivermectin in genetically-epileptic chickens. *Neuropharmacology* **25**, 1085–1088.

Crofton, K. M., and Reiter, L. W. (1984). Effects of two pyrethroid insecticides on motor activity and the acoustic startle response in the rat. *Toxicol. Appl. Pharmacol.* **75**, 318–328.

Curtis, D. R., Duggan, A. W., and Johnston, G. A. R. (1971). The specificity of strychnine as a glycine antagonist in the mammalian spinal cord. *Exp. Brain Res.* **12**, 547–565.

Cutkomp, L. K. (1943). Toxicity of rotenone and derris extract administered orally to birds. *J. Pharmacol. Exp. Ther.* **77**, 238–245.

Danilin, V. A., and Shabaeva, T. V. (1969). A case of anabasine poisoning. *Klin. Med. (Moscow)* **40**, 128–129.

Dankó, M., Cseri, J., and Varga, E. (1981). Parameters of the potential changes induced by cevadine on striated frog muscle membrane. *Acta Physiol. Sci. Hung.* **58**, 103–118.

Danysz, J. (1893). Application of artificial cultures of pathogenic microbes to the destruction of rodents (field rats and mice) in large-scale agriculture. *C. R. Hebd. Seances Acad. Sci.* **117**, 869–872 (in French).

Dathan, J. G., Orr-Ewing, J., McCall, A. J., and Taylor, J. (1947). *Salmonella enteritidis* infection associated with use of anti-rodent "virus." *Lancet* **1**, 711–713.

David, M., Commissaris, R. L., Cassella, J. V., Yang, S., Dember, L., and Harty, T. P. (1986). Differential effects of dopamine agonists on acoustically and electrically elicited startle responses: Comparison to effects of strychnine. *Brain Res.* **371**, 58–69.

De Barjac, H., Larget, I., Bénichou, L., Cosmao, V., Viviani, G., Ripouteau, H., and Pappion, S. (1980). "Safety Tests of the Serotype H-14 of *Bacillus thuringiensis* in Mammals," WHO/VBC/80.761. World Health Organ., Geneva (in French).

Decker, W. J., Baker, H. E., Tamulinas, S. H., and Korndorffer, W. E. (1982). Two deaths resulting from apparent parenteral injection of strychnine. *Vet. Hum. Toxicol.* **24**, 161–162.

Devaud, L. L., Szot, P., and Murray, T. F. (1986). PK 11195 antagonism of pyrethroid-induced proconvulsant activity. *Eur. J. Pharmacol.* **121**, 269–273.

DeWilde, A.-R., Heyndrickx, A., and Carton, D. (1986). A case of fatal rotenone poisoning in a child. *J. Forensic Sci.* **31**, 1492–1498.

Dittrich, K., Bayer, M. J., and Wanke, L. A. (1984). A fatal case of strychnine poisoning. *J. Emerg. Med.* **1**, 327–330.

Dixson, T. (1887). *Ricinus communis. Aust. Med. Gaz.* **6**, 155–157.

Drexler, G., and Sieghart, W. (1984). Evidence for association of a high affinity binding site for [^{3}H]avermectin B_{1a}. *Eur. J. Pharmacol.* **99**, 269–277.

Dyball, R. E. J. (1982). Inhibition by decamethrin and resmethrin of hormone release from the isolated rat neurohypophysis—a model mammalian neurosecretory system. *Pestic. Biochem. Physiol.* **17**, 42–47.

Dyer, R. S. (1985). The use of sensory evoked potentials in toxicology. *J. Appl. Toxicol.* **5**, 24–40.

Eadsforth, C. V., Bragt, P. C., and van Sittert, N.J. (1988). Human dose-excretion studies with pyrethroid insecticides cypermethrin and alpha-cypermethrin: Relevance for biological monitoring. *Xenobiotica* **18**, 603–614.

Ebe, T. (1969). Light and electron microscope studies on experimental pneumonitis induced by blasticidin-S, with special reference to alveolar regeneration. *Arch. Histol. Jpn.* **30**, 149–182.

Eberle, J. (1830). "A Treatise of the Materia Medica and Therapeutics," Vol. II, p. 97. John Grigg, Philadelphia, Pennsylvania.

Edmunds, M., Sheehan, T. M. T., and Van't Hoff, W. (1986). Strychnine poisoning: Clinical and toxicological observations on a non-fatal case. *J. Toxicol. Clin. Toxicol.* **24**, 245–255.

Eells, J. T., and Dubocovich, M. L. (1988). Pyrethroid insecticides evoke neurotransmitter release from rabbit striatal slices. *J. Pharmacol. Exptl. Ther.* **246**, 514–521.

Eiklid, K., Olsnes, S., and Phil, A. (1980). Entry of lethal doses of abrin, ricin and modeccin into the cytosol of HeLa cells. *Exp. Cell Res.* **126**, 321–326.

Eldefrawi, A. T., Bakry, N. M., Eldefrawi, M. E., Tsai, M-G., and Albuquerque, E.X. (1980). Nereistoxin interaction with the acetylcholine receptorionic channel complex. *Mol. Pharmacol.* **17**, 172–179.

Elliott, M. (1969). Structural requirements for pyrethrin-like activity. *Chem. Ind. (London)* **24**, 776–791.

Elliott, M. (1971). The relationship between the structure and the activity of pyrethroids. *Bull. W. H. O.* **44**, 315–324.

Elliott, M. (1977). "Synthetic Pyrethroids," ACS Symp. Ser. No. 42. Am. Chem. Soc., Washington, D.C.

Elliott, M., Farnham, A. W., Janes, N. F., and Soderlund, D. M. (1978). Insecticidal activity of the pyrethrins and related compounds. Part XI. Relative potencies of isomeric cyano-substituted 3-phenoxybenzyl esters. *Pestic. Sci.* **9**, 112–116.

Endo, Y., and Tsurugi, K. (1987). RNA *N*-glycosidase activity of ricin A-chain. *J. Biol. Chem.* **262**, 8128–8130.

Endo, Y., Mitsui, K., Motizuki, M., and Tsurugi, K. (1987). The mechanism of action of ricin and related toxic lectins on eukaryotic ribosomes. *J. Biol. Chem.* **262**, 5908–5912.

Ernster, L., Dallner, G., and Azzone, G. F. (1963). Differential effects of rotenone and amytal on mitochondrial electron and energy transfer. *J. Biol. Chem.* **238**, 1124–1131.

Eschar, Y. (1961). Insecticide poisoning. Based on material from the Kaplan Hospital. *Isr. Med. J.* **20**, 85–94.

Faingold, C. L., Hoffmann, W. E., and Caspary, D. M. (1985). Comparative effects of convulsant drugs on the sensory responses of neurones in the amygdala and brainstem reticular formation. *Neuropharmacology* **24**, 1221–1230.

Faulkner, J. M. (1933). Nicotine poisoning by absorption through the skin. *JAMA, J. Am. Med. Assoc.* **100**, 1664–1665.

Feinberg, S. M. (1934). Pyrethrum sensitization. Its importance and relation to pollen allergy. *JAMA, J. Am. Med. Assoc.* **102**, 1557–1558.

Fcurt, S. D., Jenkins, J. H., Hayes, F. A., and Crockford, J. A. (1958). Pharmacology and toxicology of nicotine with special reference to species variation. *Science* **127**, 1054.

Figley, K. D., and Rawling, F. F. A. (1950). Castor bean: An industrial hazard as a contaminant of green coffee dust and used burlap bags. *J. Allergy* **21**, 545–553.

Finnegan, J. K., Larson, P. S., and Haag, H. B. (1947). Studies on the fate of nicotine in the body. V. Observations on relation of nicotine dosage to per cent excreted in urine, rate of excretion, and rate of detoxication. *J. Pharmacol. Exp. Ther.* **91**, 357–361.

Fisher, R., and Rosner, L. (1959). Insecticide safety. Toxicology of the microbial insecticide, Thuricide. *J. Agric. Food Chem.* **7**, 686–688.

Flannigan, S. A., and Tucker, S. B. (1985a). Variation in cutaneous perfusion due to synthetic pyrethroid exposure. *Br. J. Ind. Med.* **42**, 773–776.

Flannigan, S. A., and Tucker, S. B. (1985b). Variation in cutaneous sensation between synthetic pyrethroid insecticides. *Contact Dermatitis* **13**, 140–147.

Flannigan, S. A., Tucker, S. B., Key, M. M., Ross, C. E., Fairchild, E. J., Grimes, B. A., and Harrist, R. B. (1985). Synthetic pyrethroid insecticides: A dermatological evaluation. *Br. J. Ind. Med.* **42**, 363–372.

Flury, F., and Zernik, F. (1935). Compilation of toxic and lethal doses of the most commonly used poisons in animals. *In* "Handbuch der Biologischen Arbeitsmethoden" (E. Abderhalden, ed.), Vol. IV, Part 7B, p. 1403. Urban & Schwarzenburg, Berlin (in German).

Food and Agriculture Organization/World Health Organization (FAO/WHO) (1967). "Joint FAO/WHO Expert Committee on Zoonoses. Third Report," WHO Tech. Rep. No. 278. World Health Organ., Geneva.

Food and Agriculture Organization/World Health Organization (FAO/WHO) (1971). "1970 Evaluations of Some Pesticide Residues in Food," Monograph prepared by the Joint Meeting of the FAO Working Party of Experts and the WHO Expert Group on Pesticide Residues, Rome, November 9–16, 1970, WHO/FOOD/ADD/71.42. Food Agric. Organ., Rome.

Food and Agricalature Organization/World Health Organization (FAO/WHO) (1977). Evaluations of some pesticide residues in food. Plant production and protection series No. 8. Food and Agriculture Organisation of the United Nations. Rome.

Food and Agriculture Organization/World Health Organization (FAO/WHO) (1979). FAO plant production and protection paper 15 (Supplement). Food and Agriculture Organisation of the United Nations. Rome.

Food and Agriculture Organization/World Health Organization (FAO/WHO) (1980). "FAO Plant Production and Protection Paper 20 (Supplement)." Food Agric. Organ. U.N., Rome.

Food and Agriculture Organization/World Health Organization (FAO/WHO) (1981). "FAO Plant Production and Protection Paper 26 (Supplement)." Food Agric. Organ. U.N., Rome.

Food and Agriculture Organization/World Health Organization (FAO/WHO) (1982). "FAO Plant Production and Protection Paper 42 (Monographs)." Food Agric. Organ. U.N., Rome.

Food and Agriculture Organization/World Health Organization (FAO/WHO) (1983). "FAO Plant Production and Protection Paper 49 (Monographs)." Food Agric. Organ. U.N., Rome.

Food and Agriculture Organization/World Health Organization (FAO/WHO) (1985). "FAO Plant Production and Protection Paper 67 (Monographs)." Food Agric. Organ. U.N., Rome.

Food and Agriculture Organization/World Health Organization (FAO/WHO) (1986). "FAO Plant Production and Protection Paper 72/2 (Toxicology)." Food Agric. Organ. U.N., Rome.

Forshaw, P. J., and Bradbury, J. E. (1983). Pharmacological effects of pyrethroids on the cardiovascular system of the rat. *Eur. J. Pharmacol.* **91**, 207–213.

Forshaw, P. J., and Ray, D. E. (1986). The effects of two pyrethroids, cismethrin and deltamethrin, on skeletal muscle and the trigeminal reflex system in the rat. *Pestic. Biochem. Physiol.* **25**, 143–151.

Forshaw P. J., and Ray, D. E. (1990). A novel action of deltamethrin on membrane resistance in mammalian skeletal muscle and non-myelinated nerve fibres. *Neuropharmacol.* **29**, 75–81.

Forshaw, P. J., Lister, T., and Ray, D. E. (1986). The effects of two types of pyrethroid on rat skeletal muscle. *Eur. J. Pharmacol.* **134**, 89–96.

Fox, I., and DeLeon, D. (1982). Evaluation of insecticides in collars and powders against the cat fur mite *Felistrophorus radofskyi* (Tenorio) on Persian cats. *J. Agric. Univ. P. R.* **66**, 139–144.

Franke, F. E., and Thomas, J. E. (1932). A note on the minimal fatal dose of nicotine for unanesthetized dogs. *Proc. Soc. Exp. Biol. Med.* **29**, 1177–1179.

Franke, F. E., and Thomas, J. E. (1933). A study of the cause of death in experimental nicotine poisoning in dogs. *J. Pharmacol. Exp. Ther.* **48**, 199–208.

Franke, F. E., and Thomas, J. E. (1936). The treatment of acute nicotine poisoning. *JAMA, J. Am. Med. Assoc.* **106**, 507–512.

Freudenthal, R. I., Thake, D. C., and Baron, R. L. (1981). "Carcinogenic Potential of Rotenone: Subchronic Oral and Peritoneal Administration to Rats and Chronic Dietary Administration to Syrian Golden Hamsters," U.S. E.P.A. Proj. Summ., EPA-600/S1-81-037. U.S. Environ. Prot. Agency, Washington, D.C.

Fukami, J., Nakatsugawa, T., and Narahashi, T. (1959). The relation between chemical structure and toxicity in rotenone derivatives. *Jpn. J. Appl. Entomol. Zool.* **3**, 259–265.

Fukami, J., Yamamoto, I., and Casida, J. E. (1967). Metabolism of rotenone *in vitro* by tissue homogenates from mammals and insects. *Science* **155**, 713–716.

Fukami, J., Shishido, T., Fukunaga, K., and Casida, J. E. (1969). Oxidative metabolism of rotenone in mammals, fish and insects and its relation to selective toxicity. *J. Agric. Food Chem.* **17**, 1217–1226.

Gaines, T. B. (1969). Acute toxicity of pesticides. *Toxicol. Appl. Pharmacol.* **14**, 515–534.

Gajana, A., Kazmi, S. J., BheemaRao, U. S., Suguna, S. G., and Chandrahas, R. K. (1978). Studies on a nematode parasite (*Romanomermis* sp.: Mermithidae) of mosquito larvae isolated in Pondicherry. *Indian J. Med. Res.* **68**, 242–247.

Gammon, D. W., Brown, M. A., and Casida, J. E. (1981). Two classes of pyrethroid action in the cockroach. *Pestic. Biochem. Physiol.* **15**, 181–191.

Gammon, D. W., Lawrence, L. J., and Casida, J. E. (1982). Pyrethroid toxicology: Protective effects of diazepam and phenobarbitol in the mouse and cockroach. *Toxicol. Appl. Pharmacol.* **66**, 290–296.

Ganz, A., Kelsey, F. E., and Geiling, E. M. K. (1951). Excretion and tissue distribution studics on radioactive nicotine. *J. Pharmacol. Exp. Ther.* **103**, 209–214.

Garcia-Estrada, H., and Fischman, C. M. (1977). An unusual casc of nicotine poisoning. *Clin. Toxicol.* **10**, 391–393.

Garry, V. F., and Moore, R. D. (1974). Use of the Cytograf to determine cytotoxicity in fibroblast cell cultures. *Oncology* **29**, 429.

Gaughan, L. C., Unai, T., and Casida, J. E. (1977). Permethrin metabolism in rats. *J. Agric. Food Chem.* **25**, 9–17.

Gehlbach, S. H., Williams, W. A., Perry, L. D., and Woodall, J. S. (1974). Green-tobacco sickness: An illness of tobacco harvesters. *JAMA, J. Am. Med. Assoc.* **229**, 1880–1883.

Gehlbach, S. H., Williams, W. A., Perry, L. D., and Freeman, J. I. (1975). Nicotine absorption by workers harvesting green tobacco. *Lancet* **1**, 478–480.

Gehlbach, S. H., Williams, W. A., and Freeman, J. I. (1979). Protective clothing as a means of reducing nicotine absorption in tobacco harvesters. *Arch. Environ. Health* **2**, 111–114.

Gerberg, E. J. (1973). Head lice: Control and nit removal. *Sci. Publ.—Pan Am. Health Organ.* **263**, 196–198.

Gies, W. J., and Meltzer, S. J. (1903). Studies on the influence of artificial respiration upon strychnine spasms and respiratory movements. *Am. J. Physiol.* **9**, 1–25.

Gilman, A. G., Goodman, L. S., Rall, T. W., and Murad, F., eds. (1985). "The Pharmacological Basis of Therapeutics," 7th ed. Macmillan, New York.

Gilmore, R. G., Hastings, P. A., Kulczycki, G. R., and Jennison, B. L. (1981). Crystalline rotenone as a selective fish toxin. *Fla. Sci.* **44**, 193–203.

Gindhart, F. D. (1939). Nicotine poisoning. *Ind. Med.* **8**, 515–516.

Glomot, R. (1982). Toxicity of deltamethrin to higher vertebrates. *In* "Deltamethrin" (R. Lhoste, ed.). Roussel Uclaf, Marseilles.

Gnadinger, C. B. (1936). "Pyrethrum Flowers," 2nd ed. McLaughlin Gormley King, Minneapolis, Minnesota.

Gold, H., Modell, W., Catell, M., Benton, J. G., and Cotlove, E. W. (1947). Action of digitalis glycosides on the central nervous system with special reference to the convulsant action of red squill. *J. Pharmacol. Exp. Ther.* **91**, 15–30.

Gorrod, J. W., and Jenner, P. (1975). The metabolism of tobacco alkaloids. *Essays Toxicol.* **6**, 35–78.

Gosalvez, M. (1983). Carcinogenesis with the insecticide rotenone. *Life Sci.* **32**, 809–816.

Gosalvez, M., and Diaz-Gil, J. J. (1978). Rotenone: A possible environmental carcinogen? *Eur. J. Cancer* **14**, 1403–1404.

Gosalvez, M., and Merchan, J. (1973). Induction of rat mammary adenomas with the respiratory inhibitor rotenone. *Cancer Res.* **33**, 3047–3050.

Gray, A. J. (1985). Pyrethroid structure–toxicity relationships in mammals. *Neurotoxicology* **3**, 25–35.

Gray, A. J., and Rickard, J. (1982a). Toxicity of pyrethroids to rats after direct injection into the central nervous system. *Neurotoxicology* **6**, 127–138.

Gray, A. J., and Rickard, J. (1982b). The toxicokinetics of deltamethrin in rats after intravenous administration of a toxic dose. *Pestic. Biochem. Physiol.* **18**, 205–215.

Gray, A. J., Connors, T. A., Hoellinger, H., and Nguyen-Hoang-Nam. (1980). The relationship between the pharmacokinetics of intravenous cismethrin and bioresmethrin and their mammalian toxicity. *Pestic. Biochem. Physiol.* **13**, 281–293.

Gray, J. A., and Gray, A. J. (1990). A pharmacological comparison of the effects of muscle relaxants on deltamethrin toxicity in rats. *Toxicol. Appl. Pharmacol.* (in press).

Griffin, C. S. (1973). Mammalian toxicology of pyrethrum. *Pyrethrum Post* **12**, 50–58.

Gutman, M., Singer, T. P., Beinert, H., and Casida, J. E. (1970a). Reaction sites of rotenone, piericidin A, and amytal in relation to the nonheme iron components of NADH dehydrogenase. *Proc. Natl. Acad. Sci. U.S.A.* **65**, 763–770.

Gutman, M., Singer, T. P., and Casida, J. E. (1970b). Studies on the respiratory chain-linked reduced nicotinamide adenine dinucleotide dehydrogenase. *J. Biol. Chem.* **245**, 1992–1997.

Gutman, M., Coles, C. J., Singer, T. P., and Casida, J. E. (1971). On the functional organization of the respiratory chain at the dehydrogenase–coenzyme Q junction. *Biochemistry* **10**, 2036–2043.

Gutman, M., Singer, T. P., and Beinert, H. (1972). Relation of the respiratory chain-linked reduced nicotinamide-adenine dinucleotide dehydrogenase to energy-coupling site 1. *Biochemistry* **11**, 556–562.

Haag, H. B. (1931). Toxicological studies of *Derris elliptica* and its constituents. I. Rotenone. *J. Pharmacol. Exp. Ther.* **43**, 193–208.

Haag, H. B. (1933). A contribution to the pharmacology of anabasine. *J. Pharmacol. Exp. Ther.* **48**, 95–104.

Haag, H. B. (1937). Studies on the physiologic action of diethylene glycol. I. The effect upon the irritating and toxic properties of cigarette smoke. *J. Lab. Clin. Med.* **22**, 341–346.

Haag, H. B. (1940). The physiologic activity of cigarette smoke solutions as related to their nicotine content. *J. Lab. Clin. Med.* **25**, 610–618.

Haag, H. B., and Larson, P. S. (1942). Studies on the fate of nicotine in the body. I. The effect of pH on the urinary excretion of nicotine by tobacco smokers. *J. Pharmacol. Exp. Ther.* **76**, 235–239.

Hackel, C. (1983). Effect of methoprene on the embryonic development of Wistar rats. *Rev. Bras. Genet.* **6**, 639–647.

Haigh, J. C., and Haigh, J. M. (1980). Immobilizing drug emergencies in humans. *Vet. Hum. Toxicol.* **22**, 1–5.

Haines, K. A., and Davis, L. G. (1948). Protection of workers applying nicotine alkaloid as a concentrated mist spray. *J. Econ. Entomol.* **41**, 513.

Hale, W. (1909). Studies on the tolerance No. 11—strychnine. *J. Pharmacol. Exp. Ther.* **1**, 39–47.

Haley, T. J. (1978). A review of the literature of rotenone 1,2,12,12a-tetrahydro-8,9-dimethoxy-(2-(1-methylethenyl)-1-benzopyrano[3,5-*B*]fluoro[2,3-*H*][1]-benzopyran-6(6*h*)-one. *J. Environ. Pathol. Toxicol.* **1**, 315–337.

Handson, L., Williams, H., and Klein, E. (1908). Account of an epidemic of enteritis caused by "Liverpool virus" rat poison. *Br. Med. J.* **2**, 1547–1550.

Hartenberg, P. (1913). High dose strychnine. Method and indications. *Presse Med.* **8**, 71–73 (in French).

Hatch, R. C., and Funnell, H. S. (1968). Strychnine levels in tissues and stomach contents of poisoned dogs: An eleven year survey. *Can. Vet. J.* **9**, 161–164.

Hatcher, R. W. (1904). Nicotine tolerance in rabbits, and the difference in the fatal dose in adult and young guinea pigs. *Am. J. Physiol.* **11**, 17–27.

Hausen, B. M., and Schulz, K. H. (1973). Chrysanthemum allergy. I. Information. *Berufs-Dermatosen* **21**, 199–214 (in German).

Hayes, F. A., Jenkins, J. H., Feurt, S. D., and Crockford, J. A. (1959). The propulsive administration of nicotine as a new approach for capturing and restraining cattle. *J. Am. Vet. Med. Assoc.* **134**, 283–286.

Hayes, W. J., Jr. (1975). "Toxicology of Pesticides." Williams & Wilkins, Baltimore, Maryland.

Hayes, W. J., Jr. (1976). Mortality in 1969 from pesticides including aerosols. *Arch. Environ. Health* **80,** 62–71.

Hayes, W. J., Jr. (1982). "Pesticides Studied in Man." Williams & Wilkins, Baltimore, Maryland.

Hayes, W. J., Jr., and Pirkle, C. I. (1966). Mortality from pesticides in 1961. *Arch. Environ. Health* **12,** 43–55.

Hayes, W. J., Jr., and Vaughn, W. K. (1977). Mortality from pesticides in the United States in 1973 and 1974. *Toxicol. Appl. Pharmacol.* **42,** 235–252.

Hazard, R., and Savini, E. (1953). Antagonism between nicotinic agents. Correlation between their toxicity and actions on ganglia. *Arch. Int. Pharmacodyn. Ther.* **92,** 471–481 (in French).

He, F., Wang, S., Liu, L., Chen, S., Zhang, Z., and Sun, J. (1989). Clinical manifestations and diagnosis of acute pyrethroid poisoning. *Arch. Toxicol.* **63,** 54–58.

Hearn, C. E. D. (1973). A review of agricultural pesticide incidents in man in England and Wales, 1952–71. *Br. J. Ind. Med.* **30,** 253–258.

Heikkila, E., Nicklas, W. J., Vyas, I., and Duvoisin, R. C. (1985). Dopeminergic toxicity of rotenone and the 1-methyl-4-phenylpyridinium ion after their stereotaxic administration to rats: Implication for the mechanism of 1-methyl-4-phenyl-1,2,3,6-tetrahydropyridine toxicity. *Neurosci. Lett.* **62,** 389–394.

Helke, C. J., Charlton, C. G., and Wiley, R. G. (1985). Suicide transport of ricin demonstrates the presence of substance P receptors on medullary somatic and autonomic motor neurones. *Brain Res.* **328,** 190–195.

Henningfield, J. E., Miyasato, K., and Jesinski, D. R. (1985). Abuse liability and pharmacodynamic characteristics of intravenous and inhaled nicotine. *J. Pharmacol. Exp. Ther.* **234,** 1–12.

Herishanu, Y., and Landau, H. (1972). Diazepam in the treatment of strychnine poisoning. *Br. J. Anaesth.* **44,** 747–748.

Hervé, J. J. (1985). Agricultural, public health and animal health usage. *In* "The Pyrethroid Insecticides" (J. P. Leahey, ed.). Taylor & Francis, London and Philadelphia.

Heubner, W., and Papierkowski, J. (1938). On the toxicity of nicotine in mice. *Naunyn-Schmiedebergs Arch. Exp. Pathol. (Pharmakol.)* **188,** 605–610 (in German).

Hewlett, A. W. (1913). A case of strychnine poisoning. *Am. J. Med. Sci.* **146,** 536–541.

Hijzen, T. H., and Slangen, J. L. (1988). Effects of type I and type II pyrethroids on the startle response in rats. *Toxicol. Lett.* **40,** 141–152.

Hirono, K. (1974a). Clinical and experimental studies on pneumonitis caused by pesticides. Part I. Clinical study. *Niigata Med. J.* **88,** 64–69 (in Japanese).

Hirono, K. (1974b). Clinical and experimental studies on pneumonitis caused by pesticides. Part II. Experimental study. *Niigata Med. J.* **88,** 70–75 (in Japanese).

Hoffmann, D., Laboie, E. J., and Hecht, S. S. (1985). Nicotine: A precursor for carcinogens. *Cancer Lett.* **26,** 67–75.

Holck, H. G., Kanan, M. A., Mills, L. M., and Smith, E. L. (1937). Studies upon the sex-difference in rats in tolerance to certain barbiturates and to nicotine. *J. Pharmacol. Exp. Ther.* **60,** 323–346.

Holland, E. A. (1938). Suicide by ingestion of derris root sp. in New Ireland. *Trans. R. Soc. Trop. Med. Hyg.* **32,** 293–294.

Holmstedt, B. (1988). Toxicity of nicotine and related compounds. *In* "The Pharmacology of Nicotine" (M. Rand and K. Thurau, eds.). IRL Press, Oxford.

Hudson, P. M., Tilson, H. A., Chen, P. H., and Hong, J. S. (1986). Neurobehavioral effects of permethrin are associated with alterations in regional levels of biogenic amine metabolites and amino acid neurotransmitters. *Neurotoxicology* **7,** 143–153.

Hull, F. E., and Whereat, A. F. (1967). The effect of rotenone on the regulation of fatty acid synthesis in heart mitochondria. *J. Biol. Chem.* **242,** 4023–4028.

Hurley, J. M., Lee, S. G., Andrews, R. E., Klowden, M. J., and Bulla, L. A. (1985). Separation of the cytolytic and mosquitocidal proteins of *Bacillus thuringiensis* subsp. *israelensis*. *Biochem. Biophys. Res. Commun.* **126,** 961–965.

Ignoffo, C. M., Chapman, H. C., Petersen, J. J., and Novotny, J. F. (1974).

Lack of susceptibility of mice and rats to mosquito nematode *Reesimermis nielseni* (Tsai and Grundmann). *Mosq. News* **34,** 425–428.

Ikezawa, H., Kato, T., Ohta, S., Hakabayashi, T., Iwata, Y. and Ono, K. (1985). Physiological actions of phosphatidylinositol-specific phospholipase C from *Bacillus thuringiensis* on KG III cells: Alkaline phosphatase release and growth inhibition. *Toxicon* **23,** 154–155 (in Japanese).

Imaizumi, K., Atsumi, K., Tanifuji, Y., Ishikawa, Y., and Hoshi, H. (1972). Clinical observations of ophthalmic disturbances due to agricultural chemicals. *Folia Ophthalmol. Jpn.* **22,** 154–156.

Innes, J. R. M., Ulland, B. M., Valerio, M. G., Petrucelli, L., Fishbein, L., Hart, E. R., Pallotta, A. J., Bates, R. R., Falk, H. L., Gart, J. J., Klein, M., Mitchell, I., and Peters, J. (1969). Bioassay of pesticides and industrial chemicals for tumorigenicity in mice: A preliminary note. *J. Natl. Cancer Inst.* (U.S.) **42,** 1101–1114.

Inukai, T. (1969). Metabolism of strychnine nitrate applied for the control of the bear. *Residue Rev.* **25,** 315–318.

Ishiguro, M., Takahashi, T., Funatsu, G., Hayashi, K., and Funatsu, M. (1964). Biochemical studies on ricin. I. Purification of ricin. *J. Biochem. (Tokyo)* **55,** 587–592.

Jacobson, M. (1969). Sex pheromone of the pink bollworm moth: Biological masking by its geometrical isomer. *Science* **163,** 190–191.

Jacoby, J., and Boyle, J. (1956). The treatment of strychnine poisoning with mephenesin. *J. Lab. Clin. Med.* **48,** 270–273.

Jacques, Y., Romey, G., Cavey, M. T., Kartalovski, B., and Lazdunski, M. (1980). Interaction of pyrethroids with the Na$^+$ channel in mammalian neuronal cells in culture. *Biochim. Biophys. Acta* **600,** 882–897.

Jenkins, J. H., Hayes, F. A., Feurt, S. D., and Crockford, J. A. (1961). A new method for the live capture of canines with applications to rabies control. *Am. J. Public Health* **51,** 902–908.

Jimenéz, A., and Vázquez, D. (1985). Plant and fungal protein and glycoprotein toxins inhibiting eukaryote protein synthesis. *Annu. Rev. Microbiol.* **39,** 649–672.

Jin, X., Wang, Y., Lin, H., Sun, W., Wu, P., and Xu, X. (1984). Toxicokinetics of ^{35}S-Padan after four routes of administration. *Zhonghua Yufangyixue Zazhi* **18,** 193–195.

Joy, R. M., Lister, T., Ray, D. E., and Seville, M. P. (1990). Characteristics of the prolonged inhibition produced by a range of pyrethroids in the rat hippocampus. *Toxicol. Appl. Pharmacol.* **103,** 528–538.

Kaijser, L., and Berglund, B. (1985). Effects of nicotine on coronary blood flow in man. *Clin. Physiol.* **5,** 541–552.

Kamel, S. H., and Afifi, A. A. (1969). Estimation of toxic doses of strychnine hydrochloride in rats and dogs. *Zentralbl. Veterinaermed., Reihe A* **16,** 465–470.

Kaneko, H., Takamatsu, Y., Okuno, Y., Abiko, J., Yoshitake, A., and Miyamoto, J. (1988). Substrate specificity for formation of cholesterol ester conjugates from fenvalerate analogues and for granuloma formation. *Xenobiotica* **18,** 11–19.

Kato, K., Takamatsu, T., and Wakatsuki, S. (1976). Studies on the effects of pesticides on living organisms. 6. Results of health examinations of farmers in Mie and Chukugo areas. *J. Jpn. Assoc. Rural Med.* **25,** 6 (in Japanese).

Kato, R., Chiesara, E., and Vassanelli, P. (1962). Metabolic differences of strychnine in the rat in relation to sex. *Jpn. J. Pharmacol.* **12,** 26–33.

Kato, R., Vassanelli, P., and Frontino, G. (1963). Metabolic factors determining a higher resistance to strychnine in guinea pigs. *Arch. Int. Pharmacodyn. Ther.* **144,** 416–422.

Kavlock, R., Chernoff, N., Baron, R., Linder, E., Carver, B., Dilley, J., and Simmon, V. (1979). Toxicity studies with decamethrin, a synthetic pyrethroid insecticide. *J. Environ. Pathol. Toxicol.* **2,** 751–765.

Keeler, R. F. (1978). Alkaloid teratogens from *Lupinus, Conium, Veratrum,* and related genera. *In* "Effects of Poisonous Plants on Livestock" (R. F. Keeler, K. R. Van Kampen, and L. F. James, eds.), pp. 397–408. Academic Press, New York.

Keeler, R. F., Crowe, M. W., and Lambert, E. A. (1984). Teratogenicity in swine of the tobacco alkaloid anabasine isolated from *Nicotiana glauca*. *Teratology* **30,** 61–69.

Kennedy, D. (1962). Notes on the casualties with poisons in New Zealand. *WHO Inf. Circ. Toxic. Pestic. Man,* No. 8, p. 5.

Kesten, B., and Laszlo, E. (1931). Dermatitis due to sensitization to contact substances. Dermatitis veneata, occupational dermatitis. *Arch. Dermatol. Syphilol.* **23,** 221–237.

Khera, K. S., Whalen, C., and Angers, G. (1982). Teratogenicity study on pyrethrum and rotenone (natural origin) and ronnel in pregnant rats. *J. Toxicol. Environ. Health* **10,** 111–119.

Kimbrough, R. D., Gaines, T. B., and Hayes, W. J., Jr. (1968). Combined effect of DDT, pyrethrum, and piperonyl butoxide on rat liver. *Arch. Environ. Health* **16,** 333–341.

Kitagawa, T., Kawasaki, T., and Munechika, H. (1982). Enzyme immunoassay of blasticidin-S with high sensitivity. *J. Biochem. (Tokyo)* **92,** 585–590.

Knack (1932). Acute nicotine poisoning. *Dtsch. Med. Wochenschr.* **58,** 1467 (in German).

Kolmodin-Hedman, B., Swensson, A., and Akerblom, M. (1982). Occupational exposure to some synthetic pyrethroids (permethrin and fenvalerate). *Arch. Toxicol.* **50,** 27–33.

Konishi, K. (1972). Nereistoxin and its relatives. *In* "Proceedings of the Second International IUPAC Congress of Pesticide Chemistry" (A. S. Tahori, ed.) Vol. 1. Gordon and Breach Science Publishers.

Krayer, O., Moe, G. K., and Mendez, R. (1944). Studies on veratrum alkaloids. VI. Protoveratrine: Its comparative toxicity and its circulatory action. *J. Pharmacol. Exp. Ther.* **82,** 167–186.

Kretzschmar, R., Meyer, H. J., and Teschendorf, H. J. (1970). Strychnine antagonistic potency of pyrone compounds of the kavaroot (*Piper methysticum* Forst.). *Experientia* **26,** 283–284.

Krieg, A., and Miltenburger, H. G. (1984). Bioinsecticides. I. *Bacillus thuringiensis. Adv. Biotechnol. Processes* **3,** 273–290.

Kristensen, M., and Bojlén, K. (1931). Ratin infection in man. *Hospitalstidende* **74,** 489–502.

Laird, M. (1985). New answers to malaria problems through vector control. *Experientia* **41,** 446–456.

Lakatos, C., Vacher, J., and Duchene-Marullaz, P. (1964). Sex differences in the toxicity of strychnine in the mouse. Pharmacodynamic applications *C.R. Seances Soc. Biol. Ses. Fil.* **158,** 544–546 (in French).

Lambert, J. R., Byrick, R. J., and Hammeke, M. D. (1981). Management of acute strychnine poisoning. *Can. Med. Assoc. J.* **124,** 1268–1270.

Larson, P. S., and Haag, H. B. (1942). Studies on the fate of nicotine in the body. II. On the fate of nicotine in the dog. *J. Pharmacol. Exp. Ther.* **76,** 240–244.

Larson, P. S., Haag, H. B., and Finnegan, J. K. (1945). On the relative toxicity of nicotine and nornicotine. *Proc. Soc. Exp. Biol. Med.* **58,** 231–232.

Larson, P. S., Finnegan, J. K., Bibb, J. C., and Haag, H. B. (1949). Species variation in the protective action of anesthesia against the acutely lethal effect of nicotine. *Fed. Proc., Fed. Am. Soc. Exp. Biol.* **8,** 313.

Larson, P. S., Haag, H. B., and Silvette, H. (1961). "Tobacco: Experimental and Clinical Studies." Williams & Wilkins, Baltimore, Maryland.

Larson, P. S., Haag, H. B., and Silvette, H. (1968). "Tobacco: Experimental and Clinical Studies," Suppl. I. Williams & Wilkins, Baltimore, Maryland.

Larson, P. S., Haag, H. B., and Silvette, H. (1971). "Tobacco: Experimental and Clinical Studies," Suppl. II. Williams & Wilkins, Baltimore, Maryland.

Larson, P. S., Haag, H. B., and Silvette, H. (1975). "Tobacco: Experimental and Clinical Studies," Suppl. III. Williams & Wilkins, Baltimore, Maryland.

Lawrence, L. J., and Casida, J. E. (1982). Pyrethroid toxicology: Mouse intracerebral structure–toxicity relationships. *Pestic. Biochem. Physiol.* **18,** 9–14.

Lawrence, L. J., Gee, K. W., and Yamamura, H. I. (1985). Interactions of pyrethroid insecticides with chloride ionophore-associated binding sites. *Neurotoxicology* **6,** 87–98.

Lazdunski, M., Barhanin, J., Borsotto, M., Frelin, C., Hugues, M., Lombet, A., Pauron, D., Renaud, J., Schmid, A., and Vigne, P. (1985). Markers of membrane ionic channels. *In* "Vascular Neuroeffector Mechanisms" (J. A. Bevan *et al.,* eds.), Elsevier, Amsterdam.

Lazutka, F. A., Vasiliauskene, A. P., and Gefen, Sh. G. (1969). Toxicological evaluation of the insecticide nicotine sulfate. *Gig. Sanit.* **34,** 30–33.

Leahey, J. P., ed. (1985). "The Pyrethroid Insecticides." Taylor & Francis, London and Philadelphia.

Leake, L. D., Buckley, D. S., Ford, M. G., and Salt, D. W. (1985). Comparative effects of pyrethroids on neurones of target and non-target organisms. *Neurotoxicology* **6,** 99–116.

LeClercq, M., Cotonat, J., and Foulhoux, P. (1986). Research on the antagonism of deltamethrin intoxication. *J. Toxicol. Clin. Exp.* **6,** 85–93 (in French).

LeCointe, P. (1936). Rotenone containing plants in Amazonia. *Rev. Bot. Appl.* **16,** 609–615 (in French).

Lehman, A. J. (1951). Chemicals in foods: A report to the Association of Food and Drug Officials on current developments. Part II. Pesticides. Section I. Introduction. *Q. Bull.—Assoc. Food Drug Off.* **15** (I), 122–123.

Lehman, A. J. (1952). Chemicals in foods: A report to the Association of Food and Drug Officials on current developments. Part II. Pesticides. Section II. Dermal toxicity. Section III. Subacute and chronic toxicity. Section IV. Biochemistry. Section V. Pathology. *Q. Bull.—Assoc. Food Drug Off.* **16** (II), 3–9; (III), 47–53; (IV), 85–91; (V), 126–132.

Lehman, A. J. (1954). A toxicological evaluation of household insecticides. *Q. Bull.—Assoc. Food Drug Off.* **18,** 3–13.

Lehman, A. J. (1965). "Summaries of Pesticide Toxicity." Assoc. Food Drug Off. U.S. Topeka, Kansas.

LeQuesne, P. M., Maxwell, I. C., and Butterworth, S. T. G. (1980). Transient facial symptoms following exposure to synthetic pyrethroids: A clinical and electrophysiological assessment. *Neurotoxicology* **2,** 1–11.

Leslie, P. G. (1942). The bacteriological classification of the principal cultures used in rat and mouse controls in Great Britain. *J. Hyg.* **42,** 552–562.

Lightbody, H. D., and Matthews, J. A. (1936). Toxicology of rotenone. *Ind. Eng. Chem.* **28,** 809–811.

Lindahl, P. E., and Öberg, K. E. (1961). The effect of rotenone on respiration and its point of attack. *Exp. Cell Res.* **23,** 228–237.

Lister, T., and Ray, D. E. (1988). The role of basal forebrain in the primary cholinergic vasodilation in rat neocortex produced by systemic administration of cismethrin. *Brain Res.* **450,** 364–368.

Lo, P. K. A., Fink, D. W., Williams, J. B., and Blodinger, J. (1985). Pharmacokinetic studies of ivermectin: Effects of formulation. *Vet. Res. Commun.* **9,** 251–268.

Lock, E. A., and Berry, P. N. (1981). Biochemical change in the rat cerebellum following cypermethrin administration. *Toxicol. Appl. Pharmacol.* **59,** 508–514.

Lockhart, L. P. (1933). Nicotine poisoning. *Br. Med. J.* **1,** 246–274.

Lombet, A., Mourre, C., and Lazdunski, M. (1988). Interaction of insecticides of the pyrethroid family with specific binding sites on the voltage-dependent sodium channel from mammalian brain. *Brain Res.* **459,** 45–53.

Lord, K. A., and Johnson, C. G. (1947). The production of dermatitis by pyrethrum and attempts to produce a non-irritant extract. *Br. J. Dermatol.* **59,** 367–375.

Loughhead, M., Braithwaite, J., and Denton, M. (1978). Life at pH 6.6. *Lancet* **2,** 952.

Lovegrove, F. T. B. (1963). Three cases of strychnine poisoning. *Med. J. Aust.* **1,** 783–784.

L'vova, T. S. (1984). Study of five promising pesticides for the mutagenic effect in mice bone marrow cells, human peripheral lymphocyte culture and the yeast *Saccharomyces cerevisiae. Tsitol. Genet.* **18,** 455–457 (in Russian).

Lysenko, O. (1985). Non-sporeforming bacteria pathogenic to insects: Incidence and mechanism. *Annu. Rev. Microbiol.* **39,** 673–695.

Maddock, W. G., and Collier, F. A. (1933). Peripheral vasoconstriction by tobacco and its relation to thromboangiitis obliterans. *Ann. Surg.* **98,** 70–81.

Malley, L. A., Cagen, S. Z., Parker, C. M., Gardiner, T. H., Van Gelder, G. A., and Rose, G. P. (1985). Effect of vitamin E and other amelioratory agents on the fenvalerate-mediated skin sensation. *Toxicol. Lett.* **29**, 51–58.

Malone, J. C., and Brown, N. C. (1968). Toxicity of various grades of pyrethrum to laboratory animals. *Pyrethrum Post* **9**, 3–8.

Marei, A. E. M., Ruzo, L. O., and Casida, J. E. (1982). Analysis and persistence of permethrin, cypermethrin, deltamethrin and fenvalerate in the fat and brain of treated rats. *J. Agric. Food Chem.* **30**, 558–562.

Maron, B. J., Krupp, J. R., and Tune, B. (1971). Strychnine poisoning successfully treated with diazepam. *J. Pediatr.* **78**, 697–699.

Martin, B. R. (1986). Nicotine receptors in the central nervous system. *In* "The Receptors" (P. M. Conn, ed.), Vol. 3, pp. 393–415. Pergamon, Oxford.

Martin, H., and Worthing, C. R., eds. (1977). "The Pesticide Manual," 5th ed. Br. Crop Prot. Counc., Malvern, Worcestershire, England.

Maryanska-Nadachowska, A., and Rudek, Z. (1983). A study on the mutagenic activity of cartap using the micronucleus test. *Folia Biol.* **31**, 75–78.

Matthews, J. A., and Lightbody, H. D. (1936). Toxicity of derris and cubé. *Ind. Eng. Chem.* **28**, 812–814.

McCord, C. P., Kilker, C. H., and Minster, D. K. (1921). Pyrethrum dermatitis. A record of the occurrence of occupational dermatoses among workers in the pyrethrum industry. *JAMA, J. Am. Med. Assoc.* **77**, 448–449.

McCorkle, F., Taylor, R., Martin, D., and Glick, B. (1980). The effect of permethrin on the immune response of chickens. *Poult. Sci.* **59**, 1568.

McKillop, C. M., Brock, J. A. C., Oliver, G. J. A., and Rhodes, C. (1987). A quantitative assessment of pyrethroid-induced paraesthesia in the guinea-pig flank model. *Toxicol. Lett.* **36**, 1–7.

McLaughlin, G. A. (1973). History of pyrethrum. *In* "Pyrethrum: The Natural Insecticide" (J. E. Casida, ed.), pp. 3–15. Academic Press, New York and London.

Meisner, H. M., and Sorensen, L. (1966). Metaphase arrest of Chinese hamster cells with rotenone. *Exp. Cell Res.* **42**, 291–295.

Mendez, R., and Montes, G. (1943). Studies on veratrum alkaloids. III. Qualitative and quantitative differences in the action of cevine and veratridine. *J. Pharmacol. Exp. Ther.* **78**, 238–248.

Merchan, J., Diaz-Gil, J. J., Figueras, M. A., Navarro, M. A., Viladiu, P., and Gosalvez, M. (1978). Morphological study of rotenone-induced breast tumors in Wistar rats. *Rev. Exp. Oncol.* **26**, 107–120.

Meretoja, T., Carlberg, G., Gripenberg, U., Linnainmaa, K., and Sorsa, M. (1977). Mutagenicity of *Bacillus thuringiensis* exotoxin. I. Mammalian tests. *Hereditas* **85**, 105–112.

Metcalf, R. L. (1955). "Organic Insecticides." Wiley (Interscience), New York.

Mian, L. S., and Mulla, M. S. (1982). Biological and environmental dynamics of insect growth regulators (IGRs) as used against Diptera of public health importance. *Residue Rev.* **84**, 27–112.

Miller, L. K., Lingg, A. J., and Bulla, L. A. (1983). Bacterial, viral, and fungal insecticides. *Science* **219**, 715–721.

Mitchell, J. C., Dupuis, G., and Towers, G. H. N. (1972). Allergic contact dermatitis from pyrethrum (*Chrysanthemum* spp.). The roles of pyrethrosin, a sesquiterpene lactone, and of pyrethrin. II. *Br. J. Dermatol.* **86**, 568–573.

Miyakado, M., Nakayama, I., Inoue, A., Hatakoshi, M., and Ohno, N. (1985). The piperaceae amides. VI. Chemistry and insecticidal properties of piperaceae amides and their synthetic analogs. *J. Pestic. Sci.* **10**, 11–17.

Miyamoto, J., Suzuki, T., and Nakae, C. (1974). Metabolism of phenothrin or 3-phenoxybenzyl *d-trans*-chrysanthemate in mammals. *Pestic. Biochem. Physiol.* **4**, 438–450.

Miyamoto, J., Hideo, K., and Yasuyoshi, O. (1986). A novel lipophilic cholesterol ester conjugate from fenvalerate; its formation and toxicological significance. *ACS Symp. Ser.* **299**, 268–281.

Møller, K. O., and Simesen, M. (1939). A case of fatal nicotine poisoning with quantitative determination of nicotine in the organs. *Dtsch. Z. Gerichtl. Med.* **31**, 55–59 (in German).

Moriya, M., Ohta, T., Watanabe, K., Miyazawa, T., Kato, K., and Shirasu, Y. (1983). Further mutagenicity studies on pesticides in bacterial reversion assay systems. *Mutat. Res.* **116**, 185–216.

Murakami, M., and Fukami, J. (1983). Compiled data on toxicity to cultured animal and human cells and the mammalian LD_{50} values of pesticides. *J. Pestic. Sci.* **8**, 367–370.

Murza, V. I., Kurchatov, G. V., and Khasanov, Y. U. (1974). Sanitary-hygienic characterization of aerial application of insecticide–microbe mixtures. *Gig. Sanit.* **39**, 104–106.

Narahashi, T. (1971). Effects of insecticides on excitable tissues. *Adv. Insect Physiol.* **8**, 1–93.

Narahashi, T. (1985). Nerve membrane ionic channels as the primary target of pyrethroids. *Neurotoxicology* **6**, 3–22.

Narahashi, T. (1986). Mechanisms of action of pyrethroids on sodium and calcium channel gating. *In* "Neuropharmacology of Pesticide Action" (M. G. Ford, G. G. Lunt, R. C. Reay, and P. N. R. Usherwood, eds.), pp. 36–40. Ellis Horwood, Chichester, U.K.

Nasrat, H. A., Al-Hachim, G. M., and Mahmood, F. A. (1986). Perinatal effects of nicotine. *Biol. Neonate* **49**, 8–14.

Nawrot, J. (1983). Principles for grain weevil (*Sitophilus granarius* L.) (Coleoptera: Curculionidae) control with use of natural chemical compounds affecting the behaviour of beetles. *Pr. Nauk. Inst. Ochr. Rosl.* **24**, 173–197 (in Polish).

Nielsen, L. E., and Pedersen, L. E. K. (1984). The effect of charatoxin, 4-methylthio-1,2-dithiolane, on the frog sartorius neuromuscular junction. *Experientia* **40**, 186–188.

Nishi, K., Nunoshiba, T., and Nishioka, H. (1985). DNA damaging capacity and mutagenicity of pyrethroids. *Sci. Eng. Rev. Doshisha Univ.* **26**, 93–99.

Obayashi, H., and Asaka, A. (1983). Photolytic products of cartap in aqueous solution. *Takeda Kenkyushoho* **42**, 338–343 (in Japanese).

O'Callaghan, W. G., Joyce, N., Counihan, H. E., Ward, M., Lavelle, P., and O'Brien, E. (1982). Unusual strychnine poisoning and its treatment: Report of eight cases. *Br. Med. J.* **285**, 478.

Ohkawa, H., Kaneko, H., Tsuji, H., and Miyamoto, J. (1979). Metabolism of fenvalerate (Sumicidin) in rats. *J. Pestic. Sci.* **4**, 143–155.

Okuno, Y., Ito, S., Seki, T., Hiromori, T., Murakami, M., Kadota, T., and Miyamoto, J. (1986). Fenvalerate-induced granulomatous changes in rats and mice. *J. Toxicol. Sci.* **11**, 53–66.

Olkkola, K. T. (1984). Does ethanol modify antidotal efficacy of oral activated charcoal: Studies *in vitro* and with experimental animals. *J. Toxicol. Clin. Toxicol.* **22**, 425–432.

Olsnes, S., Refsnes, K., and Pihl, A. (1974). Mechanism of action of the toxic lectins abrin and ricin. *Nature (London)* **249**, 627–631.

Orechoff, A., and Menschikoff, G. (1931). On the alkaloids from *Anabasis aphylla* I. (First description). *Ber. Dtsch. Chem. Ges.* **64**, 266–274 (in German).

Orsós, F. (1936). Vital reactions of the nervous system during intoxication. *Dtsch. Z. Gerichtl. Med.* **23**, 212–225 (in German).

Osborne, T. B., Mendel, L. B., and Harris, I. F. (1905). A study of the proteins of the castor bean, with special reference to the isolation of ricin. *Am. J. Physiol.* **14**, 258–286.

Pall, H. S., Williams, A. C., Waring, R., and Elias, E. (1987). Motorneurone disease as a manifestation of pesticide toxicity. *Lancet* **2**, 685.

Parker, C. M., Piccirillo, V. J., Kurtz, S. L., Garner, F. M., Gardiner, T. H., and Van Gelder, G. A. (1984). Six month feeding study of fenvalerate in dogs. *Fundam. Appl. Toxicol.* **4**, 577–586.

Parker, C. M., Albert, J. R., Van Gelder, G. A., Patterson, D. R., and Taylor, J. L. (1985). Neuropharmacologic and neuropathologic effect of fenvalerate in mice and rats. *Fundam. Appl. Toxicol.* **5**, 278–286.

Parkin, P. J., and LeQuesne, P. M. (1982). Effect of a synthetic pyrethroid deltamethrin on excitability changes following a nerve impulse. *J. Neurol., Neurosurg. Psychiatry* **45**, 337–342.

Pensa, P., and Ceccarelli, B. (1968). Ultrastructure of spinal cord synapses during strychnine intoxication. *Experientia* **24**, 1025–1026.

Perlman, H. H., and Dannenberg, A. M. (1942). Excretion of nicotine in breast milk and urine from cigarette smoking—its effect on lactation and the nursling. *JAMA, J. Am. Med. Assoc.* **120**, 1003–1008.

Perper, J. A. (1985). Fatal strychnine poisoning—a case report and review of the literature. *J. Forensic Sci.* **30,** 1248–1255.

Pilcher, J. D., and Sollmann, T. (1915). Studies on the vasomotor centre. XVIII. The effects of *Veratrum viride* and cevadin (veratrin). *J. Pharmacol. Exp. Ther.* **7,** 295–300.

Pivovarov, Yu. P., Ivashina, S. A., and Padalkin, V. P. (1977). Hygienic assessment of investigation of insecticide preparations. *Gig. Sanit.* **8,** 45–48.

Plimmer, J. R., Inscoe, M. N., and McGovern, T. P. (1982). Insect attractants. *Annu. Rev. Pharmacol. Toxicol.* **22,** 297–320.

Pluijmen, M., Drevon, G., Montesano, R., Malaveille, G., Hautefeuille, A., and Bartsch, H. (1984). Lack of mutagenicity of synthetic pyrethroids in *Salmonella typhimurium* strains and in V-79 Chinese hamster cells. *Mutat. Res.* **137,** 7–15.

Poe, C. F., Suchy, J. F., and Sitt, N. F. (1936). Toxicity of strychnine for male and female rats of different ages. *J. Pharmacol. Exp. Ther.* **58,** 239–242.

Poulos, L., Athanaselis, S., and Cottselinis, A. (1982). Acute intoxication with cypermethrin (NRDC149). *J. Toxicol. Clin. Toxicol.* **19,** 519–520.

Prasada Rao, K. S., Chetty, C. S., and Desaiah, D. (1984). *In vitro* effects of pyrethroid on rat brain and liver ATPase activities. *J. Toxicol. Environ. Health* **14,** 257–265.

Priest, R. E. (1938). Strychnine poisoning successfully treated with sodium amytal. *JAMA, J. Am. Med. Assoc.* **110,** 1440.

Pycock, C. J., and Kerwin, R. W. (1981). The status of glycine as a supraspinal neurotransmitter. *Life Sci.* **28,** 2679–2686.

Racouchot, J. (1939). Rotenone containing plants. Occupational dermatitis. *Arch. Mal. Prof. Hyg. Toxicol. Ind.* **2,** 149–151 (in French).

Ramirez, M. A. (1930). An etiologic factor in vasomotor rhinitis and asthma. *J. Allergy* **1,** 149–155.

Randall, L. O., Heise, G. A., Schallek, W., Bagon, R. E., Banziger, R., Boris, A., Moe, R. A., and Abrams, W. B. (1961). Pharmacological and clinical studies on Valium (T.M.), a new psychotherapeutic agent of the benzodiazepine class. *Curr. Ther. Res.* **3,** 405–425.

Rashatwar, S. S., and Matsumara, F. (1985). Interaction of DDT and pyrethroids with calmodulin and its significance in the expression of enzyme activities of phosphodiesterase. *Biochem. Pharmacol.* **34,** 1689–1694.

Ray, D. E. (1980). An EEG investigation of decamethrin-induced choreoathetosis in the rat. *Exp. Brain Res.* **38,** 221–227.

Ray, D. E. (1982a). Changes in brain blood flow associated with deltamethrin-induced choreoathetosis in the rat. *Exp. Brain Res.* **45,** 269–276.

Ray, D. E. (1982b). The contrasting actions of two pyrethroids (deltamethrin and cismethrin) in the rat. *Neurobehav. Toxicol. Teratol.* **4,** 801–804.

Ray, D. E., and Cremer, J. E. (1979). The action of decamethrin (a synthetic pyrethroid) in the rat. *Pestic. Biochem. Physiol.* **10,** 333–340.

Rhodes, C., Jones, B. K., Croucher, A., Hutson, D. H., Logan, C. J., Hopkins, R., Hall, B. E., and Vickers, J. A. (1984). The bioaccumulation and biotransformation of *cis,trans*-cypermethrin in the rat. *Pestic. Sci.* **15,** 471–480.

Rickard, J., and Brodie, M. E. (1985). Correlation of blood and brain levels of the neurotoxic pyrethroid deltamethrin with the onset of symptoms in rats. *Pestic. Biochem. Physiol.* **23,** 143–156.

Rickett, F. E., and Tyszkiewicz, K. (1973). Pyrethrum dermatitis. II. The allergenicity of pyrethrum oleoresin and its cross-reactions with the saline extract of pyrethrum flowers. *Pestic. Sci.* **4,** 801–810.

Rickett, F. E., Tyszkiewicz, K., and Brown, N. C. (1972). Pyrethrum dermatitis. I. The allergenic properties of various extracts of pyrethrum flowers. *Pestic. Sci.* **3,** 57–66.

Romey, G., and Lazdunski, M. (1982). Lipid-soluble toxins thought to be specific for Na$^+$ channels block Ca^{2+} channels in neuronal cells. *Nature (London)* **297,** 79–80.

Rose, G. P., and Dewar, A. J. (1983). Intoxication with four synthetic pyrethroids fails to show any correlation between neuromuscular dysfunction and neurobiochemical abnormalities in rats. *Arch. Toxicol.* **53,** 297–316.

Rotenberg, K. S. (1982). The pharmacokinetics of nicotine. *Pharm. Int.* **3,** 91–93.

Ruddon, R. W., and Cohen, A. M. (1970). Alteration of enzyme activity in rat liver following the acute and chronic administration of nicotine. *Toxicol. Appl. Pharmacol.* **16,** 613–625.

Ruigt, G. S. F., and van den Bercken, J. (1986). Action of pyrethroids on a nerve–muscle preparation of the clawed frog, *Xenopus laevis*. *Pestic. Biochem. Physiol.* **25,** 176–187.

Ruppert, H. (1942). Tachyphylaxis of isolobinin and nicotine in the central nervous system. *Naunyn-Schmiedebergs Arch. Exp. Pathol. Pharmakol.* **199,** 497–507 (in German).

Ruzo, L. O., Unai, T., and Casida, J. E. (1978). Decamethrin metabolism in rats. *J. Agric. Food Chem.* **26,** 918–925.

Sagaragli, G. P., and Mannaioni, P. F. (1974). Pharmacokinetic observations on a case of massive strychnine poisoning. *Clin. Toxicol.* **6,** 533–554.

Sakai, H. (1983). Bancol (Bensultap). *Jap. Pestic. Inform.* **45,** 21–24.

Salgado, V. L., Irving, S. N., and Miller, T. A. (1983). The importance of nerve terminal depolarization in pyrethroid poisoning of insects. *Pestic. Biochem. Physiol.* **20,** 169–182.

Salm, H. (1952). Fatalities after attempted abortion with Movellan tablets. *Dtsch. Gesundheitswes.* **7,** 50–53 (in German).

Samples, J. R., and Buettner, H. (1983). Corneal ulcer caused by a biologic insecticide (*Bacillus thuringiensis*). *Am. J. Ophthalmol.* **95,** 258–260.

Santi, R., and Tóth, C. E. (1965). Toxicology of rotenone. *Farmaco, Ed. Sci.* **20,** 270–279.

Santi, R., Ferrari, M., and Tóth, E. (1966). Pharmacological properties of rotenone. *Farmaco, Ed. Sci.* **21,** 689–703.

Sattelle, D. B., Harrow, I. D., David, J. A., Pelhate, M., Callec, J. J., Gepner, J. I., and Hall, L. M. (1985). Nereistoxin: actions on a CNS acetylcholine receptor/ion channel in the cockroach *Periplaneta americana*. *J. Exp. Biol.* **118,** 37–52.

Saxena, K., and Scheman, A. (1985). Suicide plan by nicotine poisoning: A review of nicotine toxicity. *Vet. Hum. Toxicol.* **27,** 495–497.

Schafer, E. W., Bowles, W. A., and Hurlbut, J. (1983). The acute oral toxicity, repellancy, and hazard potential of 998 chemicals to one or more species of wild and domestic birds. *Arch. Environ. Contam. Toxicol.* **12,** 355–382.

Schievelbein, H. (1982). Nicotine, resorption and fate. *Pharmacol. Ther.* **18,** 233–248.

Schmidt, M. (1931). Nicotine poisoning (suicide attempt). *Samml. Vergiftungsfaellen* **2A**(92), 15–16 (in German).

Schopp, R. T., and DeClue, J. W. (1980). Paralytic properties of 4-*N,N*-dimethylamino-1,2-dithiolane (nereistoxin). *Arch. Int. Pharmacodyn.* **248,** 166–176.

Schrader, G. (1937). Strychnine intoxication. *Samml. Vergiftungsfaellen* **8C** (39), 39–56 (in German).

Schwartz, L. (1934). Dermatitis due to pyrethrum contained in an insecticide. *Public Health Bull.* **215,** 51–54.

Schwarz, F. (1954). Fatal strychnine poisoning by laxatives in a 1½ year old boy. *Samml. Vergiftungsfaellen* **14,** 451–453. (in German).

Schwarz, M., Sonnet, P. E., and Wakabayashi, N. (1970). Insect juvenile hormone: Activity of selected terpenoid compounds. *Science* **167,** 191–192.

Scott, G. C., Pickett, J. A., Smith, M. C., Woodcock, C. M., Harris, P. G. W., Hammon, R. P., and Koetecha, H. D. (1984). Seed treatment for controlling slugs in winter wheat. *Proc. Br. Crop Prot. Conf.—Pesta Dis.*, pp. 133–138.

Shadduck, J. (1980). "*Bacillus thuringiensis* Serotype H-14 Maximum Challenge and Eye Irritation Safety Tests in Mammals," WHO/VBC/80.763. World Health Organ., Geneva.

Shanes, A. J. (1952). The ultraviolet spectra and neurophysiological effects of "veratrine" alkaloids. *J. Pharmacol. Exp. Ther.* **105,** 216–231.

Sharma, C. B. S. R., and Sahu, R. K. (1977). I. A preliminary study on the response of root meristems to exotoxin from *Bacillus thuringiensis*, a constituent of a microbial insecticide, Thuricide. *Mutat. Res.* **46,** 19–26.

Shepard, H. H. (1951). "The Chemistry and Action of Insecticides," 1st ed. McGraw-Hill, New York.

Sherby, S. M., Eldefrawi, A. T., David, J. A., Sattelle, D. B., and Eldefrawi, M. E. (1986). Interactions of charatoxins and nereistoxin with the nicotinic acetylcholine receptors of insect CNS and *torpedo* electric organ. *Arch. Insect Biochem. Physiol.* **3**, 431–445.

Sherby, S. M., Eldefrawi, A. T., Deshpande, S. S., Albuquerque, E. X., and Eldefrawi, M. E. (1986). Effects of pyrethroids on nicotinic acetylcholine receptor binding and function. *Pestic. Biochem. Physiol.* **26**, 107–115.

Shimkin, M. B., and Anderson, H. H. (1936). Acute toxicities of rotenone and mixed pyrethrins in mammals. *Proc. Soc. Exp. Biol. Med.* **34**, 135–138.

Shono, T., Ohsawa, K., and Casida, J. E. (1979). Metabolism of *trans-* and *cis*-cypermethrin and decamethrin by microsomal enzymes. *J. Agric. Food Chem.* **27**, 316–325.

Shorey, H. H. (1976). "Animal Communication by Pheromones." Academic Press, New York.

Shorey, H. H., and McKelvey, J. J., Jr., eds. (1977). "Chemical Control of Insect Behaviour: Theory and Application." Wiley, New York.

Siddall, J. B., and Slade, M. (1971). Absence of acute oral toxicity of *Hyalophora cecropia* juvenile-hormone in mice. *Nature (London) New Biol.* **229**, 158.

Silvette, H., Hoff, E. C., Larson, P. S., and Haag, H. B. (1962). The actions of nicotine on central nervous system functions. *Pharmacol. Rev.* **14**, 137–173.

Simmons, S. W. (1959). The use of DDT in human medicine. *In* "DDT: The Insecticide Dichlorodiphenyl-Trichloroethane and Its Significance" (P. Müller, ed.), Vol. 2, pp. 249–502. Birkhaeuser, Basel.

Simonsen, J. L., and Owen, L. N. (1947). The terpenes. *In* "The Simpler Acyclic and Monocyclic Terpenes and Their Derivatives," Vol. 1. Cambridge Univ. Press, London.

Singh, G. J. P., and Gill, S. S. (1985). Myotoxic and neurotoxic activity of *Bacillus thuringiensis* var. *israelensis* crystal toxin. *Pestic. Biochem. Physiol.* **24**, 406–414.

Sláma, K. (1971). Insect juvenile hormone analogues. *Annu. Rev. Biochem.* **40**, 1079–1102.

Sláma, K., Romaňuk, M., and Šorn, F. (1974). "Insect Hormones and Bioanalogues." Springer-Verlag, New York.

Slotkin, T. A., Greer, N., Faust, J., Cho, H., and Seidler, F. J. (1986). Effects of maternal nicotine injections on brain development in the rat: Ornithine decarboxylase activity, nucleic acids and proteins in discrete brain regions. *Brain Res. Bull.* **17**, 41–50.

Smith, C. R. (1931). Neonicotine and isomeric pyridylpiperidines. *J. Am. Chem. Soc.* **53**, 277–283.

Smith, G. S. (1951). Fatal case of nicotine poisoning. *Br. Med. J.* **2**, 1522.

Snell, M. A. (1952). Castor bean pomace exposure. *Arch. Ind. Hyg.* **6**, 113–115.

Soderlund, D. M. (1985). Pyrethroid–receptor interactions: Stereospecific binding and effects on sodium channels in mouse brain preparation. *Neurotoxicology* **6**, 35–46.

Sollmann, T. (1901). "A Text-Book of Pharmacology and Some Allied Sciences." Saunders, Philadelphia, Pennsylvania.

Sollmann, T. (1957). "A Manual of Pharmacology and Its Applications to Therapeutics and Toxicology," 8th ed. Saunders, Philadelphia, Pennsylvania.

Springfield, A. C., Carlson, G. P., and DeFeo, J. J. (1973). Liver enlargement and modification of hepatic microsomal drug metabolism in rats by pyrethrum. *Toxicol. Appl. Pharmacol.* **24**, 298–308.

Staatz, C. G., and Hosko, N. H. (1985). Effect of pyrethroid insecticides on EEG activity of conscious, immobilized rats. *Pestic. Biochem. Physiol.* **24**, 231–239.

Staatz, C. G., Bloom, A. S., and Lech, J. J. (1982). A pharmacological study of pyrethroid neurotoxicity in mice. *Pestic. Biochem. Physiol.* **17**, 287–292.

Staatz-Benson, C. G., and Hosko, M. J. (1986). Interaction of pyrethroids with mammalian spinal neurons. *Pestic. Biochem. Physiol.* **25**, 19–30.

Staub, H. (1920). A fatal infection with mouse typhoid ("mouse virus"). *Schweiz. Med. Wochenschr.* **50**, 114–115 (in German).

Stefanovich, V., Gore, I., Kajiyama, G., and Iwanaga, Y. (1969). The effect of nicotine on dietary atherogenesis in rabbits. *Exp. Mol. Pathol.* **11**, 71–81.

Stelzer, K. J., and Gordon, M. A. (1984). Effects of pyrethroids on lympho-

cyte mitogenic responsiveness. *Res. Commun. Chem. Pathol. Pharmacol.* **46**, 137–150.

Stewart, P. M., and Catterall, J. R. (1985). Chronic nicotine ingestion and atrial fibrillation. *Br. Heart J.* **54**, 222–223.

Stirpe, F., and Barbieri, L. (1986). Ribosome-inactivating proteins up to date. *FEBS Lett.* **195**, 1–5.

Storey, B. T. (1981). Inhibitors of energy-coupling site 1 of the mitochondrial respiratory chain. *In* "Inhibitors of Mitochondrial Functions" (M. Erecinska and D. F. Wilson, eds.), pp. 101–108. Int. Encycl. Pharmacol. Ther. Sect. 107. Pergamon, Oxford.

Sudan, B. J. L., Brouillard, C., Sterboul, J., and Sainte-Laudy, J. (1984). Nicotine as a hapten in seborrhoeic dermatitis. *Contact Dermatitis* **11**, 196–197.

Suga, K. (1972). Environmental pollution and eye damage. *Jpn. Rev. Clin. Ophthalmol.* **66**, 537–539 (in Japanese).

Sugimoto, T. (1972a). Studies on the reduction of ocular damage caused by blasticidin-S, a fungicidal antibiotic. *Med. Biol.* **85**, 73–176 (in Japanese).

Sugimoto, T. (1972b). Studies on ocular disturbance by improved blasticidin-S dust formulation. *J. Jpn. Assoc. Rural Med.* **21**, 316–317 (in Japanese).

Sugimoto, T. (1978). Reduction of eye irritation caused by blasticidin S, a fungicidal antibiotic. *Kurume Igakkai Zasshi* **41**, 103–113. (in Japanese).

Suh, D., Kim, D., Hong, D., and Hong, S. (1970). Acute intoxication due to agricultural chemicals. *Taehan Naekwa Hakkoe Chapchi* **13**, 197–206 (in Korean).

Suzuki, S. (1977). Chronic administration of blasticidin and alkaline phosphatase. *Toho Igakkai Zasshi* **24**, 877–900.

Sweetman, H. L. (1936). "The Biological Control of Insects." Comstock, Ithaca, New York.

Sweitzer, S. E. (1936). Scabies: Further observations on its treatment with pyrethrum ointment. *J. Lancet* **56**, 467–468.

Sweitzer, S. E., and Tedder, J. W. (1935). Pyrethrum in treatment of scabies. *Minn. Med.* **18**, 793–795.

Swiss, E. E., and Bauer, R. O. (1951). Acute toxicity of veratrum derivatives. *Proc. Soc. Exp. Biol. Med.* **76**, 847–849.

Swissman, N., and Jacoby, J. (1964). Strychnine poisoning and its treatment. *Clin. Pharmacol. Ther.* **5**, 136–140.

Symons, A. J. C., and Boyle, A. K. (1963). Accidental strychnine poisoning: A case report. *Br. J. Anaesth.* **35**, 54–56.

Szabad, J., and Bennettova, B. (1986). Analysis of the genotoxic activities of 5 compounds affecting insect fertility. *Mutat. Res.* **173**, 197–200.

Takano, Y. (1972). On the clinical cases of pesticide intoxication during the last 5 years in Akita Prefecture. *J. Jpn. Assoc. Rural Med.* **21**, 240–241 (in Japanese).

Taylor, J. (1956). Bacterial rodenticides and infection with *Salmonella enteritidis. Lancet* **1**, 630–663.

Teitelbaum, D. T., and Ott, J. E. (1970). Acute strychnine intoxication. *Clin. Toxicol.* **3**, 267–273.

Thiebault, J. J., Bost, J., and Foulhoux, P. (1985). Experimental intoxication by deltamethrin in the dog and its treatment. *Collect. Med. Leg. Toxicol. Med.* **131**, 47–62 (in French).

Thomas, W. E., and Ellar, D. J. (1983). *Bacillus thuringiensis* var. *israelensis* crystal δ-endotoxin: Effects on insect and mammalian cells *in vitro* and *in vivo. J. Cell Sci.* **60**, 181–197.

Tiess, D., and Nagel, K.-H. (1966). Fatal acute nicotine intoxication with "Nikotin 95/98%." Analysis of poison in fresh, frozen and formalin-fixed tissues. *Arch. Toxicol.* **22**, 68–79 (in German).

Tonking, H. E. (1936). Pyrethrum dermatitis in Kenya. *East Afr. Med. J.* **13**, 7–14.

Tucker, R. K., and Haegele, M. A. (1971). Comparative acute oral toxicity of pesticides to six species of birds. *Toxicol. Appl. Pharmacol.* **20**, 57–65.

Tucker, S. B., Flannigan, S. A., and Smolensky, M. H. (1983). Comparison of therapeutic agents for synthetic pyrethroid exposure. *Contact Dermatitis* **9**, 316.

Tumlinson, M., Gueldner, R. C., Hardee, D. D., Thompson, A. C., Hedin, P. S., and Minyard, J. P. (1970). The boll weevil sex attractant. *In* "Chemicals Controlling Insect Behavior" (M. Beroza, ed.), pp. 41–59. Academic Press, New York.

Turner, D. M. (1969). The metabolism of ^{14}C nicotine in the cat. *Biochem. J.* **115**, 889–896.

Ugen, K. E., and Scott, W. J. (1985). Potentiation of acetazolamide induced ectrodactyly in Wistar rats by vasoactive agents and physical clamping of the uterus. *Teratology* **31**, 273–278.

Unai, T., Cheng, H. M., Yamamoto, I., and Casida, J. E. (1973). Chemical and biological O,O-demethylation of rotenone derivatives. *Agric. Biol. Chem.* **37**, 1937–1944.

van den Bercken, J., Akkermann, L. M. A., and Van der Zalm, J. J. (1973). DDT-like action of allethrin in the sensory nervous system of *Xenopus laevis. Eur. J. Pharmacol.* **21**, 95–106.

Verbiscar, A. J., Patel, J., Banigan, T. F., and Schatz, R. A. (1986). Scilliroside and other scilla compounds in red squill. *J. Agric. Food Chem.* **34**, 973–979.

Verschoyle, R. D., and Aldridge, W. N. (1980). Structure–activity relationships of some pyrethroids in rats. *Arch. Toxicol.* **45**, 325–329.

Verschoyle, R. D., and Barnes, J. M. (1972). Toxicity of natural and synthetic pyrethrins to rats. *Pestic. Biochem. Physiol.* **2**, 308–311.

Vijverberg, H. P. M., and de Weille, J. R. (1985). The interaction of pyrethroids with voltage-dependent Na channels. *Neurotoxicology* **6**, 23–34.

Vijverberg, H. P. M., Ruigt, G. S. F., and van den Bercken, J. (1982). Structure-related effects of pyrethroid insecticides on the lateral-line sense organ and on pheripheral nerves of the clawed frog, *Xenopus laevis. Pestic. Biochem. Physiol.* **18**, 315–324.

Volle, R. L. (1980). Nicotinic ganglion-stimulating agents. *In* "Handbuch der Experimentellen Pharmakologie" (D. A. Kharkevich *et al.*, eds.), Vol. 53, pp. 281–312. Springer-Verlag, Berlin.

Wall, P. D., and Horwitz, N. H. (1951). Observations on the physiological action of strychnine. *J. Neurophysiol.* **14**, 257–263.

Warren, R. E., Rubenstein, D., Ellar, D. J., Kramer, J. M. and Gilbert, R. J. (1984). *Bacillus thuringiensis* var. *israelensis:* Protoxin activation and safety. *Lancet* **1**, 678–679.

Waters, M. D., Sandhu, S. S., Simon, V. F., Mortelmans, K. E., Mitchell, A. D., Jorgenson, T. A., Jones, D. C. L., Valencia, R., and Garrett, N. E. (1982). Study of pesticide genotoxicity. *Basic Life Sci.* **21**, 275–326.

Wehrlin, H. (1938). Acute nicotine intoxication during insecticide spraying. *Schweiz. Med. Wochenschr.* **68**, 1191–1192 (in German).

Weiss, S., and Hatcher, R. A. (1922). Studies on strychnin. *J. Pharmacol. Exp. Ther.* **19**, 419–482.

Wenzel, D. G., and Richards, M. H. (1970). Effects of chronic nicotine, acute hypoxia, and their interactions on myocardial enzymes. *Toxicol. Appl. Pharmacol.* **16**, 656–667.

White, I. N. H., Verschoyle, R. D., Moradian, M. H., and Barnes, J. M. (1976). The relationship between brain levels of cismethrin and bioresmethrin in female rats and neurotoxic effects. *Pestic. Biochem. Physiol.* **6**, 491–500.

Whiteley, H. R., and Schnepf, H. E. (1986). The molecular biology of parasporal crystal body formation in *Bacillus thuringiensis. Annu. Rev. Microbiol.* **40**, 549–576.

Wigglesworth, V. B. (1935). Functions of corpus allatum in insects. *Nature (London)* **136**, 338–339.

Wigglesworth, V. B. (1936). The function of the corpus allatum in the growth and reproduction of *Rhodnius prolixus* (Hemiptera). *Q. J. Microsc. Sci. [N.S.]* **79**, 91–121.

Wigglesworth, V. B. (1970). "Insect Hormones." Freeman, San Francisco, California.

Wiley, R. G., Talman, W. T., and Reis, D. J. (1983). Ricin transport distinguishes between central and peripheral neurones. *Brain Res.* **269**, 357–360.

Williams, C. M. (1956). The juvenile hormone of insects. *Nature (London)* **178**, 212–213.

Wilson, D. J. B. (1930). Nicotine poisoning by absorption through the skin. *Br. Med. J.* **2**, 601–602.

Wilson, R. H., and DeEds, F. (1936). Chronic nicotine toxicity. I. Feeding of nicotine sulfate, tannate, and bentonite. *J. Ind. Hyg. Toxicol.* **18**, 553–564.

Wodzicki, K. (1973). Prospects for biological control of rodent populations. *Bull. W. H. O.* **48**, 461–467.

Wood, D. L., Silverstein, R. M., and Nakajima, M., eds. (1970). "Control of Insect Behavior by Natural Products." Academic Press, New York.

World Health Organization (WHO) (1967). "Safe Use of Pesticides in Public Health," WHO Tech. Rep. Ser. No. 356. World Health Organ., Geneva.

World Health Organization (WHO) (1982). "Data Sheet on the Biological Control Agent *Bacillus thuringiensis* serotype. H-14," WHO/ VBC/79.750. Rev. I. VBC/BCDS/79.01. World Health Organ., Geneva.

Wreschner, H. (1921). Misuse and dangers in the handling of bacterial rat and mouse control agents. *Z. Hyg. Infektionskr.* **93**, 35–42 (in German).

Wright, C. D. P., Forshaw, P. J., and Ray, D. E. (1988). Classification of the actions of two pyrethroid insecticides in the rat, using the trigeminal reflex and skeletal muscle as test systems. *Pestic. Biochem. Physiol.* **30**, 79–86.

Wright, D. J. (1986). Biological activity and mode of action of avermectins. *In* "Neuropharmacology of Pesticide Action" (M. G. Ford, G. G. Lunt, R. C. Reay, and P. N. R. Usherwood, eds.), pp. 174–202. Ellis Horwood, Chichester, U.K.

Wright, J. E., and Smalley, H. E. (1977). Biological activity of insect juvenile hormone analogues against the stable fly and toxicity studies in domestic animals. *Arch. Environ. Contam. Toxicol.* **5**, 191–197.

Yamamoto, T., Iwasaki, Y., and Konno, H. (1983). Retrograde axoplasmic transport of toxic lectins is useful for transganglionic tracings of the peripheral nerve. *Brain Res.* **274**, 325–328.

Yamasaki, R. B., and Klocke, J. A. (1987). Structure–bioactivity relationships of azadirachtin, a potential insect control agent. *J. Agric. Food Chem.* **35**, 467–471.

Yonehara, H. (1984). Blasticidin S: Properties, biosynthesis, and fermentation. *Drugs Pharm. Sci.*, 651–663.

Young, A. B., and Snyder, S. H. (1973). Strychnine binding associated with glycine receptors of the central nervous system. *Proc. Natl. Acad. Sci. U.S.A.* **70**, 2832–2836.

Zerbest, G. H. (1944). Unusual hazard in a fertilizer factory. *Ind. Med.* **13**, 552.

Zhu, Q., Liu, X., Yu, Y., and Liu, F. (1986). Toxicity test for fenvalerate. *Zhonghua Yufangyixue Zazhi* **20**, 238–239 (in Chinese).

Zielinska, Z. M., Chmurzynska, W., Fedorowicz, M., Grzelakowska-Sztabert, B., and Laskowska-Bozek, H. (1981). Effects of juvenile hormone I and its analogs in animal cells cultured *in vitro. Sci. Pap., Inst. Org. Phys. Chem. Wroclaw Tech. Univ.* **22**, 497–500.

CHAPTER 14

Solvents, Fumigants, and Related Compounds

P. J. Gehring, R. J. Nolan, P. G. Watanabe, and A. M. Schumann

The Dow Chemical Company

14.1 INTRODUCTION

With very few exceptions, the insecticidal oils as well as the propellants and solvents used with other pesticides are relatively simple hydrocarbons and halohydrocarbons. All have some power to dissolve active ingredients, and this property is critical for those used as solvents. Most propellants assist in dissolving active ingredients and, at the least, mix freely with the accompanying solvent. Oils frequently are used alone as insecticides and herbicides, and in at least one instance an oil is used as a fungicide.

The main feature distinguishing propellants from solvents and oils is vapor pressure. The propellants are gases at ordinary temperatures and atmospheric pressure; when compressed to liquid form, they provide the pressure necessary to expel the contents of a bomb, often in such a way that the stream breaks into a fine aerosol. Solvents have a much lower vapor pressure but still evaporate promptly when applied as a thin film. Some petroleum distillates used as solvents, such as kerosene, may also be used as spray oils. However, spray oils often are less volatile. Extraction and measurement showed that about two-thirds of the heavy oil absorbed by the cortex of citrus leaves remained there 3 weeks later, and about one-third of the absorbed oil remained on the tree after 6 months.

The kind of danger that the compounds under discussion present to people is largely a function of their vapor pressures. Propellants, and to a lesser extent some solvents, are dangerous if inhaled in high concentrations because they are likely to sensitize the heart and precipitate fatal ventricular fibrillation. Although solvents may cause narcosis if inhaled or ingested, the injury that solvents and oils have produced most commonly is chemical pneumonitis, following their ingestion and aspiration.

14.2 PROPELLANTS

For many years, halohydrocarbons of low molecular weight, often spoken of as "Freons," have been used extensively as propellants in pressurized containers to disperse aerosols, not only of insecticides but also of paints, hair sprays, and a wide range of other products. These compounds provide pressure within the range of temperature tolerated by people and have the added advantages of being nonflammable solvents of low toxicity. The only toxicological disadvantage is that they, like similar compounds used for other purposes, may sensitize the myocardium and lead to fatal ventricular fibrillation. Potency for producing ventricular fibrillation varies with the solvent or propellant *per se* (Clark and Tinston, 1982; Simaan and Aviado, 1975). On occasion, there have been suggestions that mixtures of these agents may be more than additive in induction of cardiac arrhythmias (Valic *et al.*, 1977). Most people killed in this way had purposely misused the preparations either by "sniffing" vapor arising from solvents or glues or by inhaling the mixture of vapor and particles resulting from discharging an aerosol bomb into a paper or plastic bag (Bass, 1970; Reinhardt *et al.*, 1971; Wyse, 1973; Roberts, 1982). However, deaths have not been confined to persons who engaged in willful misuse. Deaths also have occurred among persons who used aerosols to treat asthma (Speizer *et al.*, 1968a,b) and among persons anesthetized by certain vapors, notably chloroform (Levy and Lewis, 1911; Levy, 1913). Although persons exposed to gases or vapors either accidentally or as the result of insufficient precautions at work may be killed by narcotic action or even by simple lack of oxygen, many such deaths are the result of cardiac arrhythmias.

Studies in animals indicate that some compounds are more likely than others to sensitize the heart and to produce arrhythmia. It is also clearly established that hypoxia or either exogenous or endogenous epinephrine predisposes the heart to sensitization. However, no satisfactory explanation for the observed dosage–response relationship is available. To be sure, it was shown very early that cardiac arrhythmias were more likely to occur at moderate than at high dosages of chloroform and could even be suppressed by high dosages (Levy and Lewis, 1911; Levy, 1913). It was also clear that the proportion of persons stricken in the course of anesthesia or treatment for asthma was quite small. The same probably is true of persons who are exposed to solvents accidentally or through willful misuse; however, absence of any record of the number of persons exposed makes the record of deaths (at least 44, 104, and 114 in the United States due to sniffing in 1969, 1973, and 1974, respectively) useless for calculating a ratio.

In the United States three sudden deaths in 1969 followed heavy exposure to pesticide solvents or propellants, and there was an additional case in 1970 (Hayes, 1976). In spite of a careful investigation of the vital statistics for 1973 and 1974, no similar case was found, whether associated with a pesticide or with any aerosol preparation that was not willfully misused (Hayes and Vaughn, 1977). In view of these findings and in the absence of other reports, it seems clear that cardiac arrhythmia is a real but rare danger to those who are heavily exposed to pesticide solvents or propellants without any willful misuse.

The toxicity of dichlorodifluoromethane is discussed below as an example of its class. It has been one of the most extensively used propellants for insecticide aerosols. However, it is a common practice to use more than one propellant in a single formulation. Information is entirely inadequate to judge the relative safety of this and other compounds used for this purpose in a wide range of aerosols.

14.2.1 DICHLORODIFLUOROMETHANE

14.2.1.1 Identity, Properties, and Uses

Chemical Name   Dichlorodifluoromethane.

Structure Cl_2CF_2. Proprietary names for dichlorodifluoromethane are Algofrene® Type 2, Arcton® 6, Arcton® 12, Freon® 12, Frigen® 12, Genetron® 12, Halocarbon® 12, Halon®, Isotron®, and Ledon® 12. The CAS registry number is 75-71-8.

Physical and Chemical Properties   Dichlorodifluoromethane has the empirical formula CCl_2F_2 and a molecular weight of 120.91. It is a colorless, nonflammable gas with a faint ether-like odor at high concentrations. The liquid has a density of 1.486 at the boiling point of $-29.8°C$; the freezing point is $-158°C$. It is soluble in alcohol and ether and quite soluble in water, 5.7 ml/100 ml at 26°C. Dichlorodifluoromethane is noncorrosive and stable up to 550°C. At 25°C, the vapor pressure is 6.43 atm.

Use   Dichlorodifluoromethane is used as an aerosol propellant and refrigerant.

14.2.1.2 Toxicity to Laboratory Animals

The LC 50 for rats exposed to dichlorodifluoromethane for 15 min was greater than 80 vol %, while the EC 50 for stimulation of the central nervous system during a 10-min exposure was 25 vol % (Clark and Tinston, 1982). Signs of exposure were tremors and muscular twitching. The EC 50 for cardiac sensitization of dogs to injection of epinephrine was 7.7 vol % for 5 min. In another experiment with dogs, exposure to 13.5 vol % for 30 sec sensitized the myocardium to injections of epinephrine but exposure to 2.5 vol %, 6 hr/day for 5 days resulted in no cardiac sensitization (Azar, 1971). Left ventricular systolic, diastolic, and mean pressures; the maximal rate or rise of left ventricular pressure; and the mean pulmonary arterial flow all decreased 4–8% in dogs exposed to 10 vol % but not in dogs exposed to 5 vol % (Simaan and Aviado, 1975).

When animals were exposed to 20 vol % for 7–8 hr/day for 12 weeks, no dogs or monkeys died and mortality in guinea pigs was not statistically greater than that in controls. During the first weeks dogs displayed generalized tremor a few minutes after initiation of exposure and later ataxia, lacrimation, and salivation. Monkeys showed only fine tremors. Guinea pigs showed slight irritation, which became less prominent as exposure continued. No cumulative or permanent deleterious effects were noted (Sayers et al., 1930).

Carcinogenicity was not observed in rats given 15–150 mg/kg dichlorodifluoromethane daily by intubation for 2 years (Sherman, 1974). No indications of embryotoxic, fetotoxic, or teratogenic changes were found in rats exposed to 20 vol % of a mixture of 90% dichlorodifluoromethane and 10% chlorodifluoromethane on days 4–16 of gestation (Paulet et al., 1974). Rabbits were unaffected by the same exposure on days 5–20 of gestation.

14.2.1.3 Toxicity to Humans

Experimental Exposure   Studies on human volunteers showed that exposure to 10,000 ppm dichlorodifluoromethane for 2.5 hr caused a 7% reduction in standardized psychomotor scores. Seventeen repetitive exposures to 1000 ppm, 8 hr/day, 5 days/week caused no untoward subjective or physiological responses (Azar et al., 1972). At 1000 ppm exposure, dichlorodifluoromethane in venous blood was 1.2 μg/ml, much less than the 22.8 μ/ml required to sensitize the heart of dogs (Azar et al., 1973).

Exposure of 10 healthy male subjects to aerosols containing dichlorodifluoromethane for 15–60 sec caused a decrease in the maximum expiratory flow volume within a few minutes of exposure with a second delayed decrease occurring in 13–30 min after exposure. In one subject, exposure to a 10:90 mixture of chlorodifluoromethane and dichlorodifluoromethane induced tachycardia and negative T waves (Valic et al., 1977). The concentration of these exposures was undesignated, but the study indicates that short exposure to high concentrations of propellants in aerosols can produce surprisingly persistent physiological effects on the heart and respiratory system. The half-life of dichlorodifluoromethane has been reported to be 9.36 min (Adir et al., 1975).

Accidental and Intentional Poisonings   Sudden deaths have resulted from high-level exposure to aerosols. These deaths appear to be associated with cardiac fibrillation. A 13-year-old boy died 1.5 hr after sniffing a cooking spray. Analysis of tissues revealed the following concentrations of dichlorodifluoromethane: blood, 1.2 μg/gm; brain, 3.5 μg/gm; heart, 180 μg/gm; kidney, 5.4 μg/gm; liver, 23 μg/gm; lung, 94 μg/gm; muscle, 0.5 μg/gm; omental fat, 13 μg/gm (Standefer, 1975). Notable is the high concentration found in the heart.

Three instances of death consistent with severe cardiac arrhythmias have been reported following heavy exposure to pesticide aerosols containing dichlorodifluoromethane (Hayes, 1976). A 29-year-old male was found dead at 5:30 a.m. after he had applied an aerosol in the trailer where he and another man lived. His companion was unaffected. A 36-year-old truck driver discharged part of an aerosol bomb inside the camper where he lived. After poor sleep, he awoke shortly before 5:00 a.m. gasping. He collapsed while being rushed to the hospital and was pronounced dead at 5:45 a.m. In the third episode, a 36-year-old telephone installer applied an insecticidal aerosol to his lawn and an insect repellent to himself and sat down to read indoors. A little later he complained of dizziness, had a seizure, and fell to the floor. He lived to reach the emergency room, where seven unsuccessful attempts were made to defibrillate his heart. In all three cases, the active ingredients of the aerosols were not capable of producing the observed effects. It does not seem likely that the threshold limit value, 1000 ppm or 4950 mg/m^3, could have been exceeded, except for a short duration.

Treatment of Poisoning   Treatment is entirely symptomatic. The electrocardiogram and vital signs should be carefully monitored and a calm, quiet environment should be provided to prevent an adrenalin surge. Dilantin may be useful in management of ventricular arrhythmias.

14.3 SOLVENTS AND PETROLEUM OILS

Petroleum is a mixture of gaseous, liquid, and solid hydrocarbons. Petroleums from different sources differ in physical properties and in the relative abundance of the four main groups of constituents: saturated straight and branched chains, saturated rings, unsaturated chains, and unsaturated rings. Individual compounds may represent only one kind of constituent or more than one in any combination. Native petroleums range in density from 0.65 to 1.06, and they range from amber fluids to black tars. Preparations made from different petroleums are not identical, even when they bear the same names. Thus, kerosenes vary greatly in the proportion of unsaturated compounds they contain.

A great variety of products are obtained from petroleum, first by fractional distillation and then, when necessary, by cracking, polymerization, alkylation, and other chemical procedures. Some of the more important products are shown in Table 14.1. Of course, innumerable secondary petroleum products, including the chlorinated hydrocarbon solvents, are synthesized using primary petroleum products as important precursors.

Table 14.1
Some Important Products of Petroleum

Products	Carbon atoms	Boiling range (°C)	Melting point (°C)
Gases	1–4		
Naphtha, gasoline, petroleum ether, benzene	5–10	70–150	
Kerosene	10–16	150–300	
Gas oil, distillate, fuel oil		250–350	
Lubricating oil	14–18		
Petrolatum	17–21		35
Paraffin	21–27		40–60
Asphalt, tar, pitch, coke		remaining residues	

Properties of petroleum products include density; melting range; boiling range; volatility; viscosity; flash point; surface tension; capacity for sulfonation, iodination, and oxidation; and sulfur content. Some of these properties are related, but not in a way that permits exact prediction of one property from another. In general, density, melting range, boiling range, viscosity, and volatility reflect molecular size. However, for oils of the same viscosity, density increases from paraffinic to naphthenic to aromatic. The boiling range offers a measure of homogeneity. Thus a kerosene with a narrow boiling range is more homogeneous than one with a wide boiling range.

Several measures (sulfonation, iodine value, aniline point) reflect the proportion of unsaturated compounds in an oil. Sulfonation, which corresponds to refinery operations, is expressed as the percentage of oil that does not react with sulfuric acid under standard conditions. It is the term most used to express degree of saturation, and the sulfonation value is an important indicator of the safety of the product for both plants and animals. The higher the sulfonation value, the safer the product. Dormant spray oils commonly have sulfonation tests of 70 to 85%, while those for summer foliage oils are from 90 to 98%. Irritation of the pulmonary epithelium of mammals by kerosene is proportional to the concentration of unsaturated compounds present. On the average, kerosenes intended for fuel are more likely to be irritating than those refined for spray oils.

Kerosene and other solvents for insecticides are not without some insecticidal action of their own and, when used as solvents for other insecticides, are not "inert ingredients," although they are often so labeled. The same or similar materials may be used alone as mosquito larvicides or for the control of insect eggs, scale insects, and mites, especially on fruit trees. Spray oils applied to plants vary greatly in boiling point and related properties, but all must have relatively high sulfonation values. The lighter oils occasionally are applied directly as a fine mist, but usually spray oils are applied as dilute emulsions.

Because kerosene was recommended for use against scale

insects on orange trees as early as 1865, one might suppose that the action of oil insecticides would be understood completely by now. This is not true. Experimental evidence has shown that petroleum oils can penetrate throughout the tracheal system of a scale insect, but they frequently are expelled almost as fast, apparently by efforts of the insect. Furthermore, suffocation of an insect is an extremely slow process when the organism is immersed in a nontoxic liquid or in nitrogen. That suffocation contributes to the death of exposed insects, mites, and their eggs has not been excluded, but it is evident that petroleum oils exert a toxic action. Insects can be killed by fumes of low-boiling fractions. Some kinds of insects are more effectively controlled by oils of high aromatic content, and others are more easily killed by those of low aromatic content. Finally, some are more susceptible to the liquid phase and thus to higher-boiling fractions (Shepard, 1951).

For mammals, all solvents are narcotics; some are more effective than others, and some have additional toxic actions. Any solvent can produce narcosis in workers if sufficiently misused. Compounds with low vapor pressures may reach an adequate concentration if presented in the form of an aerosol.

14.3.1 KEROSENE

14.3.1.1 Identity, Properties, and Uses

Chemical Name and Structure Kerosene is a mixture of petroleum aromatic and aliphatic hydrocarbons, chiefly of the methane series, having from 10 to 16 carbon atoms per molecule.

Synonyms Kerosene is the common name. "Coal oil" is used occasionally, as is "Deobase," a deodorized product prepared from kerosene. The CAS registry number is 800-820-6.

Physical and Chemical Properties Kerosene is a pale yellow or clear oily, low-viscosity liquid usually with a characteristic odor. Highly refined kerosene may be almost odorless. Being of variable composition, it has a broad boiling range, 175–325°C; the flash range is 65 to 85°C. Kerosene is miscible with nonpolar organic solvents and virtually insoluble in water.

History, Formulations, and Uses Kerosene is commonly used as a solvent for insecticidal formulations, both solutions and emulsions. Kerosene *per se* has been known to have insecticidal activity for a long time, having been used to control scale as early as 1865. It is still used as an ovicide and to control scale and mites on fruit trees. Occasionally, it has been used as a herbicide. Kerosene is a commonly used fuel for heating.

14.3.1.2 Toxicity to Laboratory Animals

Although the single oral dose lethality, if not aspirated into the lungs as well, is low, ingestion of kerosene with concurrent or subsequent aspiration is quite hazardous. For example, single oral dose LD 50 values without aspiration have been reported as 30 ml/kg for rats (Ashkenazi and Berman, 1961) and 28 and 20 ml/kg for rabbits and guinea pigs, respectively (Deichmann *et al.*, 1944). Gerarde (1959) estimated the LD 50 for intratracheally administered kerosene as 0.2 ml/kg and severe pneumonitis has been reported when 0.25 ml/kg was administered via this route (Lesser *et al.*, 1943; Richardson and Pratt-Thomas, 1951). Aspiration of kerosene has been estimated to be 18–140 times more lethal than ingestion in the absence of aspiration.

Kerosene is absorbed from the gastrointestinal tract. Even though aspiration was impossible, concentrations of aromatics and aliphatics as high as 144 and 917 ppm were found in blood and tissues (Gerarde, 1959; Ashkenazi and Berman, 1961). The lungs of rats dosed at 18 ml/kg via gavage showed moderate changes at sacrifice; marked pathology was observed in the lungs of rats given 30–40 ml/kg, as well as liver and kidney damage. Large doses of kerosene also cause depression leading to coma and death.

To assess whether systemically absorbed kerosene may cause significant untoward pulmonary effects, dogs with gastrotromies and esophageal transections with proximal fistulas were given 20 ml/kg kerosene via the gastronomy tube (Dice *et al.*, 1982). No radiological or histological evidence of pulmonary changes was found. As well as indicating that aspiration, not systemic absorption, constitutes the predominant hazard, this result suggests that while kerosene is absorbed from the gastrointestinal tract it appears to be readily detoxified.

Aspiration of increasing amounts of kerosene leads to progressively severe hemorrhagic pneumonitis, with the hilar and dependent portions of the lung being affected most (Gerarde, 1959). Experiments using baboons indicated that secondary bacterial infection following kerosene-induced pneumonitis is not a factor in the pathological response and probably rarely occurs (Wolfsdorf, 1976).

Inhalation of atmospheres containing kerosene is not normally hazardous because of its low vapor pressure. At room temperature, the saturated vapor concentration is about 100 mg/m^3. No adverse effects were seen in rats exposed to a saturated atmosphere for 8 hr (Carpenter *et al.*, 1976). Nonetheless, erosions of the tracheal epithelium, inflammatory infiltration, infiltration of eosinophils, and thickening of interalveolar septa were observed in guinea pigs exposed to an undefined amount of kerosene (Sanabria *et al.*, 1984). In another study, the ciliary membrane of the trachea was swollen and disrupted with deep infiltration of eosinophils into the epithelium and lamina propria in guinea pigs exposed to aerosols 15 min daily for 21 days (Noa and Sanabria, 1984). Tracheal concentrations of acetylcholinesterase decreased by 55% in guinea pigs exposed to a kerosene aerosol of 20.4 mg/liter for 20 min (Casac'o *et al.*, 1985). Finally, 4 of 10 male rats, 1 of 10 female rats, 1 of 10 male mice, and 0 of 10 female mice were killed by exposure to a kerosene aerosol of 5.3 mg/liter for 4 hr; no animals were killed by exposure to 3.4 mg/liter (Dow Chemical Company, 1983).

Dermal absorption of kerosene is negligible, but excessive

skin contact can produce scaling, cracking, and blistering. Eye contact is innocuous.

14.3.1.3 Toxicity to Humans

Accidental and Intentional Poisoning The use of kerosene sprays in closed or poorly ventilated spaces may lead to fullness of the head, headache, blurred vision, dizziness, unsteady gait, and nausea. More massive exposure may cause collapse, nervous twitching, and coma, apparently before the victim is aware of overexposure and seeks fresh air. Thus, systematically, kerosene acts as a narcotic, producing depression that may or may not be preceded by an excitement phase.

Actually, most poisoning by kerosene has occurred in infants who ingested it alone or as a solvent for something else. What is thought to be the first case involved the death of a 15-month-old boy who died 4 hr after drinking "coal-oil" (Hamilton, 1897). At one time, kerosene was a major cause of poisoning among children in the United States (Bologna and Woody, 1948; Bain, 1954; Soule and Foley, 1957) and in some other countries (Phelan, 1963). A population study conducted in England reported that 13% of the childhood poisoning cases (2098) between 1977 and 1981 were caused by ingestion of petroleum distillates, indicating that continued concern is justified (Pearn *et al.*, 1984).

Ingestion frequently results in immediate gagging, coughing, and frequently vomiting and thus often leads to aspiration of the oil. The initial symptoms may be followed by deep drowsiness. In the more serious cases, bronchopneumonia, often with fever, may develop promptly. Chest signs are often few or absent, even when X ray of the chest reveals extensive bronchopneumonia, although rhonchi have been reported by Majeed *et al.* (1981) to be detectable in 75% of children with pulmonary involvement caused by kerosene poisoning. Liver and kidney damage may be manifested by hepatomegaly and by albumin, cells, and casts in the urine (Nunn and Martin, 1934; Lesser *et al.,*1943; Reed *et al.*, 1950; Foley *et al.*, 1954; Press *et al.*, 1962; Isbister, 1963; Baldachin and Melmed, 1964; Cachia and Fenech, 1964).

Depression *per se* is apparently never fatal, although it may be alarming in kerosene poisoning (Bologna and Woody, 1948). Coma and other major central nervous system effects are frequently present in cases that result from fumes and are serious enough to come to medical attention. However, such serious effects are reported in only 6% or less of cases involving ingestion (McNally, 1956; Verhulst and Page, 1961; Cachia and Fenech, 1964). In one series of 204 cases, 4% of the children were semiconscious, but none had convulsions, 40% were lethargic, and 28% had gastrointestinal symptoms; however, all had respiratory symptoms, and 3% died (McNally, 1956). Ingestion of kerosene has been known to produce rapid death by gross aspiration and occlusion of the respiratory system. Even when death does not occur promptly, there is abundant evidence that the pneumonia commonly seen in children who swallow kerosene usually results from aspiration. The

aspiration usually occurs at the moment of ingestion or as the result of vomiting within the first hour (Bologna and Woody, 1948).

Use Experience Where not misused, kerosene is quite safe. However, like many other oils, kerosene is a local irritant and may cause a maculopapular eruption of the exposed skin. The irritation tends to increase and later decrease with repeated exposure over a long period.

Atypical Cases of Various Origins A case of fatal hypoplastic anemia was attributed to years of occupational exposure to kerosene used as a degreasing agent for machine parts (Johnson, 1955), Three nonfatal cases of bone marrow depression were attributed to use of kerosene as a therapeutic agent, either rubbed on the skin or ingested with sugar (Hiebel *et al.*, 1963), and one fatal case was attributed to external, therapeutic use (Cavanagh and Wilner, 1939).

Dosage Response Although kerosene is a common cause of poisoning, especially in children, the amount taken is seldom known. Survival has been reported following the ingestion of 1 liter (Sollmann, 1948), but death has followed the ingestion of doses as small as 30 ml, especially after kerosene was aspirated (Bologna and Woody, 1948). The lowest air concentration capable of producing acute symptoms by inhalation is not known.

Laboratory Findings Leukocytosis and albuminuria or casts (generally in severe cases only) may be present. It may be possible to recognize kerosene in stomach contents by its characteristic odor. This odor will be negligible or absent in poisoning by deodorized kerosene. X-ray and liver and kidney function tests should be used to follow the progress of visceral damage.

Pathology Bronchopneumonia, visceral congestion, acute pulmonary edema, and hemorrhage characterize the direct irritant effect of aspirated kerosene. Evidence of inflammation of the upper gastrointestinal tract may be seen in those who die early. There is frequently some enlargement of the liver.

Differential Diagnosis The case history will usually establish the diagnosis. The characteristic odor may or may not be present. When there is doubt, poisoning by alcohol and other solvents and by a wide range of narcotic agents may be considered, as may diabetic coma.

Treatment of Poisoning The injury caused by inhalation of kerosene fumes seldom requires any treatment except prompt removal from exposure. Experimentally, disodium cromoglycate has been reported to inhibit bronchoconstriction induced in rabbits by inhalation of atmospheres containing kerosene (Casac'o *et al.*, 1983).

If kerosene containing no insecticide has been ingested, gastric lavage may be done mainly as a precaution against regurgitation and aspiration from the gastrointestinal tract. In two related series of cases, complications were more common in patients who received routine gastric lavage than in those who received no lavage (Cachia and Fenech, 1964). Another more carefully designed study showed that gastric lavage was not harmful to patients but there was no conclusive evidence that it was beneficial (Press *et al.*, 1962). This is encouraging in connection with cases in which the ingested kerosene was the solvent for an insecticide that should be removed rapidly and thoroughly. If attempted, the gastric lavage should be done very early before narcosis sets in and every other possible precaution, including use of an intratracheal tube with inflated balloon, should be taken so that the lavage itself does not lead to aspiration of the kerosene (Reed *et al.*, 1950). Emetics are contraindicated (Foley *et al.*, 1954). Oil laxatives should be avoided (Gerarde, 1959), especially if the kerosene was the vehicle for an insecticide. A saline laxative may be helpful. Sedatives and stimulants may be used symptomatically in moderation. Antibiotic therapy does not benefit kerosene pneumonia as such, but it may be of some benefit in preventing bacterial invasion. Oxygen should be used promptly if the patient shows any respiratory difficulty or the slightest cyanosis. Cortisone and related drugs have been used for treating chemical pneumonitis caused by kerosene and other oils, but the value of this treatment remains to be determined. There seems to be no doubt that the inflammatory reaction is suppressed and symptoms are relieved, but there is some indication that this merely postpones the removal of oil from the lung and healing of the injury (Verhulst and Page, 1961). Thus, the value of adrenocortical steroids for the treatment of kerosene pneumonitis can be decided only after further carefully controlled study. Liver damage may be minimized by the use of a diet low in fat and adequate in carbohydrate. The usefulness of lipotropic drugs has not been investigated in this connection. Kidney involvement is rarely sufficient to merit special treatment, but for those rare cases where the kidneys are seriously involved, the treatment should be the same as for toxic nephritis of other etiology.

Kerosene dermatitis requires no special treatment and will regress spontaneously if exposure is discontinued. Cleanliness will help to prevent its occurrence.

14.3.2 TETRALIN

14.3.2.1 Identity, Properties, and Uses

Chemical Name   1,2,3,4-Tetrahydronaphthalene.

Structure   See Fig. 14.1.

Synonyms   The trade name Tetralin® often is used as a common name. Another trade name for the compound is Tetracap®. The CAS registry number is 91-60-1.

Physical and Chemical Properties   Tetralin has the empirical formula $C_{10}H_{12}$ and a molecular weight of 132.21. It is

Figure 14.1   *o-*, *m-*, and *p*-Xylene, tetralin, β-tetralol, and isophorone.

a colorless liquid with an odor resembling that of a mixture of benzene and methanol. At 20°C it has a density of 0.9702. It has a melting point of −35.79°C, a boiling point of 207.57°C, and a flash point of 77.22°C. Tetralin is insoluble in water but soluble in ethanol, butanol, acetone, benzene, ether, chloroform, petroleum ether, and Decalin. The addition of an antioxidant, such as hydroquinone, to the liquid will prevent the possibility of explosion when the compound is in prolonged, direct contact with air.

Use   Tetralin is used as an insecticidal solvent, as a solvent for naphthalene and various other industrial substances, and as a substitute for turpentine in some household products.

14.3.2.2 Toxicity to Laboratory Animals

Basic Findings   The oral LD 50 of tetralin in rats is 2860 mg/kg and the dermal LD 50 in rabbits is 17,300 mg/kg. Inhalation of saturated vapor for 8 hr is fatal to rats (Smyth *et al.*, 1951).

Aspiration of tetralin causes pulmonary edema and hemorrhage at the point of contact (Gerarde, 1960).

Repeated oral doses of tetralin produce intense diarrhea, and application to the skin produces dermatitis, indicating the irritant properties of the compound (Cardani, 1942). Regardless of route, sufficient exposure produces loss of weight and tremor, and there may be other neurological effects (Cardani, 1942; Badinand *et al.*, 1947). The most disturbing feature of animal experiments is the report of cataract following respiratory exposure or oral intubation (Badinand *et al.*, 1947; Basile, 1939). However, Fitzhugh and Buschke (1949) were unable to produce cataracts in rats fed tetralin at a dietary level of 20,000 ppm for 2 months; α-tetralol was also ineffective, but β-tetralol (see Fig. 14.1) was a powerful cataractogen. Because α-tetralol and β-tetralol have been shown to be metabolites of tetralin, it may be that reported differences in the susceptibility of different species to the cataractogenic effects of tetralin depend on differences in their metabolism of the compound. Naphthalene is well recognized as a cataractogenic compound (Gehring, 1971).

Absorption, Distribution, Metabolism, and Excretion
Williams (1959) reviewed early evidence that the reduced ring of tetralin is more readily metabolized than the aromatic ring. More recent studies have confirmed that oxidation is preferentially on the alicyclic ring. In rabbits, the main urinary metabolite was the glucuronide of α-tetralol (52.4%). Other conjugated metabolites were β-tetralol (25.3%), 4-hydroxy-α-tetralone (6.1%), and cis-tetralin-1,2-diol (0.4%) (Elliott and Hanam, 1968). Using rat liver homogenates, it was shown that conversion of tetralin to tetralol requires NADPH and that tetralin hydroperoxide is a probable intermediate (Chen and Lin, 1968). Further study confirmed this possibility and indicated that tetralin hydroxylation proceeds via a radical mechanism similar to that of lipid peroxidation (Lin and Chen, 1969).

When radioactive tetralin was fed to rabbits, 87–90% of the activity was excreted in the urine in 2 days and 0.5–3.7% on the third day. The feces contained only 0.6–1.8%. No radioactivity was found in the breath, and negligible amounts were retained in the tissues. About 90–99% of the dose was accounted for (Elliott and Hanam, 1968).

14.3.2.3 Toxicity to Humans

Accidental and Intentional Poisoning A 26-year-old woman intentionally ingested about 250 ml of Cuprex, which contained 31.5% tetralin, 0.03% copper oleate, 52.7% paraffin oil, and 15.7% acetone. The preparation is recommended for external application to combat human lice. During the 36 hr prior to admission, she vomited several times, had one episode of melena, and noticed that her urine was green in color. She also developed abdominal and bilateral costovertebral pain. On admission, the patient had protein and casts in her urine and numerous physical and laboratory findings indicating mild liver damage. At the time of discharge on hospital day 14, all laboratory tests were normal. Examination of 1900 ml of green-gray urine collected during the first 24 hr in hospital revealed glucuronides of 1,2,3,4-tetrahydro-1-naphthol and of 1,2,3,4-tetrahydro-2-naphthol plus the former and the parent compound in unconjugated form. One other metabolite was similar to the 1-naphthol by mass spectometry but was not identified. Many unidentified chromatographic peaks may have represented additional metabolites (Drayer and Reidenberg, 1973).

Use Experience Experience in the use of tetralin as an industrial solvent has been described in detail by Browning (1965). Briefly, dermal exposure to tetralin has caused eczematous dermatitis, but only rarely, and exposure to tetralin fumes in poorly ventilated places has produced narcotic effects including marked restlessness, eye irritation, headache, malaise, asthenia, nausea, and vomiting.

Laboratory Findings Although it was noticed at least as early as 1919 that persons heavily exposed to tetralin produce green urine, the chemical nature of the color apparently remains unknown. At least in some animal experiments the urine was not green but greenish brown. Thus the colors produced by humans and animals may be different.

Treatment of Poisoning Treatment is symptomatic.

14.3.3 XYLENE

14.3.3.1 Identity, Properties, and Uses

Chemical Name Dimethylbenzene. The commercial product is a mixture of three isomers: ortho (o)-, meta (m)-, and para (p)-xylene. m-Xylene predominates.

Structure See Fig. 14.1.

Synonyms Xylene is the common name of the compound and of the commercial mixture. Other names include dimethylbenzene, xylol, and aromatic oil. The CAS registry number for the mixture is 1330-20-7; for the o, m, and p isomers the numbers are 95-47-6, 108-38-3, and 106-42-3, respectively.

Physical and Chemical Properties Xylene has the empirical formula C_8H_{10} and a molecular weight of 106.16. It is a colorless, low-viscosity, flammable liquid with a density of 0.86–0.88, depending on the isomeric mixture. Xylene has a characteristic odor detectable at a concentration of about 1 ppm (Carpenter et al., 1975). Also dependent on the isomeric mixture, the boiling point ranges from 138 to 144°C and flash points range from 28 to 46°C. Vapor pressures for o-, m-, and p-xylene are 10 mm Hg at 32.1°C, 28.3°C and 27.3°C, respectively. Xylene is practically insoluble in water but miscible with many organic solvents such as alcohol and ether.

History, Formulations, and Uses Xylene was first isolated from crude wood distillate in 1850 and first obtained from coal tar in 1870. A typical commercial coal-derived xylene consists of 10–15% o-, 45–70% m-, and 20–26% p-xylene and 6–10% ethylbenzene. Xylene is used as a solvent for pesticide formulations, as a raw material for the production of industrial chemicals, and as a cleaning and sterilizing agent.

14.3.3.2 Toxicity to Laboratory Animals

Basic Findings The acute toxicity of xylene is low. The oral LD 50 for rats has been reported to be 4.3 g/kg and 10 ml/kg (Wolf et al., 1956; Hine and Zuiderma, 1950). Mice are more sensitive to xylene; the oral LD 50 was determined to be 1590 mg/kg (Schumacher and Grandjean, 1960). Lethal vapor concentrations for mice have been reported to be 6900 ppm for o-xylene, 11,500 ppm for m-xylene and 3450–8050 ppm for p-xylene (Cameron et al., 1938). Narcotic effects were observed in mice at vapor concentrations 3450–4600, 2300–3450, and 2,300 ppm of o-, m-, and p-xylene, respectively. The LT 50 was 92 min for rats that inhaled mixed xylenes at a concentration of 46,000 mg/m³ (10,580 ppm), which is near saturation at room temperature (Wolf *et al.*, 1956). For a 4-hr exposure the LC 50 was 29,000 mg/m^3 (6670 ppm) in rats (Carpenter *et al.*, 1975). High respiratory doses cause narcosis in rats; in cats anesthesia is preceded by salivation, ataxia, and tonic and clonic spasms suggesting an effect on the central nervous system.

Topical application of xylene causes erythema, edema, and exfoliation of large patches of rabbit skin. It causes slight conjunctival irritation and very slight, transient injury of the cornea of rabbits subsequent to installation into the eye (Wolf *et al.*, 1956).

Carpenter *et al.* (1975) observed no untoward effects in dogs or rats exposed to atmospheres containing 3500 mg/m^3 (810 ppm) of mixed xylenes for 6 hr/day, 5 days/week for 13 weeks. It is generally agreed that xylene is much safer than benzene with respect to causation of untoward hematopoietic effects.

In the National Toxicology Program bioassay, mixed xylenes (60% *m*-, 14% *p*-, and 9% *o*-xylene and 17% ethylbenzene) in corn oil were administered by gavage to mice and rats 5 days/week for 103 weeks. Mice received daily doses of 500 or 1000 mg/kg; rats received 250 or 500 mg/kg. No gross or histopathological lesions were related to these treatments; tumor incidence was similar for treated and control groups of either species [National Toxicology Program (NTP), 1986b]. There was no evidence for carcinogenicity. When tested for mutagenicity, *o*-, *m*-, and *p*-xylene were negative by assay in the Ames system using *Salmonella typhimurium* strains TA1535, TA1537, TA1538, TA98, and TA100 with or without metabolic activation by S9 fraction derived from livers of rats either untreated or induced with Aroclor 1254 (Bos *et al.*, 1981). Xylene did not change the number of sister chromatid exchanges or the number of chromosomal aberrations in human lymphocytes *in vitro* (Gerner-Smidt and Friedrich, 1978).

Teratogenicity has been evaluated for a xylene mixture (9.1% *o*, 60.2% *m*, 13.6% *p*, and 17.0% ethylbenzene) in pregnant albino CD-1 mice given the mixture at dosages of 2.4, 3.0, and 3.6 ml/kg/day by gavage on days 6–15 of gestation (Marks *et al.*, 1982). At these near-lethal doses, xylene produced a significant increase in malformations, with cleft palate being the major malformation observed. Exposure of CFY rats to 1000 mg/m^3 (230 ppm) xylene for 24 hr/day from day 9 to 14 of gestation was not teratogenic, although there was an increase in skeletal anomalies consisting of extra ribs and fused sternebrae (Hudak and Ungvary, 1978).

Absorption, Distribution, Metabolism, and Excretion   Following exposure of rabbits to an atmosphere of about 3000 mg/m^3 (690 ppm) for 3 hr/day, 6 days/week for 130 days, xylene was found at slightly higher average concentration in the adrenal (148 ppm), bone marrow (130 ppm), spleen (115 ppm), and brain (100 ppm) than in blood (91 ppm) or in other organs (Fabre *et al.*, 1960a). In rats, guinea pigs, and rabbits, all three isomers are oxidized on the methyl group to form the corresponding toluic acid or on the ring to form phenols (Fabre *et al.*, 1960b). There was no evidence that both methyl groups were oxidized; unconjugated 3,5-dimethylphenol and its glucuronide were isolated from urine. In rats exposed to atmospheres of *m*-xylene and ethylbenzene, methylhippuric acid, dimethylphenol, and methylbenzene alcohol were identified in urine as metabolites of *m*-xylene (Elovaara *et al.*, 1984).

Biochemical Effects   Xylene at an intraperitoneal dosage of 1000 mg/kg produced in guinea pigs an increase in serum ornithine carbamoyltransferase and a moderate accumulation of lipid in the liver but no necrosis (DiVincenzo and Krasavage, 1974).

In rats exposed to 1000, 1500, and 2000 ppm *p*-xylene for 4 hr, dosage-dependent increases were measured in serum concentrations of glutamic-pyruvic transaminase (GPT), glutamic-oxaloacetic transaminase (GOT), glucose-6-phosphate dehydrogenase (G-6-PDH), isocitrate dehydrogenase (ICD), lactate dehydrogenase (LDH), glutathione reductase, and 5'-nucleotidase (Patel *et al.*, 1979). GPT and GOT were elevated by even the lowest exposure. Surprisingly, serum cholinesterase was increased by all exposure concentrations at the termination of the exposure, although there was no increase after 24 hr.

Rats exposed 6 hr/day for 3 days to 2000 ppm of a xylene mixture of the *o, m,* and *p* isomers showed an increase in hepatic cytochrome P-450 and NADPH-cytochrome *c* reductase (Toftgard and Nilsen, 1982). The *p* isomer was less potent in inducing this effect that the other isomers or the mixture. Microsomes from lung and kidney also showed increases in cytochrome P-450 for the xylene mixture and isomers except the *p* isomer failed to induce cytochrome P-450 in microsomes from kidney.

14.3.3.3 Toxicity to Humans

Experimental Exposure   Astrand *et al.* (1978) assessed the uptake of a mixture of xylenes and ethylbenzene during rest and exercise by 12 subjects exposed to either 435 mg/m^3 (100 ppm) or 870 mg/m^3 (200 ppm). About 60% of the xylene supplied to the lungs was taken up; the ratio of the concentration in arterial blood in milligrams per kilogram to that in aleveolar air in milligrams per liter was 30 : 40. Only about 4–5% of that taken up was expired. In another study, sedentary volunteers were exposed to an atmosphere containing about 100 ppm *m*-xylene for 6 hr/day over 5 successive days (Riihimaki *et al.*, 1979). About 60% of the xylene supplied to the lungs was taken up and nearly quantitatively excreted in the urine as methylhippuric acid. Four percent was expired as unchanged xylene, and a small amount (1–2%) was excreted in the urine as 2,4-dimethylphenol. In the body, most of the xylene was found in the extracellular compartment bound to serum protein. Subsequent to exposure, the elimination of xylene was biphasic with elimination half-times of 1 and 20 hr. Presumably, the slow elimination phase occurred from tissues with high xylene solubility or poor perfusion, such as adipose tissue.

Gamberale *et al.* (1978) assessed central nervous system function in healthy subjects exposed to atmospheres containing 435 or 1300 mg/m^3 (100 or 300 ppm) xylene mixture (*p*-

xylene 12.8%, *o*-xylene 12.1%, *m*-xylene 54.4%, and ethylbenzene 20.7%) for 70 min. In 15 sedentary subjects no change in performance was revealed in tests of numerical ability, reaction time, memory, or critical flicker fusion. Eight subjects whose uptake of xylene was increased by physical work and exposure to the higher concentration experienced a performance decrement. These subjects took up approximately 1200 mg xylene versus 540 mg taken up by the sedentary subjects.

All of the six volunteers were able to detect the odor of mixed xylenes at a concentration of 60 mg/m³; four could detect 6 mg/m³, but none could detect 0.6 mg/m³. The odor threshold was calculated as 4.5 mg/m³ or about 1 ppm for a 10-sec exposure. In a 15-min exposure period, the only common sign of discomfort at 2000 mg/m³ (460 ppm) was eye irritation in four of six subjects. Some transitory olfactory fatigue occurred, with recovery in 10 min (Carpenter *et al.*, 1975).

Impaired body balance and increased reaction times were reported in subjects exposed to 100–400 ppm *m*-xylene; however, with repetitive exposures these decrements disappear within a few day (Riihimaki and Savolainen, 1980). Exposure to 200 ppm *m*-xylene tended to improve psychophysiological performance in another study (Savolainen *et al.*, 1982). Finally, 16 men exposed to 70 ppm for 4 hr experienced no change in nervous system function (Olson *et al.*, 1985).

Use Experience   Serum concentrations of liver enzymes were determined for Swedish paint industry workers exposed to a mixture of organic solvents including xylene (Lundberg and Hakansson, 1985). Mean xylene exposure for 44 individuals was 82 mg/m³ (19 ppm) with a range of 1 to 6070 mg/m³; five workers were exposed to a mean concentration of 865 mg/m³ (199 ppm). Serum alanine aminotransferase, aspartate aminotransferase, ornithine carbamoyltransferase, and γ-glutamyltransferase activities were not elevated by these exposures.

The experimental assessments attest to the relatively low toxicity of xylene in humans as well as the adequacy of the threshold limit value (TLV) of 100 ppm recommended by the ACGIH. The extreme irritation produced by contact of xylene with mucous membranes and skin provides motivation to avoid excessive exposure. Occupational experience reveals complaints of dermatitis, eczema, and irritation of the eyes and respiratory tract but rarely serious illness (Browning, 1965). It is likely that untoward effects on the hematopoietic system reported in the past as being caused by xylene resulted from benzene contamination of commercial xylene.

Treatment of Poisoning   Treatment is symptomatic.

14.4 FUMIGANTS

We continue the common practice of grouping together as fumigants and nematocides several groups of compounds that have little in common except relatively high vapor pressures

and useful toxicity to one or more pests. Some of the compounds are gases at room temperature. Although others are liquids or solids, their activity against pests depends on their vapors. The toxicity of many of the compounds follows Ferguson's principle, being lethal at thermodynamic activities between 0.1 and 1.0. In contrast to these physically active compounds, some fumigants are simply volatile chemical poisons active at thermodynamic levels far below 0.1.

14.5 CYANIDES, NITRILES, AND THIOCYANATES

In 1815 Gay-Lussac recognized that prussic acid contained what he called a compound radical. In naming this radical, he accepted the view of his colleagues that the term should be derived from the Greek word for dark blue, referring in this instance to the intense dark blue color of Prussian blue (ferric ferrocyanide). Although *cyanosis* is derived from the same Greek word, it must be noted that cyanide ordinarily does not produce cyanosis but leaves the venous blood fully oxygenated and the patient pinker than normal.

The toxicity of hydrogen cyanide and of other compounds such as cyanogen and simple salts of cyanide, which in contact with water rapidly yield the cyanide ion, depends on that ion. The toxicity of halogenated cyanogens, some organic nitriles, and organic thiocyanates also depends on the cyanide ion. The toxicity of these hydrogen cyanide precursors in mice corresponds quite well with the concentrations of cyanide which they produce in the brains of these animals (Ohkawa *et al.*, 1972). However, these compounds that release cyanide relatively slowly may have a variety of toxic actions, each of which depends on the particular intact molecule. For example, almost exactly the same concentrations (300–400 mg/m³) of hydrogen cyanide and of cyanogen chloride are rapidly fatal to humans, but hydrogen cyanide may be tolerated for ½ hr at 50 mg/m³ without immediate or late effects whereas cyanogen chloride is an intolerable irritant at 50 mg/m³. Intermediate concentrations of cyanogen chloride may produce cyanide poisoning complicated by pulmonary edema.

The reactions characteristic of the intact molecules range all the way from the obvious irritancy of cyanogen chloride to effects that are either ill-defined or incompletely explained. It has been suspected that acute poisoning by acrylonitrile is not caused exclusively by cyanide (Brieger *et al.*, 1952). Therefore the question has been raised whether medical management adequate to treat cyanide poisoning will be adequate to treat poisoning for acrylonitrile. There is no doubt that standard treatment for cyanide poisoning is beneficial against acute lethal poisoning by acrylonitrile (Willhite and Smith, 1981), but that is not the whole story. The ability of acrylonitrile under certain circumstances to destroy human epidermis is most likely a local effect of the unmetabolized molecule, although evidence supporting this interpretation is still incomplete.

The various compounds that yield cyanide slowly do so at different rates and sometimes in response to different enzymes;

the situation is made more complex by the fact that they have different solubilities and are absorbed more or less readily by the skin. Microsomal mixed-function oxidases in mouse liver liberate hydrogen cyanide from several organic nitriles. Some organic thiocyanates (e.g., isobornyl thiocyanoacetate) react readily with glutathione to produce hydrogen cyanide. The reaction between glutathione and a variety of organic thiocyanates is catalyzed by glutathione *S*-transferases, of which four from mouse liver have been resolved chromatographically (Ohkawa *et al.*, 1972).

Cyanide and cyanogenic compounds that have been used as pesticides include hydrogen cyanide, various metal salts of cyanide, cyanogen chloride, some organic nitriles, and several organic thiocyanates (see Fig. 14.2). In addition, there are several organic nitriles that have no cyanide action in mammals, presumably because these animals lack enzymes to release the cyanide group fairly rapidly.

14.5.1 HYDROGEN CYANIDE AND THE CYANIDE ION

14.5.1.1 Identity, Properties, and Uses

Chemical Name Hydrocyanic acid.

Structure See Fig. 14.2.

Synonyms The aqueous solution of hydrogen cyanide is known as prussic acid. A trade name for the compound is Cylon®. The CAS registry number is 74-90-8.

Physical and Chemical Properties Hydrogen cyanide has the empirical formula CHN and a molecular weight of 27.03. It is a colorless gas or liquid with a characteristic almond-like odor. It burns with a blue flame. The density of the gas is 0.941; that of the liquid is 0.687. The compound solidifies at −13.4°C and boils at 25.6°C. It is miscible with alcohol and water and is slightly miscible with ether. It is very weakly acid, though it does not turn litmus red.

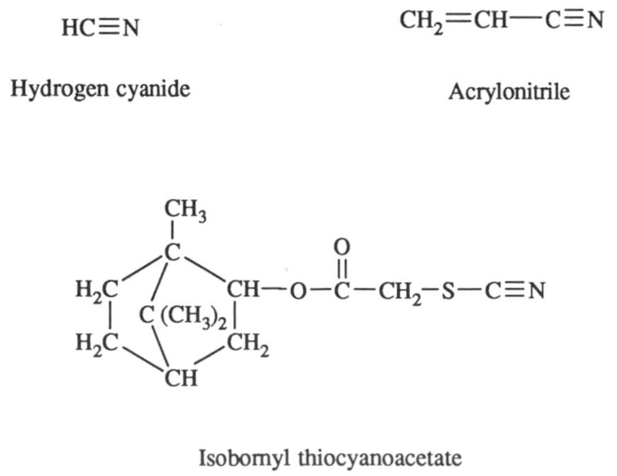

$$HC{\equiv}N \qquad\qquad CH_2{=}CH{-}C{\equiv}N$$

Hydrogen cyanide   Acrylonitrile

Isobornyl thiocyanoacetate

Figure 14.2 Examples of cyanide, nitrile, and thiocyanate fumigants.

History, Formulations, and Uses Hydrogen cyanide is an insecticidal fumigant used mainly for stored products, especially grains and flour in mills, warehouses, and ships. It also has been used extensively for combating scale insects on citrus while each tree is covered by a gas-proof tent. Hydrogen cyanide was first used as an insectical fumigant in 1886.

14.5.1.2 Toxicity to Laboratory Animals

Basic Findings In mice the LD 50 values for hydrocyanic acid administered as solutions by different routes were oral, 4.17; intraperitoneal, 2.99; intramuscular, 2.7; and intravenous, 1.1 mg/kg. The values for rabbits were intraperitoneal, 1.57; intramuscular, 1.10; and intravenous, 0.82 mg/kg (Evans, 1964).

The oral LD 50 of potassium cyanide in rats is 8.5 mg/kg (Way *et al.*, 1966) or 10 mg/kg (Hayes, 1967). The intraperitoneal LD 50 in mice is 5.99 mg/kg (Ohkawa *et al.*, 1972). When administered as potassium cyanide by stomach tube to rats, the LD 50 of the cyanide ion is about 3.4–4.0 mg/kg.

In a very unusual experiment in which the total amount of cyanide absorbed was measured chemically, it was found that the fatal, *absorbed* dosages in two dogs killed by inhalation were 1.11 and 1.55 mg/kg, and those in three dogs killed by ingestion were 1.06, 1.14, and 1.40 mg/kg (Gettler and Baine, 1938).

The cyanide ion is detoxified so effectively if intake is gradual that rats were able to consume potassium cyanide at a rate of 250 mg/kg/day without injury (see Table 2.2 in Hayes, 1975) when the compound was mixed evenly into their dry diet (Hayes, 1967). This certainly is one of the most dramatic examples of the importance of the schedule of dosage in determining toxicity.

Effects on Reproduction Congenital malformations were induced by infusion of a high dose of sodium cyanide in the golden hamster (Doherty *et al.*, 1982). Infusion of NaCN at a dose of 0.133 mmol/kg/hr during days 6–9 of gestation caused all litters to be resorbed and some maternal deaths. A slightly lower dose of 0.126–0.1295 mmol/kg/hr caused neural tube defects with varying signs of maternal toxicity. The relevance of these results in animals needs to be interpreted, considering the fact that the total dose administered constituted 30–40 times a single-dose LD 50 in hamsters. These studies also demonstrated that concurrent administration of sodium thiosulfate ameliorated the toxic as well as teratogenic effects.

Absorption, Distribution, Metabolism, and Excretion Cyanide is absorbed by all portals, including the skin. However, skin absorption is of minor importance in humans, as indicated by the effectiveness of appropriate air-purifying masks.

The cyanide ion is metabolized mainly to thiocyanate (Lang, 1894; Wood and Cooley, 1956). The cyanide ion is exhaled as hydrogen cyanide (Boxer and Rickards, 1952) and is also metabolized to a lesser degree to other compounds, including carbon dioxide and formate (Boxer and Rickards, 1952) and 2-iminothiazolidine-2-carboxylic acid (Wood and Cooley, 1956). Studies, including those with [^{35}S]cystine, showed that all the 2-iminothiazolidine-2-carboxylic acid was formed by the apparently nonenzymatic reaction of cyanide with cystine (Wood and Cooley, 1956).

All of the metabolism of cyanide represents a true detoxication. The oral and parenteral LD 50 values of the main metabolite in both rats and mice are > 480 mg/kg (Spector, 1955). From the study of Ohkawa *et al.* (1972), the intraperitoneal LD 50 values for hydrogen cyanide and sodium thiocyanate in mice were calculated as 2.5 and 535 mg/kg, respectively; the corresponding values for the CN^- and SCN^- ions were 2.4 and 383 mg/kg. Thiocyanate is cleared from the blood very efficiently. Although the amount excreted corresponded closely to the amount of potassium cyanide ingested (over a range of 3–270 ppm in drinking water), there was no increase in the concentration of thiocyanate in the plasma (Takizawa *et al.*, 1977).

Cyanide and thiocyanate are converted from one to the other, and they reach a dynamic equilibrium in surviving animals (Boxer and Rickards, 1952).

Following intraperitoneal injection of ^{14}C-labeled cyanide in mice, 72.2% of the radioactivity was excreted in the urine and feces and 25.1% was exhaled; 2.7% was retained in the body at the end of 30 days. The peak of respiratory excretion was at 6–10 minutes, and the peak urinary and fecal excretion was during 6–24 hr after dosing (Tolbert and Hughes, 1959).

Biochemical Effects   Because cyanide is a "classic" poison, its main action (inhibition of cytochrome oxidase) was discussed in Section 4.1.2.1.

It seems likely that the antidotal action of methemoglobin *in vivo* depends on the total amount of it in the body being greater than the total amount of cytochrome oxidase. Albaum *et al.* (1946) were handicapped in their *in vitro* studies by lacking a preparation of purified cytochrome oxidase. However, by using a brain homogenate containing cytochrome oxidase inhibited by cyanide, they estimated that methemoglobin added at methemoglobin/cytochrome oxidase ratios of 10:1, 20:1, and 30:1 restored the normal oxidase activity to the extent of 11, 26, and 49%, respectively.

Pathology   The pathology associated with poisoning by cyanide was reviewed by Haymaker *et al.* (1952) in connection with a report of an original study on 23 dogs, each of which received a single exposure. No significant change was found in animals that died within 3 hr. In most of those that survived longer, the gray matter suffered heavily and almost exclusively, certain structures being far more susceptible than others. In one instance the white matter was affected exclusively, there being demyelination and necrosis in all lobes; this animal, unlike any other, had had a methemoglobin level of about 70% for several hours prior to poisoning.

In rats, apparently the white matter is relatively more sus-

ceptible. In the course of recovery, remyelination occurs in the central nervous system, but it is slow and incomplete compared to that in the peripheral nerves (Hirano *et al.*, 1968).

Treatment of Poisoning in Animals   The clear benefit offered by each of the main drugs used for treating cyanide poisoning (nitrite, sodium thiosulfate, and oxygen) and the even greater benefit offered by their combined use are illustrated in Fig. 14.3. The present treatment differs from that proposed by Chen *et al.* (1934), which was based on their exemplary studies on dogs, only by some increase in dosage and the addition of oxygen. Cope (1961) was mainly responsible for introducing the use of oxygen in the treatment of cyanide poisoning. The rationale was based partly on Cope's own exploration of small doses of cyanide in volunteers as part of a pulmonary function test and partly on his own and others' studies with larger dosages in animals.

It has been reported that amyl nitrate can reverse both cardiovascular and respiratory failure in poisoned dogs sooner than can be explained by the formation of methemoglobin; the effect was attributed to inhibition of histamine-induced venous pooling (Vick *et al.*, 1973).

14.5.1.3 Toxicity to Humans

The cyanide ion has essentially the same toxicity, regardless of the route by which it is absorbed. However, accidental or intentional poisoning (excluding executions) is more likely to involve ingestion of a cyanide salt, whereas occupational poisoning is more likely to involve inhalation of hydrogen cyanide, whether it is volatilized from liquid or is generated at the site of use by the action of a mineral acid on potassium or sodium cyanate.

Accidental and Intentional Poisoning   Most nonoccupational deaths caused by cyanide are the result of suicide. However, there are examples of persons other than applicators who were poisoned because they remained in a fumigated space or were permitted to return to it before it had been ventilated adequately (Castello *et al.*, 1969). A large dosage of cyanide,

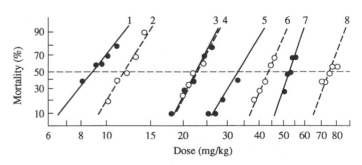

Figure 14.3   Dosage–mortality regression lines for KCN in the presence of 1, air; 2, oxygen; 3, $NaNO_2$; 4, $NaNO_2$ and oxygen; 5, $Na_2S_2O_3$; 6, $Na_2S_2O_3$ and oxygen; 7, $NaNO_2$ and $Na_2S_2O_3$; 8, $NaNO_2$, $Na_2S_2O_3$, and oxygen. Reproduced with permission from Way *et al.* (1966).

whether oral or respiratory, is followed by almost instantaneous collapse and cessation of respiration. A dosage only a little above the threshold of danger causes only headache, weakness, confusion, and sometimes nausea and vomiting. Respiration and heart rate are stimulated at first, but respiration later becomes slow and gasping. The heart may continue for some time after respiration stops. While respiration is active, the venous blood remains oxygenated and the patient's color florid; in fact this condition may persist if death is sudden. If respiration is extremely poor or if it stops some moments before the heart, the blood will become dark and the patient cyanotic.

Use Experience   Use experience when cyanide is employed by trained operators is really quite good. However, the reward of carelessness is so dramatic that cyanide has—and deserves—a bad reputation. Certainly a number of pest control applicators have been killed by it (Hayes and Vaughn, 1977). That occupational poisoning by cyanide is no more common than it is undoubtedly depends on the training of those who use it.

Atypical Cases of Various Origins   Chronic poisoning by cyanide is certainly atypical in the sense of being rare, and many industrial physicians question its existence. A staunch supporter of the existence of such a condition due to repeated exposure to cyanide, especially in plating and case-hardening, was Hamilton (1925; Hamilton and Hardy, 1974). It was pointed out that a somewhat similar clinical picture sometimes was produced when hypertension was treated with sodium or potassium thiocyanate, especially when the blood level of thiocyanate exceeded the 80 to 120 or 140 ppm required for successful therapy (Wald *et al.*, 1939; Barker *et al.*, 1941). The similarity extends even to enlargement of the thyroid, sometimes seen as a complication of thiocyanate therapy and in some persons repeatedly exposed to cyanide (Hamilton and Hardy, 1949; Hardy *et al.*, 1950).

Most aspects of chronic cyanide poisoning, except thyroid involvement, were illustrated in a case in which it was possible to reproduce the symptoms by thiocyanate. A 39-year-old man was repeatedly exposed to cyanide when he plunged very hot iron into a hardening bath. He suffered from loss of appetite, nervousness, dizziness, headache, nausea, and occasional vomiting, and he lost 6 kg in one-half year. The illness disappeared entirely when he was away from work for 2 or 3 weeks for military service or holidays, but it returned within 1 month after resumption of his old work with cyanide. During a period of recovery, the patient's symptoms were reproduced by six daily intravenous injections, each containing 1400 mg of sodium thiocyanate, which the patient was permitted to think was a treatment. The symptoms disappeared in 2–3 days after sodium chloride injections were substituted for sodium thiocyanate. Nothing happened during several initial injections of sodium chloride used as a placebo, but symptoms began after the fourth injection of thiocyanate, reached a maximum after the sixth injection, and disappeared 2–3 days after the injections were returned to sodium chloride. The patient spontaneously

reported after the sixth thiocyanate injection that the symptoms were like those he experienced while at work. The serum levels of thiocyanate increased after each injection and decreased somewhat before the next; during the most severe symptoms the levels ranged from 140 to 210 ppm (von Wuthrich, 1954).

Apparently no study has been made to learn whether persons susceptible to this kind of effect develop higher serum thiocyanate levels than other persons working in the same environment. However, blood thiocyanate levels of 150–200 ppm were considered toxic in patients treated for hypertension (Wald *et al.*, 1939; Barker *et al.*, 1941), and levels of 200–600 were very toxic to dogs (Lindberg *et al.*, 1941). Furthermore, wide individual variations and some temporal variations in the same persons were noted in the dosage of thiocyanate necessary to reach a therapeutic level for hypertension and to avoid a toxic level (Wald *et al.*, 1939).

Dietary consumption of cyanogenic substances in foodstuffs has been implicated in acute toxicity (Montgomcry, 1979; Lasch and El Shawa, 1981). Although numerous experimental studies in animals have shown neuropathologic effects, there is only circumstantial evidence linking human disease to chronic cyanide exposure. While it is acknowledged that the etiology of the ataxic neuropathy in West Africa was probably multifactorial, heavy exposure to cyanide or cyanogens from cassava appeared to be contributory (Wilson, 1973; Osuntokun, 1973).

Dosage Response   Using methods developed in animal studies, Gettler and Baine (1938) estimated that the *absorbed* dosages (as HCN) in four fatal cases of cyanide ingestion were 0.54, 1.10, 1.40, and 3.60 mg/kg and that the corresponding degrees of absorption were 81.9, 19.5, 18.1, and 15.7% respectively. In one instance, ingestion of about 50 mg of sodium cyanide led to vomiting followed by complete recovery (Curry, 1963).

For humans, a concentration of 300 mg/m^3 is immediately fatal. Concentrations of 120–150 mg/m^3 for 0.5–1 hr may be fatal, but 50–60 mg/m^3 is tolerated for this period. Even concentrations of 20–40 mg/m^3 produce some effects after several hours (Dudley and Neal, 1942). The threshold limit value (10 mg/m^3) would permit occupational exposure to cyanide as CN at the rate of 1.67 mg/kg/day. Of course, each day's dosage would be distributed over 8 hr and would not be concentrated in a few moments, as is true of dosages that have proved fatal.

Laboratory Findings   It is a curious fact that blood levels in fatal cyanide poisoning usually are higher following ingestion (3.2–160 ppm) than following inhalation (0.5–15 ppm) (Gettler and Baine, 1938; Curry, 1963; Bonnichsen and Maehly, 1966). However, it may be noted that the values of Gettler and Baine (1938) for dogs killed by ingestion and inhalation do not correspond to the relationship reported in humans; the two ranges were 7–10 and 5–17 ppm, respectively.

It is of interest that the blood level of 9.2 ppm reported by Hayes and Vaughn (1977) was associated with suicidal ingestion of cyanide and not inhalation of the gas as an occupational accident. Levels as high as 0.15 ppm may occur in the blood of healthy adults. Recovery has occurred in persons whose blood levels reached 7.5 ppm. Concentrations of cyanide in the viscera are usually but not always lower than those in the blood (Bonnichsen and Maehly, 1966).

Treatment of Poisoning Antidotes useful for treatment of poisoning by cyanide were discussed in detail in Section 8.2.3.5. The first large series of human cases treated by present methods was that of Chen and Rose (1952).

14.5.2 ACRYLONITRILE

14.5.2.1 Identity, Properties, and Uses

Chemical Name Acrylonitrile.

Structure See Fig. 14.2.

Synonyms Acrylonitrile is the common name in use. Other names for the compound include cyanoethylene, propenenitrile, and vinyl cyanide. Trade names include Fumigrain® and Ventox®. Code designations include ENT-54 and TL-314. The CAS registry number is 107-13-1.

Physical and Chemical Properties Acrylonitrile has the empirical formula C_3H_3N and a molecular weight of 53.06. It is a colorless, explosive, flammable liquid with a density of 0.806. It has a freezing point of $-83.55°C$, a boiling point of 77.3–77.5°C, and a flash point of 0°C. The vapor pressure is 105 torr at 25°C. Acrylonitrile is miscible with water (75 gm/kg at 25°C) and with most organic solvents. It may polymerize spontaneously, especially in the absence of oxygen or after exposure to light. It polymerizes violently in the presence of concentrated alkali.

History and Use Acrylonitrile was introduced as an insecticidal fumigant in 1939. It is highly potent, but of limited use because of its high cost and flammability. It occasionally is used on grain, dried fruit, walnuts, and tobacco, and it sometimes is used as a spot fumigant in flour mills and bakeries.

14.5.2.2 Toxicity to Laboratory Animals

Basic Findings An intragastric dose of acrylonitrile at the rate of 72 mg/kg was fatal to mice; the lethal dose was estimated to be >20 mg/kg. The lethal intraperitoneal dosage was estimated as 15 mg/kg (McOmie, 1949). Magos (1962) found that the subcutaneous LD 50 in rats was 95.8 mg/kg, a value not consistent with those just mentioned. The dermal LD 50 in guinea pigs was 368 mg/kg (Roudabush et al., 1965).

In a very thorough study of the effect of a single exposure to acrylonitrile vapor (Dudley and Neal, 1942), it was found that dogs were most susceptible, guinea pigs least susceptible, and rats, rabbits, cats, and monkeys intermediate. Some dogs were killed by a concentration of 240 mg/m³ for 4 hr and one was killed by 140 mg/m³. Three dogs showed slight salivation at the end of 4 hr of exposure to 63 mg/m³ (30 ppm) but no other

effect. In rats a straight-line log time–log dosage relation was demonstrated for fatal poisoning. Poisoned animals, except guinea pigs, showed an initial brief stimulation of breathing followed by rapid shallow breathing. The skin became reddened. As death approached, breathing became slow and gasping. General convulsions followed by coma preceded death. Soon after death the skin appeared darkened and grayish; the blood was dark and quite liquid. Animals that recovered did so in 12–24 hr. Acrylonitrile acted as a mucous membrane and pulmonary irritant in guinea pigs; those that died usually did so 3–6 days after exposure, apparently from lung edema.

Although the prophylactic and antidotal administration of sodium nitrite and sodium thiosulfate has protected mice from lethal intraperitoneal doses of acrylonitrile (Willhite and Smith, 1981), other studies in other species have not demonstrated that the classic cyanide antidotes are an effective means of protection from a lethal dose of acrylonitrile (Magos, 1962; Dudley and Neal, 1942). Consideration of these data collectively indicates that the acute lethal toxicity of acrylonitrile may depend partly on the molecule itself in addition to the cyanide it releases on metabolism. To further support his conclusion, Magos (1962) found that nitrite was not antidotal in rats, even though a substantial proportion (55.8%) of methemoglobin was bound to cyanide in rats killed by acrylonitrile. He emphasized that this proportion was less than 72.4%, the corresponding value in rats that survived potassium cyanide poisoning, and much less than the 85.6% binding found in rats killed by potassium cyanide. Magos also reported that cytochrome oxidase was less inhibited (71.5%) in rats killed by acrylonitrile than in those that survived (84.0%), or failed to survive (92.2%), poisoning by potassium cyanide. This would tend to negate the argument that methemoglobin in the blood has a better opportunity to intercept preformed cyanide before it reaches a critical tissue than would be true of cyanide that must be released by metabolism.

Pharmacokinetics/Metabolism Acrylonitrile is readily absorbed in animals following ingestion or inhalation. Dermal absorption is poor and occurs at about 1% of that of the lungs [Environmental Protection Agency (EPA), 1983]. Following absorption of radiolabeled acrylonitrile, the radioactivity disappears in a biphasic manner, with a half-life for the first phase of 3.5–3.8 hr and the second phase of 50–77 hr. The predominant route of elimination is through the urine (Sapota, 1982; Ahmed et al., 1982; EPA, 1983). Acrylonitrile is metabolized extensively by two pathways. Conjugation with glutathione to form cyanoethyl glutathione and the subsequent products involving mercapturic acid formation and oxidation via cyanoethylene oxide to cyanide and thiocyanate result in the major metabolic products (Kopecky et al., 1980; Langvardt et al., 1980; Delbressine et al., 1981; Ghanayem and Ahmed, 1982). Numerous studies have indicated the potential for acrylonitrile to interact with and bind to proteins, RNA, and DNA (Guengerich et al., 1981; Geiger et al., 1983; Farooqui and Ahmed, 1983; Solomon et al., 1984), but specific DNA–acrylonitrile adducts formed in vivo have yet to be identified.

Effects on Organs and Tissues   Acute and chronic toxic effects, as learned from animal experiments, seem to involve mostly the neuroendocrine system, stomach, duodenum, and possibly the liver. Szabo *et al.* (1976, 1984) reported that subacute and chronic ingestion of acrylonitrile caused decreased plasma levels of corticosterone and aldosterone and time-dependent changes in adrenal weight in rats consuming concentrations of 500–2000 ppm in water for several weeks.

Numerous chronic toxicity studies have been performed to elucidate the chronic toxicity and carcinogenicity of acrylonitrile in experimental animals. Sprague–Dawley rats exposed to vapors of acrylonitrile for 2 years at a concentration of 20 or 80 ppm showed a variety of toxic effects characterized by decreased body weight, early mortality, unthrifty appearance, and earlier-onset and more frequently observed palpable tumors. Tumors occurred in both groups in the central nervous system, tongue, Zymbal gland, small intestine, and mammary gland. Rats ingesting water containing 35, 100, or 300 ppm acrylonitrile for 2 years showed similar effects (EPA, 1983).

Subsequent studies designed to confirm the earlier studies and to determine whether similar effects occur at lower doses were conducted by intubation and drinking water to administer acrylonitrile to another strain of rat. Intubation doses were 0.1 and 10.0 mg/kg. Tumors of the central nervous system, Zymbal gland, mammary gland, forestomach, and intestine were significantly increased at 10 mg/kg/day but not at 0.1 mg/kg/day. In the drinking-water studies Fischer 344 rats received 1, 3, 10, 30, or 100 ppm and Sprague–Dawley rats received 1 or 100 ppm acrylonitrile. Central nervous system, mammary, Zymbal gland, and forestomach tumors were noted in groups receiving 10–100 ppm acrylonitrile. The incidence of tumors was not increased in rats receiving 1 or 3 ppm.

While metabolic studies suggest that acrylonitrile is metabolized to reactive species, whether this results in mammalian mutagenicity is less certain. Numerous mutagenicity tests have been conducted both *in vitro* and *in vivo* (summarized in EPA, 1983; Lambotte-Vandepaer and Duverger-van Bogaert, 1984). Considering these data collectively indicates that certain *in vitro* bacterial tests are positive but the more relevant tests in whole animals are generally negative. Therefore, whether acrylonitrile has a significant mutagenic potential in animals remains speculative at this time.

Effects on Reproduction   Pregnant rats were exposed to 0, 40, or 80 ppm acrylonitrile by inhalation for 6 hr/day on days 6–15 of gestation. Findings suggestive of a teratogenic effect were seen in offspring of rats inhaling 80 ppm (a maternally toxic dose) but not 40 ppm (also maternally toxic; Murray *et al.,* 1978). Murray *et al.* (1978) also reported that administration of acrylonitrile by gavage to rats on days 6–15 of gestation produced malformations and other evidence of embryotoxicity at 65 mg/kg/day (maternally toxic) and fewer but similar effects at 25 mg/kg/day. A dose of 10 mg/kg/day was the no-effect level for maternal rats or offspring. Willhite *et al.* (1981) reported teratogenic effects in hamsters following administration of maternally toxic doses of acrylonitrile (80–120 mg/kg,

ip) on day 8 of gestation. This effect was ameliorated by prior treatment with sodium thiosulfate, suggesting that liberation of cyanide may contribute to the teratogenic response.

Treatment of Poisoning in Animals   Sodium nitrite was effective in rats and rabbits (Dudley and Neal, 1942). In mice, sodium nitrite or thiosulfate was effective in preventing death following an intraperitoneal injection of a lethal dose of acrylonitrile (Willhite and Smith, 1981). However, McLaughlin *et al.* (1976) did not find the above antidotal regimen effective and instead found cysteine hydrochloride most effective in mice, rats, rabbits, and dogs. More recently, Buchter *et al.* (1984) showed *N*-acetylcysteine to be most effective in treating rats following inhalation of high concentrations of acrylonitrile. In summary, it appears that the cyanide antidotes, sodium nitrite and sodium thiosulfate, can be effective following oral or intraperitoneal administration and that cysteine and *N*-acetylcysteine are helpful following inhalation exposure. It may be speculated that a combination of therapy including *N*-acetylcysteine, nitrite, and thiosulfate may be most effective in preventing lethality following acute acrylonitrile intoxication.

14.5.2.3 Toxicity to Humans

Accidental and Intentional Poisoning   Two completely different kinds of potentially fatal poisoning have been attributed to acrylonitrile. One is clearly cyanide poisoning, although it may differ from that produced by hydrogen cyanide or alkali cyanides by being more insidious in onset and clinical course. The essential difference lies in the time required to release cyanide ion from acrylonitrile by metabolism (see Section 14.5). A further delaying factor in a high proportion of cases was the slow rate at which a fatal dose was absorbed by inhalation of a low concentration of the vapor. This second factor would be absent in respiratory exposure to higher concentrations or in ingestion. In fact, if the concentration of vapor is sufficient, the interval from first exposure to onset may be only a few moments.

The second form of poisoning apparently is unrelated to anything that has followed exposure to simple cyanide, although it has occurred following laboratory or industrial exposure to acrylonitrile alone or following exposure to acrylonitrile mixed with carbon tetrachloride used for fumigation. Thus the severe dermatitis that constitutes the second form of poisoning may be caused by the intact acrylonitrile molecule. There seems to be no reason to incriminate the carbon tetrachloride because it does not produce the effect when encountered alone and because the injury produced by acrylonitrile alone seems the same as that produced by the mixture.

Cyanide poisoning resulting from absorption and metabolism of acrylonitrile has caused the death of at least one person who was left in a house during fumigation and was, of course, dead when the tent was removed. In other instances, illness began insidiously as much as 24 hr after the first exposure and progressed in such an undramatic fashion that medical attention was sought very late or not at all. A disproportionate number of those who died were either infants (Grunske, 1949; Davis *et al.*, 1973) or persons over 60 already suffering from a serious chronic disease (Davis *et al.*, 1973).

A case will illustrate some characteristics of this form of poisoning. The home of a 67-year-old man with a history of essential hypertension and resection of the colon was fumigated with a mixture of acrylonitrile and methylene chloride. He returned to the house at 9:00 a.m. the day after the fumigation had been completed and ventilation had been started. During the afternoon his eyes were reddened. However, it was not until 11:00 p.m. that he felt ill, noted excessive sweating, and suffered nausea and vomiting. During the early hours of the morning he became irrational. He was taken to the hospital, where he was admitted at 4:10 a.m. and died 35 min later. Autopsy revealed arteriosclerotic heart disease, emphysema, healed hypertensive cystic infarcts of the basal ganglia and the pons, and, on analysis, a cyanide level of 0.75 ppm in the blood. During the early morning, when the victim was seriously ill, his mother and the family dog had vomited and the dog had convulsions, leaving no doubt about the toxicity of the air in the house (Davis *et al.*, 1973).

Poisoning by acrylonitrile need not be either delayed or protracted. This is illustrated by an episode in which, through a technical error, about 10 liters of the substance came out of a pipe into the pump room of a tanker. The captain and three crew members escaped by climbing up a ladder about 10 m high. On reaching the top, they felt sick and had sore throats, but all were conscious. The crew members were taken to a hospital, where they were treated with oxygen and recovered without ever experiencing serious injury. The captain refused to go to the hospital and returned to the pump room wearing a "filter" mask. About 10 min later he returned to his cabin, saying that he had inhaled gas, and collapsed. His clothes were not wet. He sniffed some amyl nitrite without effect. Breathing became difficult, and about 15 min later he lost consciousness. Mouth-to-mouth artificial respiration was administered, but edema of the lungs and convulsions developed, and he died (Van Luijt, 1963).

Fatal poisoning followed the application of about 50 ml of an acrylonitrile formulation to the scalp of a 10-year-old girl to treat head lice; the child went to bed but soon developed typical signs and symptoms and died about 4 hr after the application (Lorz, 1950).

In three of the four cases reported by Radimer *et al.* (1974), patients were hospitalized with blisters covering almost the entire skin and visible mucous membrane surfaces. Antibiotics, corticosteroids, fluids, and electrolytes produced no improvement, and all died of septic shock and gastrointestinal hemorrhage 21–28 days after the first exposure. The fourth case was that of the 10-year-old son of one of the other patients. Two weeks after first exposure, he developed widespread pruritic eruptions but survived. Treatment included topical and parenteral corticosteroid application. In all four cases biopsy showed that the blisters involved a separation between the dermis and the necrotic epidermis.

Probably the first evidence of the severe specific irritant effects of acrylonitrile on human skin was reported by Dudley and Neal (1942). In this instance, a chemist's hands were contaminated by small amounts of the liquid. A diffuse erythema of both hands and wrists developed within 24 hr, and blisters appeared on the fingertips on the third day. Healing was incomplete on the tenth day. In other instances workers developed large blisters resembling second-degree burns when they wore leather shoes for several hours after the shoes had absorbed acrylonitrile. Contrary to the view expressed by Radimer *et al.* (1974), the cases of epidermal necrolysis involving the entire body probably were the result of the local action of unmetabolized acrylonitrile, and the delays in onset were associated with prolonged exposure to otherwise nontoxic concentrations. It is of interest that no mention was made of lung involvement in the human cases, suggesting that the most susceptible tissue in humans is the skin, whereas it is the lungs in guinea pigs.

Apparently, epidermal necrolysis involving extensive skin areas has not occurred in industry. This raises several questions, including whether the three fatal cases discussed above involved exposure to higher ambient air concentrations than have occurred in industry and whether the critical exposure depended on locally high concentrations associated with vapor absorbed in foam rubber or other materials in mattresses. The published record gives no hint of contact toxicity but may not rule it out.

Use Experience Judging from experience in Florida from 1957 to 1971, the safety record of acrylonitrile as a pesticide is very poor. According to Davis *et al.* (1973), there were 24 misadventures in the use of acrylonitrile involving 41 nonfatal casualties and eight deaths between January 1957 and October 1971. A fatal case of poisoning of an infant who was returned too soon to a house that had been fumigated was reported from Germany (Grunske, 1949). Thus the problem is not restricted geographically. Even if these cases are the only ones that have resulted from the fumigation of homes, one may conclude that the pest control record involving the use of only a little acrylonitrile is far worse than the industrial record involving tremendous amounts of the compound. In fact, most of the reported cases associated with the manufacture of acrylonitrile are really cases of poisoning by cyanide used in the process.

Although a number of violations of good practice are recorded or implied by the report of Davis *et al.* (1973), it is not clear from that report or others whether acrylonitrile could be used safely under the practical conditions of pest control if the operators were properly trained and sufficiently disciplined.

Epidemiologic evidence concerning the carcinogenic potential of acrylonitrile is mixed. Ten studies have been conducted (reviewed in EPA, 1983). Six report no evidence of carcinogenic risk associated with exposure to acrylonitrile. However, all suffer from limitations in design or methodology. Of the four that suggest some association between acrylonitrile and human cancer, all suffer from limitations or confounding variables, and there do not appear to be plausible and consistent findings that collectively strengthen any one study.

Therefore, while definitive evidence of human carcinogenic activity escapes the epidemiologist, the multiple animal studies indicating carcinogenic activity strengthen the suspicion. However, as occupational limits continue to be lowered, it may be doubtful whether definitive evidence of human carcinogenicity will surface in the future.

Treatment of Poisoning Treatment of systemic poisoning beginning within about a day or less after first exposure to acrylonitrile should be the same as that for hydrogen cyanide, except that every effort should be made to remove acrylonitrile from the skin or from the gastrointestinal tract if either is thought to be contaminated (Vogel and Kirkendall, 1984). Actually, not enough cases have been treated to give one the confidence that is justified in treating simple cyanide poisoning. The fact that acrylonitrile poisoning tends to progress more slowly at first should improve the opportunity for treatment, but this delay may be associated with other factors that remain ill defined and complicate the treatment. Under the circumstances, it seems reasonable to add cysteine hydrochloride to the regimen. There is no evidence that it interferes with the nitrite–thiosulfate–oxygen method.

The treatment of epidermal necrolysis and related conditions caused by acrylonitrile is entirely symptomatic. Although corticosteroids have been used, the rationale for this use is obscure.

14.5.3 ISOBORNYL THIOCYANOACETATE

14.5.3.1 Identity, Properties, and Uses

Chemical Name 1,7,7-Trimethylbicyclo[2,2,1]hept-2-ylthiocyanatoacetate.

Structure See Fig. 14.2.

Synonyms Another name for the compound is terpinyl thiocyanoacetate. A trade name is Thanite®. The CAS registry number is 115-31-1.

Physical and Chemical Properties Isobornyl thiocyanoacetate has the empirical formula $C_{13}H_{19}NO_2S$ and a molecular weight of 253.36. It is a yellow, oily liquid with a turpentine-like odor. The boiling point is 95°C; the flash point is 82°C. The compound is very soluble in alcohol, benzene, chloroform, and ether but is practically insoluble in water. It is stable under normal storage conditions.

History, Formulations, and Use Introduced in 1945, isobornyl thiocyanoacetate is used mainly in domestic and livestock fly sprays. The technical product contains 82% or more of the compound and about 18% related terpene esters.

14.5.3.2 Toxicity to Laboratory Animals

Basic Findings The oral LD 50 of isobornyl thiocyanoacetate is 1000 mg/kg in rats (Lehman, 1951, 1952) and 722 mg/kg in

rabbits (Draize *et al.*, 1944). The dermal LD 50 in rabbits in 6880 mg/kg (Lehman, 1951, 1952).

In spite of its low acute toxicity, this compound produces, after a few hours of a delay, typical cyanide effects including restlessness, dyspnea, cyanosis, tonic convulsions, profound depression, and death.

A repeated dermal dose of just over 1000 mg/kg/day was fatal to rabbits after only four to five doses (Lehman, 1951, 1952).

14.5.3.3 Toxicity to Humans

Experimental Exposure To demonstrate the safety of isobornyl thiocyanoacetate as a household aerosol insecticide, volunteers entered a chamber where they were exposed to a dense fog of a 5% solution of the technical material in refined kerosene. No more than 10 persons were in the chamber at once. Analysis showed the concentration in the chamber to be 60 mg/m³. The study was carried out in three series. The first involved only four subjects and brief exposures. The second involved 65 people (44 men and 21 women); each subject was exposed 10 times for 30 min each during a 14-day period. In the third series, 223 people (114 men and 109 women) received a total of thirteen 30-min exposures on a slightly different schedule. The only untoward effects mentioned were irritation of the nose, throat, and eyes. In most instances the irritation subsided as soon as exposure stopped, but in some cases irritation of the nose and throat continued for 30 min after exposure. No changes traceable to the exposures were found in the course of rather extensive physical and laboratory examination before and after exposure. Patch tests revealed no evidence of primary irritation or sensitization of the skin by technical isobornyl thiocyanoacetate. It was concluded that the exposures were safe, even though they were more intense than would reasonably be expected in spray application (Keplinger, 1963).

Therapeutic Use Gerberg (1973) mentioned that "thanite" had been used for control of head lice but provided no details. Sollmann (1957) suggested that a 5% emulsion be worked into a lather on the skin and be allowed to remain 5–10 min. He reported that this treatment might produce mild irritation of the skin but apparently does not sensitize.

Accidental and Intentional Poisoning The fatal case of poisoning by isobornyl thiocyanoacetate listed by Hayes and Pirkle (1966) involved a 56-year-old man who accidently ingested the compound, which he mistook for paregoric. The dosage could not be determined. The illness, characterized by shock and unconsciousness, led to death in 8 hr. Treatment was entirely symptomatic. Autopsy findings included mucosal erosion of the esophagus, hyperemia of the stomach and intestines, pulmonary edema, bilateral pleural effusion, and ascites.

Treatment of Poisoning Poisoning associated with ingestion is due in part to release of the cyanide ion; therefore, a moderate level of treatment appropriate for cyanide should be used. However, the thiocyanate molecule itself is toxic; therefore, diuresis and perhaps dialysis should be used to promote its excretion.

14.6 MISCELLANEOUS FUMIGANTS

The compound discussed under this section that produces the best-defined biochemical lesion is carbon disulfide. The modes of action of the other compounds are understood poorly, but enough information is available to conclude that these compounds do not act in a similar way. The compounds discussed in the following section are shown in Fig. 14.4.

14.6.1 CARBON DISULFIDE

14.6.1.1 Identity, Properties, and Uses

Chemical Name   Carbon disulfide.

Structure   See Fig. 14.4.

Synonyms   Other names for the compound include carbon bisulfide and dithiocarbonic anhydride. The CAS registry number is 75-15-0.

Physical and Chemical Properties   Carbon disulfide has the empirical formula CS_2 and a molecular weight of 76.14. It is a colorless to yellowish mobile liquid. Minute amounts of the compound occur in coal tar and crude petroleum. Though impurities may give it a foul smell, the compound in pure form has a sweet odor. Carbon disulfide has a liquid density of 1.263. Its vapor density is 2.67 times that of air. It solidifies at $-108.6°C$ and boils at $46.5°C$. The closed-cup flash point is $-22°C$. The vapor pressure is 3.71 torr at $25°C$. The vapor is extremely flammable and ignites spontaneously at $100°C$. The explosive range is 1–50% (v/v) in air. Conversion factor is 1 mg/m^3 = 0.321 ppm in air.

History, Formulations, and Uses   Carbon disulfide was first used as an insecticide in 1854. It is used for the fumigation of

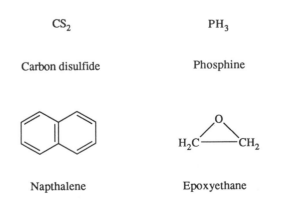

Figure 14.4   Some miscellaneous fumigants.

stored grain and nursery stock and for the treatment of soil against nematodes. For soil treatment, it is generally formulated as emulsions or solutions in thiocarbonates. For grain treatment, admixture with carbon tetrachloride is common to reduce fire hazard.

14.6.1.2 Toxicity to Laboratory Animals

Basic Findings   Carbon disulfide was more toxic to 1-day-old than to 20-day-old rats. The LD 50 for intraperitoneally administered carbon disulfide was 583 mg/kg in 1-day-old rats and 1545 mg/kg in 20-day-old rats (Green and Hunter, 1985).

In a study to determine whether the kind of illness observed in workers exposed to carbon disulfide could be reproduced experimentally, eight dogs were exposed to 400 ppm carbon disulfide in air 8 hr per day, 5 days per week, for 10–15 weeks. When removed from the chamber, the dogs were drowsy and staggered and stumbled as if drunk. They were very thirsty but did not eat for hours after leaving the chamber. Although they slept most of the time they were in the chamber, they were excited and noisy at night in their kennels. The dogs also developed many clinical and pathological signs analogous to those in workers: marked behavioral changes and toxic disease of nerve cells of the cortex of the brain were observed in all of them. Rigidity and tremor (parkinsonism) and choreatic movements were seen frequently, as was disease of the nerve cells of the basal ganglia. Motor weakness, flaccid paralysis, and nerve tenderness were the most frequent signs observed; the peripheral nerves showed axonal degeneration while the myelin sheath was well preserved. Cardiovascular changes included electrocardiographic abnormalities, especially inversion of the T wave, retinal angiospasms, and artherosclerosis of the veins of the cortex of the brain (Lewey, 1941).

Degenerative changes were also observed in the brains of rats and mice exposed for 8 hr/day to 1090 or 114 mg/m^3 carbon disulfide for periods up to 20 weeks (Wiley *et al.*, 1936). However, the complete range of injuries observed in these animals (unlike the injuries in dogs) had little resemblance to the illness observed in overexposed workers.

Absorption, Distribution, Metabolism, and Excretion   Carbon disulfide is readily absorbed from the gastrointestinal and respiratory tracts. When anesthetized rats were ventilated with air containing 640 ppm (2 mg/liter) carbon disulfide, the concentration of free carbon disulfide in the blood reached an apparent steady-state level of 12.7 μg/ml of blood within 90 min. Concentrations of free carbon disulfide in the fat and brain continued to increase throughout the 8-hr exposure period, whereas concentrations of carbon disulfide in the skeletal muscle, liver, and kidneys reached an apparent plateau after 4 hr and levels in the heart reached a plateau after 2 hr. The highest concentrations of free carbon disulfide were found in the fat and adrenals (50–60 μg/gm). Concentrations of free carbon disulfide in the kidneys and liver were similar to those in the blood (8–15 μg/ml), while the brain, heart, and skeletal muscle contained less than 5 μg/gm. When the exposure was terminated, free carbon disulfide was rapidly cleared from the blood. Approximately 40% of the free carbon disulfide was cleared from the blood with a half-life of 6 min and the remainder was cleared with a half-life of 83 min. Following a 2.5-hr exposure at 640 ppm, the rats excreted 5.3 mg of carbon disulfide in the expired air, which represented about 10% of the carbon disulfide they would have inhaled (McKenna and DiStefano, 1977).

In the body, carbon disulfide combines with amino acids and thiols to form dithiocarbamates and trithiocarbonates; these release carbon disulfide when treated with strong acid and are referred to as acid-labile carbon disulfide. The formation and elimination of acid-labile carbon disulfide are much slower than the absorption and elimination of free carbon disulfide. Levels of acid-labile carbon disulfide in the blood and most tissues continued to increase throughout an 8-hr inhalation exposure, and it was estimated that the concentration of acid-labile carbon disulfide in the blood would require 47 hr to reach steady state. Following the exposure, acid-labile carbon disulfide was cleared from the blood in a biexponential manner; the half-lives for the rapid and slow phases were 2.2 and 42.7 hr (Lam and DiStefano, 1982).

Carbon disulfide vapor is absorbed to some extent through the skin. When the whole body of rabbits was exposed to 1550 ppm carbon disulfide, concentrations of it in the exhaled breath increased gradually and reached a maximum of 2.5 ppm at the end of the 3-hr exposure. Concentrations of carbon disulfide in the air exhaled by these rabbits were nearly proportional to the exposure concentration and increased slightly during eight consecutive daily exposures (Cohen *et al.,* 1958).

Expired air was the principal route of elimination for ^{14}C-labeled carbon disulfide in the rat. Following intraperitoneal doses ranging from 4.7 to 19 mg/kg, between 67 and 87% of the administered radioactivity was excreted via the lungs. The fate of carbon disulfide was clearly dose dependent. As the intraperitoneal dose was increased from 4.7 to 19 mg/kg, the percentage of the dose excreted as carbon disulfide increased from 30 to 73% and the percentages excreted as carbonyl sulfide (COS) and carbon dioxide decreased from 25 to 7% and 11 to 7%, respectively. Saturation of carbon disulfide metabolism appears to be the explanation for the dose dependence. Rats pretreated with phenobarbital, a known inducer of drug-metabolizing enzymes, excreted a smaller fraction of the dose as carbon disulfide and a larger fraction as carbonyl sulfide and carbon dioxide (Dalvi and Neal, 1978). Twice as much ^{35}S-derived as ^{14}C-derived radioactivity was bound to liver microsomes incubated with ^{35}S- and ^{14}C-labeled carbon disulfide. This suggests that a reactive sulfur-containing metabolite of carbon disulfide is responsible for the centrilobular hepatocellar degeneration and loss of microsomal enzyme activity observed in rats (De Matteis, 1974).

Formation of a reactive intermediate during the microsomally mediated metabolism of carbon disulfide is clearly important in the hepatotoxicity induced by carbon disulfide in rats. Three mechanisms have been proposed to explain the central and peripheral neurotoxicity produced by carbon disulfide. Carbon disulfide can react with thiols or amines on proteins and disrupt normal metabolism. Carbon disulfide can also react with the free amine group pyridoxamine and produce a neuropathy similar to that observed in vitamin B_6 deficiency. In addition, dithiocarbamate formed by the reactions of carbon disulfide with amines can chelate copper and zinc cations and inhibit critical enzymes such as dopamine-β-hydroxylase. A more extensive review of the role of metabolism in the toxicity of carbon disulfide is provided by Bus (1985).

Effects on Organs and Tissues Carbon disulfide has been shown to produce a wide variety of lesions in experimental animals. Lesions in the central nervous system produced by carbon disulfide have been described in the cerebral cortex, cerebellum, basal ganglia, corpora quadrigemina, vestibular nuclei, and spinal cord. In the peripheral nervous system, a Wallerian degeneration of the axon was found with no evidence of demyelination. Carbon disulfide given by intraperitoneal injection produced an ischemic-like myocardial lesion in the rat, but a good animal model for the cardiovascular disease observed in workers exposed to carbon disulfide is not available. Centrilobular hepatocellular degeneration occurs in rats, especially those pretreated with phenobarbital, but this is of uncertain significance in the absence of similar toxicity in humans. Renal lesions involving the glomerulus and an inflammatory fibrotic lesion originating in the interstitial tissue have been described. Degenerative testicular changes involving the seminiferous tubules were observed in rats given repeated intraperitoneal injections of carbon disulfide. Altered thyroid and adrenal functions that have been described in the rat could be involved in the reproductive and cardiovascular effects of carbon disulfide. Blisters and other dermal lesions, similar to those observed in humans, were produced when carbon disulfide was applied to the rabbit ear and evaporation was retarded. Additional details concerning these lesions are provided in the excellent review by Beauchamp *et al.* (1983).

No evidence of mutagenicity was found when carbon disulfide was tested with and without metabolic activation in *Salmonella typhimurium* strains TA98 and 100 and in *Escherichia coli* WP2 *uvrA* at concentrations up to 1000 μ*M* or in *Drosophilia melanogaster* at concentrations up to 800 ppm in air (Donner *et al.*, 1981). No definitive long-term toxicity studies have been conducted with laboratory animals; thus, conclusions about the possible carcinogenicity of carbon disulfide must await further testing.

Reproduction Fetotoxicity, as evidenced by an increased number of resorptions, was observed in rabbits given carbon disulfide at 250, 75, or 25 mg/kg/day on days 6–19 of gestation. The number of malformations was increased in rabbits given 250 mg/kg/day, but this dose level was also maternally toxic (Jones-Price *et al.,* 1984b). The incidences of malformations and resorptions in rats given carbon disulfide at 600, 400, 200, or 100 mg/kg/day on days 6–15 of gestation were similar to incidence in nonexposed rats. Doses of 200 mg/kg/day and above were maternally and fetotoxic, as evidenced by reduced body weight gain by the dams and decreased mean fetal body weights (Jones-Price *et al.*, 1984a). No evidence of teratogenicity or maternal toxicity was observed when rats and rabbits were exposed for 6–7 hr/day to 20 or 40 ppm carbon disulfide in air on days 1–19 (rats) or 1–24 (rabbits) of gestation (Hardin *et al.*, 1981).

In a two-generation study of unusual design, carbon disulfide was found to sensitize the rat so that congenital malformations occurred at lower exposure levels in the second generation. Hydrocephalus, microcephalus, clubfoot, tail deformations, and hypognathia were observed in pups of the first generation when the dams were exposed for 8 hr/day throughout gestation to 64 and 32 ppm but not 3.1 or 0.01 ppm carbon disulfide. When females from the first generation were mated and exposed to carbon disulfide throughout gestation, congenital malformations were observed not only in rats exposed to 64 and 32 ppm but also in those exposed to 3.1 and 0.01 ppm carbon disulfide. Exploratory behavior and locomotion were also altered in pups of the second generation whose mothers were exposed to 3.1 and 0.01 ppm carbon disulfide (Tobacova *et al.*, 1983). These data suggest that carbon disulfide can produce congenital abnormalities in the rat; however, because of the inconsistency with previous studies, additional data on the status of the dams and experience with this study design are needed in order to evaluate these findings.

Time to mount and ejaculate and number of sperm per ejaculation were decreased in rats exposed to 600 but not 300 ppm carbon disulfide for 5 hr/day, 5 days/week, for up to 10 weeks. The testes appeared histologically normal, as were plasma levels of testosterone, follicle-stimulating hormone, and luteinizing hormone. These data suggest that carbon disulfide may interfere with processes regulating sperm transport and ejaculation but that it does not exert a direct effect on the testes (Zenick *et al.*, 1984a).

Factors Influencing Toxicity   Although neither alcohol (7–10 mg/kg body weight) nor carbon disulfide (260 ppm) alone had any effect on the acquisition of a conditioned response in the rat, combined exposure to these agents disrupted the acquisition of a conditioned avoidance response. This was interpreted as evidence that the combined exposure disrupted normal integrative CNS function (Opacka *et al.*, 1984). Coexposure to hydrogen disulfide at 50 ppm had no effect on the development of neurotoxicity, as measured by decreases in nerve conduction velocity, in rats exposed to 500 ppm carbon disulfide (Gagnaire *et al.*, 1986).

14.6.1.3 Toxicity to Humans

Most of what is known about the toxicity of carbon disulfide to humans has been learned in the industrial context. More detail than can be presented here may be found in the excellent review on carbon disulfide by Beauchamp *et al.* (1983) and in the book entitled "Toxicology of Carbon Disulfide" edited by Brieger and Teisinger (1967).

Experimental Exposure   Five men inhaled carbon disulfide vapor at a concentration of 20 or 25 ppm for as long as 2.1 hr.

They did not notice any immediate or late effect, and their heart rate, respiration, and blood pressure were unaffected. Equilibrium between the blood and the inspired concentration was reached after 60–90 min, after which the absorption of carbon disulfide was greatly reduced. When the exposure was stopped, carbon disulfide was rapidly cleared from the blood for the first 60 min and its elimination was considered to be complete after 3–8 hr. However, only 6–10% of the retained carbon disulfide was eliminated via the lungs, and urinary excretion accounted for only another 0.57%. The remaining 85–90% was considered to have been metabolized to inorganic and organic sulfur compounds (McKee *et al.*, 1943).

No complaints or objective signs of carbon disulfide intoxication were found·when six volunteers were exposed for four 50-min periods to 20 and 10 ppm carbon disulfide while at rest and 10 and 3 ppm carbon disulfide while doing 50 watts of physical exercise. Pulmonary retention of carbon disulfide ranged from 27.7 to 41.0% and was found to increase with increases in body fat and minute ventilation but decrease with increases in respiratory frequency and length of exposure. Between 5.4 and 37.9% of the carbon disulfide retained during the exposure was eliminated in the expired air. The concentration of carbon disulfide in the expired air decreased in a biexponential manner; the half-lives for the rapid initial and slower terminal phases were 1.1 and 110 min, respectively. Approximately 1.4% of the carbon disulfide retained during the exposure was metabolized and excreted in the urine as 2-thiothiazolidine-4-carboxylic acid. The rate of excretion of this metabolite in urine, based on a specimen collected immediately following the exposure, was proportional to the amount of carbon disulfide retained and represents a means of monitoring exposure to carbon disulfide (Rosier *et al.*, 1987a,b).

Accidental and Intentional Poisoning   Accidents associated with the use of carbon disulfide as a pesticide have occurred in occupational situations, even though they were not the result of occupational exposure *per se*. One case illustrates the possibility of a fatal outcome from exposure to a carbon disulfide mixture commonly used to fumigate grain. The other case, although acute, illustrates some of the strange mental disturbances that may be encountered. The death listed by Hayes and Vaughn (1977) as caused by carbon disulfide was actually the result of exposure to the residual vapor from a mixture of that compound and carbon tetrachloride used about 24 hr earlier to fumigate a grain elevator. The victim was a 32-year-old farmer who had come to the elevator on business. He and another man were found unconscious in the loading pit below the elevator. The victim was dead on arrival at the hospital; the other man survived. Autopsy revealed an extremely severe degree of pulmonary congestion and edema and a moderate degree of cerebral edema. It may be noted that the densities of carbon disulfide vapor and of air saturated with it are 2.67 and 1.74, respectively; the corresponding values for carbon tetrachloride are 5.3 and 1.64. It is not unexpected, therefore, that the vapor of both compounds would tend to collect in a pit under a grain elevator where a mixture of the materials had been used for fumigation.

In another case, a 42-year-old woman, who over a period of years had used carbon disulfide to control insects in warehouses, accidentally drank about 5 ml of the liquid from a soft-drink bottle. She induced vomiting by sticking her finger down her throat, but about 5 hr after ingestion she felt numbness of the lips and nausea and she vomited again. Twelve hours after ingestion, a hot feeling in the upper abdomen and intermittent agitation led to her hospitalization. Examination revealed accentuated tendon reflexes, bilateral positive Babinski reaction, and hyperesthesia in addition to the agitation. By 16 hr after ingestion, transient sinus tachycardia and sharp P waves appeared in the electrocardiogram, and there were some abnormalities of the electroencephalogram from the second through the sixth day of illness. Except for dizziness while walking, the patient seemed normal by the second day of hospitalization. However, about midnight of the fifth day she came to a nurse's station carrying a grapefruit and expressing very confused ideas about it and about God. The same illusion and delusion returned several times for about a week. The only other finding at this time was some loss of memory. Following discharge, the patient remained normal for 8 days and then for 2 days experienced an intermittent return of agitation, illusions, and delusions. By a little over 2 months after ingestion she was entirely healthy (Yamada, 1977).

One of the greatest potential dangers associated with the use of carbon disulfide as a pesticide lies in its flammability rather than in its toxicity. An example of this kind of accident occurred on November 16, 1973, near Yountville, California. One of two tanks on a truck was being loaded from a railroad car. Because of faulty couplings, some of the gas leaked out and was ignited by an unknown heat source, perhaps the muffler or manifold on the truck. The gas exploded, burned, and destroyed the tanks and the truck. The driver, who was sprayed by carbon disulfide and set on fire, was able to jump into a ditch of water and escaped serious injury.

Use Experience Safety experience with carbon disulfide used as a fumigant has been good. The medical case literature contained only one paper alleging adverse health effects of the use of carbon disulfide among grain fumigators. The low incidence of reported adverse effects may be due to a trend to use this particular compound (suitably mixed with other fumigants to reduce the risk of fire or explosion) for the treatment of small lots of grain, including the stores on individual farms. If carbon disulfide is used carefully and only occasionally, the danger of its cumulative effects are avoided.

Clinical symptoms attributed to carbon disulfide were described in seven men, 31–56 years old, who had been exposed to fumigants used to treat grain. Six of the men reported using "80-20" (fumigant mixture containing 80% carbon tetrachloride and 20% carbon disulfide) and malathion for periods ranging from 8.5 to 17 years. Exposures occurred while they were mixing and applying the fumigants and/or sampling and transferring treated grain. No major accidents or unusual work practices were described. Clinical manifestations included cogwheel rigidity, resting and action tremor, peripheral neuro-

pathy, pyramidal tract signs, and an EEG pattern of sleep apnea (Peters *et al.*, 1982). These symptoms were consistent with those that might be produced by carbon disulfide; however, the individual cases did not present a consistent pattern of symptoms. The exposures were poorly defined and, based on the details provided, it is questionable whether the exposures to carbon disulfide were of sufficient magnitude to have produced these symptoms. Therefore, at present, the symptoms in these individuals should be regarded as being of unknown etiology.

The picture in industry has been quite different, and at about the turn of the century, dramatic cases of acute poisoning were reported. Browning (1965) cited an official report of 1899 to the effect that the windows of a vulcanizing room had to be barred to prevent men from jumping out during attacks of mania. These early cases resulting from heavy, relatively brief, repeated exposure were characterized by mental derangement resembling that of alcoholic intoxication but with the acute mania progressing to depression, apathy, loss of memory, hallucinations, and delusions of persecution. The disorder sometimes cleared only after many months or not at all.

As industrial conditions leading to acute poisoning were brought under control, it became apparent that less dramatic, "chronic" poisoning was occurring among workers with prolonged exposures to lower concentrations of carbon disulfide. Prolonged exposure may involve the central nervous system, the peripheral nervous system, the cardiovascular system, the gastrointestinal system, the kidneys, and various other organs, and the range of reported effects is so large that it is difficult to imagine they all have a single cause. Carbon disulfide damages blood vessels and produces or promotes atherosclerosis. This may in part explain the renal, cerebral, and/or cardiac atherosclerosis as well as spasms and microscopic aneurysms of the retinal vessels that have been reported. The relationship, if any, between circulatory deficiencies and the other conditions caused by carbon disulfide is less obvious. Central nervous effects not easily traceable to atherosclerosis include (*a*) psychotic reactions; (*b*) amblyopia; (*c*) a parkinsonian syndrome characterized by muscular spasticity, tremors, speech disturbance, loss of memory, and intense mental depression; and (*d*) a syndrome characterized by intense, involuntary, choreic or athetotic muscular movements. Poisoning of the peripheral nerves usually involves motor weakness resulting in ataxia and difficulty in swallowing and speaking; it also may involve sensory loss. Some investigators consider that myopathy is a separate entity and that the tremor may be due to weakness rather than an indication of central nervous disorder. Sexual disorders may occur, but these too may depend on general weakness. The gastrointestinal syndrome may involve gastric or duodenal ulcer or gastritis with achlorhydria.

Epidemiologic studies indicate that individuals exposed to carbon disulfide primarily while working in viscose rayon production between 1940 and 1960 have 2.5-3-fold excess mortality due to coronary heart disease (Tiller *et al.*, 1968), an increased incidence of chest pain and angina (Oliver and Weber, 1984), small but statistically significant deceases in sensory and motor nerve conduction velocities (Johnson *et al.*,

1983), alterations in the retinal microvasculature (Sugimoto *et al.*, 1976), and impaired color discrimination (Raitta *et al.*, 1981).

Dosage Response Exposure to 4800 ppm for 30 min may be fatal to humans, and unconsciousness may occur after a few breaths at higher concentrations. At 2000–3000 ppm, light intoxication, paresthesia, and irregular breathing occurred within 0.5–1 hr. Exposure to 320–390 ppm was bearable for several hours but headaches and an unpleasant feeling developed after 8 hr of exposure. Exposure to 160–230 ppm was reported to cause no symptoms of acute toxicity (Teisinger, 1983). The threshold limit value of 10 ppm (10 mg/m^3) indicates that occupational intake at the rate of 4.3 mg/kg/day would be without effect.

Treatment of Poisoning Treatment is almost entirely symptomatic. The prognosis is generally good if the patient was removed from the exposure promptly. However, the prognosis for a complete recovery is dubious if the peripheral or central nervous system is affected.

14.6.2 PHOSPHINE

14.6.2.1 Identity, Properties, and Uses

Chemical Name Hydrogen phosphide.

Structure See Fig. 14.4.

Synonyms Other names are hydrogen phosphide, phosphoretted hydrogen, and phosphorus trihydride. Trade names for phosphine and preparations to generate it include Cleophos®, Delica Gastoxin®, Detia-GasEx-T and Ex-B®, and Phostoxin®. The CAS registry number is 7803-51-2.

Physical and Chemical Properties Phosphine has the empirical formula H_3P and a molecular weight of 34.00. It is a colorless gas with an odor of carbide or decaying fish. The odor threshold for the pure gas is about 2 ppm, but because of odorous impurities produced from metal phosphides, the odor threshold for the pesticide is about 0.02 ppm. Phosphine has a vapor density of 1.17 at 25°C and 760 mm Hg, a melting point of −133°C, and a boiling point of −87.7°C. The solubility in water at 17°C is 26 ml/100 ml. Phosphine is spontaneously flammable if a trace of P_2H_4 is present. The lowest explosion limit is 26,150–27,060 mg/m^3. It combines violently with oxygen and halogens.

Formulations and Uses Phosphine is a fumigant for grain and other stored products. The gas is liberated by the interaction of aluminum phosphide with water. Good commercial formulations of aluminum phosphide include about 40% ammonium carbonate, which liberates ammonia and carbon dioxide in the presence of water, resulting in a gas mixture that is not flammable or explosive. Formulations are provided in the

form of 3-gm tablets, 0.6-gm pellets, and 34-gm crepe paper bags. In any case, 3 gm of formulation generates 1 gm of phosphine. Tablets or pellets are inserted by probe or otherwise at a rate of 1–3 gm/metric ton into grain containing at least 10% moisture. Stacked goods in a gas-tight space may be fumigated by placing gas-permeable bags or other preparations in trays near the produce at a rate of 0.75–1.5 gm/m^3. Phosphine in the form of zinc phosphide (Zn_3P_2) is also used in the control of rodents and moles by placing the tablets in outdoor burrows, the openings of which then are closed.

14.6.2.2 Toxicity to Laboratory Animals

Symptomatology Animals exposed to high concentrations of phosphine soon developed lassitude, immobility, then deepened restlessness with attempts to escape, ataxia, pallor, epileptiform convulsions, and death in 0.5 hr or less. Apnea precedes cardiac arrest. Differences between species are minor. The illness produced by intermediate concentrations is similar, except that the onset is less prompt and the progression slower. At the lowest concentration leading to death (7.5 mg/m^3), the first several exposures of 6 hr each produce no detectable injury. Even after mild signs develop, they regress in some animals when exposure is interrupted for a day during a weekend. However, as exposure is resumed, the signs listed above appear and progress to death. Some cats vomit during this kind of illness (Klimmer, 1969).

Dosage Response Klimmer (1969) showed that when rats were exposed to concentrations of phosphine ranging from 7.5 to 564 mg/m^3, the product of concentration and time to death was remarkably constant, falling in the range 216–337 if time is expressed in hours. Extrapolation of the straight line shown in Fig. 14.5 predicts that a concentration of about 0.2 mg/m^3 would be uniformly fatal in 820 hr of exposure, but actually rats tolerated a concentration of 3.75 mg/m^3 for 820 hr without

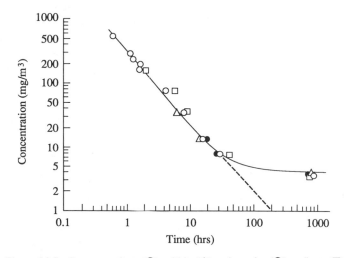

Figure 14.5 Response of rats (○), rabbits (△), guinea pigs (●), and cats (□) to phosphine. Each point indicates the concentration of phosphine to which a group of animals was exposed and the average time to death. With the exception of the concentration 3.48 mg/m^3, all animals survived for 820 hr. From data of Klimmer (1969).

clinical injury. It is clear that the toxicity of phosphine exemplifies the typical second and third segments of the logtime–logdosage curve. Thus, at concentrations of 7.5 mg/m³ and above, the effects of phosphine are almost perfectly cumulative, but at concentrations of 3.75 mg/m³ and below, there is no clinical evidence of accumulation and only questionable laboratory evidence of mild kidney injury. Values for cats, guinea pigs, and rabbits fell along the same logdosage–logtime curve, indicating astonishingly little species variation (see Fig. 14.5).

Using tabular values for respiratory volume and assuming complete absorption of phosphine, one can calculate from Klimmer's result that the total dosage received by rats killed by a concentration of 7.5 mg/m³ was about 8.9 mg/kg. Using the same assumptions, a total dosage of about 122 mg/kg over a 34-day period was tolerated by rats at a concentration of 3.75 mg/m³.

The LC 50 for phosphine in albino rats reported by Muthu *et al.* (1980) was 220–360 mg hr/m³ and is in excellent agreement with the data from Klimmer (1969). The 4-hr LC·50 reported by Waritz and Brown (1975) for phosphine in Charles River CD rats (15 μg/liter or 60 mg hr/m³) was somewhat lower than that found by Klimmer (1969). Clinical signs observed in rats exposed 4 hr/day for 12 days at one-third the LC 50 were indicative of mild respiratory irritation (i.e., lacrimation, salivation, dyspnea, and red ears) and piloerection. Weight gain was depressed during the exposure period but returned to normal during the recovery period. No gross or histopathological effects were observed in these rats that were attributable to phosphine (Waritz and Brown, 1975).

The oral LD 50 for zinc phosphide in rats is about 40 mg/kg (Dieke and Richter, 1946) and is equivalent to 10 mg phosphine/kg if all the phosphide is converted to phosphine. The oral LD 50 for zinc phosphide is in reasonable agreement with the quantity of inhaled phosphine estimated to be lethal to rats (8.9 gm/kg; see above). The oral LD 50 for zinc phosphide in the chicken was 25 mg/kg and was cited by Shivanandappa *et al.* (1979) as evidence that zinc phosphide was more toxic to domestic fowl than to rodents.

Rats showed no ill effect when they were fed grain that had been fumigated with phosphine at excessive rates, even though the grain was not cleaned (Kadkol and Jayaraj, 1968). Chronic ingestion of diets fumigated at 10 times the recommended concentration were essentially nontoxic to rats (Hackenberg, 1972).

Absorption, Distribution, Metabolism, and Excretion Inhaled phosphine is freely absorbed by the lungs. The effectiveness of proper gas masks in preventing toxicity excludes the possibility of significant absorption through skin. If tablets of aluminum phosphide or zinc phosphide are swallowed, the phosphine released from them is absorbed by the gastrointestinal mucosa. Evolution of phosphine was enhanced by acid as toxicity occurred more quickly and at lower dose levels if the zinc phosphide was administered with food or dilute hydrochloric acid. Regardless of the route of absorption, some phosphine is excreted by the lungs.

No published articles were found on the qualitative or quantitative distribution and metabolism of phosphine, but its effects on a wide range of organs suggest wide distribution in the body.

Residues of $^{32}PH_3$, mostly hypophosphite and phosphite, remain in the grain after proper ventilation. These residues were not removed by heating at baking temperatures and were incorporated into the tissues of mice that ate the fumigated flour. Excreta from these mice were highly radioactive at first, but the activity disappeared about 3 weeks after feeding was stopped (Robinson and Bond, 1970).

Mode of Action Exposure to high concentrations of phosphine leads in both humans and animals to a profound fall in blood pressure and to death in a state of collapse. Lower concentrations cause pulmonary edema, which may be fatal. Even lower concentrations (7.5 mg/m³) lead to respiratory failure while the heart continues to beat. It seems likely that the most sensitive tissue is the respiratory center. However, severe disorders of the kidney, liver, heart, and brain may be observed, especially if respiratory failure is alleviated by artificial respiration. Some of these actions may be secondary effects of anoxia or uremia. However, there is little doubt that all tissues are affected directly to some degree by phosphine itself.

Early studies cited by Klimmer (1969) suggested that phosphine was a blood poison, but this hypothesis is not supported by clinical observations in cases of fatal poisoning (Stephenson, 1967; Wilson *et al.*, 1980; Singh *et al.*, 1985). Loewenthal (1949) interpreted the pathology of the brain and liver as indicating "complex osmotic and permeability disturbances," but Peters (cited by Klimmer, 1969) considered the changes in the brain of rats as typical of those caused by anoxia.

Pretreatment of rats for 102 hr at a concentration of 1 ppm did not result in either sensitization or tolerance, as indicated by more rapid or slower death following exposure to 205 ppm (Klimmer, 1969). Similarly, tolerance to the effects of phosphine was not observed in men handling treated wheat (Jones *et al.*, 1964).

In the absence of oxygen, phosphine is virtually nontoxic to insects (Bond *et al.*, 1969). Phosphine is a potent *in vitro* inhibitor of cytochrome-*c* oxidase, the terminal electron acceptor in the mitochondrial electron transport chain; however, activities of this enzyme in phosphine-treated insects showed little inhibition (Price, 1980). In contrast, *in vitro* and *in vivo* inhibition of catalase was observed in beetles treated with phosphine, and the degree of inhibition of catalase activity paralleled their sensitivity to phosphine. Interestingly, the resistant strains of insects were found to take up less phosphine than sensitive strains (Price and Dance, 1983).

Laboratory Findings If poisoning occurs over a period of days, it may be possible to demonstrate a moderate anemia, a clear reduction of bromsulfophthalein secretion, and slight albuminuria. The color of the blood may be brownish; the reason for this is not known, but methemoglobin is not the cause. Mild, often transient albuminuria without clinical effects may be present in animals exposed to a concentration of 3.75 mg/m^3 (Klimmer, 1969).

Pathology Animals killed rapidly by high concentrations of phosphine may show pulmonary edema but little else (Klimmer, 1969; Waritz and Brown, 1975; Muthu *et al.*, 1980). Rats killed more slowly by phosphine may show pulmonary edema; petechial hemorrhages of the mucosa; a slight diffuse fatty infiltration of the liver; and cloudy swelling, isolated fatty infiltration, and isolated necrosis of the tubular epithelium of the kidney. The brain may show striking dilation of the perivascular spaces, changes in the nuclei of ganglion cells with a glial reaction, disintegrating Purkinje cells with multiplication of the Bergmann glia, edema of the white matter of the cerebellum, and occasional damage to capillary endothelium. The changes are similar in different species, except that the glial reaction apparently is absent in cats and guinea pigs (Klimmer, 1969).

No gross or histopathologic effects were observed in rats after 12 daily 4-hr exposures to one-third of the LC 50 (Waritz and Brown, 1975).

14.6.2.3 Toxicity to Humans

Accidental and Intentional Poisoning Probably the most instructive case of human poisoning by phosphine is that reported by Zipf *et al.* (1967). It involved a 25-year-old man who one morning, with suicidal intent, swallowed six tablets of aluminum phosphide dissolved in water. If all of the material had been retained permanently, it would have been sufficient to release about 6000 mg of phosphine. The man reported later that immediately after taking the poison he felt severe substernal and upper abdominal pain accompanied by an intolerable burning sensation of the whole body. Doubled up by pain, he lay on a pile of straw, vomited severely, and with a feeling of great anxiety screamed repeatedly. He lost consciousness, but his screams had brought immediate help. He was taken to the hospital, where he was found to be unconscious, pulseless, and without measurable blood pressure. In spite of his near-terminal state, he was resuscitated, and as soon as possible a massive gastric lavage was carried out using a solution of potassium permanganate and magnesium sulfate.

By evening the blood pressure was raised to 100 mm Hg and maintained. His state of consciousness cleared slowly. Production of urine had stopped but it returned during the night. On the day after ingestion, urine production was 350 ml. There was hematuria, leukocyturia, and proteinuria. Production decreased again on the third day with no improvement on the fourth day, when blood nitrogen was 6.0 mEq/liter. The patient's condition caused his transfer to a more specialized hospital, where he survived after a prolonged, stormy course.

Briefly, from the fourth day on, uremia was the primary clinical difficulty. It was accompanied by transitory glycosuria

and complicated by pulmonary edema, which began during the fourth day and was controlled only with difficulty. It increased again on the sixth day. Other complications included damage to the heart (abnormal ECG from day 4 to day 49; cardiac dilation in response to pulmonary edema from day 4 to day 19; loud systolic murmur on day 6; loud pericardial friction rub from day 9 to day 16; and auricular fibrillation with absolute ventricular arrhythmia from day 11 to day 16), brain (EEG changes), and liver (scleral icterus and hepatomegaly first recorded on day 4). Pericarditis was present and thought to be of uremic origin.

The use of hemodialysis on days 5–11 of poisoning brought about a decisive turn in the course of the disease. The patient became alert, and pulmonary edema subsided. The marked improvement in serum nitrogen and potassium levels was temporary after the first treatment but sustained after the second. During the second hemodialysis on day 11, the patient developed psychomotor unrest, trancelike states lasting 30–60 sec, vivid optical hallucinations, and other difficulties. When the velocity of dialysis was reduced, the cerebral symptomatology regressed rapidly. When the second dialysis was complete, the pericardial friction rub and pulmonary edema had diminished. It was not until this time that the odor of phosphine disappeared from the breath.

The pulmonary edema and icterus and the grosser indications of cardiac and cerebral disorder showed some improvement soon after the second hemodialysis, and they subsided after 3 weeks. The uremia also subsided after 3 weeks. Hepatomegaly disappeared by day 40, and the ECG and EEG became approximately normal by this time also. The patient still exhibited slight disturbances of thought and memory, as well as a tendency to depressive psychosis. Because of the persistence of this latter difficulty and a renewed danger of suicide, he was transferred to a mental hospital on day 75.

Respiratory exposure to phosphine produces a different picture, as illustrated by the death of three people who lived in a house immediately adjoining a granary. The husband suffered vomiting and pallor on the day the grain was treated. On the following day, his wife had similar symptoms, and a 5-year-old girl who was often in the same room vomited. The cause of difficulty was not recognized, and the next morning the two adults died in their bedroom. The child was hospitalized but died in spite of treatment with cortisone and other drugs. Autopsy revealed pulmonary edema in each instance. The concentration of phosphine found in the bedrooms where the adults died was 1.2 mg/m^3 (Hallermann and Pribilla, 1959), but it may have been higher when the injury was done.

Use Experience Careless use of phosphine has led to tragedy. Gessner (1937) reported that 12 people became sick and one died because they lived near a warehouse in which moist aluminum phosphide was stored. The concentration of phosphide reaching the victims was unknown. Other tragedies to third parties have involved the occupants of houses located near a fumigated structure (Hallermann and Pribilla, 1959), persons who returned too early to a fumigated structure (Sovljanski *et al.*, 1969), children who played for an hour on wheat that had been fumigated in the open (Heyndrickx *et al.*, 1976), a youth who climbed into a boxcar of grain that was being fumigated and went to sleep, and a family who used phosphine-generating pellets for rat control inside their home (Hayes and Vaughn, 1977).

Modrzejewski and Myslak (1967) reported that concentrations varying between 1.0 and 10 mg/m³ produced vertigo, headache, nausea, vomiting, and "psychomotor stimulation" in all of five workers exposed. In addition, four of the men experienced dyspnea and bronchial catarrh, and three developed fever and suffered enlargement of the liver with bilirubinemia.

A study of 67 grain fumigators in New South Wales showed that levels as high as 47 mg/m³, but usually not over 12 mg/m³ for periods of 8 hr or more, led to vertigo, headache, staggering gait, nausea, vomiting, diarrhea, epigastric or retrosternal pain, tightness in the chest, dyspnea, and palpitations. Although some of the men were incapacitated for several days, none presented any signs on physical examination. In half the cases, symptoms began almost immediately; in the remainder there was a delay of several hours to 2 days. There was no evidence of cumulative effects and no tendency to develop immunity. Concentrations of 0.3 ppm (0.4 mg/m³) or less sometimes produced headache but no other symptoms in the course of ordinary intermittent exposure of several months duration (Jones *et al.*, 1964).

Atypical Cases of Various Origins It seems desirable to mention an atypical case originally diagnosed as phosphine poisoning, even though careful study of the brain established an entirely different diagnosis and excluded the possibility that phosphine played a significant role. The patient was a 54-year-old man who became acutely ill while fumigating grain with phosphine. He complained of headache and nausea, followed by repeated vomiting. Three days later his hearing became impaired and his speech thick. Although he deteriorated progressively in attention, comprehension, and behavior, it was not until a month after the onset that he was referred to a neurosurgeon. Mild hemiparesis on the right and the results of an arteriogram and a pneumoencephalogram indicated a deep lesion of the left cerebral hemisphere. Thirty-two days after onset and while preparations were being made for cranial exploration, the patient died suddenly. Autopsy showed that death was caused by cerebral hemorrhage. Detailed study showed that both the large recent and small earlier hemorrhages were the result of the invasion of blood vessels by a granuomlatous disease that had existed certainly for months and perhaps for years and that its progression accounted for the patient's initial symptoms as well as his death. It was pointed out that the brain did not give evidence of hypoxia, which is characteristic of poisoning by phosphine, and that the patient's symptoms and especially his prolonged survival and sudden death were not consistent with phosphine poisoning (Courville, 1964).

Dosage Response In the case of suicide by ingestion of phosphide described by Zipf *et al.* (1967), the intake was equivalent to a dosage of about 86 mg/kg in terms of phosphine. However, vomiting was prompt and violent, and gastric lavage was performed within a short time. There was no way to determine the retained dosage, but it must have been considerably less than what was ingested. Singh *et al.* (1985) described a series of 15 cases in which 1.5–9.0 gm of aluminum phosphide were ingested. Eleven of these patient died, but death was not related to either the amount of phosphide ingested or the interval between ingestion and hospitalization, and the only factor which differentiated nonsurvivors from survivors was persistent shock that did not respond to dopamine infusions.

The threshold limit value of 0.4 mg/m³ (3 ppm) indicates that occupational intake at the rate of 0.057 mg/kg/day is considered safe.

Laboratory Findings Phosphine in the exhaled air can be recognized by its characteristic carbide or garliclike odor following either inhalation or oral exposures. Black stomach contents with garliclike odor are observed following ingestion. Elevated serum transaminase activity, bilirubin, and blood urea nitrogen and occult blood, bile, and glucose in the urine indicate involvement of the liver and kidneys. Electrocardiogram, sputum Gram stain and culture, differential white cell count, and arterial blood gas analysis are recommended by Proctor *et al.* (1978) to differentiate phosphine poisoning from cardiogenic pulmonary edema, severe viral or bacterial pneumonia, and adult respiratory distress syndrome.

Pathology Following primary respiratory exposure to phosphine, the major finding at autopsy is pulmonary edema (Wilson *et al.*, 1980). Following ingestion of a phosphide, injury to the lungs is secondary to the excretion of phosphine. Other pathological changes that have been observed following ingestion of phosphides or inhalation of phosphine include hemorrhage of the gastric and duodenal mucosa, central congestions and centrolobular necrosis of the liver, congestion of the spleen, focal myocardial necrosis, and patchy necrosis of the proximal portion of the convoluted tubules in the kidney (Wilson *et al.*, 1980; Singh *et al.*, 1985). The pathology is characteristic of hypoxia but is not diagnostic. Hyperemia, edema, and small perivascular hemorrhages of the brain have also been reported by Hallermann and Pribilla (1959).

Treatment of Poisoning No specific treatment is known for poisoning by phosphine. If phosphine has been inhaled, immediate hospitalization and observation for 72 hr for delayed onset of severe pulmonary edema is advised (Proctor *et al.*, 1978). Gastric lavage is indicated if aluminum phosphide or zinc phosphide has been ingested. Depending on the presenting signs, attention must be given to maintenance of blood pressure or control of pulmonary edema. The use of oxygen under pressure may be indicated. If pulmonary edema persists or recurs, steroids may be administered on a short-term basis

(2–4 days) to decrease pulmonary inflammation. Treat central nervous system effects symptomatically.

In a case in which uremia was the major problem, hemodialysis was almost certainly lifesaving (Zipf *et al.,* 1967).

14.6.3 NAPHTHALENE

14.6.3.1 Identity, Properties, and Uses

Chemical Name   Naphthalene.

Structure   See Fig. 14.4.

Synonyms   Naphthalene is also known as naphthalin, naphthene, tar camphor, and white tar. The CAS registry number is 91-20-3.

Physical and Chemical Properties   Naphthalene has the empirical formula $C_{10}H_8$ and a molecular weight of 128.16. It forms colorless flaky crystals with a mothball odor. It is the most abundant single constituent of coal tar. The density of naphthalene is 1.162, the melting point is 80°C, and the boiling point is 218°C. The open- and closed-cup flash points are 80 and 79°C, respectively. It has a vapor pressure of 4.92×10^{-2} mm Hg at 20°C and the odor threshold in air is 0.08 ppm (Amoore and Hautala, 1983). Naphthalene is slightly soluble in water but readily soluble in most organic solvents, especially 1,2-dichloroethane, ether, hydronaphthalenes, and fixed and volatile oils. It is flammable but otherwise stable.

History and Uses   Naphthalene has long been used as a household fumigant against clothes moths. Only pure grades, free from dust, should be used. Naphthalene is used less today than in the past; it has been replaced by a less toxic substance, paradichlorobenzene, which, if ingested, may produce local gastrointestinal tract irritation but requires no therapy except possibly a demulcent, and treatment for nausea and vomiting if severe (Gossel and Bricker, 1984).

14.6.3.2 Toxicity to Laboratory Animals

The oral LD 50 values for naphthalene in male and female rats are 2200 and 2400 mg/kg, respectively. The dermal LD 50 value was found to exceed 2500 mg/kg (Gaines, 1969). The oral LD 50 values for male and female CD1 mice are 533 and 710 mg/kg, respectively (Shopp *et al.,* 1984). In the majority of cases death occurred within 5 hr, the mice developed ptosis with clear red secretions around the eye, and death followed depressed breathing and ataxia.

In mice given 27, 53, or 267 mg naphthalene/kg/day by gavage in corn oil for 14 days, there was 5–10% mortality and decrease in body weight in both sexes at the 267 mg/kg dose level only. At the high dose level, males also had decreased thymus weights and females had decreased spleen and increased lung weights. Other organ weights, serum enzymes and electrolytes, and immunological function were unaffected

at these dose levels. In mice given 5.3, 53, or 133 mg naphthalene/kg/day by gavage in corn oil for 90 days, spleen weights were reduced in females at the 133 mg/kg dose level; otherwise there were no effects on mortality, body or organ weights, serum enzymes or electrolytes, or immunological function (ibid). Selective but reversible damage to the nonciliated bronchiolar epithelial (Clara) cells was observed in the lungs of C57Bk/6J mice given 128 and 256 mg naphthalene/kg by intraperitoneal injection (Mahvi *et al.,* 1977).

An 83% drop in hemoglobin occurred in dogs given an accumulated dose of 1800 mg naphthalene/kg over 5 days. Plasma collected 2 days after ingestion of naphthalene produced Heinz bodies when incubated for 1 hr with normal dog erythrocytes (Zuelzer and Apt. 1949). Cataracts were produced in rabbits fed 1000 mg/kg/day for 46 days, but not by direct application of a 10% solution of naphthalene in oil into the eyes or by intraperitoneal injections of 500 mg/kg/day (Ghetti and Mariani, 1956).

Absorption, Distribution, Metabolism, and Excretion
Naphthalene is readily absorbed when inhaled or ingested. Although not studied in animals, dermal absorption in humans is significant.

Radioactivity was widely distributed in the tissues of pullets and swine given single oral doses of 0.44 and 2.46 mg ^{14}C-labeled naphthalene, respectively (Eisele, 1985). The highest concentrations of ^{14}C were found in the kidney and fat of pullets and the fat of swine sacrificed 24 hr after a single oral dose of [^{14}C]naphthalene. Concentrations of radioactivity in the kidneys and fat of chickens decreased with an apparent half-life of 6–7 days and in the fat of swine with an apparent half-life of 4.4 days.

In the presence of microsomes, synthetic 1,2-naphthalene oxide is converted to all major naphthalene metabolities and is evidence that formation of the epoxide is an obligatory step in the metabolism of naphthalene. The predominant metabolite is 1-naphthol. Soluble liver enzymes catalyze the addition of glutathione to the 1,2-epoxide to form a conjugate identical to that from naphthalene (Jerina *et al.,* 1970).

Biochemical Effects   Naphthalene was not hemolytic in human blood *in vitro* or in rabbits *in vivo.* The hemolytic power of naphthalene metabolites *in vitro* decreased in the order α-naphthol > β-naphthol > α-naphthoquinone > β-naphthoquinone. In rabbits, β-napthol was weakly hemolytic and β-naphthol and the quinones were inactive (Mackell *et al.,* 1951).

Effects on Organs and Tissues   Naphthalene gave negative results in *Salmonella* (McMann *et al.,* 1975) and *Escherichia coli* (Ho and Ho, 1981) when tested for mutagenic activity.

Effects on Reproduction   Naphthalene was not teratogenic in Sprague-Dawley rats when given at a dosage of 395 mg/kg/day by intraperitoneal injection on days 1–15 of gestation (Hardin *et al.,* 1981). No effect on postpartum survival was observed in

CD1 mice given 300 mg/kg/day *per os* on days 7–15 of gestation (Plasterer *et al.*, 1985).

14.6.3.3 Toxicity to Humans

Therapeutic Uses Naphthalene has been used as an anthelmintic, especially against *Oxyuris* (Sollman, 1957); see Dosage Response in this section.

Accidental and Intentional Poisoning Most naphthalene poisoning has occurred in children who found and sucked or chewed mothballs. The condition is characterized by hemolytic anemia, but nonspecific symptoms (headache, listlessness, anorexia, vomiting, diarrhea, and the gastrointestinal disturbances) generally appear before there is any objective evidence of hemolysis. Evidence for anemia includes pallor and many changes discussed under Laboratory Findings. Pain may be prominent or apparently absent. If present, it may be midabdominal at first but later have the distribution of urethral pain. Urination may be frequent and painful and later suppressed (Nash, 1903; Zuelzer and Apt, 1949). The liver and/or spleen may be palpable.

The greatest threat to life from naphthalene poisoning involves newborn infants, who may develop kernicterus from exposure to heavily treated clothing (Valaes *et al.*, 1963; Naiman and Kosoy, 1964).

Another complication may be blockage of kidney tubules with consequent oliguria and azotemia (MacGregor, 1954; Gidron and Leurer, 1956). Hemoglobin deposits have been noted in the kidney tubules at autopsy (Schafer, 1951). The possibility that kidney damage may persist and even progress after initial recovery is raised by a case listed by Hayes and Vaughn (1977). This involved a confused 85-year-old man who mistook mothballs for candy. He was hospitalized for gastroenteritis, albuminuria, and severe debility. The odor of naphthalene was noted on his breath, and the mothballs were found hidden in a drawer at home. Although the amount and duration of intake were unknown, it was thought he had consumed at least half a package over a period of 4–5 days. In 10 days he recovered enough to be sent home, but there he grew progressively weaker over a period of 10 days and, following 2 days of acute illness, he was readmitted. He was semicomatose and had many abnormal findings, including a blood urea nitrogen value of 98 mg %. It is of interest that his hemoglobin was normal. In spite of treatment, the patient's condition deteriorated, the azotemia increased, bronchopneumonia developed, and the patient died on the sixth hospital day. The massive dose and the slowness with which naphthalene is known to be excreted are what suggest the possibility of continuing kidney damage, but the patient's age and his general arteriosclerosis that had been recognized for several years make it uncertain whether to attribute the second illness directly to naphthalene.

A rare but interesting form of naphthalene poisoning has involved transplacental transfer of naphthalene or its oxidation products. In two instances young women developed the habit of sucking on mothballs during the last trimester of pregnancy.

Hemolytic anemia was discovered in one of them a few days before delivery and in the other in the course of studying her infant. No abnormality was noted in the babies at birth, but jaundice was noted in one after 7 hr and in the other on the third day. The mothers and babies recovered (Zinkham and Childs, 1958; Anziulewicz *et al.*, 1959).

At least four infants were poisoned by exposure to naphthalene vapor released into the air of their rooms by placing a cough remedy consisting of benzyl cinnamate, benzyl benzoate, camphor, naphthalene, and volatile oil into boiling water (Hanssler, 1964; Irle, 1964). In a larger number of cases exposure of infants was through clothing or bedclothes that had been stored with naphthalene (Schafer, 1951; Cock, 1957; Dawson *et al.*, 1958; Valaes *et al.*, 1963; Naiman and Kosoy, 1964; Grigor *et al.*, 1966). In some instances the poisoning was attributed to dermal absorption (Cock, 1957). Valaes *et al.* (1963) attributed absorption in such instances to inhalation of the vapor, the odor of which was evident from the clothing. Although they discounted the importance of dermal absorption, they offered no valid supporting evidence for doing so. The probable importance of dermal absorption in these instances was pointed out (Jacobziner and Raybin, 1964). In other cases it has been suggested that the application of oil to the skin promoted the absorption of naphthalene (Schafer, 1951).

When naphthalene was administered as a drug, very few patients experienced untoward effects. Much later it was found that one factor contributing to the high susceptibility of a few persons is an inherited deficiency of glucose-6-phosphate dehydrogenase (G-6-PD). This explains the greater susceptibility of males and of Oriental, Negro, or Mediterranean ethnic groups. However, as is true of hemolytic conditions caused by other agents influenced by G-6-PD, naphthalene has caused hemolysis in persons whose G-6-PD level was normal, but the condition tended to be milder in these normal people (Valaes *et al.*, 1963).

It must be recalled that acute hemolytic anemia may be caused in susceptible people by some drugs (notably primaquin) and some foods (notably fava beans); it also can occur without any demonstrable cause. Diagnosis of naphthalene poisoning therefore requires proof of adequate exposure.

Use Experience Exposure to concentrated naphthalene vapor may cause vomiting, optic neuritis, and hematuria, but no effects of prolonged industrial exposures have been reported. The ordinary use of naphthalene mothballs is safe also, even though odor of the vapor is perceptible. Danger from naphthalene is almost exclusively to children or others who eat mothballs or to babies whose clothing has been stored in naphthalene.

Atypical Cases of Various Origins A chronic scaling dermatitis, which gradually cleared each time the patient was hospitalized but recurred within a day or two each time he returned home, was attributed to naphthalene after direct testing indicated susceptibility. Following this insight, the man carefully avoided naphthalene and had had no further recurrence for 7 years when a report of the case was published (Fanburg, 1940).

Dosage Response Prochownik (1911) reported a fatal case of naphthalene poisoning but pointed out that he had previously used the drug without difficulty for 8 years as a treatment for oxyuriasis. The 6-year-old boy who died had taken seven of ten 250-mg powders, a total dosage of about 80 mg/kg, in the course of 2 days. It was pointed out that the dosage administered lay within the range recommended by some five authorities.

A 33-year-old woman became seriously ill after taking seven of eight 400-mg doses within 2 days, but she recovered. The total dosage was about 47 mg/kg (Heine, 1913). In a number of cases, patients who recovered were thought to have eaten a single mothball or part of one (Nash, 1903; Zuelzer and Apt, 1949). Mothballs now weigh about 2600 mg, and this may have been true in the past.

Persons who became ill after receiving naphthalene as therapy obviously were abnormally susceptible to it, and dosage–response data for such cases reflect this abnormal susceptibility and very likely an underlying deficiency of G-6-PD. In cases of suicide where no measurement of G-6-PD was made, the patients may have been genetically normal; in any event, Gidron and Leurer (1956) reported two attempted suicides with doses of 6,000 and 10,000 mg of naphthalene. One patient recovered and the other, perhaps because of treatment, did not become sick. For the 16-year-old girl, the dosage was about 113 mg/kg; in the other patient the dosage was not less than 140 mg/kg.

A typical dose of naphthalene formerly used to treat intestinal worms was 100–500 mg for adults and 50 mg for 1.5-year-old children, given three times a day for a total of 10 days (Prochownik, 1911; Sollman, 1957).

The threshold limit value (50 mg/m³) indicates that an occupational intake of 7 mg/kg/day is considered safe.

Laboratory Findings The most important metabolite of naphthalene in human urine is α-naphthol; β-naphthol and α- and β-naphthoquinone occur in smaller concentrations. The concentrations may be sufficient that the urine smells of naphthalene, a condition which may persist 12 days or more after ingestion stops (Mackell *et al.*, 1951).

Blood findings include a rapid fall in erythrocyte count, hemoglobin, and hematocrit followed by a temporary increase in reticulocytes and normoblasts in the peripheral blood. During a hemolytic crisis, the fragility of the remaining cells is increased. Oxyhemoglobin and methemoglobin are present in the plasma. Red cells may contain Heinz bodies and the cells may be fragmented. Icterus may develop. The urine may be wine-colored, brown, or black. The color may vary from patient to patient or during the course of illness. This is a direct indication of the complex nature of the breakdown products formed from hemoglobin.

In most but not all persons poisoned by naphthalene, a deficiency of G-6-PD can be demonstrated by suitable tests.

Treatment of Poisoning If poisoning is at all serious, the patient should receive one or more transfusions. Other treatment also is symptomatic.

A patient who had ingested naphthalene with suicidal intent and who was treated promptly with 100 mg of cortisone daily developed Heinz bodies and excreted naphthalene derivatives but did not become ill (Gidron and Leurer, 1956). The value of cortisone in naphthalene poisoning remains to be confirmed.

14.6.4 EPOXYETHANE

14.6.4.1 Identity, Properties, and Uses

Chemical Name 1,2-Epoxyethane.

Structure See Fig. 14.4.

Synonyms Epoxyethane (BSI) is also known commonly as ethylene oxide (ESA, ISO, JMAF). Other names include ETO, ETOX, EO, dihydrooxirene, dimethylene oxide, ethene oxide, ethylene (oxide D), oxane, and oxirane. Trade names include Amprolene®, Anprolene®, Anproline®, Oxyfume®, Oxyfume® 12, T-Gas®, and Carboxide®, a mixture of epoxyethane and carbon dioxide. The CAS registry number is 75-21-8.

Physical and Chemical Properties Epoxyethane has the empirical formula C_2H_4O and a molecular weight of 44.05. It is a colorless, flammable gas at room temperature. It has a density of 0.8969, a melting point of −113°C, and a boiling point of 10.4°C. Its vapor pressure is 1095 torr at 20°C. The odor threshold is 300 ppm in air (Amoore and Hautala, 1983). Epoxyethane is miscible with water and most organic solvents. The explosion limits are 3–100% by volume in air. It is relatively noncorrosive.

History, Formulations, and Uses Introduced as a pesticide in 1928, epoxyethane is an insecticidal fumigant for stored food products, bedding, carpets, and clothing. It also is used as an agricultural fungicide and to sterilize heat-sensitive medical devices.

To render epoxyethane nonflammable at all concentrations, at least 7.15 parts of carbon dioxide to 1 part epoxyethane are required. (Other components besides carbon dioxide may be used.) A ratio of 9 parts carbon dioxide to 1 part epoxyethane (such as Carboxide®) is a common formulation.

14.6.4.2 Toxicity to Laboratory Animals

Basic Findings The 4-hr inhalation LC 50 values were 2630 mg/m³ (1460 ppm) in rats, 1504 mg/m³ in mice, and 1730 mg/m³ in dogs (Jacobson *et al.*, 1956). Oral LD 50 values for epoxyethane administered as a 1% aqueous solution were 330 and 270 mg/kg in rats and guinea pigs, respectively (Smyth *et al.*, 1941). The compound was more toxic as a 10% solution in olive oil; 200 mg/kg killed all rats, but all survived 100 mg/kg. In fact, rats survived 15 doses in 21 days administered at a rate of 100 mg/kg/day, although this produced marked loss of body weight, gastric irritation, and slight liver damage. Rats that received 22 oral doses in 30 days at rates of 30 mg/kg/day or less showed no adverse effects as judged by growth, hematology, blood urea nitrogen, organ weight, and gross and microscopic morphology (Hollingsworth *et al.*, 1956a). When small cotton pads moistened with 10 or 50% aqueous solutions of epoxyethane were applied to the shaved skin of rabbits, hyperemia and edema resulted when the duration of skin contact was 6 min or more. The intensity of the response was roughly proportional to the concentration and length of the exposure. Exposures for only 60 min led to ulceration and eventual scarring (Hollingsworth *et al.*, 1956b).

Daily 7-hr inhalation exposures to 841 ppm epoxyethane were irritating to the respiratory tract of rats, guinea pigs, mice, rabbits, and a female monkcy. All animals died after eight or fewer exposures in 10 days. two or three days of exposure at this concentration produced pulmonary congestion, edema, and hemorrhage; fatty degeneration of the liver; cloudy swelling of the convoluted tubules in the kidney; and fatty vacuoles in the adrenal cortex of rats and guinea pigs. Growth was markedly depressed in rats, mice, rabbits, and monkeys exposed for 7 hr/day to 357 ppm epoxyethane; all mice were dead after 33 exposures and most of the rats after 42 exposures. Secondary respiratory infection was the main cause of these deaths. During the later portion of the study, some rats, rabbits, and monkeys developed a sensory and motor polyneuropathy confined to the hindquarters and leading to muscle atrophy. The polyneuropathy was completely reversible in these species, as determined by observation for 100 or more days after exposure stopped. Guinea pigs exposed to 357 ppm showed less pulmonary response than the other species and no neurological response. All survived 123 7-hr exposures at 357 ppm, but appreciable tubular degeneration and replacement with fibrosis were observed in the testis of male guinea pigs. Guinea pigs were essentially unaffected by repeated exposure to 204 ppm. Rats, mice, rabbits, and monkey eventually showed similar but milder effects, as they had shown at 357 ppm. Guinea pigs, rats, and monkeys tolerated 122 7-hr exposures to 113 ppm without injury, although a slight depression in growth and a moderate increase in lung weight were observed in the rats. Rats, mice, rabbits, and guinea pigs suffered no adverse effects of 127 7-hr exposures to 49 ppm epoxyethane, as judged by general appearance, behavior, mortality, growth, final body and organ weights, and gross and microscopic examination of the tissue (Hollingsworth *et al.*, 1956a).

In summary, epoxyethane is an irritant, a central nervous system depressant, and a protoplasmic poison. Sufficient exposure may cause deep anesthesia with respiratory arrest. Single or repeated exposure at lower concentrations may cause delayed death from lung edema, secondary respiratory infection, and/or kidney and liver injury.

Wistar rats exposed for 6 hr to 500 ppm epoxyethane three times a week for 13 weeks developed ataxia in the hind limbs. Axonal degeneration of mylenated fibers in the hind leg was observed in these rats with no involvement of the nerve cell body (Ohnishi *et al.*, 1985).

In mice exposed by inhalation for 5 hr/day, 5 days/week, for 10 weeks to 250, 100, 50, 10, or 0 ppm epoxyethane in air, clinical significant pathological findings were limited to the group exposed to 250 ppm. These findings included minimal decreases in red blood cell count, packed cell volume, and hemoglobin; decreased testicular and spleen weights; and increased liver weight. Abnormal pinch and righting reflexes, posture, and locomotion were also observed in mice exposed to 250 ppm. However, histological sections of the liver, testis, bone marrow, brain, and spleen taken from these mice were normal (Snellings *et al.*, 1984b).

The toxicity of food and other materials treated with epoxyethane may not be due to residues of the parent compound temporarily remaining after treatment; the injury may be entirely different from that produced by excessive exposure to the fumigant itself. This is illustrated by the appearance of fatal hemorrhagic diathesis among certain strains of male mice soon after starting to use bedding sterilized with epoxyethane. The condition could not be reproduced by the fumigant alone. However, it was shown that, at the temperature and pressure used for sterilization, epoxyethane reacted with water to form ethylene glycol and that the condition was reproduced to a large extent by ethylene glycol (Allen *et al.*, 1962). A similar hemorrhagic diathesis, confined almost entirely to males, occurred in another mouse colony when epoxyethane-treated bedding was used (Reyniers *et al.*, 1964).

Injury may be due in part to the destruction of an essential component of the diet rather than production of a toxicant. Thus, a treated diet that led to weight loss and death of rats was distinctly improved when supplemented with thiamine after sterilization (Hawk and Mickelsen, 1955). Many other investigations dealing with the production of toxicants or destruction of vitamins by epoxyethane were reviewed by Lindgren *et al.* (1968).

Most, if not all, injury to animals by epoxyethane-fumigated feed or bedding has followed treatment suitable for sterilization and is far in excess of treatments necessary for insect control. No change in appearance, behavior, growth, mortality, organ weights, and gross and microscopic morphology, compared to controls, was observed in a 2-year study in rats fed fumigated feed, in which the initial concentration of epoxyethane varied from 500 to 1900 ppm (Baer and Griepentrog, 1969).

Absorption, Distribution, Metabolism, and Excretion   Inhaled epoxyethane is well absorbed. The absorption of inhaled epoxyethane was limited by alveolar ventilation in resting rats (Filser and Bolt, 1984) and mice (Ehrenberg *et al.*, 1974). In mice, the highest concentrations of radioactivity were found in the liver and kidneys following a 75-min inhalation exposure to 2.2 ppm [^{14}C]epoxyethane. Concentrations of radioactivity in the testes, spleen, lungs, and brain were approximately equal to the level expected if [^{14}C]epoxyethane was evenly distributed in the body. The radioactivity was rapidly cleared from the tissue and eliminated in the urine. The biological half-life of epoxyethane was about 9 min. Most (90%) of the urinary radioactivity was excreted within 24 hr, and after 48 hr the urine accounted for 60–106% of the radioactivity estimated to have been absorbed (Ehrenberg *et al.*, 1974). The apparent volume of distribution for intravenously administered epoxyethane in the dog was between 0.8 and 1.0 liter/kg; this is consistent with epoxyethane being evenly distributed in the body water. The half-life for the disappearance of epoxyethane in the dog was approximately 30 min (Martis *et al.*, 1982).

Effects on Reproduction   Rats and rabbits were exposed to 150 ppm epoxyethane for 7 hr/day on days 1–16 or 7–16 of gestation. Maternal toxicity consisting of decreased body weight and increased spleen and kidney weights was observed in the rats. Evidence of fetotoxicity in rats consisted of reduced fetal body weight, crown–rump length, and ossification. No evidence of maternal or fetal toxicity was observed in rabbits, and no evidence of teratogenicity was observed in either rabbits or rats. An increased number of resorptions and a decreased number of corpora lutea were observed in female rats exposed to 150 ppm epoxyethane for 3 weeks prior to breeding and throughout gestation. These data led Hardin *et al.* (1983) to conclude that epoxyethane was fetotoxic but not teratogenic to rats and that it might impair reproductive potential by impairing oocyte maturation or ovulation. Snellings *et al.* (1982b) exposed rats for 6 hr/day to 100 ppm epoxyethane on days 6–15 of gestation and found that fetal body weights were reduced but that epoxyethane was neither lethal to embryos or fetuses nor teratogenic in the rat under these conditions.

In a one-generation study in which male and female rats were mated following 12 weeks of exposure (6 hr/day, 7 days/week) to 100, 33, or 10 ppm epoxyethane, the major effects observed were fewer pups per litter, fewer implantation sites per pregnant female, and fewer pups born per implantation site in rats exposed to 100 ppm epoxyethane. Compared to the controls, more of the rats in the 100-ppm exposure group had gestation periods that were longer than 22 days. No effects on the growth or survival of the pups during the lactational period were observed, even though the dams were exposed to epoxyethane during this period (Snellings *et al.*, 1982a). Exposure of male rats to 255 ppm (6 hr/day, 5 days/week) epoxyethane for 2 or 11 weeks prior to mating resulted in a significant reduction in number of live embryos, i.e., a positive dominant-lethal effect (Generoso *et al.*, 1983). By mating mice at various days after a 4-day exposure period it was demonstrated that the most sensitive period was 4.5–7.5 days postexposure, indicating that sperm in late spermatids to early spermatozoa were the most sensitive. The response was clearly nonlinear. The incidence of dominant lethals following four consecutive inhalation exposures for 6 hr/day was 62% at 500 ppm, 28% at 400 ppm, and a marginal 4% at 300 ppm epoxyethane. Short exposures to high concentrations were also more effective in inducing dominant lethals than longer exposures at lower concentrations; the incidences of dominant lethals were 76, 32, and 11% in mice exposed for 1.5

hr at 1200 ppm, 3 hr at 600 ppm, and 6 hr at 300 ppm, respectively (Generoso *et al.*, 1986).

Effects on Organs and Tissues   Epoxyethane is mutagenic in a variety of bacterial systems in both the presence and absence of an exogenous metabolic system, in *Drosophila melanogaster,* and in mammalian cells. It was positive in tests for unscheduled DNA synthesis (UDS), dominant lethal mutations, chromosomal abnormalities in bone marrow and peripheral lymphocytes, micronuclei, and sister chromatid exchange (SCE) [see International Agency for Research on Cancer (IARC), 1985].

Epoxyethane was found to increase the incidence of selected tumors in rats exposed by inhalation to 100, 33, 10, or 0 ppm in air for 6 hr/day, 5 days/week, for 2 years. Tumors increased in incidence by exposure to epoxyethane included mononuclear leukemia in females (58% at 100 ppm, 29% at 33 ppm, 20% at 10 ppm, and 8 and 11% in the two control groups) and males (30% at 100 ppm, 31% at 33 ppm, 18% at 10 ppm, and 10 and 16% in the two control groups), peritoneal mesothelioma in males (13, 10, 4, and 2% at 100, 33, 10, and 0 ppm, respectively), and primary brain tumors in females (8, 3, 0, and 2% at 100, 33, 10, and 0 ppm, respectively) and males (8, 4, 0, and 0% at 100, 33, 10, and 0 ppm, respectively) (Snellings *et al.*, 1984a). The same types of tumors had increased incidences in male rats exposed to 300 or 100 ppm epoxyethane in air 7 hr/day, 5 days/week, for 2 years (Lynch *et al.*, 1984). Interpretation of these studies is complicated by an outbreak of viral sialodacryoadenitis (Snellings *et al.*, 1984a) and *Mycoplasma pulmonis* (Lynch *et al.*, 1984) that led to increased early mortality among the rats exposed to epoxyethane.

Orally and subcutaneously administered epoxyethane increased the incidence of tumors at the site of administration. Twice-weekly oral doses for 107 weeks of epoxyethane dissolved in salad oil increased the number of squamous cell carcinomas of the forestomach in female rats. The incidences of stomach tumors in rats given 30 and 7.5 mg epoxyethane/kg and in the two control groups were 62, 16, 0, and 0%, respectively (Dunkelberg, 1982). Weekly subcutaneous injections for 95 weeks of epoxyethane dissolved in tricaprylin increased the number of local tumors, mostly fibrosarcomas, in female mice. The incidences of all subcutaneous sarcomas were 0% in controls; 2% in mice given tricaprylin alone; and 22, 16, and 5% in mice given 1, 0.3, and 0.1 mg epoxyethane/mouse, respectively (Dunkelberg, 1981). No increase in tumors was observed in a lifetime study involving thrice-weekly application of a 10% solution of epoxyethane in acetone (approximately 100 mg solution per application) to the clipped dorsal skin of mice (Van Duuren *et al.*, 1965).

Biochemical Effects   Sexton and Henson recognized in 1950 that the injury produced by epoxyethane was similar to that produced by mustard gases. Biochemically, epoxyethane behaves as a cytotoxic alkylating agent and it has been shown to become covalently bound to DNA and hemoglobin

(Segerback, 1983). The second-order rate constant for the reaction of epoxyethane with the histidine N-3 in hemoglobin (Hb) was determined to be 0.14×10^{-4} (gm Hb)$^{-1}$ hr^{-1} (Callemann *et al.*, 1978).

14.6.4.3 Toxicity to Humans

Experimental Exposure A total of 51 tests were carried out on eight volunteers who permitted concentrated epoxyethane or different aqueous solutions of it to be placed on small areas of their forearms for intervals of different durations. Exposure to 40–60% solutions for as little as 0.75–1.0 min produced second-degree burns. Stronger or weaker solutions required longer to produce the same effect. A 1% solution produced no effects after a 20–25-min exposure, first-degree burns when the exposure was for 50 or 60 min, and second-degree burns when the contact was for 75 min or more. The injury resembled that produced by mustard gases in several respects: a latent period before the appearance of erythema and vesication, the formation of large blebs, marked desquamation, and the formation of residual pigment. Undiluted epoxyethane produced no burns, but it rapidly evaporated when sprayed on the skin and produced an immediate painful frosting. The central area was pale and surrounded by a zone of erythema. An itching urticarial wheal developed over the entire injured area; the wheal disappeared within 4 hr, and the itching stopped spontaneously. There were no aftereffects. Three of the volunteers became sensitized to the chemical at points of previous contact; sensitization required 19–20 days to develop (Sexton and Henson, 1950).

Accidental and Intentional Poisoning The cases tabulated by Hayes and Pirkle (1966) involved a 65-year-old man who was trapped in a railroad car during fumigation with Carboxide®. He was not occupationally involved. Autopsy revealed acute pulmonary edema.

A 43-year-old female licensed practical nurse, while sterilizing heat-sensitive medical items, accidentally dropped and broke an ampule containing 17 gm epoxyethane. While disposing of the broken ampule, she began to experience nausea and stomach spasms. The exposure was estimated to have been of 2–3 min duration and not to have exceeded 500 ppm. Upon leaving the contaminated room, she became pale, lightheaded, and passed out for approximately 3–4 min. Convulsive movements of her arms and legs were noted during a 1-min period of apnea. She was given oxygen, began breathing, and awoke instantly without confusion or nausea. Approximately 3 min later she again felt nausea, stomach spasms, and lightheadedness and became apneic and passed out. Twitching of the extremities occurred and she was given oxygen again. Arterial blood gases, chest X rays, and routine laboratory measurements performed at that time were normal. A final convulsive episode milder than the previous ones occurred prior to discharge. During the 24 hr following discharge she continued to complain of random muscle twitches, nausea, and malaise.

She complained of malaise and inability to perform minor tasks for up to 2 weeks after discharge. A neurological evaluation conducted 3 weeks postexposure was normal, and at a 2-month follow-up the patient was asymptomatic without recurrence of any symptoms (Salinas *et al.*, 1981).

Four cases of epoxyethane toxicity were described that resulted from a leaking sterilizer in a hospital. The first individual had 3 weeks experience and worked up to 70 hr/week. He noted conjuctival and mucous membrane irritation and transient blunting of his senses of smell and taste. Near the end of a work shift he developed headache, nausea, vomiting, and lethargy, followed by recurrent major motor seizures at 20–30-min intervals. Between seizures he was febrile and responded with semipurposeful movements to deep pain. Brain scans, cerebral spinal fluid, and routine laboratory tests were normal. He continued to have convulsions during the first 2 days of hospitalization despite anticonvulsant therapy. Thereafter, he had no further seizures, he became afebrile, and his mental status rapidly cleared and was judged normal after 1 week.

A second operator had worked as a sterilizer for 2 years when he began to have headaches, acral numbness, limb weakness, and increased fatigability. His mentation and cranial nerve function were normal, but he had mild weakness of intrinsic hand and foot muscles, slow and clumsy alternating hand movements, heal–shin ataxia, and a wide-based unsteady gait. Vibratory sense was absent in the feet and decreased at the knees, hips, and sacrum. Pinprick sensation and sense of finger and toe joint position were slightly decreased. Ankle jerk reflex was absent and the muscle stretch reflex reduced. Changes in nerve conduction velocity, amplitude, and latency were compatible with generalized sensorimotor polyneuropathy.

The third individual had been an operator for 4 years when he began to have trouble with memory, thinking, fatigability, difficult swallowing, cramps, and numbness and weakness in the extremities. He became confused when giving his medical history and had slurred speech, mild bifacial weakness, clumsy alternating movement of the hands, heel–shin ataxia, and a wide-based gait. Vibratory sense was diminished at the toes, but joint position and pinprick sensation were normal. Muscle stretch reflex was absent at ankle, trace at knee, and decreased in upper extremities. Nerve conduction studies were compatible with a sensorimotor polyneuropathy. He reported that 3 years previously he had had similar symptoms that cleared spontaneously.

The fourth operator was asymptomatic, but motor and sensory nerve conduction velocities were compatible with a sensorimotor polyneuropathy. There was marked improvement of all subjective symptoms in 2 weeks after the exposure was terminated. Nerve conduction remained normal in the first operator but did not improve in operators three and four. Operator two took a position with no exposure to epoxyethane and his condition significantly improved. It was later determined that the sterilizer had been leaking for 3 weeks, and it was estimated that the epoxyethane concentration exceeded 700 ppm at times because the operators reported intermittently smelling epoxyethane (Gross *et al., 1979*).

The dermal effects of epoxyethane were illustrated by an accident at a new plant in which the hands, forearms, lower trunk, and legs of six men were drenched with a 1% aqueous solution of epoxyethane. It was warm, and because the men suspected no danger they simply removed their pants and continued to work in their shorts. Three of the men suffered nausea and vomiting 3–4 hr after the exposure and vesications on the wetted skin surfaces beginning 5 or more hours postexposure. Some of the blebs that developed were as large as lemons. Serous drainage was profuse, and healing required about 2 weeks. The other three men had no systemic symptoms and little or no dermatitis (Sexton and Henson, 1949).

A case was reported in which a patient developed erythema and vesicular lesions from contact with an oxygen mask sterilized with epoxyethane. Subsequent patch tests demonstrated that the patient was sensitive to epoxyethane and ethylene chloride but not to ethylene glycol or to a piece of the gas mask given longer to off-gas (Alomar *et al., 1981*).

Use Experience Evidence is accumulating that epoxyethane may be carcinogenic under conditions of exposure which were previously considered safe and in the absence of any recognized overexposure. Hogstedt *et al.* (1979) described a mortality study involving three cohorts: 89 production workers with full-time exposure, 86 maintenance workers with intermittent exposure, and 66 employees with no exposure to epoxyethane. Concentrations of epoxyethane in the plant were estimated to average 13.8, 6–28, and 0.6–6 ppm in 1941–1947, 1950–1963, and the 1970s, respectively. Overall mortality was increased (23/13.5) in the full-time exposure group but not the maintenance and nonexposed groups. The increased mortality in the full-time exposure group was due to increased incidences of leukemia (2/0.14), stomach cancer (3/0.4), and circulatory disease (12/6.3). Although not identified statistically, the nonexposed cohort also had a nearly twofold increase (6/3.5) in mortality due to circulatory disease. Morgan *et al.* (1981) described a retrospective cohort study involving 767 chemical workers at an outside production facility with estimated epoxyethane exposures of less than 10 ppm. Overall mortality and cancers of all types were lower than expected in this group; however, excesses of pancreatic cancer (3/0.8), brain and CNS cancer (2/0.7), and Hodgkin's disease (2/0.35) were noted, but no leukemia was observed. Thiess *et al.* (1981) described mortality in 602 former and current employees of an alkylene oxide production facility. Current exposures were less than 4 ppm, but records of treated cases of intoxication suggested that concentrations were considerably higher in the past. There was no increase in overall mortality, but the incidence of cancers of all types was slightly higher than expected (14/9.4) than in the in-plant cohort. In addition, the incidences of stomach (4/2.7) and brain (1/0.07) cancer and myeloid leukemia (1/0.15) were greater than expected. These studies suggest that there may be a casual relationship between exposure to epoxyethane and leuke-

mia (IARC, 1982), but because of their small size, uncertainties about the actual epoxyethane exposures, and concurrent exposure to other suspected carcinogens, additional epidemiology studies are needed.

An increased incidence of spontaneous abortions was found in staff members of about 80 Finnish hospitals who were involved in sterilizing instruments with epoxyethane. The adjusted rate of spontaneous abortions was 16.1% in the group exposed to epoxyethane during pregnancy, versus 7.8% if no epoxyethane exposure occurred during pregnancy. Exposure data are not available, but peak concentrations up to 250 ppm and 8-hr time-weighted average concentrations of 0.1–0.5 ppm have been measured in sterilizing units of many Finnish hospitals (Hemminki *et al., 1982*).

Increased incidences of sister chromatid exchanges (Stolley *et al., 1984*) and chromosome aberrations (Galloway *et al., 1986*) were observed in lymphocytes from individuals with occupational exposure to epoxyethane. The utility of these data is limited by the small number of individuals in the affected groups (two to six) and uncertainties about the magnitude of the exposures.

Biomonitoring The concentration of epoxyethane was determined in venous blood, alveolar air, and room air collected during and at the end of the work shift from ten individuals who operated a hospital sterilizer. The average concentrations of epoxyethane in the alveolar air and venous blood were 0.24 and 3 times the concentration in the room air. This suggests that 76% of the inhaled epoxyethane was retained. Thus an individual with an alveolar ventilation of 10 liters/min would absorb 7.0–7.3 mg of epoxyethane during an 8-hr exposure at the current TLV of 1 ppm (2 mg/m^3). In addition, concentrations of epoxyethane in alveolar air and venous blood should not exceed 0.4–0.5 and 6.6–8.5 μg/liter, respectively, if exposure is controlled within the current guideline of 1 ppm (Brugnone *et al., 1986*).

Air and blood analysis can be used to define the exposure at a particular point in time, but measuring alkylated amino acid residues in hemoglobin may provide a means of quantifying individual exposures integrated over a period of several months. Epoxyethane reacts with hemoglobin to form N-3-(2-hydroxyethyl) histidine, and individuals with weekly occupational exposures to epoxyethane in the range of 40–1560 ppm hr (i.e., exposure concentration × hours exposed) were found to have 2.6–14.3 nmol N-3-(2-hydroxyethyl) histidine/gm hemoglobin (Calleman *et al., 1978*). Larger amounts of N-3-(2-hydroxyethyl) histidine were found in the individuals with the larger exposures; however, the data were too variable to establish a quantitative relationship between exposure and amount of N-3-(2-hydroxyethyl) histidine bound to hemoglobin.

Dosage Response The threshold limit value of 1 ppm (2 mg/m^3) indicates that occupational exposure to 0.286 mg/kg/day is considered safe.

Treatment of Poisoning There are no specific antidotes and treatment is symptomatic. However, if high levels are inhaled, immediate hospitalization and observation for 72 hr for delayed onset of pulmonary edema are advisable.

14.7 HALOGENATED HYDROCARBON FUMIGANTS AND NEMATOCIDES

Chloropicrin was proposed as an insecticide in 1907. A number of other halogenated hydrocarbon fumigants were introduced and became well known before World War II. Narcosis is the primary toxic effect of this class of compounds. Several of them have been used as general anesthetics. Even the best general anesthetic has some side effects, often nausea, vomiting, and headache. These side effects usually appear as anesthesia wears off, or they may occur in the course of occupational or accidental exposure not sufficient to cause anesthesia.

Halogenated hydrocarbon fumigants that are too toxic to have been considered as anesthetics may have distinctly less narcotic action than the others but do have other, sometimes quite separate, toxic actions, including irritancy to the lung or injury to the liver, kidney, brain, or heart.

There is an apparent tendency for bromine-substituted hydrocarbon fumigants to be more toxic than the corresponding chlorine-substituted compounds. However, no safe generalization seems to be available. For reasons that remain obscure, a

slight chemical difference may determine a large difference in toxicity. For example, Klaassen and Plaa (1966, 1967) found 1,1,1-trichloroethane to be the least toxic and 1,1,2-trichloroethane to be the most toxic of seven compounds they studied in mice and dogs.

Some of the halogenated hydrocarbon fumigants commonly are employed as mixtures, either to take advantage of the combined insect toxicity of two or more compounds or, more generally, to take advantage of the high toxicity of one compound while rendering it nonflammable by mixing it with a less toxic but fire-suppressant compound. So far, none of the mixtures used has shown mammalian toxicity substantially different either quantitatively or qualitatively from what would be predicted from the toxicities of the constituents. The possibility that interaction between constituents might occur was specifically investigated in connection with three of the most widely used mixtures; although statistically significant potentiating effects were found, the differences were so small as to be of no practical importance from an industrial hygiene viewpoint (McCollister *et al.*, 1956).

The compounds discussed in the following sections are shown in Fig. 14.6. They are arranged with the small molecules first and the larger ones last.

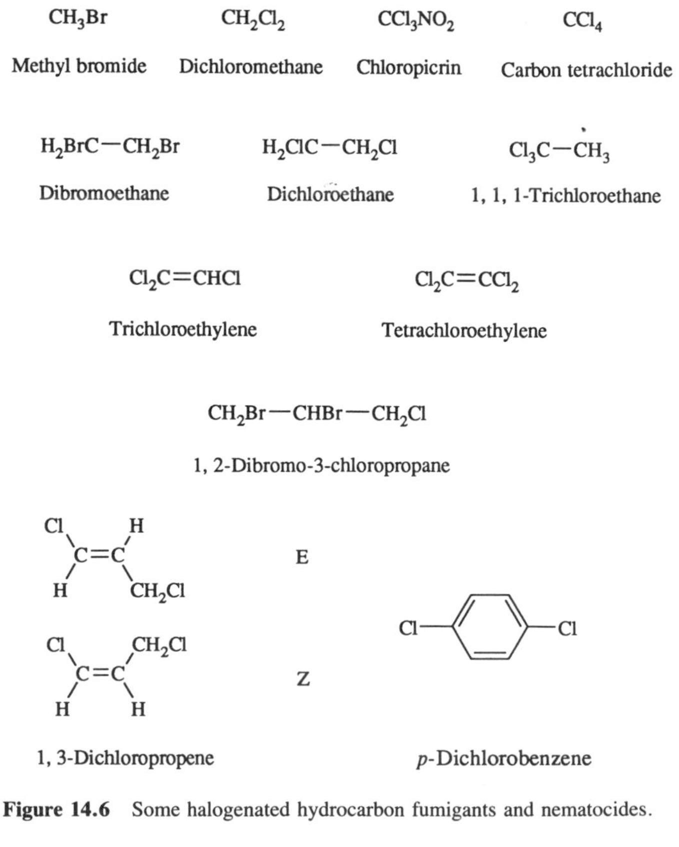

14.7.1 METHYL BROMIDE

14.7.1.1 Identity, Properties, and Uses

Chemical Name Bromomethane.

Structure See Fig. 14.6.

Synonyms Other names for methyl bromide are MBX and monobromoethane. Trade names include Dowfume MC-2®, Dowfume MC-2® Soil Fumigant, Dowfume MC-33®, and Embafume®. The CAS registry number is 74-83-9.

Physical and Chemical Properties Methyl bromide has the empirical formula CH_3Br and a molecular weight of 94.95. It is a colorless gas with a burning taste and a sweet chloroform-like odor at high concentrations. It is nonflammable in air but does burn in oxygen. Methyl bromide has a melting point of $-93.6°C$ and a boiling point of $3.56°C$. The vapor pressure at 20°C is 1420 mm Hg. The solubility in water at 20°C is 1.75 gm/100 gm. Methyl bromide is freely soluble in alcohol, chloroform, ether, carbon disulfide, carbon tetrachloride, and benzene. It is stable and noncorrosive.

History and Use Methyl bromide was introduced as an insecticide in 1932. It is used widely as a fumigant for all types of dry foodstuffs, especially produce contained in bags or packages. It is used in mills, warehouses, ships, and freight cars. It is a soil fumigant used in greenhouses and fields for control of nematodes, fungi, and weeds. Methyl bromide is mixed with ethylene dibromide and carbon tetrachloride when

Figure 14.6 Some halogenated hydrocarbon fumigants and nematocides.

it is applied to large, unencased bulk produce, but this use is limited.

14.7.1.2 Toxicity to Animals

Basic Findings The acute toxicity of methyl bromide vapor was first evaluated by Sayers *et al.* (1929) in guinea pigs and later by Irish *et al.* (1940) in rats and rabbits. These early studies defined the lung and the nervous system as target organs. The lung injury was characterized by irritation, edema, and resultant bronchial pneumonia. Straight-line relationships were observed when log concentration was plotted against log time for immediately fatal, delayed fatal, and tolerated exposures. Guinea pigs that died during exposure to high concentrations of methyl bromide fell on their sides, struggled to breathe, and died quickly. Those exposed to lower concentrations for 4 hr showed delayed weakness, rapid pulse, roughened fur, and signs of lung irritation and pneumonia; they died sometimes several days after exposure (Sayers *et al.*, 1929).

Steep dosage–response relationships characterize the toxicity of methyl bromide. All rabbits given an oral dose of 63.9 mg/kg died, whereas all those receiving 56.1 mg/kg or less survived (Dudley *et al.*, 1940). For rats exposed to methyl bromide vapor for 8 hr, 100% survival and 100% lethality occurred at approximately 240 and 470 ppm, respectively (Irish *et al.*, 1940). Consistent with this observation, an 8-hr LC 50 (and 95% confidence limits) of 302 (267–340) ppm has been reported by Honma *et al.* (1985). Severe hemorrhage was noted in the lungs of dead rats. Following exposure of mice to methyl bromide vapor for 1 hr, little evidence of substantial pulmonary lesions was observed, the nervous system appeared to be affected only at lethal concentrations, and the liver was the primary target organ (Alexeeff *et al.*, 1985). The 1-hr LC 50 for mice was determined in this study to be approximately 1200 ppm, with the LC 10 and LC 90 range contained within a doubling of the exposure concentration.

The neurotoxic effects of methyl bromide are striking. Central neuronal degeneration has been reported in mice and rats exposed to 160 ppm methyl bromide for up to 30 exposures (Eustis *et al.*, 1986). Hurtt *et al.* (1986) also reported cerebellar and cerebral neuronal degeneration in rats exposed to 175–325 ppm methyl bromide 6 hr/day for 5 days. Significantly lower levels of norepinephrine have been observed in various brain regions of rats exposed to 100 ppm methyl bromide for 24 hr or to 10 ppm for 3 weeks continuously (Honma *et al.*, 1982). No evidence of neurotoxic effects was observed by Anger *et al.* (1981) in rats exposed for 36 weeks to 55 ppm or for 4 weeks to 65 ppm methyl bromide (6–7.5 hr/day, 4–5 days/week).

Rabbits appear more sensitive than rats to the neurotoxic effects of methyl bromide. Decreased eyeblink reflex and hind limb paralysis associated with decreased sciatic and ulnar nerve conduction velocities were observed in rabbits exposed for 4 weeks to 65 ppm methyl bromide (Anger *et al.*, 1981). Only partial recovery was observed in these rabbits 6–8 weeks after cessation of exposure (Russo *et al.*, 1984). In contrast, no detrimental effects were observed on the nervous system of

rabbits exposed to 27 ppm methyl bromide, 7.5 hr/day, 4 days/week, for 8 months (Russo *et al.*, 1984).

Absorption, Distribution, Metabolism, and Excretion

The disposition of [^{14}C]methyl bromide has been evaluated in rats by several investigators after oral and ip administration (23.7 mg/kg) or inhalation exposure (1.6–310 ppm for 6–8 hr) (Medinsky *et al.*, 1984, 1985; Bond *et al.*, 1985; and Honma *et al.*, 1985). Methyl bromide is extensively metabolized and rapidly eliminated. Following oral or inhalation exposure, 75–85% of the body burden was eliminated by rats 65–72 hr postexposure. Depending on the route of exposure, 30–50% of the absorbed methyl bromide was recovered as ^{14}CO$_2$, 16–40% was recovered as metabolized methyl bromide in the urine, and only 4–20% was recovered in the expired air as parent compound. Medinsky *et al.* (1984) observed extensive biliary excretion of ^{14}C activity as indicated by the fact that 46% of the dose was recovered in bile within 24 hr following oral administration of [^{14}C]methyl bromide. However, subsequent reabsorption was observed, resulting in only 2% of the dose being recovered in the feces over the 72-hr postexposure collection interval.

Major organs of distribution of radioactivity observed immediately after exposure include fat, lung, liver, adrenals, and kidney; concentrations of one-third to one-tenth less were found in the brain (Bond *et al.*, 1985; Honma *et al.*, 1985). More than 90% of the tissue radioactivity was attributed to metabolized methyl bromide. Tissue clearance half-lives ranged from approximately 0.5 hr (Honma *et al.*, 1985) to approximately 1.5–8 hr (Bond *et al.*, 1985). While glutathione conjugation was indicated by reduced concentrations of glutathione or nonprotein sulfhydryls in the liver of rodents exposed to methyl bromide (Roycroft *et al.*, 1981; Alexeeff *et al.*, 1985), distinct conjugates have not been identified to date.

Honma *et al.* (1985) explored the relationship between methyl bromide metabolism and CNS toxicity. Time course studies of methyl bromide, bromine, and methanol indicate that the observed CNS toxicity is probably not attributable to the methyl bromide hydrolysis products bromine and methanol, but rather to the alkyl halide molecule itself. These observations are consistent with the data and hypotheses of Irish *et al.* (1940) and Kolb *et al.* (1952).

Biochemical Effects Methyl bromide reacts *in vitro* with a number of SH enzymes and causes progressive and irreversible inhibition (Lewis, 1948). Winteringham *et al.* (1958) concluded that, at least in houseflies, the biochemical picture was not consistent with SH enzyme inhibition as an explanation of death. Interestingly, they found that initial immobilization of flies was apparently due to a reversible breakdown of ATP and that temporary recovery was associated with a return toward normal levels of ATP. The later collapse and death of the flies were not accompanied by renewed breakdown of ATP and remained unexplained.

Whereas the relation of the inhibition of SH enzymes to the toxicity of methyl bromide remains obscure, there can be no doubt that the action of methyl bromide is chemical as distinct from physical. In view of the vapor pressure of the compound, the concentration necessary to kill 50% of a population of the grain weevil *Calandra granaria* indicated that the thermodynamic activity was only 0.0004 (Ferguson and Pirie, 1948).

Effects on Organs and Tissues The carcinogenic potential of methyl bromide has not yet been thoroughly evaluated. Squamous cell carcinoma was observed in 13 of 20 rats receiving 50 mg methyl bromide/kg body weight by gavage for 90 days (Danse *et al.*, 1984). However, this response was accompanied by severe gastric toxicity due to the reactivity of methyl bromide and was characterized by ulceration, diffuse epithelial hyperplasia, and hyperkeratosis of the forestomach. Although methyl bromide has been positive in several genetic toxicity test systems and negative in others, it is considered to have low mutagenic potency (Djalali-Behzad *et al.*, 1981; Kramers *et al.*, 1985; McGregor, 1981; Simmon *et al.*, 1977). Thus, in spite of the potential initiating activity of methyl bromide, Danse *et al.* (1984) conclude that cellular injury and compensatory hyperplasia probably play a predominant role in the observed tumorigenic response and that the risk of cancer from subpromotional doses is very small.

Effects on Reproduction Methyl bromide was not teratogenic to rats exposed to 20 or 70 ppm for 7 hr/day, 5 days/week, for 3 weeks prior to mating and daily through gestation day 19 (Hardin *et al.*, 1981). In the same study, rabbits exposed to 70 ppm methyl bromide showed severe neurotoxicity and mortality. However at 20 ppm, no maternal toxicity, fetotoxicity, or teratogenic effects were elicited.

Treatment of Poisoning in Animals In a study of rats, mice, and rabbits that had been exposed to LD 50 doses of methyl bromide, cysteine had not only a prophylactic effect but also a therapeutic effect when administered subcutaneously within 30 min after poisoning (Mizyukova and Bakhishev, 1971). In both mice and rabbits, glutathione was slightly more effective than BAL when both were given before an otherwise fatal respiratory exposure to methyl bromide; at a dosage of 750 mg/kg, glutathione prevented death in all mice tested (Ueda and Kaai, 1971; Kawai and Ueda, 1972). However, Edson, as quoted by Winteringham and Barnes (1955), reported that BAL was useless when administered to rats already poisoned by methyl bromide.

14.7.1.3 Toxicity to Humans

Accidental and Intentional Poisoning Von Oettingen (1955) tabulated 47 fatal and 206 nonfatal cases of poisoning by methyl bromide arising mainly from its manufacture or from its use as a fumigant or as a fire-extinguishing fluid. Use as a fumigant led to 11 of the fatal and 44 of the nonfatal cases. More recent cases associated with fumigation have been reported by Rathus and Landy (1961), Drawneek *et al.* (1964), Collins (1965), Brodniewicz (1967), Hine (1969), Araki *et al.* (1971), Takahashi *et al.* (1973), Nakakita (1973), Garcia Rico *et al.* (1974),

Toyonaga and Tokuda (1976), Ushio and Osotsuka (1977a,b), Shield *et al.* (1977), Takayama and Numajiri (1979), Zatuchni and Hong (1981), Marraccini *et al.* (1983), and Behrens and Dukes (1986).

High concentrations of methyl bromide can produce rapid unconsciousness during exposure, leading to a prompt "anesthetic" death (Garcia Rico *et al.*, 1974). However, anesthesia plays no part in the great majority of cases, which are characterized by delayed onset, a great variety of symptoms, and delayed recovery, if death does not occur. The delay in onset usually is several hours, but a delay of only a few minutes (Araki *et al.*, 1971) and a delay of 48 hr have been observed. In fatal cases with delayed onset, death generally occurs within 4–6 hr but sometimes after 24–48 hr. In rare instances, death may be delayed as much as 18 days (Davay, 1972). The cause of death in these cases usually is circulatory failure.

The most common initial symptoms in fatal or nonfatal cases with delayed onset are malaise, headache, visual disturbances, nausea, and vomiting. Later, a great variety of central nervous system manifestations appear, including numbness, ataxia, tremor, myoclonus, exaggerated (or absent) deep reflexes, positive Romberg's sign, paroxysmal abnormalities of the EEG, great agitation, change of personality, coma, and clonic, tonic (often Jacksonian) convulsions. Whereas convulsions generally occur in fatal cases (and many nonfatal ones too), death usually is the result of pulmonary edema leading to respiratory failure or cardiovascular collapse.

When death does not intervene, recovery may occur in a few days or hospitalization may be required for many weeks and the patient may be left with gross, permanent disability (Rathus and Landy, 1961; Ohsawa *et al.*, 1978).

There is no reason to doubt that dermal exposure can produce systemic illness, and severe illness occurred in a case involving gross contamination of the skin (Longley and Jones, 1965). However, the occurrence of severe systemic illness without significant respiratory involvement is no proof of a lack of respiratory exposure; such cases have occurred when exposure was exclusively respiratory (Shield *et al.*, 1977).

Use Experience What has been said about accidents emphasizes the very real hazard of using methyl bromide as a fumigant.

The early literature contains accounts of similar cases associated with manufacturing. One form of injury—that is, the formation of large blisters by direct toxic action of methyl bromide on the skin—has occurred from industrial exposure (Watrous, 1942). This effect generally occurs only when evaporation is retarded and is especially likely following prolonged exposure to contaminated clothing and shoes, including rubber articles. Blistering apparently has not resulted from fumigation.

A number of deaths and other serious poisonings caused by methyl bromide used as a fumigant involved leakage of the gas from the space being treated into an occupied work or other area where no warning had been posted (State of California, 1958; Hine, 1969).

Neurobehavioral deficits have been suggested in California soil and structural fumagators using methyl bromide (Anger *et al.*, 1986). However, implications with respect to low-level exposure (≤2.3 ppm, 1.5–8 hr/day) are tenuous due to questions regarding the extent of prior exposure and appropriateness of the available control cohort.

Dosage Response   Partly because most cases of poisoning by methyl bromide have involved respiratory exposure, there apparently is no information on the dosages involved. The threshold limit value (5 ppm; 20 mg/m³) would permit an occupational exposure of about 2.9 mg/kg/day.

Laboratory Findings   Hine (1969) reported blood bromide levels of 400 and 250 ppm in two fatal cases. Patients who presented with severe, moderate, and mild symptoms had blood levels of 220, 180, and 120 ppm, respectively. Blood bromide on hospital admission may be as low as 24 ppm or as high as 400 ppm in nonfatal cases (Rathus and Landy, 1961). In an extremely severe but nonfatal case, the serum level was 328 ppm and the urinary level 296 ppm (Ushio and Osotsuka, 1977b). Finally, a serum bromide level of 550 ppm was found in a man who suffered repeated epileptic convulsions and, after partial recovery, was left with disabling, unilateral nerve involvement (Longley and Jones, 1965).

An average urinary bromide concentration of 23 ppm was found in people working in an atmosphere containing methyl bromide at a bromide concentration of 4–5 ppm. This was not associated with symptoms (Momotani *et al.*, 1976).

According to Drawneek *et al.* (1964), serum bromide levels over 50 ppm may, in the absence of any illness, be accompanied by mild euphoria leading to carelessness in the handling of methyl bromide.

Among workers exposed for a few months to 11 years, subjective symptoms could not be related to blood bromine levels in the range 4–23 ppm. However, slight electroencephalographic changes and a small increase in serum transaminase levels were related to these bromide concentrations (Verberk *et al.*, 1979).

Methyl bromide itself can be measured in expired air, and the gas chromatographic method is sensitive to 6 ppm in air. Unfortunately, human data obtained by this method are not available (Stewart, 1974). Presumably, the same chromatographic method could also be applied to blood samples. However, the only common measurement is for inorganic bromide derived metabolically from the organic compound. This measurement is meaningful insofar as exposure to more than minimal amounts of preformed inorganic bromides can be excluded. Bromides occur naturally in soil and in food. A blood bromine level of 50 ppm may be considered normal. However, any increase above this level due to absorption of methyl bromide is an indication of potentially hazardous exposure from which the person must be withdrawn immediately. Yet volunteers who took a full dosage (5 doses/day) of a popular bromide headache remedy reached blood bromide levels of approximately 50 ppm after 1 day and 270–310 ppm after 7 days.

When dosage was stopped, blood levels fell promptly but only gradually; the average was 70 ppm 24 days after the last dose. It was estimated that blood bromide levels of 700–800 ppm are not uncommon among those who habitually use bromide headache remedies. When inorganic bromides are prescribed, blood levels greater than 1000 ppm were achieved regularly and levels of 1500 ppm usually did not cause concern (Gay, 1962).

Treatment of Poisoning   Treatment is symptomatic.

In a poisoned man suffering from action myoclonus, the condition was controlled by diazepam (60 mg/day). However, because of severe somnolence, the treatment was changed to clonazepam at 3–4 mg/kg. This treatment was effective; the somnolence disappeared, and the myoclonus decreased conspicuously (Toyonaga and Tokuda, 1976). Clonazepam produced mild improvement in another case with action myoclonus (Shield *et al.*, 1977). Although BAL has been used for treating methyl bromide poisoning (Rathus and Landy, 1961), there is no evidence that it was beneficial. Treatment of a poisoning case with acetylcysteine was concluded to be not harmful and possibly beneficial (Zatuchni and Hong, 1981).

14.7.2 DICHLOROMETHANE

14.7.2.1 Identity, Properties, and Uses

Chemical Name   Dichloromethane.

Structure   See Fig. 14.6.

Synonyms   Dichloromethane also is known as methylene chloride, methylene bichloride, and methylene dichloride. The CAS registry number is 75-09-2.

Physical and Chemical Properties   Dichloromethane has the empirical formula CH_2Cl_2 and a molecular weight of 84.94. It is a colorless liquid with a density of 1.3255 at 20°C. It solidifies at −95°C and boils at 39.75°C. It is about 2% soluble in water and miscible with alcohol, ether, and dimethylformamide. The vapor is nonflammable and nonexplosive.

Use   Fruit-ripening agent.

14.7.2.2 Toxicity to Laboratory Animals

Basic Findings   Rats of different ages showed relatively little difference in susceptibility to dichloromethane, compared with the corresponding differences for some other solvents. The oral LD 50 values for 14-day-old rats, young adults, and older adults were 2385, 2120, and 3047 mg/kg, respectively (Kimura *et al.*, 1971). A rabbit that received dichloromethane subcutaneously at a rate of 2700 mg/kg died; a few that received smaller doses survived. Dogs that received dichloromethane orally at doses of 3000 mg/kg or greater died, whereas the few that received doses of 2750 mg/kg or less survived. Small numbers of dogs were killed by an intravenous dosage of 200 mg/kg but others survived 175 mg/kg or less (Barsoum and Saad, 1934).

The intraperitoneal LD 50 in mice was 1990 mg/kg (Klaassen and Plaa, 1966).

Reported LC 50 values for a standard 7–8-hr exposure in mice range from 8000 to 15,000 ppm (Svirbely *et al.*, 1947; von Oettingen *et al.*, 1949).

The potential for dichloromethane to produce renal or hepatic injury on acute or subacute exposure is low (Plaa and Larson, 1965; Gehring, 1968; Condie *et al.*, 1983). The time required to produce hepatic injury as determined by a significant SGPT elevation, upon acute exposure to 13,500 ppm dichloromethane vapor, exceeded the time to produce anesthesia and was similar to that producing death (Gehring, 1968). When administered in the lethal range, dichloromethane did produce some renal histological change, characterized by hydropic degeneration with minimal necrosis of the convoluted tubules (Klaassen and Plaa, 1966).

Two of four dogs showed slight to moderate fatty degeneration of the liver following six 4-hr exposures at a concentration of 9800 ppm, which caused slight to moderate narcosis during exposure. Guinea pigs also developed liver injury after repeated exposure. Rats, rabbits, and monkeys did not develop liver injury when exposed to the same concentration 4 hr/day, 5 days/week, for 7.5 weeks. However, some rats and rabbits died of acute pulmonary edema. Guinea pigs grew slowly, but rats, rabbits, and dogs showed no adverse effect when exposed to 4885 ppm 7 hr/day, 5 days/week, for 6 months. The possibility of liver damage was studied with particular care in the dogs, but no evidence of such injury was found (Heppel *et al.*, 1944).

Although an air concentration of 2450 ppm had no depressant effect on young male rats as judged by ordinary inspection, it greatly diminished their running activity during exposure as measured by a standard revolving drum (Heppel and Neal, 1944).

Depressed motor activity and REM sleep at 5000 and 1000 ppm dichloromethane vapor, respectively, as well as decreased peripheral nerve conduction velocity after injection of dichloromethane, have been reported in rats by Winneke (1981).

Repeated application of dichloromethane to the ears of rabbits caused hyperemia followed by scaly exfoliation (Heppel *et al.*, 1944).

Installation of dichloromethane directly into eyes of rabbits produced inflammation of the conjunctiva and eyelid which persisted for 2 weeks, keratitis and iritis, and a 59% increase in corneal thickness at 6 hr which returned to normal by 9 days (Ballantyne *et al.*, 1976).

Absorption, Distribution, Metabolism, and Excretion The concentration of dichloromethane in the blood of rabbits just after 1 hr of exposure to vapor at a level of 10,000 ppm ranged from 87 to 171 ppm (Heppel *et al.*, 1944).

In dogs subjected to anesthesia for 7 hr at a concentration of 15,000 ppm, the blood level approached a steady state (430

ppm) within 1.5–2 hr; the highest level reached temporarily by any dog within the 7-hr exposure period was 566 ppm. Dogs exposed to 40,000 ppm died soon after reaching blood levels of 620–940 ppm and without reaching a steady state (von Oettingen *et al.*, 1949).

Two pathways have been associated with the metabolism of dichloromethane. The mixed-function oxidase (MFO) pathway involves an initial oxidative dehalogenation of dichloromethane by cytochrome P-450, resulting in the production of carbon monoxide (CO) and chloride ion (Kubic and Anders, 1975, 1978) as well as appreciable amounts of CO_2 (Gargas *et al.*, 1986; Reitz *et al.*, 1986) via the proposed intermediate formyl chloride. A second metabolic pathway is localized in the cytosol, is catalyzed without consumption of glutathione, is dependent on glutathione transferase, and produces CO_2 and chloride ion via the proposed intermediates formaldehyde and formic acid (Ahmed and Anders, 1976, 1978). Disposition studies in the rat confirmed the saturable nature of the MFO pathway (McKenna and Zempel, 1981; McKenna *et al.*, 1982). Gargas *et al.* (1986) have characterized the MFO pathway as high affinity, low capacity and the cytosolic pathway as low affinity, high capacity. Thus, metabolism via the MFO pathway will predominate at subsaturating concentrations. The MFO pathway is thought to involve detoxication, whereas the cytosolid pathway appears to be associated with intoxication (Andersen *et al.*, 1987; Green and Purchase, 1987). The development of a physiologically based pharmacokinetic model allows for determinations of internal doses to target tissues across species and routes of exposure (Andersen *et al.*, 1987).

Overall, dichloromethane is extensively distributed in the rat, with highest concentrations observed in fat, brain, liver, kidneys, and adrenal tissue (Carlson and Hultengren, 1975; DiVincenzo and Hamilton, 1975). A half-life of elimination from the blood of rats of approximately 15 min has been reported by McKenna *et al.* (1982). No observable changes in pharmacokinetics resulted from repeated oral dosing of rats and mice for 2 weeks (Angelo *et al.*, 1986a,b).

Pharmacological Effects Von Oettingen *et al.* (1949) made an extremely thorough clinical study of dichloromethane in dogs both at an anesthetic concentration and at a level that was fatal in 90–300 min. Anesthesia was of poor quality. A concentration of 15,000 ppm, which eliminated the corneal reflex in about 26 min and produced complete muscular relaxation in 32 min, continued to produce frequent tremors, walking movements, twitching, and rhythmic contractions of the diaphragm. Even at this anesthetic concentration, while respiration, heart rate, and arterial blood pressure were stable, there was a moderate increase in venous blood pressure during the last 3 hr of a 7-hr exposure, suggesting some depression of cardiac muscle. Regarding the fatal level of exposure, it was concluded that the fall in arterial blood pressure, rise in venous pressure, and slowing of the heart were probably due to depression of the medullary centers and later depression of the cardiac muscle. Respiratory depression involved the medullary centers at first, but later there was a temporary hypoxic stimulation when circulatory failure already was well advanced. The heart usually stopped before the respiration.

Biochemical Effects   The fact that dichloromethane is metabolized in part to carbon monoxide was discovered in humans and later confirmed in several experimental animal species. Other solvents (methyl, ethyl, and isopropyl alcohols and toluene) inhibited the formation of carboxyhemoglobin in rats and monkeys exposed to dichloromethane, but in some instances the inhibition was manifest only when the solvents were given intraperitoneally. No evidence of potentiation of the formation of carboxyhemoglobin was found (Ciuchta et al., 1979).

Effects on Organs and Tissues   The chronic toxicity of dichloromethane has been evaluated in rats, hamsters, and mice. Studies in rats include inhalation of dichloromethane at concentrations ranging from 50 to 4000 ppm 6 hr/day, 5 days/week, for 2 years (Burek et al., 1984; NTP, 1986a; Nitschke et al., 1988a), as well as consumption of dichloromethane in the drinking water for 2 years at concentrations corresponding to 0, 5, 50, 125, and 250 mg/kg/day (Serota et al., 1986a). An increase in the normally high spontaneous incidence of benign mammary gland tumors in female (and to a lesser extent male) rats have been observed at concentrations of 500 ppm and greater. No progression toward malignancy has been observed in the mammary tissue. A low but statistically significant increase in a variety of ventral neck region sarcomas, in and around the salivary glands of male rats only, was observed at 3500 ppm, with a trend at 1500 ppm (Burek et al., 1984). This finding was not confirmed in other studies in rats, mice, or hamsters. Dichloromethane was not tumorigenic in rats exposed via the drinking water (Serota et al., 1986a). A no-observed-effect level for chronic toxicity has been reported to be 200 ppm dichloromethane vapor (Nitschke et al., 1988a).

No toxicologic or oncogenic effects were observed in hamsters exposed via inhalation to concentrations of dichloromethane as high as 3500 ppm (Burek et al., 1984).

Increased incidences of spontaneous lung and liver tumors were reported in male and female B6C3F1 mice exposed to 0, 2000, or 4000 ppm dichloromethane 6 hr/day, 5 days/week, for 2 years (NTP, 1986a). Exposure of this strain to dichloromethane in the drinking water for 2 years at a concentration of 0, 60, 125, 185, or 250 mg/kg/day did not result in a tumorigenic response (Serota et al., 1986b).

Dichloromethane has been found to be weakly mutagenic in microorganisms and has been associated with the induction of chromosomal aberrations at high concentrations in cell culture. In contrast, dichloromethane has produced largely negative results in other mammalian cell systems in vitro as well as in whole-animal assays. These studies have been reviewed by Broome and Sivac (1987) and Green and Purchase (1987).

Pulmonary injury, characterized by Clara cell damage, and a hepatostimulatory effect have been observed after acute exposure to tumorigenic concentrations of dichloromethane in

B6C3F1 mice, but not in rats (Green et al., 1986a; Eisenbrandt and Reitz, 1986). Since dichloromethane does not appear to be directly genotoxic in vivo but does produce altered homeostasis in the lung and liver of the mice, tissues susceptible to spontaneous tumor development, it is probable that dichloromethane affects a later stage of the tumorigenic process. Review of the mechanistic and pharmacokinetic data for dichloromethane (Greene and Purchase, 1987) indicates a very low likelihood that this material poses a carcinogenic threat to humans under current use conditions.

Effects on Reproduction   No teratogenic effects have been noted in pregnant rats (Hardin and Manson, 1980) or rats and mice (Schwetz et al., 1975) exposed to 4500 and 1250 ppm dichloromethane vapor during gestation, respectively. Exposure of rats to inhaled concentrations of dichloromethane as high as 1500 ppm for 6 hr/day did not affect any reproductive parameters over two generations (Nitschke et al., 1988b).

14.7.2.3 Toxicity to Humans

Experimental Exposure   Each of four volunteers who immersed one thumb in methylene chloride for 30 min noted a mild burning sensation within 5–10 min. The sensation reached its maximum, described as mild to moderate, in 15–20 min. After thumbs were withdrawn from the solvent, the burning continued without decrease for about 10 min before gradually subsiding within 1 hr. The marked edema present after exposure subsided within 1–2 hr. Evidence for dermal absorption of the compound by these people is discussed under Laboratory Findings (Stewart and Dodd, 1964).

Four other volunteers inhaled dichloromethane from accurately measured atmospheres using a mouthpiece equipped with valves that permitted continuous measurement of the vapor in the expired air, both during and after exposure. Respiratory absorption and respiratory excretion each consisted of segments which were attributed to equilibration of the dead space of the lung with the atmosphere, equilibration of alveolar air with the blood, equilibration of the blood with aqueous body tissues, and equilibration of these tissues with body fat (Riley et al., 1966).

In yet another study (Stewart et al., 1972a,b), 11 healthy men inhaled dichloromethane vapor at concentrations of approximately 500 and 1000 ppm for 1 or 2 hr. Again, the analytical findings concerning the expiration of the solvent and its metabolism to carbon monoxide are discussed under Laboratory Findings. None of the volunteers developed any symptom or sign of intoxication when exposed for an hour to an average concentration of 514 ppm, but this exposure did cause a change in the visual evoked response that was considered indicative of a change in sensory processes consistent with early CNS depression. Exposure to 868 ppm (following 1 hr of 514 ppm) promptly caused lightheadedness in some persons that persisted for the remainder of the 1-hr exposure and 5 min after the end of exposure.

Therapeutic Use According to a well-documented review by Gwathmey and Baskerville (1914), dichloromethane was introduced as a general anesthetic in 1867 by Richardson. He reported that the vapor was pleasant to inhale and not irritating. Anesthesia was rapid with a short but rather severe spasmodic stage. Insensibility was perfect and recovery rapid and usually without bad symptoms. However, although one physician used it 1800 times without a single accident, some others were not so fortunate. By 1914 it was considered not to be a safe anesthetic.

Accidental and Intentional Poisoning Apparently no poisoning has been reported as a result of the use of dichloromethane as an agricultural chemical. An industrial accident reported by Moskowitz and Shapiro (1952) indicates the kind of illness excessive exposure is likely to produce. The accident occurred in a factory where an oleoresin was extracted from plant material by dichloromethane in a single workroom measuring 9 × 15 × 18 m high. When the foreman of the day shift entered this small factory one morning at 7:15 a.m., he found all four workers on the night shift unconscious. One was pronounced dead when an ambulance arrived. The others were semiconscious or drowsy when they reached the hospital about 7:30 a.m., and they were fully conscious by 10:00 a.m. The dead man was found in the single, large workroom of the factory. Those who survived were found in the dressing room and a lavatory in the basement of an adjoining building connected to the basement of the factory by an open corridor. One of the survivors was a chemical worker, who remembered that he left the plant about 4:30 a.m. for the dressing room where he was found unconscious. Two of the workers were firemen normally stationed in a third building, who entered the contaminated area about 6:30 a.m. and a little later, respectively, to clean up in preparation for going home. Thus the survivors had been anesthetized for approximately 3, 1, and <1 hr, respectively, when removed to fresh air. They had no memory of smelling dichloromethane, but the foreman detected a strong odor when he came in from outdoors.

All of the survivors were coughing when they reached the hospital, but rales and other objective evidence of respiratory tract irritation were detected in only two. Some ran a slight fever for a day or two, and one complained of eye irritation. All had moderate leukocytosis and moderate depression of red cell count and hemoglobin level. The men were discharged in 4–8 days.

The density of air saturated with dichloromethane vapor at room temperature is 1.97. The circumstances of this accident make it clear that the vapor had settled in the lower part of the workroom and the interconnected basements. The factory had lost solvent at an average rate of 446 liters/day from vents directly into the workroom. The accident, which occurred in winter, apparently was due to a critical reduction of ventilation rather than to any unusual release of solvent. After the accident, all vents of tanks and percolators were connected to pipes leading outdoors and ending 1.82 m above the roof. Additional ventilation was provided in the factory, and other safety measures were taken.

More typical of the usual effects of dichloromethane were the cases of two painters who experienced headache, faintness, giddiness, irritability, numbness and tingling of the extremities, loss of appetite, and apathy when they used the compound to remove the paint from the walls of a large closed room (Collier, 1936).

As would be expected, sedative concentrations of dichloromethane can temporarily alter both human and animal task performance. These effects were reviewed by Winneke (1981). Twenty-nine workers exposed to concentrations of less than 100 ppm were evaluated to determine whether there was any evidence of neuropsychological damage (Cherry et al., 1981). No evidence of long-term damage attributed to dichloromethane was found on clinical examination and evaluation of motor conduction velocities of ulnar and median nerves, ECG, or a psychological test battery designed to detect minimal brain damage.

Laboratory Findings Analysis of the lungs of the man found dead in a factory workroom revealed a concentration of 265 ppm (Moskowitz and Shapiro, 1952).

The first sample of expired air from a man who had been anesthetized accidentally by dichloromethane contained about 550 ppm. From this and other measurements and from the dynamics of excretion measured in volunteers, it was estimated that the atmosphere to which he had been exposed contained 8000–10,000 ppm (Riley et al., 1966).

Immersion of only one thumb in dichloromethane for 30 min produced a mean peak breath concentration of 3.1 ppm; by 2 hr after exposure the mean value was 0.69 ppm. Dichloromethane was absorbed more readily than four other solvents tested in the same way, the highest mean peak value for any one of these (1,1,1-trichloroethane) being 1.0 ppm (Stewart and Dodd, 1964).

The discovery that carbon monoxide is a metabolite of dichloromethane in humans was the result of the chance observation that a physician had much higher than expected levels of carboxyhemoglobin on each of two mornings following his use of varnish remover the evening before. A marked increase in carboxyhemoglobin was then produced when the same man was exposed under controlled conditions to only 213 ppm for only 1 hr. Subsequent studies with a total of 11 volunteers who did not smoke showed that all of them produced carbon monoxide as a metabolite of dichloromethane. The highest carboxyhemoglobin level recorded following 1 hr of exposure at a level of 515 ppm was 4.6%. However, 2 hr of exposure at a mean level of 691 ppm led to a level as high as 8.4%. Two hours of exposure to 986 ppm produced a maximal carboxyhemoglobin level of 14.8% and a mean peak level of 10.17%. These values may be compared to 7.9%, the equilibrium carboxyhemoglobin level following exposure to the threshold limit of carbon monoxide itself (50 ppm). Presumably because carbon monoxide was still being metabolized from dichloromethane, the rate of decrease of carboxyhemoglobin after it reached a peak was much slower after exposure to the solvent than after exposure to carbon monoxide itself (Stewart *et al.*, 1972a,b).

A group of workers exposed to 180–200 ppm dichloromethane had carboxyhemoglobin levels of about 4.5% in their alevolar air at the beginning of their workday. The level rose to about 9% after 8 hr and then decreased exponentially. The 24-hr time-weighted average was 7.2%, compared with 2.7 and 3.8% for persons exposed to 35 and 50 ppm, respectively, of carbon monoxide (Ratney *et al.*, 1974).

Humans exposed for a single 7.5-hr period to 50, 100, 150, and 200 ppm dichloromethane showed peak blood carboxyhemoglobin values of 1.9, 3.4, 5.3, and 6.8%, respectively (DiVincenzo and Kaplan, 1981). Five daily exposures produced only marginal increases in blood carboxyhemoglobin above that seen after a single exposure.

Epidemiology Two epidemiology studies have been conducted in workers exposed for varying lengths of time to various concentrations (up to and exceeding 20 years at 8-hr time-weighted average concentrations ranging from approximately 20 to 475 ppm) (Ott *et al.*, 1983; Hearne *et al.*, 1987). No significant excesses in malignant disease or ischemic heart disease compared with control cohorts were observed in either study, except for a suggestive increase in tumors of the pancreas (Hearne *et al.*, 1987). These authors, however, suggest numerous risk factors other than dichloromethane which may have affected the incidence of pancreatic cancer, and they plan to continue monitoring the study population.

Dosage Response The odor of dichloromethane is moderately strong but not particularly objectionable at about 1000 ppm (Stewart *et al.*, 1972a).

Exposure at the ACGIH threshold limit value (100 ppm) would permit occupational exposure at the rate of 50 mg/kg/day. The ACGIH has proposed lowering the current threshold limit value to 50 ppm in response to the animal tumorigenicity issue.

Treatment of Poisoning Treatment is symptomatic.

14.7.3 CHLOROPICRIN

14.7.3.1 Identity, Properties, and Uses

Chemical Name Trichloronitromethane or nitrochloroform.

Structure See Fig. 14.6.

Synonyms Chloropicrin is the common name. As a war gas, the compound was known as aquinite, Klop, and vomiting gas. As a fumigant, it is known as Acquinite®, Chlor-O-Pic®, Larvacide 100®, Nemax®, and Picfume®. Code designations include G-25, NC, NCl-C00533, PS, and S-1. The CAS registry number is 76-06-2.

Physical and Chemical Properties Chloropicrin has the empirical formula CCl_3NO_2 and a molecular weight of 164.39. It is a colorless, slightly oily liquid with an intense odor. It has a density of 1.648 at 25°C. It solidifies at −64°C and −69.2°C (corr.) and boils at 112.4°C. The vapor pressure is 23.8 torr at 25°C. The solubility in water is 1.62 gm/liter at 25°C. Chloropicrin is miscible with acetone, benzene, carbon tetrachloride, diethyl ether, methanol, and carbon disulfide. It is noncorrosive to copper, brass, and bronze but does corrode iron, zinc, and other light metals. It is flammable.

History and Use Chloropicrin was first patented as an insecticide in 1908. It is used to fumigate stored grain and to treat soil against nematodes. It is generally applied at rates of 32–80 g/m³. During World War I chloropicrin was used as a lachrymatory gas.

14.7.3.2 Toxicity to Laboratory Animals

Basic Findings Chloropicrin is intensely irritating. The intraperitoneal LD 50 in mice was 25 mg/kg (Fridman *et al.*, 1976). According to Tatken and Lewis (1983), the following additional acute toxicity values have been reported: an oral LD 50 of 250 mg/kg in rats; a 10-min LC 50 of 1600 mg/m³ in mice; and lethality within 20 min on inhalation of 800 mg/m³ in cats, rabbits, and dogs (1 ppm = 7 mg/m³). Moderate to severe degeneration of the respiratory and olfactory epithelium, as well as fibrosing peribronchitis and peribronchiolitis of the lung, was observed in mice exposed to 8 ppm chlorpicrin vapor 6 hr/day for 5 days (Buckley *et al.*, 1984).

Chlorpicrin was found to be weakly mutagenic in bacteria (Moriya *et al.*, 1983) but did not induce mutation in *Drosophila melanogaster* on feeding or injection (Valencia *et al.*, 1985).

Treatment of Poisoning in Animals Intravenous injection with chloropicrin at a dosage of 15 mg/kg killed all of 14 rabbits within 15–240 min; clinical and autopsy findings were typical of acute pulmonary edema. Fifteen rabbits injected subcutaneously with an antihistamine (*N*-dimethylamino-2-propyl-1-thiodiphenylamine) at a rate of 20 mg/kg 30–40 min before intravenous chloropicrin at 15 mg/kg survived without any sign of pulmonary edema (Halpern and Cruchaud, 1947). It certainly would be of interest to learn whether an antihistamine would be of any value if administered after chloropicrin, especially after the onset of symptoms.

14.7.3.3 Toxicity to Humans

Chloropicrin, which was first prepared in 1848, was well known from industrial uses before it was employed as a combat gas in World War I. In this connection, it was used partly because of its inherent toxicity. The concentrations of chlorine, chloropicrin, and phosgene that are lethal in 10 min are 5600, 2000, and 500 mg/m³, respectively. However, the main reason for using chloropicrin was its irritating properties. It is adsorbed on charcoal, but it was not removed from the air by certain World War I gas masks designed specifically for chlorine and/or phosgene. The lacrimation, coughing, and vomiting produced by chloropicrin could cause troops wearing masks to remove them and thus expose themselves to even greater danger, especially from phosgene (Prentiss, 1937).

Accidental and Intentional Poisoning There have been at least two episodes in which people living near the site of chloropicrin use were affected by it. In Japan, some people who lived near a site where leaf tobacco was fumigated complained of excessive lacrimation, cough, vertigo, headache, nausea, vomiting, and fatigue at the time of exposure. In most instances symptoms lasted for several hours to as much as 3 days after exposure. A few persons reported that their difficulties lasted more than a month. Complaints were received from some persons living over 100 m away from the site of application (Okada *et al.*, 1970). Persistence of symptoms after substantial exposure is not unexpected. Persons exposed to chloropicrin as a war gas often experienced nausea. vomiting, and diarrhea lasting for weeks (Prentiss, 1937).

In another instance, the soil of a portion (approximately 100 × 130 m) of a large field was fumigated with a mixture of methyl bromide and chloropicrin, and the area was covered with plastic. One side of the treated area was contiguous with a residential area. The application was made during daylight, but there apparently was no difficulty until a light wind arose at about 9:00 p.m. Everyone who reported any symptoms reported eye irritation, and this began an average of 2.5 hr after each person noticed the odor. Nausea was reported by 20% of those affected and coughing and sore throat by 11% each. Other symptoms reported by 3–6% of persons reporting any symptom included vomiting, dizziness, drowsiness, wheezing, blurred vision, skin irritation, headache, and a bad taste in the mouth. Three of the residents were treated as outpatients at a local hospital. The attack rate among residents of the street nearest the treated area was 53%. Again, some persons were affected at a distance greater than 100 m. Although the material applied to the field was a mixture, the character and timing of the effects indicated that chloropicrin was the cause of symptoms (Murray *et al.*, 1974).

Dosage Response Chloropicrin is lethal in 10 min at 2000 mg/m³, intolerable at 50 mg/m³, and causes lacrimation at 2 mg/m³ (Prentiss, 1937). The odor can be detected at 7.3 mg/m³ (Sutton, 1963). The threshold limit value (0.7 mg/m³) would permit an occupational dosage of 0.1 mg/kg/day.

Treatment of Poisoning Treatment is symptomatic. The prophylactic value of an antihistamine in one animal experiment suggests the cautious trial of one of these compounds in case of impending pulmonary edema. Proctor *et al.* (1978) recommend

maintaining PO_2 above 60 mm Hg by instituting the following measures stepwise as needed: (1) administration of 60–100%

oxygen; (2) intubation and mechanical ventilation; (3) positive and expiratory pressure breathing. Fluid balance must be maintained; use of a diuretic may be required. Steroids may be administered as a short-term basis (two to four days) to decrease the inflammatory response of the lung.

14.7.4 CARBON TETRACHLORIDE

14.7.4.1 Identity, Properties, and Uses

Chemical Name Tetrachloromethane.

Structure See Fig. 14.6.

Synonyms Carbon tetrachloride is the name in general use, although the compound is also known as perchloromethane. Trade names include Benzinoform® and Necatorina®. A code designation is ENT-4.705. The CAS registry number is 56-23-5.

Physical and Chemical Properties Carbon tetrachloride has the empirical formula CCl_4 and a molecular weight of 153.84. It is a colorless liquid with a sweetish odor. The density at 25°C is 1.589. It solidifies at −23°C and boils at 76.7°C. The vapor pressure is 114.5 torr at 25°C. The solubility of carbon tetrachloride in water is 0.28 gm/kg at 25°C. It is miscible with alcohol, benzene, chloroform, ether, carbon disulfide, petroleum ether, and oils. It is nonflammable and noncorrosive. It is inert generally but is decomposed by water at high temperatures.

History, Formulations, and Uses Carbon tetrachloride was introduced as a fumigant about 1908. It is used primarily for the fumigation of stored grain. Because it is not highly toxic to insects, it is often used in admixture with more potent insecticides such as ethylene dichloride, ethylene dibromide, acrylonitrile, carbon disulfide, and methyl bromide. The low toxicity is overcome by long exposure periods, usually 7–14 days. The usual rate of application is in the range 350–375 ml/metric ton of grain. Since the compound penetrates to great depths, it is especially useful for the fumigation of deep grain silos. Carbon tetrachloride has not been found to combine chemically with the constituents of food crops. Residue in wheat germ within a high fat content was found to be less than 50% of that found in bran (Conroy *et al.*, 1957).

14.7.4.2 Toxicity to Laboratory Animals

Basic Findings The oral LD 50 of carbon tetrachloride in the rat was reported to be 2800 mg/kg (Smyth *et al.*, 1970) and 5720 mg/kg (Garner and McLean, 1969). Oral LD 50 values of 5400, 10,170, and 23,358 mg/kg, respectively, were found in rats fed a regular diet, those fed a regular diet but starved 18 hr before and 4 hr after dosing, and those fed a diet containing no protein (McLean and McLean, 1966).

In dogs, the 24-hr intraperitioneal LD 50 value was 1510 mg/kg. In mice, the corresponding value was higher (4290 mg/kg). The ED 50 values for liver dysfunction as measured by SGPT were only 30 and 15.6 mg/kg in dogs and mice, respectively. The potency ratio, a measure of the hepatotoxicity of the compound compared to its anesthetic power, was 79 in dogs and 280 in mice, compared to 5.0 and 6.4 for chloroform in the two species and compared to values <3.6 for several other chlorinated hydrocarbons (Klaassen and Plaa, 1967). The corresponding LD 50 and ED 50 values for mice were 4677 and 29 mg/kg, and the potency ratio was 160 (Gehring, 1968).

Male rats fed carbon tetrachoride for 6 weeks at a rate of 25 mg/kg/day grew slowly, but females grew normally. A dosage 13.5 mg/kg/day for 6 weeks increased the concentrations of total lipids and of triglycerides in the liver, but 7.4 mg/kg/day did not. An intake of 10 mg/kg/day was tolerated for 2 years without interfering with growth, fertility, reproduction, or several biochemical tests (Alumot *et al.*, 1976).

The minimal concentrations and durations of exposure to carbon tetrachloride that killed rats have been defined; when plotted, they formed a straight logtime–logdosage curve. The same was true of lower exposures producing nonfatal injury and maximal exposures causing no effect (Adams *et al.*, 1952).

At a concentration of 8500 ppm, carbon tetrachloride killed 50% of mice in 690 min. At this concentration, the LT 50 was between 680 and 850 min and the ET 50 values for anesthesia and increased SGPT activity were 21.0 and 0.155 min, respectively. The potency ratio based on anesthetic effect was 136, but based on mortality it was ≥4,390 (Gehring, 1968).

When animals were exposed 7 hr/day, 5 days/week, for 6 months, the maximal vapor concentrations without adverse effect for different species were 25 ppm for monkeys, 10 ppm for rabbits, and 5 ppm for both rats and guinea pigs (Adams *et al.*, 1952).

Rats that had received daily exposure to concentrations of 50–400 ppm showed distinctly less liver and kidney damage than controls following exposure for 30 min to 20,000 ppm (Smyth *et al.*, 1936). A similar effect was observed in connection with relatively large, repeated doses. Using a dosage such that each administration killed about 5% of the mice, it was found that when administrations were repeated every 2 weeks, more mice died sooner than when administrations were repeated every other day (Sarkisov *et al.*, 1969). This suggests not a cumulative effect but the existence of some condition during recovery that confers substantially decreased susceptibility. The mechanism for this tolerance is unclear, but it may involve diminished activation, enhanced detoxification, selection of resistant cells, or a combination of factors.

Schwetz *et al.* (1974) exposed pregnant rats to 300 and 100 ppm carbon tetrachloride for 7 hr/day on days 6–15 of gestation. Signs of maternal toxicity included decreased body weight and increased liver weight, as well as elevated serum SGPT activity and the appearance of pale, mottled livers, both of which returned to normal within 6 days after the last exposure. Only simple growth delays were noted in the offspring, indicating slight embryotoxicity and fetotoxicity. Carbon tetrachloride was found not to be teratogenic, indicating that the fetus is not uniquely susceptible to this material.

In people poisoned by carbon tetrachloride, it is often dysfunction of the kidney rather than of the liver that is critical to survival. In many laboratory animals the kidney is less affected than the liver (Rush *et al.*, 1984). However, the kidney is susceptible to injury by the compound in the cat (Cantarow *et al.*, 1938) and in at least one species of toad (*Bufo melanostictus*) (Biswas and Mukherji, 1968).

After receiving a dose of 6 ml of carbon tetrachloride, ducks showed no adverse effect, and cockerels showed only light narcosis and anorexia for 48–72 hr. No evidence was found that the birds metabolize the compound (Fowler, 1970b). No evidence of lipid peroxidation was found in chickens (Nachtomi and Alumot, 1972).

Absorption, Distribution, Metabolism, and Excretion   In dogs, no absorption of carbon tetrachloride from the ligated stomach could be detected. Much of a large dose placed in the intestine was excreted in the feces, but essentially all of a 3-ml dose was absorbed. The compound appeared in the expired air only a very few minutes after an intestinal dose and reached a maximal concentration in about 1 hr. When carbon tetrachloride was placed in the intestine alone, none of it could be detected in the clear lymph from the thoracic duct; however, when it was administered with milk (fat), its concentration in the chyle was 460, 600, and 750 ppm in three experiments. The average concentration in the portal blood was 200 ppm. Thus, administration with fat permitted a substantial proportion of carbon tetrachloride to avoid a single passage through the liver, to reach a higher concentration in the systemic blood, and to produce central nervous system effects. Whereas alcohol increased the absorption of carbon tetrachloride with which it was administered, the degree of the increase was trivial and insufficient to explain the potentiation of carbon tetrachloride poisoning by alcohol (Robbins, 1929).

The distribution of carbon tetrachloride in the tissues reflects their fat content. The concentration in the liver becomes relatively greater as that organ becomes progressively fatty. The highest concentration is found in body fat. Other tissues that show concentrations greater than that of the blood are nervous tissue, bone marrow, and adrenals. After prolonged exposure, the liver, kidney, and spleen also may contain concentrations somewhat higher than those in the blood (Robbins, 1929; McCollister *et al.*, 1951; Fabre *et al.*, 1961).

During exposures lasting 139 or more minutes, monkeys absorbed an average of 30% of the carbon tetrachloride they inhaled. Absorption of ^{14}C-labeled carbon tetrachloride vapor from the skin was much less. The blood concentration of a monkey after only dermal exposure to an air concentration of 1150 ppm for 270 min was equivalent to that found after 24 min of inhalation of 46 ppm (McCollister *et al.*, 1951).

Carbon tetrachloride is metabolized predominantly in the liver by select NADPH-dependent cytochrome P-450 isoenzymes (Seawright and McClean, 1967; Uehleke *et al.*, 1973; Sipes *et al.*, 1977; English and Anders, 1985). Reported metabolites of carbon tetrachloride include chloroform, phosgene, trichloromethyl free radical, electrophilic chlorine, trichloromethyl peroxy radical, hexachloroethane, dichloromethyl carbene, CO_2 and CO (discussed by Reynolds et al., 1984; Rush et al., 1984). Nonuniform loss of cytochrome P-450-dependent activities and isoenzymes results from apparent reactive intermediate binding and deactivation of the enzyme system (Head et al., 1981; Noguchi et al., 1982a,b; English and Anders, 1985).

The tissues of poisoned rabbits contain carbon tetrachloride, chloroform, hexachloroethane, and two unidentified metabolites. Although hexachloroethane is hepatotoxic, it probably is not primarily responsible for the toxicity of carbon tetrachloride (Fowler, 1969). Carbon tetrachloride, chloroform, and hexachloroethane were found in the bile (Fowler, 1970a). Chloroform, as well as carbon tetrachloride, was detected in the breath of dogs treated with the latter compound (Butler, 1961).

After respiratory exposure of monkeys was stopped, at least 51% of the retained activity was exhaled within 1800 hr; most was unmetabolized carbon tetrachloride, but a part was in the form of carbon dioxide. Excretion of unchanged carbon tetrachloride was still detectable 28 days after exposure ended (McCollister et al., 1951).

The urine of monkeys also contained ^{14}C that had entered the metabolic pool and was excreted in the form of urea and carbonates. In addition, the urine contained unidentified metabolites (McCollister et al., 1951).

Dose-dependent pharmacokinetics was observed in rats 0–24 hr following gavage administration of [^{14}C]carbon tetrachloride at doses ranging from 15 mg/kg (nontoxic) to 4000 mg/kg (severely hepatotoxic) (Reynolds et al., 1984). Twenty percent of the dose was eliminated in expired air as parent compound at 15 mg/kg, compared with 70–90% at 46–4000 mg/kg. Correspondingly, 28% of the dose was metabolized to $^{14}CO_2$ at 15 mg/kg, 12% at 46 mg/kg, and only <3% at 308–4000 mg/kg. Reynolds et al. hypothesize that the diminished capacity of the rat to metabolize carbon tetrachloride at doses ≥46 mg/kg may be related to either less efficient first-pass removal of absorbed carbon tetrachloride by the liver or impairment of metabolism due to hepatotoxicity.

Biochemical Effects   In his masterful chapter on toxicology of the liver, Plaa (1980) pointed out that for 50 years investigators have had a special interest in unraveling the mechanisms involved in the liver injury produced by carbon tetrachloride, and they often have used the compound as a reference substance when examining other hepatotoxins. Under these circumstances it is not astonishing that the chapter constituted a review of the hepatotoxicity of carbon tetrachloride. It contains a history of concepts of liver injury and far more fully referenced detail than can be given here. The following findings seem to have the greatest relevance to human poisoning by the compound.

Necrosis and accumulation of triglycerides, the two liver changes characteristic of carbon tetrachloride, are not caused by the same mechanism. There is a very real question whether abnormal accumulation of fat is damaging in itself. Further evidence of separable injuries to the liver by carbon tetrachloride was given by Popp et al. (1978).

The early inhibition of protein synthesis in the rat is confined to the centrilobular and midzonal areas of the liver and does not occur in the duodenum, ileum, pancreas, or kidney. Apparently, this detail has not been explored in the kidney of a species especially susceptible to kidney damage by carbon tetrachloride.

The fact that the hepatotoxicity of carbon tetrachloride is increased by a wide range of factors that promote its metabolism and is decreased by many factors that inhibit its metabolism has led to the firm conviction that one or more metabolites, and not the parent compound, are responsible for its injury to the liver. The clinical importance of ethanol as a promoter of carbon tetrachloride hepatotoxicity has been recognized for a long time. It was first theorized that alcohol promoted absorption of the ingested compound. However, alcohol is effective regardless of the route of exposure to carbon tetrachloride. It is now certain that ethanol promotes the toxicity of carbon tetrachloride mainly by promoting its metabolism. Acetone and several alcohols, especially isopropanol, have a marked potentiating effect and might be important in some industrial situations. Chlordecone, as well, markedly potentiates the hepatotoxicity and lethality of carbon tetrachloride in rats and mice (Curtis et al., 1979; Klingensmith and Mehendale, 1982; Agarwal and Mehendale, 1983). The extent to which this effect may be related to enhanced bioactivation of carbon tetrachloride versus observed perturbations of hepatocellular calcium homeostasis is presently unresolved (Agarwal and Mehendale, 1984; Fariss and Reed, 1985).

Evidence that carbon tetrachloride leads to lipid peroxidation includes the production of conjugated dienes both in vitro and in vivo and the fact that antioxidants, especially vitamin E, can prevent the appearance of fatty livers and necrosis in animals treated with carbon tetrachloride. However, no conjugated dienes could be found after administration of chloroform in doses that resulted in fatty livers and necrosis. This casts doubt on the general applicability of lipid peroxidation as a cause of liver necrosis associated with all halogenated hydrocarbons capable of producing it. Furthermore, some investigators (Green et al., 1969) have been unable to confirm either increased lipid peroxidation or the protective action of vitamin E in rats poisoned by carbon tetrachloride. However, additional evidence for lipid peroxidation was demonstrated by the production of pentane in rats treated with carbon tetrachloride and some other halomethanes. Comparing different compounds, there was a good relationship ($r = 0.987$) between the amount of pentane produced and the bond dissociation energies. There also was a good correlation ($r = 0.96$) between pentane production in vivo and conjugated diene formation in the liver (Sagai and Tappel, 1979).

Five minutes after intravenous injection of [^{14}C]- or [^{36}Cl]carbon tetrachloride, liver lipids, especially phospholipids, were labeled. Labeling of microsomal lipids was one-fourth to one-seventh that of the mitochondrial lipids but was much greater than labeling of the microsomal proteins.

There was a slight decline in the degree of labeling between 5 and 15 min, after which the level of radioactivity remained constant. For a time after dosing and while the degree of binding remained constant, the amount of free carbon tetrachloride greatly exceeded the amount bound, indicating that the number of binding sites is limited (Gordis, 1969; Rao and Rechnagel, 1969). Derangement of the synthesis of microsomal phospholipids and proteins also begins promptly (within 10–15 min after dosing) and becomes maximal within 60 min (Halbreich and Mager, 1969). These findings are compatible with the idea that the metabolites are free radicals and indicate that other toxicologic processes acting in concert with lipid peroxidation are probably involved in the mechanism of necrosis.

Carbon tetrachloride impairs the NADPH-dependent oxidative enzymes in rat liver microsomes by causing irreversible damage to cytochrome P-450 and not by acting as a competitive inhibitor (Sasame et al., 1968). It is of interest that chloroform failed to damage cytochrome P-450 significantly, and this raises a question about the relationship of this damage to necrosis. With carbon tetrachloride, the decrease in cytochrome P-450 is associated with a loss of heme component (Greene et al., 1969). These biochemical changes undoubtedly account for the observed interference of carbon tetrachloride with ability to metabolize other substances, for example, hexobarbital (Lal et al., 1970) and a number of other drugs (Feuer and Granda, 1970).

A study of many enzymes in the liver and in the plasma of animals at intervals following exposure to carbon tetrachloride showed that the relationship between each circulating and tissue enzyme was a function of time. At the 8- and 16-hr sampling periods, activities of glutamic-oxaloacetic transaminase and aldolase (all commonly used in following the clinical course of human patients poisoned by the compound) were significantly elevated in the liver as well as in the serum. This suggested a considerable net increase in liver enzyme activity. At other times and for other enzymes, "normal" hepatic enzyme levels accompanied gross increases of activity in the serum. This, too, suggested increased production of enzymes (Dinman and Bernstein, 1968a; Kroener and Staib, 1968). High levels of enzymes persisted into the period when the liver was undergoing regeneration (Dinman and Bernstein, 1968b; Musser and Spooner, 1968). Bel et al. (1968) considered changes in the serum ornithine carbamoyltransferase activity, the most sensitive indicator of impending liver necrosis.

An extensive review of chemical injury of microsomes by carbon tetrachloride and some other compounds is that of De Matteis (1978).

Effects on Organs and Tissues The International Agency for Research on Cancer (IARC) reviewed the available carcinogenicity data for carbon tetrachloride in 1972, 1979, and, most recently, 1982 and concluded that there is sufficient evidence for carcinogenicity to animals (IARC, 1982). Many of the older studies were complicated by inappropriate numbers of animals or lack of appropriate control groups; however, association of carbon tetrachloride with hepatomas has been consistent. Mice appear markedly more sensitive to the development of hepatic tumors than rats (Weisburger, 1977). Results of genetic toxicity assays have generally been negative (Marsalis and Butterworth, 1980; Bermudez et al., 1982; IARC, 1982; Barbin et al., 1983), suggesting that hepatic injury may play a predominant enhancing role in carbon tetrachloride tumorigenesis in rodents.

Pathology Centrilobular necrosis of the liver is the lesion most characteristic of poisoning by carbon tetrachloride in most experimental animals. With repeated respiratory exposure to concentrations of about 100–200 ppm, this necrosis occurred cell by cell and was accompanied by replacement of new cells that were somewhat more resistant to injury. If exposure was discontinued after many months, recovery was complete. At higher exposure levels, replacement of hepatocytes was accompanied by fibrosis leading to cirrhosis, which was reversible but only very slowly. Although rats exposed to 100 mg/m³ or more showed no kidney dysfunction, they did show limited tubal damage. Other morphological changes not resulting in recognized functional change and occurring mainly in guinea pigs included granular swelling of the adrenals, minor degenerative changes of ganglion cells in the retina, abnormal occurrence of fat in the peripheral nerves, and limited degenerative changes of the ocular muscles (Smyth et al., 1936).

In the rat, the cells of livers regenerating after partial hepatectomy are less sensitive to carbon tetrachloride than are the cells of normal livers (Georgijew et al., 1968).

Cirrhosis also occurs in mice (Edwards and Dalton, 1942), dogs (Lamson and Wing, 1926), and pigs (White, 1939) following exposure to carbon tetrachloride.

As viewed with the electron microscope, the distinctive changes in the rat liver produced by carbon tetrachloride consist of depletion of vesiculation of the rough endoplasmic reticulum, formation of clumps of tangled smooth membranes, and vacuolization of the Golgi apparatus as well as loss of polysomes and accumulation of fat. Different chemical classes of hepatotoxins produce distinctly different ultrastructural changes in the liver (Ganote and Rosenthal, 1968; Meldolesi, 1968). During regeneration, the free polysomes reappear much sooner than the membrane-bound ones (Michel et al., 1968).

Definite renal tubular lesions, including tubular necrosis, casts, and deposition of calcium, were observed regularly in cats poisoned by carbon tetrachoride (Cantarow et al., 1938). Mitochondria and not endoplasmic reticulum, as in the liver, appears to be the primary subcellular site of carbon tetrachloride toxicity in the kidney (Rush et al., 1984).

Treatment of Poisoning in Animals Dogs in coma and convulsions caused by carbon tetrachloride recovered normal behavior within 10–20 min after intravenous injection of calcium chloride. Relapses were treated by additional calcium, and permanent recovery was eventually achieved (Minot, 1927). The survival of poisoned cats was improved by calcium (Cantarow et al., 1938).

With the exception of this work on calcium, little study seems to have been made of therapeutic measures. It may be that the very rapid binding of a metabolite of carbon tetrachloride to the lipids and proteins of liver and perhaps kidney precludes specific therapy after absorption of the compound has occurred. However, this is unproved. It might be useful to explore in animals the possible therapeutic value of some measures that have been shown to have prophylactic value in poisoning by carbon tetrachloride. These include dietary protein deficiency (McLean and McLean, 1966), hypothermia (Larson and Plaa, 1965), pregnancy (Douglas and Clower, 1968; Clower *et al.,* 1968), or treatment with vitamin E (Hove, 1948; Meldolesi, 1968; Gallagher, 1961), various other antioxidants (Gallagher, 1961), phenoxybenzamine (Brody *et al.,* 1961), promethazine (Slater and Sawyer, 1969; Serratoni *et al.,* 1969), propylgallate (Ugazio and Torrielli, 1968), intravenous trypan blue (Petrelli and Stenger, 1969), or reserpine (Douglas and Clower, 1968; Clower *et al.,* 1968).

14.7.4.3 Toxicity to Humans

Experimental Exposure When carbon tetrachloride was being introduced as an anthelmintic, a murderer under sentence of death volunteered to take the compound. He received 6 ml about 1 hr after a midday meal; he apparently had no symptom but did pass four ascarid worms. The same dose was repeated 13 days later on an empty stomach; this time he felt a little giddy and sleepy 4.75 hr after the dose, but the symptoms soon disappeared. The execution took place a week after the second dose. No hookworms or ascarids were found at autopsy, and microscopic examination of the organs revealed no sign of degeneration of any kind (Nicholls and Hampton, 1922).

Wells (1925) measured the excretion of carbon tetrachloride in expired breath after he had taken 3 ml by mouth and again after a slightly smaller dose administered by duodenal tube. In each instance the dose produced some dizziness and increased peristalsis. Respiratory excretion (indicated by odor of the breath as well as by chemical analysis) began within 10 min after duodenal administration and reached a maximum in 15 min. Excretion decreased rapidly in both tests but was still measurable a little over 35 hr after administration.

Volunteers were exposed to carbon tetrachloride vapor (50 ppm) for 70 min and to lower concentrations for 180 min in order to determine the relationship between exposure and concentration of the compound in the exhaled breath (Stewart *et al.,* 1961b). The average concentration in breath just after the highest exposure was about 15 ppm, and it fell exponentially thereafter.

In three volunteers, immersion of one thumb in carbon tetrachloride caused a burning sensation that subsided about 10 min after exposure stopped. Erythema was produced but cleared in 1–2 hr. The compound was detected in the alveolar air within 10 min after immersion of the thumb; the concentration rose steadily throughout the remainder of the 30-min exposure and for 10–30 min following exposure and then fell exponentially. The average peak concentration in the breath was 0.64 ppm (4 mg/m³) (Stewart and Dodd, 1964).

Therapeutic Use An extensive and successful study of carbon tetrachloride for combating hookwork in dogs and other animals (Hall, 1921) was followed by extensive use of the compound for the same purpose in people (Lambert, 1922; Nicholls and Hampton, 1922). Side effects were not a serious problem, being distinctly less than those caused by the anthelmintics, notably chenopodium, previously in use for the same purpose. In preliminary tests leading to treatment of over 20,000 people, it was found that the incidence of sleepiness, headache, and vomiting could be minimized by administering 30 gm of magnesium sulfate 3 hr after administration of the carbon tetrachloride. It was noted that alcohol was contraindicated. The severest symptoms occurred in those who took an alcoholic drink within several hours, either before or after the carbon tetrachloride. At the time, this effect was attributed to increased absorption of the drug. The same explanation was applied to the constipating effect of food taken just before or after the drug. The dose selected for children was 0.2 ml per year of age, with an adult dose of 3–4 ml, depending on body size. The dose was given on an empty stomach and followed in 3 hr by 30 gm of magnesium sulfate. It was concluded that when this regimen was carried out under strict control, no symptoms were produced (Lambert, 1922).

Later in the same campaign there were six deaths attributed to carbon tetrachloride. One was in a young boy who proved to have a congenital malformation of the intestine, which it was thought would have led to death before maturity. One was in a woman addicted to alcohol. The other four were in children heavily infested with *Ascaris lumbricoides.* However, deaths were rare, and none occurred in a consecutive series of 100,000 treatments (Lambert, 1933). Other investigators also emphasized the importance of alcohol, ascariasis, dietary fat, and calcium deficiency as factors contributing to the toxicity of carbon tetrachloride (Lamson *et al.,* 1928). The reason carbon tetrachloride was replaced was not its danger but the equal effectiveness of tetrachloroethylene, which has a more pronounced taste and greater anesthetic effect but lacks really objectionable side effects.

None of the explanations that have been offered for the danger of administering carbon tetrachloride to persons heavily infested with *A. lumbricoides* are entirely satisfactory, but there is no reason to doubt the clinical observation.

Accidental and Intentional Poisoning Carbon tetrachloride poisoning is characterized by different syndromes, depending in part on dosage, route, and duration of exposure. Most cases fall somewhere within a spectrum, at one extreme of which are cases of simple narcosis, fatal or otherwise, almost always resulting from a single brief respiratory exposure to a high vapor concentration. At the other extreme are cases of kidney and/or liver failure without initial narcosis and characterized by gradual onset following repeated, sometimes unrecognized, respiratory exposure. These conditions and the intermediate condition in which some degree of narcosis and gastroenteritis is followed by failure of the kidney and/or liver can be understood in terms of animal experiments. The narcotic effects undoubtedly conform to Ferguson's principle (see Section 4.1.1.2 in Hayes, 1975), whereas kidney or liver injury is the result of potentially cumulative chemical action that may progress at blood levels too low to produce anesthesia. The variation in clinical course following ingestion results largely from variation in the amount and composition of material in the gastrointestinal tract at the time of ingestion or soon thereafter. The presence of food of any kind tends to reduce the cathartic action of carbon tetrachloride and thus to increase the absorbed dose. The presence of fat directs much of the absorption of carbon tetrachloride to the lymph, thus avoiding the initial pass through the liver; this results in relatively more unmetabolized carbon tetrachloride in the general circulation and may, therefore, promote anesthesia.

Apparently unexplained is the fact that the relative importance of kidney and liver injury varies from case to case, although kidney injury generally is more critical—far more important than in any animal model that has been studied thoroughly.

Beyond the spectrum of illnesses just discussed are a few cases of sudden death caused by ventricular fibrillation in hearts sensitized by carbon tetrachloride. This property of myocardial sensitization is poorly understood but is possessed by a number of other hydrocarbons, especially halogenated hydrocarbons (see Section 14.2).

The great majority of cases of poisoning by carbon tetrachloride have involved respiratory exposure associated with its use as a cleaning fluid or accidental or suicidal ingestion of preparations intended for that use. Use of the compound as a pesticide has caused few cases, mainly because relatively few people have any contact with it as a pesticide. However, cases associated with pesticides have shown the same spectrum of clinical effects seen with other uses of the compound. They range from the typical effects of respiratory exposure to the grain fumigant to the effects of ingestion. A case listed by Hayes and Vaughn (1977) involved a 64-year-old man who, having consumed some wine, turned to a product called "Wevil-Kill" that had been stored in a whiskey bottle.

Cases exemplifying this spectrum of clinical effects may be found in books by Moeschlin (1965), Johnstone (1942), and Johnstone and Miller (1960), in a paper by Jacobziner and Raybin (1964), and in a very large number of reports referenced by von Oettingen (1955).

Use Experience   Use experience with carbon tetrachloride has always been better in larger factories than in smaller establishments and far better in both than in association with occasional use of the compound in homes and shops. Even so, when 100 ppm was considered a safe level of continuing exposure, a substantial proportion of workers showed increased icterus index, indirect Van de Berg reaction, increased circulating lymphocytes and monocytes, restriction of the visual fields, and reduced blood calcium (Smyth *et al.*, 1936).

Atypical Cases of Various Origins   A 59-year-old man was severely poisoned by respiratory exposure to carbon tetrachloride following the ingestion of alcohol. Seven years later he was

found to have hepatocellular carcinoma superimposed on cirrhosis of undetermined type (Tracey and Sherlock, 1968).

Dosage Response   Most deaths caused by known doses of carbon tetrachloride have involved therapeutic use complicated either by ingestion of alcohol, recent administration of an anesthetic, or the presence of *Ascaris* (Lamson *et al.*, 1928). It must be emphasized, however, that thousands of people received the same dosages without serious untoward effect. The dosage has varied from about 32 mg/kg in infants to 90–100 mg/kg in adults. The most common side effect was sleepiness; headache lasting several days was fairly common; vomiting was uncommon. A volunteer experienced no untoward effect after ingesting 136 mg/kg and experienced only slight, temporary giddiness and sleepiness following the same dosage 13 days later (Nicholls and Hampton, 1922).

The present threshold limit value of 5 ppm permits an occupational intake of 4.5 mg/kg/day.

Laboratory Findings   Carbon tetrachloride often may be smelled on the breath of persons poisoned by it, or it may be measured by infrared or gas chromatographic analysis (Stewart *et al.*, 1961b, 1963).

In addition, laboratory tests are likely to indicate kidney and liver damage.

The presence of conjugated dienes in the liver of a man who died 2 days after drinking 500 ml of carbon tetrachloride was evidence that the compound produces lipid peroxidation in people (Hashimoto *et al.*, 1968).

Treatment of Poisoning   Although treatment is symptomatic, special attention should be given to the use of mannitol to minimize kidney damage. Stewart *et al.* (1963) recommended that infusion of this drug should be started before laboratory confirmation of poisoning is possible. The dose during the first 6-hr period is 50 gm, followed by 25 gm every 6 hr for at least 5 days unless oliguria appears and proves refractory to a total of 75 gm of mannitol after its onset. In the absence of oliguria, mannitol should be continued until the concentration of carbon tetrachloride in the expired air has fallen to a low level. If oliguria does develop, hemodialysis may be lifesaving.

Calcium has been inadequately tested in the treatment of carbon tetrachloride poisoning in humans, but its value in dogs poisoned by carbon tetrachloride and in people poisoned by dichloroethane suggests that a trial would be justified.

14.7.5 1,2-DIBROMOETHANE

14.7.5.1 Identity, Properties, and Uses

Chemical Name   1,2-Dibromoethane.

Structure   See Fig. 14.6.

Synonyms   1,2-Dibromoethane is also known as ethylene dibromide and EDB. The CAS registry number is 106-93-4.

Physical and Chemical Properties 1,2-Dibromoethane has the empirical formula $C_2H_4Br_2$ and a molecular weight of 187.88. It is a heavy, colorless liquid with a chloroform-like odor. The density of the liquid at 20°C is 2.172. The compound solidifies at 9°C and boils at 131–132°C. Its vapor pressure is 11 torr at 25°C. 1,2-Dibromoethane has a solubility of 4.3 gm/kg in water at 30°C and is miscible in alcohol and ether. It is stable and nonflammable.

History, Formulations, and Uses 1,2-Dibromoethane was introduced as an insecticide in 1925 and first produced commercially in 1946. It has been used as a fumigant for stored grain, fruits, and vegetables; for the treatment of soil against nematodes; and for spot treatment in flour mills. The compound was sometimes mixed with carbon tetrachloride or dichloropropene to increase the spectrum of activity. However, since the use of dibromoethane as a fumigant is now restricted in the United States, its primary use today is as a scavenger in gasoline containing tetraethyllead.

14.7.5.2 Toxicity to Laboratory Animals

Basic Findings Oral LD 50 values were 146 and 117 mg/kg in male and female rats, respectively; 420 mg/kg in mice; 55 mg/kg in rabbits; and 110 mg/kg in guinea pigs (Rowe *et al.*, 1952). The dermal LD 50 in rabbits was about 450 mg/kg following 24-hr exposure with an impermeable cover (Rowe *et al.*, 1952).

Undiluted dibromoethane caused obvious pain and conjunctival irritation. In spite of superficial necrosis of the cornea, healing was complete within 48 hr. A 10% solution in propylene glycol produced a more severe response than did the undiluted material. Healing was not apparent for 48 hr and required about 12 days. Prompt washing of the injured eye was always beneficial. Dermal exposure of rabbits to 10% or to more concentrated formulations often killed them. If allowed to evaporate, a 1% solution produced erythema followed by superficial exfoliation. When the same solution was bandaged repeatedly onto the shaved abdomen, it caused erythema and edema progressing to necrosis and sloughing of the superficial layers of skin. Healing was complete without scarring within 7 days after exposure stopped.

Dibromoethane is irritating to mucous membranes. Animals anesthetized by it often resist and those that regain consciousness after even light, brief anesthesia often die within 15 – 18 hr (Lucas, 1928).

Following single inhalation exposures such that less than half of the rats survived, deaths occurred within 24 hr and were due to respiratory or cardiac failure. Deaths from inhalation exposures of lower intensities usually were delayed, sometimes as much as 12 days, and were caused by pneumonitis. Separate parallel straight-line relationships were obtained when the logarithm of the exposure concentration was plotted against the statistically determined logarithm of the length of the exposure producing 99.99, 50, or 0.01% mortality and the no-effect levels. The dosage–response relationship was quite steep; only 2 of 20 rats died following a 1-hr exposure at 400 ppm but 16 or 25 rats died after being exposed for 2 hr at this concentration. Mortality was 50% following daily 7-hr exposures to 50 ppm but the rats tolerated 151 exposures in 213 days to 25 ppm (190 mg/m³) without adverse effect, as judged by general appearance and behavior, growth, and final body and organ weights.

Repeated inhalation exposure of rats to 40 ppm dibromoethane for 6 hr/day, 5 days/week, for up to 13 weeks resulted in decreased body weight gain and in increased liver and kidney weights. The only histologic change observed in these rats was a reversible hyperplasia and nonkeratinizing squamous metaplasia of the nasal respiratory epithelium. Slight hyperplasia of the nasal epithelium was observed in rats repeatedly exposed to 10 ppm, although this regimen had no effect on body weight gain or organ weights. The no-observed-effect level for rats in this study was 3 ppm (Nitschke *et al.*, 1981). Similar nasal lesions and dose response were observed when rats and mice were exposed 6 hr/day, 5 days/week, for 13 weeks to 3, 15, or 75 ppm dibromoethane (Reznik *et al.*, 1980b).

Absorption, Distribution, Metabolism, and Excretion Toxicity studies show that acutely toxic quantities of dibromoethane can be absorbed from the skin and from the respiratory and gastrointestinal tracts.

Anesthetized rats retained 58% of the dibromoethane they inhaled, and no unchanged dibromoethane was eliminated in the expired air (Stott and McKenna, 1984). Following intraperitoneal administration of [¹⁴C]dibromoethane to guinea pigs at a rate of 30 mg/kg, 66% of the administered radioactivity was excreted in the urine and less than 3% was eliminated in the feces within 72 hr (Plotnick and Conner, 1976). Rats given 40 mg/kg of [¹⁴C]dibromoethane by gavage eliminated 40% of the radioactivity in the urine in 24 hr. No unchanged dibromoethane was found in the urine. Another 5% of the dose was excreted in the bile in 2.5 hr and between 5 and 8% of the radioactivity was excreted in the expired air (Edwards *et al.*, 1970).

The metabolism of dibromoethane is mediated by enzymes located in the microsomal and cytosolic fractions of the cell. Microsomal metabolism of dibromoethane leads to the formation of bromoacetaldehyde, a highly reactive metabolite that can either spontaneously lose bromide to yield ethylene or covalently bind to various cellular nucleophiles. The metabolism of dibromoethane by the cytosolic fraction is mediated by glutathione transferase and leads to the formation of *S*-2-bromoethylglutathione, which spontaneously loses bromine and rearranges to form a reactive half mustard. Data obtained with tetradeuterated dibromoethane and inhibitors of the microsomal pathway indicate that the hepatotoxicity and mutagenicity of dibromoethane are due to *S*-2-bromoethylglutathione formed by the cytosolic pathway even though the microsomal pathway is qualitatively more important and also leads to reactive metabolites (Van Bladeren, 1983; White *et al.*, 1983).

Biochemical Effects Following oral administration, [^{14}C]dibromoethane was incorporated into DNA, RNA, and proteins of rat liver (Nachtomi and Sarma, 1977). Oral administration of dibromoethane to rats at dose levels that did not produce necrosis (i.e., 75 and 100 mg/kg) stimulated DNA synthesis and induced 16% of the cells in the liver to undergo mitosis (Nachtomi and Farber, 1978).

Effects on Organs and Tissues Dibromoethane has been shown to be mutagenic in a variety of bacterial systems, mammalian cells, and *Drosophila melanogaster*. It was positive in tests for sister chromatid exchange but has repeatedly been negative in dominant lethal assays (see Sax, 1984). The mutagenicity of dibromoethane has been shown to be dependent on metabolism; its activity is greatly enhanced by the addition of cytosolic enzymes and glutathione.

Tumors at the portal of entry have been a consistent finding in long-term rodent studies with dibromoethane. Nasal carcinomas and adenocarcinomas were observed in rats and mice exposed by inhalation to 40 or 10 ppm dibromoethane 7 hr/day, 5 days/week, for up to 103 weeks. In addition to the nasal tumors, the incidence of tumors in the spleen, mammary gland, mesentery, and subcutaneous tissue was increased by this treatment. These exposures also caused hepatic necrosis, toxic nephropathy, and testicular and retinal degeneration in the rats and hyperplasia of the respiratory epithelium in the mice (NTP, 1982). Oral administration of dibromoethane at dose levels ranging from 40 to 107 mg/kg/day produced squamous cell carcinoma of the forestomach in rats and mice. The incidence of hepatocellular carcinomas and hemangiosarcomas in rats and lung tumors in mice was also increased by dibromoethane (NCI, 1978a). Repeated application of dibromoethane in a two-stage carcinogenesis assay in which phorbol myristate acetate was used as a promoter increased the incidence of skin papillomas and carcinomas and lung tumors in mice (Van Duuren *et al.*, 1979).

Effects on Reproduction Intraperitoneal administration of 55 mg dibromoethane/kg/day on days 1–15 of gestation was judged to be maternally toxic but neither fetotoxic nor teratogenic in the rat (Hardin *et al.*, 1981). No evidence of developmental toxicity was observed in rats or mice exposed by inhalation on days 6–10 of gestation to concentrations of dibromoethane that were not overtly toxic to the dams (Short *et al.*, 1978). Exposure to 80 ppm dibromoethane 6 hr/day, 5 days/week, for 10 weeks resulted in 20% mortality in male and female rats. In addition, testicular atrophy, reduced serum testosterone concentrations, and decreased ability to impregnate unexposed females was noted in males. Females exposed to 80 ppm dibromoethane remained in diestrus and failed to begin to cycle until 3–4 days after the exposures ended. No effects on reproduction were observed in rats exposed to concentrations of dibromoethane that were not overtly toxic (i.e., 39 and 10 ppm; Short *et al.*, 1979).

Interactions Inclusion of 0.05% disulfiram in the diet of rats exposed by inhalation to 20 ppm dibromoethane greatly increased both the toxicity and the number and types of tumors produced by dibromoethane (Wong *et al.*, 1982).

14.7.5.3 Toxicity to Humans

Accidental and Intentional Poisoning A depressed 43-year-old female alcoholic was admitted to the hospital complaining of abdominal pain, nausea, vomiting, and diarrhea, all of which began soon after she ingested 4.5 ml of dibromoethane in capsular form 48 hr earlier. Approximately 36 hr after ingestion, the patient had noticed her urine turned dark and became scant. She was anuric on admission. Examination revealed mild icterus and marked agitation; the pulse was 140 and the respiration 24. Laboratory studies confirmed the presence of jaundice; several liver tests were abnormal, and there was moderate anemia, but azotemia had not yet developed. In spite of supportive treatment, the patient's condition deteriorated rapidly and she died 4 hr after admission (Olmstead, 1960).

Two fatalities occurred in connection with the cleaning of a 28.5-m^3 nurse tank at a small fertilizer–pesticide storage and distribution center in California. The first case involved a 31-year-old, 90-kg male, who collapsed 5 min after entering the tank and was in the tank for 45 min. After being removed from the tank, he was intermittently comatose, vomiting, and complained of burning eyes and throat. He was washed with a fire hose and transported by ambulance. In the ambulance he was combative and incoherent, reeked of a chemical odor, and was given oxygen and atropine for an episode of bradycardia. One hour later in the emergency room he was lethargic, coughing, had vomiting and diarrhea, and had a strong chemical odor. His blood pressure was 140/100, pulse 120, and respiration 24. Physical examination revealed inflammation of the conjunctivae and pharynx, cyanotic nail beds, an abrasion of the left flank, and decreased response to pain. An ECG indicated sinus bradycardia. the chest X ray was normal. Arterial blood gas values measured while he breathed room air were PaO$_2$ 99 mm Hg, PaCo$_2$ 36 mm Hg, and pH 7.29, suggesting mild acidosis. Abnormal laboratory findings were: hematocrit, 50.0%; white blood cell (WBC) count, 15,100/μl; serum chloride, 110 mEq/liter; anion gap, 17.6; blood glucose, 279 mg/dl; and creatinine, 1.5 mg/dl. Serum bromide, measured 2 hr after the exposure, was 830 mg/liter. He was treated with intranasal oxygen, nasogastric lavage, intravenous fluids, and morphine for back and thorax pain and was transported by helicopter to a nearby burn center because of anticipated chemical burns of the airways. En route, he alternated between being awake and lethargic. The pilot complained of difficulty flying due to the strong odor from the patient. Five hours after exposure, the patient was semicomatose, arousable only by painful stimuli, and had a notable metabolic acidosis (pH 7.18) despite intravenous administration of 90 mEq of sodium bicarbonate. Approximately 6 hr postexposure, the WBC count was 28,700/μl, with 20% band forms, and the anion gap was 15.5. Serum phosphorus was low (1.3 mg/dl), while serum calcium (9.3 mg/dl) and uric acid (17.6 mg/dl) were elevated. Serum lactate dehydrogenase (366 IU/liter), aspartate aminotransferase (158 IU/liter), creatinine phosphokinase (1555 IU/liter), and pseudocholinesterase (18.6 IU/liter) were also elevated. Approximately 12 hr after exposure, the patient suddenly became combative, turned ashen, and died of cardiopulmonary arrest. Autopsy findings included bilateral pulmonary edema, cyanosis of the face and body, and severe congestion of the viscera including the brain. Histopathologic examination revealed focal interstitial inflammation and edema of the myocardium. The bromide level in a postmortem whole-blood specimen was 24 mg/liter.

The second case was a 49-year-old male, weighing 105 kg, who climbed into the nurse tank to rescue his co-worker. He collapsed and was in the tank for 20–30 min before being rescued. Once outside the tank he became delirious, combative, vomited, and complained of burning eyes. He was washed with a fire hose and transported to the hospital. One hour later he was alert but somewhat confused. His blood pressure was 105/95, pulse 80, and respiration 24. Physical examination, ECG, chest X ray, and blood gases were normal. Abnormal laboratory tests included hematocrit, 50%; WBC, 17,900; serum potassium, 2.9 mEq/liter; serum chloride, 108 mEq/liter; and anion gap, 18. In the emergency room, the patient experienced nausea, vomiting, abdominal cramps, and severe diarrhea. His sensorium cleared rapidly and he was washed with soap and water and transferred to intensive care.

By 24 hr, the urine output was less than 5 ml/hr. He was alert and asymptomatic except for the erythema and blister that had appeared on his trunk and legs. Abnormal laboratory values at this time included serum urea nitrogen, 33 mg/dl; creatinine, 3.5 mg/dl; serum uric acid, 13.2 mg/dl; bilirubin, 4.0 mg/dl; lactate dehydrogenase, 1220 IU/liter; lactate, 8.9 mmol/liter; and serum bromide, 500 mg/liter. Forty-eight hours postexposure, the patient was stuporous and had a blood pressure of 80/20, severe metabolic acidosis, and progressive renal failure. Hemodialysis with sodium acetate was performed for 4 hr but the patient again became acidemic and was treated with intravenous sodium bicarbonate, fluids, dopamine, and further hemodialysis. He became more obtunded and hepatomegaly with right abdominal tenderness developed. Laboratory tests indicated progressive liver damage. In spite of continued treatment, the patient became severely acidemic (blood pH 7.06), developed supraventricular tachycardia and then asystole, and died 64 hr after entering the tank. Bromide level in a postmorten whole-blood specimen was 136 mg/liter. Due to postmortem autolysis, the autopsy was not informative.

When inspected approximately 2 hr after the accident, the bottom of the nurse tank was covered by about 7.5 cm of liquid containing 1–3% dibromoethane. Air collected from the tank 20 hr after the accident contained 28 ppm (215 mg/m^3) dibromoethane. Oxygen content in these sample was 21% and no other airborne toxin was detected. It was noted that short exposures to 28 ppm dibromoethane in air are not fatal to animals, and the fatalities were attributed to the brief (20–60 min) dermal exposure (Letz *et al.*, 1984).

Use Experience   Peoples *et al.* (1978) reviewed the minor mishaps reported in connection with the use of dibromoethane in California during 1975 and 1976. There were 16 cases, five with suspected systemic effects of mild irritation of the eyes or skin or both from splashes of the liquid. Failure to remove the fumigant promptly and thoroughly led to chemical burns, but proper removal was effective in preventing injury.

Normal sperm levels were found in 59 male workers from a chemical plant in which time-weighted dibromoethane concentrations were below 5 ppm (Ter Harr, 1980). Fertility, as determined by a retrospective analysis of births, was normal among male employees of three chemical plants producing dibromoethane but significantly less than expected at a fourth plant. Dibromoethane levels were controlled to below 5 ppm at all plants; thus, the difference could not be explained on the basis of differences of exposure. The lower than expected number of births may have been related to the prevalence of vasectomy, which was higher at this than the other three plants (Wong *et al.*, 1979). A mortality study was conducted involving 161 employees exposed to dibromoethane while working in two production units operated from 1942 to 1969 and from the mid-1920s to 1976, respectively. No increase in overall mortality or deaths from malignant neoplasms was observed at either unit. Although the sample size was small, there was no evidence that dibromoethane is a human carcinogen. Moreover, far fewer malignant neoplasms were observed than predicted by direct extrapolation of the animal data (Ott *et al.*, 1980).

Dosage Response   A dosage of about 15.5 mg/kg was fatal, but the patient was an alcohol abuser.

Because of its carcinogenic action in animals, dibromoethane is awaiting reassignment of a threshold limit value.

Pathology   In the suicide described by Olmstead (1960), autopsy revealed massive centrilobular necrosis of the liver and focal damage of the proximal renal tubules.

Treatment of Poisoning   Treatment is symptomatic.

14.7.6 1,2-DICHLOROETHANE

14.7.6.1 Identity, Properties, and Uses

Chemical Name   1,2-Dichloroethane.

Structure   See Fig. 14.6.

Synonyms   1,2-Dichloroethane is also known as Dutch liquid, EDC (JMAF), ethylene chloride, ethylene dichloride, and *sym*-dichloroethane. A trade name for the compound is Brocide®. A code designation is ENT-1,656. The CAS registry number is 107-06-2.

Physical and Chemical Properties   1,2-Dichloroethane has the empirical formula $C_2H_4Cl_2$ and a molecular weight of 98.96. It is a heavy liquid with a chloroform-like odor and a sweet taste. Its vapors are irritating, and its flame appears smoky. The liquid has a density of 1.2569. It solidifies at $-40°C$ and boils at $83-84°C$. Its flash point is $15°C$. The vapor pressure is 78 torr at $20°C$. 1,2-Dichloroethane has a solubility in water of 4.3 gm/liter at room temperature. It is miscible with alcohol, chloroform, and ether. It is stable, resistant to oxidation, and noncorrosive.

History, Formulations, and Uses   1,2-Dichloroethane was first used as an anesthetic in 1848–1849. Its insecticidal properties were recognized in 1927. A fumigant for stored products, the compound is mixed with 25% carbon tetrachoride to reduce the hazard of fire. The usual application rate is 0.13–0.225 kg/m³. The compound alone is also used as an industrial solvent.

14.7.6.2 Toxicity to Laboratory Animals

Basic Findings   The acute oral toxicity of dichloroethane was 680 mg/kg in rats (McCollister *et al.*, 1956), 700 mg/kg in mice (Heppel *et al.*, 1945), and 1142 mg/kg in rabbits (Kagramanov, 1970). In mice the intraperitoneal LD 50 was 370 mg/kg, and in rats the subcutaneous value was 700 mg/kg (Heppel *et al.*, 1945).

Rats were maintained for 2 years on diets fumigated with 1,2-dichloroethane and bred seven times during this period. Initial concentrations of 1,2-dichloroethane in the diet were 500 and 250 ppm, and it was estimated that the amount of fumigant actually consumed was 60–70% of the residue initially present or approximately 15.9 and 7.9 mg/kg. Growth, fertility, reproduction, and biochemical tests in both female and male rats were unaffected at these levels (Alumot *et al.*, 1976).

Calculated inhalation LC 50 values for rats lay along a straight line when the exposure concentration was plotted against the length of the exposure on logarithmic scales, and this line included a point for exposure at 1000 ppm for 7.2 hr. Essentially all rats died if exposed to 3000 ppm for 7.5 hr or to higher concentrations for briefer periods. The toxic effects of single respiratory exposures consisted of central nervous system depression, pulmonary irritation, and injury to the liver, kidneys, and adrenals (Heppel *et al.*, 1946; Spencer *et al.*, 1951).

When four animal species were exposed to vapor 7 hr/day, 5 days/week, for 8 months, the maximal concentrations without adverse effect were: dogs, 400 ppm; monkeys and rabbits, 200 ppm; and guinea pigs, 100 ppm (Heppel *et al.*, 1946). Only slightly different levels of tolerance were reported by Spencer *et al.* (1951) as follows: rabbits, 400 ppm; rat, 200 ppm; and both monkey and guinea pig, 100 ppm.

Very similar results were obtained in a study in which rats, guinea pigs, and rabbits were exposed for 6 hr/day, 5 days/week. 1,2-Dichloroethane was toxic to all species at a concentration of 500 ppm, while the animals tolerated exposure to 100 ppm (405 mg/m³) for 17 weeks. It is of interest that the 1,1- isomer was only one-fifth as toxic (Hofmann *et al.*, 1971).

Absorption, Distribution, Metabolism, and Excretion   1,2-Dichloroethane is readily absorbed from the gastrointestinal and respiratory tracts. Blood 1,2-dichloroethane levels plateau in the rat at 8.3 μg/ml after a 2–3-hr exposure at 150 ppm. Steady-state blood concentrations in the rat increased exponentially as the exposure concentration increased; after 6 hr of exposure at 50, 150, and 250 ppm, blood 1,2-dichloroethane levels were 14, 8.3, and 31.3 μg/ml, respectively. During a 6-hr, 150-ppm exposure, the rats were calculated to have absorbed 113 mg 1,2-dichloroethane/kg, or about 70% of the 1,2-dichloroethane they would have inhaled if the minute ventilation was 0.76 liter/min/kg body weight. 1,2-Dichloroethane was rapidly cleared from the blood ($t_{1/2} < 1$ hr) even following oral doses (<50 mg/kg) and inhalation exposures (<150 ppm) that result in nonlinear kinetics. Urine was the principal route of elimination; approximately 85% of the radioactivity recovered following an oral exposure to 150 mg/kg or a 6-hr inhalation exposure to 150 ppm of 1,2-[¹⁴C]dichloroethane was excreted in the urine as thiodiacetic acid and thiodiacetic acid sulfoxide. Another 29% of the oral dose, but only 1.8% of the inhaled 1,2-[¹⁴C]dichloroethane, was excreted unchanged via the lungs (Reitz *et al.*, 1982; Spreafico *et al.*, 1980).

The metabolism of 1,2-dichloroethane is mediated by enzymes located in the microsomal and cytosolic fraction of the liver. The microsomal pathway is mediated by cytochrome P-450 and is quantitatively more important in terms of both total metabolism and irreversible binding of 1,2-[¹⁴C]dichloroethane to proteins. The cytosolic pathway is mediated by glutathione transferase and is responsible for the mutagenicity of 1,2-[¹⁴C]-dichloroethane and for its binding to DNA (Guengerich *et al.*, 1980). The absorption and metabolism of inhaled 1,2-dichloroethane was enhanced in rats pretreated with phenobarbital, a classical inducer of cytochrome P-450 and of drug metabolism. Pretreatment of rats with disulfiram, which inhibits cytochrome P-450-mediated metabolism, significantly decreased the absorption and metabolism of inhaled 1,2-[¹⁴C]-dichloroethane. Pretreatment of rats with butylated hydroxyanisole, which induces glutathione transferase activity, had little effect on the absorption and metabolism of inhaled 1,2-[¹⁴C]dichloroethane (Igwe *et al.*, 1986).

Liver microsomes isolated from rats given 2 gm ethanol/day for 3 weeks or fed diets low in carbohydrates metabolized more 1,2-dichloroethane, while pretreatment with classical inducers of drug metabolism (e.g., phenobarbital, polychlorinated biphenyl, and 3-methylchloranthrene) did not increase 1,2-dichloroethane metabolism (Sato and Nakajima, 1985).

Biochemical Effects   1,2-[¹⁴C]Dichloroethane has been shown to bind covalently to DNA and other cellular macromolecules. Higher levels of binding were observed in the stomach following oral than inhalation administration; however, the observed differences in binding between tissues and routes of administration are inadequate to explain the difference in toxicity (Reitz *et al.*, 1982). Large doses of 1,2-dichloroethane (e.g., 200 mg/kg ip) caused persistent hepatic DNA damage, which was measured as an increase in single-stranded DNA (Storer *et al.*, 1984). Oral administration of 1,2-dichloroethane at 750 mg/kg caused a reduction of cytochrome P-450 content and microsomal enzyme activity in the liver of rats (Kokarovtseva, 1979).

Effects on Organs and Tissues ECG recordings of rats eventually killed by dichloroethane showed a stable bradycardia and a slowing of auriculoventricular conductivity. Respiratory arrest preceded cardiac arrest.

1,2-Dichloroethane has been found repeatedly to be weakly mutagenic in the Ames test with *Salmonella*. The mutagenicity is highly dependent on metabolic activation and is increased by the addition of cytosolic enzymes and glutathione (Davidson *et al.*, 1982). 1,2-Dichloroethane produced sex-linked recessive lethal mutations in *Drosophila melanogaster* (King *et al.*, 1979) and was mutagenic when tested in a mammalian cell line using the Chinese hamster ovary cell (Tan and Hsie, 1981).

1,2-Dichloroethane has been reported to be carcinogenic in rodents following oral but not inhalation exposure. When given by gavage to mice at time-weighted average dose levels of 195 and 97 mg/kg/day for males and 299 and 149 mg/kg/day for females, 1,2-dichloroethane caused an increase in alveolar/bronchiolar adenomas in both sexes; hepatocellular carcinomas in males; and mammary adenocarcinomas, endrometrial tumors, and squamous cell carcinomas of the forestomach in females. When given by gavage to rats at time-weighted average dose levels of 97 and 47 mg/kg, 1,2-dichloroethane produced squamous cell carcinoma of the forestomach, hemangiosarcomas, and subcutaneous fibromas in males and mammary gland adenocarcinomas in females (NCI, 1978b). In contrast, no increase in tumors was observed in mice or rats exposed by inhalation 7 hr/day, 5 days/week, for 78 weeks to 150 ppm 1,2-dichloroethane (Maltoni *et al.*, 1980). The reason for the difference in response for the two routes is not known. In both studies, the maximum tolerated dose was clearly exceeded and the dose levels had to be reduced due to mortality in the treated groups.

Effects on Reproduction 1,2-Dichloroethane was not teratogenic in rats inhaling 100 ppm or in rabbits inhaling 100 or 300 ppm for 7 hr/day throughout the period of major organogenesis. Of the 16 rats exposed to 300 ppm, 10 died, which demonstrates that the 300 ppm exposure concentration was maternally toxic. Symptoms which preceded death included lethargy, ataxia, decreases in body weight and food consumption, and vaginal bleeding. In addition, 3 of the 19 pregnant rabbits exposed to 300 ppm and 4 of the 21 rabbits exposed to 100 ppm died during the study. No pathological changes were observed on gross necropsy. Reproduction was not affected in rats exposed to up to 150 ppm 1,2-dichloroethane by inhalation 6 hr/day for 176 days (Rao *et al.*, 1980). Similarly, 1,2-dichloroethane was not

teratogenic when given to mice via the drinking water at doses of up to 50 mg/kg/day. The 50 mg/kg/day dose level also had no effect on reproduction, as evidenced by the absence of effects on fertility, gestation, viability and lactation indices, and pup survival and weight gain. In addition, the 50 mg/kg/day dose level failed to produce a dominant lethal effect in two generations (Lane *et al.*, 1982).

Treatment of Poisoning in Animals Large doses of activated charcoal reduced the enteral absorption and toxicity of 1,2-dichloroethane, while liquid paraffin and castor oil showed no protective effect (Laass, 1980). Acetylcysteine given by intravenous or intramuscular injection dramatically decreased lethality of 1,2-dichloroethane in mice, rats, and rabbits (Kokarovtseva, 1980).

14.7.6.3 Toxicity to Humans

Therapeutic Use As reviewed by Gwathmey and Baskerville (1914), 1,2-dichloroethane ("Dutch liquid") has been employed as a general anesthetic instead of chloroform, especially in ophthalmic surgery.

Accidental and Intentional Poisoning Following ingestion of 1,2-dichloroethane, simple narcosis was notably absent. Gastroenteritis was followed by signs of liver and kidney injury, and intestinal hemorrhages appeared in some cases. Death usually was the result of cardiocirculatory collapse and occurred 17–120 hr after ingestion (Hubbs and Prusmack, 1955; Martin *et al.*, 1968; Schoenborn *et al.*, 1970; Yodaiken and Babcock, 1973; Zhizhonkov, 1976). In one case, the first symptom (slight dizziness) did not begin until about 4 hr after intake (Zhizhonkov, 1976). In another case onset was delayed only 1.75 hr but was violent; the patient became severely ill and fell to the floor. Immediate examination revealed severe shock, cyanosis, pulmonary edema, and light coma (Hubbs and Prusmack, 1955). In a third case, the patient was already sleepy, cyanotic, and bradycardiac when he arrived at a clinic only 1 hr after taking the poison (Schoenborn *et al.*, 1970).

Some cases in young children also exemplify the delayed, sudden onset of really serious illness, but even icterus and coma did not preclude recovery without sequelae (Jacobziner and Raybin, 1961).

Three workers who spent about 4 hr washing yarn in an open vat became dizzy and nauseated and vomited profusely. They complained of weakness, trembling, and cramplike epigastric pain. When examined about an hour after onset, all were still vomiting frequently, all had red macerated hands, and at least one had rales in both lungs and a palpable liver. The absence of narcosis at any time was noteworthy. Partial recovery was prompt, but occasional nausea persisted for several days. The men were discharged in a week but their hands healed only after several more weeks (Wirtschafter and Schwartz, 1939).

Common clinical manifestations in 27 patients with acute dichloroethane poisoning were headache, vertigo, abdominal pain, nausea, and vomiting. Some patients also had hepatomegaly, icteric skin and sclera, and increased serum bilirubin levels. In addition, increased heart rate and decreased cardiac output and circulating blood volume were frequently observed in these patients (Andriukin, 1979).

In a case-controlled study, no association was found between exposure to chemicals including 1,2-dichloroethane and the incidence of primary brain tumors among employees of a Texas petrochemical plant (Austin and Schnatter, 1983). A positive association was observed, in a cohort study, between exposure to ethylene oxide and 1,2-dichloroethane and excess mortality due to circulatory disease and tumors. However, the increase in cancer and mortality could not be attributed to exposure to any particular chemical (Hogstedt *et al.,* 1979). In another study, an increased incidence of colon cancer was found in Iowa cities in which the concentration of 1,2-dichloroethane in the drinking water was greater than 0.1 μg/liter. However, the levels of 1,2-dichloroethane in the drinking water were interpreted as indicators of possible contamination of other types rather than as being casually related to the colon cancer (Isacson *et al.,* 1985).

Dosage Response   Oral doses of 50 ml (Schoenborn *et al.,* 1970), 40 ml (Martin *et al.,* 1968), 30 ml (Zhizhonkov, 1976), and 14 ml (Yodaiken and Babcock, 1973) were fatal. The ingestion of 30 ml (about 540 mg/kg) was accidental, and the man induced vomiting and then received gastric lavage to no avail. On the contrary, a 1.5-year-old survived drinking an estimated 25 ml of a "nerve medicine" containing the chemical. Nine hours after ingestion there were no clinical or EEG changes; by 19 hr, agitation and readiness for convulsion were reflected in the EEG, but these signs cleared following infusion diuresis. Serum transaminases remained normal throughout (Rohmann *et al.,* 1969).

The threshold limit value of 10 ppm (40 mg/m^3) would permit an occupational dosage of 5.7 mg/kg/day.

Laboratory Findings   Laboratory evidence of both liver and kidney injury may be found, depending on the severity of the case. In three cases of poisoning from 4 hr of respiratory and dermal exposure, low blood glucose was a prominent feature, even after the men were essentially well and were eating a high-carbohydrate diet (Wirtschafter and Schwartz, 1939).

Pathology   Pathology has included intense necrotic and hemorrhagic enteritis, widespread petechial hemorrhages, centrilobular or midzonal fatty degeneration and necrosis of the liver, tubular and glomerular degeneration of the kidney, pulmonary congestion or edema, and edema and satellitosis of the brain (Hubbs and Prusmack, 1955). A clinical impression of intravascular clotting in a few cases was not sustained by gross or microscopic examination at autopsy (Schoenborn *et al.,* 1970).

Treatment of Poisoning   Treatment is primarily symptomatic. Kindler (1979) reported that hyperventilation induced by administration increased the respiratory elimination and therefore decreased complications and fatality in cases of poisoning

with a number of chlorinated solvents, including 1,2-dichloroethane. Administration of acetylcysteine was found to be of no major benefit by Luzhnikov *et al.* (1985) in the treatment of an acute case of 1,2-dichlorethane poisoning.

14.7.7 1,1,1-TRICHLOROETHANE

14.7.7.1 Identity, Properties, and Uses

Chemical Name   1,1,1-Trichloroethane.

Structure   See Fig. 14.6.

Synonyms   1,1,1-Trichloroethane is also known as methyl chloroform. A trade name for the compound is Chlorothene®. The CAS registry number is 75-51-6.

Physical and Chemical Properties   1,1,1-Trichloroethane has the empirical formula $C_2H_3Cl_3$ and a molecular weight of 133.42. It is a nonflammable liquid with a density of 1.3376. It solidifies at −32.5°C and boils at 74.1°C. It is insoluble in water but soluble in acetone, benzene, carbon tetrachloride, methanol, and ether.

Use   1,1,1-Trichloroethane is an insecticidal fumigant. It is also used for degreasing metal and plastic.

14.7.7.2 Toxicity to Laboratory Animals

Basic Findings   The oral LD 50 values of 1,1,1-trichloroethane for rats (male), mice, rabbits, and guinea pigs were 12,300, 11,240, 5660, and 9470 mg/kg, respectively. The oral toxicity of the compound with added inhibitors was virtually the same (Torkelson *et al.,* 1958). The intraperitoneal LD 50 was 4147 mg/kg in dogs (Klaassen and Plaa, 1967) and 5083 mg/kg (Klaassen and Plaa, 1966) or 4696 mg/kg (Gehring, 1968) in mice.

Dermal toxicity is low. Rabbits were not killed by a single dosage of 4000 mg/kg applied under a cuff for 24 hr or by repeated daily applications of 500 mg/kg/day for 90 days. The latter regimen did produce reversible local irritation (Torkelson *et al.,* 1958).

Rats exposed to 1,1,1-trichloroethane vapor at a concentration of 10,000 ppm for 1 hr showed various degrees of anesthesia ranging from ataxia to semiconsciousness. When this exposure was repeated 5 days/week for 70 days, the rats tended to become acclimated, showing less effect during the latter part of each week. A similar acclimatization was observed in dogs. Based on appearance, growth, mortality, gross pathology, and microscopic changes, the only effect of the repeated exposure in rats was a very slight increase in liver weight.

Guinea pigs, which were the most susceptible animals tested, showed an increase in liver weight, centrilobular fatty change, and inflammation of the lungs when exposed 3 hr/day, 5 days/week, for 3 months at a concentration of 1000 ppm.

Rats, guinea pigs, rabbits, and monkeys were unaffected by

exposure 7 hr/day, 5 days/week, for 6 months at a concentration of 500 ppm (Torkelson *et al.*, 1958).

A series of straight lines were obtained when log concentration was plotted against log time of exposure for specified responses to both single and repeated doses (Adams *et al.*, 1950; Torkelson *et al.*, 1958).

When 1,1,1-trichloroethane was explored as an anesthetic in rats, dogs, and monkeys, no hepatic impairment was found in dogs and no liver or kidney damage was found in rats, except in one animal after nine anesthesias. The ECG was not significantly changed in the dog and monkey, but the blood pressure of the dog was markedly depressed and oxygen uptake was depressed in the monkey. The average dosage necessary to produce respiratory failure exceeded the dosage necessary to induce anesthesia by a factor of 1.77 in dogs and 2.15 in monkeys (Krantz *et al.*, 1959).

All investigators agree that the main effect of single or repeated doses is an anesthetic one. Minor liver damage is produced by repeated doses that approach anesthetic effects.

Absorption, Distribution, Metabolism, and Excretion The initial pathway of 1,1,1-trichloroethane biotransformation involves oxidation via the microsomal cytochrome P-450 mixed-function oxidase system (Ivanetich and Van Den Honert, 1981). The low systemic toxicity of 1,1,1-trichloroethane to animals and humans appears related to its very limited extent of metabolism. When 1,1,1,-[^{14}C]trichloroethane was injected intraperitoneally into rats at a dose of approximately 700 mg/kg, 98.7% of the dose was accounted for as parent compound in the expired air. An average of 0.5% was converted to $^{14}CO_2$. Much of the remainder was excreted as the glucuronide of 2,2,2-trichloroethanol (Hake *et al.*, 1960).

Following inhalation of 150 or 1500 ppm 1,1,1-[^{14}C]trichloroethane for 6 hr, rats and mice eliminated more than 96% of their end-exposure body burden within 24 hr (Schumann *et al.*, 1982a). The major route of elimination was exhalation of parent compound, constituting 87–97% of the body burden in mice and 94–98% in rats at 150 and 1500 ppm, respectively. The remaining ^{14}C activity (2–13%) was recovered as metabolized 1,1,1-trichloroethane in the expired air ($^{14}CO_2$) and as nonvolatile radioactivity in the urine, feces, carcass, and cage wash. Mice metabolized two to three times more 1,1,1-trichloroethane on a body-weight basis than did rats. Markedly higher concentrations of ^{14}C activity were recovered in the fat of both species than in the liver and kidney; however, it was cleared rapidly so that by 24 hr <2% of the initial radioactivity remained. Prior long-term exposure to 1,1,1-trichloroethane had little effect on its disposition compared to single exposure (Schumann *et al.*, 1982b).

A unified physiologically based pharmacokinetic model for 1,1,1-trichloroethane has been developed and allows comparison of body burden and target tissue dose across species and across routes of exposure (Reitz *et al.*, 1987).

Effects on Organs and Tissues By comparison of LD 50 values and corresponding ED 50 values for liver injury, it was

shown that 1,1,1-trichloroethane has only a slight tendency to injure the liver of mice or dogs (Klaassen and Plaa, 1966, 1967; Gehring, 1968). The compound does not injure the kidney (Klaassen and Plaa, 1966, 1967).

An attempt to anesthetize two dogs with 1,1,1-trichloroethane without premedication led to sudden death, presumably of cardiac origin. Administration of the compound to dogs already anesthetized by barbital produced ventricular extrasystoles and ventricular tachycardia in all of them. Maximal sensitization of the heart to epinephrine occurred after a dosage of 334–535 mg/kg, being less at higher dosages. The compound was considered less sensitizing than chloroform but more sensitizing than cyclopropane (Rennick *et al.*, 1949).

Increased cardiac sensitization to epinephrine has been demonstrated in dogs and rabbits at 1,1,1-trichloroethane concentrations of approximately 5000 ppm or greater (Carlson, 1981; Clark and Tinston, 1973; Reinhardt *et al.*, 1973). Exposure of rabbits to 5600 ppm 1,1,1-trichloroethane for 60 min, without epinephrine challenge, did not induce cardiac arrythmias (Carlson, 1981).

Herd *et al.* (1974), confirming the initial observation of Krantz *et al.* (1959), demonstrated diminished arterial blood pressure in anesthetized dogs exposed to 8000–25,000 ppm 1,1,1-trichloroethane. Phenylephrine reversed the decrease in total peripherial resistance, and exogenous calcium reversed the decline in myocardial contractility. The threshold concentration of 1,1,1-trichloroethane vapor required to produce a decrease in blood pressure in the anesthetized dog was 4000–5000 ppm (Kobayashi *et al.*, 1983). Delayed cardiotoxicity from acute exposure to 1,1,1-trichloroethane has not been demonstrated.

The behavioral effects of 1,1,1-trichloroethane have been assessed in a variety of test systems evaluating locomotor activity, coordination, unconditioned reflex and conditioned avoidance tests, a despair swimming test, and fixed ratio responding (Wooverton and Balster, 1981; Mullin and Krivanek, 1982; DeCeaurriz *et al.*, 1983; Kjellstrand *et al.*, 1985; Moser and Balster, 1985; Moser *et al.*, 1985). 1,1,1-Trichloroethane concentrations of approximately 2000 ppm or greater were required to produce effects when they occurred. These effects appeared related to the CNS sedative properties of 1,1,1-trichloroethane rather than any induction of organic brain damage.

1,1,1-Trichloroethane did not produce a carcinogenic response in mice receiving daily time-weighted average doses of 2807 and 5615 mg/kg by gavage for 78 weeks or in rats similarly exposed to doses of 750 and 1500 mg/kg (NCI, 1977a). However, high mortality precluded definitive conclusions. Male and female rats were exposed by Quast *et al.* (1978) to 0, 875, or 1750 ppm of 1,1,1-trichloroethane vapor, 6 hr/day, 5 days/week, for 12 months, followed by observation for up to 31 months of age. Focal hepatotoxicity was observed in female rats at 1750 ppm; however, no tumorigenic effects were observed in either sex. In a subsequent study, male and female rats and mice were exposed to 0, 150, 500, or 1500 ppm of a formulation containing 94% 1,1,1-trichloroethane, 6 hr/day, 5 days/week, for 2 years (Quast *et al.*, 1987). Parameters measured during the study included mortality, in-life clinical signs of toxicity, hematology, urinalysis, clinical chemistry, body weight, organ weights, gross pathology, and histopathology. There were no indications of an oncogenic effect in either species following 2 years of exposure to 1,1,1-trichloroethane. The only treatment-related effects observed consisted of decreased body weights in female rats at 1500 ppm. In addition, very slight microscopic hepatic effects were found in male and female rats in the 1500 ppm exposure group at 6, 12, and 18 months of study. These effects were characterized by altered cytoplasmic staining around the central vein and the general appearance of smaller hepatocytes in the portal region. However, hepatic necrosis was not observed. The minimal hepatic effects were not descernible after 2 years due to normal geriatric changes present in aged rats. No toxicologic effects were detected in rats exposed to 150 or 1500 ppm or in mice exposed to the highest concentration tested, 1500 ppm.

Effects on Reproduction 1,1,1-Trichloroethane was not teratogenic in rats or mice exposed by inhalation to a concentration of 875 ppm for 7 hr/day on days 6–15 of gestation (Schwetz *et al.*, 1974). York *et al.* (1982) exposed female rats to 2100 ppm 1,1,1-trichloroethane vapor 2 weeks before mating and throughout day 20 of gestation. Slight fetotoxicity was observed in some of the fetuses, although no malformations were produced. The offspring which were born and reared showed no significant treatment-related effects on body weight, survival, neurobehavior, or incidence of gross lesions at 12 months of age. No adverse effects on fertility, gestation, viability, or teratogenicity occurred in mice exposed to 0, 100, 300, or 1000 mg of 1,1,1-trichloromethane/kg body weight administered via drinking water for two gnerations (Lane *et al.*, 1982).

14.7.7.3 Toxicity to Humans

Experimental Exposure Tauber (1880) reported that under the supervision of a colleague he inhaled about 20 gm of 1,1,1-trichloroethane, which caused anesthesia without excitation, with little effect on pulse and respiration, and with rapid recovery, marred only by one episode of vomiting soon after awakening and a sense of dullness lasting about an hour.

After the anesthetic properties of 1,1,1-trichlorocthane had been studied in animals, it was used to anesthetize a 30-year-old volunteer. Induction was smooth, and anesthesia was maintained uneventfully for 30 min. There were no significant electrocardiographic changes. The blood pressure dropped to 70% of the preanesthetic level. Recovery was slow but uneventful. The person complained of being tired for several hours after the anesthesia (Krantz *et al.*, 1959).

When as many as four people at a time were exposed to measured concentrations of 1,1,1-trichloroethane, the odor was noted at average concentrations of 506 and 546 ppm but tended to disappear in the course of a 7.5-hr exposure. No subjective or objective changes were detected. An average concentration of 920 ppm had a strong odor to two of four volunteers, and in the course of exposure as short as 70 min, it produced lightheadedness and slight but definite incoordination. Recovery required

only 5–10 min. Results of tests of liver function and other clinical laboratory tests remained normal. An average concentration of 1900 ppm produced obvious disturbance of equilibrium in only 5 min. Exposure of seven men for 15 min to an atmosphere in which the concentration of 1,1,1-trichloroethane vapor was rapidly increased from 0 to 2650 ppm resulted in two men being unable to stand and three others being very lightheaded but able to stand; in fact, one of the latter was able to stand on one foot with eyes closed and hands to the sides (Torkelson *et al.*, 1958; Stewart *et al.*, 1961d).

Five men were exposed to commercial grade 1,1,1-trichloroethane vapor at a concentration of 500 ppm for 6.5–7 hr/day for 5 consecutive days to simulate a work week. Six other volunteers were exposed to the same concentration for 6.5–7 hr on separate days. During the first 5 min of the first exposure, the odor was considered strong by most of the men but mild by the others. Within 6 hr, half of the men could no longer detect the odor. The subjective responses were mild, inconsistently present, and of doubtful clinical significance. The only objective response was decreased ability of two men to stand on one foot with eyes closed and hands to the sides during exposure. Clinical laboratory tests were normal (Stewart *et al.*, 1969). The analytical results are discussed under Laboratory Findings.

Exposure to 600 ppm for only 3 hr was tolerated by six volunteers without subjective or objective damage (Gazzaniga *et al.*, 1969).

No statistically significant disturbance of motor function, coordination, equilibrium, or behavior pattern was detected among six male university students exposed to 1,1,1-trichloroethane vapor at an average concentration of 450 ppm for 4 hr in the morning and, after an interval of 1.5 hr, for 4 hr in the afternoon (Salvini *et al.*, 1971).

When each of the six persons immersed one thumb in 1,1,1-trichloroethane for 30 min, a slight prickling or burning sensation was noted in 10 min. This sensation did not increase. After each thumb was withdrawn from the solvent, a mild erythema was noted that subsided in 30–60 min. The solvent was detected in the breath within 10 min after exposure started, and the level reached concentrations of 0.19–1.02 ppm in different volunteers. When a volunteer immersed an entire hand in the solvent for 30 min, the pain was somewhat more intense; the greatest concentration reached in the alveolar breath was 21.5 ppm, compared to 1.0 ppm for the same man when he immersed only his thumb, which displaced 25 times less solvent (Stewart and Dodd, 1964). This would seem to indicate a greater rate of absorption per unit area of total hand surface than of thumb surface because the surface of the thumb is about 8.55 times less than that of the hand.

The pharmacokinetics of inhaled 1,1,1-trichloroethane were defined in six male volunteers following single 6-hr exposures to 350 and 35 ppm (Nolan *et al.*, 1984). Approximately 25% of the 1,1,1-trichloroethane inhaled during the 6-hr exposure was absorbed. Over 91% of the absorbed 1,1,1-trichloroethane was excreted unchanged by the lungs, 5–6% was metabolized and excreted predominantly in the urine as trichloroethanol and trichloroacetic acid, and less than 1% remained in the body after 9 days. Over the exposure concentration range evaluated, the pharmacokinetics of 1,1,1-trichloroethane were found to be first order.

Accidental and Intentional Poisoning Two cases of workers found dead in tanks they were cleaning have been described by Hatfield and Maykoski (1970) and Bonventre et al. (1977). In other cases, a 17-year-old male garage employee died using 1,1,1-trichloroethane for upholstery cleaning, as did a 20-year-old male electrician apprentice who used 1,1,1-trichloroethane as a degreasing solvent from an open bowl in a closed room (Jones and Winter, 1983). Northfield (1981) described the deaths of a 15-year-old male who used 1,1,1-trichloroethane in an open metal degreasing tank and of a 16-year-old male believed to have been abusing 1,1,1-trichloroethane in duties involving the use of the solvent in a centrifuge to degrease small metal parts. Respiratory or cardiac depression, ventricular fibrillation, and/or anoxia were the likely causes of death. In the case of the upholstery cleaner (Jones and Winter, 1983), inhalation of vomit was a primary contributing factor. In sniffing deaths, ventricular fibrillation is the most likely mechanism of death (Bass, 1970).

Dosage Response In a case in which a man was found dead in a tank he had been cleaning, reconstruction of the accident revealed a concentration of 1,1,1-trichloroethane of 62,000 ppm (Hatfield and Maykoski, 1970). In a different accident, concentrations of 73,000–94,000 ppm 1,1,1-trichloroethane at 8–15 cm, respectively, below the rim of the open metal degreasing tank were achievable on disturbing the liquid solvent and the vapor equilibrium above it (Northfield, 1981). The ACGIH threshold limit value of 350 ppm for 1,1,1-trichloroethane would allow occupational intake of 270 mg/kg/day.

Laboratory Findings The reported concentrations of 1,1,1-trichloroethane in the blood of poisoning victims include the following: 60 and 240 ppm for the men found dead in separate tank-cleaning incidents (Hatfield and Maykoski, 1970; Bonventre et al., 1977); 18 ppm for the upholstery cleaner and 42 ppm for the apprentice electrician (Jones and Winter, 1983); and 270 ppm for the solvent abuse case reported by Northfield (1981). Two people who died from sniffing the compound had blood levels of 130 and 720 ppm 1,1,1-trichloroethane (Hall and Hine, 1966). The blood concentration of men exposed to 955 ppm for 73 min reached 7–10 ppm at 65 min after the start of the exposure (Stewart et al., 1961d). However, only 9 min after the exposure was stopped, the blood concentration of men who had been exposed from 0 ppm to an almost anesthetic vapor concentration (2650 ppm) in 15 min was only 5 ppm. The end exposure concentration of 1,1,1-trichloroethane in the blood of human volunteers who inhaled 350 ppm for 6 hr was 1.8 ppm, 90% of which had been attained by 1.5 hr after initiation of exposure (Nolan et al., 1984).

Measurement of urinary urobilinogen was considered the most sensitive test of liver stress produced by markedly excessive exposure to 1,1,1-trichloroethane (Stewart et al., 1961d).

Treatment of Poisoning Treatment is symptomatic.

14.7.8 TRICHLOROETHYLENE

14.7.8.1 Identity, Properties, and Uses

Chemical Name Trichloroethylene.

Structure See Fig. 14.6.

Synonyms Other names for trichloroethylene include ethinyl trichloride, ethylene trichloride, and trichloroethene. Trade names include Algylen®, Benzinol®, Blacosolv®, Dukerson®, Gemalgene®, Germalgene®, Trethylene®, TriClene®, Trichloran®, Trichloren®, Trilene®, Triline®, and Trimar®. The CAS registry number is 79-01-6.

Physical and Chemical Properties Trichloroethylene has the empirical formula C_2HCl_3 and a molecular weight of 131.40. It is a colorless, nonflammable, mobile liquid with an odor resembling that of chloroform. It has a density of 1.4649 and a vapor density of 4.53 (air = 1.00). It solidifies at −84.8°C and boils at 86.7°C. The vapor pressure is 58 mm Hg at 20°C. Trichloroethylene is practically insoluble in water but soluble in ether, alcohol, and chloroform. It is relatively stable but may decompose slowly with formation of HCl in the presence of light and moisture. In the presence of heat it forms dichloroacetylene, a much more toxic material.

History and Use Trichloroethylene was discovered in 1864. Its use as an industrial solvent and degreasing agent for machinery began soon thereafter in Germany and Great Britain. Around 1911 the narcotic properties of the compound were discovered, and the use of trichloroethylene as an anesthetic began to be tested. Its use as an insecticide began in 1920. An account of the history of the compound is given in a review by Defalque (1961). Today, trichloroethylene is used in the preparation of insecticidal fumigants. It also has many industrial uses; as a solvent for oils, fats, waxes, and other substances, it is employed in both extraction and degreasing processes. It is also used in medicine to a limited extent as a general surgical anesthetic.

14.7.8.2 Toxicity to Laboratory Animals

Basic Findings The oral LD 50 for trichloroethylene was 4920 mg/kg in the rat (Smyth et al., 1969) and 2402 and 2443 mg/kg in male and female mice, respectively (Tucker et al., 1982). In the mouse and dog the intraperitoneal LD 50 values were 3222 and 2783, respectively (Klaassen and Plaa, 1967). One or more dogs survived oral dosages as high as 6000 mg/kg and an intravenous dosage of 125 mg/kg but were killed by 150 mg/kg intravenously (Barsoum and Saad, 1934).

When rats inhaled different concentrations of trichloroethylene for single periods of different durations, the results fell along a series of straight lines when log concentration was plotted against log time for exposures that were uniformly fatal and for the largest nonfatal exposures. The largest exposures that were nonfatal were almost identical to the largest ones that caused no detectable organic injury. A concentration of about 17,000 ppm was required to kill all rats in 7 hr, but all survived 3000 ppm for the same period. Rats tolerated without adverse effect 151 exposures at 200 ppm for 7 hr/day, 5 days/week. Comparable values for approximately 6-month exposures were 400 ppm for monkeys, 200 ppm for rabbits, and 100 ppm for guinea pigs. The only toxic effects of importance associated with single exposures were anesthetic ones. In fact, the capacity to cause organic injury was minor, even for repeated exposures (Adams et al., 1951).

Absorption, Distribution, Metabolism, and Excretion The initial reaction in the biotransformation of trichloroethylene involves oxidation via the cytochrome P-450 mixed-function oxidase system (Costa et al., 1980; Miller and Guengerich, 1982) resulting in the formation of a reactive species capable of binding to and deactivating cytochrome P-450 (Henschler et al., 1979; Koizumi et al., 1983; Pessayre et al., 1979). Gas uptake studies in rats using closed recirculating inhalation chamber technology have shown the metabolism of trichloroethylene to be a saturable process that is first-order at low concentrations and progresses to zero-order at high concentrations (Andersen et al., 1980; Filser and Bolt, 1979).

Disposition studies in laboratory rodents have further characterized the saturable nature of the metabolism of trichloroethylene. Rats expired a greater percentage of their end-exposure body burden as unmetabolized [^{14}C]trichloroethylene, 21.1% at 600 ppm versus 2.1% at 10 ppm, over a 50-hr interval following a 6-hr inhalation exposure (Stott et al., 1982). Upon gavage administration, rats expired approximately 1% of a single oral dose of 10 mg/kg as unmetabolized [^{14}C]trichloroethylene, compared to 43–50% at 500 mg/kg (Prout et al., 1985). Mice metabolize trichloroethylene more rapidly than do rats. Higher doses of trichloroethylene are therefore required to saturate metabolism in the mouse, resulting in less dramatic dose-dependent shifts in the fate of this material compared to that in the rat over comparable dose ranges (Dekant et al., 1986a; Prout et al., 1985; Stott et al., 1982). Based on total urinary metabolites, a trichloroethylene dose of 2400 mg/kg was required to produce clear evidence of saturated metabolism in the mouse, compared to 500 mg/kg in the rat (Buben and O'Flaherty, 1985; Prout et al., 1985).

Dekant et al. (1984) identified the following metabolites in rat urine after a single oral trichloroethylene dose of 200 mg/kg: trichloroethanol, free (11.7%) and as the glucuronide (61.9%); trichloroacetic acid (15.3); dichloroacetic acid (2.0%); oxalic acid (1.3%); and N-(hydroxyacetyl)aminoethanol (HAAE) (7.2%). Under the same experimental conditions, the primary metabolite of trichloroethylene in mouse urine was trichloroethanol, free and conjugated (94.3%), followed by HAAE (4.1%), oxalic acid (0.7%), and traces of dichloro- and trichloroacetic acid. Similar results were reported by Green and Prout (1985) in that 85–92% of the radioactivity in 24-hr urine of rats and mice was recovered as trichloroethanol glucuronide (<2% free) following 10–2000 mg/kg; however, 6–12% was recovered as trichloroacetic acid. CO_2, chloral, chloroform, CO, glyoxylic acid, and/or trichloroethylene epoxide have also been reported as trichloroethylene metabolites in various in vivo and in vitro experiments (Barrett and Johnston, 1939; Barrett et al., 1939; Butler, 1949; Dekant et al., 1984; Miller and Guengerich, 1982; Parchman and Magee, 1982; Soucek and Vlachova, 1960).

Rats and mice metabolize trichloroethylene in a qualitatively similar fashion; however, the greater rate of metabolism in mice resulted in (a) a 4-fold greater burden of metabolized trichloroethylene per kilogram of body weight (600 ppm/hr and 2000 mg/kg oral dose) and (b) 4- and 7-fold higher blood concentrations of trichloroethanol and trichloroacetic acid in mice versus rats (1000 mg/kg oral dose), respectively (Green and Prout, 1985; Prout et al., 1985; Stott et al., 1982). Humans also metabolize trichloroethylene to trichloroethanol and trichloroacetic acid, but more slowly than either mice or rats, which is thought to have important implications with respect to the greater sensitivity of the mouse to toxic effects of trichloroethylene (Elcombe, 1985; Ertle et al., 1972; Ikeda and Imamura, 1973; Kimmerle and Eben, 1973; Monster et al., 1976; Nomiyama and Nomiyama, 1979) (see Effects on Organs and Tissues). Hepatic toxicity was shown to be linearly related to metabolized trichloroethylene in mice (Buben and O'Flaherty, 1985; Dekant et al., 1986a; Prout et al., 1985).

The proposed pathways of trichloroethylene metabolism have been discussed by several authors [Dekant et al., 1984; Green and Prout, 1985; Prout et al., 1985; World Health Organization (WHO), 1985]. Trichloroethylene is metabolized by the cytochrome P-450 mixed-function oxidase system to chloral (trichloroacetaldehyde), which is subsequently oxidized to trichloroacetic acid or reduced to trichloroethanol (free and conjugated). There is still considerable confusion, however, about the intermediate involved in the formation of chloral. The existence of trichloroethylene epoxide has been postulated, and it is hypothesized that intramolecular rearrangement of chlorine is catalyzed by the iron of cytochrome P-450 acting as a Lewis acid. The transient epoxide is not believed to exist in appreciable amounts as a free species, since alternative pathways leading to CO, CO_2, and mono- and dichloroacetic acid would predominate (Henschler et al., 1979). Miller and Guengerich (1982) have suggested that epoxide formation is not an obligatory intermediate and alternatively suggest an oxygenated trichloroethylene–cytochrome P-450 transition state leading to chloral formation. CO_2 likely arises from further metabolism of trichloroacetic acid, while dichloroacetic acid, glyoxylic acid, oxalic acid, and HAAE are formed by various oxidative, reductive, and conjugative pathways from trichloroethylene epoxide and/or the proposed oxygenated enzyme–trichloroethylene complex.

It is clear that the production from trichloroethylene of

molecules with three chlorines on one carbon is due to intramolecular rearrangement, for the specific activities of excreted trichloroacetic acid and trichloroethanol were the same as those of the administered [^{36}Cl]trichloroethylene. Virtually no (0.37%) trichloroacetic acid was excreted when trichloroethanol was administered to rats (Daniel, 1963).

Metabolites of trichloroethylene are excreted very slowly, at least in part because some of the parent compound is stored in fat and is released for metabolism only slowly. This possibility is supported by a finding in human patients anesthetized under highly controlled conditions, namely that the concentration of anesthetic in venous blood collected from the antecubital fossa required at least an hour to approach the arterial concentration in more obese patients but only about 30 min in slim patients and even less time if the collections were made from veins on the back of the hand (Clayton and Parkhouse, 1962). However, this is not the full story. Excretion of trichloroacetate in humans is inherently slow, as was demonstrated in volunteers injected intravenously with the sodium salt (Powell, 1945).

It was pointed out in 1958 by Prerovska and colleagues (cited by Mikiskova and Mikiska, 1966) that patients who had ingested trichloroethylene tended to remain in coma during the first 1 or 2 days, when they were excreting large amounts of trichloroethanol in the urine, but that they often awoke by the third or fourth day, when the excretion of trichloroethanol had already dropped to a low level but the excretion of trichloroacetic acid was just reaching its maximum. The authors concluded that the narcotic state was due not only to trichloroethylene but also to the trichloroethanol formed by metabolism. Based on a study of guinea pigs injected intraperitoneally, Mikiskova and Mikiska (1966) concluded that trichloroethylene and trichloroethanol do not differ qualitatively in any way in their effects on four measured electrophysiological responses, but trichloroethanol is at least three and probably five or six times more effective at the same injected dose. Because intoxicated people excrete one-third to one-half of retained trichloroethylene as trichloroethanol, it was concluded that enough of the latter was formed to contribute substantially to prolonging and even to deepening the depressant effect of trichloroethylene itself.

The other main metabolite is neither narcotic nor very toxic. In fact, the toxicity of tricloroacetic acid is essentially the same as that of acetic acid (Woodard et al., 1941). As much as 3000 mg of sodium trichloroacetate has been injected intravenously into volunteers without injury (Powell, 1945).

Biochemical Effects Rats pretreated with phenobarbital and to a lesser extent other inducers of liver microsomal enzymes showed prolonged anesthesia, increased excretion of trichlorinated urinary metabolites, increased morphologic injury to the liver, and elevation of SGOT, compared to controls exposed to the same anesthetic concentration of vapor (Moslen et al., 1976). This finding is consistent with the importance of metabolism (bioactivation) in the toxicologic process.

The effects of high dosages of trichloroethylene on micro-somal enzymes of the liver are reported to be extremely complex, involving inhibition, stimulation, induction, and destruction (Koizumi et al., 1983; Pessayre et al., 1979). Green and Prout (1985) evaluated the influence of daily 1000 mg/kg oral doses of trichloroethylene on its own metabolism in mice after 10 and 180 days. The overall extent of metabolism of trichloroethylene was not altered; however, the amount of trichloroacetic acid excreted in the urine at 10 and 180 days was double that after a single exposure. An equivalent percentage decrease in trichloroethanol glucuronide suggests stimulation of the oxidative metabolism of chloral to trichloroacetic acid at the expense of the reductive pathway to trichloroethanol.

Effects on Organs and Tissues The potency ratios (LD 50/SGPT ED 50) for trichloroethylene in mouse and dog were only 1.4 and 3.3, indicating a very limited capacity of the compound for liver injury (Klaassen and Plaa, 1966, 1967). This is consistent with the earlier report of Kylin et al. (1962).

The toxicity of trichloroethylene has been reviewed by Kimbrough et al. (1985) and the World Health Organization (1985). A central tissue in the safety evaluation of trichloroethylene is its tumorigenic potential in mice and the relevance of this potential for humans. Trichloroethylene has been shown to increase the incidence of various types of spontaneous tumors in different strains of mice. When purified trichloroethylene was administered by gavage to B6C3F1 mice 5 days/week for 103 weeks at a dose of 1000 mg/kg/day, the incidence of hepatocellular adenoma/carcinoma was increased in male mice from 23 to 76% and in female mice from 8 to 39% in controls compared to treated groups, respectively (NTP, 1983). This result confirmed an earlier report of hepatic tumorigenicity in the same strain of mouse receiving time-weighted average doses of technical grade (epoxide-stabilized) trichloroethylene of up to 2400 mg/kg (NCI, 1976).

Interestingly, no increase in hepatic or other tumors was observed in Swiss mice exposed to purified trichloroethylene at 2400 mg/kg for 18 months followed by an additional 6-month observation period prior to sacrifice (Henschler et al., 1984). In an earlier study, Henschler et al. (1980) reported an increase in the spontaneous incidence of lymphoma in female but not male NMRI mice exposed for 18 months to 0, 100, and 500 ppm trichloroethylene vapor 6 hr/day, 5 days/week. The NMRI strain of mouse has a high and variable spontaneous incidence of lymphoma, which led the authors to speculate that trichloroethylene or nonspecific factors such as stress may have influenced the spontaneous incidence of lymphoma via a nongenetic mechanism such as immune suppression rather than via a true carcinogenic (directly genotoxic) effect.

An additional apparent strain-specific site of tumorigenesis was observed in the lungs of female ICR mice (Fukuda et al., 1983). The female mice were exposed to 0, 50, 150, or 450 ppm trichloroethylene vapor 7 hr/day, 5 days/week, for 104 weeks. The incidence of total lung tumors (adenomas and adenocarcinomas) was not statistically different in the exposed and control groups. However, the incidence of adenocarcinoma in the lung increased from 2% at 0 ppm to 6% at 50 ppm, 16% at 150 ppm, and 15% at 450 ppm, with the values at the two highest exposure concentrations being statistically different from the control value. Enhancement of spontaneous pulmonary tumors by trichloroethylene in this strain of mouse may be associated with recurrent cytotoxicity, as high doses of trichloroethylene are known to induce Clara cell and type II alveolar cell damage in this species (Forket *et al.*, 1985). No tumorigenic effects were seen at other sites.

Other species clearly appear less sensitive to the tumorigenic effects of trichloroethylene. Although early mortality complicated the interpretation of the study, trichloroethylene was not tumorigenic in male or female rats administered time-weighted doses of 550 or 1100 mg/kg by gavage, 5 days/week for 78 weeks (NCI, 1976). In a repeat study, rats were exposed by gavage to trichloroethylene at dosages of 0, 500, or 1000 mg/kg, 5 days/week for 103 weeks (NTP, 1983). Three renal adenocarcinomas were detected in the high-dose male rats, compared with none in the control group. This sex- and site-specific response was statistically significant only upon correction for decreased survival due in part to the toxicity of trichloroethylene and to gavage errors. It is noteworthy, from a mechanistic viewpoint, that the response in the kidney was accompanied by chronic toxic nephrosis induced by the high doses of trichloroethylene administered. No tumorigenic effects were observed in rats (Fukuda *et al.*, 1983) or in rats or hamsters (Henschler *et al.*, 1980) upon chronic inhalation exposure under the conditions previously described.

Mechanistic studies conducted with trichloroethylene and integrated with the animal bioassay data provide insight into the tumorigenic potential (or lack thereof) of this material for humans. The mutagenic potential of trichloroethylene has been extensively evaluated in a broad spectrum of *in vitro* and *in vivo* test systems (see reviews by Kimbrough *et al.*, 1985; WHO, 1985). Many of the studies are complicated by the presence of mutagenic epoxide stabilizers; however, even these results provide evidence of only weak activity. The predominant results with purified trichloroethylene further support the view that if trichloroethylene is mutagenic, it is likely to be so weak as not to be a predominant factor in the toxicity of this material. This is consistent with the lack of demonstrated DNA adduct formation in target tissue of trichloroethylene-exposed rodents (Berman, 1983; Parchman and Magee, 1982; Stott *et al.*, 1982).

In the apparent absence of marked genotoxic activity, trichloroethylene probably exerts its tumor-enhancing effect via an epigenetic mechanism(s) (Stott *et al.*, 1982). A plausible explanation for the hepatotumorigenic effects seen in mice (but not rats) is the fact that trichloroethylene is a hepatic peroxisome proliferating agent in the mouse (Elcombe, 1985; Elcombe *et al.*, 1985; Goldsworthy and Popp, 1987). The causative peroxisome proliferating agent has been identified as the trichloroethylene metabolite trichloroacetic acid (Elcombe, 1985). The relationship between peroxisome proliferation and neoplastic transformation is thought to involve "reactive O_2"

cytotoxicity and/or genotoxicity (Reddy *et al.*, 1980, 1982). Thus, a practical threshold can be envisioned whereby doses of trichloroethylene that do not produce peroxisomes should preclude tumor formation. Studies of the *in vitro* metabolism of trichloroethylene to trichloroacetic acid have shown that mouse hepatocytes are 30 times more active in trichloroacetic acid production than rat hepatocytes, and rat hepatocytes are 3 times more active than human cells (Elcombe, 1985). These observations are consistent with the whole-animal disposition studies previously discussed. Furthermore, human cells appear intrinsically less sensitive to peroxisomal proliferation. Trichloroacetic acid did not increase peroxisomal β-oxidation in human cells *in vitro*, in contrast to the situation in the rodent (Elcombe, 1985). Overall, it appears that under current use conditions, trichloroethylene poses little carcinogenic hazard for humans.

Although it involves a chemical derivative and a striking example of species susceptibility, it should be noted that when trichloroethylene was used to extract soybean meal in the presence of heat and the extracted meal was used as cattle feed, the animals developed hemorrhages. The disease was reproduced experimentally after its relationship to extraction was suspected from cases on farms. It was shown that the whole beans or beans extracted with naphtha are not toxic and that trichloroethylene itself did not produce hemorrhagic disease (Stockman, 1916).

After more than three decades, cases continued to appear; it was recognized that blood dyscrasia was the basis of the hemorrhage (Pritchard *et al.*, 1952), but no progress had been made in identifying the chemical responsible. Having shown that trichloroethylene reacts with protein of soybeans and that, of various amino acids tested, only cysteine reacts with this solvent, McKinney *et al.* (1957) synthesized *S*-(dichlorovinyl)-L-cysteine and showed that, when fed to calves at a rate of 0.22 mg/kg/day, this compound produced typical thrombocytopenia leading to death in 60 days. Higher dosages produced death more rapidly. Later, *S*-(dichlorovinyl)-L-glutathione was synthesized and shown to have the same action but to require a larger dosage. An *intravenous* dosage of 0.40 mg/kg/day rendered a calf moribund in 49 days (McKinney *et al.*, 1959).

Effects on Reproduction The reproductive function of male and female rats exposed to trichloroethylene at 0, 10, 100, or 1000 mg/kg/day was not directly affected at any dose level (Manson *et al.*, 1984; Zenick *et al.*, 1984b). Female rats were exposed 2 weeks before and throughout mating to gestation day 21. Five of 23 female rats died and decreased neonatal survival was observed secondary to maternal toxicity at 1000 mg/kg. No adverse effects were observed at 10 or 100 mg/kg, which led Manson *et al.* (1984) to conclude that oral exposure to trichloroethylene at doses below those causing limited maternal toxicity have no influence on pregnancy outcome. Male rats were exposed to the dose levels indicated above for 5 days/week for 6 weeks, and reproductive performance was evaluated at weeks 1 and 5 of treatment and 4 weeks postexposure (Zenick *et* *al.*, 1984b). Other than impaired copulatory behavior at week 1, which appeared related to the narcotic effects of trichloroethylene at 1000 mg/kg/day and which returned to normal by week 5, no direct adverse effects on the male reproductive system were observed.

Trichloroethylene did not cause significant maternal, embryonal, or fetal toxicity, nor was it teratogenic in either female rats or mice exposed to 300 ppm vapor 7 hr/day for days 6–15 of gestation (Schwetz *et al.*, 1975). Dorfmueller *et al.* (1979) exposed female rats to 1800 ppm trichloroethylene vapor 6 hr/day for 2 weeks before mating and/or during pregnancy through gestation day 20. Skeletal and soft tissue variations indicative of delayed development, not malformations, were observed in the group exposed during pregnancy only. Trichloroethylene was determined not to be teratogenic nor to have caused behavior deficits. Exposure of rats and rabbits to 500 ppm trichloroethylene vapor for 3 weeks prior to gestation and/or during gestation resulted in no adverse effects on fetal development (Beliles *et al.*, 1980). Thus, the fetus does not appear to be uniquely susceptible to the toxicity of trichloroethylene.

14.7.8.3 Toxicity to Humans

Experimental Exposure Three volunteers each placed one thumb in trichloroethylene for 30 min. They experienced a burning sensation on the dorsum of their thumbs within 3–18 min, and this burning became moderately severe within 5 min after onset in two persons but remained mild in one. The pain became more intense for several minutes just after the thumbs were removed from the solvent, and tingling persisted for 30 min. Erythema subsided within 2 hr. The compound was measurable in the breath of some volunteers within 10 min after exposure started and in all within 20 min. The mean peak breath concentration was 0.5 ppm (Stewart and Dodd, 1964).

Eight men inhaled trichloroethylene at concentrations of 0, 100, 300, and 1000 ppm for 2 hr. Each man received the different concentrations in random order. Five tests of visual-motor performance were administered to each volunteer three times during each 2-hr session, and one additional test was administered immediately before and immediately after exposure. At a concentration of 1000 ppm, the compound adversely affected performance in tests of depth perception, steadiness, and manual skill but had no statistically significant effect on performance in three other standard tests. The small increase in errors associated with 100 and 300 ppm were not statistically significant (Vernon and Ferguson, 1969). The results were confirmed by a second series of tests, which also showed that a small intake of alcohol (35 mg/man, leading to blood levels of 0.02–0.03%) markedly augmented the adverse effects of trichloroethylene (Ferguson and Vernon, 1970). The more sensitive of these tests apparently gave a more reproducible result than the measurement of optokinetic nystagmus, which Kylin *et al.* (1967) had showed was reduced for a time in some but not all volunteers exposed to 1000 ppm trichloroethylene for 2 hr. On the other hand, Stopps and McLaughlin (1967) reported that they could detect a slight decline in performance on some of their psychomotor tests at a level of exposure as low as 200 ppm (but not 100 ppm) for 2.75 hr. However, only one volunteer was involved, and even at 500 ppm it was questionable whether the degree of some of the measured changes was statistically significant.

Two to six men participated in separate tests involving inhalation of commercial grade trichloroethylene vapor at a concentration of 100 ppm for 4 hr or at about 200 ppm for different periods, including 7 hr/day for 5 consecutive days. Some persons regarded the odor of trichloroethylene as strong and others thought it moderately strong when they first entered a chamber containing 200 ppm, but after 6.5 hr none could detect the odor. Ability to detect the odor diminished progressively during a week of daily exposure; even on the second day all persons had lost ability to detect the odor within 30–60 min after entering the chamber. Ability to detect the odor was restored immediately by one breath of uncontaminated air. When asked specifically about a whole series of possible untoward effects, some of the volunteers reported dryness of the throat or mild eye irritation during their first day in the chamber. However, the significance of these complaints was uncertain because they were not repeated during subsequent exposures. On the contrary, toward the end of the week, volunteers complained of feeling fatigued, and some of them felt sleepy while doing monotonous tasks during exposure. No volunteer showed any untoward objective response; all neurological tests were unequivocally normal, although half of the subjects reported that it required mental effort to balance on one foot with eyes closed and hands to the sides (Stewart *et al.*, 1970a). Analytical results arising from this study are discussed under Laboratory Findings.

Six naive volunteers were exposed to trichloroethylene aerosol and vapor for 8 hr in one day (two 4-hr exposures separated by a 1.5-hr interval); the concentration varied from 90 to 130 ppm. A slight sense of dizziness and transient eye irritation occurred during maximal fluctuations in concentration. Although there was no objective disturbance of motor function, coordination, equilibrium, or behavior, there was a statistically significant decrement in performance of standard tests of perception, memory, complex reaction time, and manual dexterity. Similar results were obtained when the study was repeated with six workers who were accustomed to the odor of the compound (Salvini *et al.*, 1971). Why these tests were apparently more sensitive than those reported earlier is unclear.

Therapeutic Use Von Oettingen (1955) reviewed and documented a number of therapeutic uses of trichloroethylene, including treatment of trigeminal neuralgia, treatment of migraine, reduction of the sensitivity of the cornea in cases of severe inflammation, naroanalysis, cleaning of wounds, prevention of attacks of angina pectoris, and general analgesia and anesthesia. Of these uses, only anesthesia and analgesia now appear to have a sound pharmacological basis, and they are the only ones that have stood the test of time. Its use as an anesthetic has been so extensive that one author (Ostlere, 1948) was able to review 40,000 administrations without finding a death attributable to the anesthetic. Trichloroethylene has potent analgesic properties but is unsatisfactory as a primary agent for general anesthesia because of slow induction and recovery rates, inadequate ability to relax skeletal muscle, and adverse effects on the cardiovascular and respiratory systems [American Medical Association (AMA), 1977]. It has been used as an analgesic in minor diagnostic and surgical procedures, in obstetrics and dentistry, and as a supplement to nitrous oxide in general anesthesia. The compound may cause all kinds of cardiac arrhythmias, but ventricular arrhythmias are more common at deep levels of anesthesia or they may be induced by administration of a catecholamine. At deep levels of anesthesia, trichloroethylene may cause ventilatory arrest. Liver injury is considered unlikely but possible. The agent occasionally causes convulsions in children and is not recommended for people with convulsive disorders. Vomiting and headache are relatively rare during the postoperative period. Although the faults of other gaseous anesthetics are not identical, they are not notably less.

Accidental and Intentional Poisoning   Apparently no case of poisoning attributed to trichloroethylene used as a fumigant has been reported. However, numerous cases reported in connection with other uses and with intentional abuse show the kind of illness that misuse of the fumigant might produce. The cases have been reviewed and documented by von Oettingen (1955), Defalque (1961), Browning (1965), and Smith (1966).

Briefly, the toxicity of trichloroethylene has been what would have been predicted from its evaluation as an anesthetic. In many cases, whether resulting from ingestion or inhalation, the only important effects have been anesthetic in character, including excitement, inebriation, headache, dizziness, tinnitus, ataxia, fatigue, and sleepiness. Exposure to higher concentrations has produced coma and sometimes convulsions. Local contact with vapor may cause conjunctivitis and irritation of the nose and even irritation of the lung. If swallowed, the compound causes, after a latent period, nausea, vomiting, diarrhea, and sometimes abdominal pain. If exposure can be reduced substantially before death occurs, the anesthesia generally wears off, and the patient survives after illness lasting a day or two. When death does occur in accidental poisoning, the circumstances often do not permit identification of the cause. However, deaths in the course of anesthesia have been caused by respiratory arrest or cardiac arrhythmia (especially ventricular fibrillation), cardiac arrest, pulmonary edema, or, more rarely, liver and/or kidney damage.

Sudden fatal ventricular fibrillation has occurred in industrial workers either during work or some minutes or hours after leaving work (Kleinfeld and Tabershaw, 1954).

It must be mentioned that trichloroethylene has been an object of addiction, notably among people who become involved in the fad of "sniffing."

Epidemiologic studies published to date on trichloroethylene have been limited by several factors including small cohort numbers, young age of the cohorts resulting in few deaths, short follow-up periods, and/or minimal quantification of exposure concentrations. Nevertheless, employee health did not appear to be adversely affected, nor was any apparent cancer hazard evident (Axelson et al., 1978; Shindell and Ulrich, 1985; Tola et al., 1980).

In a few cases, chronic illness originally attributed to trichloroethylene apparently resulted from a degradation product. One example was the finding that dichloroacetylene was formed when trichloroethylene was administered to patients by a closed-system anesthesia machine containing soda lime that became hot and thus caused decomposition of the anesthetic. The dichloroacetylene formed was toxic for the cranial nerves, especially the fifth. Even when illness is truly chronic and the likelihood that a contaminant is the cause is recognized, as in the case reported by Mitchell and Parsons-Smith (1969), it may be difficult to identify the offending agent. However, sufficient analytical study or even sufficient inquiry usually will reveal the true cause. For example, it was pointed out by Lloyd (1969) that the circumstances (visible vapor) reported in the case just mentioned indicated a temperature high enough to cause degradation of trichloroethylene.

Laboratory Findings   Five male volunteers were exposed to 70 ppm trichloroethylene by inhalation, 4 hr/day for 5 consecutive days (Monster et al., 1979a). The daily uptake of trichloroethylene was calculated to be 6.6 mg/kg of lean body mass in 4 hr. Of the estimated total dose, 78% was recovered after the last exposure: 11% of the total dose recovered as exhaled trichloroethylene; 43% and 2% eliminated as trichloroethanol in the urine and expired air, respectively; and 24% as trichloroacetic acid excreted in the urine.

Upon a single 4-hr inhalation exposure to 70 or 140 ppm, end-exposure concentrations of trichloroethylene in the expired air of approximately 0.2 and 0.4 mg/liter were observed, respectively, in four male volunteers (Monster et al., 1976). The concentration of trichloroethylene in the expired air declined in a multiphasic manner. An initial rapid phase was evident in which the concentration declined to approximately one-tenth of the end-exposure concentration in 5 min. Thereafter, trichloroethylene was more slowly eliminated so that at 68 hr its concentration in the expired air was approximately 1000-fold less than the end-exposure value. The concentration of trichloroethylene in the blood followed a similar time course, and the postexposure quotient of blood concentration (mg/liter) and expired air concentration (mg/liter) remained a nearly constant value of 23 (Monster and Boersma, 1975; Monster et al., 1979a).

Maximal blood concentrations of trichloroethanol were observed within approximately 30 min postexposure and declined rapidly with a half-life of 10–12 hr. In contrast, trichloroacetic acid concentrations continued to rise in the blood, reaching a peak approximately 40–60 hr postexposure, and then declined slowly with a half-life of 70–100 hr (Monster et al., 1976).

Following the repeated daily exposure regimen of 70 ppm previously described, the concentration of trichloroethylene in blood was two times greater 18 hr after the fifth exposure than 18 hr after the first exposure (Monster et al., 1979a).

Concentrations of trichloroethanol in the blood increased from 0 to 3.4 mg/liter on the first day of exposure and from 1.1 to 4.2 mg/liter on the fifth exposure day. During the exposure-free interval, the half-life of clearance of trichloroethanol was 8–10 hr. The concentration of trichloroacetic acid in the blood increased during and between exposures. The concentration after the first exposure was 5 mg/liter of blood and reached a maximum of 31 mg/liter on the fifth to sixth day. Thereafter, the half-life of trichloroacetic acid clearance from the blood was 70–90 hr. The 24-hr (8–8 a.m.) urinary excretion of trichloroethanol was 142 mg the first day and 217 mg on the fifth day. Ten mg of trichloroacetic acid was excreted into the urine on the first day and 82 mg on the fifth day (Monster *et al.*, 1979a).

Urinary concentrations of trichloroacetic acid as high as 800 and 920 ppm have been found following nonfatal ingestion of trichloroethylene (Uhl and Haag, 1958). The concentration of trichloroacetic acid in the urine is exposure and time dependent. The highest value recorded from a woman who had been unconscious for an hour was only 320 ppm (Frant and Westendorp, 1950). On the contrary, a concentration of 780 ppm was found in the urine of a female worker who, although genuinely sick and complaining of vomiting, abdominal cramps, weakness, and weight loss, had been working steadily and went to a physician of her own volition. Reoperation of the machine she had been using produced trichloroethylene vapor concentrations of 260–280 ppm in the breathing zone (Milby, 1968). Bardodeg (1968) reported that symptoms were present when the urinary level of trichloroethanol reached 400 ppm. This value is consistent with recent reports. It probably is not consistent with the view of Ahlmark and Forssman (1951), who considered that exposure giving rise to urinary concentrations of trichloroacetic acid as high as 20 ppm probably gave rise to definite complaints only in exceptional cases. Effects occurred in about one-half of the persons excreting 40–75 ppm and in almost all those excreting over 100 ppm. When the urinary excretion exceeded 200 ppm, symptoms were often so intense that sick leave was requested.

Not only is part of the compound exhaled during exposure, but also this form of excretion continues for longer periods. Eighty-eight hours following exposure to 200 ppm for 7 hr/day for 5 days, the average concentration of trichloroethylene in the expired breath still averaged about 0.2 ppm (Stewart *et al.*, 1970a). Similar results were reported by Malchy and Parkhouse (1969) in studies of trichloroethylene anesthesia, and these results approximate those of Monster *et al.* (1979a).

During respiratory exposure, the concentration of trichloroethylene in the expired breath increased rapidly during the first few minutes. The highest concentration (76 ppm at an ambient concentration of 200 ppm) was detected within 3 hr after exposure began. During consecutive exposures, there was a slight but definite accumulation of the compound that approached an equilibrium on the second day. There was little individual variation (Stewart *et al.*, 1970a). There was a reasonably close straight-line relationship between the concentrations of trichloroethylene in alveolar air and in the blood (Kylin *et al.*, 1967).

In a study of volunteers, Stewart *et al.* (1970a) noted a striking difference in the combined excretion of trichloroacetic acid and trichloroethanol in different persons following identical respiratory exposure. However, consecutive 24-hr urine specimens associated with exposure to 200 ppm trichloroethylene for 7 days showed a progressive increase in the excretion of these metabolites in all persons. The average combined excretion during the first day after exposure was 400 mg. Excretion decreased exponentially after the last exposure, but detectable concentrations were still present 12 days later.

Heavy, even excessive, occupational exposure does not lead to significant liver injury. Normal values were found in various laboratory tests of liver function in workers whose average concentrations of urinary trichloroacetic acid varied from 219 to 505 ppm in different years (Tolot *et al.*, 1964).

The current ACGIH threshold limit value for trichloroethylene is 50 ppm (270 mg/m^3), which would permit occupational exposure at a rate of 38.5 mg/kg/day.

Pathology In general, pathology is quite nonspecific, as one would expect with an anesthetic. In one case, a very striking parchment-like appearance of the exposed skin (face, hands, and forearms) was attributed to desiccation and extraction of subcutaneous fat of a woman who was found dead with her head and forearms over the rim of a degreasing basin (Derobert, 1952).

Treatment of Poisoning Treatment of poisoning by trichloroethylene is symptomatic. In studies with eight volunteers exposed to an average concentration of approximately 190 ppm, Bartonicek (1963) showed that excretion of trichloroethanol was significantly reduced by intravenous administration of either fructose or sodium lactate. Because of the contribution of trichloroethanol to the toxicity of trichloroethylene, it was proposed that infusions of 10% fructose and 5% sodium lactate should be administered to patients for several hours as soon as possible after their hospitalization. In an entirely similar way, Bartonicek and Teisinger (1962) showed that divided doses of disulfiram totaling 3000–3500 mg decreased the metabolism and increased the exhalation of trichloroethylene inhaled by four women.

14.7.9 TETRACHLOROETHYLENE

14.7.9.1 Identity, Properties, and Uses

Chemical Name Tetrachloroethylene.

Structure See Fig. 14.6.

Synonyms Tetrachloroethylene is the name most generally used. Other names for the compound include ethylene tetrachloride, perchloroethylene, tetra, and tetrachloroethene. Trade names include Ankilostin®, Dikadene®, Dowper®, Nema®, Perclene®, Tetracap®, and Tetropil®. A code designation is ENT-1,860. The CAS registry number is 127-18-4.

Physical and Chemical Properties Tetrachloroethylene has the empirical formula C_2Cl_4 and a molecular weight of 165.85. It is a colorless, nonflammable liquid with a density of 1.6230. It solidifies at $-22°C$ and boils at $121°C$. The vapor pressure at $25°C$ is 19 mm Hg. Tetrachloroethylene is practically insoluble in water but is miscible with alcohol, ether, chloroform, and benzene.

Use Tetrachloroethylene is used as a fumigant for insects and rodents. It also is an industrial solvent for a number of purposes, particularly dry cleaning and degreasing. In people, tetrachloroethylene has been used as an anthelmintic.

14.7.9.2 Toxicity to Laboratory Animals

Basic Findings The oral LD 50 of undiluted tetrachloroethylene in mice was 0.109 ml/mouse (about 8424 mg/kg) (Dybling and Dybling, 1946). Pozzani et al. (1959) reported an acute oral LD 50 of 2600 mg/kg for rats. More recently, acute oral LD 50 values of 3835 and 3005 mg/kg for male and female rats, respectively, observed over a 16-day interval were reported (Hayes et al., 1986). The intraperitoneal LD 50 of tetrachloroethylene for mice ranged from about 4643 to 5672 mg/kg (Gehring, 1968; Klaassen and Plaa, 1966), and an intraperitoneal LD 50 of 3408 mg/kg was reported for dogs (Klaassen and Plaa, 1967).

The few dogs tested survived oral dosages as high as 6000 mg/kg. However, dogs were killed by an intravenous dosage of 85 mg/kg; the few that received 75 mg/kg or less survived (Barsoum and Saad, 1934).

Hayes et al. (1986) exposed rats to tetrachloroethylene in their drinking water at concentrations producing doses of 0, 14, 400, and 1400 mg/kg/day for 90 consecutive days. Body weights were significantly lower and serum 5'-nucleotidase activity significantly elevated (suggesting possible hepatotoxicity) in males receiving 1400 mg/kg/day and in females receiving 400 or 1400 mg/kg/day. However, other serum indicators of hepatic function, as well as urine analysis and hematology, were not affected by treatment. Ratios of liver and kidney weight to body weight were higher in both sexes at 1400 mg/kg/day and the ratio of kidney to body weight was higher in the males at 400 mg/kg/day. No gross pathological effects were observed in this study.

Rats died within a few minutes of inhaling a vapor concentration of 30,000 ppm tetrachloroethylene and in about 30 min at 19,000 ppm (Carpenter, 1937). Death was narcotic in nature. A series of essentially straight lines was obtained when log concentration was plotted against log time for exposures to tetrachloroethylene that were just sufficient to cause lethality in rats, just small enough to be survived by all rats, and just small enough to cause no organic injury (Rowe et al., 1952). A concentration of 2000 ppm was tolerated for up to 14 hr, and 3000 ppm was tolerated for 4 hr with no deaths. Unconsciousness was produced in rats within a few minutes at concentrations of 6000 ppm or greater and after several hours at 3000 ppm, but unconsciousness was not observed at 2000 ppm.

Rats, rabbits, and monkeys withstood 7-hr exposures to 400 ppm tetrachloroethylene vapor 5 days/week for 6 months without apparent adverse effects on mortality, growth, body and organ weights, and periodic clinical chemistry determinations. However, guinea pigs could tolerate repeated 7-hr exposures at concentrations no higher than 100 ppm (Rowe et al., 1952).

An 8-hr LC 50 of 5040 ppm tetrachloroethylene for rats was reported by Pozzani et al. (1959). In a more recent report, the highest concentration of tetrachloroethylene that did not result in lethality in rats or mice following a single 4-hr exposure and 16-day observation period was approximately 2450 ppm (NTP, 1986c).

Absorption, Distribution, Metabolism, and Excretion Tetrachloroethylene is well absorbed by the inhalation and oral routes of exposure and more slowly through the skin (Pegg et al., 1979; Schumann et al., 1980; Stewart and Dodd, 1964; Tsuruta, 1975). Once absorbed, the highest concentrations of tetrachloroethylene are found in adipose tissue, reflecting its high lipid solubility (Savolainen et al., 1977). This solvent is metabolized by the microsomal cytochrome P-450 mixed-function oxidase system in a dose-dependent manner. Gas uptake studies using rats exposed in a closed inhalation chamber system indicate that tetrachloroethylene is very slowly metabolized in this species, with first-order pharmacokinetics evident at low concentrations and zero-order (metabolic saturation) pharmacokinetics predominating at higher exposure concentrations (Filser and Bolt, 1979).

Animal disposition data confirm the limited extent of metabolism of tetrachloroethylene in the rat, as well as its saturable nature. Pegg et al. (1979) recovered 72 and 90% of the body burden as unmetabolized parent compound in the expired air 72 hr after oral administration of 1 and 500 mg/kg, respectively, of [^{14}C]tetrachloroethylene in rats, and 68 and 88% as expired parent compound over the same time interval following inhalation of 10 and 600 ppm [^{14}C]tetrachloroethylene for 6 hr. The remaining dose was recovered as nonvolatile (metabolized) radioactivity in the urine, feces, and carcass and as expired $^{14}CO_2$. The disposition and elimination pharmacokinetics of [^{14}C]tetrachloroethylene in rats following a 12-hr drinking-water exposure resulting in a dose of 8.1 mg/kg was not substantially different from that observed after gavage or inhalation exposure (Frantz and Watanabe, 1983). Approximately 88% of the body burden was eliminated as expired parent compound in a monophasic manner with a half-life of 7.1 hr.

In contrast, tetrachloroethylene is more rapidly metabolized by the mouse. Only 12% of the body burden was expired as parent compound in the mouse over 72 hr after exposure to 10 ppm [^{14}C]tetrachloroethylene vapor for 6 hr (Schumann et al., 1980). The remaining 88% of the body burden was recovered as nonvolatile (metabolized) radioactivity in the urine (63%), feces (6.8%), carcass (3.0%), and cage wash (7.7%) and as expired $^{14}CO_2$ (7.9%). At a high metabolically saturating dose (500 mg/kg, oral), the predominant route of elimination in mice shifted to exhalation of parent compound (82.6% of the body burden). Thus, mice were found to metabolize (bioactivate) 8.5- and 1.6-fold more tetrachloroethylene on a body weight basis than the rat following inhalation of 10 ppm for 6 hr or a single oral dose of 500 mg/kg (Schumann *et al.*, 1980).

Based on the appearance of total urinary metabolites versus dose, the metabolism of tetrachloroethylene deviated from linearity at 500 mg/kg in mice exposed by gavage to 0, 20, 100, 200, 500, 1000, 1500, or 2000 mg/kg or tetrachloroethylene for 6 weeks (Buben and O'Flaherty, 1985). Furthermore, plots of hepatotoxicity data against total urinary metabolites were linear, confirming the observation of Moslen *et al.* (1977) and Schumann *et al.* (1980) that the hepatotoxicity of tetrachloroethylene is related to the extent of its metabolism.

The production of a type I binding spectrum with rat hepatic microsomes *in vitro* indicates that tetrachloroethylene binds to the active site of the cytochrome P-450 mixed-function oxidase system (Costa and Ivanetich, 1980). Metabolites identified in tetrachloroethylene-treated animals suggest initial oxidation by cytochrome P-450 to the transient electrophile tetrachloroethylene epoxide. Although the epoxide has never been isolated in biological materials (e.g., blood, tissue, or urine), it is presumed to rearrange spontaneously with intramolecular migration of a chlorine atom to trichloroacetyl chloride, which rapidly hydrolyzes to trichloroacetic acid (Daniel, 1963; Henschler and Hoos, 1982; Odum *et al.*, 1987; Yllner, 1961). Trichloroacetic acid has been identified *in vitro* using rat hepatocytes (Costa and Ivanetich, 1984) and in the isolated perfused liver (Bonse *et al.*, 1975).

Dekant *et al.* (1986b) exposed female rats and mice to a high, metabolically saturating oral dose of 800 mg/kg of [^{14}C]tetrachloroethylene and recovered 2.3 and 7.1% of the dose in the urine, respectively. The following metabolites, expressed as a percentage of the total urinary radioactivity, were identified: trichloroacetic acid (54% in rats, 57.8% in mice); trichloroacetic acid conjugate (1.8%, 1.3%); oxalic acid (8.0%, 2.9%); trichloroethanol, free and conjugated (8.7%, 8.0%); dichloroacetic acid (5.1%, 4.4%); and *N*-trichloroacetyl-aminoethanol (5.4%, 5.7%). Trichloroacetic acid, oxalic acid, dichloroacetic acid, ethylene glycol, chlorine, and/or CO_2 have been identified by other investigators as metabolites of tetrachloroethylene (Buben and O'Flaherty, 1985; Daniel, 1963; Pegg *et al.*, 1979; Schumann *et al.*, 1980; Yllner, 1961).

It was generally assumed that the metabolism of tetrachloroethylene occurred exclusively via cytochrome P-450-mediated oxidative pathways. Consistent with this hypothesis, Pegg *et al.* (1979) did not observe depletion of hepatic nonprotein sulfhydryls, suggesting that tetrachloroethylene was not metabolized or detoxified by conjugation with glutathione. However, Dekant *et al.* (1986b) identified as a minor metabolite the tetrachloroethylene–mercapturic acid conjugate 1,1,2-trichlorovinyl-*N*-acetylcysteine in the urine of rats and mice (1.6 and 0.5% of total urinary radioactivity, respectively) following a high metabolically saturating oral dose of 800 mg/kg [^{14}C]tetrachloroethylene. Odum and Green (1987) also identified a mercapturic acid conjugate of tetrachloroethylene in the bile of rats dosed orally with 1500 mg/kg and in the urine of

rats and mice exposed by inhalation to 400 ppm for 6 hr. The urinary concentration of the mercapturic acid conjugate was 10 times lower in the mouse than the rat. This metabolite appears to be a substrate for activation to a reactive electrophile by renal β-lyase, and the K_m of this enzyme was five times higher and the V_{max} five times lower in the mouse than the rat. At present it is not known whether this quantitatively minor metabolic pathway operates *in vivo* at low substrate concentrations or whether it represents a "spillover" pathway at concentrations of tetrachloroethylene that saturate the microsomal mixed-function oxidase system.

Effects on Organs and Tissues   The intravenous potency ratios (LD 50/SGPT ED 50) of Plaa (Plaa *et al.*, 1958; Klaassen and Plaa, 1967) were 0.98 and 2.8 for tetrachloroethylene in the mouse and dog, respectively, indicating a relatively slight tendency of tetrachloroethylene to produce liver injury. The same investigators found that the compound caused significant kidney dysfunction, as evidenced by reduced excretion of PSP, but only at near-lethal doses. Histological effect on the kidney was minimal. The very low level of hepatotoxicity was confirmed by Gehring (1968) in mice exposed to tetrachloroethylene vapor. A more marked hepatotoxicity following inhalation in mice was reported by Kylin *et al.* (1962). Fatty infiltration was observed 1 and 3 days after a single 4-hr exposure to 400 ppm tetrachloroethylene, but necrosis was not observed even after exposure to 1600 ppm.

Drew *et al.* (1978) exposed rats for 4 hrs to 500, 1000, or 2000 ppm tetrachloroethylene and measured the serum enzymes SGOT, SGPT, glucose-6-phosphatase (G6P), and ornithine carbamoyltransferase. All four enzymes, classical indicators of hepatic injury, were markedly elevated at 2000 ppm, less so at 1000 ppm, and largely unaffected by exposure to 500 ppm. Liver/body weight, liver triglycerides, G6P, and SGPT values were significantly elevated in mice at doses of 100, 100, 500, and 500 mg/kg/day and greater, respectively (Buben and O'Flaherty, 1985). The mice had been administered 0, 20, 100, 200, 500, 1000, 1500, or 2000 mg tetrachloroethylene/kg/day, 5 days/week, for 6 weeks.

Reichert (1983) reviewed the biological actions of tetrachloroethylene in mammalian species, which serves as a useful adjunct to the present discussion. The chronic toxicity of tetrachloroethylene in laboratory animals, in particular its tumorigenic potential and human health implications (or lack thereof), has been extensively evaluated over the past decade. Rampy *et al.* (1978) exposed male and female Sprague–Dawley rats to 0, 300, or 600 ppm tetrachloroethylene vapor 6 hr/day, 5 days/week, for 12 months. The rats were then allowed to survive until sacrifice 31 months after the start of the study. Clinical signs of toxicity were not observed and mean body weights were similar among all groups. Mortality was slightly greater in high-dose males than in controls, which was thought to be due to earlier onset of spontaneous chronic renal disease. Tetrachloroethylene was not tumorigenic in the rat under these exposure conditions.

Following chronic oral administration of tetrachloroethylene to rats and mice by gastric intubation, an increase in the spontaneous incidence of hepatocellular carcinoma was reported in mice (NCI, 1977b). Male and female B6C3F1 mice received time-weighted average doses of 536 and 1072 mg/kg (males) and 386 and 772 mg/kg (females) 5 days/week for 78 weeks and were sacrificed at 90 weeks. Male and female Osborne-Mendel rats received time-weighted average doses of approximately 475 and 950 mg/kg for a similar duration of dosing (78 weeks) and were sacrificed at 110 weeks. The incidence of hepatocellular carcinoma was increased from a spontaneous incidence of approximately 10% in both sexes of untreated plus vehicle control mice to 40 and 65% for low-dose and 40 and 56% for high-dose female and male mice, respectively. In addition, toxic nephropathy was observed in nearly all treated mice but not in the controls. Toxic nephropathy was also observed in more than 85% of the treated male rats, in 50–80% of the treated female rats, but not in control rats. Tetrachloroethylene was not tumorigenic in rats, although diminished survival prevented definitive conclusions by the investigators (NCI, 1977b).

In a subsequent study, male and female B6C3F1 mice and Fischer 344 rats were exposed by inhalation 6 hr/day, 5 days/week, for 103 weeks to tetrachloroethylene concentrations of 0, 100, or 200 ppm (mice) or 0, 200, or 400 ppm (rats) (NTP, 1986c). Again, the spontaneous incidence of hepatocellular carcinomas plus adenomas was elevated in exposed mice, and the following incidences for control, low-dose, and high-dose mice were reported: males, 35, 63, and 82%; females, 8, 34, and 76%. In rats the high spontaneous incidence of mononuclear cell leukemia was increased from a control value of 36% to 60 and 58% in females at 200 and 400 ppm and from 36% to 74 and 74% in the male rats at 0, 200, and 400 ppm tetrachloroethylene, respectively. Two renal tubular cell adenocarcinomas were also observed in the male rats (but not females) exposed to 400 ppm, compared to none at 0 or 200 ppm. This response was not statistically significant, however, biological relevance has been suggested (NTP, 1986c). Renal tubular cell hyperplasia and/or karyomegaly was reported at varying instances in rats and mice, suggesting long-term renal toxicity during the course of the study.

Studies designed to assess the macromolecular interactions of tetrachloroethylene have provided valuable insight for interpreting the chronic bioassay results. Tetrachloroethylene has in most cases given negative results, or at worst infrequent weak positive results, when tested in *in vitro* or *in vivo* genetic toxicity (mutagenicity) assays (e.g., bacteria, mammalian cells in culture, *Drosophila,* and whole-animal assays) (Beliles *et al.,* 1980; Bronzetti *et al.,* 1983; Callen *et al.,* 1980; Henschler and Bonse, 1977; Ikeda *et al.,* 1980; NTP, 1986c; Reichert, 1983; Shimada *et al.,* 1985). Furthermore, tetrachloroethylene was not detected bound to hepatic DNA of B6C3F1 mice following a single oral dose of 500 mg/kg or inhalation of 600 ppm [^{14}C]tetrachloroethylene for 6 hr (Schumann *et al.,* 1980).

Tetrachloroethylene has been shown to induce peroxisomal proliferation in mouse liver, but not in rat liver, by virtue of its more extensive metabolism to the known peroxisome-proliferating agent trichloroacetic acid in the mouse compared to the rat (Goldsworthy and Popp, 1987; Green *et al.,* 1986b; Odum *et al.,* 1987). It is probable that (*a*) resultant peroxisome-mediated oxidative damage to mouse hepatic DNA under these conditions (see previous discussion for tetrachloroethylene), (*b*) the genetic predisposition for hepatic tumor development, and (*c*) elevated rates of toxicity-induced hepatic DNA synthesis by tetrachloroethylene in this strain of mouse (Schumann *et al.,* 1980) act in concert in promoting B6C3F1 mouse liver tumors.

With respect to the low, not statistically significant incidence of male rat kidney tumors, Goldsworthy *et al.* (1987) observed increased protein droplet formation in renal proximal convoluted tubular cells in male rats exposed orally to 1000 mg tetrachloroethylene/kg/day for 10 days. In addition, renal tubular cell proliferation was observed in the male rats. Protein droplet formation and cell replication in treated females did not differ from observations in controls. A marked morphologic correlation existed between protein droplet formation and the male rat-specific protein α-2μ-globulin. The early morphologic and toxic changes of tetrachloroethylene-induced nephrotoxicity may be predominant events in the tumorigenic process and are similar to those observed with some other male rat-specific renal tumorigens such as unleaded gasoline (Short *et al.,* 1986).

However, a direct genotoxic effect in the rat kidney cannot be ruled out at this time. The cysteine conjugate of tetrachloroethylene has been shown *in vitro* to be activated by renal β-lyase to an electrophilic sulfur-containing metabolite which is positive in the Ames bacterial mutagenicity assay (Dekant *et al.,* 1986c; Green and Odum, 1985). The extent to which the low-level mercapturic acid conjugate of tetrachloroethylene identified in rats and mice (see the preceding section on Absorption, Distribution, Metabolism, and Excretion) is bioactivated via renal β-lyase and whether, if activated, the reactive intermediate reaches renal tubular cell DNA are presently unknown. In light of the very low renal tumor incidence observed and its sex and species specificity, it is probable that renal tubular cell toxicity (whether acting in concert with a low-level genotoxic insult or the low spontaneous renal tumor rate) is a predominant factor which, if precluded by low-dose exposure, would likely preclude tumor formation.

The toxicologic relevance for humans of the observed increase in rat mononuclear cell leukemia is highly suspect due to the high and variable spontaneous incidence of this lesion in the Fischer 344 rat. Furthermore, this lesion has not been induced in other strains of rats or mice chronically exposed to tetrachloroethylene.

Upon evaluation of the entire data base, coupled with available, though limited human epidemiology data (see below), it is not likely that tetrachloroethylene poses significant carcinogenic risk for humans under current use conditions.

Effects on Reproduction Daily exposure to vapor concentrations as high as 470 ppm did not impair the reproduction of rats (Carpenter, 1937).

Schwetz *et al.* (1975) exposed mice and rats to 300 ppm

tetrachloroethylene vapor 7 hr/day on days 6–15 of gestation. It was concluded that tetrachloroethylene was not teratogenic in either species. The same conclusion was reached by Beliles *et al.* (1980) for rats and rabbits exposed by inhalation to 500 ppm tetrachloroethylene 7 hr/day, 5 days/week, before mating and/or daily during gestation. Additional studies have been reviewed by John *et al.* (1984), who concluded that the animal studies showed no teratogenic potential for this compound, and fetal toxicity is evident only at high, maternally toxic exposure concentrations. Subtle neonatal behavioral changes seen in one study at 900 ppm but not 100 ppm were variable with age, poorly correlated with exposure to tetrachloroethylene, and not observed in a subsequent study at 1000 ppm (see John *et al.*, 1984). Thus, the current ACGIH threshold limit value of 50 ppm for human exposure would appear to provide adequate protection with respect to reproductive outcome.

14.7.9.3 Toxicity to Humans

Experimental Exposure Concentrations of tetrachloroethylene of 2000 ppm or more produced very light narcosis in four unacclimatized subjects within a few minutes. After their return to fresh air, nausea, vertigo, and ringing in the ears were reported. Exposure to 1000 ppm produced very light inebriation in 45 min but no narcosis in 1 hr and 35 min. A concentration of 500 ppm produced only slight discomfort in 2 hr; symptoms included increased salivation, sweetish metallic taste, slight irritation of the eyes, tightness in the frontal sinuses, increased sweating of the hands, increased nasal secretion, and in one man slight nausea. The odor of tetrachloroethylene was detected by men entering a concentration of 50 ppm from fresh air (Carpenter, 1937).

Tetrachloroethylene was explored as a general anesthetic in 4 volunteers and 14 selected patients; one volunteer was anesthetized 3 times, making a total of 20 inductions. Briefly, it was found that tetrachloroethylene has the advantage of being nonflammable and nonexplosive and of being capable of producing a moderate depth of surgical anesthesia even in fully oxygenated patients. No toxicity was encountered in the small series of human inductions. However, it was found that tetrachloroethylene was difficult to vaporize and that this probably contributed to the production of first- or second-degree burns in 4 of the 20 administrations. It was considered that the observed irritation of mucous membranes indicated that the compound would offer no improvement in regard to postanesthetic pulmonary complications compared to compounds already in use. Furthermore tetrachloroethylene was not capable of producing full muscle relaxation, and it produced excessive secretions. It was concluded that the disadvantages outweighed the advantages (Foot *et al.*, 1943).

Two to six volunteers were exposed to various concentrations of tetrachloroethylene vapor to help determine a satisfactory industrial limit. They found the compound more irritating than others had reported, even though the material was redistilled and 99.9% pure. It was concluded that concentrations of about 1000 ppm were painful and highly disagreeable, and concentrations of about 600 ppm were appreciably irritating to the eyes and nose. Concentrations above 200 ppm (206–356 ppm) produced lightheadedness, a burning sensation in the eyes, congestion of the frontal sinuses, thickness of the tongue, tightness about the mouth, and irresponsibility; coordination required mental effort; nausea occurred in one subject after about 30 min but disappeared before the end of a 2-hr exposure; recovery usually occurred within an hour but one man did not feel well for several hours after a 2-hr exposure. Concentrations in the range 83–130 ppm were not objectionable (Rowe *et al.*, 1952).

Studies involving male volunteers were carried out to determine the relationship between the intensity and duration of exposure and the concentration of tetrachloroethylene in blood and expired air (Monster *et al.*, 1979b; Stewart *et al.*, 1961c). The results are discussed under Laboratory Findings.

Sixteen healthy men and one woman volunteered to inhale tetrachloroethylene vapor for 7 hr at continuously monitored concentrations averaging 100 ppm (670 mg/m^3), and five of the men were exposed in this way for five consecutive days, simulating a work week. All of these people judged the odor to be moderately strong when they first entered the chamber, but their ability to detect the odor gradually diminished, especially during the first several hours. All of those with repeated exposures could smell the compound at the beginning of each exposure, but fatigue set in more rapidly as the week progressed. Within the first 2 hr of exposure, some of the volunteers complained of one or more of the following: frontal headache; mild irritation of the eyes, nose, or throat; a sensation of flushing; lightheadedness; sleepiness; and difficulty in speaking. The symptoms did not become progressively greater, and the irritation tended to subside before the end of the exposure. Those who were repeatedly exposed had fewer subjective complaints than the others, but some reported mild headache or mild irritation. The only untoward objective response was a decreased ability of three of the people to stand on one foot with eyes closed and hands to the sides. They were able to perform normally when given a second chance. Ability to read and to reason was unimpaired (Stewart *et al.*, 1970b).

Five volunteers each placed one thumb in tetrachloroethylene for 40 min. A mild burning sensation was noted by all subjects within 5–10 min; the burning reached its maximum within 15–20 min but continued for 10 min after exposure was stopped and then gradually subsided within an hour. A marked erythema developed during exposure but subsided within an hour or two after exposure stopped. The compound was detected in the exhaled breath within 10 min after exposure started. The degree of absorption as measured by concentration in the breath was slightly less than that of other chlorinated hydrocarbons tested under the same conditions, but the rate at which expiration of the compound declined after exposure was lower than for any of the others (Stewart and Dodd, 1964).

Therapeutic Use As a result of their studies in dogs, Hall and Shillinger (1925) suggested that tetrachloroethylene be tested cautiously for treatment of hookworm disease in humans. It was tested and found to be as effective as carbon tetrachloride but safer. Later, tetrachloroethylene was shown to be effective in oxyuriasis (infestation with *Enterobius vermicularis*) (Wright *et al.*, 1937).

According to a recent evaluation, a single oral dose cures 50% or more of infestations by *Necator americanus* and about 25% of those by *Archylostoma duodenale* (AMA, 1977). Although alcohol should be avoided by patients who receive tetrachloroethylene, the danger of combining the two is very small compared with the danger of combining alcohol and carbon tetrachloride. Manson (1934) reported that tetrachloroethylene had been given to alcoholics without adverse results. Maplestone and Chopra (1933) considered that one of the advantages of tetrachloroethylene was that it could be administered as an alcoholic solution.

Accidental and Intentional Poisoning   Apparently no accidents associated with the use of tetrachloroethylene as a fumigant have been reported. Accidents associated with its use as a cleaning agent illustrate its potential for injury but also its relative safety.

The fatal cases reviewed by Browning (1965), as well as those reported more recently, had in common repeated exposure to unmeasured but obviously high concentrations. In several cases death was attributed to pulmonary edema, but in all instances there was some evidence of liver and kidney damage. Multiple hemorrhagic foci have been detected at autopsy. In a case reported by Treuse and Zimmermann (1969), it is difficult to believe that the observed hemoptysis and massive hematotemesis did not contribute importantly to death, which was attributed to cardiovascular failure.

As might be expected from a compound that has been used as an anesthetic, unconsciousness caused by tetrachloroethylene is not always followed by serious illness. This was illustrated by the case of a 25-year-old man who started cleaning a tank car with this solvent. He wore a chemical respirator, but within 5 min the odor became so strong inside the mask that he left the tank. In spite of this warning, he soon returned to the tank and 10 min later was discovered unconscious. Thirty minutes after his removal he was drowsy but well oriented. His vital signs were normal, and his neurological findings were normal except for inability to remain balanced on one foot with his eyes closed. As predicted from the concentration of solvent in his breath samples, the patient developed a slight increase of SGOT on days 3 and 4 and a delayed elevation of urobilinogen, both indicating transient liver dysfunction (Stewart, 1969). A similar case was reported by Stewart *et al.* (1961a).

In 44 cases of industrial overexposure to tetrachloroethylene reported to HM Factory Inspectorate in the United Kingdom from 1961 to 1980, 17 resulted in unconsciousness and 3 were fatal (McCarthy and Jones, 1983). The frequency of signs and symptoms reported include the following: 22 with central nervous system depression; 9 with nausea and vomiting; 9 with respiratory symptoms (cough, breathlessness, chest tightness);

and 1 with a very marginally raised SGPT in an otherwise asymptomatic 46-year-old man.

Use Experience   Brown and Kaplan (1987) published the results of a retrospective cohort mortality study of 1690 dry cleaning workers, from four labor unions, with solvent exposure for at least 1 year prior to 1960. As had been a complicating factor in prior reports, the workers evaluated in the dry cleaning industry had experienced exposure to multiple solvents such as, but not limited to, benzene, carbon tetrachloride, and/or petroleum derivatives (various types of Stoddard solvents). However, Brown and Kaplan (1987) were able to identify a subcohort of 615 workers exposed to tetrachloroethylene as the primary, and presumably only, solvent. Compared to U.S. rates, the mortality of the total exposed cohort was 86% of that expected, indicating a healthy worker effect. Total cancer deaths were greater in the exposed cohort (142 observed versus 122.9 expected) when compared to the U.S. population but nearly identical to the expected number (140) when compared to the rates in states where the unions were located. No liver cancer deaths were observed, whereas 3.5 were expected. Only urinary tract cancer (kidney and bladder) showed a statistically significant elevation (12 versus 4.7 expected) in the total cohort. However, in the tetrachloroethylene-only exposed cohort this effect disappeared (only 1 urinary tract cancer death versus 1.3 expected). Thus, analysis of workers exposed to tetrachloroethylene as the primary solvent suggests strongly that prior associations between tetrachloroethylene and excess risk for urinary tract cancer (see discussion, Brown and Kaplan, 1987) were confounded by exposure to other synthetic or petroleum solvents.

Dosage Response   When doses of 6 ml or more were given for treatment of hookworm, a few patients developed giddiness, faintness, and weakness (Fernando *et al.*, 1939). Narcosis was seen very rarely but has occurred quite unpredictably after as little as 3 ml taken by a healthy, well-developed man (Kendrick, 1929; Sandground, 1941).

The usual therapeutic dosage is 0.12 ml/kg with a maximal dose of 5.0 ml (about 116 mg/kg). The drug should be given early in the morning following a low-bulk, low-fat evening meal and no breakfast. No laxative should be given, and alcohol should be avoided (AMA, 1977).

The ACGIH threshold limit value of 50 ppm (335 mg/m^3) for tetrachloroethylene would permit occupational exposure at the rate of 48 mg/kg/day.

Laboratory Findings   Tetrachloroethylene can be measured with specificity, accuracy, and high sensitivity in the expired breath. Following 7 hr of exposure to 100 ppm, the concentration of the solvent decreased exponentially; a small residual amount was still present 16 hr after exposure. During consecutive exposures, there was a slight but definite accumulation of the solvent; a steady state was approached but was not completely reached in 5 days. The highest breath concentration was about 32 ppm (217 mg/m³). The difference in tetrachloroethylene breath concentrations between identically exposed individuals was astonishingly small, but the concentration tended to become higher for heavy people (77–85 kg) than for lighter ones (57–62 kg). This trend was apparent about 100 hr after exposure, and it became more marked by 300 hr (Stewart *et al.*, 1970b).

Six male volunteers were exposed to 72 or 144 ppm tetrachloroethylene for 4 hr (Monster *et al.*, 1979b). End-exposure concentrations of tetrachloroethylene in the blood and expired air appeared proportional to the exposure concentrations. In the postexposure period, the quotient of the blood and exhaled air concentrations remained nearly constant at 23. The blood levels of tetrachloroethylene measured 2 and 20 hr after termination of exposure were approximately 37 and 5%, respectively, of the end-exposure values (end-exposure values of 3 and 6 mg/liter for the 72 ppm and 144 ppm exposure groups, respectively, were estimated from the graphically depicted data). Exhalation of parent compound was the major route of elimination, with only approximately 1–2% of the absorbed tetrachloroethylene recovered in the urine as trichloroacetic acid. The markedly lower extent of metabolism (bioactivation) of tetrachloroethylene by humans compared to the rat, which is less than that for the mouse, correlates with the lower tissue injury-related toxicity potential in humans versus rodents, as discussed previously.

A workman who lost consciousness 3.5 hr after he started using a 50%:50% tetrachloroethylene:Stoddart solvent solution for cleaning had a breath level of 84 ppm tetrachloroethylene when first sampled 36 min after exposure stopped (Stewart *et al.*, 1961a). It was later reconstructed that the concentration to which the man had been exposed ranged from 25 to 1470 ppm. Approximately 20 min after exposure stopped, volunteers who had been exposed to an average concentration of 194 ppm for 187 min (long enough to approach an apparent steady state-concentration in their blood of 2.5 ppm) had an average breath concentration of 27 ppm tetrachloroethylene (Stewart *et al.*, 1961c). Those exposed in a similar way to a vapor concentration of 101 ppm had breath levels of 16 ppm. Both the workmen and the volunteers excreted tetrachloroethylene very slowly. Following exposure for 3 hr to a concentration of 194 ppm tetrachloroethylene, the compound was measurable in the breath for at least 110 hr and found to be present at a concentration of 0.3 ppm. The pattern of decrease after exposure was stopped was exponential.

Liver function tests may become minimally abnormal by day 3 or as late as 9 days after excessive exposure and remain abnormal for 2 weeks or more. This occurred in a man who lost consciousness momentarily but never developed anorexia, nausea, vomiting, jaundice, or neurological symptoms and was fully alert within an hour of his removal from tetrachloroethylene vapor (Stewart *et al.*, 1961a; Stewart, 1969).

In one fatal case, the initial chest X ray suggested diffuse bronchopneumonia, allergic-toxic lung, or acute miliary tuberculosis (Treuse and Zimmermann, 1969).

Treatment of Poisoning Treatment is symptomatic.

14.7.10 DIBROMOCHLOROPROPANE

14.7.10.1 Identity, Properties, and Uses

Chemical Name 1,2-Dibromo-3-chloropropane.

Structure See Fig. 14.6.

Synonyms Dibromochloropropane is the name commonly used, although JMAF has approved the acronym DBCP. Trade names include Femafume®, Fumazone®, and Nemagon®. The CAS registry number is 96-2-8.

Physical and Chemical Properties Dibromochloropropane has the empirical formula $C_3H_5Br_2Cl$ and a molecular weight of 236.36. It forms a brown liquid with a pungent odor that boils at 196°C. The vapor pressure at 21°C is 0.8 mm Hg. Dibromochloropropane is slightly miscible with water and miscible with oils, isopropyl alcohol, acetone, methanol, and dichloropropane. It is stable in neutral and acidic media but is converted by alkali to 2-bromoallyl alcohol. It corrodes aluminum and magnesium and their alloys, but it will not corrode steel or copper alloys unless it contains more than 0.02% water.

History and Use Dibromochloropropane was introduced in 1955 as a soil fumigant and nematocide. The application rate was 10–125 kg/ha.

14.7.10.2 Toxicity to Laboratory Animals

Basic Findings In 1961, Torkelson *et al.* published a study demonstrating the acute and chronic toxicological effects of DBCP to four animal species: rats, guinea pigs, rabbits, and monkeys. The LD 50 of DBCP by oral intubation was 150–370 mg/kg body weight in male rats, 260–620 mg/kg body weight in female rats, and 150–300 mg/kg in male guinea pigs. Based on these results, the acute oral toxicity of DBCP was considered moderate. The percutaneous LD 50 was 1400 mg/kg body weight. The inhalation LC 50 values in rats over various time intervals (with 95% confidence limits) were: 1 hr, 368 ppm; 2 hr, 232 ppm (202–265); 4 hr, 154 ppm (135–177); and 8 hr, 103 ppm (90–118). Rats exhibited slight to moderate CNS depression when exposed to DBCP vapor, and respiratory irritation was evident at concentrations of 60 ppm and higher. Torkelson *et al.* (1961) also found that when DBCP was applied to rabbit skin, a single dose of 0.5 ml was slightly irritating; when applied to the rabbit eye, a single dose of 0.1 ml of DBCP caused slight transient irritation that cleared completely 48 hr after application.

In repeated inhalation exposure studies, male and female rats were exposed to DBCP vapors at 5, 10, 20, or 40 ppm for 50 exposures over a 7-week period. At the 5 ppm level, some male rats exhibited a decrease in testicular weight, and at the 10 ppm and higher exposures, gross lesions in the lungs, intestinal mucosa, kidneys, and testes developed. At the 20 and 40 ppm levels, the testes atrophied. Inhalation exposures of rabbits and guinea pigs to 12 ppm DBCP for 50–66 times over 70–92 days produced atrophy and degeneration of the testes (Torkelson *et al.*, 1961).

In another experiment described by Torkelson *et al.* (1961), rats were fed a diet containing DBCP at levels of 0, 5, 20, 150, 450, or 1350 ppm for 90 days. At the 1350 ppm level rats showed poor growth, decreased activity, increased mortality, and increased liver and kidney weights. Lesser changes were seen in rats at the 450 ppm level. Rats fed 150 ppm (7.4 mg/kg/day) or less remained in good condition for 90 days.

No further investigations were reported until Rakhmatullaev (1971) demonstrated decreased testicular weight and decreased sperm mobility in rats given DBCP orally at 5 mg/kg/day for 8 months. Subsequently, Reznik and Sprinchan (1975) reported that daily oral administration of DBCP to rats at 10 mg/kg for 4–5 months produced atypical estrous cycles in females and reductions in sperm count and mobility in male rats. Rao *et al.* (1982, 1983) exposed rats and rabbits by inhalation to 0, 0.1, 1, or 10 ppm DBCP for 8–14 weeks. Rabbits demonstrated decreased sperm counts at 1 and 10 ppm DBCP; both rats and rabbits exhibited significant decreases in testicular weight at the high exposures. Rats exposed to 0.1 and 1 ppm and rabbits exposed to 0.1 ppm DBCP did not show any testicular injury.

Absorption, Distribution, Metabolism, and Excretion In rats given a single oral dose of 20 mg/kg of DBCP, only a trace (0.04%) of the ^{14}C activity was excreted in the expired air as unchanged DBCP, but some was metabolized to CO_2. Essentially all (98.8%) was absorbed from the gut and 90% of the absorbed dose was excreted in 3 days. During the first 24 hr, 49, 14, and 16.5% of the dose were excreted in the urine, feces, and expired air, respectively. Urinary excretion was primarily in the form of glutathione conjugates (Kato *et al.*, 1979a).

A preferential accumulation of the radiocarbon in the liver and kidneys was apparent. Based on extensive studies, Kato *et al.* (1979b) concluded that in the tissues DBCP was covalently bound to protein following oxidation to a reactive intermediate in the presence of microsomal enzymes. The authors proposed that an epoxide could be one of the reactive intermediates (Kato *et al.*, 1980). Later, Suzuki and Lee (1981) investigated the ability of DBCP to induce epoxide-metabolizing enzymes in rats treated with a single oral dose of 125 mg/kg. In these rats a significant increase in aryl hydrocarbon hydroxylase and epoxide hydrolase activity was observed in the testes, kidney, and stomach. The authors concluded that DBCP induces epoxide-metabolizing enzymes via the *de novo* synthesis of new hemoproteins.

Effects on Reproduction Dibromochloropropane was not teratogenic to rats when given orally on days 6–15 of gestation

at levels of 12.5, 25, or 50 mg/kg/day. The two highest levels were toxic, resulting in reduced maternal and fetal weights (Ruddick and Newsome, 1979). Oral doses of DBCP given to rabbits at 15 mg/kg in water and to rats at 15 mg/kg in corn oil did not significantly effect fertility (Amann and Berndtson, 1986; Foote *et al.*, 1986). When male rats were exposed to DBCP vapor at a concentration of 10 ppm for 14 weeks, they were able to fertilize females, but the proportion of resorptions was increased over control levels, suggesting a dominant lethal effect (Rao *et al.*, 1983). Rabbits were more sensitive than rats; male rabbits exposed to 1 or 10 ppm DBCP showed testicular atrophy, loss of spermatogenic cells, and complete infertility at the high exposure level (Rao *et al.*, 1982). Reel *et al.* (1984) confirmed the reproductive toxicity potential of DBCP at 100 mg/kg/day by gavage in a continuous breeding design in mice.

The potential for DBCP to reduce male fertility by acting at a site in the genital tract beyond the testes was evaluated in rats. Doses of 10–40 mg/kg/day for 7 days given subcutaneously caused reduction in the metabolism of glucose to CO_2 by epididymal sperm. Thus DBCP may cause nearly immediate infertility via a direct effect on posttesticular sperm (Kluwe *et al.*, 1983).

Mutagenic Effects of DBCP Rosenkranz (1975) found DBCP to be a direct mutagen in short-term microbial assays. DBCP blocked growth of *E. coli polA*, and it was mutagenic for *Salmonella typhimurium* strain TA1530. DBCP did not induce mutations in *S. typhimurium* strain TA1538. These results indicate that DBCP causes base substitution but not frameshift mutations in bacteria.

In vivo mammalian genetic toxicity tests have been conducted for chromosomal effects. Aberrations were found cytologically in spermatogonia and bone marrow of orally exposed rats (Kapp, 1978), and an increase in YFF bodies, an indication of Y-chromosome nondisjunction, in the sperm of DBCP-exposed men has been reported (Kapp *et al.*, 1979). The latter needs independent confirmation because Y chromosome counts were made on ejaculates with extremely low sperm counts, the control sample was from a different location, and the statistical methodology is subject to question.

Three separate studies in male rats have demonstrated positive dominant lethal results whether the animals were exposed orally (Teramoto *et al.*, 1980; Saito-Suzuki *et al.*, 1982) or by inhalation (Rao *et al.*, 1982). Dominant lethal tests to date have been negative in the mouse (Teramoto *et al.*, 1980; Generoso *et al.*, 1985), but a report of unscheduled DNA synthesis in premeiotic spermatocytes of prepubertal mice (Lee and Suzuki, 1979) suggests the vulnerability of mouse germ cell DNA to DBCP-induced damage. In addition, chromosomal aberrations in cultured Chinese hamster cells (Tezuka *et al.*, 1980) and sex-linked recessive lethal mutations in *Drosophila melanogaster* males (Inoue *et al.*, 1982) have been reported.

Russell *et al.* (1986) undertook to determine whether DBCP would induce heritable gene mutations in the mouse specific-locus test. Oral administration of DBCP at 80 mg/kg/day to mice did not induce mutations in spermatogonial stem cells. In contrast to these results, Saski *et al.* (1986) reported positive results with DBCP in the mouse spot test, which is another method for detecting genetic alterations in somatic cells.

Effects on Organs and Tissues   Olson *et al.* (1973) studied the chronic toxic effects of DBCP in rats and mice. Fifty animals of each sex for each dose were used. Rats received oral doses of DBCP of 24 and 12 mg/kg/day, 5 days per week. These doses were increased to 30 and 15 mg/kg/day after 14 weeks. Male mice initially received 160 and 80 mg/kg/day, increasing to 260 and 130 mg/kg/day. Initial doses in females were 120 and 60 mg/kg/day. At the conclusion of the study (54 weeks in rats, 42 weeks in mice), gastric squamous carcinoma was evident in a high percentage of both male and female rats and mice. In addition, mammary adenocarcinomas developed in female rats. These results have been confirmed in subsequent studies in which DBCP was administered to rats and mice in the diet and by gavage (cited in Whorton and Foliari, 1983).

Van Duuren *et al.* (1979) studied the chronic toxic effects of dermal applications of DBCP in mice. Thirty animals were included in each experimental group. A single dose of 69 mg was applied to the shaved skin of mice, followed 14 days later by 5 mg of the tumor promoter phorbol myristate acetate three times per week. By 61 weeks, a significant increase in papillomas was found in treated animals. In a second phase of the study, repeated dermal doses of 35 or 11.7 mg/mouse were applied three times per week for 63–84 weeks. At both levels, excess lung and stomach tumors were observed. The incidence of skin papillomas was not increased in the repeated-dose bioassay.

Reznik *et al.* (1980a) found an excess in nasal cavity tumors in rats chronically exposed by inhalation to 0.6 and 3.0 ppm DBCP, 6 hr/day, 5 days/week, for 103 weeks. Both sexes at both doses developed significant increases in nasal cavity tumors. A higher percentage of tumors were malignant in the high-dose groups than in the low-dose groups.

14.7.10.3 Toxicity to Humans

Accidental and Intentional Poisoning   A 54-year-old woman entered the hospital with complaints of severe continuous cramping, epigastric and right upper quadrant pain, fever, anorexia, nausea, vomiting, and diarrhea of 24–48 hr duration. Initial physical examination revealed an enlarged tender liver, mild jaundice, and slight fever. Laboratory findings on admission showed a mild anemia, increased white count with a shift to the left, and albumin and occult blood in the urine. More extensive studies the next day confirmed major dysfunction of the liver and kidneys. In spite of appropriate treatment, the patient's hospital course was characterized by rapid deterioration, and she died within 2 days. Autopsy revealed massive, mainly centrilobular liver necrosis and acute proximal tubular necrosis of the kidneys. During life, the patient had said that she became sick after spraying her lawn with a formulation of DBCP. Exposure to the compound was established by measur-

ing it by gas chromatography at a concentration of 21.5 ppm in a specimen of liver taken at autopsy. Although the hospital summary and autopsy report made no mention of suicide, it seems doubtful that such a high level of DBCP would remain in the liver 4 days after the reported environmental exposure. The patient's indefiniteness about the time of onset and her delay in seeking medical attention point to the same conclusion (Hayes, 1982). An earlier example in which chemical analysis served to reveal suicide in a case where poisoning was initially blamed on environmental exposure was reported by Stewart (1974).

Use Experience   In 1977, a small group of workers in a chemical plant in northern California became aware that few of them had fathered children recently. When oligospermia or azoospermia were found in all five men, an investigation was initiated (Whorton *et al.*, 1977). A common factor in all the affected workers was exposure to DBCP. Extensive investigation showed the following: of the 107 men exposed to DBCP, 13.1% were azoospermic, 16.6% were severely oligospermic, and 15.8% were mildly oligospermic, whereas among the 35 nonexposed workers, 2.9% were azoospermic, none were severely oligospermic, and 5.7% were mildly oligospermic (Whorton *et al.*, 1979; Milby and Whorton, 1980). Furthermore, some of the azoospermic workers who were exposed to DBCP had elevated serum levels of follicle-stimulating hormone (FSH) and luteinizing hormone (LH). An analysis of semen from DBCP-exposed workers showed a positive correlation between the length of exposure to DBCP and the extent of reduction in sperm production (Marshall *et al.*, 1978). Testicular biopsies in 10 affected workers showed seminiferous tubules to be the site of damage. In severely affected men, the seminiferous tubules were devoid of spermatogenic cells, with only Sertoli cells remaining. In the less severely affected, there was a decrease in the amount of cellularity within the seminiferous tubules (Biava *et al.*, 1978).

Based on the 1977 findings, other investigations of DBCP-exposed workers were initiated. Data from eight worker exposure surveys are summarized in Table 14.2. Information on actual absorbed dose of DBCP, by both inhalation and skin absorption, is not available in any of these studies. However, all the studies have revealed that occupational exposures to DBCP has adverse effects on testicular function, as 15.7% of the subjects were azoospermic and another 22.1% were oligospermic. Based on studies of other populations, one would normally expect a group of 500 workers to have 9–10% oligospermic and at most 1% azoospermic men.

A study by Egnatz *et al.* (1980) conducted several years after cessation of DBCP production found normal testicular function in the 232 DBCP-exposed workers examined. The chemical plant investigated had produced DBCP from 1957 through 1975. Examinations were performed at least 20 months after termination of DBCP production. In a subgroup directly exposed to DBCP within 5 years of the study, 4 of 26 employees had sperm counts below 10 million/ml. Duration of exposure was highly correlated with decreases in sperm count

Table 14.2
Summary of DBCP Worker Surveys[a]

Study population	Number of subjects[b]	Number of men with sperm count results (million/ml)			Reference
		0	0.1–9	10–19	
California factory workers	114	15	8	12	Whorton *et al.* (1977)
Colorado factory workers	64	5	2	7	Lipschultz *et al.* (1980)
Alabama factory workers	71	1	6	5	Lipschultz *et al.* (1980)
Arkansas factory workers	86	30	(17)[c]	(3)	Lanham (1981)
California DBCP applicators	74	6	8	(7)	Glass *et al.* (1979)
Israeli factory workers	23	12	6	0	Potashnik *et al.* (1978)
Southeast United States DBCP users	53	2	12	8	Sandifer *et al.* (1979)
Mexican factory workers	23	9	(11)		Marquez (1978)
Totals of exposed population	508	80	70	42	
		(15.7%)	(13.8%)	(8.3%)	
Composite control	90	2.2	1.1	1.2	Milby and Whorton (1980)

[a] Adapted from Whorton and Foliari (1983).
[b] Variable exposures.
[c] Numbers in parentheses represent estimates extrapolated from the data presented.

and increases in FSH. The subgroup's mean values for sperm count, FSH, LH, and testosterone were within normal limits. The authors interpreted the overall data as indicative of a testicular effect from DBCP that was reversible over time.

Follow-up studies of workers exposed to DBCP reported improved sperm production in some adversely affected men, which appeared to be dose related. Whorton and Milby (1980) reported normal sperm concentrations in six of the nine originally oligospermic men 1 year after exposure was terminated, but there was no change in any of the azoospermic men. In all cases with subsequent normospermia the exposure to DBCP was less than 4 years. Conversely, none of the men exposed for 4 years or more showed signs of improved sperm production. Potashnik (1983) reported increases in sperm counts 4 years after exposure ended in both oligospermic and azoospermic men who had been exposed for shorter periods of time. Lantz *et al.* (1981) reported increases in sperm density of all the exposed oligospermic men they tested 18–21 months after exposure ended. None of the men in their study had been exposed to DBCP for more than 2.5 years, and most had been exposed for much shorter periods of time.

Eaton *et al.* (1986) reported on 44 men whose exposure to DBCP in a formulation plant was first described in 1977. Five to 8 years after the initial effects of DBCP exposure were discovered and all exposures terminated, there appeared to be no major changes in testicular function of most of the exposed men as measured by sperm concentrations or serum FSH levels. Recovery of sperm production in two of eight originally azoospermic workers was observed, and no increase in sperm production could be detected in men who had low sperm counts in 1977.

Lanham (1987), on the contrary, has reported a much higher return of testicular function 9 years after termination of DBCP exposure in a group of workers who had potential exposure to

DBCP for up to 18 months. Of 30 workers who were found to be azoospermic in 1977, 26 have participated in periodic testing. The sperm counts for seven have remained at zero. Of the 19 who have had return of function, 15 have reached levels of more than 20 million sperm/ml, and one elected to have a vasectomy early in his recovery phase. The longest interval from end of exposure to return of sperm production was 82 months. Seventeen workers were found to be oligospermic (less than 20 million sperm/ml) at their initial examination in 1977. Fourteen of these have participated in periodic testing and all have reached levels greater than 20 million sperm/ml. Three workers were lost to follow-up. FSH levels, which were elevated in azoospermic and oligospermic workers, returned to normal in those who recovered function with the exception of three who were azoospermic and now are oligospermic. Elevated FSH levels in the seven who remain azoospermic continue to be elevated.

Treatment of Poisoning Treatment is symptomatic.

14.7.11 1,3-DICHLOROPROPENE

14.7.11.1 Identity, Properties, and Uses

Chemical Name 1,3-Dichloro-1-propene. The pesticide is a mixture of *trans* (E) and *cis* (Z) isomers.

Structure See Fig 14.6.

Synonyms 1,3-Dichloropropene is also known as α-chloroallyl chloride and 1,3-dichloropropylene. The CAS registry number for 1,3-dichloropropene is 542-75-6. The number for the trans isomer is 10061-02-6; that for the cis isomer is 10061-01-5. Commercial formulations, containing varying amounts of a mixture of cis and trans isomers, have historically been marketed under the trademarks Dorlone® (admixture with 1,2-dibromoethane), D-D® Soil Fumigant, Nemex®, Telone®, and Vidden D®. More recent trademarks include Vorlex® (admixture with isothiocyanate), Di-Trapex®, D-D® Super, Telone® II Soil Fumigant, and Telone® C-17 Soil Fugicide and Nematicide (admixture with chloropicrin).

Physical and Chemical Properties   1,3-Dichloropropene has the empirical formula $C_3H_4Cl_2$ and a molecular weight of 110.98. It is a white to amber-colored liquid with a sweet penetrating odor. The density at 25°C is 1.217. The boiling points of the cis and trans isomers are 104°C and 112°C, respectively. The flash point is 28°C. The solubility in water at 20°C is 1 gm/kg. The compound is miscible with acetone, benzene, carbon tetrachloride, heptane, and methanol.

History, Formulations, and Uses   Introduced in 1945, 1,3-dichloropropene is a soil fumigant for the control of nematodes in numerous food and nonfood crops.

14.7.11.2 Toxicity to Laboratory Animals

Basic Findings   The oral LD 50 of 1,3-dichloropropene in rats ranges from 130 to 713 mg/kg in males and 110 to 510 mg/kg in females, depending on the vehicle and strain used. The dermal LD 50 has been reported as greater than 1211 mg/kg in both sexes of rats (unoccluded); 1000 and 13000–2000 mg/kg in male and female rats, respectively (occluded); and 333–540 mg/kg for both sexes of rabbits (occluded) (Torkelson and Oyen, 1977; Toyoshima *et al.*, 1978; Jeffrey, 1987a,b; Jones and Collier, 1986a,b). The acute 4-hr LC 50 value for 1,3-dichloropropene vapor in rats was 855–1035 ppm for males and 904 ppm for females (Streeter *et al.*, 1987). Exposed animals had a distinct "garlic" odor and suffered eye and nasal irritation. Brief exposure to concentrations in excess of 2700 ppm vapor also caused severe lung, liver, and kidney injury (Torkelson and Oyen, 1977).

1,3-Dichloropropene is irritating to the skin of rabbits, causing a moderate erythema and moderate to severe edema immediately following a 4-hr dermal exposure period and may cause a marked redness and slight to moderate chemosis of the conjunctivae immediately following instillation of 0.1 ml into the eyes of rabbits. These effects are gradually reversible, and in most instances washing with water was effective in averting injury (Jeffrey, 1987c,d; Torkelson and Oyen, 1977). Similar results have been reported for a formulation of 1,3-dichloropropene containing approximately 30% 1,2-dichloropropane (D-D®) (Hine *et al.*, 1953). 1,3-Dichloropropene also tested positive in a guinea pig skin sensitization assay (Jeffrey, 1987e).

Repeated oral gavage dosing of male and female rats with 1,3-dichloropropene at 1, 3, 10, or 30 mg/kg/day, 6 days/week, for 13 weeks resulted in elevated kidney weights of all top-dose animals and of males administered 10 mg/kg/day. However, no gross or microscopic pathologic changes or alterations in hematologic indices, urinalysis, or serum enzymes occurred in treated rats (Till *et al.*, 1973).

In an inhalation study conducted in 1958, exposure of male and female rats, guinea pigs, rabbits, and dogs (females only) to 1 or 3 ppm 1,3-dichloropropene vapor 7 hr/day, 5 days/week, for 6 months was reported to result in a slight, reversible change in the kidneys of male rats in the high exposure group (Torkelson and Oyen, 1977). No effects were observed in female rats or other animals exposed to 1 ppm vapor. More recent studies in which both sexes of rats and mice were exposed (6 hr/day, 5 days/week) to mixed-isomer vapor concentrations of 5, 10, or 30 ppm for 30 days; 10, 30, or 90 ppm for 13 weeks; and 10, 30, 90, or 150 ppm for 13 weeks have not substantiated these earlier findings. Instead, these studies, conducted with more recent formulations, have identified the nasal mucosa and urinary bladder as potential target tissues of inhaled 1,3-dichloropropene (Coate, 1979a,b; Stott *et al.*, 1985). Nasal effects consisted of degeneration of olfactory epithelium and/or hyperplasia of respiratory epithelium in both sexes of rats (≥30 ppm) and mice (>90 ppm) and respiratory metaplasia in olfactory regions of mice (150 ppm). Bladder effects consisted of hyperplasia of the transitional epithelium in female mice only (≥90 ppm). A similar exposure of rats and mice to 5, 15, or 50 ppm D-D® for 12 weeks resulted in liver and kidney weight changes in high-exposure male and female rats, respectively, and diffuse hepatocellular swelling in high-exposure male mice (urinary bladders were not examined) (Parker *et al.*, 1982).

Absorption, Distribution, Metabolism, and Excretion
Toxicity and pharmacokinetic data indicate that 1,3-dichloropropene is absorbed from the skin, respiratory tract, and gastrointestinal tract. Following absorption, both the cis and trans isomers are rapidly eliminated from the bloodstream of rats (half-life < 30 min) (Stott and Kastl, 1985). The predominant routes of excretion of radioactivity in male and female rats following a single oral dose of cis, trans, or racemic (males only) 1,3-dichloropropene were via the urine (cis, 82–84%; trans, 56–61%; racemic, 51–61%), feces (cis or trans, 2–3%; racemic, 17–21%), and expiration of CO_2 (cis, 2–5%; trans, 23–24%; racemic, 15–18%) (Hutson *et al.*, 1971; Dietz *et al.*, 1984a,b). A relatively small amount of mixed cis and trans isomers was found to bind macromolecules in the forestomach and, to a lesser extent, in the glandular stomach of treated rats and mice (Dietz *et al.*, 1984a,b). Macromolecular binding correlated with a dose- and time-related depression in the nonprotein sulfhydryl content of stomach and liver tissues of these animals.

Excretion and distribution of 1,3-dichloropropene were independent of dose in rats administered up to 50 mg/kg, with greater than 80% of the administered dosages being excreted within 24 hr of dosing. A similar pattern of excretion and distribution occurred in mice administered up to 100 mg/kg racemic compound (Dietz *et al.*, 1984b). Excretion in rats occurred primarily as the mercapturic acid conjugate of 1,3-dichloropropene and its corresponding sulfoxide via the urine (Climie *et al.*, 1979; Dietz *et al.*, 1984a,b). The mercapturic acid conjugate has also been identified in the urine of investigators and applicators exposed to mixed-isomer vapors of 1,3-

dichloropropene under field application conditions (Osterloh *et al.*, 1984).

Effects on Organs and Tissues Initial studies of the mutagenic potential of mixed-isomer formulations of 1,3-dichloropropene and gas chromatographically purified cis and trans isomers found 1,3-dichloropropene to be mutagenic to *S. typhimurium* (strains TA100 and TA1535) in the absence of added liver homogenate (Eder *et al.*, 1982; Stolzenberg and Hine, 1980; Neudecker *et al.*, 1977; De Lorenzo *et al.*, 1977). Mutagenic activity was decreased on addition of microsomes or glutathione to the assay (Creedy *et al.*, 1984). Subsequent studies of the bacterial mutagenicity of 1,3-dichloropropene using material which was purified by silicic acid absorption chromatography were negative (Talcott and King, 1984; Watson *et al.*, 1987). A weakly positive response could be obtained in the presence of liver microsomes but this was abolished by the addition of cytosolic enzymes, presumably glutathione transferase. Thus, it appears that earlier positive mutagenicity findings were a result of the presence of mutagenic stabilizing agents present in 1,3-dichloropropene formulations and/or the formation of mutagenic oxidation products of 1,3-dichloropropene generated during gas chromatographic purification operations (Watson *et al.*, 1987).

Consistent with the inactivation of 1,3-dichloropropene and/or its oxidation products by glutathione, negative results have been obtained for a racemic formulation of 1,3-dichloropropene in the Chinese hamster ovary hypoxanthine–guanine phosphoribosyltransferase (HGPRT) forward mutation assay, rat hepatocyte unscheduled DNA synthesis assay, and mouse bone marrow micronucleus test (Mendrala, 1985; 1986; Gollapudi *et al.*, 1985). In contrast, gas chromatographically purified cis and trans isomers induced unscheduled DNA synthesis in HeLa cells *in vitro* (Schiffmann *et al.*, 1983).

Chronic toxicity and oncogenicity studies of 1,3-dichloropropene have been conducted. cis-1,3-Dichloropropene was negative in a mouse skin initiation–promotion bioassay when tested with 7,12-dimethylbenzanthracene and phorbol myristate and was not carcinogenic following repeated dermal application of 122 mg to the backs of Ha : ICR Swiss mice three times a week for up to 85 weeks (Van Duuren *et al.*, 1979). However, an increase in local fibrosarcomas was reported in mice following repeated subcutaneous injections (once a week) for up to 83 weeks. Administration of a mixed-isomer formulation of 1,3-dichloropropene to rats (25 or 50 mg/kg/day) and mice (50 or 100 mg/kg/day) via gavage, 3 days/week, for up to 2 years resulted in increases in several benign and malignant tumor types in both species (NTP, 1985; Yang *et al.*, 1986). These included forestomach and liver tumors in male rats (50 or 25 mg/kg/day or both); forestomach tumors in female rats (50 mg/kg/day); and forestomach, lung, and urinary bladder tumors in female mice (50 or 100 mg/kg/day or both). The gavage bioassay in male mice was judged to be an "inadequate study of carcinogenicity" due to excessive early mortality of controls.

Inhalation exposure of rats and mice to 5, 20, or 60 ppm 1,3-dichloropropene 6 hr/day, 5 days/week, for 2 years resulted in nontumorigenic lesions of the nasal mucosa in both sexes of rats and mice exposed to 60 ppm and female mice exposed to 20 ppm, the urinary bladder epithelium of both sexes of mice exposed to 60 ppm, and the forestomach of male mice exposed to 60 ppm (Stott *et al.*, 1987; Lomax *et al.*, 1987). Slight changes in the morphology of renal and hepatic tissues of male and female mice, respectively, exposed to 60 ppm were also observed. However, in contrast to the results of the oral gavage bioassay, an increased incidence of benign lung tumors in male mice in the high exposure group was the only tumorigenic response observed.

Effects on Reproduction Mixed-isomer vapors of 1,3-dichloropropene were not embryotoxic or teratogenic in bred rats or inseminated rabbits exposed to 20, 60, or 120 ppm vapors for 6 hr/day during gestation days 6–15 (rats) or 6–18 (rabbits) (Hanley *et al.*, 1987). Maternal toxicity was evidenced at all exposure levels. Exposure of male and female rats to 14, 32 or 96 ppm D-D®, 6 hours/day for 10 weeks did not affect animal mating behavior or fertility (Clark, 1980). Further, exposure of male and female rats to 10, 30, or 90 ppm 1,3-dichloropropene vapors for two generations did not adversely affect reproduction or neonatal growth or survival, even though 90 ppm proved to be a toxic exposure level (Breslin *et al.*, 1987). Consistent with these results, no treatment-related changes in testes weight, sperm count, or sperm morphology occurred in mice 30 days after being injected ip with 1,3-dichloropropene at 10, 19, 38, 75, 150, 300, or 600 mg/kg/day for 5 days (Osterloh *et al.*, 1983).

Pathology Major target tissues of 1,3-dichloropropene following an acute, high-dose oral or inhalation exposure are the liver, kidneys, and lungs (inhalation) in rats and guinea pigs. Following a more prolonged lower-level exposure, the stomach, liver, and nasal mucosa of rats and the stomach, nasal mucosa, lungs, and urinary bladder of mice may be affected.

14.7.11.3 Toxicity to Humans

Experimental Exposure Seven of ten volunteers detected 1,3-dichloropropene at an air concentration of 3 ppm; some reported fatigue of the sense of smell after a few minutes. The same proportion of volunteers detected 1 ppm, but the odor was noticeably fainter (Torkelson and Oyen, 1977). In a population of 22 persons, the concentration at which odor was detected was 4.4 ± 3.1 ppm (mean ± SD) (Rick and McCarty, 1987).

Accidental and Intentional Poisoning Forty-six people were treated for exposure to 1,3-dichloropropene fumes following a traffic accident in 1975 involving spillage of 4500 liters of a formulated product. Twenty-four of these, three of whom had lost consciousness, were hospitalized overnight with symptoms including headache, irritation of mucous membranes, and chest discomfort. All patients took showers and were given intravenous fluids and three received oxygen and corticosteroids because of chest pain and cough. Eleven of 41 persons tested had slightly higher than average sperm SGOT and/or SGPT values, which reverted to normal within 48–72 hr, except for five who still had slightly higher than average SGOT values. Follow-up interviews with patients 1–2 weeks later revealed symptoms including headache, abdominal and chest discomfort, and malaise. One was diagnosed as having had pneumonia. Symptoms were reported more frequently in those most heavily exposed to the fumes. Patient interviews conducted approximately 2 years after the accident revealed complaints of headache, chest pain or discomfort, and "personality changes" (fatigue, irritability, difficulty in concentrating, or decreased libido). Two had undergone cardiac catheterizations but their arteriograms were normal. There was no correlation of these long-persisting symptoms with intensity of exposure (Flessel *et al.*, 1978).

The only fatality reported to involve 1,3-dichloropropene occurred following the accidental ingestion of D-D® (Gosselin *et al.*, 1976). The victim experienced abdominal pain and vomiting, became semicomatose, exhibited muscular twitching, and died despite gastric lavage and therapy for pulmonary edema.

Use Experience 1,3-Dichloropropene causes edema, redness, and necrosis of the skin (Torkelson and Oyen, 1977) and in one documented case was believed to have caused contact hypersensitivity in a repeatedly exposed farmer (Nater and Gooskens, 1976). A fertility study of 64 employees engaged in the production of chlorinated three-carbon compounds, including 1,3-dichloropropene, revealed no effects on hormone levels (LH, FSH, testosterone), sperm count, sperm motility, and percentage of normal and abnormal sperm regardless of duration or magnitude of exposure (Venable *et al.*, 1980). Yang (1986) has reviewed the human toxicity data for 1,3-dichloropropene.

Treatment of Poisoning Treatment is symptomatic.

14.7.12 *p*-DICHLOROBENZENE

14.7.12.1 Identity, Properties, and Uses

Chemical Name 1,4-Dichlorobenzene.

Structure See Fig. 14.6.

Synonyms *p*-Dichlorobenzene is also known as paracide, PDB, and PDCB. Trade names include Paradow®, Paramoth®, Paranuggets®, and Parazene®. The CAS registry number is 106-46-7.

Physical and Chemical Properties *p*-Dichlorobenzene has the empirical formula $C_6H_4Cl_2$ and a molecular weight of 147.01. It forms colorless crystals with a strong odor. The density is 1.4581. The vapor pressure is 1.0 torr at 25°C. *p*-Dichlorobenzene is soluble in water (80 mg/liter at 25°C) and

readily soluble in organic solvents. It is stable and noncorrosive.

History and Use Introduced in 1913, *p*-dichlorobenzene is a fumigant for moths in clothes and for mites in fungal cultures.

14.7.12.2 Toxicity to Laboratory Animals

Basic Findings The intraperitoneal LD 50 of *p*-dichlorobenzene in rats is 2562 mg/kg (Zupko and Edwards, 1949). This is consistent with the finding that an oral dosage of 4000 mg/kg was fatal to rats, but all survived 1000 mg/kg (Hollingsworth *et al.*, 1956b). Guinea pigs were killed by 2800 mg/kg, but all survived 1600 mg/kg without symptoms (Sollman, 1919).

Rats that received 138 doses by stomach tube in the course of 192 days at a rate of 376 mg/kg/day showed a slight increase in the weights of liver and kidney and slight focal necrosis and cirrhosis of the liver. At 188 mg/kg/day, changes were still perceptible, but no adverse effect was detected in rats maintained on 18.8 mg/kg/day (Hollingsworth *et al.*, 1956b).

When rats, guinea pigs, and rabbits were exposed for 30 min a day to an initial nominal concentration of 16,640 ppm (100,000 mg/m³), a few showed simple eye and nose irritation, but most showed intense irritation, muscle twitches, loss of righting reflex, horizontal and vertical nystagmus, and rapid labored breathing. Recovery after each exposure required only 30–120 min in most animals, but a few died. This treatment led to a granulocytopenia and some tendency to increased lymphocytes, so that there was little effect on total white count (Zupko and Edwards, 1949).

When rats, guinea pigs, and rabbits were exposed for 8 hr/day, 5 days/week, for as many as 69 exposure days to a measured average concentration of 798 ppm (4800 mg/m³), some of the animals died and all exhibited weakness, tremors, weight loss, eye irritation, and coma. Rabbits that survived 62 exposures apparently recovered completely within 17 days. When rats and guinea pigs were exposed 7 hr/day, 5 days/week, for 6 months to an average concentration of 341 ppm (2050 mg/m³), the only positive findings included slight growth depression, slight increase in liver and kidney weights, and slight histological changes. Similar exposure of rats, guinea pigs, rabbits, and one monkey to an average concentration of 158 ppm (950 mg/m³) produced similar but less pronounced changes in rats and guinea pigs only. When the same five species were exposed to a measured concentration of 96 ppm (580 mg/m³) for 6 months or more, no adverse effect was detected in any of them, as judged by gross appearance, behavior, growth, organ weight, hematological studies, and clinical findings (Hollingsworth *et al.*, 1956b).

p-Dichlorobenzene was found to be nonsensitizing in guinea pigs (Landsteiner and Jacobs, 1936).

Absorption, Distribution, Metabolism, and Excretion The *p* distribution, excretion, and biotransformation of [^{14}C]-dichlorobenzene was studied in rats after repeated inhalation, oral, and subcutaneous doses (Hawkins *et al.*, 1980). Following repeated daily exposures for 10 days to 1000 ppm *p*-dichlorobenzene vapor for 3 hr/day or administration of oral or subcutaneous doses of 250 mg/kg/day, tissue concentration of ^{14}C activity did not increase after 6 days of exposure but tended to decrease. During a 5-day postexposure interval after the last dose, 91–97% of the excreted radioactivity was recovered in the urine, 1–6% in the feces, and 0.2–6.4% in the expired air. In rats with cannulated bile ducts, 46–63% of the dose was recovered in the bile and appeared to be reabsorbed in the intact animal (enterohepatic circulation) and ultimately excreted in the urine. Sulfate and glucuronide conjugates of 2,5-dichlorophenol represented 46–54% and 31–34% of the urinary radioactivity, along with dihydroxydichlorobenzene and a mercapturic acid of *p*-dichlorobenzene as minor components. The glucuronide of 2,5-dichlorophenol (30–42%) was the major radiolabeled component in the bile. Kimura *et al.* (1979) also identified 2,5-dichlorophenol as the major urinary metabolite in rats after an oral *p*-dichlorobenzene dose of 200 mg/kg. 2,5-Dichlorophenyl methyl sulfoxide and 2,5-dichlorophenyl methyl sulfone were identified in the blood and as minor components in the urine.

After repeated daily inhalation or oral exposures, the highest concentrations of radioactivity in rats occurred in fat (10–40 times greater) compared to kidneys, liver, and lungs (Hawkins *et al.*, 1980). Concentrations of radioactivity in fat had declined from 2400 ppm 1 hr after the last of 10 inhalation exposures to 5 ppm at 120 hr postexposure. Similar results were reported by Kimura *et al.* (1979) after single oral administration of 200 mg/kg *p*-dichlorobenzene in rats.

Biochemical Effects   *p*-Dichlorobenzene was one of several halogenated benzenes studied by Reid and Krishna (1973). It caused the least liver pathology, but this was consistent with the overall conclusion that the degree of liver necrosis was proportional to the degree of covalent binding of active metabolites of these compounds to liver proteins.

Having noted that hexachlorobenzene causes porphyria in humans and rats, Rimington and Ziegler (1963) investigated nine other compounds, including *p*-dichlorobenzene. All of the lower chlorinated benzenes were able to induce hepatic porphyria in rats but did not induce photosensitivity (390–410 nm). Urinary coproporphyrin excretion increased first; later porphobilinogen and δ-aminolevulic acid increased, but the exact pattern of porphyria was different for different compounds. Dosage with *p*-dichlorobenzene at a maximal rate of 770 mg/kg/day for 5 days caused at least a 9-fold increase in urinary coproporphyrin, a 37-fold increase in uroporphyrin, a 204-fold increase in porphobilinogen, and an 8-fold increase in δ-aminolevulic acid compared to control values. On the contrary, Carlson (1977) reported negative results, almost certainly as a result of the smaller dosage used (maximum of 200 mg/kg/day orally for 120 days).

Effects on Organs and Tissues   Repeated, 8-hr exposures of rabbits to vapor concentrations of 4600–4800 mg/m³ (765–800

ppm) produced tremor and toxic eye ground changes but no change of the ocular lens. The same was true of oral doses that produced weakness, tremor, and weight loss. The eye ground and systemic changes were reversible when dosing was stopped. Respiratory exposure was maintained as long as 83 days, and oral dosing at a rate of 500 mg/kg was continued as long as a year. Naphthalene at the same dosages did produce cataracts quite promptly (Pike, 1944; Hollingsworth *et al.*, 1956b).

An inhalation toxicity study was reported by Loeser and Litchfield (1983) in which male and female rats and mice were exposed to 0, 75, or 500 ppm *p*-dichlorobenzene vapor 5 hr/day, 5 days/week, for 57 weeks (mice) or 78 weeks (rats). The animals were then allowed to survive until they were sacrificed, 18 weeks postexposure for the mice and 36 weeks postexposure for the rats. Male mice were removed from the study after 57 weeks of exposure due to high mortality (80%) resulting from fighting and a possible respiratory infection. Mortality of female mice was comparable to that of the control group. Aside from a high background of respiratory disease in all groups of mice, no treatment-related histopathologic changes or carcinogenic effects were observed in the *p*-dichlorobenzene-exposed female mice. In rats, mortality was comparable to the control value, liver and kidney weights were increased at 500 ppm, and 75 ppm was considered to be without toxicologic effect. No tumorigenic response was observed in either sex of rat (Loeser and Litchfield, 1983).

Subsequently, *p*-dichlorobenzene was administered by gavage, 5 days/week for 2 years, at doses of 0, 150, and 300 mg/kg/day to male rats (Fischer 344) and 0, 300, and 600 mg/kg/day to female rats and male and female B6C3F1 mice (NTP, 1987). Under conditions that resulted in recurrent renal toxicity (male > female), *p*-dichlorobenzene increased the incidence of renal tubular cell adenocarcinomas in male rats (1/50, 3/50, and 7/50 at 0, 150, and 300 mg/kg/day, respectively) but not in female rats. *p*-Dichlorobenzene increased the incidence of hepatocellular carcinomas in high-dose male (14/50, 11/49, 32/50) and female mice (5/50, 5/48, 19/50) and produced an increase in pheochromocytomas, only one of which was malignant, in high-dose male mice (0/47, 2/48, 4/49).

The pathological changes elicited in the male rat kidney (see below) and the male rat-specific low-incidence renal tumor response suggest that *p*-dichlorobenzene might be acting via an epigenetic (not directly genotoxic) mechanism similar to that reported for unleaded gasoline (Short *et al.*, 1986). Similarly, the degenerative hepatic effects observed in the mouse liver during treatment (NTP, 1987) suggest that the enhancement of the spontaneous liver tumor incidence in this species may simply result from promotional effects of recurrent degenerative/regenerative processes. These hypotheses are attractive, since *p*-dichlorobenzene has produced largely negative results in genetic toxicity assays such as bacterial mutagenicity, mammalian cell mutagenicity, chromosomal aberration (*in vivo* and *in vitro*), and DNA repair assays (Loeser and Litchfield, 1983; NTP, 1987; Perocco *et al.*, 1983). Thus, exposure of humans to *p*-dichlorobenzene, at doses below those which would be expected to produce tissue injury, would not be likely to pose a significant chronic health hazard.

Pathology *p*-Dichlorobenzene at a subcutaneous dosage of 25 mg/kg occasionally produced slight centrilobular liver necrosis in rats similar to the more extensive necrosis produced by the more toxic *o*- isomer (Cameron and Thomas, 1937). Similar changes were found in guinea pigs and rabbits exposed to concentrated vapor (Berliner, 1939). Hollingsworth *et al.* (1956b) also found the major histological change in the liver, although some changes were found in the kidneys. On the contrary, the major changes observed by Zupko and Edwards (1949) were in the kidneys. Repeated respiratory exposure of rats, guinea pigs, and rabbits that produced marked lung injury and was fatal to some animals also produced little effect on the liver but marked injury to the tubules and glomeruli of the kidneys of all three species. Exposures that lasted only 30 min were initiated by placing crystals of *p*-dichlorobenzene on a hot plate inside the chamber at a rate of 100,000 mg/m^3 (16,640 ppm). Whether the procedure used for vaporization could have led to chemical reaction so that the difference in pathology was due to a difference in compounds is unclear.

Administration of *p*-dichlorobenzene to male rats (0, 150, or 300 mg/kg/day orally for 2 years) caused epithelial hyperplasia of the renal pelvis (1/50, 30/50, 31/50, respectively), mineralization of the collecting tubules in the renal medulla (4/50, 46/50, 47/50), and focal hyperplasia of the renal tubular epithelium (0/50, 1/50, 9/50). The kidneys of female rats receiving 0, 300, and 600 mg/kg/day orally for 2 years were markedly less affected. In mice (0, 300, and 600 mg/kg/day, orally, for 2 years), hepatic degeneration and necrosis was produced in 60–75% of the low-dose males and high-dose males and females (NTP, 1987).

Reproductive Effects The fetotoxic potential of inhaled *p*-dichlorobenzene was evaluated in pregnant rabbits by Hayes *et al.* (1985) and in rats by Hodge *et al.* (1977). The rabbits were exposed to 0, 100, 300, or 800 ppm *p*-dichlorobenzene 6 hr/day on days 6–18 of gestation and the rats to 0, 75, 200, or 500 ppm on days 6–15 of gestation. Slight maternal toxicity was observed in rabbits exposed to 800 ppm, as indicated by a significant decrease in weight gain during the first 3 days of exposure. *p*-Dichlorobenzene was not teratogenic or fetotoxic in rats or rabbits at concentrations as high as 500 and 800 ppm, respectively.

During a dominant lethal study in mice exposed to 0, 75, 225, or 450 ppm *p*-dichlorobenzene vapor, 6 hr/day, 5 days/week, there was no reduction in the fertility of male mice (Loeser and Litchfield, 1983).

14.7.12.3 Toxicity to Humans

Accidental and Intentional Poisoning Apparently there has been no case of poisoning of a person by *p*-dichlorobenzene showing the signs and clinical course one would expect from animal tests. The reasons almost certainly are the low acute toxicity of the compound and the irritant character of the vapor, which discourages prolonged exposure, either single or repeated. Except for the violation of formal logic, there would be some reason to classify all the reported cases as "atypical." After all, with the exception of some groups of cases reported in a single paper, few of the cases have much in common. Actually, it is some of the single cases associated with large doses and perhaps involving some element of hypersensitivity that are most convincing. On the other hand, it is to be expected that a compound used extensively by the general public would be blamed for some cases of illness for which no satisfactory explanation is available.

A 3-year-old boy developed hemolytic anemia complicated by jaundice and oliguria after he played with and presumably ingested *p*-dichlorobenzene crystals. Four abnormal phenols, including a trace of 2,5-dichlorophenol, were found in the urine (Hallowell, 1959). A similar but much milder case involved a 21-year-old woman who ate one or two air-freshener blocks per week during all but the last week or so of pregnancy, when she was found to have a refractory anemia. The patient's hemoglobin rose steadily after withdrawal of the chemical. Labor and the baby girl it produced were normal (Campbell and Davidson, 1970). The massiveness of the dosage and the absence of any liver or kidney involvement in this case were remarkable. No measurement of G-6-PD activity was made in either case.

A 69-year-old man had a bout of dyspnea while seated in a chair which his wife had treated earlier in the same day with *p*-dichlorobenzene crystals. Within 24–48 hr a petechial and purpuric rash gradually appeared on his hands, forearms, feet, and legs. The hands and feet became swollen. Acute glomerular nephritis appeared as a complication during hospitalization. Five months later an indirect basophil degranulation test was strongly positive when tested against the insecticide. A control run later was negative for aspirin, phenacetin, and caffeine, the only drugs the patient had used (Nalbandian and Pearce, 1965).

Women only 25 and 27 years old developed cataracts 6 and 12 months, respectively, after they had experienced illnesses characterized by weight loss and jaundice. Each entire illness was attributed to relatively heavy exposure of the women to *p*-dichlorobenzene in their homes prior to onset. The fact that liver changes constituted the main pathology in animals killed by constant exposure to concentrated vapor was considered evidence that the women's jaundice was caused by the compound. Cataract was produced in one of four rabbits (Berliner, 1939). The purity of the *p*-dichlorobenzene tested was not stated.

A 53-year-old woman who experienced a productive cough and progressive dyspnea over a period of about 4 years was shown by biopsy to be suffering from a granulomatous reaction with foreign-body giant cells containing crystals. The condition was attributed to the woman's unusually extensive use of *p*-dichlorobenzene in her home for 12–15 years. The woman's husband, living in the same house, had no respiratory complaints. Chemical analysis of the crystals was unsuccessful (Weller and Crellin, 1953). Although the woman's use of the compound was most unusual, it is difficult to imagine that her exposure exceeded that of many workers, none of whom has suffered from pneumoconiosis. No attention was given to the possibility that the crystals were some other material.

Four cases diagnosed as subacute yellow atrophy with jaundice and a tendency to connective tissue formation were attributed to *p*-dichlorobenzene (Cotter, 1953). Exposure was substantial in the two patients who survived—one apparently with complete recovery—but was vague in the two fatal cases, a man and his wife. The diagnosis was acute yellow atrophy in the husband and Laennec's cirrhosis in the wife, but no details of the autopsy results were given. No attempt was made to confirm the chemical composition of the material said to be *p*-dichlorobenzene.

Perrin (1941) associated the slight weakness, dizziness, moderate hypochromic anemia, and relative granulocytopenia in a 62-year-old man with his not unusual exposure to *p*-dichlorobenzene at home. After use of the compound was discontinued, the patient recovered gradually. With this idea fixed in mind, several more or less similar cases were found that were thought to recall "myelotoxicoses benzoliques."

Swelling of the hands, feet, and ankles of an athletic young woman occurred while she slept for one night with some exposure to fumes of *p*-dichlorobenzene she had used the day before in storing winter clothing. The condition was not severe enough to prevent playing golf, and it disappeared in about 3 days (Claytor, 1935).

A 68-year-old woman noted tiredness and decreasing tolerance for exercise about 1 month after the end of 3 weeks of intense exposure to *p*-dichlorobenzene and naphthalene. Her symptoms gradually became worse, and 2 months after onset she entered the hospital, where a diagnosis of aplastic anemia was made. It was possible to stabilize her condition and discharge her in 2 weeks. She required about one unit of packed blood cells per month to maintain a hematocrit of 30%. Ecchymoses and petechiae recurred intermittently during the first several months and then disappeared. Complaints of skin tightness were made at about the time of hospitalization, but it was about 8 months later when there was enough physical evidence to justify a diagnosis of Schulman's syndrome. No conclusion was reached regarding the relationship of this syndrome to the earlier aplastic anemia or to the fumigants (Harden and Baetjer, 1978). The editor of the journal in which the report was published pointed out that the relationship between aplastic anemia and the fumigants·probably was merely circumstantial in view of the tremendous tonnage of both compounds that have been dispensed over a period of 25 years without previous reports of a similar case.

The case tabulated by Hayes (1976) involved a 64-year-old woman whose death after 1 month of congestive heart failure was attributed to *p*-dichlorobenzene and specifically to nephrosis, which had been present for 6 months. No information beyond that on the death certificate was obtained. The circumstances of exposure are unknown and the validity of the case is questionable (Hayes, 1982).

Use Experience   Except for irritation of the eyes and nose before industrial hygiene was improved, relatively pure *p*-dichlorobenzene has been a source of no difficulty in industry. Pike (1944) and Hollingsworth *et al.* (1956b) specifically pointed out the lack of visual disturbance, including cataract, attributable to this substance. Workers develop some acclimatization to the compound and become able to tolerate levels as high as 725 ppm that ordinary people could not accept without a gas mask. This acclimatization is lost in the absence of intermittent exposure to high concentrations (Hollingsworth *et al.*, 1956b).

On the contrary, eight workers who inhaled mists of *p*-dichlorobenzene and nitrogen-containing contaminants developed anorexia, inflammation of the mucosa, and methemoglobinemia (Wallgren, 1953). It would seem that the contaminants may have been responsible.

Atypical Cases of Various Origins   Two cases of chronic leukemia, two cases of acute myeloblastic leukemia, and one case of myeloproliferative syndrome were reported in persons exposed to *o*-dichlorobenzene or to a mixture of isomers in which the *o*- isomer was predominant (Girarde *et al.*, 1969). Although exposure to benzene was denied, the possibility of some contaminant is suggested by the absence of similar reports from other places where dichlorobenzene is used extensively.

Dosage Response   There is no definite information on dosage in the cases attributed to *p*-dichlorobenzene, but in some of them it was massive, as in the case where one or two air-freshener blocks were eaten per week.

p-Dichlorobenzene is irritating to the eyes and nose of most people at concentrations between 50 and 160 ppm (300 and 962 mg/m^3). People detect a faint odor at 15–30 ppm, and the odor is strong at 30–60 ppm (Hollingsworth *et al.*, 1956b). The ACGIH threshold limit value for occupational exposure of 75 ppm (450 mg/m^3) permits exposure at the rate of 64 mg/kg/day.

Laboratory Findings   Among workers manufacturing or packaging *p*-dichlorobenzene, the concentration of dichlorophenol in the urine at the end of the work shift varied from 10 to 233 ppm. These values correlated well with the concentrations of *p*-dichlorobenzene in the air where the persons worked (Pagnotto and Walkley, 1965).

The identity of *p*-dichlorobenzene in samples from people in Tokyo was confirmed by gas chromatography–mass spectrometry. The concentration in 34 samples of fat ranged from 0.2 to 11.7 ppm and averaged 2.3 ppm. In six blood samples from different people, the range was 0.004–0.016 ppm, and the average was 0.0095 ppm. The mean concentration in fat was almost the same as that for polychlorinated biphenyls, but the concentration of *p*-dichlorobenzene in blood was about three times greater than that for PCBs (Morita and Ohi, 1975).

Treatment of Poisoning   Treatment is symptomatic.

ACKNOWLEDGMENTS

The authors gratefully acknowledge the contributions of the following individuals: Ms. Jean K. Shuler and Ms. Brenda D. Caldwell for their clerical assistance; Dr. K. S. Rao and Dr. William T. Stott for their technical assistance; and Dr. Wayland J. Hayes, Jr., whose original work served as a basis for this revision.

REFERENCES

Adams, E. M., Spencer, H. C., Rowe, V. K., and Irish, D. D. (1950). Vapor toxicity of 1,1,1-trichloroethane (methyl chloroform) determined by experiments on laboratory animals. *Arch. Ind. Hyg. Occup. Med.* **1,** 225–236.

Adams, E. M., Spencer, H. C., Rowe, V. K., McCollister D. D., and Irish, D. D. (1951). Vapor toxicity of trichloroethylene determined by experiments on laboratory animals. *Arch. Ind. Hyg. Occup. Med.* **4,** 469–481.

Adams, E. M., Spencer, H. C., Rowe, V. K., McCollister D. D. and Irish, D. D. (1952). Vapor toxicity of carbon tetrachloride determined by experiments on laboratory animals. *Arch. Ind. Hyg. Occup. Med.* **6,** 50–66.

Adir, J., Blake, D. A., and Mergner, G. M. (1975). Pharmacokinetics of fluorocarbon 11 and 12 in dogs and humans. *J. Clin. Pharmacol.* **15,** 760–770.

Agarwal, A. K., and Mehendale, H. M. (1983). Potentiation of CCl_4 hepatotoxicity and lethality of chlordecone in female rats. *Toxicology* **26,** 231–242.

Agarwal, A. K., and Mehendale, H. M. (1984). Perturbation of calcium homeostasis by CCl_4 in rats pretreated with chlordecone and phenobarbital. *Environ. Health Perspect.* **57,** 289–291.

Ahlmark, A., and Forssman, S. (1951). Evaluating trichloroethylene exposures by urinalyses for trichloroacetic acid. *Arch. Ind. Hyg. Occup. Med.* **3,** 386–398.

Ahmed, A. E., and Anders, M. W. (1976). Metabolism of dihalomethane to formaldehyde and inorganic chloride. *Drug. Metab. Dispos.* **4,** 357–361.

Ahmed, A. E., and Anders, M. W. (1978). Metabolism of dichloromethane to formaldehyde and inorganic halide. II. Studies on the mechanism of the reaction. *Biochem. Pharmacol.* **27,** 2021–2025.

Ahmed, A. E., Farooqui, M. Y. H., Upreti, R. K., and El-Shabrawy, O. (1982). Distribution and covalent interactions of [1-^{14}C]acrylonitrile in the rat. *Toxicology* **23,** 159–175.

Albaum, H. G., Tepperman, J., and Bodansky, O. (1946). A spectrophotometric study of the competition of methemoglobin and cytochrome oxidase for cyanide *in vitro. J. Biol. Chem.* **163,** 641–647.

Alexeeff, G. V., Kilgore, W. W., Munoz, P., and Watt, D. (1985). Determination of acute toxic effects in mice following exposure to methylbromide. *J. Toxicol. Environ. Health* **15,** 109–123.

Allen, R. C., Meier, H., and Hoag, W. G. (1962). Ethylene glycol produced by ethylene oxide sterilization and its effect on blood clotting factors in an inbred strain of mice. *Nature (London)* **193,** 387–388.

Alomar, A., Camarasa, J. M. G., Noguera, J., and Aspinolea, F. (1981). Ethylene oxide dermatitis. *Contact Dermatitis* **7,** 205–207.

Alumot, E., Nachtomi, E., Mandel, E., Holstein, P., Bondi, A., and Herzberg, M. (1976). Tolerance and acceptable daily intake of chlorinated fumigants in the rat diet. *Food Cosmet Toxicol.* **14,** 105–110.

Amann, R. P., and Berndtson, W. E. (1986). Assessment of procedures for screening agents for effects on male reproduction: Effects of dibromochloropropane (DBCP) on the rat. *Fundam. Appl. Toxicol.* **7,** 244–255.

American Medical Association (AMA) (1977). "AMA Drug Evaluations." Publishing Sciences Group, Littleton, Massachusetts.

Amoore, H. E., and Hautala, E. (1983). Odor as an aid to chemical safety: Odor thresholds compared with threshold limit values and volatilities for 214 industrial chemicals in air and water dilution. *J. Appl. Toxicol.* **3,** 272–290.

Andersen, M. E., Gargas, M. L., Jones, R. A., and Jenkins, L. J., Jr. (1980). Determination of the kinetic constants for metabolism of inhaled toxicants *in vivo* using gas uptake measurements. *Toxicol. Appl. Pharmacol.* **54,** 100–116.

Andersen, M. E., Clewell, H. J., Gargas, M. L., Smith, F. A., and Reitz, R. H. (1987). Physiologically based pharmacokinetics and the risk assessment process for methylene chloride. *Toxicol. Appl. Pharmacol.* **87,** 185–205.

Andriukin, A. A. (1979). Toxic effect of dichloroethane on the cardiovascular system. *Klin. Med. (Moscow)* **57,** 43–47 (in Russian).

Angelo, M. J., Pritchard, A. B., Hawkins, D. R., Walker, A. R., and Roberts, A. (1986a). The pharmacokinetics of dichloromethane. I. Disposition in $B_6C_3F_1$ mice following intravenous and oral administration. *Food Chem. Toxicol.* **24**(a), 965–974.

Angelo, M. J., Pritchard, A. B., Hawkins, D. R., Walker, A. R., and Roberts, A. (1986b). The pharmacokinetics of dichloromethane. II. Disposition in Fischer 344 rats following intravenous and oral administration. *Food Chem. Toxicol.* **24**(9), 975–980.

Anger, W. K., Setzer, J. V., Russo, J. M., Brightwell, W. S., Wait, R. G., and Johnson, B. L. (1981). Neurobehavioral effects of methylbromide exposures. *Scand. J. Work Environ. Health* **7,** Suppl. 4, 40–47.

Anger, W. K., Moody, L., Burg, J., Brightwell, W. S., Taylor, B. J., Russo, J. M., Dickerson, N., Setzer, J. V., Johnson, B. L., and Hicks, K. (1986). Neurobehavioral evaluation of soil and structural fumigators using methyl bromide and sulfuryl fluoride. *Neurotoxicology* **7**(3), 137–156.

Anziulewicz, J. A., Dick, H. J., and Chiarulli, E. E. (1959). Transplacental naphthalene poisoning. *Am. J. Obstet. Gynecol.* **78,** 519–521.

Araki, S., Ushio, K., Suwa, K., Abe, A., and Uehara, K. (1971). Methyl bromide poisoning: A report based on fourteen cases. *Jpn. J. Ind. Health* **13,** 507–513.

Ashkenazi, A. E., and Berman, S. E. (1961). Experimental kerosene poisoning in rats: Use of ^{14}C-labelled hendecane as indicator of absorption. *Pediatrics* **28,** 642–649.

Astrand, I., Engström, J., and Ovrum, P. (1978). Exposure to xylene and ethylbenzene. I. Uptake, distribution and elimination in man. *Scand. J. Work Environ. Health* **4,** 185–194.

Austin, S. G., and Schnatter, A. R. (1983). A case-control study of chemical exposures and brain tumors in petrochemical workers. *J. Occup. Med.* **25,** 313–320.

Axelson, O., Andersson, K., Hogstedt, C., Holmberg, B., Molina, G., and de Verdier, A. (1978). A short study of trichloroethylene exposure and cancer mortality. *J. Occup. Med.* **20,** 194–196.

Azar, A. (1971). Cardiovascular effects of fluorocarbon exposure. *Aerosp. Med. Res. Lab. [Tech. Rep.] AMRL-TR (U.S.)* **AMRL-TR-71-120,** 41–56.

Azar, A., Reinhart, C. F., Maxfield, M. E., Smith, P. E., Jr., and Mullin, L. S. (1972). Experimental human exposure to fluorocarbon 12 (dichlorodifluoromethane). *Am. Ind. Hyg. Assoc. J.* **33,** 207–216.

Azar, A., Trochimowicz, H. J., Terrill, J. B., and Mullin, L. S. (1973). Blood levels of fluorocarbon related to cardiac sensitization. *Am. Ind. Hyg. Assoc. J.* **34,** 102–109.

Badinand, A., Paufique, L., and Rodier, J. (1947). Experimental intoxication with Tetraline. *Arch. Mal. Prof. Med. Trav. Secur. Soc.* **8,** 124 (in French).

Baer, F., and Griepentrog, F. (1969). Long-tern experiment on the feeding of rats with feed fumigated with ethylene oxide. *Bundesgesundheitsblatt* **12,** 106–107 (in German).

Bain, K. (1954). Death due to accidental poisoning in young children. *J. Pediatr.* **44,** 616–623.

Ballantyne, B., Gazzard, M. F., and Swanston, D. W. (1976). The ophthalmic toxicity of dichloromethane. *Toxicology* **6,** 173–187.

Barbin, A., Bereziat, J. C., and Bartsch, H. (1983). Evaluation of DNA damage by the alkaline elution technique in liver, kidneys and lungs of rats and hamsters treated with *N*-nitrosodialkylamines. *Carcinogenesis (London)* **4,** 541–545.

Barbodeg, Z. (1968). Exposure to trichloroethylene by means of uninalysis. *Med. Welt.* **19**, 1636–1638 (in German).

Barker, M. H., Lindberg, H. A., and Wald, M. H. (1941). Further experiences with thiocyanates. Chemical and experimental observations. *JAMA, J. Am. Med. Assoc.* **117**, 1591–1594.

Barrett, H. M., and Johnston, J. H. (1939). The fate of trichloroethylene in the organism. *J. Biol. Chem.* **127**, 765–770.

Barrett, H. M., Cunningham, J. G., and Johnston, J. H. (1939). A study of the fate in the organism of some chlorinated hydrocarbons. *J. Ind. Hyg. Toxicol.* **21**, 479–490.

Barsoum, G. S., and Saad, K. (1934). Relative toxicity of certain chlorine derivatives of the aliphatic series. *Q. J. Pharm. Pharmacol.* **7**, 205–214.

Bartonicek, V. (1963). The effect of some substances on the elimination of trichloroethylene metabolites. *Arch. Int. Pharmacodyn. Ther.* **144**, 69–85.

Bartonicek, V., and Teisinger, J. (1962). Effect of tetraethyl thiuram disulfide (disulfiram) on metabolism of trichloroethylene in man. *Br. J. Ind. Med.* **19**, 216–221.

Basile, G. (1939). Experiments on the action of some hydrogenation products of naphthalene (Tetralin and Decalin) on the lens and its posterior capsule of the rabbit. *Boll. Ocul.* **18**, 951–957.

Bass, M. (1970). Sudden sniffing death. *JAMA, J. Am. Med. Assoc.* **212**, 2075–2079.

Beauchamp, R. O., Jr., Bus, J. S., Popp, J. A., Boreiko, C. J., and Goldberg, L. (1983). A critical review of the literature on carbon disulfide toxicity. *CRC Crit. Rev. Toxicol.* **11**, 169–278.

Behrens, R. H., and Dukes, D. C. D. (1986). Fatal methylbromide poisoning. *Br. J. Ind. Med.* **43**, 561–562.

Bel, A., Levrat, R., Nesmoz, J., Lewontey, A., and Delorme, G. (1968). Comparative evolution of ornithine-carbamyl-transferase (OCT) and serum transaminases in acute carbon tetrachloride intoxication in the rat. *Rev. Int. Hepatol.* **18**, 651–661.

Beliles, R. P., Brusick, D. J., and Mecler, F. J. (1980). "Teratogenic–Mutagenic Risk of Workplace Contaminants: Trichloroethylene, Perchloroethylene, and Carbon Disulfide" (Contract No. 210-77-0047). U. S. Department of Health, Education, and Welfare, Washington, D.C.

Berliner, M. L. (1939). Cataract following inhalation of paradichlorobenzene vapor. *Arch. Ophthalmol. (Chicago)* **22**, 1023–1034.

Berman, K. (1983). Interactions of trichloroethylene with DNA *in vitro* and with RNA and DNA of various mouse tissues *in vivo. Arch. Toxicol.* **54**, 181–193.

Bermudez, E., Mirsalis, J. C., and Eales, H. C. (1982). Detection of DNA damage in primary cultures of rat hepatocytes following *in vivo* and *in vitro* exposure to genotoxic agents. *Environ. Mutagen.* **4**, 667–679.

Biava, C. G., Smuckler, E. A., and Whorton, D. (1978). The testicular morphology of individuals exposed to dibromochloropropane. *Exp. Mol. Pathol.* **29**, 448–458.

Biswas, N. M., and Mukherji, M. (1968). Histochemical changes in the kidney of the toad (*Bufo melanostictus*) after carbon tetrachloride intoxication. *Anat. Anz.* **123**, 100–104.

Bologna, N. A., and Woody, N. C. (1948). Kerosene poisoning. *New Orleans Med. Surg. J.* **101**, 256–260.

Bond, E. J., Robinson, J. R., and Buckland, C. T. (1969). The toxic action of phosphine. Absorption and symptoms of poisoning in insects. *J. Stored Prod. Res.* **5**, 289–298.

Bond, J. A., Dutcher, J. S., Medinsky, M. A., Henderson, R. F., and Birnbaum, L. S. (1985). Disposition of [^{14}C]methyl bromide in rats after inhalation. *Toxicol. Appl. Pharmacol.* **78**, 259–267.

Bonnichsen, R., and Maehly, A. C. (1966). Poisoning by volatile compounds. III. Hydrocyanic acid. *J. Forensic Sci.* **11**, 516–528.

Bonse, G., Urban, T., Reichert, D., and Henschler, D. (1975). Chemical reactivity, metabolic oxirane formation, and biological reactivity of chlorinated ethylenes in the isolated perfused rat liver preparation. *Biochem. Pharmacol.* **24**, 1829–1834.

Bonventre, J., Brennan, O., Jason, D., Henderson, A., and Bastos, M. L. (1977). Two deaths following accidental inhalation of dichloromethane and 1,1,1-trichloromethane. *J. Anal. Toxicol.* **1**, 158–160.

Bos, R. P., Brouns, R. M. E., van Doorn, R., Theuws, J. L. G., and Henderson, P. T. (1981). Non-mutagenicity of toluene, *o-, m-,* and *p*-xylene, *o*-methylbenzylalcohol, and *o*-methylbenzylsulfate in the Ames assay. *Mutat. Res.* **88**, 273–279.

Boxer, G. E., and Rickards, J. C. (1952). Detoxication of cyanide by cystine. *J. Biol. Chem.* **218**, 449–457.

Breslin, W. J., Kirk, H. D., Streeter, C. M., Quast, J. F., and Szabo, J. R. (1987). "TELONE® II Soil Fumigant: 2-Generation Inhalation Reproduction Study in Fischer 344 Rats." Report of The Dow Chemical Company, Midland, Michigan.

Brieger, H., and Teisinger, J. eds. (1967). "Toxicology of Carbon Disulfide." Excerpta Medica, Amsterdam.

Brodniewicz, A. (1967). Poisoning of seamen with methyl bromide due to fumigation of a Polish cargo ship in Haiphong (Viet-Nam). *Arh. Hig. Rada Toksikol.* **18**, 19–24.

Brody, T. M., Calvert, D. N., and Schneider, A. F. (1961). Alteration of carbon tetrachloride-induced pathologic changes in the rat by spinal transection, adrenalectomy, and adrenergic blocking agents. *J. Pharmacol. Exp. Ther.* **131**, 341–345.

Bronzetti, G., Bauer, C., Corsi, C., Del Carratore, R., Galli, A., Nieri, R., and Paolini, M. (1983). Genetic and biochemical studies on perchloroethylene *in vitro* and *in vivo. Mutat. Res.* **116**, 323–331.

Broome, M. G., and Sivak, A. (1987). An evaluation of short-term genotoxicity test results with dichloromethane. *Food Chem. Toxicol.*

Brown, D. P., and Kaplan, S. D. (1987). Retrospective cohort mortality study of dry cleaner workers using perchloroethylene. *J. Occup. Med.* **29**, 535–541.

Browning, E. (1965). "Toxicity and Metabolism of Industrial Solvents." Elsevier, Amsterdam.

Brugnone, F., Perbellini, L., Faccini, G. B., Pasini, F., Bartolucci, G. B., and DeRosa, E. (1986). Ethylene oxide exposure: Biological monitoring by analysis of alveolar air and blood. *Int. Arch. Occup. Environ. Health* **58**, 105–112.

Buben, J. A., and O'Flaherty, E. J. (1985). Delineation of the role of metabolism in the hepatotoxicity of trichloroethylene and perchloroethylene: A dose–effect study. *Toxicol. Appl. Pharmacol.* **78**, 105–122.

Buchter, A., Peter, H., and Bolt, H. M. (1984). *N*-Acetylcysteine as antidote in accidental acrylonitrile intoxications. *Int. Arch. Occup. Environ. Health* **53**, 311–319 (in German).

Buckley, L. A., Jiang, X. Z., James, R. A., Morgan, K. T., and Barrow, C. S. (1984). Respiratory tract lesions induced by sensory irritants at the RD50 concentration. *Toxicol. Appl. Pharmacol.* **74**, 417–429.

Burek, J. D., Nitschke, K. D., Bell, T. J., Wackerle, D. L., Childs, R. C., Beyer, J. E., Dittenber, D. A., Rampy, L. W., and McKenna, M. J. (1984). Methylene chloride: A two-year inhalation toxicity and oncogenicity study in rats and hamsters. *Fundam. Appl. Toxicol.* **4**, 30–47.

Bus, J. S. (1985). The relationship between carbon disulfide metabolism and toxicity. *Neurotoxicology* **6**, 73–80.

Butler, T. C. (1949). Metabolic transformations of trichloroethylene. *J. Pharmacol. Exp. Ther.* **97**, 84–91.

Butler, T. C. (1961). Reduction of carbon tetrachloride *in vivo* and reduction of carbon tetrachloride and chloroform *in vitro* by tissues and tissue constituents. *J. Pharmacol. Exp. Ther.* **134**, 311–319.

Cachia, E. A., and Fenech, F. F. (1964). Kerosene poisoning in children. *Arch. Dis. Child.* **39**, 502–504.

Calleman, C. J., Ehrenberg, L., Jansson, B., Osterman-Golkar, S., Segerback, D., Svensson, K., and Wachtmeister, C. A. (1978). Monitoring and risk assessment by means of alkyl groups in hemoglobin in persons occupationally exposed to ethylene oxide. *J. Environ. Pathol. Toxicol.* **2**, 427–442.

Callen, D. F., Wolf, C. R., and Philpot, R. M. (1980). Cytochrome P-450 mediated genetic activity and cytotoxicity of seven halogenated aliphatic hydrocarbons in *Saccharomyces cerevisiae. Mutat. Res.* **77**, 55–63.

Cameron, G. R., and Thomas, J. C. (1937). The toxicity of certain chlorine derivatives of benzene, with special reference to *o*-dichlorobenzene. *J. Pathol. Bacteriol.* **44**, 281–296.

Cameron, G. R., Paterson, J. L., deSarom, G. S., and Thomas, J. C. (1938). The toxicity of some methyl derivatives of benzene with special reference to pseudocumene and heavy coal tar naphtha. *J. Pathol. Bacteriol.* **46,** 95–107.

Campbell, D. M., and Davidson, R. J. L. (1970). Toxic haemolytic anaemia in pregnancy due to a pica for paradichlorobenzene. *J. Obstet. Gynaecol. Br. Commonw.* **77,** 657–659.

Cantarow, A., Stewart, H. L., and Morgan, D. R. (1938). Experimental carbon tetrachloride poisoning in the cat. I. The influence of calcium administration. *J. Pharmacol. Exp. Ther.* **63,** 153–172.

Cardani, A. (1942). Experimental study of the toxicity of Tetralin and Decalin. *Med. Lav.* **33,** 145 (in Italian).

Carlson, A., and Hultengren, M. (1975). Exposure to methylene chloride. II. Metabolism of ^{14}C-labelled methylene chloride in the rat. *Scand. J. Work Environ. Health* **1,** 104–108.

Carlson, G. P. (1977). Chlorinated benzene induction of hepatic porphyria. *Experientia* **33,** 1627–1629.

Carlson, G. P. (1981). Effect of alterations in drug metabolism in epinephrine-induced cardiac arrhythmias in rabbits exposed to methylchloroform. *Toxicol. Lett.* **9,** 307–313.

Carpenter, C. P. (1937). The chronic toxicity of tetrachloroethylene. *J. Ind. Hyg. Toxicol.* **19,** 323–336.

Carpenter, C. P., Kinkead, E. R., Sullivan, D. L., Jr., and King, J. M. (1975). Petroleum hydrocarbon toxicity studies. V. Animal and human response to vapors of mixed xylenes. *Toxicol. Appl. Pharmacol.* **33,** 543–558.

Carpenter, C. P., Geary, D. L., Jr., Myers, D. J., Nuchreiner, D. J., Sullivan, L. J., and King, J. M. (1976). Petroleum hydrocarbon toxicity studies. XI. Animal and human response to vapors of deodorized kerosene. *Toxicol. Appl. Pharmacol.* **36,** 443–456.

Casac'o, A., Arruzazabala, L., Gonzalez, R., and Rodriguez de la Vega, A. (1983). Disodium chromoglycate inhibits bronchoconstriction by kerosene aerosol in rabbits. *Allergol. Immunopathol.* **11,** 335–337.

Casac'o, A., Garcia, M., Gonzalez, R., and Rodriguez de la Vega, A. (1985). Induction of acetylcholinesterase inhibition in the guinea pig trachea by kerosene. *Respiration* **48,** 46–49.

Castello, C., Giussani, A., and Berti, A. (1969). Poisoning by hydrocyanic acid; clinical and therapeutic considerations and presentation of a case. *Minerva Anestesiol.* **35,** 437–447 (in Italian).

Cavanagh, J. R., and Wilner, P. R. (1939). Aplastic anemia due to kerosene. *Med. Ann. D.C.* **8,** 140–144.

Chen, C., and Lin, C. C. (1968). Mechanism of aliphatic hydroxylation. Tetralin hydroperoxide as an intermediate in the hydroxylation of Tetralin in rat liver homogenate. *Biochim. Biophys. Acta* **170,** 366–374.

Chen, K. K., and Rose, C. L. (1952). Nitrite and thiosulfate therapy in cyanide poisoning. *JAMA, J. Am. Med. Assoc.* **149,** 113–119.

Chen, K. K., Rose, C. L., and Clowes, G. H. A. (1934). Comparative values of several antidotes in cyanide poisoning. *Am. J. Med. Sci.* **188,** 767–781.

Cherry, N., Venables, H., Waldron, H., and Wells, G. (1981). Some observations on workers exposed to methylene chloride. *Br. J. Ind. Med.* **38,** 351–355.

Ciuchta, H. P., Savell, G. M., and Spiker, R. C. (1979). The effect of alcohols and toluene upon methylene chloride-induced carboxyhemoglobin in the rat and monkey. *Toxicol. Appl. Pharmacol.* **49,** 347–354.

Clark, D. G. (1980). "D-D: A 10 Week Inhalation Study of Mating Behaviour, Fertility, and Toxicity in Male and Female Rats." Report of The Shell Toxicology Laboratory, Tunstall, U. K.

Clark, D. G., and Tinston, D. J. (1973). Correlation of the cardiac sensitizing potential of halogenated hydrocarbons with their physicochemical properties. *Br. J. Pharmacol.* **49,** 355–357.

Clark, D. G., and Tinston, D. J. (1982). Acute inhalation of some halogenated and non-halogenated hydrocarbons. *Hum. Toxicol.* **1,** 239–247.

Clayton, J. I., and Parkhouse, J. (1962). Blood trichloroethylene concentrations during anaesthesia under controlled conditions. *Br. J. Anaesth.* **34,** 141–148.

Claytor, T. A. (1935). Dangers of dichlorobenzene. *JAMA, J. Am. Med. Assoc.* **104,** 1028.

Climie, I., Hutson, D., Morrison, B., and Stoydin, G. (1979). Glutathione

conjugation in the detoxication of (Z)-1,3-dichlorophene (a component of the nematocide D-D) in the rat. *Xenobiotica* **9,** 149–156.

Clower, B. R., Couglas, B. H., and Williams, W. L. (1968). Effects of pretreatment with epinephrine and reserpine on carbon tetrachloride-induced hepatic damage. *Eur. J. Pharmacol.* **4,** 325–330.

Coate, W. B. (1979a). "Subacute Inhalation Study in Rats and Mice: TELONE II." Report of The Dow Chemical Company, Midland, Michigan.

Coate, W. B. (1979b). "90-day Inhalation Study in Rats and Mice: TELONE II." Report of The Dow Chemical Company, Midland, Michigan.

Cock, T. D. (1957). Acute hemolytic anemia in the neonatal period. *Am. J. Dis. Child.* **94,** 77–79.

Cohen, E. E., Paulus, H. J., Kennan, R. G., and Scheel, L. D. (1958). Skin absorption of carbon disulfide vapor in rabbits. I. Associated changes in blood protein and zinc. *AMA Arch. Ind. Health* **17,** 164–169.

Collier, H. (1936). Methylene dichloride intoxication in industry. *Lancet* **1,** 594–595.

Collins, R. P. (1965). Methyl bromide. A bizarre neurological disorder. *Calif. Med.* **103,** 112–116.

Condie, L. W., Smallwood, C. L., and Laurie, R. D. (1983). Comparative renal and hepatotoxicity of halomethanes: Bromodichloromethane, bromoform, chloroform, dibromochloromethane and methylene chloride. *Drug Chem. Toxicol.* **6**(6), 563–78.

Conroy, H. W., Walkden, H. H., and Farrell, E. (1957). Residues in foods and feeds resulting from fumigation of grains with the commoner liquid formulations of carbon disulfide, carbon tetrachloride, ethylene dichloride, and ethylene dibromide. *J. Assoc. Off. Agric. Chem.* **40,** 163–192.

Cope, C. (1961). The importance of oxygen in the treatment of cyanide poisoning. *JAMA, J. Am. Med. Assoc.* **175,** 1061–1064.

Costa, A. K., and Ivanetich, K. M. (1980). Tetrachloroethylene metabolism by the hepatic microsomal cytochrome P-450 system. *Biochem. Pharmacol.* **29,** 2863–2869.

Costa, A. K., and Ivanetich, K. M. (1984). Chlorinated ethylenes: Their metabolism and effect on DNA repair in rat hepatocytes. *Carcinogenesis (London)* **5,** 1629–1636.

Costa, A. K., Katz, I. D., and Ivanetich, K. M. (1980). Trichloroethylene: Its interaction with hepatic microsomal cytochrome P-450 in vitro. *Biochem. Pharmacol.* **29**(3), 433–439.

Cotter, L. H. (1953). Paradichlorobenzene poisoning from insecticides. *N.Y. State J. Med.* **53,** 1690–1692.

Courville, C. B. (1964). Confusion of presumed toxic gas poisoning for fatal granulomatous meningo-encephalitis resulting in a severe progressive arteritis and gross cerebral hemorrhages. Report of a fatal case assessed as hydrogen phosphide (phosphene) poisoning. *Bull. Los Angeles Neurol. Soc.* **29,** 291–294.

Creedy, C., Brooks, T., Dean, B., Hutson, D., and Wright, A. (1984). The protective action of glutathione on the microbial mutagenicity of the Z- and E-isomers of 1,3-dichloropropene. *Chem.-Biol. Interact.* **50,** 39–48.

Curry, A. S. (1963). Cyanide poisoning. *Acta Pharmacol. Toxicol.* **20,** 291–294.

Curtis, L. R., Williams, W. L., and Mehendale, H. M. (1979). Potentiation of carbon tetrachloride following pre-exposure to chlordecone (Kepone) in the male rat. *Toxicol. Appl. Pharmacol.* **51,** 283–293.

Dalvi, R. R., and Neal, R. A. (1978). Metabolism *in vivo* of carbon disulphide to carbonyl sulfide and carbon dioxide in the rat. *Biochem. Pharmacol.* **27,** 1608–1609.

Daniel, J. W. (1963). The metabolism of ^{36}Cl-labeled trichloroethylene and tetrachloroethylene in the rat. *Biochem. Pharmacol.* **12,** 795–802.

Danse, L. H. J. C., Van Velsen, F. L., and Van der Heijden, C. A. (1984). Methylbromide: Carcinogenic effects in the rat forestomach. *Toxicol. Appl. Pharmacol.* **72,** 262–271.

Davay, G. G. (1972). Methyl bromide poisoning. *Indian J. Ind. Med.* **18,** 78–85.

Davidson, I. W. F., Sumner, D. D., and Parker, J. C. (1982). Ethylene dichloride: A review of its mutagenic and carcinogenic potential. *Drug Chem. Toxicol.* **5,** 319–388.

Davis, J. H., Davies, J. E., Raffonelli, A., and Reich, G. (1973). The investigation of fatal acrylonitrile intoxications. *In* "Pesticides and the Environment: A Continuing Controversy" (W. B. Deichmann, ed.), pp. 547–555. Intercontinental Medical Book Corp., New York.

Dawson, J. P., Thayer, W. W., and Desforges, J. F. (1958). Acute hemolytic anemia in the newborn infant due to naphthalene poisoning. Report of two cases, with investigations into the mechanism of the disease. *Blood* **13**, 1113–1125.

DeCeaurriz, J., Desiles, J. P., Bonnet, P., Marignac, B., Muller, J., and Guenier, J. P. (1983). Concentration-dependent behavioral changes in mice following short-term inhalation exposure to various industrial solvents. *Toxicol. Appl. Pharmacol.* **67**, 383–389.

DeCeaurriz, J., Micillino, J. C., Marignac, B., Bonnet, P., Muller, J., and Guenier, J. P. (1984). Quantitative evaluation of sensory irritating and neurobehavioral properties of aliphatic ketones in mice. *Food Chem. Toxicol.* **22**, 545–550.

Defalque, R. J. (1961). Pharmacology and toxicology of trichloroethylene. A critical review of the world literature. *Clin. Pharmacol. Ther.*, **2**, 665–688.

Deichmann, W. B., Kitzmiller, K. V., Witherup, S., and Johansmann, R. (1944). Kerosene intoxication. *Ann. Intern. Med.* **21**, 803–823.

Dekant, W., Metzler, M., and Henschler, D. (1984). Novel metabolites of trichloroethylene through dechlorination reactions in rats, mice and humans. *Biochem. Pharmacol.* **33**, 2021–2028.

Dekant, W., Schulz, A., Metzler, M., and Henschler, D. (1986a). Absorption, elimination and metabolism of trichloroethylene: A quantitative comparison between rats and mice. *Xenobiotica* **16**, 143–152.

Dekant, W., Metzler, M., and Henschler, D. (1986b). Identification of S-1,2,2-trichlorovinyl-N-acetylcysteine as a urinary metabolite of tetrachloroethylene: Bioactivation through conjugations as a possible explanation of its nephrocarcinogenicity. *J. Biochem. Toxicol.* **1**, 57–72.

Dekant, W., Vamvakas, S., Berthold, K., Schmidt, S., Wild, D., and Henschler, D. (1986c). Bacterial β-lyase mediated cleavage and mutagenicity of cysteine conjugates derived from the nephrocarcinogenic alkenes trichloroethylene, tetrachloroethylene and hexachlorobutadiene. *Chem.-Biol. Interact.* **60**, 31–45.

Delbressine, L. P. C., van Bladeren, P. J., Hoogeterp, J. J., Beaumont, A. H. G. M., Breimer, D. D., Seutter-Berlage, F., and van der Gen, A. (1981). Formation of mercapturic acids from acrylonitrile, crotononitrile, and cinnamonitrile by direct conjugation and via an intermediate oxidation process. *Drug Metab. Dispos.* **9**, 246–249.

De Lorenzo, F., Degl'Innocenti, S., Ruocco, A., Silengo, L., and Cotese, R. (1977). Mutagenicity of pesticides containing 1,3-dichloropropene. *Cancer Res.* **37**, 1915–1917.

De Matteis, F. (1974). Covalent binding of sulfur to microsomes and loss of cytochrome P-450 during the oxidative desulfuration of several chemicals. *Mol. Pharmacol.* **10**, 849–854.

De Matteis, F. (1978). Loss of microsomal components in drug-induced liver damage, in cholestasis and after administration of chemicals which stimulate heme catabolism. *Pharmacol. Ther., Part A* **2**, 693–725.

Derobert, L. (1952). Death during a toxicomaniac inhalation with trichloroethylene. *Ann. Med. Leg.* **36**, 293–294 (in French).

Dice, W. H., Ward, G., Kelley, J., and Kilpatrick, W. R. (1982). Pulmonary toxicity following gastrointestinal ingestion of kerosene. *Ann. Emerg. Med.* **11**, 138–142.

Dieke, S. H., and Richter, C. P. (1946). Comparative assays of rodenticides on wild Norway rats. *Public Health Rep.* **61**, 672.

Dietz, F., Hermann, E., and Ramsey, J. (1984a). The pharmacokinetics of ¹⁴C-1,3-dichloropropene in rats and mice following oral administration. *Toxicologist* **4**, 147 (Abstr. No. 585).

Dietz, F., Dittenber, D., Kirk, H., and Ramsey, J. (1984b). Non-protein sulfhydryl content and macromolecular binding in rats and mice following administration of 1,3-dichloropropene. *Toxicologist* **4**, 147 (Abstr. No. 586).

Dinman, B. D., and Bernstein, I. A. (1968a). Acute carbon tetrachloride hepatotoxicity. IV. Liver and serum enzyme activity during acute damage phase. *Arch. Environ. Health* **10**, 770–776.

Dinman, B. D., and Bernstein, I. A. (1968b). Acute carbon tetrachloride hepatotoxicity. V. Enzymatic activity and structural concomitants during the regenerative phase. *Arch. Environ. Health* **16**, 777–784.

DiVincenzo, G. D., and Hamilton, M. L. (1975). Fate and distribution of [¹⁴C]methylene chloride in the rat. *Toxicol. Appl. Pharmacol.* **32**, 385–393.

DiVincenzo, G. D., and Kaplan, C. J. (1981). Uptake, metabolism, and elimination of methylene chloride vapor by humans. *Toxicol. Appl. Pharmacol.* **59**, 130–140.

DiVincenzo, G. D., and Krasavage, W. J. (1974). Serum ornithine carbamyl transferase as a liver response test to organic solvents. *Am. Ind. Hyg. Assoc. J.* **35**, 21–29.

Djalali-Behzad, G., Hussain, S., Osterman-Golkar, S., and Segerback, D. (1981). Estimation of genetic risks of alkylating agents. VI. Exposure of mice and bacteria to methyl bromide. *Mutat. Res.* **84**, 1–9.

Doherty, P. A., Ferm, V. H., and Smith, R. P. (1982). Congenital malformations induced by infusion of sodium cyanide in the golden hamster. *Toxicol. Appl. Pharmacol.* **64**, 456–464.

Donner, M., Falck, K., Hemminki, K., and Sorsa, M. (1981). Carbon disulfide is not mutagenic in bacteria or *Drosophila*. *Mutat. Res.* **91**, 163–166.

Dorfmueller, M. A., Henne, S. P., York, R. G., Bornschein, R. L., and Manson, J. M. (1979). Evaluation of teratogenicity and behavioral toxicity with inhalation exposure of maternal rats to trichloroethylene. *Toxicology* **14**, 153–166.

Douglas, B. H., and Clower, B. R. (1968). Hepatotoxic effect of carbon tetrachloride during pregnancy. *Am. J. Obstet. Gynecol.* **102**, 236–239.

Dow Chemical Company (1983). Toxicology Research Laboratory, Midland, Michigan (unpublished data).

Draize, J. F., Woodard, G., and Calvery, H. O. (1944). Methods for the study of irritation and toxicity of substances applied topically to the skin and mucous membranes. *J. Pharmacol. Exp. Ther.* **82**, 377–390.

Drawneek, W., O'Brien, M. J., Goldsmith, H. J., and Bourdillon, R. E. (1964). Industrial methyl-bromide poisoning of fumigators. *Lancet* **2**, 855–866.

Drayer, D. E., and Reidenberg, M. M. (1973). Metabolism of Tetralin and toxicity of Cuprex in man. *Drug Metab. Dispos.* **1**, 577–579.

Drew, R. T., Patel, J. M., and Lin, F. N. (1978). Changes in serum enzymes in rats after inhalation of organic solvents singly and in combination. *Toxicol. Appl. Pharmacol.* **45**, 809–820.

Dudley, H. C., and Neal, P. A. (1942). Toxicology of acrylonitrile (vinyl cyanide). I. Study of the acute toxicity. *J. Ind. Hyg. Toxicol.* **24**, 27–36.

Dudley, H. C., Miller, J. W., Neal, P. A., and Sayers, R. R. (1940). Studies on foodstuffs fumigated with methyl bromide. *Public Health Rep.* **55**, 2251–2282.

Dunkelberg, H. (1981). Carcinogenic activity of ethylene oxide and its reaction products 2-chloroethanol, 2-bromoethanol, ethylene glycol and diethylene glycol. I. Carcinogenicity of ethylene oxide in comparison with 1,2-propylene oxide after subcutaneous administration in mice. *Zentralbl. Bakteriol., Parasitenkd., Infektionskr. Hyg., Abt. 1: Orig. Reine B* **174**, 383–404 (in German).

Dunkelberg, H. (1982). Carcinogenicity of ethylene oxide and 1,2-propylene oxide upon intragastric administration to rats. *Br. J. Cancer* **46**, 924–933.

Dybling, F., and Dybling, O. (1946). The toxic effect of tetrachloromethane and tetrachloroethylene in oily solution. *Acta Pharmacol.* **2**, 223–226.

Eaton, M., Schenker, M., Whorton, D., Samuels, S., Perkins, C., and Overstreet, J. (1986). Seven-year follow-up of workers exposed to 1,2-dibromo-3-chloropropane. *J. Occup. Med.* **28**, 1145–1150.

Eder, E., Neudecker, T., Lutz, D., and Henschler, D. (1982). Correlation of alkylating and mutagenic activities of allyl and allylic compounds: Standard alkylation test vs. kinetic investigation. *Chem.-Biol. Interact.* **38**, 303–315.

Edwards, J. E., and Dalton, A. J. (1942). Induction of cirrhosis of the liver and hepatomas in mice with carbon tetrachloride. *J. Natl. Cancer Inst. (U. S.)* **3**, 19–41.

Edwards, K., Jackson, H., and Jones, A. R. (1970). Studies with alkylating esters. II. A chemical interpretation through metabolic studies of the anti-fertility effects of ethylene dimethanesulphonate and ethylene dibromide. *Biomed. Pharmacol.* **19**, 1783–1789.

Egnatz, D. G., Ott, M. G., Townsend, J. C., Olson, R. D., and Jones, D. B. (1980). DBCP and testicular function in chemical workers: An epidemiological survey in Midland. *J. Occup. Med.* **22**, 727–732.

Ehrenberg, L., Hiesche, K. D., Osterman-Golkar, S., and Wennberg, I. (1974). Evaluation of genetic risks of alkylation agents: Tissue doses in the mouse from air contaminated with ethylene oxide. *Mutat. Res.* **14**, 83–103.

Eisele, G. R. (1985). Naphthalene distribution in tissues of laying pullets, swine and dairy cattle. *Bull. Environ. Contam. Toxicol.* **35**, 549–556.

Eisenbrandt, D. L., and Reitz, R. H. (1986). Acute toxicity of methylene chloride: Tumorigenic implications for $B_6C_3F_1$ mice. *Toxicologist* **6**(1), 164.

Elcombe, C. R. (1985). Species differences in carcinogenicity and peroxisome proliferation due to trichloroethylene: A biochemical human hazard assessment. *Arch. Toxicol., Suppl.* **8**, 6–17.

Elcombe, C. R., Rose, M. S., and Pratt, I. S. (1985). Biochemical, histological, and ultrastructural changes in rat and mouse liver following the administration of trichloroethylene: Possible relevance to species differences in hepatocarcinogenicity. *Toxicol. Appl. Pharmacol.* **79**, 365–376.

Elliott, T. H., and Hanam, J. (1968). The metabolism of Tetralin. *Biochem. J.* **108**, 551–559.

Elovaara, E., Engström, K., and Vainio, H. (1984). Metabolism and disposition of simultaneously inhaled *m*-xylene and ethylbenzene in the rat. *Toxicol. Appl. Pharmacol.* **75**, 466–478.

English, J. C., and Anders, M. W. (1985). Evidence for the metabolism of *N*-nitrosodimethylamine and carbon tetrachloride by a common isozyme of cytochrome P-450. *Drug Metab. Dispos.* **13**, 449–452.

Environmental Protection Agency (EPA) (1983). "Health Assessment Document for Acrylonitrile," Final Report, EPA-600-8-82-007F. Office of Health and Environmental Assessment, Washington, D. C.

Ertle, T., Henschler, D., Muller, G., and Spassovski, M. (1972). Metabolism of trichloroethylene in man. I. The significance of trichloroethanol in long-term exposure conditions. *Arch. Toxicol.* **29**, 177–188.

Eustis, S. L., Haber, S. B., Drew, R. T., and Yang, R. S. H. (1986). Pathology of methyl bromide toxicity. *Toxicologist* **6**(1), 54.

Fabre, R., Truhaut, R., and Laham, S. (1960a). Toxicologic research on benzene replacement solvents. IV. Studies of xylenes. *Arch. Mal. Prof.* **21**, 301–313 (in French).

Fabre, R., Truhaut, R., and Laham, S. (1960b). Research on comparative metabolism of xylenes or dimethylbenzenes. *Arch. Mal. Prof.* **21**, 314–328 (in French).

Fabre, R., Truhaut, R., and Laham, S. (1961). Toxicologic research on carbon tetrachloride. *Proc. Int. Congr. Occup. Health, 13th, 1960* (in French).

Fanburg, S. J. (1940). Exfoliative dermatitis due to naphthalene. Report on an eruption resembling mycosis fungoides. *Arch. Dermatol. Syphilol.* **42**, 53–58.

Fariss, M. W., and Reed, D. J. (1985). Mechanism of chemical induced toxicity. II. Role of extracellular calcium. *Toxicol. Appl. Pharmacol.* **79**, 296–306.

Farooqui, M. Y. H., and Ahmed, A. E. (1983). *In vivo* interactions of acrylonitrile with macromolecules in rats. *Chem.-Biol. Interact.* **47**, 363–371.

Ferguson, J., and Pirie, H. (1948). The toxicity of vapours to the grain weevil. *Ann. Appl. Biol.* **35**, 532–550.

Ferguson, R. K., and Vernon, R. J. (1970). Trichloroethylene in combination with CNS drugs. Effects on visual–motor tests. *Arch. Environ. Health* **20**, 462–467.

Fernando, P. B., D'Silva, M., Stork, G. M. B., and Sinnatamby, G. R. (1939). Tetrachloroethylene in the treatment of hookworm disease with special reference to toxicity. *Ind. J. Med. Res.* **26**, 759–783.

Feuer, G., and Granda, V. (1970). Antagonistic effect of foreign compounds on microsomal enzymes of the liver of the rats. *Toxicol. Appl. Pharmacol.* **16**, 626–637.

Filser, J. G., and Bolt, H. M. (1979). Pharmacokinetics of halogenated ethylenes in rats. *Arch. Toxicol.* **42**, 123–136.

Filser, J. G., and Bolt, H. M. (1984). Inhalation pharmacokinetics based on gas uptake studies. VI. Comparative evaluation of ethylene oxide and butadiene monoxide as exhaled reactive metabolites of ethylene and 1,3-butadiene in rats. *Arch. Toxicol.* **55**, 219–223.

Fitzhugh, O. G., and Buschke, W. H. (1949). Production of cataracts in rats by beta-tetralol and other derivatives of naphthalene. *Arch. Ophthalmol. (Chicago)* **41**, 572–582.

Flessel, P., Goldsmith, J., Kahn, E., Wesolowski, J., Maddy, K., and Peoples, S. (1978). Acute and possible long-term effects of 1,3-dichloropropene—California. *Morbid. Mortal. Wkly. Rep.* **27**, 50–55.

Foley, J. C., Dreyer, N. B., Soule, A. B., and Woll, E. (1954). Kerosene poisoning in young children. *Radiology (Easton, Pa.)* **62**, 817–829.

Foot, E. B., Bishop, K., and Apgar, V. A. (1943). Tetrachloroethylene as an anesthetic agent. *Anesthesiology* **4**, 283–292.

Foote, R. H., Schermerhorn, E. C., and Simkin, M. E. (1986). Measurement of semen quality, fertility, and reproductive hormones to assess dibromochloropropane (DBCP) effects in live rabbits. *Fundam. Appl. Toxicol.* **6**, 628–637.

Forket, P. G., Sylvestre, P. L., and Poland, J. S. (1985). Lung injury induced by trichloroethylene. *Toxicology* **35**, 143–160.

Fowler, J. S. L. (1969). Carbon tetrachloride metabolism in the rabbit. *Br. J. Pharmacol.* **37**, 733–737.

Fowler, J. S. L. (1970a). Carbon tetrachloride metabolism in sheep and in *Fasciola hepatica*. *Br. J. Pharmacol.* **39**, 599–607.

Fowler, J. S. L. (1970b). Chlorinated hydrocarbon toxicity in the fowl and the duck. *J. Comp. Pathol.* **80**, 465–471.

Frant, R., and Westendorp, J. (1950). Medical control on exposure of industrial workers to trichloroethylene. *Arch. Ind. Hyg. Occup. Med.* **1**, 308–318.

Frantz, S. W., and Watanabe, P. G. (1983). Tetrachloroethylene: Balance and tissue distribution in male Sprague-Dawley rats by drinking water administration. *Toxicol. Appl. Pharmacol.* **69**, 66–72.

Friborska, A. (1969). The phosphatases of peripheral white blood cells in workers exposed to trichloroethylene and perchloroethylene. *Br. J. Ind. Med.* **26**, 159–161 (in French).

Fridman, A. L., Zalesov, V. S., Surkov, V. D., Kratynskaya, L. V., and Plaksina, A. N. (1976). Synthesis and study of the physiological activity of aliphatic nitro compounds. X. Relation among structure, toxicity, and antimicrobial activity in a series of nitroalkanes and their α-halo derivatives. *Khim.-Farm. Zh.* **10**, 53–56 (in Russian).

Fukuda, K., Takemoto, K., and Tsuruta, H. (1983). Inhalation carcinogenicity of trichloroethylene in mice and rats. *Ind. Health* **21**, 243–254.

Gagnaire, F., Simon, P., Bonnet, P., and DeCeaurriz, J. (1986). The influence of simultaneous exposure to carbon disulfide and hydrogen sulfide on the peripheral nerve toxicity and metabolism of carbon disulfide in rats. *Toxicol. Lett.* **34**, 175–183.

Gaines, T. B. (1969). Acute toxicity of pesticides. *Toxicol. Appl. Pharmacol.* **14**, 515–534.

Gallagher, C. H. (1961). Protection by antioxidants against lethal doses of carbon tetrachloride. *Nature (London)* **192**, 881–882.

Galloway, S. M., Berry, P. K., Nichols, W. W., Wolman, S. R., Soper, K. A., Stolley, P. D., and Archer, P. (1986). Chromosome aberrations in individuals occupationally exposed to ethylene oxide, and in a large control population. *Mutat. Res.* **170**, 55–74.

Gamberale, F., Annwall, G., and Hultengren, M. (1978). Exposure to xylene and ethylbenzene. III. Effects on central nervous functions. *Scand. J. Work Environ. Health* **4**, 204–211.

Ganote, C. E., and Rosenthal, A. S. (1968). Characteristic lesions of methylazoxy-methanol-induced liver damage. A comparative ultrastructural study with dimethylnitrosamine, hydrazine sulfate and carbon tetrachloride. *Lab. Invest.* **19**, 382–398.

Garcia Rico, A. M., Garces Bruses, J., Mas Marfany, J., and Nolla Pandes, R. (1974). Collective acute poisoning by methyl bromide. *Med. Clin. North Am.* **63**, 291–296.

Gargas, M. L., Clewell, H. J., and Andersen, M. E. (1986). Metabolism of inhaled dihalomethanes *in vivo:* Differentiation of kinetic constants for two independent pathways. *Toxicol. Appl. Pharmacol.* **82,** 211–223.

Garner, R. C., and McLean, A. E. M. (1969). Increased susceptibility to carbon tetrachloride poisoning in the rat after pretreatment with oral phenobarbitone. *Biochem. Pharmacol.* **18,** 645–650.

Gay, H. H. (1962). Blood and urinary levels following exposure to bromides. *Ind. Med. Surg.* **31,** 438–439.

Gazzaniga, G., Binaschi, S., Sportelli, A., and Riva, M. (1969). The elimination in the alveolar air in man of 1,1,1-trichloroethane following exposure to 600 ppm for 3 hours. *Boll. Soc. Ital. Biol. Sper.* **45,** 97–99 (in Italian).

Gehring, P. J. (1968). Hepatotoxic potency of various chlorinated hydrocarbon vapors relative to their narcotic and lethal potencies in mice. *Toxicol. Appl. Pharmacol.* **13,** 287–298.

Gehring, P. J. (1971). Cataractogenic activity of chemicals. *CRC Crit. Rev. Toxicol.* **1,** 93–118.

Geiger, L. E., Hogy, L. L., and Guengerich, F. P. (1983). Metabolism of acrylonitrile by isolated rat hepatocytes. *Cancer Res.* **43,** 3080–3087.

Generoso, W. M., Cumming, R. B., Bandy, J. A., and Cain, K. T. (1983). Increased dominant-lethal effects due to prolonged exposure of mice to inhaled ethylene oxide. *Mutat. Res.* **119,** 377–379.

Generoso, W. M., Cain, K. T., and Hughes, L. A. (1985). Tests for dominant-lethal effects of 1,2-dibromo-3-chloropropane (DBCP) in male and female mice. *Mutat. Res.* **156,** 103–108.

Generoso, W. M., Cain, K. T., Hughes, L. A., Sega, G. A., Branden, P. W., Gosslee, D. G., and Shelby, M. D. (1986). Ethylene oxide dose and dose-rate effects in the mouse dominant-lethal test. *Environ. Mutagen.* **8,** 1–7.

Georgijew, A., Kalczak, M., and Wegiel, J. (1968). Some observations on the effect of CCl₄ on normal and regenerating liver. *Pol. Med. J.* **7,** 1431–1437.

Gerarde, H. W. (1959). Toxicological studies on hydrocarbons. V. Kerosine. *Toxicol. Appl. Pharmacol.* **1,** 462–474.

Gerarde, H. W. (1960). "Toxicology and Biochemistry of Aromatic Hydrocarbons." Am. Elsevier, New York.

Gerberg, E. J. (1973). Head lice: Control and nit removal. *Sci. Publ.—Pan Am. Health Organ.* **263,** 196–198.

Gerner-Smidt, P., and Friedrich, U. (1978). The mutagenic effect of benzene, toluene and xylene studied in SCE technique. *Mutat. Res.* **58,** 313–316.

Gessner, O. (1937). Lethal hydrogen-phosphide poisoning caused by fumigation of grain weevils with Delicia (aluminum phosphide). *Samml. Vergiftungsfallen* **9**(B79), 13 (in German).

Gettler, A. O., and Baine, J. O. (1938). The toxicology of cyanide. *Am. J. Med. Sci.* **195,** 182–198.

Ghanayem, B. I., and Ahmed, A. E. (1982). *In vivo* biotransformation and biliary excretion of 1-¹⁴C-acrylonitrile in rats. *Arch. Toxicol.* **50,** 175–185.

Ghetti, G., and Mariani, L. (1956). Eye changes due to naphthalene. *Med. Lav.* **47,** 533–538 (in Italian).

Gidron, E., and Luerer, J. (1956). Naphthalene poisoning. *Lancet* **1,** 228–230.

Girarde, R., Tolot, F., Martin, P., and Bourret, J. (1969). Serious blood diseases and exposure to chlorinated derivatives of benzene (with reference to 4 cases). *J. Med. Lyon.* **50,** 771–773 (in German).

Glass, R. I., Lyness, R. N., Mengle, D. C., Powell, K. E., and Kahn, E. (1979). Sperm count depression in pesticide applicators exposed to dibromochloropropane. *Am. J. Epidemiol.* **109,** 346–351.

Goldsworthy, T. L., and Popp, J. A. (1987). Chlorinated hydrocarbon-induced peroxisomal enzyme activity in relation to species and organ carcinogenicity. *Toxicol. Appl. Pharmacol.* **88,** 225–233.

Goldsworthy, T. L., Lyglit, O., and Popp, J. A. (1987). Relationship between alpha-2μ-globulin (α2μ), protein droplet accumulation and cell replication in male and female rats exposed to chlorinated hydrocarbons. *Proc. 78th Annu. Meet. Am. Assoc. Cancer Res.* Vol. 28, p. 87.

Gollapudi, B. B., Bruce, R. J., and Hinze, C. A. (1985). "Evaluation of TELONE II Soil Fumigant in the Mouse Bone Marrow Micronucleus Test." Report of The Dow Chemical Company, Midland, Michigan.

Gordis, E. (1969). Lipid metabolites of carbon tetrachloride. *J. Clin. Invest.* **48,** 203–209.

Gossel, T. A., and Bricker, J. D. (1984). "Principles of Clinical Toxicology," pp. 194–195. Raven Press, New York.

Gosselin, R., Hodge, H., Smith, R., and Gleason, M. (1976). "Clinical Toxicology of Commercial Products," 4th ed., pp. 119–121. Wilkins & Williams, Baltimore, Maryland.

Green, E. C., and Hunter, A. (1985). Toxicity of carbon disulfide in developing rats: LD50 values and effects on the hepatic mixed-function oxidase enzyme system. *Toxicol. Appl. Pharmacol.* **78,** 130–138.

Green, J., Bunyan, J., Cawthorne, M. S., and Diplock, A. T. (1969). Vitamin E and hepatotoxic agents. 1. Carbon tetrachloride and lipid peroxidation of the rat. *Br. J. Nutr.* **23,** 297–307.

Green, T., and Odum, J. (1985). Structure/activity studies of the nephrotoxic and mutagenic action of cysteine conjugates of chloro- and fluoroalkenes. *Chem.-Biol. Interact.* **54,** 15–31.

Green, T., and Prout, M. S. (1985). Species differences in response to trichloroethylene. II. Biotransformation in rats and mice. *Toxicol. Appl. Pharmacol.* **79,** 401–411.

Green, T., and Purchase, I. F. H. (1987). "The Assessment of Carcinogenic Hazard for Human Beings Exposed to Methylene Chloride," Tech. Rep. No. 26. Eur. Chem. Ind. Ecol. Toxicol. Cent., Brussels, Belgium.

Green, T., Foster, J. R., and Hext, P. M. (1986a). The effects of dichloromethane exposure on the lungs and livers of rats and mice. *Toxicologist* **6** (1), 314.

Green, T., Odum, J., Foster, J. R., and Hext, P. M. (1986b). Perchloroethylene induced hepatic peroxisome proliferation in mice and renal hyaline droplet formation in rats. *Toxicologist* **6,** 314.

Greene, F. E., Stripp, B., and Gillette, J. R. (1969). The effect of carbon tetrachloride on heme components and ethylmorphine metabolism in rat liver microsomes. *Biochem. Pharmacol.* **18,** 1531–1533.

Grigor, W. G., Robin, H., and Harley, J. D. (1966). An Australian variant on "full moon disease." *Med. J. Aust.* **2,** 1229–1230.

Gross, J. A., Haas, M. L., and Thomas, T. R. (1979). Ethylene oxide neurotoxicity: Report of four cases and review of the literature. *Neurology* **29,** 978–983.

Grunske, F. (1949). Ventox and Ventox poisoning. *Dtsch. Med. Wochenschr.* **74,** 1081 (in German).

Guengerich, F. P., Crawford, W. M., Jr., Domoradzki, J. Y., MacDonald, T. L., and Watanabe, P. G. (1980). *In vitro* activation of 1,2-dichloroethane by microsomal and cytosolic enzymes. *Toxicol. Appl. Pharmacol.* **55,** 303–307.

Guengerich, F. P., Geiger, L. E., Hogy, L. L., and Wright, P. L. (1981). In vitro metabolism of acrylonitrile to 2-cyanoethylene oxide, reaction with glutathione, and irreversible binding to proteins and nucleic acids. *Cancer Res.* **41,** 4925–4933.

Gwathmey, J. T., and Baskerville, C. (1914). "Anesthesia." Appleton, New York.

Hackenberg, U. (1972). Chronic ingestion by rats of standard diet treated with aluminum phosphide. *Toxicol. Appl. Pharmacol.* **23,** 147–158.

Hake, C. L., Waggoner, T. B., Robertson, D. N., and Rowe, V. K. (1960). The metabolism of 1,1,1-trichloroethane by the rat. *Arch. Environ. Health* **1,** 101–105.

Halbreich, A., and Mager, J. (1969). Early effects of carbon tetrachloride on the synthesis of phospholipids in the rat liver and their possible pathogenetic role in fatty liver induction. *Biochim. Biophys. Acta* **187,** 584–587.

Hall, F. B., and Hine, C. H. (1966). Trichloroethane intoxication: A report of two cases. *J. Forensic Sci.* **11,** 404–413.

Hall, M. C. (1921). The use of carbon tetrachloride for the removal of hookworm. *JAMA, J. Am. Med. Assoc.* **79,** 2055–2057.

Hall, M. C., and Shillinger, J. E. (1925). Tetrachlorethylene, a new anthelmintic. *Am. J. Trop. Med.* **5,** 229–237.

Hallermann, W., and Pribilla, O. (1959). Lethal poisonings with hydrogen phosphide. *Arch. Toxikol.* **17,** 219–242 (in German).

Hallowell, M. (1959). Acute haemolytic anemia following the ingestion of paradichlorobenzene. *Arch. Dis. Child.* **34,** 74–75.

Halpern, B., and Cruchaud, S. (1947). Preventive action of the *N*-dimethylamino-2-propyl-1-thiodiphenylamine antihistaminic on acute experimental pulmonary edema induced by the administration of a toxic gas: Chloropicrin. *C. R. Hebd. Seances Acad. Sci.* **225,** 1194–1196 (in French).

Hamilton, A. (1925). "Industrial Poisons in the United States." Macmillan, New York.

Hamilton, A., and Hardy, H. L. (1949). "Industrial Toxicology," 2nd ed. Harper (Hoeber), New York.

Hamilton, A., and Hardy, H. L. (1974). "Industrial Toxicology," 3rd ed. Publishing Sciences Group, Acton, Massachusetts.

Hamilton, W. C. (1897). Death from drinking coal oil. *Med. News* **71,** 214–215.

Hanley, T. R., John-Greene, J. A., Young, J. T., Calhoun, L. L., and Rao, K. S. (1987). Evaluation of the effects of inhalation exposure to 1,3-dichloropropene on fetal development in rats and rabbits. *Fundam. Appl. Toxicol.* **8,** 562–570.

Hanssler, H. (1964). Life-threatening naphthalene poisoning in an infant caused by Vaporine fumes. *Dtsch. Med. Wochenschr.* **89,** 1794–1795 (in German).

Harden, R. A., and Baetjer, A. M. (1978). Aplastic anemia following exposure to paradichlorobenzene and naphthalene. *J. Occup. Med.* **20,** 820–822.

Hardin, B. D., and Manson, J. M. (1980). Absence of dichloromethane teratogenicity with inhalation exposure in rats. *Toxicol. Appl. Pharmacol.* **52,** 22–28.

Hardin, B. D., Bond, G. P., Sikov, M. R., Andres, F. D., Beliles, R. P., and Niemeier, R. W. (1981). Testing of selected workplace chemicals for teratogenic potential. *Scand. J. Work Environ. Health* **7,** Suppl. 4, 66–75.

Hardin, B. D., Niemeier, R. W., Sikov, M. R., and Hackett, P. L. (1983). Reproductive–toxicologic assessment of the epoxides ethylene oxide, propylene oxide, butylene oxide, and styrene oxide. *Scand. J. Work. Environ. Health* **9,** 94–102.

Hardy, H. L., Jefferies, W. M., Wasserman, M. M., and Waddell, W. R. (1950). Thiocyanate effect following industrial cyanide exposure; report of 2 cases. *N. Engl. J. Med.* **242,** 968–972.

Hashimoto, S., Glende, E. A., Jr., and Recknagel, R. O. (1968). Hepatic lipid peroxidation in acute fatal human carbon tetrachloride poisoning. *N. Engl. J. Med.* **279,** 1082–1085.

Hatfield, T. R., and Maykoski, R. T. (1970). A fatal methylchloroform (trichloroethane) poisoning. *Arch. Environ. Health* **20,** 279–281.

Hawk, E. A., and Mickelsen, O. (1955). Nutritional changes in diets exposed to ethylene oxide. *Science* **121,** 442–444.

Hawkins, D. R., Chasseaud, L. F., Woodhouse, R. N., and Cresswell, D. G. (1980). The distribution, excretion and biotransformation of *p*-dichloro[^{14}C]benzene in rats after repeated inhalation, oral and subcutaneous doses. *Xenobiotica* **10,** 81–95.

Hayes, J. R., Condie, L. W., and Borzelleca, J. F. (1986). The subchronic toxicity of tetrachloroethylene (perchloroethylene) administered in the drinking water of rats. *Fundam. Appl. Toxicol.* **7,** 119–125.

Hayes, W. C., Hanley, T. R., Jr., Gushow, T. S., Johnson, K. A., and John, J. A. (1985). Teratogenic potential of inhaled dichlorobenzenes in rats and rabbits. *Fundam. Appl. Toxicol.* **5,** 190–202.

Hayes, W. J., Jr. (1967). The 90-dose LD 50 and a chronicity factor as measures of toxicity. *Toxicol. Appl. Pharmacol.* **11,** 327–335.

Hayes, W. J., Jr. (1975). "Toxicology of Pesticides." Williams & Wilkins, Baltimore, Maryland.

Hayes, W. J., Jr. (1976). Mortality in 1969 from pesticides including aerosols. *Arch. Environ. Health* **31,** 61–72.

Hayes, W. J., Jr. (1982). "Pesticides Studied in Man." Williams & Wilkins, Baltimore, Maryland.

Hayes, W. J., Jr., and Pirkle, C. I. (1966). Mortality from pesticides in 1961. *Arch. Environ. Health* **12,** 43–55.

Hayes, W. J., Jr., and Vaughn, W. K. (1977). Mortality from pesticides in the United States in 1973 and 1974. *Toxicol. Appl. Pharmacol.* **42,** 235–252.

Haymaker, W., Ginzler, A. M., and Ferguson, R. L. (1952). Residual neuropathological effects of cyanide poisoning. A study of the central nervous system of 23 dogs exposed to cyanide compounds. *Mil. Surg.* **111,** 231–246.

Head, B., Moody, D. E., Woo, C. H., and Smuckler, E. A. (1981). Altera-

tions of specific forms of cytochrome P-450 in rat liver during acute carbon tetrachloride intoxication. *Toxicol. Appl. Pharmacol.* **61,** 286–295.

Hearne, T. F., Grose, F., Pifer, J. W., Friedlander, B. R., and Raleigh, R. L. (1987). Methylene chloride mortality study: Dose–response characterization and animal model comparison. *J. Occup. Med.* **29**(3), 217–228.

Heine, L. (1913). A case of naphthalene poisoning. *Med. Klin. (Munich)* **9,** 62–63 (in German).

Hemminki, K., Mutnaen, P., Saloniemi, I., Niemi, M.-L., and Vainio, H. (1982). Spontaneous abortions in hospital staff engaged in sterilizing instruments with chemical agents. *Br. Med. J.* **285,** 1461–1463.

Henschler, D., and Bonse, G. (1977). Metabolic activation of chlorinated ethylenes: Dependence of mutagenic effect on electrophilic reactivity of the metabolically formed epoxides. *Arch. Toxicol.* **39,** 7–12.

Henschler, D., and Hoos, R. (1982). Metabolic activation deactivation mechanisms of di-, tri-, and tetrachloroethylenes. *In* "Biological Reactive Intermediates" (R. Snyder, D. V. Parke, D. J. Jallow, C. G. Gibson, and C. M. Witmer, eds.), Vol. 2, Part A, pp. 659–666. Plenum, New York.

Henschler, D., Hoos, W. R., Fetz, H., Dallmeier, E., and Metzler, M. (1979). Reactions of trichloroethylene epoxide in aqueous systems. *Biochem. Pharmacol.* **28,** 543–548.

Henschler, D., Romen, W., Elsasser, H. M., Reichert, D., Eder, E., and Radawan, Z. (1980). Carcinogenicity study of trichloroethylene by long-term inhalation in three animal species. *Arch. Toxicol.* **43,** 237–248.

Henschler, D., Elsasser, H., Roman, W., and Eder, E. (1984). Carcinogenicity study of trichloroethylene with and without epoxide stabilizers in mice. *J. Cancer Res. Clin. Oncol.* **107,** 149–156.

Heppel, L. A., Neal, P. A., Endicott, K. M., and Porterfield, V. T. (1944). Toxicology of dichloroethane. I. Effect on the cornea. *Arch. Ophthalmol. (Chicago)* **32,** 391–394.

Heppel, L. A., Neal, P. A., Perrin, T. L., Endicott, K. M., and Porterfield, V. T. (1945). The toxicology of 1,2-dichloroethane (ethylene dichloride). III. Its acute toxicity and the effect of protective agents. *J. Pharmacol. Exp. Ther.* **84,** 53–63.

Heppel, L. A., Neal, P. A., Perrin, T. L., Endicott, K. M., and Porterfield, V. T. (1946). The toxicology of 1,2-dichloroethane (ethylene dichloride). V. The effects of daily inhalations. *J. Ind. Hyg. Toxicol.* **28,** 113–120.

Herd, P. A., Lipsky, M., and Martin, H. F. (1974). Cardiovascular effects of 1,1,1-trichloroethane. *Arch. Environ. Health* **28,** 227–233.

Heyndrickx, A., Van Peteghem, C., Van den Heede, M., and Lauwaert, R. (1976). A double fatality with children due to fumigated wheat. *Eur. J. Toxicol.* **9,** 113–118.

Hiebel, J. H., Gant, H. L., Schwartz, S. O., and Friedman, I. A. (1963). Bone marrow depression following exposure to kerosene. A report of 3 cases. *Am. J. Med. Sci.* **246,** 185–191.

Hine, C. H. (1969). Methyl bromide poisoning. *J. Occup. Med.* **11,** 1–10.

Hine, C. H., and Zuiderma, H. (1970). The toxicological properties of hydrocarbon solvents. *Ind. Med. Surg.* **39,** 215–220.

Hine, C. H., Anderson, H. H., Moon, H. D., Kodama, J. K., Morse, M., and Jacobsen, N. W. (1953). Toxicology and safe handling of CBP-55 (technical 1-chloro-3-bromopropene-1). *AMA Arch. Ind. Hyg. Occup. Med.* **7,** 118–136.

Hirano, A., Levine, S., and Zimmerman, H. M. (1968). Remyelination in the central nervous system after cyanide intoxication. *J. Neuropathol. Exp. Neurol.* **27,** 234–245.

Ho, Y. L., and Ho, S. K. (1981). Screening of carcinogens with the prophage clt × 857 induction test. *Cancer Res.* **41,** 532–536.

Hodge, M. C. E., Palmer, S., Wilson, J., and Bennett, I. P. (1977). "Para-Dichlorobenzene: Teratogenicity Study in Rats," Unpublished report. Imperial Chemical Industries Ltd., Central Toxicology Laboratory, Alderley Park, Macclesfield, Cheshire, U. K. (reviewed in Loeser and Litchfield, 1983).

Hofmann, H. T., Birnsteil, H., and Jobst, P. (1971). Inhalation toxicity from ethylidene chloride and ethylene dichloride. *Arch. Toxikol.* **27,** 248–265 (in German).

Hogstedt, C., Rohlen, O., Brendtsson, B. S., Axelson, O., and Ehrenberg, L. (1979). A cohort study of mortality and cancer incidence in ethylene oxide production workers. *Br. J. Ind. Med.* **36,** 276–280.

Hollingsworth, R. L., Rowe, V. K., Oyen, F., McCollister, D. D., and Spencer, H. C. (1956a). Toxicity of ethylene oxide determined on experimental animals. *Arch. Ind. Health* **13,** 217–227.

Hollingsworth, R. L., Rowe, V. K., Oyen, F., Hoyle, H. R., and Spencer, J. C. (1956b). Toxicity of paradichlorobenzene. Determinations on experimental animals and human subjects. *Arch. Ind. Health* **14,** 138–147.

Honma, T., Sudd, A., Miyagawa, M., Sato, M., and Hasegawa, H. (1982). Significant changes in monoamines in rat brain induced by exposure to methyl bromide. *Neurobehav. Toxicol. Teratol.* **4**(5), 521–524.

Honma, T., Miyagawa, M., Sato, M., and Hasegawa, H. (1985). Neurotoxicity and metabolism of methyl bromide in rats. *Toxicol. Appl. Pharmacol.* **81,** 183–191.

Hougaard, K., Ingvar, M., Wieloch, T., and Siesjo, B. K. (1984). Cerebral metabolic and circulatory effects of 1,1,1-trichlorethane, a neurotoxic industrial solvent. I. Effects on local cerebral glucose consumption and blood flow during acute exposure. *Neurochem. Pathol.* **2,** 39–53.

Hove, E. L. (1948). Interrelation between α-tocopherol and protein metabolism. III. The protective effect of vitamin E and certain nitrogenous compounds against CCl₄ poisoning in rats. *Arch. Biochem.* **17,** 467–473.

Hubbs, R. S., and Prusmack, J. J. (1955). Ethylene dichloride poisoning. *JAMA, J. Am. Med. Assoc.* **159,** 673–675.

Hudak, A., and Ungvary, G. (1978). Embryotoxic effects of benzene and its methyl derivatives: Toluene, xylene. *Toxicology* **11,** 55–63.

Hurtt, M. E., Morgan, K. T., and Working, P. K. (1986). Histopathology of acute responses in rats exposed by inhalation to methyl bromide. *Pharmacologist* **28**(3), 207.

Hutson, D., Moss, J., and Pickering, B. (1971). The excretion and retention of components of the soil fumigant D-D® and their metabolites in the rat. *Food Cosmet. Toxicol.* **9,** 677–680.

Igwe, O. J., Que Hee, S. S., and Wagner, W. D. (1986). Inhalation pharmacokinetics of 1,2-dichloroethane after different dietary pretreatments of male Sprague-Dawley rats. *Arch. Toxicol.* **59,** 127–134.

Ikeda, M., and Imamura, T. (1973). Biological half-life of trichloroethylene and tetrachloroethylene in human subjects. *Int. Arch. Arbeitsmed.* **31,** 209–224.

Ikeda, M., Koizumi, A., Watanabe, T., and Sato, K. (1980). Cytogenetic and cytokinetic investigations on lymphocytes from workers occupationally exposed to tetrachloroethylene. *Toxicol. Lett.* **5,** 251–256.

Inoue, T., Miyazawa, N., Tanahashi, M., Morima, M., and Shirasu, Y. (1982). Induction of sex-linked recessive lethal mutations in *Drosophila melanogaster* males by gaseous 1,2-dibromo-3-chloropropane (DBCP). *Mutat. Res.* **105,** 89–94.

International Agency for Research on Cancer (IARC) (1982). "Monographs on the Evaluation of the Carcinogenic Risk of Chemicals to Humans," IARC Monogr., Suppl. 4. Int. Agency Res. Cancer, Lyon, France.

International Agency for Research on Cancer (IARC) (1985). "Monographs on the Evaluation of the Carcinogenic Risks of Chemicals to Humans," Vol. 36, pp. 189–226. Int. Agency Res. Cancer, Lyon, France.

Irish, D. D., Adams, E. M., Spencer, H. C., and Rowe, V. K. (1940). Response attending exposure of laboratory animals to vapors of methyl bromide. *J. Ind. Hyg. Toxicol.* **22,** 218–230.

Irle, U. (1964). Acute hematoxylin anemia caused by naphthalene inhalation in two premature infants and one neonate. *Dtsch. Med. Wochenschr.* **89,** 1798–1800 (in German).

Isacson, P., Bean, J. A., Splinter, R., Olson, D. B., and Kohler, J. (1985). Drinking water and cancer incidence in Iowa. III. Association of cancer with indices of contamination. *Am. J. Epidemiol.* **121,** 856–869.

Isbister, C. (1963). Poisoning in childhood, with particular reference to kerosene poisoning. *Med. J. Aust.* **2,** 652–656.

Ivanetich, K. M., and Van Den Honert, L. H. (1981). Chloroethanes: Their metabolism by hepatic cytochromes P450 in vitro. *Carcinogenesis (London)* **2,** 697–702.

Jacobson, P. L., Hackley, E. B., and Feinsilver, L. (1956). The toxicity of inhaled ethylene oxide and propylene oxide vapors. *Arch. Ind. Health* **13,** 237–244.

Jacobziner, H., and Raybin, H. W. (1961). Ethylene dichloride poisoning. *Arch. Pediatr.* **78,** 490–495.

Jacobziner, H., and Raybin, H. W. (1964). Naphthalene poisoning. *N.Y. State J. Med.* **64,** 1762–1763.

Jay, M. K., Swift, T. R., and Hull, D. S. (1982). Possible relationship of ethylene oxide exposure to cataract formation. *Am. J. Ophthalmol.* **93,** 727–732.

Jeffrey, M. M. (1987a). "TELONE II Soil Fumigant: Acute Oral Toxicity Study in Fischer 344 Rats." Report of The Dow Chemical Company, Midland, Michigan.

Jeffrey, M. M. (1987b). "TELONE II Soil Fumigant: Acute Dermal Toxicity Study in New Zealand White Rabbits." Report of The Dow Chemical Company, Midland, Michigan.

Jeffrey, M. M. (1987c). "TELONE II Soil Fumigant: Primary Dermal Irritation Study in New Zealand White Rabbits." Report of The Dow Chemical Company, Midland, Michigan.

Jeffrey, M. M. (1987d). "TELONE II Soil Fumigant: Primary Eye Irritation Study in New Zealand White Rabbits." Report of The Dow Chemical Company, Midland, Michigan.

Jeffrey, M. M. (1987e). "TELONE II Soil Fumigant: Dermal Sensitization Potential in the Hartley Albino Guinea Pig." Report of The Dow Chemical Company, Midland, Michigan.

Jerina, D. M., Daly, J. W., Witkop, B., Zaltzman-Nirenberg, P., and Udenfriend, S. (1970). 1,2-Naphthalene oxide as an intermediate in the microsomal hydroxylation of naphthalene. *Biochemistry* **9,** 147–156.

John, J. A., Wroblewski, D. J., and Schwetz, B. A. (1984). Teratogenicity of experimental and occupational exposure to industrial chemicals. *In* "Issues and Reviews in Teratology" (H. Kalter, ed.), Vol. 2, pp. 267–324. Plenum, New York.

Johnson, B. L., Boyd, J., Burg, J. R., Lee, S. T., Xintaras, C., and Albright, B. E. (1983). Effects on the peripheral nervous system of workers: Exposure to carbon disulfide. *Neurotoxicology* **4,** 53–66.

Johnson, D. E. (1955). Hypoplastic anemia following chronic exposure to kerosene. *J. Am. Med. Women's Assoc.* **10,** 421–424.

Johnstone, R. T. (1942). "Occupational Diseases, Diagnosis, Medicolegal Aspects and Treatment." Saunders, Philadelphia, Pennsylvania.

Johnstone, R. T., and Miller, S. E. (1960). "Occupational Diseases and Industrial Medicine." Saunders, Philadelphia, Pennsylvania.

Jones, A. T., Jones, R. C., and Longley, E. O. (1964). Environmental and clinical aspects of fumigation of bulk wheat with aluminum phosphide. *Am. Ind. Hyg. Assoc. J.* **25,** 376–379.

Jones, J. R., and Collier, T. A. (1986a). "TELONE II: Acute Oral Toxicity in the Rat." Report of The Dow Chemical Company, Midland, Michigan.

Jones, J. R., and Collier, T. A. (1986b). "Telone II: Acute Dermal Toxicity Test in the Rat." Report of The Dow Chemical Company, Midland, Michigan.

Jones, R. D., and Winter, D. P. (1983). Two case reports of deaths on industrial premises attributed to 1,1,1-trichloroethane. *Arch. Environ. Health* **38,** 59–61.

Jones-Price, C., Wolkowski-Tyl, R., Marr, M. C., and Kimmel, C. A. (1984a). "Teratologic Evaluation of Carbon Disulfide (CAS No. 75-15-0) Administered to New Zealand White Rabbits on Gestational Days 6 through 15," Rep. FDA/NCTR-83/79.

Jones-Price, C., Wolkowski-Tyl, R., Marr, M. C., and Kimmel, C. A. (1984b). "Teratologic Evaluation of Carbon Disulfide (CAS No. 75-15-0) Administered to CD Rats on Gestational Days 6 through 19," Rep. FDA/NCTR-84/78.

Kadkol, S. B., and Jayaraj, P. (1968). Effects of phosphine fumigated rice on the growth of albino rats. *J. Food Sci. Technol.* **5,** 6–7.

Kagramanov, B. G. (1970). A case of pulmonary edema in peroral poisoning with dichloroethane. *Azerb. Med. Zh.* **47,** 79–81 (in Russian).

Kapp, R. W., Jr. (1978). Mutagenicity of 1,2-dibromo-3-chloropropane (DBCP) in in vivo cytogenetics study in the rat. *Toxicol. Appl. Pharmacol.* **48,** A46.

Kapp, R. W., Jr., Picciano, D. J., and Jacobson, C. B. (1979). Y-chromosome nondisjunction in dibromochloropropane-exposed workmen. *Mutat. Res.* **64,** 47–51.

Kato, Y., Matano, O., and Goto, S. (1979a). Covalent binding of DBCP to proteins in vitro. *Toxicol. Lett.* **3,** 299–302.

Kato, Y., Sato, K., Makai, S., Matano, O., and Goto, S. (1979b). Metabolic fate of 1,2-dibromo-3-chloropropane (DBCP) in rats. *J. Pestic. Sci.* **4,** 195–203.

Kato, Y., Sato, K., Matano, O., and Goto, S. (1980). Metabolic fate of DBCP in rats. 2. Alkylation of cellular macromolecules by reactive metabolic intermediates of DBCP. *J. Pestic. Sci.* **5,** 45–53.

Kawai, M., and Ueda, K. (1972). Effect of glutathione on acute intoxication due to methyl bromide. *J. Jpn. Assoc. Rural Med.* **21,** 314–315 (in Japanese).

Kendrick, J. F. (1929). The treatment of hookworm disease with tetrachloroethylene. *Am. J. Trop. Med.* **9,** 483–488.

Keplinger, M. L. (1963). Use of humans to evaluate safety of chemicals. *Arch. Environ. Health* **6,** 342–349.

Kimbrough, R. D., Mitchell, F. L., and Houk, V. N. (1985). Trichloroethylene: An update. *J. Toxicol. Environ. Health* **15,** 369–383.

Kimmerle, G., and Eben, A. (1973). Metabolism, excretion and toxicology of trichloroethylene after inhalation. 2. Experimental human exposure. *Arch. Toxicol.* **30,** 127–138.

Kimura, E. T., Ebert, D. M., and Dodge, P. W. (1971). Acute toxicity and limits of solvent residue for sixteen organic solvents. *Toxicol. Appl. Pharmacol.* **19,** 699–704.

Kimura, R., Hayashi, T., Sato, M., Aimoto, T., and Murata, T. (1979). Identification of sulfur-containing metabolites of *p*-dichlorobenzene and their disposition in rats. *J. Pharm. Dyn.* **2,** 237–244.

Kindler, U. (1979). Poison elimination by hyperventilation. *In* "Human Toxicology. Acute Poisoning and Poison Information" (S. Okonek, G. Fülgraff, and R. Frey, eds.), 2nd Int Symp., pp. 60–64. Fischer, Stuttgart.

King, M. T., Beikirch, H., Eckhardt, K., Gocke, E., and Wild, D. (1979). Mutagenicity studies with x-ray contrast media, analgesics, antipyretics, antirheumatics and some other pharmaceutical drugs in bacterial, *Drosophila* and mammalian test systems. *Mutat. Res.* **66,** 33–43.

Kjellstrand, P., Holmquist, B., Jonsson, I., Romare, S., and Mansson, L. (1985). Effects of organic solvents on motor activity in mice. *Toxicology* **35,** 35–46.

Klaassen, C. D., and Plaa, G. L. (1966). Relative effects of various chlorinated hydrocarbons on liver and kidney function in mice. *Toxicol. Appl. Pharmacol.* **9,** 139–151.

Klaassen, C. D., and Plaa, G. L. (1967). Relative effects of various chlorinated hydrocarbons on liver and kidney function in dogs. *Toxicol. Appl. Pharmacol.* **10,** 119–131.

Kleinfield, M., and Tabershaw, I. (1954). Trichloroethylene toxicity. Report of five cases. *AMA Arch. Ind. Hyg.* **10,** 134–141.

Klimmer, O. R. (1969). Effect of hydrogen phosphide (PH₃). *Arch. Toxikol.* **24,** 164–187 (in German).

Klingensmith, J. S., and Mehendale, H. M. (1982). Potentiation of CCl₄ lethality by chlordecone. *Toxicol. Lett.* **11,** 149–154.

Kluwe, W. M., Gupta, B. N., and Lamb, J. C. IV. (1983). The comparative effects of 1,2-dibromo-3-chloropropane (DBCP) and its metabolites, 3-chloro-1,2-propaneoxide (epichlorohydrin), and oxalic acid on the urogenital system of male rats. *Toxicol. Appl. Pharmacol.* **70,** 67–86.

Kobayashi, H., Hobara, T., Hirota, H., and Sakai, T. (1983). Neural control of blood pressure following 1,1,1-trichloroethane inhalation: A role of sympathetic nervous system. *Arch. Environ. Health* **38,** 93–98.

Koizumi, A., Kumai, M., and Ikeda, M. (1983). Dose-dependent induction and suppression of liver mixed-function oxidase system in chlorinated hydrocarbon solvent metabolism. *J. Appl. Toxicol.* **3,** 208–217.

Kokarovtseva, M. G. (1979). Effect of dichloroethane on the hydroxylating and conjugating activities of cytoplasmic membrane in liver. *Ukr. Biokhim. Zh.* **51,** 10–13 (in Russian).

Kokarovtseva, M. G. (1980). Acetylcysteine as a detoxicating agent in acute poisonings with 1,2-dichloroethane. *Vrach. Delo* **3,** 106–108 (in Russian).

Kolb, R. W., Schneiter, R., Floyd, E. P., and Byers, D. H. (1952). Disinfective action of methyl bromide, methanol, and hydrogen bromide on anthrax spores. *AMA Arch. Ind. Hyg. Occup. Med.* **5,** 354–364.

Kopecky, J., Gut, I., Nerudova, J., Zacharadova, D., and Holecek, V. (1980). Two routes of acrylonitrile metabolism. *J. Hyg. Epidemiol., Microbiol., Immunol.* **3,** 356–362.

Kramers, P. G. N., Voogd, C. E., Knaap, A. G. A. C., and Van der Heijden, C. A. (1985). Mutagenicity of methyl bromide in a series of short-term tests. *Mutat. Res.* **155,** 41–47.

Krantz, J. C., Park, C. S., and Ling, J. S. (1959). Anesthesia LX: The anesthetic properties of 1,1,1-trichloroethane. *Anesthesiology* **20,** 635–640.

Krasavage, W. J., O'Donouoghue, L., and DiVincenzo, G. D. (1982). *In* "Patty's Industrial Hygiene and Toxicology" (G. D. Clayton and F. E. Clayton, eds.), Vol. IIC. Wiley, New York.

Kroener, H., and Staib, W. (1968). Liver enzymes in acute carbon tetrachloride poisoning: A contribution to the mechanism of serum enzyme changes. *Z. Klin. Chem. Klin. Biochem.* **6,** 318–321.

Kubic, V. L., and Anders, M. W. (1975). Metabolism of dihalomethanes to carbon monoxide. II. *In vitro* studies. *Drug Metab. Dispos.* **3,** 104–112.

Kubic, V. L., and Anders, M. W. (1978). Metabolism of dihalomethanes to carbon monoxide. III. Studies on the mechanism of reaction. *Biochem. Pharmacol.* **27,** 2349–2355.

Kylin, B., Reichard, H., Sumegi, I., and Yllner, S. (1962). Hepatoxic effect of tri- and tetrachloroethylene on mice. *Nature (London)* **193,** 395.

Kylin, B., Axel, K., Ehrner-Samuel, H., and Lindborg, A. (1967). Effect of inhaled trichloroethylene on the CNS as measured by optokinetic nystagmus. *Arch. Environ. Health* **15,** 48–52.

Laass, W. (1980). Therapy of acute oral poisonings by organic solvents: Treatment by activated charcoal in combination with laxatives. *Arch. Toxicol.* **4,** 406–409.

Lal, H., Puri, S. K., and Fuller, G. C. (1970). Impairment of hepatic drug metabolism by carbon tetrachloride inhalation. *Toxicol. Appl. Pharmacol.* **16,** 35–39.

Lam, C.-W., and DiStefano, V. (1982). Behaviour and characterization of blood carbon disulfide in rats after inhalation. *Toxicol. Appl. Pharmacol.* **64,** 327–334.

Lambert, S. M. (1922). Carbon tetrachloride in the treatment of hookworm disease. Observations in twenty thousand cases. *JAMA, J. Am. Med. Assoc.* **79,** 2055–2057.

Lambert, S. M. (1933). Hookworm disease in the South Pacific. Ten years of tetrachlorides. *JAMA, J. Am. Med. Assoc.* **100,** 247–248.

Lambotte-Vandepaer, M., and Duverger-van Bogaert, M. (1984). Genotoxic properties of acrylonitrile. *Mutat. Res.* **134,** 49–59.

Lamson, P. D., and Wing, R. (1926). Early cirrhosis of the liver produced in dogs by carbon tetrachloride. *J. Pharmacol. Exp. Ther.* **29,** 191–202.

Lamson, P. D., Minot, A. S., and Robbins, B. H. (1928). The prevention and treatment of carbon tetrachloride intoxication. *JAMA, J. Am. Med. Assoc.* **90,** 345–349.

Landsteiner, K., and Jacobs, J. (1936). Studies on the sensitization of animals with simple chemical compounds. *J. Exp. Med.* **64,** 625–639.

Lane, R. W., Riddle, B. L., and Borzelleca, J. F. (1982). Effects of 1,2-dichloroethane and 1,1,1-trichloroethane in drinking water on reproduction and development in mice. *Toxicol. Appl. Pharmacol.* **63,** 409–421.

Lang, S. (1894). Conversion of acetonitrile and its homologs in the animal organism. *Arch. Exp. Pathol. Pharmacol.* **34,** 247 (in German).

Langvardt, P. W., Putzig, C. L., Braun, W. H., and Young, J. D. (1980). Identification of the major urinary metabolites of acrylonitrile in the rat. *Toxicol. Environ. Health* **6,** 273–282.

Lanham, J. M. (1981). Effects of 1,2-dibromo-3-chloropropane (DBCP) on an exposed work population. *Toxicologist* **1,** 102–103 (abstr.).

Lanham, J. M. (1987). Nine-year follow-up of workers exposed to 1,2-dibromo-3-chloropropane. *J. Occup. Med.* **29,** 488–490.

Lantz, G. D., Cunningham, G. R., Huckins, C., and Lipshults, L. I. (1981). Recovery from severe oligospermia after exposure to dibromochloropropane. *Fertil. Steril.* **35,** 46–53.

Larson, R. E., and Plaa, G. L. (1965). A correlation of the effects of cervical cordotomy, hypothermia, and catecholamines on carbon tetrachloride-induced hepatic necrosis. *J. Pharmacol. Exp. Ther.* **147,** 103–111.

Lasch, E. E., and El Shawa, R. (1981). Multiple cases of cyanide poisoning by apricot kernels in children from Gaza. *Pediatrics* **68,** 5–7.

Lehman, A. J. (1951). Chemicals in foods: A report to the Association of Food and Drug Officials on current developments. Part II. Pesticides. Section I. Introduction. *Q. Bull.—Assoc. Food Drug Off.* **15** (I), 122–133.

Lehman, A. J. (1952). Chemicals in foods: A report to the Association of Food and Drug Officials on current developments. Part II. Pesticides. Section II. Dermal toxicity. Section III. Subacute and chronic toxicity. Section IV. Biochemistry. Section V. Pathology. *Q. Bull.—Assoc. Food Drug Off.* **16**, (II), 3–9; (III), 47–53; (IV), 85–91; (V), 126–132.

Lesser, L. I., Weens, H. S., and McKey, J. D. (1943). Pulmonary manifestations following ingestion of kerosene. *J. Pediatr.* **23**, 352–364.

Letz, G. A., Pond, S. M., Osterloh, J. D., Wade, R. L., and Becker, C. E. (1984). Two fatalities after acute occupational exposure to ethylene dibromide. *JAMA, J. Am. Med. Assoc.* **252**, 2428–2431.

Levy, A. G. (1913). The exciting causes of ventricular fibrillation in animals under chloroform anesthesia. *Heart* **4**, 319–378.

Levy, A. G., and Lewis, T. (1911). Heart irregularities resulting from the inhalation of low percentages of chloroform vapour, and their relationship to ventricular fibrillation. *Heart* **3**, 99–112.

Lewey, F. H. (1941). Experimental chronic carbon disulfide poisoning in dogs. A clinical and pathological study. *J. Ind. Hyg. Toxicol.* **23**, 415–436.

Lewis, S. E. (1948). Inhibition of SH enzymes by methyl bromide. *Nature (London)* **161**, 692–693.

Lin, C. C., and Chen, C. (1969). The effects of carbon tetrachloride and some antioxidants on the hydroxylation of Tetralin by rat liver homogenate. *Biochim. Biophys. Acta* **192**, 133–135.

Lindberg, H. A., Wald, M. H., and Barker, M. H. (1941). Observations on the pathologic effects of thiocyanate. An experimental study. *Am. Heart J.* **21**, 605–616.

Lindgren, D. L., Sinclair, W. B., and Vincent, L. E. (1968). Residues in raw and processed foods resulting from post-harvest insecticidal treatments. *Res. Rev.* **21**, 1–121.

Lipshultz, L. I., Ross, C. E., and Whorton, M. D. (1980). Dibromochloropropane and its effects on testicular function in man. *J. Urol.* **124**, 464–468.

Lloyd, E. L. (1969). Trichloroethylene neuropathy. *Br. Med. J.* **2**, 118–119.

Loeser, E., and Litchfield, M. H. (1983). Review of recent toxicology studies on *p*-dichlorobenzene. *Food Cosmet. Toxicol.* **21**, 825–832.

Loewenthal, M. (1949). Hydrogen-phosphide poisoning. *Schweiz. Z. Pathol. Bakteriol.* **12**, 313–350 (in German).

Lomax, L. G., Calhoun, L. L., Stott, W. T., and Frauson, L. E. (1987). "Technical Grade 1,3-dichloropropene: Two-Year Chronic Toxicity Oncogenicity Study in Fischer 344 rats," Report of The Dow Chemical Company, Midland, Michigan.

Longley, E. O., and Jones, A. T. (1965). Methyl bromide poisoning in man. *Ind. Med. Surg.* **34**, 499–502.

Lorz, H. (1950). Percutaneous poisoning with acrylonitrile (Ventox). *Dtsch. Med. Wochenschr.* **75**, 1087–1088 (in German).

Lucas, G. H. W. (1928). A study of the fate and toxicity of bromine and chlorine containing anesthetics. *J. Pharmacol. Exp. Ther.* **34**, 223–237.

Lundberg, I., and Hakansson, M. (1985). Normal serum activities of liver enzymes in Swedish paint industry workers with heavy exposure to organic solvents. *Br. J. Ind. Med.* **42**, 596–600.

Luzhnikov, E. A., Lisovik, Z. A., and Novikovskaya, T. V. (1985). 1,2-Dichloroethane metabolism in man after acute poisoning. *Sud.-Med. Ekspert.* **28**, 47–49.

Lynch, D. W., Lewis, T. R., Moorman, W. J., Burg, J. R., Groth, D. H., Khan, A., Ackerman, L. J., and Cockrell, B. Y. (1984). Carcinogenic and toxicologic effects of inhaled ethylene oxide and propylene oxide in F344 rats. *Toxicol. Appl. Pharmacol.* **76**, 69–84.

MacGregor, R. R. (1954). Naphthalene poisoning from the ingestion of moth balls. *Can. Med. Assoc. J.* **70**, 313–314.

Mackell, J. V., Rieders, F., Brieger, W., and Bauer, E. L. (1951). Acute hemolytic anemia due to ingestion of moth balls. *Pediatrics* **7**, 722–728.

Magos, L. (1962). A study of acrylonitrile poisoning in relation to methaemoglobin–CN complex formation. *Br. J. Ind. Med.* **19**, 283–286.

Mahvi, D., Bank, H. B., and Harley, R. (1977). Morphology of a naphthalene-induced bronchiolar lesion. *Am. J. Pathol.* **86**, 559–566.

Majeed, H. A., Bassyouni, H., Kalaowy, M., and Farwana, S. (1981). Kerosene poisoning in children: A children-radiological study of 205 cases. *Ann. Trop. Paediatr.* **1**, 123–130.

Malchy, H., and Parkhouse, J. (1969). Respiratory studies with trichloroethylene. *Can. Anaesth. Soc. J.* **16**, 119–134.

Maltoni, C., Valgimigli, L., and Scarnato, C. (1980). Long-term carcinogenic bioassays on ethylene dichloride administered by inhalation to rats and mice. *Banbury Rep.* **5**, 3–29.

Manson, D. (1934). A comparative record of anthelmintic treatment with tetrachlorethylene and oil of chenopodium. *Indian Med. Gaz.* **69**, 500–507.

Manson, J. M., Murphy, M., Richdale, N., and Smith, M. K. (1984). Effects of oral exposure to trichloroethylene on female reproductive function. *Toxicology* **32**, 229–242.

Maplestone, P. A., and Chopra, R. N. (1933). The toxicity of tetrachlorethylene to cats. *Indian Med. Gaz.* **68**, 554–556.

Marks, T. A., Ledoux, T. A., and Moore, J. A. (1982). Teratogenicity of a commercial xylene mixture in the mouse. *J. Toxicol. Environ. Health* **9**, 97–105.

Marquez, M. E. (1978). 1,2-Dibromo-3-chloropropane (DBCP), nematocide with sterilizing action in man. *SPM* **20**, 195–200.

Marraccini, J. V., Thomas, G. E., Ongley, J. P., and Pfaffenberger, C. D. (1983). Death and injury caused by methyl bromide, an insecticide fumigant. *J. Forensic Sci.* **28**(3), 601–607.

Marsalis, J. C., and Butterworth, B. E. (1980). Detection of unscheduled DNA synthesis in hepatocytes isolated from rats treated with genotoxic agents: An *in vivo–in vitro* assay for potential carcinogens and mutagens. *Carcinogenesis (N.Y.)* **1**, 621–625.

Marshall, S., Whorton, M. D., Krauss, R. M., and Palmer, W. S. (1978). Effect of pesticides on testicular function. *Urology* **11**, 257–259.

Martin, G., Knorpp, K., Huth, K., Heinrich, F., and Mittermayer, C. (1968). Clinical aspects, pathogenesis, and treatment of ethylene dichloride poisoning. *Dtsch. Med. Wochenschr.* **93**, 2002, 2004–2006, 2009–2010 (in German).

Martis, L., Kroes, R., Darby, T. D., and Woods, E. F. (1982). Disposition kinetics of ethylene oxide, ethylene glycol, and 2-chloroethanol in the dog. *J. Toxicol. Environ. Health* **10**, 847–856.

McCarthy, T. B., and Jones, R. D. (1983). Industrial gassing poisonings due to trichloroethylene, perchloroethylene, and 1,1,1-trichloroethane, 1961–1980. *Br. J. Ind. Med.* **40**, 450–455.

McCollister, D. D., Beamer, W. H., Atchinson, G. J., and Spencer, H. C. (1951). The absorption, distribution and elimination of radioactive carbon tetrachloride by monkeys upon exposure to low vapor concentrations. *J. Pharmacol. Exp. Ther.* **102**, 112–124.

McCollister, D. D., Hollingsworth, R. L., Oyen, F., and Rowe, V. K. (1956). Comparative inhalation toxicity of fumigant mixtures. Individual and joint effects of ethylene dichloride, carbon tetrachloride, and ethylene dibromide. *AMA Arch. Ind. Health* **13**, 1–7.

McGregor, D. B. (1981). "Tier II Mutagenic Screening of 13 NIOSH Priority Compounds. Individual Compound Report: Methyl Bromide," NIOSH Contract 210-78-0026; Rep. No. 32. U. S. Govt. Printing Office, Washington, D. C.

McKee, R. W., Kiper, C., Fountain, J. H., Riskin, A. M., and Drinker, P. (1943). A solvent vapor carbon disulfide. Absorption, elimination, metabolism, and mode of action. *JAMA, J. Am. Med. Assoc.* **122**, 217–222.

McKenna, M. J., and DiStefano, V. (1977). Carbon disulfide. I. The metabolism of inhaled carbon disulfide. *J. Pharmacol. Exp. Ther.* **202**, 245–252.

McKenna, M. J., and Zempel, J. A. (1981). The dose-dependent metabolism of [^{14}C]methylene chloride following oral administration to rats. *Food Cosmet. Toxicol.* **19**, 73–78.

McKenna, M. J., Zempel, J. A., and Braun, W. H. (1982). The pharmacokinetics of inhaled methylene chloride in rats. *Toxicol. Appl. Pharmacol.* **65**, 1–10.

McKinney, L. L., Weakley, F. B., Eldridge, A. C., Campbell, R. E., Cowan, J. C., Picken, J. C., Jr., and Biester, H. E. (1957). S-(Dichlorovinyl)-L-cysteine: An agent causing fatal aplastic anemia in calves. *J. Am. Chem. Soc.* **79**, 3932–3933.

McKinney, L. L., Picken, J. C. Jr., Weakley, F. B., Eldridge, A. C., Campbell, R. E., Cowan, J. C., and Biester, H. E. (1959). Possible toxic factor of trichloroethylene-extracted soybean oil meal. *J. Am. Chem. Soc.* **81**, 909–915.

McLaughlin, M., Krivanek, N. D., and Trochimowicz, H. J. (1976). Evaluation of antidotes for acrylonitrile poisoning. *Toxicol. Appl. Pharmacol.* **37**, 133–134.

McLean, A. E. M., and McLean, E. K. (1966). The effect of diet and 1,1,1-trichloro-2,2-bis-(*p*-chlorophenyl)ethane (DDT) on microsomal hydroxylating enzymes and on sensitivity of rats to carbon tetrachloride poisoning. *Biochem. J.* **100**, 564–571.

McMann, J., Choi, E., Yamasaki, E., and Ames, B. N. (1975). Detection of carcinogens as mutagens in the *Salmonella*/microsomal test: Assay of 300 chemicals. *Proc. Natl. Acad. Sci. U.S.A.* **12**, 5133–5139.

McNally, W. D. (1956). Kerosene poisoning in children: A study of 204 cases. *J. Pediatr.* **48**, 296–299.

McOmie, W. A. (1949). Comparative toxicity of methacrylonitrile and acrylonitrile. *J. Ind. Hyg. Toxicol.* **31**, 113–116.

Medinsky, M. A., Bond, J. A., Dutcher, J. S., and Birnbaum, L. S. (1984). Disposition of [14C]methyl bromide in Fischer 344 rats after oral or intraperitoneal administration. *Toxicology* **32**, 187–196.

Medinsky, M. A., Dutcher, J. S., Bond, J. A., Henderson, R. F., Mauderly, J. L., Snipes, M. B., Mewhinney, J. A., Cheng, Y. S., and Birnbaum, L. S. (1985). Uptake and excretion of [14C]methyl bromide as influenced by exposure concentration. *Toxicol. Appl. Pharmacol.* **78**, 215–225.

Meldolesi, J. (1968). Protective effects of alpha-tocopherol on the hepatotoxicity of carbon tetrachloride: An electron microscopy study. *Exp. Mol. Pathol.* **9**, 141–147.

Mendrala, A. L. (1985). "Evaluation of TELONE II in the Rat Hepatocyte Unscheduled DNA Synthesis Assay." Report of The Dow Chemical Company, Midland, Michigan.

Mendrala, A. L. (1986). "The Evaluation of TELONE II Soil Fumigant in the Chinese Hamster Ovary Cell/Hypoxanthine (Guanine) Phosphoribosyl Transferase (CHO/HGPRT) Forward Mutation Assay." Report of The Dow Chemical Company, Midland, Michigan.

Michel, S., Richter, G., Tschisgale, M., and Brux, B. (1968). Behavior of free and membrane-bound rat-liver ribosomes after experimental damage by CCl. *Acta Biol. Med. Ger.* **21**, 603–614 (in German).

Mikiskova, H., and Mikiska, A. (1966). Trichloroethanol in trichloroethylene poisoning. *Br. J. Ind. Med.* **23**, 116–125.

Milby, T. H., and Whorton, D. (1980). Epidemiological assessment of occupationally related sperm count suppression. *J. Occup. Med.* **22**, 77–82.

Miller, R. E., and Guengerich, F. P. (1982). Oxidation of trichloroethylene by liver microsomal cytochrome P-450: Evidence for chloride migration in a transition state not involving trichloroethylene oxide. *Biochemistry* **21**, 1090–1097.

Minot, A. S. (1927). The relation of calcium to the toxicity of carbon tetrachloride in dogs. *Proc. Soc. Exp. Biol. Med.* **24**, 617–620.

Mitchell, A. B. S., and Parsons-Smith, B. G. (1969). Trichloroethylene neuropathy. *Br. Med. J.* **1**, 422–423.

Mizyukova, I. G., and Bakhishev, G. N. (1971). Specific treatment of acute poisoning with methyl bromide. *Vrach. Delo* **7**, 128–131 (in Russian).

Modrzejewski, J., and Myslak, Z. (1967). Phosphine poisoning during the fight against corn vermin in a port elevator. *J. Med. Pracy* **18**, 78–82 (in Polish).

Moeschlin, S. (1965). "Poisoning: Diagnosis and Treatment," 1st Am. ed. Grune & Stratton, New York.

Momotani, H., Kshizu, S., Sato, M., and Morinobu, S. (1976). Bromine determination in urine of persons exposed to methyl bromide. *Jpn. J. Ind. Health* **81**, 141 (in Japanese).

Monster, A. C., and Boersma, G. (1975). Simultaneous determination of trichloroethylene and metabolites in blood and exhaled air by gas chromatography. *Int. Arch. Occup. Environ. Health* **35**, 155–163.

Monster, A. C., Boersma, G., and Duba, W. C. (1976). Pharmacokinetics of trichloroethylene in volunteers: Influence of workload and exposure concentration. *Int. Arch. Occup. Environ. Health* **38**, 87–102.

Monster, A. C., Boersma, G., and Duba, W. C. (1979a). Kinetics of trichloroethylene in repeated exposure of volunteers. *Int. Arch. Occup. Environ. Health* **42**, 283–292.

Monster, A. C., Boersma, G., and Steenweg, H. (1979b). Kinetics of tetrachloroethylene in volunteers; influence of exposure concentration and workload. *Int. Arch. Occup. Environ. Med.* **42**, 303–309.

Montgomery, R. D. (1979). Cyanogenetic glucosides. *Hand Clin. Neurol.* **36**, 515–527.

Morgan, R. W., Claxton, K. W., Divine, B. J., Kaplan, S. D., and Harris, V. B. (1981). Mortality among ethylene oxide workers. *J. Occup. Med.* **23**, 767–770.

Morita, M., and Ohi, G. (1975). Para-dichlorobenzene in human tissue and atmosphere in Tokyo metropolitan area. *Environ. Pollut.* **8**, 269–274.

Moriya, M., Ohta, T., Watanabe, K., Miyazawa, T., Kato, K., and Shirasu, Y. (1983). Further mutagenicity studies on pesticides in bacterial reversion assay systems. *Mutat. Res.* **116**, 185–216.

Moser, V. C., and Balster, R. L. (1985). Acute motor and lethal effects of inhaled 1,1,1-trichloroethane, halothane ethanol in mice: Effects of exposure duration. *Toxicol. Appl. Pharmacol.* **77**, 285–291.

Moser, V. C., Scimeca, J. A., and Balster, R. L. (1985). Minimal tolerance to the effects of 1,1,1-trichloroethane on fixed-ratio responding in mice. *Neurotoxicology* **6**, 35–42.

Moskowitz, S., and Shapiro, H. (1952). Fatal exposure to methylene chloride vapor. *AMA Arch. Ind. Hyg. Occup. Med.* **6**, 116–123.

Moslen, M. T., Reynolds, E. S., and Szabo, S. (1976). Correlations between the chemically induced potentiation of trichloroethylene hepatotoxicity and its metabolism. *Fed. Proc., Fed. Am. Soc. Exp. Biol.* **35**, 375.

Moslen, M. T., Reynolds, E. S., and Szabo, S. (1977). Enhancement of the metabolism and hepatotoxicity of trichloroethylene and perchloroethylene. *Biochem. Pharmacol.* **26**, 369–375.

Mullin, L. S., and Krivanek, N. D. (1982). Comparison of unconditioned reflex and conditioned avoidance tests in rats exposed by inhalation to carbon monoxide, 1,1,1-trichloroethane, toluene or ethanol. *Neurotoxicology* **3**, 126–137.

Murray, F. J., Schwetz, B. A., Nitschke, K. D., John, J. A., Norris, J. M., and Gehring, P. J. (1978). Teratogenicity of acrylonitrile given to rats by gavage or by inhalation. *Food Cosmet. Toxicol.* **16**, 547–551.

Murray, R. A., Mahoney, L. E., and Sachs, R. R. (1974). Illness associated with soil fumigation: California. *Morbid. Mortal. Wkly. Rep.* **23**, 217–218.

Musser, A. W., and Spooner, G. H. (1968). Serum ornithine carbamyl transferase levels and hepatocellular damage in rats treated with carbon tetrachloride. *Arch. Pathol.* **86**, 606–609.

Muthu, M., Krishnakumaari, M. K., Muralidhara, and Majumder, S. K. (1980). A study on the acute inhalation toxicity of phosphine to albino rats. *Bull. Environ. Contam. Toxicol.* **24**, 404–410.

Nachtomi, E., and Alumot, E. (1972). Comparison of ethylene dibromide and carbon tetrachloride toxicity in rats and chicks: Blood and liver levels; lipid peroxidation. *Exp. Mol. Pathol.* **16**, 71–78.

Nachtomi, E., and Sarma, D. S. R. (1977). Repair of rat liver DNA *in vivo* damaged by ethylene dibromide. *Biochem. Pharmacol.* **26**, 1941–1945.

Naiman, J. L., and Kosoy, M. H. (1964). Red cell glucose-6-phosphate dehydrogenase deficiency—a newly recognized cause of neonatal jaundice and kernicterus in Canada. *Can. Med. Assoc. J.* **91**, 1243–1249.

Nakakita, H. (1973). Toxicity and residue of some grain fumigants. *Bochu Kagaku* **38**, 43–66 (in Japanese).

Nalbandian, R. M., and Pearce, J. F. (1965). Allergic purpura induced by exposure to *p*-dichlorobenzene. *JAMA, J. Am. Med. Assoc.* **194**, 828–829.

Nash, F. L. (1903). Naphthalene poisoning. *Br. Med. J.* **1**, 251.

Nater, J. P., and Gooskens, V. H. J. (1976). Occupational dermatosis due to a soil fumigant. *Contact Dermatitis* **2**, 227–229.

National Cancer Institute (NCI) (1976). "Carcinogenesis Bioassay of Trichloroethylene," Tech. Support Ser. No. 2, DHEW Publ. No. (NIH) 76-802. U.S. Dept. of Health, Education, and Welfare, Washington, D.C.

National Cancer Institute (NCI) (1977a). "Bioassay of 1,1,1-Trichloroethane for Possible Carcinogenicity," Carcinogenesis Tech. Rep. Ser. No. 3. U.S. Govt. Printing Office, Washington, D.C.

National Cancer Institute (NCI) (1977b). "Bioassay of Tetrachloroethylene for Possible Carcinogenicity," DHEW Publ. No. (NIH) 77-813. U.S. Dept. of Health, Education, and Welfare, Washington, D.C.

National Cancer Institute (NCI) (1978a). "Bioassay of 1,2-Dichloroethane for Possible Carcinogenicity," Carcinogenesis Tech. Rep. Ser. Vol 86, DHEW Publ. No. (NIH) 78-1336. U.S. Govt. Printing Office, Washington, D.C.

National Cancer Institute (NCI) (1978b). "Bioassay of 1,2-Dibromoethane for Possible Carcinogenicity," Carcinogenesis Tech. Rep. Ser. Vol 55, DHEW Publ. No. (NIH) 78-1361. U.S. Govt. Printing Office, Washington, D.C.

National Research Council (1980). "Drinking Water and Health," Vol. 3. Natl. Acad. Press, Washington, D.C.

National Toxicology Program (NTP) (1982). "Carcinogenesis Bioassay of 1,2-Dibromoethane (CAS No. 106-93-4) in F344 Rats and B6C3F1 Mice (Inhalation Study)," DHHS Publ. No. (NIH) 82-1766. U.S. Govt. Printing Office, Washington, D.C.

National Toxicology Program (NTP) (1983). "NTP Technical Report on the Carcinogenesis Studies of Trichloroethylene (without Epichlorohydrin) in F344/N rats and $B_6C_3F_1$·Mice (Gavage Studies)," NIH Publ. No. 83-1799. U.S. Dept. of Health and Human Services, Research Triangle Park, North Carolina.

National Toxicology Program (NTP) (1985). "Toxicology and Carcinogenesis Studies of Telone II® in F344/N Rats and B6C3F1 Mice (Gavage Studies)," Tech. Rep. No. 269. U.S. Govt. Printing Office, Washington, D.C.

National Toxicology Program (NTP) (1986a). "The Toxicology and Carcinogenesis Studies of Dichloromethane in F344/N Rats and $B_6C_3F_1$ Mice (Inhalation Studies)," Tech. Rep. Ser. No. 306, Final Report—January. U.S. Dept. of Health and Human Services, Research Triangle Park, North Carolina.

National Toxicology Program (NTP) (1986b). "Toxicology and Carcinogenesis Studies of Xylenes (Mixed) in F-344 Rats and B6C3F1 Mice," Tech. Rep. Ser. No. 327. Natl. Toxicol. Program, Research Triangle Park, North Carolina.

National Toxicology Program (NTP) (1986c). "Toxicology and Carcinogenesis Studies of Tetrachloroethylene in F344/N Rats and $B_6C_3F_1$ Mice," Tech. Rep. Ser. No. 311, NIH Publ. No. 86-2567. U.S. Dept. of Health and Human Services, Research Triangle Park, North Carolina.

National Toxicology Program (NTP) (1987). "Toxicology and Carcinogenesis Studies of 1,4-Dichlorobenzene in F344/N Rats and $B_6C_3F_1$ Mice (Gavage Studies)," Tech. Rep. Ser. No. 319. Natl. Toxicol. Program, Research Triangle Park, North Carolina.

Neudecker, T., Stefani, A., and Henschler, D. (1977). *In vitro* mutagenicity of soil nematocide 1,3-dichloropropene. *Experientia* 33, 1084–1085.

Nicholls, L., and Hampton, G. G. (1922). Treatment of human hookworm infection with carbon tetrachloride. *Br. Med. J.* 2, 8–11.

Nitschke, K. D., Kociba, R. J., Keyes, D. G., and McKenna, M. J. (1981). A thirteen week repeated inhalation study of ethylene dibromide in rats. *Fundam. Appl. Toxicol.* 1, 437–442.

Nitschke, K. D., Burek, J. D., Bell, T. J., Kociba, R. J., Rampy, L. W., and McKenna, M. J. (1988a). Methylene chloride: A two-year inhalation toxicity and oncogenicity study in rats. *Fundam. Appl. Toxicol.* 11, 48–59.

Nitschke, K. D., Eisenbrandt, D. L., Lomax, L. G., and Rao, K. S. (1987b). Methylene chloride: Two-generation inhalation reproduction study in Fischer 344 rats. *Fundam. Appl. Toxicol.* 11, 60–67.

Noa, N., and Sanabria, J. (1984). Tracheal ultrastructure in kerosene treated guinea pigs. A preliminary report. *Allergol. Immunopathol.* 12, 33–36.

Noguchi, T., Fong, K. L., Lai, E. K., Olson, L., and McCoy, P. B. (1982a). Selective early loss of polypeptides in liver microsomes of CCl_4-treated rats. Relationship to cytochrome P-450 content. *Biochem. Pharmacol.* 31, 609–614.

Noguchi, T., Fong, K. L., Lai, E. K., Alexander, S. S., King, M. M., Olson, L., Poyer, J. L., and McCay, P. B. (1982b). Specificity of a phenobarbital-induced cytochrome P-450 for metabolism of carbon tetrachloride to the trichloromethyl radical. *Biochem. Pharmacol.* 31, 615–624.

Nolan, R. J., Freshour, N. L., Rick, D. L., McCarty, L. P., and Saunders, J. H. (1984). Kinetics and metabolism of inhaled methyl chloroform (1,1,1-trichloroethane) in male volunteers. *Fundam. Appl. Toxicol.* 4, 654–662.

Nomiyama, H., and Nomiyama, K. (1979). Host and agent factors modifying metabolism of trichloroethylene. *Ind. Health* 17, 21–28.

Northfield, R. R. (1981). Avoidable deaths due to acute exposure to 1,1,1-trichloroethane. *J. Soc. Occup. Med.* 31, 164–166.

Nunn, J. A., and Martin, F. M. (1934). Gasoline and kerosene poisoning in children. *JAMA, J. Am. Med. Assoc.* 103, 472–474.

Odum, J., and Green, T. (1987). Perchloroethylene metabolism by the glutathione conjugation pathway. *Toxicologist* 7, 269.

Odum, J., Green, T., Foster, J. R., and Hext, P. M. (1987). Species differences in peroxisome proliferation and metabolism after inhalation exposure to perchloroethylene. *Toxicologist* 7, 190.

Ohkawa, H., Ohkawa, R., Yamamoto, I., and Casida, J. E. (1972). Enzymatic mechanisms and toxicological significance of hydrogen cyanide liberation from various organothiocyanates and organonitriles in mice and houseflies. *Pestic. Biochem. Physiol.* 2, 95–112.

Ohnishi, A., Inoue, N., Yamamoto, T., Murai, Y., Hori, H., Koga, M., Tanaka, I., and Akiyama, T. (1985). Ethylene oxide induces central–peripheral distal axonal degeneration of the lumbar primary neurons in rats. *Br. J. Ind. Med.* 42, 373–379.

Ohsawa, M., Naruse, K., Inoue, S., Furukawa, T., and Maruyama, K. (1978). A case of intention myoclonus by intoxication due to methyl bromide. *Clin. Neurol. (Rinsho Shinkeigaky)* 18, 443 (in Japanese).

Okada, E., Takahashi, K., and Nakamura, H. (1970). A study of chloropicrin intoxication. *Nippon Naika Gakkai Zasshi* 59, 1214–1221 (in Japanese).

Oliver, C. O., and Weber, R. P. (1984). Chest pain in rubber chemical workers exposed to carbon disulphide and methemoglobin formers. *Br. J. Ind. Med.* 41, 296–304.

Olmstead, E. V. (1960). Pathological changes in ethylene dibromide poisoning. *AMA Arch. Ind. Health* 21, 525–529.

Olson, B. A., Gamberale, F., and Iregren, A. (1985). Coexposure to toluene and *p*-xylene in man: Central nervous functions. *Br. J. Ind. Med.* 42, 117–122.

Olson, W. A., Habermann, R. T., Weisburger, E. K., Ward, J. M., and Weisburger, J. H. (1973). Induction of stomach cancer in rats and mice by halogenated aliphatic fumigants. *J. Natl. Cancer Inst. (U.S.)* 51, 1993–1995.

Opacka, J., Baranski, B., and Wronska-Nofer, T. (1984). Effect of alcohol intake on some disturbances induced by chronic exposure to carbon disulphide in rats. I. Behavioral alterations. *Toxicol. Lett.* 23, 91–97.

Osterloh, J. D., Letz, G., Pond, S., and Becker, C. (1983). An assessment of the potential testicular toxicity of 10 pesticides using the mouse-sperm morphology assay. *Mutat. Test.* 116, 407–415.

Osterloh, J. D., Cohen, B. S., Popendorf, W., and Pond, S. M. (1984). Urinary excretion of the *N*-acetyl cysteine conjugate of *cis*-1,3-dichloropropene by exposed individuals. *Arch. Environ. Health* 39, 271–275.

Ostlere, G. (1948). Role of trichloroethylene in general anesthesia. *Br. Med. J.* 1, 195–196.

Osuntokun, B. O. (1973). Ataxic neuropathy associated with high cassava diets in West Africa. *Int. Dev. Res. Cent. [Monogr.] IDRC* **IDRC-010e.**

Ott, M. G., Scharnweber, H. C., and Langner, R. R. (1980). Mortality experience of 161 employees exposed to ethylene dibromide in two production units. *Br. J. Ind. Med.* 37, 163–168.

Ott, M. G., Skory, L. K., Holder, B. B., Bronson, J. M., and Williams, P. R. (1983). Health evaluation of employees occupationally exposed to methylene chloride. *Scand. J. Work Environ. Health* 9, Suppl. 1, 1–38.

Pagnotto, L. D., and Walkley, J. E. (1965). Urinary dichlorophenol as an index of *para*-dichlorobenzene exposure. *Am. Ind. Hyg. Assoc. J.* 26, 137–142.

Parchman, L. G., and Magee, P. N. (1982). Metabolism of ^{14}C-trichloroethylene to $^{14}CO_2$ and interaction of a metabolite with liver DNA in rats and mice. *J. Toxicol. Environ. Health* 9, 797–813.

Parker, C., Coate, W., and Voelker, R. (1982). Subchronic inhalation toxicity of 1,3-dichloropropene/1,2-dichloropropane (D-D®) in mice and rats. *J. Toxicol. Environ. Health* 9, 899–910.

Patel, J. M., Harper, C., Gupta, B. N., and Drew, R. T. (1979). Changes in serum enzymes after inhalation exposure of *p*-xylene. *Bull. Environ. Contam. Toxicol.* 21, 17–24.

Paulet, G., Debrousses, S., and Vidal, F. (1974). Absence of teratogenic effect of fluorocarbons in the rat and rabbit. *Arch. Mal. Prof. Med. Trav. Secur. Soc.* **35,** 658–662 (in French).

Pearn, J., Nixon, J., Ansford, A., and Corcoran, A. (1984). Accidental poisoning in childhood: Five year urban population study with 15 year analysis of fatality. *Br. Med. J.* **288,** 44–46.

Pegg, D. G., Zempel, J. A., Braun, W. H., and Watanabe, P. G. (1979). Disposition of tetrachloro(^{14}C)ethylene following oral and inhalation exposure in rats. *Toxicol. Appl. Pharmacol.* **51,** 465–474.

Peoples, S. A., Maddy, K. T., and Riddle, L. C. (1978). Human occupational health problems from exposure to ethylene dibromide in California in 1975 and 1976. *Vet. Hum. Toxicol.* **20,** 241–244.

Perocco, P., Bolognesi, S., and Alberghini, W. (1983). Toxic activity of 17 industrial solvents and halogenated compounds on human lymphocytes cultured *in vitro. Toxicol. Lett.* **16,** 69–76.

Perrin, M. (1941). Possible harmfulness of paradichlorobenzene used for "anti-mites" purposes. *Bull. Acad. Med.* **125,** 302–304 (in French).

Pessayre, D., Allemand, H., Wandscheer, J. C., Descatoire, V., Artigou, J. Y., and Benhamou, J. P. (1979). Inhibition, activation, destruction, and induction of drug-metabolizing enzymes by trichloroethylene. *Toxicol. Appl. Pharmacol.* **49,** 355–363.

Peters, H. A., Levine, R. L., Matthews, C. G., Sauter, S. L., and Rankin, J. H. (1982). Carbon disulfide-induced neuropsychiatric changes in grain storage workers. *Am. J. Ind. Med.* **3,** 373–391.

Petrelli, M., and Stenger, R. J. (1969). The effect of trypan blue on the hepatotoxicity of carbon tetrachloride in the rat. *Exp. Mol. Pathol.* **10,** 115–128.

Pfeiffer, E. H., and Dunkelberg, H. (1980). Mutagenicity of ethylene oxide and propylene oxide and of the glycols and halohydrins formed from them during the fumigation of foodstuffs. *Food Cosmet. Toxicol.* **18,** 115–118.

Phelan, P. D. (1963). Accidental poisoning in childhood. *Med. J. Aust.* **2,** 656–657.

Pike, M. H. (1944). Ocular pathology due to organic compounds. *J. Mich. State Med. Soc.* **43,** 581–584.

Plaa, G. L. (1980). Toxicology of the liver. *In* "Toxicology: The Basic Science of Poisons" (L. J. Casarett and J. Doull, eds.), pp. 170–189. Macmillan, New York.

Plaa, G. L., and Larson, R. E. (1965). Relative nephrotoxic properties of chlorinated methane, ethane and ethylene derivatives in mice. *Toxicol. Appl. Pharmacol.* **7,** 37–44.

Plaa, G. L., Evans, E. A., and Hine, C. H. (1958). Relative hepatoxicity of seven halogenated hydrocarbons. *J. Pharmacol. Exp. Ther.* **123,** 224–229.

Plasterer, M. R., Bradshaw, W. S., Booth, G. M., Carter, M. W., Schuler, R. L., and Hardin, B. D. (1985). Developmental toxicity of nine selected compounds following prenatal exposure in the mouse: Naphthalene, nitrophenol, sodium selenite, dimethyl phthalate, ethylenethiourea, and four glycol ether derivatives. *J. Toxicol. Environ. Health* **15,** 25–38.

Plotnick, H. B., and Conner, W. L. (1976). Tissue distribution of ^{14}C-labeled ethylene dibromide in the guinea pig. *Res. Commun. Chem. Pathol. Pharmacol.* **13,** 251–258.

Popp, J. A., Shinozuka, H., and Farber, E. (1978). The protective effects of diethyldithiocarbamate and cycloheximide on the multiple hepatic lesions induced by carbon tetrachloride in the rat. *Toxicol. Appl. Pharmacol.* **45,** 549–564.

Potashnik, G. (1983). A four-year reassessment of workers with dibromochloropropane-induced testicular dysfunction. *Andrologia* **15,** 164–170.

Potashnik, G., Ben Aderet, N., Israeli, R., Yanai-Inbar, I., and Sober, I. (1978). Suppressive effect of 1,2-dibromo-3-chloropropane on human spermatogenesis. *Fertil. Steril.* **30,** 444–447.

Powell, J. F. (1945). Trichloroethylene: Absorption, elimination and metabolism. *Br. J. Ind. Med.* **2,** 142–145.

Pozzani, U. C., Weil, C. S., and Carpenter, C. P. (1959). The toxicological basis of threshold limit values. 5. The experimental inhalation of vapor mixtures by rats, with notes upon the relationship between single dose inhalation and single oral data. *Am. Ind. Hyg. Assoc. J.* **20,** 364–369.

Prentiss, A. M. (1937). "Chemicals in War. A Treatise on Chemical Warfare." McGraw-Hill, New York.

Press, E., Adams, W. C., Chittenden, R. F., Christian, J. R., Grayson, R., Stewart, C. C., and Everist, B. W. (1962). Evaluation of gastric lavage and other factors in the treatment of accidental ingestion of petroleum distillate products. *Pediatrics* **29,** 648–678.

Price, R. P. (1980). Some aspects of the inhibition of cytochrome-*c* oxidase by phosphine in susceptible and resistant strains of *Rhyzoopertha dominica. Insect Biochem.* **10,** 65–71.

Price, R. P., and Dance, J. S. (1983). Some biochemical aspects of phosphine action and resistance in three species of stored product beetles. 277–288.

Pritchard, W. R., Rehfeld, C. E., and Sautter, J. H. (1952). Aplastic anemia of cattle associated with ingestion of trichloroethylene-extracted soybean oil meal (Stockman disease, Duren disease, Brabant disease). I. Clinical and laboratory investigation of field cases. *J. Am. Vet. Med. Assoc.* **121,** 1–8.

Prochownik (1911). A case of naphthalene poisoning with lethal outcome. *Ther. Monatsh.* **25,** 489–490 (in German).

Proctor, N. H., Hughes, J. P., and Wesenberg, G. J. (1978). The chemical hazards. *In* "Chemical Hazards of the Workplace" (N. H. Proctor and J. P. Hughes, eds.), pp. 171–172, 399–401, 415–416. Lippincott, Philadelphia, Pennsylvania.

Prout, M. S., Provan, W. M., and Green, T. (1985). Species differences in response to trichloroethylene. I. Pharmacokinetics in rats and mice. *Toxicol. Appl. Pharmacol.* **79,** 389–400.

Quast, J. F., Rampy, L. W., Balmer, M. F., Leong, B. D. J., and Gehring, P. J. (1978). "Toxicological and Carcinogenic Evaluation of a 1,1,1-Trichloroethane Formulation by Chronic Inhalation in Rats." Available from The Dow Chemical Co., Health and Environmental Sciences, Midland, Michigan.

Quast, J. F., Calhoun, L. L., and Frauson, L. E. (1987). Chlorothene VG: A chronic inhalation toxicity and oncogenicity study in Fischer 344 rats and $B_6C_3F_1$ mice. *Fundam. Appl. Toxicol.* (submitted for publication).

Radimer, G. F., Davis, J. H., and Ackerman, A. B. (1974). Fumigant-induced toxic epidermal necrolysis. *Arch. Dermatol.* **110,** 103–104.

Raitta, C., Henrik, T., Tolonen, M., Nurminen, M., Helpio, E., and Malström, S. (1981). Impaired color discrimination among viscose rayon workers exposed to carbon disulfide. *J. Occup. Med.* **23,** 189–192.

Rakhmatullaev, N. N. (1971). Hygienic characteristics of the nematocide Nemagon (dibromochloropropane) in relation to water pollution control. *Hyg. Sanit. (USSR)* **36,** 344–348 (in Russian).

Rampy, L. W., Quast, J. F., Leong, B. K. J., and Gehring, P. J. (1978). Results of long-term inhalation toxicity studies on rats of 1,1,1-trichloroethane and perchloroethylene formulations. *In* "Proceedings of the First International Congress of Toxicology" (G. L. Plaa and W. A. M. Duncan, eds.). Academic Press, New York.

Rao, K. S., and Rechnagel, R. O. (1969). Early incorporation of carbon-labeled carbon tetrachloride into rat liver particulate lipids and proteins. *Exp. Mol. Pathol.* **10,** 219–228.

Rao, K. S., Murray, J. S., Deacon, M. M., John, J. A., Calhoun, L. L., and Young, J. T. (1980). Teratogenicity and reproduction studies in animals inhaling ethylene dichloride. *Banbury Rep.* **5,** 149–161.

Rao, K. S., Burek, J. D., Murray, F. J., John, J. A., Schwetz, B. A., Murray, J. S., Bell, T. S., Beyer, J. E., Potts, W. J., and Parker, C. M. (1982). Toxicologic and reproductive effects of inhaled 1,2-dibromo-3-chloropropane in rabbits. *Fundam. Appl. Toxicol.* **2,** 241–251.

Rao, K. S., Burek, J. D., Murray, F. J., John, J. A., Schwetz, B. A., Murray, J. S., Battjes, J. E., Bell, T. S., Potts, W. J., and Parker, C. M. (1983). Toxicologic and reproductive effects of inhaled 1,2-dibromo-3-chloropropane in rats. *Fundam. Appl. Toxicol.* **3,** 104–110.

Rathus, E. M., and Landy, R. J. (1961). Methyl bromide poisoning. *Br. J. Ind. Med.* **18,** 53–57.

Ratney, R. S., Wegman, D. H., and Elkins, H. B. (1974). *In vivo* conversion of methylene chloride to carbon monoxide. *Arch. Environ. Health* **28,** 223–226.

Reddy, J. K., Azarnoff, D. L., and Hignite, C. E. (1980). Hypolipidemic hepatic peroxisome proliferators from a novel class of chemical carcinogens. *Nature (London)* **283,** 397–398.

Reddy, J. K., Lalwani, N. D., Reddy, M. K., and Qureshi, S. A. (1982). Excessive accumulation of autofluorescent lipofuscin in the liver during hepatocarcinogenesis by methyl clofenapate and other hypolipidemic peroxisome proliferators. *Cancer Res.* **42,** 259–266.

Reed, E. S., Leikin, S., and Kerman, H. D. (1950). Kerosene intoxication. *Am. J. Dis. Child.* **79,** 623–632.

Reel, J. R., Wolkowski-Tyl, R., Lawton, A. D., Feldman, D. B., and Lamb, J. L. (1984). "Dibromochloropropane: Reproduction and Fertility Assessment in CD-1 mice When Administered by Gavage," NTP-84-263. Natl. Toxicol. Program, Natl. Inst. Environ. Health Sci., Research Triangle Park, North Carolina.

Reichert, D. (1983). Biological actions and interactions of tetrachloroethylene. *Mutat. Res.* **123,** 411–429.

Reid, W. D., and Krishna, G. (1973). Centrolobular hepatic necrosis related to covalent binding of metabolites of halogenated aromatic hydrocarbons. *Exp. Mol. Pathol.* **18,** 80–99.

Reinhardt, C. F., Azar, A., Maxfield, M. E., Smith, P. E., Jr., and Mullin, L. S. (1971). Cardiac arrhythmias and aerosol "sniffing." *Arch. Environ. Health* **22,** 265–279.

Reinhardt, C. F., Mullin, L. S., and Maxfield, M. E. (1973). Epinephrine induced cardiac arrhythmia potential of some common industrial solvents. *J. Occup. Med.* **15,** 953–955.

Reitz, R. H., Fox, T. R., Ramsey, J. C., Quast, J. F., Langvardt, P. W., and Watanabe, P. G. (1982). Pharmacokinetics and macromolecular interactions of ethylene dichloride in rats after inhalation or gavage. *Toxicol. Appl. Pharmacol.* **62,** 190–204.

Reitz, R. H., Smith, F. A., and Andersen, M. E. (1986). *In vivo* metabolism of ^{14}C-methylene chloride. *Toxicologist* **6**(1), 260.

Reitz, R. H., Nolan, R. J., and Schumann, A. M. (1987). Methylchloroform pharmacokinetics in rats, mice and men after inhalation or consumption in drinking water. *Toxicol. Appl. Pharmacol.*

Rennick, B. R., Malton, S. D., Moe, G. K., and Seevers, M. H. (1949). Induction of idioventricular rhythms by 1,1,1-trichlorethane and epinephrine. *Fed. Proc., Fed. Am. Soc. Exp. Biol.* **8,** 327.

Reyniers, J. A., Sacksteder, M. R., and Ashburn, L. L. (1964). Multiple tumors in female germfree inbred albino mice exposed to bedding treated with ethylene oxide. *J. Natl. Cancer Inst. (U.S.)* **32,** 1045–1057.

Reynolds, E. S., Treinen, R. J., Farrish, H. H., and Moslen, M. T. (1984). Metabolism of ^{14}C-carbon tetrachloride to exhaled, excreted and bound metabolites. Dose-response, time-course and pharmacokinetics. *Biochem. Pharmacol.* **33,** 3363–3374.

Reznik, G., Reznik-Schuller, H., Ward, J. M., and Stinson, S. F. (1980a). Morphology of nasal-cavity tumors in rats after chronic inhalation of 1,2-dibromo-3-chloropropane. *Br. J. Cancer* **42,** 772–781.

Reznik, G., Stinson, S. F., and Ward, J. M. (1980b). Respiratory pathology in rats and mice after inhalation of 1,2-dibromo-3-chloropropane or 1,2-dibromoethane for 13 weeks. *Arch. Toxicol.* **46,** 233–240.

Reznik, Y. B., and Sprinchan, G. K. (1975). Experimental data on the gonadotoxic effect of Nemagon. *Gig. Sanit.* **6,** 101–102.

Richardson, J. A., and Pratt-Thomas, H. R. (1951). Toxic effects of varying doses of kerosene administered by different routes. *Am. J. Med. Sci.* **221,** 531–536.

Rick, D. L., and McCarty, L. P. (1987). The determination of the odor threshold of vapor and gases. *Am. Ind. Hyg. Assoc. J.*

Riihimaki, V., and Savolainen, K. (1980). Human exposure to *m*-xylene. Kinetics and acute effects on the central nervous system. *Ann. Occup. Hyg.* **23,** 411–422.

Riihimaki, V., Pfaffi, P., Savolainen, K., and Perkari, K. (1979). Kinetics of *m*-xylene in man. General features of absorption, distribution and excretion in repetitive inhalation exposure. *Scand. J. Work Environ. Health* **5,** 217–231.

Riley, E. C., Fassett, D. W., and Sutton, W. L. (1966). Methylene chloride vapor in expired air of human subjects. *Am. Ind. Hyg. Assoc. J.* **27,** 341–348.

Rimington, C., and Ziegler, G. (1963). Experimental porphyria in rats induced by chlorinated benzenes. *Biochem. Pharmacol.* **12,** 1387–1397.

Robbins, B. H. (1929). The absorption, distribution and excretion of carbon tetrachloride in dogs under various conditions. *J. Pharmacol. Exp. Ther.* **37,** 203–216.

Roberts, D. J. (1982). Abuse of aerosol products by inhalation. *Hum. Toxicol.* **1,** 231–238.

Robinson, J. R., and Bond, E. J. (1970). The toxic action of phosphine: Studies with 32-PH$_3$; terminal residues in biological materials. *J. Stored Prod. Res.* **6,** 133–136.

Rohmann, E., Zinn, D., and Kuelz, J. (1969). Electroencephalographic observations in childhood poisoning and their therapeutic consequences. *Kinderaerztl. Prax.* **37,** 209–216 (in German).

Rosenkranz, H. S. (1975). Genetic activity of 1,2-dibromo-3-chloropropane, a widely used fumigant. *Bull. Environ. Contam. Toxicol.* **14,** 8–12.

Rosier, J., Veulemans, H., Masschelein, R., Vanhoorne, and Van Peteghem, C. (1987a). Experimental human exposure to carbon disulfide. I. Respiratory uptake and elimination of carbon disulfide under rest and physical exercise. *Int. Arch Occup. Environ. Health* **59,** 233–242.

Rosier, J., Veulemans, H., Masschelein, R., Vanhoorne, and Van Peteghem, C. (1987b). Experimental human exposure to carbon disulfide. II. Urinary excretion of 2-thiothiazolidine-4-carboxylic acid (TTCA) during and after exposure. *Int. Arch Occup. Environ. Health* **59,** 243–250.

Roudabush, R. L., Terhaar, C. J., Fassett, D. W., and Dziuba, S. P. (1965). Comparative acute effects of some chemicals on the skin of rabbits and guinea pigs. *Toxicol. Appl. Pharmacol.* **7,** 559–565.

Rowe, V. K., Spencer, H. C., McCollister, D. D., Hollingsworth, R. L., and Adams, E. M. (1952). Toxicity of ethylene dibromide determined on experimental animals. *AMA Arch. Ind. Hyg. Occup. Med.* **6,** 158–173.

Roycroft, J. H., Jskot, R. H., Grose, E. C., and Gardner, D. E. (1981). The effects of inhalation exposure of methyl bromide in the rat. *Toxicologist* **1** (1), 79.

Ruddick, J. A., and Newsome, W. H. (1979). A teratogenicity and tissue distribution study on dibromochloropropane in the rat. *Bull. Environ. Contam. Toxicol.* **21,** 483–487.

Rush, G. F., Smith, J. H., Newton, J. F., and Hook, J. B. (1984). Chemically induced nephrotoxicity: Role of metabolic activation. *CRC Crit. Rev. Toxicol.* **13**(2), 99–160.

Russell, L. B., Hunsicker, P. R., and Cacheiro, N. L. A. (1986). Mouse specific-locus test for the induction of heritable gene mutations by dibromochloropropane (DBCP). *Mutat. Res.* **170,** 161–168.

Russo, J. M., Anger, W. K., Setzer, J. V., and Brightwell, W. S. (1984). Neurobehavioral assessment of chronic low-level methyl bromide exposure in the rabbit. *J. Toxicol. Environ. Health* **14,** 247–255.

Sagai, M., and Tappel, A. L. (1979). Lipid peroxidation induced by some halomethanes as measured by *in vivo* pentane production in the rat. *Toxicol. Appl. Pharmacol.* **49,** 283–291.

Saito-Suzuki, R., Termaoto, S., and Shirasu, Y. (1982). Dominant lethal studies in rats with 1,2-dibromo-3-chloropropane and its structurally related compounds. *Mutat. Res.* **101,** 321–327.

Salinas, E., Sasich, L., Hall, D. H., and Kennedy, R. M. (1981). Acute ethylene oxide intoxication. *Drug Intell. Clin. Pharm.* **15,** 384–396.

Salvini, M., Binaschi, S., and Riva, M. (1971). Evaluation of the psychophysiological functions of humans exposed to the threshold limit value of 1,1,1-trichloroethane. *Br. J. Ind. Med.* **28,** 286–292.

Sanabria, J., Noa, M., Casaco, A., and Gonzalez, R. (1984). Morphological alterations of respiratory tract in guinea pig treated with kerosene aerosol. *Allergol. Immunopathol* **12,** 213–215 (in Spanish).

Sandground, J. H. (1941). Coma following medication with tetrachlorethylene. *JAMA, J. Am. Med. Assoc.* **117,** 440–441.

Sandifer, S. H., Wilkins, R. T., Loanholt, C. B., Lane, L. G., and Eldridge, J. C. (1979). Spermatogenesis in agricultural workers exposed to dibromochloropropane (DBCP). *Bull. Environ. Contam. Toxicol.* **23,** 703–710.

Sapota, A. (1982). The disposition of [^{14}C]acrylonitrile in rats. *Xenobiotica* **12,** 259–264.

Sarkisov, D. S., Krymskii, L. D., Dzarakhov, K. I., and Rubetskoi, L. S. (1969). The paradoxical effect of the action of carbon tetrachloride at various frequencies of administration. *Byull. Eksp. Biol. Med.* **68,** 115–117 (in Russian).

Sasame, H. A., Castro, J. A., and Gillette, J. R. (1968). Studies on the destruction of liver microsomal cytochrome P-450 by carbon tetrachloride administration. *Biochem. Pharmacol.* **17**, 1759–1768.

Saski, Y. F., Imanishi, H., Watanabe, M., Sekiguchi, A., Morina, M., Shirasu, Y., and Tutikawa, K. (1986). Mutagenicity of 1,2-dibromo-3-chloropropane (DBCP) in the mouse spot test. *Mutat. Res.* **174**, 145–147.

Sato, A., and Nakajima, T. (1985). Enhanced metabolism of volatile hydrocarbons in rat liver following food deprivation, restricted carbohydrate intake, and administration of ethanol, phenobarbital, polychlorinated byphenyls, and 3-methylcholanthrene. *Xenobiotica* **15**, 67–75.

Savolainen, H., Pfaffli, P., Tengen, M., and Vainio, H. (1977). Biochemical and behavioral effects of inhalation exposure to tetrachloroethylene and dichloromethane. *J. Neuropathol. Environ. Neurol.* **36**, 941–949.

Savolainen, K., Riihimaki, V., Laine, A., and Kekoni, J. (1982). Short-term exposure of human subjects to *m*-xylene and 1,1,1-trichloroethane. *Arch. Toxicol., Suppl.* **5**, 96–99.

Sax, N. I. (1984). "Dangerous Properties of Industrial Materials," Spec. Bull. EDB. Van Nostrand-Reinhold, New York.

Sayers, R. R., Yant, W. P., Thomas, B. G. H., and Berger, L. B. (1929). "Physiological Response Attending Exposure to Vapors of Methyl Bromide and Ethyl Chloride," Public Health Bull. No. 185. U.S. Govt. Printing Office, Washington, D.C.

Sayers, R. R., Yant, W. P., Choruyak, J., and Shoaf, H. W. (1930). Toxicity of dichlorodifluoromethane: A new refrigerant. *Rep. Invest.—U.S., Bur. Mines* RI-3013, 1–15 (cited in National Research Council, 1980).

Schafer, W. B. (1951). Acute hemolytic anemia related to naphthalene. Report of a case in a newborn infant. *Pediatrics* **7**, 172–174.

Schiffmann, D., Eder, E., Neudecker, T., and Henschler, D. (1983). Induction of unscheduled DNA synthesis in HeLa cells by allylic compounds. *Cancer Lett.* **20**, 263–269.

Schoenborn, H., Prellwitz, W., and Braun, P. (1970). Consumption coagulopathy in ethylene dichloride poisoning. *Klin. Wochenschr.* **48**, 822–824 (in German).

Schumacher, H., and Grandjean, E. (1960). Vergleichende Untersuchungen uber die narkotische wirksamkeit und die akute toxicitat von neun losungsmitteln. *Arch. Gewerbepathol. Gewerhehyg.* **18**, 109–119 (in German).

Schumann, A. M., Quast, J. F., and Watanabe, P. G. (1980). The pharmacokinetics and macromolecular interactions of perchloroethylene in mice and rats as related to oncogenicity. *Toxicol. Appl. Pharmacol.* **55**, 207–219.

Schumann, A. M., Fox, T. R., and Watanabe, P. G. (1982a). ^{14}C-Methyl chloroform (1,1,1-trichloroethane): Pharmacokinetics in rats and mice following inhalation exposure. *Toxicol. Appl. Pharmacol.* **62**, 390–401.

Schumann, A. M., Fox, T. R., and Watanabe, P. G. (1982b). A comparison of the fate of inhaled methyl chloroform (1,1,1-trichloroethane) following single or repeated exposure in rats and mice. *Fundam. Appl. Toxicol.* **2**, 27–32.

Schwetz, B. A., Leong, B. K. J., and Gehring, P. J. (1974). Embryo- and fetotoxicity of inhaled carbon tetrachloride, 1,1-dichloroethane and methylethyl ketone in rats. *Toxicol. Appl. Pharmacol.* **28**, 452–464.

Schwetz, B. A., Leong, B. K. J., and Gehring, P. J. (1975). The effect of maternally inhaled trichloroethylene, perchloroethylene, methylchloroform, and methylene chloride in mice and rats. *Toxicol. Appl. Pharmacol.* **32**, 84–96.

Seawright, A. A., and McClean, A. E. M. (1967). The effects of diet on carbon tetrachloride metabolism. *Biochem. J.* **105**, 1055.

Segerback, D. (1983). Alkylation of DNA and hemoglobin in the mouse following exposure to ethene and ethene oxide. *Chem.-Biol. Interact.* **45**, 139–151.

Serota, D. G., Thakur, A. K., Ulland, B. M., Kirschman, J. C., Brown, N. M., and Coots, R. H. (1986a). A two-year drinking water study of dichloromethane in rodents. I. Rats. *Food Chem. Toxicol.* **24**, 951–958.

Serota, D. G., Thakur, A. K., Ulland, B. M., Kirschman, J. C., Brown, N. M., Coots, R. H., and Morgareidge, K. (1986b). A two-year drinking water study of dichloromethane in rodents. II. Mice. *Food Chem. Toxicol.* **24**, 959–963.

Serratoni, F. T., Schnitzer, B., and Smith, E. B. (1969). Promethazine protec-

tion in carbon tetrachloride liver injury, an electron microscopic study. *Arch. Pathol.* **87**, 46–51.

Sexton, R. J., and Henson, E. H. (1949). Dermatological injuries by ethylene oxide. *J. Ind. Hyg. Toxicol.* **31**, 297–300.

Sexton, R. J., and Henson, E. V. (1950). Experimental ethylene oxide human skin injuries. *Arch. Ind. Hyg. Occup. Med.* **2**, 549–564.

Sherman, H. (1974). "Long-term Feeding Studies in Rats and Dogs With Dichlorodifluoromethane (Freon 12 Food Freezant)," Haskell Lab. Rep. No. 24-74. Haskell Lab. Toxicol. Ind. Med., E. I. duPont de Nemours and Company, Newark, Delaware.

Shield, L. K., Coleman, T. L., and Markesbery, W. R. (1977). Methyl bromide intoxication: Neurologic features, including simulation of Reye syndrome. *Neurology* **27**, 959–962.

Shimada, T., Swanson, A. F., Leber, P., and Williams, G. M. (1985). Activities of chlorinated ethane and ethylene compounds in the *Salmonella*/rat microsome mutagenesis and rat hepatocyte/DNA repair assays under vapor phase exposure conditions. *Cell Biol. Toxicol.* **1**, 159–219.

Shindell, S., and Ulrich, S. (1985). A cohort study of employees of a manufacturing plant using trichloroethylene. *J. Occup. Med.* **27**, 577–579.

Shivanandappa, T., Ramesh, H. P., and Krishnakumari, M. K. (1979). Rodenticidal poisoning of non-target animals: Acute oral toxicity of zinc phosphide to poultry. *Bull. Environ. Contam. Toxicol.* **23**, 452–455.

Shopp, G. M., White, K. L., Jr., Holsapple, M. P., Barnes, D. W., Duke, S. S., Anderson, A. C., Condie, L. W., Jr., Hayes, J. R., and Brozellieca, J. F. (1984). Naphthalene toxicity in CD-1 mice: General toxicology and immunotoxicology. *Fundam. Appl. Toxicol.* **4**, 406–419.

Short, B. G., Burnett, V. L., and Swenberg, J. A. (1986). Histopathology and cell proliferation induced by 2,2,4-trimethylpentane in the male rat kidney. *Toxicol. Pathol.* **14**, 194–203.

Short, R. D., Minor, J. L., Winston, J. M., Seifter, J., and Lee, C. C. (1978). Inhalation of ethylene dibromide during gestation by rats and mice. *Toxicol. Appl. Pharmacol.* **46**, 173–182.

Short, R. D., Winston, M., Hong, C. B., Minor, J. L., Lee, C. C., and Seifter, J. (1979). Effects of ethylene dibromide on reproduction in male and female rats. *Toxicol. Appl. Pharmacol.* **49**, 97–105.

Simaan, J. A., and Aviado, D. M. (1975). Hemodynamic effects of aerosol propellants. I. Cardiac depression in the dog. *Toxicology* **5**, 127–138.

Simmon, V. F., Kauhanen, K., and Tardiff, R. G. (1977). Mutagenic activity of chemicals identified in drinking water. *In* "Progress in Genetic Toxicology" (D. Scott, B. A. Bridges, and F. H. Sobels, eds.), pp. 249–258, Elsevier, Amsterdam.

Singh, S., Dilawari, J. B., Vashist, R., Malhotra, H. S., and Sharma, B. K. (1985). Aluminum phosphide ingestion. *Br. Med. J.* **290**, 1110–1111.

Sipes, I. G., Krishna, G., and Gillette, J. R. (1977). Bioactivation of carbon tetrachloride, chloroform, and bromotrichloromethane: Role of cytochrome P-450. *Life Sci.* **20**, 1541–1548.

Slater, T. F., and Sawyer, B. C. (1969). The effects of carbon tetrachloride on rat liver microsomes during the first hour of poisoning *in vivo*, and the modifying actions of promethazine. *Biochem. J.* **111**, 317–324.

Smith, G. F. (1966). Trichloroethylene: A review. *Br. J. Ind. Med.* **23**, 249–262.

Smyth, H. F., and Seaton, J. (1940). Acute response of guinea pigs and rats to inhalation of vapors of isophorone. *J. Ind. Hyg. Toxicol.* **22**, 477–483.

Smyth, H. F., Jr., Smith, H. F., Jr., and Carpenter, C. P. (1936). The chronic toxicity of carbon tetrachloride: Animal exposures and field studies. *J. Ind. Hyg. Toxicol.* **18**, 277–298.

Smyth, H. F., Jr., Seaton, J., and Fischer, L. (1941). The single dose toxicity of some glycols and derivatives. *J. Ind. Hyg. Toxicol.* **23**, 259–268.

Smyth, H. F., Jr., Seaton, J., and Fischer, L. (1942). Response of guinea pigs and rats to repeated inhalation of vapors of mesityl oxide and isophorone. *J. Ind. Hyg. Toxicol.* **24** 46–50.

Smyth, H. F., Jr., Carpenter, C. P., and Weil, C. S. (1951). Range-finding toxicity data. List IV. *AMA Arch. Ind. Hyg. Occup. Med.* **4**, 119–122.

Smyth, H. F., Jr., Carpenter, C. P., Weil, C. S., Pozzani, U. C., Striegel, J. A., and Nycum, J. S. (1969). Range-finding toxicity data. List VII. *Am. Ind. Hyg. Assoc. J.* **30**, 470–476.

Smyth, H. F., Jr., Weil, C. S., West, J. S., and Carpenter, C. P. (1970). An exploration of joint toxic action. II. Equitoxic versus equivolume mixtures. *Toxicol. Appl. Pharmacol.* **17,** 498–503.

Snellings, W. M., Zelenak, J. P., and Weil, W. S. (1982a). Effects on reproduction in Fischer 344 rats exposed to ethylene oxide by inhalation for one generation. *Toxicol. Appl. Pharmacol.* **63,** 382–388.

Snellings, W. M., Maponpot, R. R., Selenak, J. P., and Laffoon, C. P. (1982b). Teratology study in Fischer 344 rats exposed to ethylene oxide by inhalation. *Toxicol. Appl. Pharmacol.* **63,** 476–481.

Snellings, W. M., Weil, S. W., and Maronpot, R. R. (1984a). A two-year inhalation study of the carcinogenic potential of ethylene oxide in Fischer 344 rats. *Toxicol. Appl. Pharmacol.* **75,** 105–117.

Snellings, W. M., Weil, S. W., and Maronpot, R. R. (1984b). A subchronic inhalation study on the toxicologic potential of ethylene oxide in B6C3F1 mice. *Toxicol. Appl. Pharmacol.* **76,** 510–518.

Sollman, T. (1919). Observations on paradichlorobenzene and para-dibromobenzene. *J. Pharmacol. Exp. Ther.* **14,** 243–250.

Sollman, T. (1948). "A Manual of Pharmacology and Its Applications to Therapeutics and Toxicology," 7th ed. Saunders, Philadelphia, Pennsylvania.

Sollman, T. (1957). "A Manual of Pharmacology and Its Applications to Toxicology and Therapeutics," 8th ed. Saunders, Philadelphia, Pennsylvania.

Solomon, J. J., Cote, I. L., Wortman, M., Decker, K., and Segal, A. (1984). In vitro alkylation of calf thymus DNA by acrylonitrile. Isolation of cyanoethyl-adducts of guanine and thymine and carboxyethyl-adducts of adenine and cytosine. *Chem.-Biol. Interact.* **51,** 167–190.

Soucek, B., and Vlachova, D. (1960). Excretion of trichloroethylene metabolites in human urine. *Br. J. Ind. Med.* **17,** 60–64.

Soule, A. B., Jr., and Foley, J. C. (1957). Poisoning from petroleum distillates. The hazards of kerosene and furniture polish. *J. Maine Med. Assoc.* **48,** 103–110.

Sovljanski, R., Tasic, M., Sovljanski, M., and Stojanovic, T. (1969). Accidental poisoning during fumigation with Phostoxin. *Arh. Hig. Rada Toksikol.* **20,** 209–212 (in Serbo-Croatian).

Spector, W. S., ed. (1955). "Handbook of Toxicology," Vol. I, WADC Tech. Rep. 55-16. Wright-Patterson Air Force Base, Ohio.

Speizer, F. E., Doll, R., and Heaf, P. J. (1968a). Observations on recent increase in mortality from asthma. *Br. Med. J.* **1,** 335–339.

Speizer, F. E., Doll, R., and Heaf, P. J. (1968b). Investigation into the use of drugs preceding death from asthma. *Br. Med. J.* **1,** 339–342.

Spencer, H. C., Rowe, V. K., Adams, E. M., McCollister, D. D., and Irish, D. D. (1951). Vapor toxicity of ethylene dichloride determined by experiments on laboratory animals. *AMA Arch. Ind. Hyg. Occup. Med.* **4,** 482–493.

Spreafico, F., Zuccato, E., Marcucci, F., Sironi, M., Paglialunga, S., Madonna, M., and Mussini, E. (1980). Pharmacokinetics of ethylene dichloride in rats treated by different routes and its long-term inhalatory toxicity. *Banbury Rep.* **5,** 107–129.

Standefer, J. C. (1975). Death associated with fluorocarbon inhalation: Report of a case. *J. Forensic Sci.* **20,** 548–551.

State of California, Department of Health (1958). Reports of occupational disease attributed to pesticides and agricultural chemicals (during 1958) (cited by World Health Organization "Information Circular on the Toxicity of Pesticides to Man," No. 7, pp. 1–2).

Stephenson, J. B. P. (1967). Zinc phosphide poisoning. *Arch. Environ. Health* **15,** 83–88.

Stewart, R. D. (1969). Acute tetrachloroethylene intoxication. *JAMA, J. Am. Med. Assoc.* **208,** 1490–1492.

Stewart, R. D. (1974). The use of breath analysis in clinical toxicology. *Essays Toxicol.* **5,** 121–147.

Stewart, R. D., and Dodd, H. C. (1964). Absorption of carbon tetrachloride, trichloroethylene, tetrachloroethylene, methylene chloride, and 1,1,1-trichloroethane through the human skin. *Am. Ind. Hyg. Assoc. J.* **25,** 439–446.

Stewart, R. D., Erley, D. S., Schaffer, A. W., and Gay, H. H. (1961a).

Accidental vapor exposure to anesthetic concentrations of a solvent containing tetrachloroethylene. *Ind. Med. Surg.* **30,** 327–330.

Stewart, R. D., Gay, H. H., Erley, D. S., Hake, C. L., and Peterson, J. E. (1961b). Human exposure to carbon tetrachloride vapor. Relation of expired air concentration to exposure and toxicity. *J. Occup. Med.* **3,** 586–590.

Stewart, R. D., Gay, H. H., Erley, D. S., Hake, C. L., and Schaffer, A. W. (1961c). Human exposure to tetrachloroethylene vapor. Relationship of expired air and blood concentrations to exposure and toxicity. *Arch. Environ. Health* **2,** 40–46.

Stewart, R. D., Gay, H. H., Erley, D. S., Hake, C. L., and Schaffer, A. W. (1961d). Human exposure to 1,1,1-trichloroethane vapor: Relationship of expired air and blood concentrations to exposure and toxicity. *Am. Ind. Hyg. Assoc. J.* **22,** 252–262.

Stewart, R. D., Bóettner, E. A., Southworth, R. S., and Cerney, J. C. (1963). Acute carbon tetrachloride intoxication. *JAMA, J. Am. Med. Assoc.* **183,** 994–997.

Stewart, R. D., Gay, H. H., Schaffer, A. W., Erley, D. S., and Rowe, V. K. (1969). Experimental human exposure to methyl chloroform vapor. *Arch. Environ. Health* **19,** 467–472.

Stewart, R. D., Dodd, H. C., Gay, H. H., and Erley, D. S. (1970a). Experimental human exposure to trichloroethylene. *Arch. Environ. Health* **20,** 64–71.

Stewart, R. D., Baretta, E. D., Dodd, H. C., and Torkelson, R. D. (1970b). Experimental human exposure to tetrachloroethylene. *Arch. Environ. Health* **20,** 224–229.

Stewart, R. D., Fischer, T. N., Hosko, M. J., Peterson, J. E., Baretta, E. D., and Dodd, H. C. (1972a). Experimental human exposure to methylene chloride. *Arch. Environ. Health* **25,** 342–348.

Stewart, R. D., Fischer, T. N., Hosko, M. J., Peterson, J. E., Baretta, E. D., and Dodd, H. C. (1972b). Carboxyhemoglobin elevation after exposure to dichloromethane. *Science* **176,** 295–296.

Stockman, S. (1916). Cases of poisoning in cattle by feeding on meal from soya bean after extraction of the oil. *J. Comp. Pathol. Ther.* **29,** 95–107.

Stolley, P. D., Soper, K. A., Galloway, S. M., Nichols, W. W., Norman, S. A., and Wolman, S. R. (1984). Sister-chromatid exchanges in association with occupational exposure to ethylene oxide. *Mutat. Res.* **129,** 89–102.

Stolzenberg, S., and Hine, C. (1980). Mutagenicity of 2- and 3-carbon halogenated compounds in the *Salmonella*/mammalian-microsome test. *Environ. Mutagen.* **2,** 59–66.

Stopps, G. J., and McLaughlin, M. (1967). Psychophysiological testing of human subjects exposed to solvent vapors. *Am. Ind. Hyg. Assoc. J.* **28,** 43–50.

Storer, R. D., Jackson, N. M., and Conolly, R. B. (1984). *In vivo* genotoxicity and acute hepatotoxicity of 1,2-dichloroethane in mice: Comparison of oral, intraperitoneal, and inhalation routes of exposure. *Cancer Res.* **44,** 4267–4271.

Stott, W. T., and McKenna, M. J. (1984). The comparative absorption and excretion of chemical vapors by the upper, lower, and intact respiratory tract of rats. *Fundam. Appl. Toxicol.* **4,** 594–602.

Stott, W. T., Quast, J. F., and Watanabe, P. G. (1982). The pharmacokinetic and macromolecular interactions of trichloroethylene in mice and rats. *Toxicol. Appl. Pharmacol.* **62,** 137–151.

Stott, W. T., Young, J., Calhoun, L., and Battjes, J. E. (1985). Telone II® soil fumigant: A 13-week inhalation study in rats and mice. *Toxicologist* **5,** 220 (Abstr. No. 877).

Stott, W. T., Kastl, P. L., and McKenna, M. J. (1986). Inhalation pharmacokinetics of technical grade 1,3-dichloropropene in rats. *Toxicol. Appl. Pharmacol.* **85,** 332–341.

Stott, W. T., Johnson, K. A., Calhoun, L. L., and Frauson, L. E. (1987). "TELONE II soil fumigant: Two-Year Inhalation Chronic Toxicity Oncogenicity Study in B6C3F1 Mice." Report of The Dow Chemical Company, Midland, Michigan.

Streeter, C. M., Battjes, J. E., and Lomax, L. G. (1987). "TELONE II Soil Fumigant: An Acute Vapor Inhalation Study in Fischer 344 Rats." Report of The Dow Chemical Company, Midland, Michigan.

Sugimoto, K., Goto, S., and Hotta, R. (1976). An epidemiological study on retinopathy due to carbon disulfide—CS$_2$ exposure level and development of retinopathy. *Int. Arch. Occup. Environ. Health* **37**, 1–8.

Sutton, W. L. (1963). Heterocyclic and miscellaneous nitrogen compounds. In "Industrial Hygiene and Toxicology" (F. A. Patty, ed.), pp. 2171–2234. Wiley (Interscience), New York.

Suzuki, K., and Lee, I. P. (1981). Induction of aryl hydrocarbon hydroxylase and epoxide hydrolase in TDT liver, kidney, testes, prostate glands, and stomach by a potent nematocide, 1,2-dibromo-3-chloropropane. *Toxicol. Appl. Pharmacol.* **58**, 151–155.

Svirbely, J. L., Highman, B., Alford, W. C., and von Oettingen, W. F. (1947). The toxicity and narcotic action of mono-chloro-mono-bromo-methane with special reference to inorganic and volatile bromide in blood, urine, and brain. *Ind. Hyg. Toxicol.* **29**, 382–389.

Szabo, S., Reynolds, E. S., Komanicky, P., Moslen, M. T., and Melby, J. C. (1976). Effect of chronic acrylonitrile ingestion on rat adrenal. *Toxicol. Appl. Pharmacol.* **37**, 133.

Szabo, S., Gallagher, G. T., Silver, E. H., Maull, E. A., Horner, H. C., Komanicky, P., Melby, J. C., McComb, D. J., and Kovacs, K. (1984). Subacute and chronic action of acrylonitrile on adrenals and gastrointestinal tract: Biochemical, functional and ultrastructural studies in the rat. *J. Appl. Toxicol.* **4**, 131–140.

Takahashi, S., Moroji, T., and Yamauchi, T. (1973). A case of methyl bromide intoxication which showed paroxysmal abnormal EEG. *Clin. Electroencephalogr.* **15**, 725.

Takayama, J., and Numarjiri, S. (1979). A serious case of methyl bromide intoxication. *Acta Paediatr. Jpn.* **83**, 332–333 (in Japanese).

Takizawa, A., Nakayama, E., Ishizu, S., Momotani, H., Sato, M., Mori, N., and Sato, M. (1977). Experimental studies on hydrogen cyanide intoxication. *Jpn. J. Hyg.* **32**, 205 (in Japanese).

Talcott, R., and King, J. (1984). Mutagenic impurities in 1,3-dichloropropene preparations. *JNCI, J. Natl. Cancer Inst.* **72**, 1113–1116.

Tan, E. L., and Hsie, A. W. (1981). Mutagenicity and cytotoxicity of haloethanes as studied in the CHO/HGPRT system. *Mutat. Res.* **90**, 183–191.

Tatken, R. T., and Lewis, R. J., Sr., eds. (1983). "Registry of Toxic Effects of Chemical Substances," 1981–1982 ed., Vol. 2. Natl. Inst. Occup. Saf. Health, Cincinnati, Ohio.

Tauber, E. (1880). Two new anesthetics. I. Monochloroethylidene chloride (methyl chloroform). II. Monochloroethylenchlorid. CH$_2$Cl-CHCl$_2$. *Zentralbl. Med. Wiss.* **18**, 775–778 (in German).

Teisinger, J. (1983). Carbon disulfide. In "Encyclopedia of Occupational Health and Safety" (L. Parmeggiani, ed.), 3rd ed., Vol. 1, pp. 393–395. International Labour Office, Geneva.

Teramoto, S., Saito, R., Aoyama, H., and Shirasu, Y. (1980). Dominant lethal mutation induced in male rats by 1,2-dibromo-3-chloropropane (DBCP). *Mutat. Res.* **77**, 71–78.

Terr Harr, G. (1980). An investigation of possible sterility and health effects from exposure to ethylene dibromide. *Banbury Rep.* **5**, 167–188.

Tezuka, H., Ando, N., Suzuki, R., Terahata, M., Moriya, M., and Shirasu, Y. (1980). Sister-chromatid exchanges and chromosomal aberrations in cultured Chinese hamster cells treated with pesticides positive in microbial reversion assays. *Mutat. Res.* **78**, 177–191.

Thiess, A. M., Frentzel-Beyme, R., Link, R., and Stocker, W. G. (1981). Mortality study on employees exposed to alkylene oxides (ethylene oxide/propylene oxide) and their derivatives. In "Prevention of Occupation Cancer" (C. R. Shaw, ed.), Occup. Saf. Health Ser. No. 46, pp. 249–259. Int. Labour Off., Geneva.

Til, H. P., Spanjers, M. T., Feron, V. J., and Reuzel, P. J. C. (1973). "Sub-Chronic (90-Day) Toxicity Study with TELONE* in Albino Rats." Report of The Dow Chemical Company, Midland, Michigan.

Tiller, J. R., Schilling, R. S. F., and Morris, J. N. (1968). Occupational toxic factor in mortality from coronary heart disease. *Br. J. Med.* **4**, 407–411.

Tobacova, S., Nikiforov, B., and Balbaveva, L. (1983). Carbon disulfide intrauterine sensitization. *J. Appl. Toxicol.* **3**, 223–229.

Toftgard, R., and Nilsen, O. G. (1982). Effects of xylene and xylene isomers on cytochrome P-450 and *in vitro* enzymatic activities in rat liver, kidney and lung. *Toxicology* **23**, 197–212.

Tola, S., Vilhunen, R., Jarvinen, E., and Korkala, M. L. (1980). A cohort study on workers exposed to trichloroethylene. *J. Occup. Med.* **22**, 737–740.

Tolbert, B. M., and Hughes, A. M. (1959). Cl4-labeled cyanide: Radioactivity excretion in mice and estimation of radiation dose to humans. *Metab. Clin. Exp.* **8**, 73–78.

Tolot, F., Viallier, J., Roullet, A., Rivoire, J., and Figueres, J. C. (1964). Hepatic toxicity of trichloroethylene. *Arch. Mal. Profess. Med. Trav. Secur. Soc.* **25**, 9–15 (in French).

Torkelson, R., and Oyen, F. (1977). The toxicity of 1,3-dichloropropene as determined by repeated exposure of laboratory animals. *Am. Ind. Hyg. Assoc. J.* **38**, 217–223.

Torkelson, T. R., Oyen, F., McCollister, D. D., and Rowe, V. K. (1958). Toxicity of 1,1,1-trichloroethane as determined on laboratory animals and human subjects. *Am. Ind. Hyg. Assoc. J.* **19**, 353–362.

Torkelson, T. R., Sadek, S. E., Rowe, V. K., Kodama, J. K., Anderson, H. H., Loquvam, C. S., and Hine, C. H. (1961). Toxicologic investigations of 1,2-dibromo-3-chloropropane. *Toxicol. Appl. Pharmacol.* **3**, 545–559.

Toyonaga, K., and Tokuda, S. (1976). Physiological examination and treatment by clonazepam of action myoclonus due to methyl bromide intoxication. *Clin. Neurol.* **16**, 830–831.

Toyoshima, S., Sato, R., and Sato, S. (1978). "The Acute Toxicity Test of TELONE II in Rats." Report of The Dow Chemical Company, Midland, Michigan.

Tracey, J. P., and Sherlock, P. (1968). Hepatoma following carbon tetrachloride poisoning. *N.Y. State J. Med.* **68**, 2202–2204.

Treuse, E., and Zimmermann, H. (1969). Fatal inhalatory poisoning through chronically acting perchloroethylene vapors. *Zentralbl. Arbeitsmed. Arbeitsschutz* **19**, 131–137 (in German).

Tsuruta, H. (1975). Percutaneous absorption of organic solvents. I. Comparative study of the *in vivo* percutaneous absorption of chlorinated solvents in mice. *Ind. Health* **13**, 227–236.

Tucker, A. N., Sanders, V. M., Barnes, D. W., Bradshaw, T. J., White, K. L., Sain, L. F., Borzelleca, J. F., and Munson, A. E. (1982). Toxicology of trichloroethylene in the mouse. *Toxicol. Appl. Pharmacol.* **62**, 351–357.

Ueda, K., and Kaai, M. (1971). Antidotal effectiveness of glutathione in acute poisoning of mice and rabbits with methyl bromide. *J. Jpn. Assoc. Rural Med.* **19**, 371–372 (in Japanese).

Uehleke, H., Hellmer, K. H., and Tabarelli-Poplawski, S. (1973). Binding of ^{14}C-carbon tetrachloride to microsomal proteins *in vitro* and formation of CHCl$_3$ by reduced liver microsomes. *Xenobiotica* **3**, 1.

Ugazio, G., and Torrielli, M. V. (1968). Action of propyl gallate in hepatic steatosis from carbon tetrachloride. *Boll. Soc. Ital. Biol. Sper.* **44**, 1166–1170 (in Italian).

Uhl, G., and Haag, T. P. (1958). Oral poisoning with trichloroethylene and its chemical demonstration. *Arch. Toxikol.* **17**, 197–203 (in German).

Ushio, K., and Osotsuka, R. (1977a). A severe case of methyl bromide intoxication. *Proc. Annu. Meet. Jpn. Assoc. Ind. Health* **50**, 260–261 (in Japanese).

Ushio, K., and Osotsuka, R. (1977b). A case of severe intoxication due to methyl bromide. *Jpn. J. Ind. Health* **19**, 355–356 (in Japanese).

Valaes, T., Doxiadis, S. A., and Fessas, P. (1963). Acute hemolysis due to naphthalene inhalation. *J. Pediatr.* **63**, 904–915.

Valencia, R., Mason, J. M., Woodruff, R. C., and Zimmering, S. (1985). Chemical mutagenesis testing in *Drosophila*. III. Results of 48 coded compounds tested for the National Toxicology Program. *Environ. Mutagen.* **7**, 325–348.

Valic, F., Skuric, Z., Bantic, Z., Rudar, M., and Hecej, M. (1977). Effects of fluorocarbon propellants on respiratory flow and ECG. *Br. J. Ind. Med.* **34**, 130–136.

Van Bladeren, P. J. (1983). Metabolic activation of xenobiotics: Ethylene dibromide and structural analogs. *J. Am. Coll. Toxicol.* **2**, 73–83.

Van Duuren, B. L., Orris, L., and Nelson, N. (1965). Carcinogenicity of epoxides, lactones, and peroxy compounds. Part II. *J. Natl. Cancer Inst. (U.S.)* **35**, 707–717.

Van Duuren, B. L., Goldschmidt, B. M., Lowewengart, G., Smith, A. C., Melchionne, S., Seldman, I., and Roth, D. (1979). Carcinogenicity of halogenated olefinic and aliphatic hydrocarbons in mice. *JNCI, J. Natl. Cancer Inst.*, **63**, 1433–1439.

Van Luijt, D. E. (1963). Fatal acrylonitrile poisoning. *Ned. Tijdschr. Geneeskd.* **2**, 2186–2188 (in Dutch).

Venable, J. R., McClimans, C. D., Flake, R. E., and Dimick, D. B. (1980). A fertility study of male employees engaged in the manufacture of glycerine. *J. Occup. Med.* **22**, 87–91.

Verberk, M. M., Rooyakkers-Beemster, T., De Vlieger, M., and Van Vliet, A. G. M. (1979). Bromine in blood, EEG and transaminases in methyl bromide workers. *Br. J. Ind. Med.* **36**, 59–62.

Verhulst, H. L., and Page, L. A. (1961). "Bulletin of the National Clearinghouse for Poison Control Centers," pp. 1–4. U.S. Govt. Printing Office, Washington, D.C.

Vernon, R. J., and Ferguson, R. K. (1969). Effects of trichloroethylene on visual-motor performance. *Arch. Environ. Health* **18**, 894–900.

Vick, J., Johnson, R., Groff, W., and Hassett, C. C. (1973). Recent studies on the therapy of cyanide poisoning. *Fed. Proc., Fed. Am. Soc. Exp. Biol.* **32**, 372.

Vogel, R. A., and Kirkendall, W. M. (1984). Acrylonitrile (vinyl cyanide) poisoning: A case report. *Tex. Med.* **80**(5), 48–51.

von Oettingen, W. F. (1955). "The Halogenated Aliphatic, Olefinic, Cyclic, Aromatic, and Aliphatic–Aromatic Hydrocarbons Including the Halogenated Insecticides, Their Toxicity and Potential Dangers," Public Health Serv. Publ. No. 414. U.S. Govt. Printing Office, Washington, D.C.

von Oettingen, W. F., Powell, C. C., Sharpless, N. E., Alford, W. C., and Pecora, L. J. (1949). "Relation Between the Toxic Action of Chlorinated Methanes and Their Chemical and Physiochemical Properties," Natl. Inst. Health Bull. No. 191. U.S. Govt. Printing Office, Washington, D.C.

von Wuthrich, F. (1954). Chronic cyanogen poisoning as industrial intoxication. *Schweiz. Med. Wochenschr.* **84**, 105–107 (in German).

Wald, M. H., Lindberg, H. A., and Barker, M. H. (1939). The toxic manifestations of the thiocyanates. *JAMA, J. Am. Med. Assoc.* **112**, 1120–1124.

Wallgren, K. (1953). Chronic poisoning in the production of insect powder. *Zentralbl. Arbeitsmed. Arbeitsschutz* **3**, 14–15 (in German).

Waritz, R. S., and Brown, R. M. (1975). Acute and subacute inhalation toxicities of phosphine, phenylphosphine and triphenylphosphine. *Am. Ind. Hyg. Assoc. J.* **36**, 452–458.

Watrous, R. M. (1942). Methyl bromide: Local and mild systemic toxic effects. *Ind. Med.* **11**, 575–579.

Watson, W. P., Brooks, T. M., Huckle, K. R., Hutson, D. H., Land, K. L., Smith, R. J., and Wright, A. S. (1987). Microbial mutagenicity studies with (Z)-1,3-dichloropropene. *Chem.-Biol. Interact.* **61**, 17–30.

Way, J. L., Gibbon, S. L., and Sheehy, M. (1966). Effect of oxygen on cyanide intoxication. I. Prophylactic protection. *J. Pharmacol. Exp. Ther.* **153**, 381–385.

Weisburger, E. K. (1977). Carcinogenicity studies of halogenated hydrocarbons. *Environ. Health Perspect.* **21**, 7–16.

Weller, R. W., and Crellin, A. J. (1953). Pulmonary granulomatosis following extensive use of paradichlorobenzene. *Arch. Intern. Med.* **91**, 408–413.

Wells, H. S. (1925). A quantitative study of the absorption and excretion of the anthelmintic dose of carbon tetrachloride. *J. Pharmacol. Exp. Ther.* **25**, 235–273.

White, E. G. (1939). The effect of carbon tetrachloride on the liver of the pig, with especial reference to experimental cirrhosis. *J. Pathol. Bacteriol.* **49**, 95–103.

White, R. D., Petry, T. W., and Sipes, I. G. (1983). The bioactivation of 1,2-dibromomethane in rat hepatocytes: Deuterium isotope effect. *Toxicol. Appl. Pharmacol.* **69**, 170–178.

Whorton, M. D., and Foliari, D. E. (1983). Mutagenicity, carcinogenicity and reproductive effect of dibromochloropropane. *Mutat. Res.* **123**, 13–30.

Whorton, M. D., and Milby, T. H. (1980). Recovery of testicular function among DBCP workers. *J. Occup. Med.* **22**, 177–179

Whorton, M. D., Krauss, R. M., Marshall, S., and Milby, T. H. (1977). Infertility in male pesticide workers. *Lancet* **2**, 1259–1261.

Whorton, M. D., Milby, T. H., Krauss, R. M., and Stubbs, H. A. (1979). Testicular function in DBCP exposed workers. *J. Occup. Med.* **21**, 161–166.

Wiley, F. H., Hueper, W. C., and von Oettingen, W. F. (1936). On the toxic effects of low concentrations of carbon disulfide. *J. Ind. Hyg. Toxicol.* **18**, 733–740.

Willhite, C. C., and Smith, R. P. (1981). The role of cyanide liberation in the acute toxicity of aliphatic nitriles. *Toxicol. Appl. Pharmacol.* **59**, 589–602.

Willhite, C. C., Ferm, V. H., and Smith, R. P. (1981). Teratogenic effects of aliphatic nitriles. *Teratology* **23**, 317–323.

Williams, R. T. (1959). "Detoxication Mechanisms," 2nd ed. Wiley, New York.

Wilson, J. (1973). "Cyanide and Human Disease," pp. 121–125.

Wilson, R., Lovejoy, F. R., Jaeger, R. J., and Landrigan, P. L. (1980). Acute phosphine poisoning aboard a grain freighter. *JAMA, J. Am. Med. Assoc.* **244**, 148–150.

Winneke, G. (1981). The neurotoxicity of dichloromethane. *Neurobehav. Toxicol. Teratol.* **3**, 391–395.

Winteringham, F. P. W., and Barnes, J. M. (1955). Comparative response of insects and mammals to certain halogenated hydrocarbons used as insecticides. *Physiol. Rev.* **35**, 701–739.

Winteringham, F. P. W., Hellyer, G. C., and McKay, M. A. (1958). Effects of methyl bromide on phosphorus metabolism in the adult housefly, *Musca domestica*. L. *Biochem. J.* **69**, 640–648.

Wirtschafter, Z. T., and Schwartz, E. D. (1939). Acute ethylene dichloride poisoning. *J. Ind. Hyg. Toxicol.* **21**, 126–131.

Wolf, M. A., Rowe, V. K., McCollister, D. D., Hollingsworth, R. L., and Oyen, F. (1956). Toxicological studies of certain alkylated benzenes and benzene. Experiments on laboratory animals. *AMA Arch. Ind. Health* **14**, 387–398.

Wolfsdorf, J. (1976). Experimental kerosene pneumonitis in primates: Relevance to the therapeutic management of childhood poisonings. *Clin. Exp. Pharmacol. Physiol.* **3**, 539–544.

Wong, L. C. K., Winston, J. M., Hong, C. B., and Plotnick, H. (1982). Carcinogenicity and toxicity of 1,2-dibromoethane in the rat. *Toxicol. Appl. Pharmacol.* **63**, 155–165.

Wong, O., Utidjian, M. D., and Karten, V. S. (1979). Retrospective evaluation of reproductive performance of workers exposed to ethylene dibromide (EDB). *J. Occup. Med.* **2**, 98–102.

Wood, J. L., and Cooley, S. L. (1956). Detoxication of cyanide by cystine. *J. Biol. Chem.* **218**, 449–457.

Woodard, G., Lange, S. W., Nelson, K. W., and Calvery, H. O. (1941). The acute oral toxicity of acetic, chloracetic, dichloracetic and trichloracetic acids. *J. Ind. Hyg. Toxicol.* **23**, 78–82.

Wooverton, W. L., and Balster, R. L. (1981). Behavioral and lethal effects of combinations of oral ethanol and inhaled 1,1,1-trichloroethane in mice. *Toxicol. Appl. Pharmacol.* **59**, 1–7.

World Health Organization (WHO) (1985). "Environmental Health Criteria 50: Trichloroethylene." World Health Organ., Geneva.

Wright, P. L., and Levinskas, G. J. (1982). Chronic oral toxicity of acrylonitrile in Fischer 344 rats. *Toxicologist* **2**, 153.

Wright, W. H., Bozicevich, J., and Gordon, L. S. (1937). Studies on oxyuriasis. V. Therapy with single doses of tetrachloroethylene. *JAMA, J. Am. Med. Assoc.* **109**, 570–573.

Wyse, D. C. (1973). Deliberate inhalation of volatile hydrocarbons: A review. *Can. Med. Assoc. J.* **108**, 71–74.

Yamada, Y. (1977). A case of acute carbon disulfide poisoning by accidental ingestion. *Jpn. J. Ind. Health* **19**, 140–141 (in Japanese).

Yang, R. S. H. (1986). 1,3-Dichloropropene. *Residue Rev.* **97**, 19–35.

Yang, R. S. H., Huff, J. E., Boorman, G. A., Haseman, J. K., and Kornreich, M. (1986). Chronic toxicology and carcinogenesis studies of TELONE II by gavage in Fischer 344 rats and B6C3F1 mice. *J. Toxicol. Environ. Health* **18**, 377–392.

Yllner, S. (1961). Urinary metabolites of ^{14}C-tetrachloroethylene in mice. *Nature (London)* **191**, 820–821.

Yodaiken, R. E., and Babcock, J. R. (1973). 1,2-Dichloroethane poisoning. *Arch. Environ. Health* **26**, 281–284.

York, R. G., Sowry, B. M., Hastings, L., and Manson, J. M. (1982). Evaluation of teratogenicity and neurotoxicity with maternal inhalation exposure to methylchloroform. *J. Toxicol. Environ. Health* **9**, 251–266.

Zatuchni, J., and Hong, K. (1981). Methyl bromide poisoning seen initially as psychosis. *Arch. Neurol. (Chicago)* **38**(8), 529–530.

Zenick, H., Blackburn, K., Hope, E., and Baldwin, D. (1984a). An evaluation of the copulatory, endocrinologic, and spermatotoxic effects of carbon disulfide in the rat. *Toxicol. Appl. Pharmacol.* **73**, 275–283.

Zenick, H., Blackburn, K., Hope, E., Richdale, N., and Smith, M. K. (1984b). Effects of trichloroethylene exposure on male reproductive function in rats. *Toxicology* **31**, 237–250.

Zhizhonkov, N. V. (1976). Acute poisoning by dichloroethane. *Vrach. Delo* **6**, 127–128 (in Russian).

Zinkham, W. H., and Childs, B. (1958). A defect of glutathione metabolism in erythrocytes from patients with a naphthalene-induced hemolytic anemia. *Pediatrics* **22**, 461–471.

Zipf, K. E., Arndt, T., and Heintz, R. (1967). Clinical observations in a case of phostoxin poisoning. *Arch. Toxikol.* **22**, 209–222 (in German).

Zuelzer, W. W., and Apt, L. (1949). Acute hemolytic anemia due to naphthalene poisoning. *JAMA, J. Am. Med. Assoc.* **141**, 185–190.

Zupko, A. G., and Edwards, L. D. (1949). A toxicological study of *p*-dichlorobenzene. *J. Am. Pharm. Assoc.* **38**, 124–131.

CHAPTER 15

Chlorinated Hydrocarbon Insecticides

Andrew G. Smith
Medical Research Council Toxicology Unit,
United Kingdom

15.1 CLASSIFICATION OF CHLORINATED HYDROCARBON INSECTICIDES

All chlorinated hydrocarbon insecticides are aryl, carbocyclic, or heterocyclic compounds of molecular weights ranging from about 291 to 545. Their cyclic structure and their greater molecular weight set them apart chemically from the chlorinated hydrocarbons used as solvents and fumigants (molecular weight < 236), which are described in Chapter 14. In a biological context the chlorinated hydrocarbon insecticides also differ from the chlorinated hydrocarbon solvents in that the former are generally stimulants of the nervous system while the latter are depressants. However, this distinction is not absolute: the γ isomer of benzene hexachloride (γ-BHC; lindane) is a stimulant, but two other isomers have an opposite effect.

The chlorinated hydrocarbon insecticides may be divided into five groups: DDT and its analogs, BHC, cyclodienes and similar compounds, toxaphene and related chemicals, and the caged structures mirex and chlordecone. There is a greater tendency of insects to develop overlapping resistance to insecticides within each group than between groups, the latter probably reflecting differences in modes of action. However, overlapping of resistance between groups does occur.

In spite of some similarity of chemical structure and pharmacological effect, the individual insecticides within each group differ widely in toxicity and in their capacity for storage. Furthermore, toxicity and storage do not always vary in a parallel way. Methoxychlor is much less toxic and much less stored than DDT, whereas endrin, which is more toxic than dieldrin, is stored far less. Thus, each compound must be judged separately.

Although the organochlorine insecticides were widely used in agriculture and malarial control programs from the 1940s to 1960s with dramatic beneficial effects, they have come into disfavor because of their persistence in the environment, wildlife, and humans. The relatively low cost of these insecticides and unavailability of complete substitutes for some uses, how- ever, ensure their continued use in many countries for some years to come.

The structures of the different chlorinated hydrocarbon insecticides are shown in the appropriate sections: DDT and analogs in Section 15.3, BHC in Section 15.4, cyclodienes in Section 15.5, toxaphene in Section 15.6, and mirex and chlordecone in Section 15.7.

15.2 TOXICOLOGY OVERVIEW

15.2.1 SYMPTOMATOLOGY

In general, the signs of poisoning produced by different chlorinated hydrocarbon insecticides are similar, that is, expressions of neuronal hyperactivity. However, there are certain differences between the effects of DDT and its analogs, on the one hand, and all other chlorinated hydrocarbon insecticides on the other. Not only is tremor characteristic of poisoning by DDT, but also the onset of poisoning by it occurs with easily detectable mild effects that progress gradually, but continuously, to the point of convulsions. In contrast, lindane, aldrin, dieldrin, endrin, toxaphene, and several related compounds frequently produce illness in which a convulsion is the first sign of injury. This is true not only in experimental animals but also in people, who sometimes report that they experienced no prodromal symptoms of any kind prior to the initial fit. As described under Effects on the Nervous System in Section 15.3.1.2, with rats the incoordination associated with tremor induced by DDT may be demonstrated by measuring how long they can stay afloat in cool water. Whereas DDT causes marked reduction in swimming time at dose levels that cause no other clinical effect, dieldrin and some other pesticides interfere with swimming only at dosages that depress food intake and reduce weight gain so that it is reasonable to assume that the animals are weak. Thus it is probable that the incoordination observed in animals and people poisoned by these insecticides, other than DDT and its analogs, is different from the tremor caused by DDT and should be referred to as ataxia or some other term.

The degree of stimulation of the nervous system appears to be related directly to the concentration of these insecticides in nerve tissue at the time. Usually the effect is rapidly reversible in animals after either single or multiple doses. Recovery occurs when the concentration of the chlorinated hydrocarbon insecticide in the nervous system falls below a critical level. It should be noted that this does not necessarily imply a loss of the chemical from the body but rather a redistribution to other tissues, such as adipose tissue, and has been studied particularly in connection with dieldrin (see Section 15.5.4.2).

15.2.2 ABSORPTION, DISTRIBUTION, METABOLISM, AND EXCRETION

15.2.2.1 Routes of Absorption

All chlorinated hydrocarbon insecticides can be absorbed through the skin as well as by the respiratory and oral routes. The importance of dermal absorption varies greatly for the different compounds. This is partly because some of them, such as methoxychlor, have such a low toxicity that a small amount absorbed by any route is of no importance; more importantly, the efficiency of dermal absorption varies for the different insecticides. For example, DDT is poorly absorbed by the skin from solutions, and the absorption of solid material is so poor that it is difficult or impossible to measure either the uptake of DDT or its effect. In contrast, even solid dieldrin, if very finely ground, is absorbed so effectively through the skin that it is about half as toxic when applied dermally as when administered by mouth. The dermal penetration of these insecticides involves not only partition coefficients but also binding to various dermal, epidermal, and serum sites. This leads to complications in interpreting experimental findings from a kinetic viewpoint (Shah *et al.*, 1981).

Because of their relatively low vapor pressure, chlorinated hydrocarbon insecticides seldom reach levels in the air above those permitted. Of course, they may be absorbed from the lung if they reach the respiratory epithelium in the form of solid or liquid aerosols of appropriate particle size.

The intestinal absorption of lipophilic substances such as these insecticides will be influenced by fiber and fat constituents of the diet as well as by the total food intake. The absorption of dieldrin, for instance, is enhanced by starvation (Heath and Vandekar, 1964).

15.2.2.2 Distribution, Metabolism, and Excretion

Chlorinated hydrocarbon insecticides have become infamous because of their tendency to accumulate in humans, animals, birds, and the general environment. After single or repeated doses, most of these chemicals eventually reach their highest concentrations in adipose tissue with somewhat lower levels in other tissues with high contents of neutral lipids, such as adre-

nals. Although storage in adipose tissue can be partly explained by the lipophilicity of these insecticides, other factors such as structural elements of the chemical and competition between binding sites in lean and adipose tissue are of great importance (Bickel, 1984). Another, perhaps even more important factor is the rate of metabolism and excretion of the parent chemical and any metabolites. For instance, DDT and its primary metabolite DDE are stored in adipose tissue of humans, whereas the closely related insecticide methoxychlor, which is metabolized much more rapidly, occurs in fat only at very low levels. Indeed, this difference has led to the increasing use of methoxychlor as an insecticide with the decline in the popularity of DDT. The isomers of BHC are stored to very different degrees in a pattern that does not correspond to their solubility in body fat (see Section 15.4.1.2) and is probably due to some extent to differential metabolism. Dieldrin is stored avidly, whereas its isomer endrin is stored so little that it has been detected in patients only after acute exposure and not even in people engaged in its manufacture (see Section 15.5.5.3). Again, this is due to differential metabolism; the unhindered *anti*-C-12 hydrogen in endrin makes this position far more susceptible to attack than any other position in either isomer (Bedford and Hutson, 1976). Metabolites of dieldrin are thus excreted at a much lower rate in bile and feces than are those from an equal dose of endrin (Cole *et al.*, 1970). Of course, in itself, storage of chemicals in adipose tissue can be viewed as a detoxification mechanism.

The specific metabolic transformations undergone by chlorinated hydrocarbon insecticides are covered in the appropriate sections. General principles of these metabolic routes are discussed in Chapter 3. In common with other lipophilic xenobiotics, chlorinated hydrocarbon insecticides can be metabolized by the microsomal cytochrome P-450 system to hydroxyl derivatives, perhaps with dehydrochlorination as observed for lindane, or by conversion to stable epoxides as in the case of the formation of dieldrin from endrin. The O-dealkylation of methoxychlor probably also involves a cytochrome P-450-mediated hydroxylation step. Other routes of metabolism involve conjugation with glutathione to give eventually mercapturates, which are usually excreted in the urine (see Section 15.4.1 for lindane), or the production of glucuronides, as in the case of the alcohol formed by reduction of chlordecone (see Section 15.7.2).

Parent insecticides are usually excreted either in the bile or possibly through the intestinal wall. Both routes may be manifested ultimately as fecal excretion. Metabolites of the chlorinated hydrocarbon insecticides can also be excreted in the urine if they are of relatively high polarity. This may have involved resorption of conjugates from the intestinal tract and transport to the liver and kidney (enterohepatic circulation), followed by further metabolic transformations. Such would be the case for glutathione conjugates excreted in bile, some of which may be reabsorbed and converted to the mercapturates for urinary excretion.

An important consideration when discussing the excretion of chlorinated hydrocarbon insecticides is their presence in milk (Jensen, 1983). The lipid content of milk (3–5%) and high blood flow to breast tissue can lead to considerable concentration of these chemicals compared to that in tissues. Thus, contamination of both cow's milk and human milk is not just a form of excretion but a unique one that could also lead to toxic effects in the recipient. Infants in countries with a large use of insecticides could be at particular risk, especially since breast feeding is recommended by the World Health Organization and other health agencies. Levels of these chemicals in human milk can be 10 times those in cow's milk. Measurement of chlorinated hydrocarbon insecticides in human milk is a convenient method for determining exposure of populations to these compounds, although it is prone to variability due to the effects of age, smoking, diet, and other factors (Jensen, 1983).

The excretion of DDT, DDE, and dieldrin in association with hair has been reported (Matthews *et al.*, 1976), probably representing their presence in hair or skin oils.

15.2.2.3 Factors Influencing Storage and Toxicity

Although the interaction of pesticides among themselves or with other chemicals is outlined in Chapter 2, it is pertinent here to discuss the interaction between chlorinated hydrocarbon insecticides. The ways in which these compounds influence the metabolism of themselves or of others of the same group is complex and still poorly understood. The results are essentially opposite in some species compared to others.

In dogs, when dieldrin and DDT are administered together, the storage of dieldrin is decreased but that of DDT is *increased* compared to the storage when each insecticide is given separately (Deichmann *et al.*, 1971a). If both aldrin and DDT are fed simultaneously to dogs, the storage of both compounds is increased such that the storage of aldrin is about the same, and the storage of DDT, and especially DDE, is somewhat greater than when each compound is given alone but at twice the dietary concentration (Deichmann *et al.*, 1969).

In the trout the situation is similar to that in dogs (Mayer *et al.*, 1970; Macek *et al.*, 1970), and in trout methoxychlor behaves like DDT when combined with other compounds (Mayer *et al.*, 1970).

In Japanese quail, the storage of DDE is increased in the presence of dieldrin but the latter remains essentially unchanged (Ludke, 1974).

In rats, when the compounds are combined, the storage of dieldrin is markedly decreased while the storage of DDT is uninfluenced (Street, 1964; Street and Chadwick, 1967; Street and Blau, 1966; Pearl and Kupfer, 1972; Street *et al.*, 1966a,b). The actions of methoxychlor and hexachlorobenzene (Avrahami and Gernert, 1972) are similar to that of DDT in reducing dieldrin storage. Hexachlorobenzene (*not* BHC) will also reduce storage of aldrin but increase the storage of DDT and mirex (Clark *et al.*, 1981). At the same time, polar urinary metabolites of the insecticides are increased from aldrin and mirex but remain unchanged from DDT. Storage of heptachlor in rats is depressed by DDT (Street *et al.*, 1966b) and excretion

of [^{14}C]dieldrin administered ip is stimulated (Pearl and Kupfer, 1972).

In guinea pigs, when DDT and dieldrin are fed together, the storage of dieldrin is little affected but that of DDT is decreased (Wagstaff and Street, 1971b).

Undoubtedly, the interaction of compounds of this type in different species depends in part on their ability to induce the microsomal drug-metabolizing enzymes in those species. However, relationships between induction, storage, and excretion of metabolites are rarely simple and there are few studies of the induction of the metabolism of one pesticide by another. Lindane and DDT have been found to be only moderately active inducers in guinea pigs although their storage is low, whereas dieldrin was a strong inducer, yet its storage is much higher than that of the other two insecticides (Wagstaff and Street, 1971b). In mice, treatment for 5 months with DDE decreased the urinary excretion of [^{14}C]DDE and increased hepatic levels (Gold and Brunk, 1986). However, there was no effect on the levels of the only metabolite detected, 1,1-dichloro - 2 - (4-chlorophenyl) - 2 - (3-hydroxy-4-chlorophenyl) ethane. It is very difficult to interpret experimental findings of this type in the context of human exposures both of the general population and of heavily exposed workers. Dose levels and routes of administration in experimental animals are usually much different from those experienced by humans. Thus there are few studies of the effects of these pesticides on their own metabolism or that of other insecticides in humans. One possible example is the finding that current and former endrin workers stored significantly lower levels of *p,p'*-DDE; in fact, the levels were below detectable limits (Jager, 1970).

Other xenobiotics and drugs will undoubtedly affect the storage, distribution, and metabolism of chlorinated hydrocarbon insecticides as described above for hexachlorobenzene. Recent progress in our understanding of the induction of the drug-metabolizing systems (e.g., cytochrome P-450 and glutathione transferase isoenzymes) in both animals and humans and the influence of age, sex, and genetics, however, should make interactions easier to predict.

The combined effect of chlorinated hydrocarbon insecticides and anticholinesterase insecticides is one form of interaction that has received special attention even though there is no evidence that it has ever been of any clinical importance. Pretreatment of experimental animals with various chlorinated insecticides (including aldrin, dieldrin, chlordane, and DDT) has afforded some protection against single doses of some anticholinesterases (Triolo and Coon, 1966a,b; Williams and Casterline, 1970; Deichmann and Keplinger, 1970; Bass *et al.*, 1972). In other instances, the toxicity of an organophosphorus insecticide is increased by pretreatment with chlorinated hydrocarbon insecticides. For example, the toxicity of fenitrothion in rats is increased by heptachlor (Mestitzová *et al.*, 1970a,b, 1971). In one case, protection by aldrin against parathion appeared after 16 hr, reached a maximum in 4 days, and lasted at least 12 days. A dose of 1 mg/kg provided significant protection (Triolo and Coon, 1966a,b). Most of these enhancing or protective effects of chlorinated hydrocarbon insecticides are probably the consequence of induction of particular routes of metabolism and should now be mostly predictable. Piperonyl butoxide, an inhibitor of cytochrome P-450, will block the protective action of chlorinated insecticides on 6-chloro-3-xylyl methylcarbamate (Williams and Casterline, 1970). Chlorinated hydrocarbon insecticides appear to have an affinity for a hydrophobic site of cholinesterase although they do not inhibit the active site of the enzyme (Mayer and Himel, 1972); whether this interferes with the approach of the substrate to the active site is not known.

Mobilization of fat in adipose tissue due to starvation or other reasons can release into the circulation stored chlorinated hydrocarbon insecticides, sometimes with marked effects.

15.2.3 MODES OF ACTION AND CAUSE OF DEATH

15.2.3.1 Effects on the Central Nervous System

Mode of Action   As discussed elsewhere (Section 4.1.2.3), there is considerable evidence to suggest that the chlorinated hydrocarbon insecticides act by altering the electrophysiological and associated enzymatic properties of nerve cell membranes, causing a change in the kinetics of Na^+ and K^+ ion flow through the membrane. Disturbances of calcium transport or Ca^{2+}-ATPase activity may also be involved, as well as phosphokinase activities (Matsumura and Patil, 1969; End *et al.*, 1981; Joy, 1982a; Shankland, 1982; Tilson and Mactutus, 1982; Woolley *et al.*, 1985; Ishikawa *et al.*, 1989). Other cell membranes may also be affected by related mechanisms. Dieldrin at a concentration of 10 μM affects liver cell membranes in a way very similar to that of the insect nervous system *in vivo* (Wang and Matsumura, 1969). DDT and some of its analogs (but not others) have been shown to inhibit Ca^{2+}-ATPase from human term placentas (Treinen and Kulkarni, 1986). Most studies have been conducted with DDT (Section 15.3.1.2) and chlorodecone and other cyclodienes (Section 15.7.2.2). Full explanations for the differences in the *in vivo* neutrotoxic effects of these two groups of chlorinated hydrocarbon insecticides are still not completely apparent, including the peripheral versus central nervous system (CNS) actions. DDT and its analogs appear to act particularly at the nerve axon by prolonging opening of the ion gates of the sodium channel (Ishikawa *et al.*, 1989), whereas cyclodienes, mirex, and lindane seem to act at presynaptic terminals. Lindane, toxaphene, and cyclodienes have been shown to inhibit *t*-butylbicyclophosphorothionate binding to brain specific sites, indicating action at the γ-aminobutyric acid (GABA)-regulated chloride channel (Casida and Lawrence, 1985; Cole and Casida, 1986). DDT, mirex, and chlordecone had no effect. Cyclodienes and lindane also inhibit GABA-induced ^{36}Cl influx into rat brain membrane microsacs (Abalis *et al.*, 1986).

Whatever the exact mechanisms, nonconvulsant doses of chlorinated hydrocarbon insecticides increase the susceptibility of animals to convulsions precipitated by many other poisons or by electroshock. One study of this relationship concluded that the convulsant effects of dieldrin may be mediated by effects on the hippocampus and other limbic structures (Swanson and Woolley, 1978). Fonseca *et al.* (1986) have demonstrated that p,p'-DDT and lindane decrease the number of muscarinic receptor sites in selective regions of rat brain.

A toxic dosage of dieldrin (50 mg/kg) led to a decrease in norepinephrine in the brain of rats 5 hr after ingestion but no change in dopamine or serotonin. When rats were maintained on a dietary level of 80 ppm (about 2.4 mg/kg/day) that they tolerated well for more than 10 weeks, norepinephrine and serotonin (but not dopamine) were depleted in certain parts of the brain soon after feeding but later returned to normal values (Wagner and Greene, 1974). A decrease in brain stem norepinephrine and acetylcholine and an increase in serotonin have been observed in rats following toxic doses of several cyclodiene insecticides (Hrdina *et al.*, 1974). Similar changes were seen with DDT (Hrdina *et al.*, 1973). It is clear that changes in the biogenic amines parallel the toxicity of chlorinated hydrocarbon insecticides, including the phenomenon of initial illness followed by clinical recovery. Whether these changes in the biogenic amines are a cause or a consequence is not clear. What is certain is that a variety of stimuli, including electrical stimuli and some insecticides, can change the production of biogenic amines in the brain (Campos and Jurupe, 1970).

The relative acute toxicities of the chlorinated hydrocarbon insecticides in animals and humans have been listed by Joy (1982a). The cyclodienes endrin, dieldrin, and isobenzan appear to be among the most toxic to humans and perhaps >10-fold more acutely toxic than DDT, which is the most potent agent in the dichlorodiphenylethane group.

Origin of Fever   Fever may be a specific result of poisoning of the temperature control center in the brain. The effect may be more common than has been recognized. What has been recognized in a few human cases is high fever of sometimes late but sudden onset, frequently followed promptly by death. This kind of fever has been observed in poisoning by BHC, dieldrin, and endrin.

Fortunately, high fever of central origin is rare, but because it is such a grave sign, it is essential to distinguish it from other kinds of fever that may be the result of poisoning. Fever may accompany convulsions in humans or larger animals simply because it may be impossible to dissipate heat as rapidly as it is generated by the violent activity, which certainly is muscular and may be metabolic also. Fever of this origin has no special prognostic significance beyond that of the convulsions that give rise to it.

Regardless of the exact cause, a moderate increase in body temperature during the early course of illness carries no serious implications (Osuntokun, 1964). However, unless fever subsides promptly after convulsions are controlled, some other basis for it must be sought.

Fever may also be a response to chemical pneumonitis following aspiration of solvents or other chemical irritants; of course, fever of this origin may occur after a formulation of any chlorinated hydrocarbon insecticide has been aspirated. It may depend in part on secondary infection. Usually it is delayed about 12 hr or more, and in relatively mild cases it may not appear until the patient has recovered from neurological manifestations.

EEG   It is clear that the electroencephalogram (EEG) is a good index of the convulsive action of chlorinated hydrocarbon insecticides (Joy, 1982a). The sequence of EEG changes following a single convulsive dose of DDT and dieldrin to cats has been reported (Joy, 1973).

Pathology   Chlorinated hydrocarbon insecticides produce little morphological change in the CNS of animals even when given in single or repeated doses sufficient to kill. The changes that do occur seem to reflect the agonal state but are not sufficient to account for death or assist in diagnosis, and they have been discussed by Joy (1982a).

15.2.3.2 Effects on the Liver

There is no doubt that DDT and a number of other chlorinated hydrocarbon insecticides cause marked changes in the livers of various rodents and that these changes progress to tumor formation in some species, especially the mouse. However, the relationship of these tumors arising in rodents to the potential induction of hepatocellular carcinoma in humans is still very obscure, as exemplified by DDT (Anderson, 1985), although the view that they are peculiar to rodents may not be completely justified, since for practical and financial reasons there have been few studies with other species.

Evidence for the carcinogenicity of chlorinated hydrocarbon insecticides has been reviewed by the International Agency for Research on Cancer (IARC) on a number of occasions during the last two decades. The IARC evaluation of these chemicals when administered by the oral route is shown in Table 15.1. Most of the insecticides produce tumors in mice, but results in rats are less conclusive. None of the chemicals have been completely negative in both rats and mice. Perhaps for this reason and the fact that their mechanism of action in liver has not yet been completely elucidated, the IARC seem reluctant to state categorically that they pose no carcinogenic risk to humans.

In connection with DDT, which has been studied the most in this group of chemicals, it has been concluded that the evidence for carcinogenicity in humans is inadequate (IARC, 1982, 1987). In mice the oral hepatocarcinogenicity has been demonstrated in several strains and shows a dose–response relationship. A dietary level of 2 ppm (about 0.3 mg DDT/kg/day) produces a significant increase of hepatomas in male but not female CF1 mice and not in either sex of BALB/c mice. Increased tumor incidence (particularly lung adenomas) has also been reported in some other organs of mice. There is now clear evidence, confirming the preliminary studies of Fitzhugh and Nelson (1947), that DDT can be hepatocarcinogenic to rats (Rossi *et al.*, 1977; Cabral *et al.*, 1982b). Results in hamsters,

Table 15.1

Summary of the Oral Hepatocarcinogenicity of Some Chlorinated Hydrocarbon Insecticides in Animals as Assessed by IARC Working Groups on the Evaluation of Carcinogenic Risk of Chemicals to Humans (1974, 1979, 1982, 1983, 1987)[a]

Chemical	Species	Evaluation
DDT	mouse	positive in both sexes and in various strains
	rat	positive
	hamster	negative
	dog	inconclusive
	monkey	inconclusive
DDE	mouse	positive
methoxychlor	mouse	positive
	rat	inconclusive
chlorobenzilate	mouse	positive
	rat	inconclusive
dicofol	mouse	positive in males
	rat	inconclusive
BHC	mouse	technical mixture, α isomer and γ isomer (lindane) positive; β isomer limted positive evidence
	rat	inconclusive
chlordane	mouse	positive
	rat	inconclusive
heptachlor	mouse	positive
	rat	inconclusive
aldrin	mouse	positive
	rat	negative or inconclusive
dieldrin	mouse	positive
	rat	negative
	dog	inconclusive
	monkey	inconclusive
endrin	mouse	inconclusive
	rat	negative or inconclusive
toxaphene	mouse	positive
	rat	negative
mirex	mouse	positive in two strains
	rat	positive
chlordecone	mouse	positive
	rat	positive

[a] Evaluations for chlorobenzilate, methoxychlor, BHC, and toxaphene in rats may have to be revised; see Sections 15.3.4, 15.3.5, 15.4.1, and 15.6.1.

dogs, and monkeys appear to be still inconclusive, although hamsters do give liver tumors with p,p'-DDE, as do mice (Cabral, 1985). There appear to have been no new studies of the hepatocarcinogenicity of DDT in dogs and monkeys since those first reported (IARC, 1974). These studies, which were inconclusive, did continue for some time (monkeys up to 7.5 years), and though the numbers were small they were no less than those which had given positive results for other potential carcinogens.

Chlorinated hydrocarbon insecticides are, in general, negative in mutagenicity tests (Wildemauwe *et al.*, 1983). Whether their tumorigenicity in rodents is due to the promotion of spontaneous initiated events is not known. It is clear, however, that DDT, BHC, and the cyclodiene insecticides are efficient promoters of the actions of recognized potent hepatocarcinogens such as diethylnitrosamine and 2-acetylaminofluorene (Peraino *et al.*, 1975; Williams and Numoto, 1984; Schulte-Hermann, 1985). The ability of these chemicals to cause tumors in the liver and promote those initiated by other carcinogens is probably tied up with the induction of microsomal and other enzyme systems. The following paragraphs are concerned with these matters.

Early Changes in the Rodent Liver Associated with Induction of Microsomal Enzymes The response of the rodent liver to DDT is entirely similar to its response to moderate dosages of BHC, chlordane, dieldrin, toxaphene (Lehman, 1951, 1952; Ortega *et al.*, 1956), and the important drug phenobarbital (Stevenson and Walker, 1969; Wright *et al.*, 1972; Thorpe and Walker, 1973). Similar early changes also were demonstrated in the livers of rats fed dimethrin, pyrethrins, and especially synergized pyrethrins (Kimbrough *et al.*, 1968) (see Chapter 13). Some of these lesions are also known to arise spontaneously (Popp *et al.*, 1985).

The earliest changes in some liver cells of rodents administered DDT involve so much increase in the smooth endoplasmic reticulum of individual cells that they enlarge, and the large granules that ordinarily are scattered throughout the cytoplasm are displaced to the periphery of the affected cell. Quite early, some of the endoplasmic reticulum forms whorls that may have fat droplets as their centers—this justifying the term "lipospheres" applied to them by Ortega *et al.* (1956, 1957). Others have referred to these inclusions as "hyaline oxyphil masses" (Lillie and Smith, 1944), "lamellar bodies" (Ito *et al.*, 1973), or "myelin whorls" (Hansell and Ecobichon, 1975). These changes are accompanied by some increase in fat droplets, not all of which become surrounded by endoplasmic reticulum. This cluster of changes (hypertrophy, margination, and lipospheres) is characteristic of the response of rodents to compounds that induce microsomal enzymes. The characteristic changes develop promptly. An increase in smooth endoplasmic reticulum and the appearance of lamellar structures have been seen as early as 4 and 7 days after dosing began (Wright *et al.*, 1972). When DDT was administered to rat dams by stomach tube for 3 days at the rate of 50 mg/kg/day, no significant induction of liver microsomal enzymes and no morphological changes in the hepatocytes of the pups were observed prior to their birth, even though residues were found in fetal tissues. The young of treated mothers did show increased smooth endoplasmic reticulum, lipid inclusions, and myelin whorls when they were 4 days old and thereafter, and no samples were collected from birth until day 4. Similar but somewhat lesser changes were produced on the same schedule by phenobarbital (75 mg/kg/day) (Hansell and Ecobichon, 1975).

The accumulation of lipid following a single large dose of dieldrin was reported to involve triglycerides only, with no increase in phospholipid or cholesterol. The increase in triglycerides was accompanied by increased incorporation of [^{14}C]glucose into glyceride–glycerol but a decrease of its incorporation into fatty acids (Bhatia and Venkitasubramanian,

1972). Presumably, more triglyceride is formed in the presence of more glyceride–glycerol.

Certain changes other than the characteristic one have been reported but not confirmed. These include enlargement and morphological change of the mitochondria (Obuchowska and Pawlowska-Tochman, 1973; Watari, 1973), increased numbers of primary lysosomes, and atrophy of the Golgi body (Watari, 1973), none of which were found by Ortega (1966).

Although microsomal enzymes may be induced in other species, their livers do not seem to show the same morphological changes as viewed by light microscopy (Laug *et al.*, 1950; Lehman, 1951, 1952; Ortega *et al.*, 1956; Stevenson and Walker, 1969) or show them to a lesser degree as viewed by electron microscopy (Wright *et al.*, 1972).

The changes in liver cells that characterize induction of microsomal enzymes in rodents are distinct from the focal necrosis that may be produced with about the same ease in the livers of rodents or of other species by fatal or near-fatal dosages of chlorinated hydrocarbon insecticides. These necrotic lesions have been described by Smith and Stohlman (1944), Lillie *et al.* (1947), Nelson *et al.* (1944), Cameron and Burgess (1945), Deichmann *et al.* (1950), and Ortega *et al.* (1956). The necrosis does not appear to progress, since if high dosages are continued the animals die, whereas if dosing is stopped and the animals survive, the necrotic cells are removed by autolysis and phagocytic action. The lesions then heal, usually without scarring (Cameron and Burgess, 1945), although this can occur (Lillie and Smith, 1944; Lillie *et al.*, 1947). An interesting indication of the defensive or adaptive nature of the characteristic liver changes is the observation that they occur only in animals that remain healthy and not in animals that are frankly intoxicated by very high dosage levels (Ferrigan *et al.*, 1965). This does not mean that rats that have developed the changes may not later show signs of poisoning.

On the other hand, there is one aspect of the morphological change in the endoplasmic reticulum that may be even more critical than marked hypertrophy of the smooth variety in determining whether tumorigenesis will occur. Williams and Rabin (1971) reported that a range of established carcinogens promoted the degranulation of rat liver rough endoplasmic reticulum *in vitro*, whereas a range of noncarcinogens were without this effect. In a parallel way, carcinogens prevented smooth microsomal membranes from binding added ribosomes in the presence of estradiol. Wright *et al.* (1977) showed that results of biochemical tests for degranulation corresponded not only to the tumorigenicity of different compounds but also to differences in the susceptibility of different species and strains and of males and females of the same strain.

The Question of Reversibility and the Relation of Dosage to Induction of Microsomal Enzymes At least in their early stages, the changes in liver cells that characterize induction of microsomal enzymes in rodents are reversible (Fitzhugh and Nelson, 1947; Ortega *et al.*, 1956; Wright *et al.*, 1972). The reversibility does not depend on cell removal but simply on reversion of the physiological and morphological condition of the cells to their original condition. Return of the liver to normal size also occurs if dosage is discontinued soon enough (Kunz *et al.*, 1966). On the other hand, normalization may be slow, especially when the inducer remains in the target tissue. Although the liver weight of rats returned to normal within 2 weeks after one or two doses of α-BHC at the rate of 200 mg/kg, the DNA content of the liver remained high, as did the proportion of the cells with tetraploid nuclei during a 7-week posttreatment period (Schulte-Hermann *et al.*, 1971). In rats fed photomirex (a degradation product of mirex) for 4 weeks (50 ppm), histological changes in the liver and thyroid could still be seen 48 weeks after return to normal diet (Chu *et al.*, 1981a,b). Consistent with these persistent changes was the finding of significant levels of photomirex remaining in the liver.

Of course, reversibility is incompatible with progression, but whether observed irreversibility will be associated with progression must be determined directly in each instance. In the following paragraphs, the question of progression is discussed only after consideration of the problem of irreversibility in general.

If dosing with chlorinated hydrocarbon insecticides or other inducers is continued long enough and at a sufficiently high level, the liver changes become irreversible, if for no other reason than that the remaining life span of the animals is too short to permit excretion of the inducing chemical or complete reversion of the liver cells to their original state. Just when this shift to irreversibility occurs remains unknown, but it seems very likely that dosages sufficient to produce irreversible morphological change also exceed the physiological adaptability of the liver. The important distinction between adaptation and injury as it relates to enzyme induction and liver morphology has been studied in relation to dieldrin (see Section 3.1.2.3). The matter has received some biochemical study, which suggested that hypoactive hypertrophic endoplasmic reticulum involves a qualitative change in the induced cytochrome P-450 (Stevens *et al.*, 1977).

Briefly, the evidence is strong that enlargement of the liver and of individual liver cells is adaptive at dosages where the increase in endoplasmic reticulum is accompanied by a parallel increase in activity of the associated enzymes and by no depression in the activity of other enzymes and that these liver changes are pathological at higher dosages where the activity of the drug-metabolizing enzymes fails to keep pace with the morphological changes or where the activities of these or other enzymes are depressed.

The relation of dosage to the induction of microsomal enzymes has been discussed previously (see Sections 2.3.8 and 7.4.3). The effects of DDT were explored by Kinoshita *et al.* (1966) and later studied more thoroughly by Hoffman *et al.* (1970). They found that, when DDT was fed to male weanling rats for only 14 days at dietary concentrations of 0.5–2048 ppm, concentrations of 0.5 and 2 ppm had no effect on the *O*-demethylation reaction used as a test, but concentrations of 4–750 ppm produced increases in the rate of metabolism propor-

tional to the log of dosage. Extrapolation of this portion of the dosage–response curve to the abscissa provided a calculated no-effect level of 3.27 ± 1.02 ppm equivalent to about 0.327 mg/kg/day. This is in reasonable agreement with other estimates of the threshold for induction of various enzymes in the rat, including some studies involving longer administration of DDT. These estimates, expressed as milligrams per kilogram per day, are approximately 0.05 (Kinoshita *et al.*, 1966; Street *et al.*, 1969), 0.5 (Schwabe and Wendling, 1967), and 0.125 (Gillett, 1968). The relationship may not be the same for different inducers in the same species or for the same inducer in different species or sexes. For example, DDT in the squirrel monkey promotes the metabolism of EPN and *p*-nitroanisole; the first requires a DDT dosage of 5.0 mg/kg/day, but the latter requires only 0.5 mg/kg/day (Cranmer *et al.*, 1972). *In vivo* administration of both chlordecone and mirex induces the V_{max} of *p*-nitroanisole metabolism by male rat microsomes and increases apparent K_m values, but with females this metabolism was reduced with either agent and the apparent K_m value was elevated by chlordecone but little affected by mirex (Ebel, 1984). Metabolism of DDT is promoted by DDT itself in the hamster (Gingell and Wallcave, 1974) but not in the mouse (Gingell and Wallcave, 1974) or in the squirrel monkey (Chadwick *et al.*, 1971b). However, most of the estimates for minimal effective dosage are of the same order of magnitude as 0.25 mg/kg/day, known to be effective in humans (Poland *et al.*, 1970), but all are more than 100 times greater than the highest dosage of people in the general population during the late 1960s (Duggan, 1968). In the study by Hoffman and his colleagues (1970), increase of the dietary level above 750 ppm produced no further increase in enzyme activity. Intake less than 128 ppm produced no increase in liver weight within the period of observation; increase was proportional to dosage within the range 128–512 ppm and was submaximal at intakes above 512 ppm.

The biochemical pattern of induction of mixed-function oxidase enzymes is similar for DDT and phenobarbital but distinctly different for 3-methylcholanthrene (Vainio, 1975). DDE, the major metabolite of DDT, was shown to induce mRNA for a cytochrome P-450 identical to that induced by phenobarbital but had a much more persistent effect (Morohashi *et al.*, 1984).

Late Changes in the Rodent Liver Associated with Induction of Microsomal Enzymes As indicated above, the earliest morphological changes caused by phenobarbital-type enzyme inducers in the rodent liver involve separate cells in the centrilobular area. If the dosage is sufficiently high and prolonged, nodules consisting entirely of hypertrophied cells may appear. At first, these microscopic nodules are distinguishable only by pattern; they have no bounding membrane and they do not compress or change in any other detectable way the smaller liver cells that surround them. Some nodules may become large enough to be seen without a microscope, and a few may exceed 1 cm in diameter. In these large nodules there is almost complete loss of lobular architecture. Nodules apparently were first described by Fitzhugh and Nelson (1947), who felt they could be regarded as adenomas or as low-grade hepatic cell carcinomas. Just why this latter term was used is not clear because neither mitosis, tissue invasion, nor metastasis was observed. Although Ortega et al. (1956) reported small nodules in the livers of rats they had dosed and although they examined tissue loaned by Fitzhugh and Nelson's laboratory, they were entirely unimpressed by the lesions, referring to them as "focal incongruities."

The classification introduced by Thorpe and Walker (1973) and Walker et al. (1973) might have been expected to lead to better agreement or at least to a clearer definition of points of difference. As a result of their studies in mice, these investigators proposed that simple nodular growths of liver parenchymal cells be called type a lesions and that areas of papilliform and adenoid growth of tumor cells, sometimes accompanied by metastases to the lungs, be called type b lesions. It was concluded by Walker et al. (1973) on the basis of earlier studies of rats and dogs in their own laboratory and also on the basis of results of others that tumorigenic action of dieldrin had been demonstrated only in mice.

However, there still is no agreement regarding the carcinogenicity of the chlorinated hydrocarbon insecticides. The views of some pathologists remain diametrically opposite. This is true despite the finding of (a) pulmonary metastases of hepatic cells in mice that had received DDT (Tomatis et al., 1972; Walker et al., 1973), β-BHC, γ-BHC, dieldrin, or phenobarbital (Thorpe and Walker, 1973); or (b) progression of liver enlargement beginning 12 weeks after cessation of ingestion of α-BHC by mice for 24 or 36 weeks (Nagasaki et al., 1974) or progressive increase in the size of liver nodules after DDT feeding was stopped (Tomatis et al., 1974b; Tomatis and Turusov, 1975); or even (c) in BHC-exposed mice the time pattern of increase in liver weight (as reflected in body weight), which gained momentum only after a delay of 4 weeks but showed a further acceleration in week 13 in spite of decreased food consumption (Tomii et al., 1972), which appears to establish without question that at least some of the liver changes produced by these compounds in rodents are malignant.

Of course, the reasons for disagreement are that tumors indistinguishable from those caused by DDT, other chlorinated hydrocarbon insecticides, and phenobarbital occasionally occur in control mice (Davis and Fitzhugh, 1962; Walker et al., 1973) and rats (Fitzhugh and Nelson, 1947; Popp et al., 1985) and, more especially, because these tumors differ from real cancers in their biochemistry and they are not malignant in the classical sense. Specifically, (a) they do not actively invade tissues, (b) their "metastases" usually do not grow even through large growths of liver cells in the lungs occasionally have been seen (Walker et al., 1973), (c) any shortening of life span that occurs may be related to the toxicity of large dosages and not to tumors per se, and finally (d) mice receiving DDT at a rate of 5.5 mg/kg/day as a result of dietary intake show a decrease in the success of transplantation and a significant increase in survival following inoculation with an otherwise

uniformly transplantable and uniformly fatal ependymoma (Laws, 1971).

Although the displacement of liver cells to the lung occasionally seen after prolonged dosage with DDT usually is referred to as metastasis, it might better be called embolism because the lesion rarely progresses and, therefore, usually lacks the clinical significance of real metastasis. Because it usually does not grow, the lesion is usually hard to find. A number of investigators have failed to mention liver cells in the spleen, lymph nodes, or lungs, and some have stated specifically that they were not found (Nagasaki, 1973).

Perhaps the most illuminating studies of the liver changes caused by various chlorinated hydrocarbon insecticides are those in which 2,7-fluorinediamine, diazoaminobenzene, or some other classical carcinogen has been used as a positive control (Wright et al., 1972; Walker et al., 1973; Kuwabara and Takayama, 1974). In each case the lesion caused by the classical carcinogen was different from that caused by the insecticide in one or more of the following ways: (a) it did not involve induction of microsomal enzymes; (b) it started as hyperplastic nodules rather than as isolated cell changes; (c) bile duct proliferation or other lesions not found in controls or in insecticide-treated animals were present; (d) the final lesion was hepatocellular carcinoma, in contrast to the adenoma caused by DDT or BHC; and (e) α-fetoprotein was formed, which did not occur in connection with DDT or BHC. Other workers also have failed to find α-fetoprotein in mice treated with a chlorinated hydrocarbon insecticide (Hanada et al., 1973).

It must be emphasized that the chlorinated hydrocarbon insecticides and phenobarbital do not produce in other animals, to the same extent, the early, visible changes in the endoplasmic reticulum that are so characteristic of some rodents and that may progress to tumor formation in them. The fact that these compounds do not lead to tumor formation in other animals might have been predicted by the fact that they do not cause in other animals the early changes, characterized by hypertrophy, margination, and lipospheres. Of course, it must also be said that the number of studies that have been conducted with nonrodent species are relatively few. In addition, chlorinated hydrocarbon insecticides may all be positive carcinogens in the mouse but not all seem to cause tumors in rats (see Table 15.1) despite considerable induction of the endoplasmic reticulum by other chemicals in the group. On the other hand, large increases in liver size after lindane treatment in CF1 mice but not B6C3F1 mice or Osborne–Mendel rats do seem to correlate with propensities for tumor formation (Oesch et al., 1982). In recent years, an epigenetic mechanism for the tumorigenicity of chlorinated hydrocarbon insecticides has become likely in which there is a disruption in intercellular communication—perhaps leading to inhibition of exchange of growth inhibitors (Maslansky and Williams, 1981; Tsushimoto et al., 1983; Wärngård et al., 1985, 1987, 1988, 1989, Zhong-Xiang et al., 1986). How this would relate to induction of microsomal enzymes, if at all, is not yet clear.

The fact that chlorinated hydrocarbon insecticides and some

other pesticides thought to act by entirely different mechanisms are not additive in their tumorigenic effects may be related to the fact that, whereas all chlorinated hydrocarbon insecticides induce microsomal enzymes, they do so in different ways, as discussed in Section 15.2.2.3. Whatever the reason, the fact remains that the effects are not additive. Experiments in rats were carried out on combinations of Aramite, DDT, methoxychlor, and thiourea (three separate tests) and Aramite, DDT, methoxychlor, and aldrin (Radomski *et al.*, 1965; Deichmann *et al.*, 1967). In the final tests, each compound was fed separately at a dosage corresponding to 50% of its liver tumor-inducing dosage, and four compounds were fed in combination in such a way as to produce a total theoretical tumorigenic dosage of 200%. The authors concluded: "Considering the increased period of survival of rats fed mixtures no. 1 and no. 2 and the lower number of liver tumors produced in these rats, one cannot help but wonder whether the feeding of these mixtures produces an antagonistic type of effect" (Deichmann *et al.*, 1967).

Discussion of Liver Changes in Rodents and Their Possible Significance for Humans   In spite of disagreement about interpretation of the liver cell changes, there is general agreement about their development and appearance. The change that can be detected first and can be produced by the smallest effective dosage involves the endoplasmic reticulum. The initial change is reversible but, even more important, it is especially pronounced in rodents. So far, there is no good evidence that anything from the first increase in endoplasmic reticulum to the final development of a highly nodular liver with occasional displacement of cells to the lung can be directly related to the health of humans.

One cannot accept uncritically the high degree of correlation between the ability of compounds to induce parenchymal liver tumors in mice and their ability to induce tumors in the liver and/or other organs of rats and hamsters. As demonstrated by Tomatis *et al.* (1973), this correlation is extremely good for compounds that are or are suspected of being carcinogens in humans but the correlation is poor for chlorinated hydrocarbon insecticides.

All available evidence indicates that humans do not appear to be susceptible to the tumorigenic action of the chlorinated hydrocarbon insecticides and phenobarbital. No increase in the occurrence of tumors has been found in heavily exposed populations. This includes groups of workers who manufacture and formulate DDT, dieldrin, aldrin, endrin, chlordane, and heptachlor and who have been examined carefully for tumors (Laws *et al.*, 1967; Jager, 1970; Vergsteeg and Jager, 1973; van Raalte, 1977; Wang and MacMahon, 1979a,b; Ditraglia *et al.*, 1981; Shindell *et al.*, 1981; Shindell and Ulrich, 1986; Ribbens, 1985).

Studies based on complete tumor registries indicate no increase of liver tumors attributable to phenobarbital among men and women who received heavy, essentially lifelong dosing with this drug for the control of epilepsy (Clemmesen *et al.*,

1974; MacMahon, 1985). In the United States, the total death rates for cancer of the liver and its biliary passages (classified individually as "primary," "secondary," and "not stated whether primary or secondary") lead to the conclusion that there has been a significant, almost constant decrease in the total rate of liver cancer deaths from 8.8 per 100,000 population in 1930 to 8.4 in 1944 (when DDT was introduced) to 5.6 in 1972. This almost constant decline in total liver cancer death rates over 42 years offers no evidence of any increase in liver cancer deaths since the introduction of the first organochlorine pesticide into the environment. The decrease in liver cancer deaths is even more significant in light of the increasing life span of the general population in the United States, which has resulted in an increased percentage of the population at risk from cancer over these years. In spite of the limitation inherent in the interpretation of such data, this record is a reminder that, more than 30 years after the introduction of DDT, there is no evidence whatsoever that DDT is carcinogenic in humans [Deichmann and MacDonald, 1976, 1977; World Health Organization (WHO), 1979; Higginson, 1985].

In the United States, the incidence of cancer is lower in rural counties than in metropolitan areas in general (Mason *et al.*, 1975). Actually, the highest nonoccupational storage of DDT in the United States has been measured in rural situations, largely as a result of local consumption of foods such as eggs that had high residues because of practices involving foods raised for local consumption only.

Sometimes it is implied that epidemiological evidence is useless for revealing the carcinogenicity of a material to humans unless it involves large numbers of people who have been exposed to the material for most or all of a lifetime. The fact is that some human carcinogens have been detected through their occurrence in high incidence in small groups for periods much less than 25 years. What is commonly considered the first recognition of chemical carcinogenesis in humans depended on the observations of a surgeon (Pott, 1775, 1790) in a small fraction of his patients. Such was the intensity of the exposure of the apprentices of chimney sweepers that cancer of the scrotum often appeared at puberty. In connection with tumors of the bladder caused mainly by β-naphthylamine but to a lesser degree by other aromatic amines, Hueper (1942, pp. 496–497) reviewed a series of cases in which the time from first exposure to recognition of symptoms was 8–41, 9–28, and 2–35 years, and in one series of 83 cases 71% of the tumors appeared from 1 to 15 years after exposure. Kleinfeld (1967) reported a 50–76% incidence of bladder cancer among several groups of workers. He also noted a sharp drop in incidence of this condition following decrease—but not discontinuation—of occupational exposure to β-naphthylamine. Thus heavy exposure to aromatic carcinogens may therefore produce cancer quickly. Hepatomegaly and induction of microsomal enzymes caused by chlorinated hydrocarbon insecticides do, however, occur in humans and may be slow to regress (Guzelian, 1985), so that for chemicals of this type other than DDT—for instance, BHC and chlordecone—it may be too soon to be absolutely sure that they are of no carcinogenic hazard to humans. For instance, a recent study of DDT, DDE, and β-BHC levels in ear wax collected from 3800 persons in the general populations of 35 Chinese counties showed a significant correlation between β-BHC levels and mortality rates from liver cancer, colon and rectal cancer, and lung cancer in males and colon cancer in females (Wang *et al.*, 1988).

In addition, it is worth remembering that in animals many of these insecticides are good promoters of liver cancer initiated by well-known carcinogens. Some of the areas of the world where DDT and lindane are used in large quantities are also areas where the risk of hepatocellular carcinoma is much greater than in the United States due to aflatoxin contamination of food or to carrying of the hepatitis B virus.

Changes in Nonmicrosomal Enzymes In addition to the important changes in microsomal enzymes caused by various chlorinated hydrocarbon insecticides, changes in nonmicrosomal enzymes have been documented. Among these enzymes are a number involved with gluconeogenesis (Karnik *et al.*, 1981). There is evidence that the first step in this process by DDT, chlordane, endrin, or heptachlor is stimulation of the cyclic AMP–adenylate cyclase system (Singhal and Kacew, 1976).

15.2.3.3 Other Toxic Effects

Besides affecting the liver and the nervous system, chlorinated hydrocarbon insecticides can cause disturbances of function in other tissues of experimental animals. These will be covered in the appropriate sections but include the thyroid (e.g., A. Singh *et al.*, 1985), which may lead to thyroid tumors (IARC, 1974, 1979, 1982, 1983). DDT and analogs have estrogenic effects (see Section 15.3.1.2) and, like the polyhalogenated aromatic chemicals, chlorinated hydrocarbon insecticides can accumulate in adrenals, causing various hormonal changes in the animal (Baggett *et al.*, 1980). Mirex will cause cataracts in fetuses and rat pups from dams treated with the chemical (Gaines and Kimbrough, 1970; Rogers and Grabowski, 1983) and many of these insecticides have effects on the immune system (Descotes, 1986), although whether this causes any adverse effects in the animal is unknown.

15.2.4 DIFFERENTIAL DIAGNOSIS

Poisoning caused by chlorinated hydrocarbon insecticides is acute whether caused by single or repeated doses. Of course, animals may be kept in a state of continuing illness by carefully chosen repeated doses. However, animals that survive recover promptly when dosage is discontinued. The same appears to be true of humans.

Human poisoning following massive accidental or suicidal exposure presents no problem of differential diagnosis. Diagnosis might be difficult if exposure were unrecognized and the illness so mild that no convulsion occurred. However, any such illness would be brief and without sequel, so a failure of diagnosis would not be too serious.

If the fact of exposure is unrecognized in a case involving one or more convulsions, the differential diagnosis must involve (*a*) poisoning by a chlorinated hydrocarbon insecticide, (*b*) poisoning by some other kind of compound, including numerous drugs, (*c*) epilepsy, (*d*) convulsions secondary to infection, and (*e*) convulsions due to toxemia of pregnancy.

If substantial exposure to any chemical is suspected, every effort should be made to obtain samples that could confirm or refute a diagnosis of poisoning. This means that samples of vomit, stomach washings, urine and feces, blood, and food the patient was eating or materials actually used in preparing that food should also be saved for chemical analysis.

When it appears that convulsions are caused by a toxicant but the identity of the material is unknown, some hint of its nature may be obtained by careful observation of the patient. Convulsions caused by chlorinated hydrocarbon insecticides tend to appear early in the course of illness. The patient is unconscious during the convulsion, which resembles an epileptic fit except that no aura is present. The patient is left in a dazed state, but even during this period the vital signs are good, the immediate recovery is striking, and there is only a slight tendency for stimulation to induce a second convulsion. Convulsions caused by strychnine involve far more tonic spasm and opisthotonos than is ordinarily seen in poisoning by chlorinated hydrocarbon insecticides, and patients poisoned by strychnine remain conscious during the attack. Most convulsions associated with poisoning by organic phosphorus compounds occur late in the course of illness and are anoxic in origin. The patient is seriously ill before the convulsions begin, and the vital signs, especially respiration, are of poor quality. Of course, if convulsions continue and the patient's course is downhill, convulsions of any origin may be seen in a person with poor respiratory and cardiac function.

The presence of significant, febrile illness before the onset of convulsions tends to point to a diagnosis of infection. Fever can occur in connection with poisoning by chlorinated hydrocarbon insecticides (see Section 15.2.3.1), but it tends to start after convulsions, not before. Convulsions associated with infection are most common in babies still too young to explore and ingest poisons. In contrast, poisoning is most common between the ages of 1 and 3 years.

Poisoning by DDT is characterized by tremor early in the illness in a way that is not true of other chlorinated hydrocarbon insecticides (see Section 15.3.1.2). With this exception, it is essentially impossible to distinguish between the acute clinical pictures produced by sufficient dosages of the different chlorinated hydrocarbon insecticides without a history of exposure or analytical results.

The only chlorinated hydrocarbon insecticide that has caused chronic poisoning—but apparently no acute poisoning—is chlordecone, for which the clinical picture is quite different (see Section 15.7.2.3).

sible that DDA was not the only chlorinated organic compound present.

Later work by many authors has amply confirmed that DDA isomers are the major urinary metabolites of p,p'-DDT and o,p'-DDT in all mammals, including humans. It may be added that in spite of great strides in analytical chemistry, the nature of all excreted metabolites may not have been elucidated fully.

The ability of phenobarbital and especially diphenylhydantoin to promote the excretion of DDT was discovered in humans (Davies *et al.*, 1969) and later confirmed in animals (Cranmer, 1970; Alary *et al.*, 1971; Fries *et al.*, 1971).

The fact that DDE is stored in tissue was first demonstrated in connection with human fat (Pearce *et al.*, 1952; Mattson *et al.*, 1953). The authors did not know whether the compound resulted from partial degradation of DDT residues on plants or whether the DDE was formed during the process of digestion or after absorption. It is now known, using modern methods, that some of our food contains DDE but that humans are capable of forming the product from DDT.

That portion of the metabolism of DDT that leads to DDA in rats was explored by Peterson and Robinson (1964), who gave evidence for the sequence of changes leading to DDA involving reduction to 1,1-dichloro-2,2-bis(4-chlorophenyl)ethane (DDD) followed by dehydrochlorination to 1-chloro-2,2-bis(4-chlorophenyl)ethene (DDMU), which was apparently converted to 2,2-bis-(4-chlorophenyl)ethanol (DDOH) via 2,2-bis(4-chlorophenyl)ethene (DDNU). The compound identified by Peterson and Robinson (1964) as a "probable" intermediate aldehyde between p,p'-DDOH and p,p'-DDA was later synthesized and shown to be highly labile (McKinney *et al.*, 1969), confirming the guess by Peterson and Robinson that it is unlikely to accumulate in tissues in measurable amounts. Kujawa *et al.* (1985) have obtained evidence for its formation from p,p'-DDD by rat liver homogenates and its presence in the urine of rats injected with DDD. Abou-Donia and Menzel (1968) identified two additional metabolites, bis(*p*-chlorophenyl)methane (DDM) and bis(*p*-chlorophenyl) methyl ketone (DBP) in chicken eggs and young chicks. Not only was DBP found to result from the metabolism of DDA with DDM as an intermediate, but DBP was the only metabolite of DDE administered directly to eggs or chicks.

Organ perfusion studies indicated that the liver is capable of biotransformation of DDT, DDE, DDD, DDMU, and other possible metabolites (Datta and Nelson, 1970). Cultures of human embryonic lung cells are capable of metabolizing DDT to DDA via DDD (North and Menzer, 1973).

When DDA was discovered, it was postulated on chemical grounds that DDE was a step in its formation (White and Sweeney, 1945); however, rats which produced both DDE and DDA from DDT were said by Peterson and Robinson (1964) to be incapable of forming DDA when fed preformed DDE. This finding was contradicted by Datta (1970) and by Datta and Nelson (1970), who claimed that ^{14}C-labeled p,p'-DDE was converted by rats to 1-chloro-2,2-bis(4-chlorophenyl)ethene (p,p'-DDMU), which then underwent further metabolism to p,p'-DDA. Datta suggested that the predominance of detoxica-

tion via DDE or DDD may depend on physiological response or the amount of toxicant used. The fact remains that DDE is stored more tenaciously than DDT.

The way in which DDE is lost from storage remained something of a mystery. In humans (Cueto and Biros, 1967), seals, and guillemots (Jansson *et al.*, 1975) part of it is excreted unchanged, but the fact that its elimination is promoted by induction of microsomal enzymes (see Use Experience in Section 15.3.1.3) strongly suggested that it undergoes metabolism, conjugation, or both. That metabolism does occur was first demonstrated by identification of two hydroxylated derivatives of DDE in the feces of wild seals and guillemots and in the bile of seals (Jansson *et al.*, 1975). When p,p'-DDE was fed to rats, the same metabolites and one other were isolated from the feces, and within the first 6 days they accounted for about 5% of the dose (Sundström *et al.*, 1975). Later, a fourth hydroxylated derivative was identified from the feces of rats fed p,p'-DDE. The compounds are *m*-hydroxy-p,p'-DDE [1,1-dichloro-2-(*p*-chloro-*m*-hydroxyphenyl)-2,2(*p*-chlorophenyl)ethylene, the major metabolite], *o*-hydroxy-p,p'-DDE, *p*-hydroxy-m,p'-DDE (the product of an NIH shift), and *p*-hydroxy-p'-DDE. A scheme involving m,p-epoxy-p,p'-DDE and o,m'-epoxy-p,p'-DDE was proposed for the formation of these metabolites as well as a fifth metabolite (Sundström, 1977). Neither the fifth metabolite nor the hypothetical intermediates have been isolated. In mice, feeding DDE increased the hepatic levels of radioactivity from [^{14}C]DDE and decreased that in the urine and feces (Gold and Brunk, 1986). The only metabolite identified was the *o*-hydroxylated product.

DDE is metabolized not only to easily excretable phenols but also to *m*-methylsulfone-p,p'-DDE. In the blubber of seals from the Baltic, this compound was found in a concentration of 4 ppm along with DDE (138 ppm), DDD (10 ppm), DDT (78 ppm), and various polychlorinated biphenyls (PCBs) and their metabolites (150 ppm) (Jensen and Jansson, 1976). Sulfur-containing metabolites of halogenated aliphatic and aromatic chemicals usually arise by initial conjugation with glutathione. The possibility of glutathione-derived conjugates of DDT seems to be a virtually unexplored field.

Because DDT causes liver tumors, particularly in mice (See Table 15.7), some of the steps in its metabolism leading to reactive intermediates were studied with liver microsomal systems. The reductive declorination of p,p-DDT to DDD can occur with a cytochrome P-450 system, especially under anaerobic conditions (Hassall, 1971; Esaac and Matsumura, 1980; Zaidi, 1987). A one-electron reduction of DDT to the 1,1-dichloro-2,2-bis(*p*-chlorophenyl)ethyl radical seems to occur, followed by abstraction of a hydrogen atom, possibly from lipid, to give DDD (Kelner *et al.*, 1986). The reduction of DDT to DDD is stimulated by thiols in an unknown manner. The formation of an intermediate radical explains binding to microsomal lipid, especially under anaerobic conditions (Baker and Van Dyke, 1984). DDD, on the other hand, needs aerobic conditions for binding, implying that further metabolism is required. Other studies with mouse liver microsomes have shown the formation of 2,2-bis(*p*chlorophenyl)-1,2-ethanediol

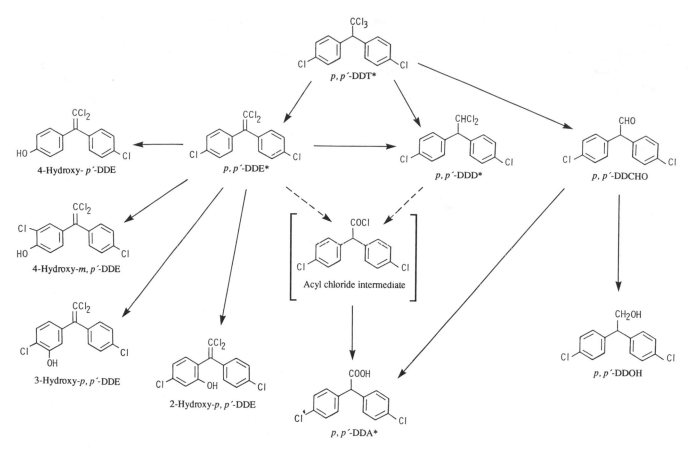

Figure 15.1 Metabolites of *p,p'*-DDT and the postulated route of metabolism in the rat. The metabolites indicated by an asterisk have been found in humans.

(DDNU-diol) from DDNU, suggesting that a reactive epoxide intermediate might be formed (Planche *et al.*, 1979). When synthesized, however, the ethylene oxide (DDNU-oxide) was not mutagenic.

In a series of papers, Gold and colleagues examined the metabolism of DDT metabolites in mice *in vivo*. The results seem to be a little different from that previously accepted for rats. It is thought that DDMU can undergo epoxidation; the resulting mutagenic epoxide is hydrolyzed and oxidized to 2-hydroxy-2,2-bis(4-chlorophenyl)acetic acid (αOH-DDA), which is excreted in the urine (Gold *et al.*, 1981; Gold and Brunk, 1982). Another route of metabolism of DDT in both the mouse and hamster (Gold and Brunk, 1982, 1983, 1984) seems to be the formation of DDA by a route involving hydroxylation on the C-1 side chain carbon of DDD (see Fig. 15.2). Loss of HCl gives an intermediate acyl chloride, 2,2-bis(4-chlorophenyl)acetyl chloride (Cl-DDA), capable of reacting with cellular proteins, DNA, etc. or losing water to give DDA.

Since this work, the metabolism of DDT in rats has been reexamined (Fawcett *et al.*, 1981, 1987) and seems to be similar to that described above for hamsters and mice. The conversion of *p,p'*-DDD to *p,p'*-DDA occurs primarily by hydroxylation leading to Cl-DDA, which on hydrolysis gives DDA. This acyl chloride may also be formed from DDE via an epoxidation route. Although DDMU is converted to DDA (Gold and

Brunk, 1984; Fawcett *et al.*, 1987), there is now considerable doubt as to whether it is an important intermediate in DDT metabolism. In addition, there is evidence to suggest that DDOH is a reduction product of DDCHO formed directly from DDT and not a precursor. A current scheme for the metabolism of *p,p'*-DDT in rats is shown in Fig. 15.1 and is still incomplete after nearly 40 years of study. However, it is possible that this will need to be amended. For instance, the role of DDOH still appears to be uncertain (Kujawa *et al.*, 1985).

The conversion of *o,p'*-DDT to *p,p'*-DDT has been reported (Klein *et al.*, 1965; French and Jefferies, 1969), but when the possibility was reinvestigated using ^{14}C-labeled *o,p'*-DDT, no conversion could be detected (Cranmer, 1972). The chromatographic peak closely resembling that of *p,p'*-DDT observed in the earlier studies undoubtedly is the result of a metabolite of *o,p'*-DDT.

The opposite conversion, namely biotransformation of *p,p'*-DDT or *p,p'*-DDD to the corresponding *o,p'*-compounds, has been reported in chicken egg and young chicks (Abou-Donia and Menzel, 1968) but has not been confirmed.

Compared to *p,p'*-DDT, the more rapid excretion of *o,p'*-DDT is explained at least in part by the observed ring hydroxylation of the parent compound in rats (Feil *et al.*, 1973) and chickens (Feil *et al.*, 1975) and of its metabolite *o,p'*-DDD in rats (Reif and Sinsheimer, 1975) and humans (Reif *et al.*, 1974)

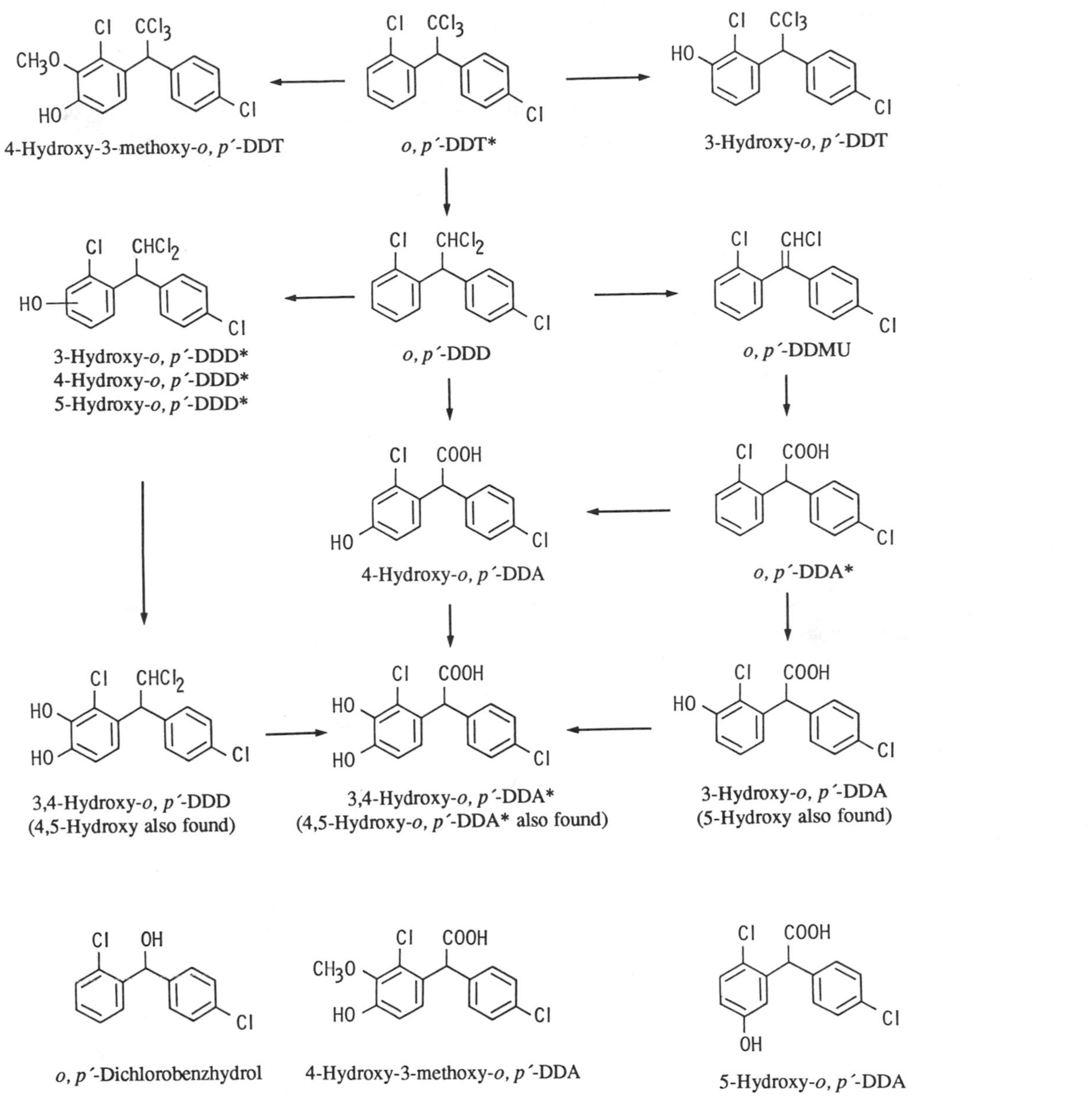

Figure 15.2 Metabolites of o,p'-DDT and the main derivative o,p'-DDD in rats. The sequence of metabolism shown may have to be evolved in light of recent investigations of p,p'-DDT metabolism. Compounds indicated by an asterisk have been found in humans, including those humans treated with large doses of o,p'-DDD. In rats, glycine and serine conjugates of o,p'-DDA have been found in the urine, and the aspartic acid conjugate of o,p'-DDA has been found in the feces.

(see Fig. 15.2). At least 13 metabolites were detected in rats and 15 in chickens. Ring hydroxylation, which has not been observed with p,p'-DDT or p,p'-DDD (but has been seen with p,p'-DDE), was present in all species. There were, however, some species differences. For example, o,p'-DDE and three hydroxylated o,p'-DDEs were found in the excreta of chickens but not in the excreta of rats. In two patients with adrenal carcinoma for which they were receiving o,p'-DDD at a rate of 2000 mg/day, as much as 46–56% of the daily intake was recovered in the urine following acid hydrolysis. Just over half of the recovered material was in the form of o,p'-DDA, but the remainder was in the form of hydroxylated derivatives, specifically m-hydroxy-, p-hydroxy-, m-hydroxy-p-methoxy-, and p-

hydroxy-m-methoxy-o,p'-DDA. Some other hydroxylated compounds were found in trace amounts. All hydroxylation had occurred on the ring that had its chlorine in the o position (Reif et al., 1974). When the metabolism of a single 100-mg oral dose of o,p'-[^{14}C]DDD was studied in rats, averages of 7.1 and 87.8% of the activity were recovered in the urine and feces, respectively, within 8 days (Reif and Sinsheimer, 1975). The high recovery indicated rapid excretion with little storage.

o,p-DDD is specifically toxic for the adrenal cortex in a number of species including humans. In vitro studies suggest that this is due to its activation in adrenal mitochondria to a metabolite which binds covalently. Unlike the situation in liver, a metabolite more polar than DDA is also produced

(Martz and Straw, 1977, 1980; Pohland and Counsell, 1985). Recently, Lund *et al.* (1988) have shown that 3-methysulfonyl-*f,f*-DDE is selectively covalently bound and toxic to the adrenal zona fasciculata of mice. A similar situation may prevail to account for the covalent binding of *o,p*-DDD in mouse lung (Lund *et al.*, 1986, 1989) and may be related to the acyl chloride formation already reported for *p,p'*-DDT in rats and mice (Fig. 15.1).

Of the compounds shown in Figs. 15.1 and 15.2, only DDT, DDD, DDE, and DDA commonly are reported in the tissues or excreta of animals, including humans. A novel finding has been the identification of conjugates of DDOH with fatty acids in the livers and spleens of rats given DDT (Leighty *et al.*, 1980). They can be removed *in vivo* by treatment with bile salts, heparin, or lecithin (Leighty, 1981).

Although microorganisms, plants, insects, and birds produce many of the same metabolites found in mammals, there are interesting differences. Nearly 20 derivatives (including mammalian metabolites) have been identified, and the chemical structures of several more are still unknown. Some aspects of nonmammalian, as well as mammalian, metabolism have been reviewed (Menzie, 1969; Klein and Korte, 1970; Fishbein, 1974; Schroeder and Dorozalska, 1975; Korte, 1979). The metabolism of microorganisms and plants, as well as that of domestic animals, may influence the composition of DDT-derived residues in human food, but there is no evidence that these residues contain a significant amount of any compound not formed from DDT by human metabolism. In view of recent developments in the field of *p,p'*-DDT metabolism, it is possible that in the future the metabolism of *o,p'*-DDT as shown in Fig. 15.2 may have to be amended.

Excretion   When large doses of DDT are ingested, some of the compound is unabsorbed and is passed in unaltered state in the feces. Only traces of unaltered DDT may be found in the feces when exposure is by any route other than oral. However, true fecal excretion of DDT metabolites was established irrespective of the route of administration (Hayes, 1965). In humans the ratio is obviously different. Although the excretion of DDT-related material in the feces of humans receiving 35 mg/person/day has been studied using colorimetry (Hayes *et al.*, 1956), this result has never been confirmed by gas chromatography, even in connection with workers whose exposure was heavy and prolonged (Hayes, 1982). Either DDT metabolites are not excreted by humans in the feces to any important degree, or they are excreted in one or more forms different from those already demonstrated in rats.

The bile appears to be the principal source of DDT metabolites in the feces of rats. When the bile duct was cannulated before intravenous injection of radioactive DDT, 65% of the dose was recovered in the bile, 2% in the urine, and only 0.3% in the feces (Jensen *et al.*, 1957), and the possibility of some contamination of the feces by urine could not be excluded.

The different routes of excretion are not unrelated. Burns *et al.* (1957) found that there was an increase in urinary excretion of radioactive material following ligation of the bile duct in rats fed radioactive DDT. This is an indirect confirmation of the finding by Jensen and his colleagues that most of the metabolites in bile are DDA or closely related to it. Although an enterohepatic circulation of the metabolites of DDT has not been proved directly, it seems likely that such a circulation exists, as has been demonstrated for ethylan. The difference between the excretion of DDT and its metabolites in rats and the slower excretion in birds seems to be the reduced ability of birds to further metabolize DDE and convert DDD to DDA (Fawcett *et al.*, 1981). The excretion of DDE in rats is dependent on dose and probably involves induction of drug-metabolizing systems (Ando, 1982).

Demonstration of excretion of DDT in milk was first published by Woodard *et al.* (1945) in connection with a dog fed at the rate of 80 mg/kg/day. Within a short time, excretion of DDT in milk was reported in rats, goats, and cows, and in 1951 it was demonstrated in women (Lang *et al.*, 1951). Telford and Guthrie (1945) reported that rats fed a diet containing 1000 ppm produced milk toxic to their young.

Since the early laboratory studies, the presence of DDT has been demonstrated repeatedly in the milk of cows. A review (Hayes, 1959a) showed that cows fed substantial, but nontoxic, residues of DDT commonly excrete 10% or slightly more of the total dose in their milk, and amounts slightly more than 30% have been observed.

The proportion of the mother's DDT intake that could be recovered from her milk varied from 12.6 to 30.2% and averaged 24.6% in rats receiving the compound from their diet at an average rate of 32.4 mg/kg/day. Under these circumstances, the dosage of the young was somewhat less than half of that of their mothers on a milligram per kilogram basis. The oral dosage of 32.4 mg/kg/day was well tolerated by both dams and pups, as was also true of an intraperitoneal dosage of 100 mg/kg/day. An intraperitoneal dosage of 200 mg/kg/day killed some dams, but most of the pups of other dams survived. All of the pups of these mothers experienced reduced milk intake and reduced weight gain. The concentration of DDT in the brains of these pups was much lower than in pups killed by oral administration of the compound, indicating that the young of mothers receiving massive dosages of DDT suffer malnutrition but not poisoning (Hayes, 1976b).

Wilson *et al.* (1946) showed that DDT was secreted from the skin of a cow maintained on an oral dosage of about 53 mg/kg/day.

Because DDA is the main form in which DDT is excreted, it might be expected that, following its direct administration, DDA would be excreted relatively efficiently, and this is true. It was found very early that, during the first several days after oral dosing, rabbits excreted DDA in the urine approximately 15 times faster than animals given DDT at an equivalent dosage. Although the rate of DDA excretion increased somewhat, the rate of excretion associated with DDT increased more rapidly, so that the values differed by a factor of only 5 after day 20 of feeding (Smith *et al.*, 1946).

Biochemical Effects   There is reason to think that the mechanism of action of DDT is its effect on membranes in the nervous system, especially axonal membranes. Certainly, action on membranes is a fundamental property of the compound. Its action on conductance in an inanimate membrane and in the membranes of the giant axons of cockroaches and lobsters is discussed in Section 4.1.2.3. The effect on axons may be related to inhibition of Na^+-, K^+-, and Mg^{2+}-adenosine triphosphatase derived from a nerve ending fraction of rabbit brain that is inhibited by DDT and is discussed in the same section. A similar enzyme that binds [^{14}C]DDT has been isolated from the synapses of rat brain (Bratowski and Matsumura, 1972). There has been considerable interest in a Ca-ATPase which may regulate calcium levels at the axon surface (Ghiasuddin and Matsumura, 1979), and DDT is known to cause prolonged opening of the ion gates of the sodium channel perhaps by affecting phosphorylation in the α-subunit protein (Ishikawa *et al.,* 1989).

At a supralethal dosage of 600 mg/kg, DDT caused in rats a marked decrease in the concentration of cortical and striatal acetylcholine and of brain stem norepinephrine and a significant increase in brain stem 3-methoxy-6-hydroxyphenylglycol and 5-hydroxyindoleacetic acid (Hrdina *et al.,* 1973; Hudson *et al.,* 1985; Tilson *et al.,* 1986). *p*-Chlorophenylalanine blocked all of the neurotoxic signs of poisoning, and other inhibitors blocked one or another but not all of the effects. It was concluded that changes in the metabolism of 5-hydroxytryptamine and norepinephrine may be responsible for DDT-induced hypothermia and acetylcholine may be related to tremors and convulsions (Hrdina *et al.,* 1973). However, the situation is complex and many factors are involved (Herr *et al.,* 1985, 1986; Hudson *et al.,* 1985). Although spinal α,-adrenoceptors have been proposed as modulating DDT-induced tremor (Herr and Tilson, 1987) attenuation of DDT-induced motor dysfunction requires blockade of α, adrenoceptors in region other than solely the spinal cord (Herr *et al.,* 1989). At a lower dose of DDT (180 mg/kg), but one which still induced convulsive tremor, acetylcholine and cyclic GMP were increased in the cerebellum (Aldridge *et al.,* 1978). In adult rats and mice there is a decrease in the cholinergic muscarinic receptors of rat brain (Eriksson *et al.,* 1984), particularly in the cerebellum (Fonseca *et al.,* 1986). A particularly interesting finding is that the palmitic acid conjugate of DDOH can also have this effect (Eriksson and Nordberg, 1986). Disturbances of brain lipid metabolism have been observed in monkeys after chronic exposure to DDT (Sanyal *et al.,* 1986). Khaikina and Shilina (1971) reported that administration of DDT to rats at only one-fifth of the LD 50 for 20 days increased by 188% the amount of 5-hydroxyindoleacetic acid excreted in their urine. This indicated a change in the metabolism of serotonin, but probably does not support a serotonin deficiency as a DDT mode of action (Chung Hwang and Van Woert, 1981).

It is evident that many of the side effects of DDT are the result of its induction of microsomal enzymes. Both the dosage response and the morphological aspects and implications of this induction are discussed in Section 15.2.3.2. Background information on the biochemical aspects of induction of microsomal enzymes by DDT and other pesticides has been reviewed earlier (see Sections 3.1.2 and 3.1.3 and Table 3.6). The following additional observations are of interest.

Oral administration of *o,p'*-DDT to dogs at a rate of 50 mg/kg/day stimulates the microsomal enzymes of the liver as indicated by increase in liver size, total protein, microsomal protein, and cytochrome P-450 concentration and by direct measurements of enzyme activity. These changes in the liver are initially accompanied by an increase in the size of the adrenals and of the cells of the zona fasciculata; these cells become vacuolated and devoid of acidophilic cytoplasm, and their nuclei become hyperchromatic and often peripheral in position. Synthesis of corticosteroids by the adrenal is not blocked (Copeland and Cranmer, 1974). Thus, the effect of a substantial dosage of *o,p'*-DDT is quite different from that of *o,p'*-DDD, although part of the metabolism of *o,p'*-DDT must be by that route.

The tissue level of DDE necessary to induce liver microsomal enzymes is lower in the rat than in the quail (and presumably other birds). Thus Bunyan *et al.* (1972), using residues in the heart as an index, found a maximal increase in cytochrome P-450 per gram of liver and a maximal activity of aniline hydroxylase levels at tissue levels of approximately 3 ppm DDE in rats and 40 ppm DDE in quail. However, at any given dietary level, higher tissue levels were reached by quail than by rats, so the dosage responses of the two were similar. These authors concluded that DDE is more important than DDT in inducing microsomal enzymes, but in humans the opposite appears to be true (see Use Experience in Section 15.3.1.3).

In squirrel monkeys (and presumably in other species) only 2 days on a vitamin C-deficient diet impairs both the induction of *O*-demethylase and the stimulation of the glucuronic acid system by DDT (5 mg/monkey/day) (Chadwick *et al.,* 1971b). In guinea pigs, maintenance of induction of microsomal enzymes requires a higher dietary level of vitamin C than does prevention of scurvy (Wagstaff and Street, 1971a).

The association of lipids with the function of microsomal enzymes is recognized generally, as is the fact that DDT induces these enzymes. Therefore, it might have been expected that DDT and essential fatty acids would interact. Tinsley and Lowry (1972) found that the growth of female rats receiving *p,p'*-DDT at a dietary level of 150 ppm was depressed if they received a diet deficient in essential fatty acids but was slightly stimulated if they received the same diet supplemented with these acids. Another parameter influenced by the same variables was the ratio of various liver lipids. The changes in fatty acid composition were related to the proliferation of hepatic smooth endoplasmic reticulum; it was suggested that DDT influenced essential fatty acid metabolism by increasing the demand for them. Sampson *et al.* (1980) found that DDT did not exacerbate aspects of essential fatty acid deficiency but did alter lipid metabolism in an unexplained way.

In contrast, a variety of diets (containing fats that may occur in the human diet and that were in approximately the same proportion as fats in typical human food in the United States had little or no influence on the storage of DDT and a wide range of pesticides fed to rats for four generations in combination at rates only 200 times those found in the Market Basket Study of food in the United States (Adams *et al.*, 1974). Fat mobilization can cause rapid release of stored DDT, but this does not seem to be associated with any major toxic effect assessed pathologically or biochemically (Mitjavila *et al.*, 1981b).

DDT has been shown *in vitro* and sometimes *in vivo* to influence some enzymes of intermediary metabolism and other miscellaneous enzymes. For instance, DDT and a variety of analogs have been shown to affect isolated rat liver mitochondria but the significance of this *in vivo* is uncertain (Ohyama *et al.*, 1982). So far evidence is lacking that the degree of this inhibition in the intact organism is sufficient to have any influence on function.

The hyperglycemia observed during much of the early part of acute poisoning may be associated with an increase in four gluconeogenic enzymes (pyruvate carboxylase, phosphoenolpyruvate carboxykinase, fructose-1,6-diphosphatase, and glucose-6-phosphatase). Increase in these enzymes in the renal cortex of rats has been observed after a single dose at a rate as low as 100 mg/kg or greater or following 45 daily doses at rates of 5 or 25 mg/kg/day. The changes are not mediated through release of corticosteroids from the adrenal glands (Kacew and Singhal, 1973). The fact that 100 mg/kg is the smallest single dosage that produced a statistically significant change in these enzymes indicates that their alteration is a complication rather than a cause of poisoning.

A review (Hayes, 1959a) of early literature indicates that high concentrations of DDT inhibit phosphatidase, muscle phosphatases, carbon anhydrase, and oxaloacetic carboxylase and increase the activity of cytochrome oxidase and succinic dehydrogenase. However, none of these changes with the possible exception of inhibition of carbonic anhydrase could be shown to have any connection with the toxic action of DDT or even with its side effects. Neal *et al.* (1944) reported a small but consistent increase in the volume of urine excreted in 24 hr when dogs were dosed orally or by insufflation at the rate of 100 mg/kg/day. No other change in the urine and no change in kidney function was demonstrated. The possibility that increased urinary output is related to the inhibition of carbonic anhydrase (Torda and Wolff, 1949) may deserve attention. However, reexamination of data from volunteers receiving 3.5 or 35 mg/person/day indicated no increase in urinary volume compared with controls (Hayes *et al.*, 1971).

On the other hand, many enzymes including plasma amylase, aldylase, glutamic-pyruvic transaminase, and isocitric dehydrogenase were not changed in squirrel monkeys given dosages from 0.05 to 50 mg/kg/day, the latter of which proved fatal within 14 weeks (Cranmer *et al.*, 1972).

Effects on the Nervous System The major toxic action of DDT is clearly on the nervous system, probably by slowing down closing of "gates" in axon sodium channels (Dubois and Bergman, 1977; Woolley, 1982, 1985; Hong *et al.*, 1986), and it requires an intact organism for full expression. The fact that DDT causes a myotonic response in muscle and substitution of a train of spikes for the normal diphasic electroneurogram (Eyzaguirre and Lilienthal, 1949) is in marked contrast to the absence of detectable injury or, in fact, any response in other isolated tissues. As early as 1945, Lewis and Richards found DDT to be inert when it was exposed to tissue cultures of heart, kidney, stomach and intestine, liver, and muscle from 7- to 9-day chick embryos and of brain and spleen from a 1-day rat. The physiology of the cells including the mitoses of fibroblasts was normal. The migration and extension of the various cells were unchanged. The authors stated that "living fibrilloblasts, as they moved about in the cultures, sometimes touched or even migrated over DDT crystals without appreciable injury to themselves during a period of several days." Some observations were carried out for periods as great as 21 days.

In spite of the importance of the nervous system, a detailed review of early literature indicates that although the presence of some specialized nervous function may be necessary for the manifestation of DDT poisoning, the mere occurrence of specialized nervous fibers in certain protozoa or the occurrence of a rather complex nervous system in mollusks is not sufficient to render these forms susceptible. Just as there is no explanation for the effect of DDT in susceptible species, so there is no explanation for the fact that certain species and even entire phyla are inherently resistant to the compound.

A review (Hayes, 1959a) of literature on the effects of DDT on the nervous system reveals that all major parts, both central and peripheral, are affected. Whereas effects on specific portions, notably the cerebellum and the motor cortex, have been viewed as of greatest importance, it probably is more accurate to emphasize the interaction of functions, all modified to some degree.

One sensitive measure of brain activity is the electrocorticogram. Farkas *et al.* (1968) found that the wave frequency showed considerable increase in resting rats that had received 20 mg/kg/day as a result of dietary intake. Rats that had received 5 mg/kg/day did not exhibit this change while at rest, but even these exhibited abnormalities when exposed to a rhythmic light stimulus. Electrical activity may become abnormal only a minute or two after administration of a large dose of DDT; four stages culminating in generalized seizures have been described by Joy (1973). Phenobarbital, but not diphenylhydantoin or trimethadione, was effective in stopping seizures.

The most characteristic effect of DDT in contrast to dieldrin, for example, is the production of tremor. Sufficient dosages of DDT produce tremor even at ambient temperatures that approach body heat. However, dosages of DDT that produce no other clinical effect make rats more sensitive to low temperatures, and this sensitivity may be demonstrated conveniently by having the rats swim to exhaustion in cool water. The ability of a rat to keep afloat is more dependent on coordination than on physical strength.

It was found that normal rats can swim for over 100 min in water 25°C or warmer but for only about 30 min at 23°C and less than 10 min at 15°C. At any given temperature, male rats could swim longer than females. Of the temperatures studied, the effect of DDT was most striking at 25°C; normal females swam for 117 min, whereas those that had received a dietary level of 50 ppm (2.62 mg/kg/day) swam only an average of 7 min. At 27°C, both groups of rats swam over 120 min, and at 37°C the swimming time of rats on a dietary level of 200 ppm approached or equaled that of normal animals. In order to expedite testing, the conditions were standardized at a water temperature of 19.9–20.2°C, and 0.006% sodium lauryl sulfate was added to the water to reduce the trapping of air in the fur, which tends to buoy up rats and permit them to swim longer. Under these conditions, the swimming time of normal animals averaged about 12 min when they were first tested but approached 16 min within a month if the animals were tested repeatedly. If DDT was fed for 2 weeks starting after the rats had become accustomed to swimming, those at a dietary level of 20 ppm showed a reduction in swimming time that was of questionable statistical significance. Those at a dietary level of 50 ppm showed a gradual decrease in swimming time during the 2-week exposure period and failed to return to the endurance of the controls in over a month after dosing was stopped. At dietary levels of 150 and 400 ppm, there was a sharp reduction in swimming time (to 7.3 and 4.0 min, respectively) on the first day of dosing, followed by a gradual decline during the remaining 13 days of dosing and then a slow, incomplete return toward normal (Hayes, 1982).

When measured by the same device 4 min after rats had swum to exhaustion, the tremor of a rat on a dietary level of 200 ppm involved much more energy than that of a normal rat, but the frequencies of the tremors were essentially identical—13–15/sec. In spite of the difference in energy, it appears likely that the tremorigenic action of DDT involves toxicity to that portion of the brain responsible for the control of ordinary shivering. In any event, the presence of tremor depends largely on the temperature of the head. This was demonstrated by Dr. Carl Rothe by placing a rat's head through a hole in a rubber sheet so that the rubber fit snugly about the neck and then varying the temperature of the head and the body relatively independently by separate sprays of either warm or cold water in front of and behind the sheet.

Like tremor, the coldness of the skin and ruffling of the fur seen in acute poisoning probably represent an indication of disturbed thermal regulation. Apparently, it was not until the work of Hrdina et al. (1975) that an increase of almost 3°C in body temperature was reported in rats following a fatal (600 mg/kg) oral dosage of DDT.

The central nervous systems of mice and hamsters are equally sensitive, the concentration of DDT in their brains at death being similar. However, after an oral dosage of 500 mg/kg, the DDT concentration of the mouse brain was twice that of the hamster. This cannot be explained by a difference in absorption, metabolism, or excretion but apparently is due to a difference in permeability of the blood–brain barriers of the two species.

When animals received DDT at a dietary level of 205 ppm for 6 weeks, the residues in fat and liver were seven to eight times higher in the mouse, a fact only partially explained by the greater food intake of mice relative to body weight. Although urinary excretion of $[^{14}C]$DDT was similar in previously unexposed hamsters and mice, this excretion was stimulated in the hamster but little affected in the mouse by previous dietary exposure to DDT (Gingell and Wallcave, 1974).

Mice also differ from rats in their hormonal regulation of the basic activity of hepatic microsomal mixed-function enzymes as well as in the response of these enzymes to inducers (Chhabra and Fouts, 1974).

Cause of Death Death from DDT poisoning is usually the result of respiratory arrest. The heart continues to beat to the end and in some instances continues a little while after respiration stops. Deichmann et al. (1950) found that the onset of hyperirritability was accompanied by an increase in the frequency and amplitude of respiration. Later, with the occurrence of tremors, the depth of respiration frequently returned to a more normal level, but the rate remained high. In some animals respiration stopped suddenly after a deep inspiration during a tonic convulsion. In other animals the rate and amplitude decreased progressively and finally ceased without any terminal spasm. Animals that die of respiratory failure caused by DDT do so after a relatively long period of muscular activity that leaves them exhausted.

It was shown by Philips and Gilman (1946) and Philips et al. (1946) that the hearts of dogs given large intravenous doses of DDT were sensitized to epinephrine. This was true not only of injected epinephrine but also of the compound released by the adrenal glands during a seizure. Stimulated in this way, the sensitized hearts of dogs developed an irreversible, fatal ventricular fibrillation. However, the hearts of monkeys were able to recover from fibrillation and resume normal rhythm. It is not clear how important sensitization of the myocardium is when DDT is administered by other routes, but ventricular fibrillation may be the cause of death in animals that die suddenly soon after onset of poisoning.

Thus, DDT not only sensitizes the myocardium in a way similar to that of halogenated hydrocarbon solvents but also, through its action on the central nervous system, produces the stimulus that increases the likelihood of fibrillation.

There is no evidence that repeated, tolerated doses of DDT sensitize the heart. Rats were fed DDT at a dietary level of 200 ppm (about 10 mg/kg/day) for 8 months, during which they received weekly intraperitoneal doses of vasopressin, a compound which causes a temporary myocardial ischemia. Electrocardiograms showed no significant increase in cardiac arrhythmias in the DDT-fed rats compared with controls. Intravenous noradrenaline given at the end of the 8-month period did not produce a greater incidence of arrhythmias in the DDT-fed rats. The same results were obtained in rabbits treated in essentially the same way (Jeyaratnam and Forshaw, 1974).

Mutation and Carcinogenesis DDT has been tested in a number of ways for possible mutational effect. Much of this work has been reviewed in detail together with most of the carcinogenicity studies shown in Table 15.7 (Coulston, 1985). For example, Shirasu et al. (1976) listed DDT as a negative chemical in microbial mutagenicity screening studies on 166 pesticides. The test system consisted of rec-assay utilizing H 17 Rec $^+$ and M 45 Rec $^-$ strains of *Bacillus subtilis* and reversion assays without metabolic activation using auxotrophic strains of *Escherichia coli* (WP 2) and *Salmonella typhimurium* (Ames series). The further studies with metabolic activation failed to reveal mutagenicity of DDT (Shirasu et al., 1977). McCann et al. (1975) and McCann and Ames (1976) reported negative results on DDE in *S. typhimurium* testing with metabolic activation.

At a dosage of 105 mg/kg it produced no increase of dominant lethals in mice (Epstein and Shafner, 1968). However, concentrations of 10 ppm or greater produced chromosome breaks and exchange figures in a marsupial somatic cell line (Palmer et al., 1972). Saturated solutions produced chromosome breaks in the root tips of onion and other plants (Vaarama, 1947). A slight mutagenic effect in mammals has been reported by Markarian (1966). Deletions plus gaps were reported to be more common in the chromosomes of mice that had received DDT. On the whole, *in vitro* tests of the mutagenicity of DDT have given only negative or dubious results (Coulston, 1985).

An unconventional test for mutagenicity involved examination of explants of pulmonary tissue from embryonic mice whose dams had been fed dietary concentrations of 10 and 50 ppm DDT. An increase of diffuse hyperplasia and focal proliferation was observed, but a dosage–response relationship was not clear. Some of the embryos were allowed to live and the experiment was repeated in subsequent generations. There was no continuing progression of the reported changes in succeeding generations (Shabad et al., 1972).

DDT causes inhibition of intercellular communication in cultured rat liver cells (Williams et al., 1981) and in hamster lung fibroblasts (Wärngård et al., 1985, 1987, 1988) like other chlorinated chemicals. The exact significance of the effect is unknown, but it does not seem to involve direct activation of protein kinase C, unlike 12-o-tetradecanoylphorbol-13-acetate (Wärngård et al., 1989). o,p'-DDT supports the growth of an estrogen-responsive tumor (Robison et al., 1985a).

The question of whether DDT is carcinogenic really seems to be restricted to its action in the liver of some rodents. This matter and its relation to the induction of liver microsomal enzymes by DDT, by other chlorinated hydrocarbon insecticide, and by phenobarbital is discussed in Section 15.2.3.2. Some of the positive findings shown in Table 15.7 have not been found in other studies [National Cancer Institute (NCI), 1978a]. However, there is still the evidence that DDT can act as a promoter of carcinogenesis initiated by aflatoxin and of other chemicals *in vitro* and *in vivo* (Peraino et al., 1975; Schulte-Hermann, 1985; Rojanapo et al., 1987).

Other Miscellaneous Effects on Organs and Tissues The effects of DDT and other chlorinated hydrocarbon insecticides on the liver are discussed in Section 15.2.3.2.

Many early reports reviewed by Hayes (1959a) indicate that large doses of DDT may have no effect on the blood or they may produce a moderate leukocytosis and a decrease in hemoglobin, with or without a decrease in the concentration of red cells. The leukocytosis probably is secondary to stimulation of the sympathetic nervous system, while the loss of hemoglobin may be nutritional in origin. Later study has not confirmed the early results. A range of hematologic parameters remained unchanged in squirrel monkeys dosed orally at rates of 0, 0.05, 0.5, 5, and 50 mg/kg/day, even though the highest dosage was fatal within 14 weeks (Cranmer et al., 1972).

Average protein-bound iodine (PBI) levels of 5.42 and 6.93 μg/%, respectively, were reported in the sera of 42 workers occupationally exposed to chlorinated hydrocarbon insecticides and 51 workers not so exposed. The difference was statistically significant even though all values fell within the normal range of 4–8 μg/% (Wassermann et al., 1971). It was not recorded whether the workers involved were from the same factory as those with 10 or more years of occupational exposure whose plasma DDT levels were reported by M. Wassermann et al (1970a). The small difference in PBI levels is difficult to evaluate. Goldman (1981) has reported that after a single large dose (100 mg/kg) to rats thyroidal ^{131}I release was completely inhibited for more than 12 hr. It was the view of Clifford and Weil (1972) that there was no evidence that occupational exposure to DDT has had any effect on human endocrine organs.

The possibility that some pesticides, including DDT, are probiotic has been discussed in Section 2.4.14. Although this general question remains open, one group of investigators has shown clearly that what at first appeared to be an immunological response really involved a quite different, predictable effect. Briefly, it was shown that guinea pigs sensitized to diphtheria toxoid were less susceptible to anaphylaxis in response to a challenge dose of the toxoid if they were pretreated with DDT at a dosage of only 10–20 mg/kg/day. Direct measurement of antitoxin production indicated little or no difference between protected and unprotected animals. Furthermore, some protection was given by DDT administered for only 3 days prior to the induction of anaphylaxis (Gabliks et al., 1973, 1975). Further study showed that DDT treatment reduced the histamine levels in the lungs of both immunized and nonimmunized animals. The number of detectable mast cells was also reduced; this was true whether the count was made in tissues from guinea pigs dosed systemically with DDT or in lungs and mesenteries from untreated animals exposed to DDT *in vitro* at concentrations ranging from 10 to 45 ppm. These results indicated that the protection offered by DDT was the result of a reduction of the amount of histamine available for sudden release in response to a challenge dose of toxoid (Askari and Gabliks, 1973). Regardless of exposure to DDT, immunization leads to an increase in detectable mast cells (Gabliks et al., 1975). DDT has been reported to cause acute renal failure in rats after intravenous infusion (Koschier et al., 1980).

Effects on Reproduction It was shown very early (Burlington and Linderman, 1950) that DDT produces a striking inhibition of testicular growth and secondary sexual characteristics of cockerels when injected subcutaneously in dosages as high as 300 mg/kg/day. Changes in the testis involve the tubules and not the interstitial tissues, and they have been attributed to an estrogen-like action of DDT.

It must be noted that the action of DDT on the testis of chickens is dosage related. Before the problem of residues became evident, DDT was used extensively for control of lice and common mites on chickens without any adverse effects on egg production or other aspects of reproduction. Many rats would be killed the first day if they were given the dosage of DDT that has been shown to affect the testis of cockerels. The report that under special conditions DDT has a gonadotoxic effect (Rybakova, 1968) is of questionable significance in view of the results of multigeneration tests in rats, mice, and dogs. Dean *et al.* (1980) were unable to demonstrate any changes in either serum androgens or testicular synthesis of testosterone in young rats after exposure to DDT despite significant induction of metabolism of testosterone by isolated hepatic microsomes.

Intraperitoneal injection of as little as 5 mg/kg of technical DDT or 1 mg/kg of *o,p'*-DDT causes a significant increase in weight of the uterus of normal immature female rats or of ovariectomized adult females. A much smaller stimulation is caused by *p,p'*-DDT. Treatment of rats with DDT, especially *o,p'*-DDT, 2 hr before injection of [6,7-^{3}H] estradiol-17 inhibited uptake of the hormone by the uterus *in vivo,* possibly by competition for binding sites. Isomers of DDD and DDE do not influence uterine weight or the binding of estradiol (Welch *et al.,* 1969). It seems unlikely that metabolic activation of *o,p'*-DDT is necessary as is true of *o,p'*-methoxychlor (Kupfer and Bulger, 1979). The action of *o,p'*-DDT on the uterus seems to be as a long-acting agonistic estrogen interacting with the same receptor as 17β-estradiol and causing the formation of the so-called induced protein (Ireland *et al.,* 1980; Robison *et al.,* 1984; Galand *et al.,* 1987). However, some differences from estradiol have been recorded (Robison *et al.,* 1985b). The lesser enantiomer of *o,p'*-DDT seems to be the active isomer (McBlain, 1987). The binding and estrogenic activity of DDT analogs in rats is only about 1/10,000 as great as that of diethylstilbestrol (Nelson, 1973).

A considerably smaller dosage of *o,p'*-DDT resulting from a dietary level of 10 ppm for 2–9 months had no effect on reproduction in ewes (Wrenn *et al.,* 1971b). In a similar way, dietary levels of *o,p'*-DDT as high as 40 ppm, giving a dosage level of about 2.1 mg/kg/day in rats, failed to interfere with reproduction and lactation in these animals, although dosage was continued through two pregnancies (Wrenn *et al.,* 1971a).

The report (Heinricks *et al.,* 1971) that *o,p'*-DDT significantly advances puberty, induces persistent vaginal estrus after a period of normal estrous cycles, and causes other reproductive abnormalities in female rats would at first appear inconsistent with the lack of effect of technical DDT or of *o,p'*-DDT on reproduction cited above. The same is true of other effects of *o,p'*-DDT demonstrated by the same investigators (Gellert *et al.,* 1972). The abnormal effects were obtained initially by injecting 1 mg of the *o,p'*-DDT subcutaneously on the second, third, and fourth days of life (counting the day of birth as zero). Because rat pups on the third day weight about 12 gm or less

each, it follows that the subcutaneous dosage was about 83.3 mg/kg/day or more, that is, about 40 times greater than the highest oral dosage of *o,p'*-isomer fed to breeding rats and about 10^5 times greater than what ordinary people get in their food.

Ottoboni (1969) found that female rats reproduced normally when fed DDT for two generations at dietary levels as high as 200 ppm (about 10 mg/kg/day except during lactation, when intake is increased about threefold). In fact, at a dietary level of 20 ppm, the dams had a significantly longer reproductive life span (14.55 months) than their littermate controls (8.91 months); the number of females becoming pregnant after the age of 17 months and the number of successful pregnancies after that age were significantly different in the two groups (Ottoboni, 1972).

In a study focused mainly on DDT in milk, the full ability of rats to reproduce at a dietary level of 200 ppm was confirmed, and the ability of dams injected intraperitoneally at levels as high as 100 mg/kg/day to rear their young was demonstrated (Hayes, 1976b).

A six-generation test of reproduction in mice showed no effect of DDT at a dietary level of 25 ppm on fertility, gestation, viability, lactation, and survival. A level of 100 ppm produced a slight reduction in lactation and survival in some generations but not all, and the effect was not progressive. A level of 250 ppm was distinctly injurious to reproduction (Keplinger *et al.,* 1970). The dietary concentrations used determine dosages of 3.33, 13.3, and 33.2 mg/kg/day in nonpregnant, nonlactating, adult, female mice. The intake is much higher in both young and lactating mice. The authors concluded that their study provided no obvious reason for continuing reproduction tests for more than three generations.

Four female dogs of unstated age that previously had received DDT at the rate of 12 mg/kg/day, 5 days/week, for 14 months were bred when they went into heat. The males involved had been fed aldrin (0.15 mg/kg/day) plus DDT (60 mg/kg/day) for 14 months prior to breeding but not during breeding. Two of the females went into heat but failed to become pregnant, and one failed to come into heat during 12 months after feeding stopped. Four of six pups born to the fourth female died within 1 week of birth; the other two were weaned successfully even though only two posterior mammae of the mother were functional (Deichmann *et al.,* 1971b). A three-generation study failed to confirm any of the injuries suggested by the study of four dogs. In the three-generation study, male and female dogs were fed technical DDT from weaning at rates of 0, 1, 5, and 10 mg/kg/day. Observations were made on 135 adult females, 63 adult males, and 650 pups. There were no statistically significant differences among controls and DDT-treated dogs in length of gestation, fertility, success of pregnancy, litter size, or lactation ability of the dams; in viability at birth, survival to weaning, sex distribution, and growth of pups; or in morbidity, mortality, organ/body weight ratios, or gross histological abnormalities in all the animals studied. The only clear difference was that DDT-treated females had their first estrus 2 or 3 months earlier than the control dogs. There was a slight increase in liver/body weight ratio in some DDT-treated animals but the difference was not statistically significant, not dosage-related, and not associated with any histological change (Ottoboni *et al.*, 1977).

When *p,p'*-DDT was administered to pregnant mice at a rate of 1 mg/kg on days 10, 12, and 17 of gestation, it was not teratogenic but did alter the gonads and decrease the fertility of the young, especially the females (McLachlan and Dixon, 1972). A single dose at the rate of 15 mg/kg or repeated doses of 2.5 mg/kg/day given during pregnancy may be embryotoxic but not teratogenic to mice (Schmidt, 1973). Why one or a few doses during pregnancy may be embryotoxic although the same dosage is harmless when administered during the entire reproductive period is of theoretical but no practical importance.

Teratogenic effects of DDT have not been seen in studies of reproduction, including those for two generations in rats, six generations in mice, and three generations in dogs.

Because of the estrogenic properties of large doses of DDT, the compound was considered as a possible cause of abortion in dairy cattle, but no evidence for a relationship was found (Macklin and Ribelin, 1971). A similar conclusion was reached regarding human abortions (O'Leary *et al.*, 1970).

Behavioral Effects Behavioral changes may be demonstrated in animals receiving DDT daily at rates too low to produce illness. Khairy (1959) was able to detect ataxia in the form of changes in gait in rats that had been fed DDT at dietary levels of 100 ppm or more for 21 days. The results were recorded in terms of the tangent, that is, the ratio of the width and length of step. At a dosage of about 5 mg/kg/day the ratio was less than normal, a change attributed to an exaggeration of the stretch reflex. At dosages of about 10, 20, and 30 mg/kg/day, the ratio was progressively increased above normal as a result of broadening of the gait and shortening of the steps. These same dosage levels did not affect problem-solving behavior or speed of locomotion. The experimental animals were found to be generally less reactive to stress than normal ones. The acoustic startle response of rats is significantly increased after a 12.5 mg/kg dose of *p,p'*-DDT but can be attenuated by phenytoin and an adrenergic receptor antagonist, phenoxybenzamine (Tilson *et al.*, 1985, 1986; Saitoh *et al.*, 1986; Herr *et al.*, 1987), which also decreased DDT-induced myoclonus (Huang and van Voert, 1978). See also Effects on the Nervous System.

Pathology Morphological changes are inadequate to account for death from DDT poisoning. Changes that occur in the liver are discussed in Section 15.2.3.2. Mild to moderate morphological changes have been reported in the kidneys of animals that had received massive single doses or repeated doses; examples are fatty degeneration, necrosis, and calcification (Lillie *et al.*, 1947; Stohlman and Lillie, 1948) or slight brown pigmentation of the convoluted tubular epithelium (Fitzhugh and Nelson, 1947). However, it sometimes has happened that a complete absence of change in the kidney has been reported in connection with other studies carried out in the same laboratories (Lillie and Smith, 1944; Nelson *et al.*, 1944).

Treatment of Poisoning in Animals The more successful studies of treatment of animals poisoned by DDT involve the nervous system. Smith and Stohlman (1944) noted the possibility that narcotics in general may exhibit an antagonism to DDT. Rats survived on a diet containing 1000 ppm DDT for 90 days when they received cyclohexanone in the same diet at the rate of 2000 ppm but were uniformly killed in a shorter period when they received DDT at the same rate but without cyclohexanone. Later, it was shown that cyclohexanone offers no protection when used as a solvent for single massive doses of DDT (Deichmann *et al.*, 1950).

Smith and Stohlman (1945) later showed that, when rats were given urethane and, to a lesser extent, sodium dilantin as required after the onset of illness, the animals were protected from poisoning. Sodium amobarbital gave slight benefit, sodium phenobarbital a doubtful benefit, and paraldehyde no protection at all. All drugs were given intraperitoneally except paraldehyde, which was given by stomach tube. The mortality of rats treated with urethane was 12.5% and that of their controls was 80%. A total dosage of 1.2–2.5 gm/kg spread over a period of 1–3 days was found most satisfactory. Sodium dilantin reduced mortality to 46.7%, compared to 96.7% for the controls. The smallest effective dosage was 200–250 mg/kg, a value very close to the LD 50, which, under the conditions of the test, was 300 mg/kg.

Läuger *et al.* (1945a,b) also found that sodium phenobarbital was of questionable value in treating rats poisoned by DDT. However, completely different results were seen in larger animals. Philips and Gilman (1946) found phenobarbital by far the most outstanding remedy they tested. In a dosage well below the anesthetic level, it not only prevented death in many instances but also controlled tremor and convulsions. Signs of illness were more readily controlled in dogs and cats than in monkeys, which required nearly a full anesthetic dosage before tremors completely disappeared.

Magnesium sulfate did not reduce mortality in poisoned dogs and cats, although it did control tremors and convulsions briefly. Sodium bromide was entirely ineffective. Mortality was reduced with urethane, but a full anesthetic dosage was required to control tremor and convulsion. Similarly, sodium barbital and sodium pentobarbital controlled symptoms only when given in full anesthetic doses and even then did not greatly reduce mortality. 5,5-Diphenylhydantoin (phenytoin), when given to rats before they received DDT, reduced the lethal action without showing a notable effect on the signs of poisoning; it was not effective in cats. More recently, Tilson *et al.* (1985, 1986) have reported that phenytoin attenuates the tremor produced in rats by DDT and permethrin but not by lindane and chlordecone.

Vaz and his colleagues (1945) were apparently the first to note the antidotal effect of calcium in DDT poisoning. Dogs were given DDT orally as a 10% oily solution at a daily dosage of 100 mg/kg until signs of intoxication appeared. The same dosage could then be repeated to produce intense symptomatology from which the animals would recover spontaneously in 12–24 hr. For the actual tests, a larger challenge dosage of DDT (150–200 mg/kg) was used. Each dose of calcium gluconate (30 ml of a 10% solution) was injected intravenously into dogs weighing 8–18 kg. Dogs that were injected with calcium gluconate daily for 4 days and challenged with a large dose of DDT on the fourth day developed no symptoms or only slight ones. Dogs receiving a single dose of calcium gluconate showed symptoms of short duration and survived following a dosage of DDT large enough to kill two controls.

Koster (1947) studied cats poisoned by the intravenous injection of a soya lecithin–corn oil emulsion of DDT. A comparison was made of several aspects of intoxication, including number of convulsions, general severity (tremors, prostration, dyspnea), duration, and mortality. Both calcium gluconate and sodium gluconate reduced mortality but not severity. Gluconic acid increased the survival time, reduced mortality, but did not reduce convulsions or severity. Calcium chloride reduced convulsions but not mortality or tremors. Molecular equivalent doses of the candidate antidotes were used. Gluconic acid and its two salts were effective against an LD 95 dosage of DDT. The lifesaving capacity of calcium gluconate at a rate of 40 mg/kg was confirmed by Judah (1949), even though he found normal blood calcium values in most poisoned but unmedicated animals. One animal showed a high calcium value, and Cameron and Burgess (1945) reported a similar result. It has been suggested that increased blood calcium may be associated with acidosis caused by the accumulation of lactate.

Calcium has, then, an antidotal action against DDT in intact animals of several species. The suppression by calcium of the effect of DDT on the isolated nerve and muscle of the rat has been demonstrated (Eyzaguirre and Lilienthal, 1949). The hypothesis has been advanced (Welsh and Gordon, 1946; Gordon and Welsh, 1948) that certain neurotoxins, including DDT, act by delaying the restoration of calcium ions to a surface complex following breaking of the chelate linkage of calcium ions to surface polar groups by an initial exciting impulse. This action of the neurotoxin is conceived as depending largely on its physical rather than on its chemical properties. The hypothesis is helpful in explaining the fact that a wide variety of chemically unrelated compounds produce repetitive responses in excitable tissue and also the fact that many compounds that show a high toxicity for arthropods and mammals are fat-soluble and chemically relatively inert. It has been pointed out that this hypothesis postulates a very localized action of calcium at the nerve cell membrane; the hypothesis is not inconsistent with the finding that the blood calcium of poisoned animals may be unchanged or even increased. On the other hand, calcium may help to offset the effects of DDT on calcium-dependent ATPases, especially in the neuronal axons (see Biochemical Effects, p. 755).

Having observed the effect of DDT on the metabolism of glucose and glycogen, Läuger and his colleagues (1945a,b) investigated the use of glucose as an antidote. All of the 10 dogs given 2000 mg of DDT per kilogram of body weight orally in the form of an oil solution died within 8–24 hr. Five of the 10 dogs treated with one or more 20-ml doses of 20%

glucose survived the same dosage of DDT. The glucose was given intravenously in most instances.

Koster (1947) found that glucose given before or after an LD 33 dosage reduced convulsions and mortality and, when given before the poison, reduced tremors, prostration, and dyspnea in cats. Glucose, unlike gluconic acid and its sodium and calcium salts, was ineffective against an LD 95 dosage except to increase the time of survival. Insulin given intramuscularly 16–25 min before DDT increased the survival time and the severity of poisoning but did not affect mortality or convulsions. When given 53–130 min before DDT, insulin reduced convulsions in animals that died but increased convulsions, tremors, and other disorders in the survivors.

15.3.1.3 Toxicity to Humans

Experimental Oral Exposure Table 15.8 summarizes the effects of one or a few carefully measured oral doses of DDT. The results are consistent with those in accidents reported by Garrett (1947) and Hsieh (1954) in which it was possible to

Table 15.8
Summary of the Effects of One or a Few Oral Doses of DDT on Volunteers

Dose (mg) and formulation	Result	Reference
250 × 9, suspension	no effect	Domenjoz (1944)
1500, butter solution	no effect, but mice killed when fed 6 and 12 hr after dose	MacCormack (1945)
500, oil solution	no clinical effect	Neal et al. (1946)
770, oil solution	no clinical effect; DDA measured in urine	Neal et al. (1946)
250, suspension	none except slight disturbance of sensitivity of mouth	Velbinger (1947a,b)
250, oil solution	variable hyperesthia of mouth	Velbinger (1947a,b)
500, oil solution	variable hyperesthia of mouth	Velbinger (1947a,b)
750, oil solution	disturbance of sensitivity of lower part of face; uncertain gait; peak reaction (6 hr after ingestion) characterized by malaise, cold moist skin, and hypersensitivity to contact; reflexes normal	Velbinger (1947a,b)
1000, oil solution	same as above; no joint pains, fatigue, fear or difficulty in seeing or hearing	Velbinger (1947a,b)
1500, oil solution	prickling of tongue and around mouth and nose beginning 2.5 hr after dose; disturbance of equilibrium; dizziness; confusion; tremor of extremities; peak reaction (10 hr after ingestion) characterized by great malaise, headache, and fatigue; delayed vomiting; almost complete recovery in 24 hr	Velbinger (1947a,b)

estimate accurately the amount ingested. It may be concluded that a single dose at the rate of 10 mg/kg produces illness in some but not all subjects even though no vomiting occurs. Smaller doses generally produce no illness, although a dosage of 6 mg/kg produced perspiration, headache, and nausea in a man who was sickly and who was hungry at the time of eating. Persons who were made sick by 10 mg/kg have not shown convulsions, but convulsions have occurred in accidents when the dosage level was 16 mg/kg or greater (Hsieh, 1954). Rarely, a dosage as high as 20 mg/kg may be taken without apparent effect (MacCormack, 1945). Dosages at least as high as 285 mg/kg have been taken accidentally without fatal result (Garrett, 1947). However, large doses lead to prompt vomiting, so the amount actually retained cannot be determined accurately.

In acute poisoning a slight decrease in hemoglobin and a moderate leukocytosis without any constant deviation in the differential white count have been observed in volunteers (Velbinger, 1947a,b). These findings are considered secondary to the neurological effects.

It has been noted in the course of tests with volunteers that dilute colloidal aqueous suspensions of DDT are odorless and tasteless (Domenjoz, 1944; Hoffman and Lendle, 1948). Saturated alcoholic solutions of DDT have a weak aromatic taste, or rather odor. Some people find these solutions slightly anesthetic to the tongue (Hoffman and Lendle, 1948). The taste of DDT in vegetable oil is so slight that many persons cannot identify capsules containing 0, 3.5, and 35 mg of DDT when they are presented separately but can arrange them in proper order when one of each is available for comparison.

The possible clinical effects of many repeated doses of DDT were first explored by Fennah (1945). Because of his interest in predicting the results of indiscriminate use, he expressed the exposures in terms of environmental levels rather than in dosage units. The exposures were clearly higher than those ordinarily encountered. In one test, lasting a total of 11.5 months, Fennah daily inhaled 100 mg of pure DDT and drank water dusted at the rate of 3240 mg/m^2. Much of the inhaled dust must have been deposited in the upper respiratory tract and swallowed. Later, for 1 month Fennah ate food all of which had been sprayed at the rate of 2160 mg/m^2 after it had been served. No ill effect of any kind was observed.

Some later studies of DDT in volunteers have been designed to explore the details of storage and excretion of the compounds in humans and to search for possible effects of doses considered to be safe. In the first of these studies, men were given 0, 3.5, and 35 mg/person/day. These administered dosages plus DDT measured in the men's food resulted in dosage levels of 0.0021–0.0034, 0.038–0.063, and 0.36–0.61 mg/kg/day, respectively, the exact value depending on the weight of each individual. Six volunteers received the highest dosage of technical DDT for 12 months, and three received it for 18 months. A smaller number of men ingested the lower dosage of technical DDT or one of the dosages of p,p'-DDT for 12–18 months. No volunteer complained of any symptom or showed by the tests any signs of illness that did not have an easily

recognizable cause clearly unrelated to the exposure of DDT. At intervals, the men were given a systems review, physical examination, and a variety of laboratory tests. Particular attention was given to the neurological examination and liver function tests, because the major effects of DDT in animals involve the nervous system and the liver (Hayes et al., 1956).

The same result was obtained in a second study in which the same dosages were given for 21 months and the volunteers were observed for a minimum of 27 additional months (Hayes et al., 1971).

In the first study, the storage of DDT was proportional to dosage, but there was a then unexplained difference in the storage of the p,p'-isomer and of technical DDT. Following dosing for 12 months, the pure material was stored in fat at an average concentration of 340 ppm, but the technical material was stored at an average of only 234 ppm. The difference was statistically significant for the 3.5 mg/person/day dosages given for 3–6 and for 7–18 months. The difference was significant for the 35 mg/person/day doses after 7–18 months of dosing but not after only 3–6 months.

Men who ate p,p'-DDT showed a definite increase in the absolute amount of DDE stored. After 6 months at a dosage of 35 mg/person/day, eight men showed an average DDE fat storage of 32.6 ± 7.0 ppm as compared to 12.3 ± 1.5 ppm for the same individuals upon entering the investigation. There was a further increase of DDE storage as exposure progressed. However, DDT was stored in so much greater concentration that the relative storage of DDE decreased sharply. Thus, after 6 months at a dosage of 35 mg/person/day, eight men stored only 14% of their total DDT-derived material in the form of DDE as compared to 65% for the same persons at the beginning of the investigation.

The storage of DDE by men who ate technical DDT presented a different picture. Until 18 months after exposure, there was no clear evidence that these men stored any more DDE after exposure than they did before. However, at 18 months the only three samples available showed DDE concentrations ranging from 28 to 85 ppm, all substantially above general population levels. Thus, both the total amount stored and the rate at which DDT converted to DDE served to distinguish the metabolism of p,p'-DDT and technical DDT in humans (Hayes et al., 1956). This was true even though later study showed that the concentration of DDE in serum increased immediately in persons ingesting technical DDT at rates of 10 and 20 mg/person/day. Of course, daily values were subject to considerable variation, but the upward slopes of the graphs recording the results were apparent in 60 days or less and apparently the graphs were straight throughout the 5-month feeding period. Under the same conditions, the level of DDT in serum increased within 1 day and continued to increase in a curvilinear fashion for 5 months (Apple et al., 1970). A similar rapid increase reaching its maximum in 30 hr after a single exposure has been observed in workers (Edmundson et al., 1969a). The more rapid excretion of o,p'-DDT was demonstrated by Morgan and Roan (1972).

In a second study in which the volunteers received 0, 3.5, and 35 mg/person/day, the storage of DDT was again propor-

Table 15.9
Storage of DDT in Volunteers

| Type of DDT | Added dosage (mg/person/day) | Concentration of DDT[a] | | | | Significance of difference (p) |
		First study[b] 11 months or more (ppm)		Second study[c] 21.5 months (ppm)		
Technical	0	8–17	(12.5 ± 4.5)	16–30	(22.0 ± 2.9)	>0.1
	3.5	26–33	(23.8 ± 1.4)	59–76	(50.2 ± 5.6)	<0.025
	35	101–367	(234 ± 21.4)	105–619	(281 ± 79.5)	>0.4
Recrystallized	35	216–466	(340 ± 36.4)	129–659	(325 ± 62.2)	>0.2

[a] Range, mean ± SEM.
[b] Hayes *et al.* (1956).
[c] Hayes *et al.* (1971).

tional to dosage. Although, in this instance also, the storage of technical DDT was less than that of *p,p'*-DDT, the difference was not statistically significant. The real but very gradual accumulation of DDE was confirmed. A steady state of storage was approached later in the second study (18.8–21.5 months) than in the earlier one (about 12 months). The second study was superior in that more men were observed for a longer period but inferior in that dosing was less regular. Because of the latter difficulty, it seems impossible to decide whether 12 months or 21.5 months is a more valid estimate of the time necessary for people to approach a steady state of storage when intake is uninterrupted and unvarying in amount. It is interesting that the storage levels eventually reached at the same dosage in the two studies were statistically indistinguishable in most instances (see Table 15.9). In the one instance in which a statistical difference existed, the greater storage by men in the second study may have been explained by the fact that some of them inadvertently received higher doses than intended.

DDT was lost slowly from storage in fat after dosing was stopped. The concentration remaining following 25.5 months of recovery was from 32 to 35% of the maximum stored for those who had received 35 mg/person/day but was 66% for those who had received only 3.5 mg/person/day, indicating slower loss at lower storage levels (Hayes *et al.*, 1971).

Morgan and Roan (1971) fed volunteers not only technical DDT but also *p,p'*-DDE and *p,p'*-DDD. They found that DDE is stored more tenaciously than the other compounds in humans, the order being *p,p'*-DDE > *p,p'*-DDT > *o,p'*-DDT ≥ *p,p'*-DDD. The slow metabolism of DDT to DDE was confirmed. It was noted that *p,p'%*-DDT is lost from storage in adipose tissue much more slowly in humans than in the monkey, dog, or rat.

Less than 18% *p,p'*-DDT and *p,p'*-DDE is carried in human erythrocytes. In plasma of ordinary fat content, less than 1% of all DDT-related compounds is carried by the chylomicrons. Instead, these compounds are carried by proteins and are undetectable in plasma from which protein has been precipitated. Following ultracentrifugation, *p,p'*-DDT and *p,p'*-DDE are found mainly in the triglyceride-rich, low-density and very low-density lipoproteins. Following continuous electrophore-

sis, these compounds are found mainly in association with plasma albumin and α-globulins (Morgan *et al.*, 1972).

DDA is the main urinary metabolite of DDT. In humans, it was found first in a volunteer by Neal *et al.* (1946), who reported that, following ingestion of 770 mg of *p,p'*-DDT, excretion rose sharply to 4.0 mg/day during the second 24-hr period, decreased rapidly on the third and fourth days, decreased gradually thereafter, but was still above baseline on day 14. Judging from a graph, the highest concentration was about 2.6 ppm.

Much later studies in volunteers who received smaller but repeated doses confirmed the very rapid rise in excretion of DDA (Roan *et al.*, 1971; Hayes *et al.*, 1971) and showed that a steady state of excretion was reached after about 6–8 months. During a 56-week period of continued dosing after equilibrium was fully established, the concentration of DDA associated with technical DDT at the rate of 35 mg/person/day varied from 0.18 to 9.21 ppm and averaged 2.98 ppm; corresponding values for *p,p'*-DDT were 0.40–6.27 ppm with a mean of 1.88 ppm. Thus technical DDT, as compared to *p,p'*-DDT, was excreted more effectively and stored less.

During the latter half of the dosing period, it was possible in the two groups receiving recrystallized and technical DDT at the rate of 35 mg/person/day to account for an average of 13 and 16%, respectively, of the daily dose in terms of urinary DDA. The excretion of DDA was relatively constant in each individual, but marked differences were observed between men receiving the same dose. For example, over the period of 56 weeks the highest rate measured for one man was 0.16 mg/hr while the lowest rate for another in the same group was 0.15 mg/hr. Their mean rates during this period were 0.089 and 0.269 mg/hr, respectively. The difference was highly significant ($P < 0.001$) (Hayes *et al.*, 1971).

Experimental Dermal Exposure Depending on dosage, oral administration of DDT to volunteers has produced either no illness or brief poisoning entirely similar to that seen in experimental animals. The oral dosage necessary to produce any clinical effect was almost always 10 mg/kg or more. It is a strange coincidence that, in two studies involving only three subjects in all, experimental dermal exposure to DDT was followed by fatigue, aching of the limbs, anxiety or irritability, and other subjective complaints. Recovery was delayed a month or more (Wigglesworth, 1945; Case, 1945). In neither study was there an independent control. Although the dosage was unmeasured, the amounts of DDT absorbed must have been much smaller than those involved in the oral tests. One of the studies involved self-experimentation by one man. A similar but somewhat more severe test on six volunteers produced no toxic or irritant effect at all (Dangerfield, 1946). In view of all other experiments and extensive practical experience, it must be concluded that the illnesses reported by Wigglesworth and Case were unrelated to DDT.

With the exceptions just mentioned, dermal exposure to DDT has been associated with no illness and usually no irritation (Domenjoz, 1944; Cameron and Burgess, 1945; Dangerfield, 1946; Chin and T'Ant, 1946; Wasicky and Unti, 1944; Draize *et al.*, 1944; Haag *et al.*, 1948; Fennah, 1945). In fact, Hoffman and Lendle (1948) reported that even subcutaneous injection of colloidal suspensions of DDT in saline in concentrations up to 30 ppm caused no irritation. Zein-el-Dine (1946) reported that DDT-impregnated clothing caused a slight, transient dermatitis, but the method of impregnation was not stated and the absence of solvent was not guaranteed. Other more thorough studies of DDT-impregnated clothing have found it nonirritating (Domenjoz, 1944; Cameron and Burgess, 1945).

Chin and T'Ant (1946) applied small pads impregnated with different formulations of DDT to the inner surface of the forearm of 32 volunteers whose cutaneous sensation had previously been measured for a period of 5 weeks. Pads impregnated with all the elements of the formulation except DDT were applied to the corresponding position on the other arm as a control. Powdered DDT and 5% solutions of DDT showed little effect. Ten percent and 20% solutions in olive oil and petroleum showed no remarkable effect on sensation of pain, cold, or heat but reduced tactile sensation in most cases so that the minimal pressure that could arouse this sensation was 1–2.5 gm/cm^2 higher than in the control.

Experimental Respiratory Exposure Neal *et al.* (1944) reported almost continuous daily exposure to aerosols sufficient to leave a white deposit of DDT on the nasal vibrissae of the volunteers. This exposure produced moderate irritation of the nose, throat, and eyes. Except for this irritation during exposure, there were no symptoms, and laboratory tests and physical examination, including neurological evaluation, failed to reveal any significant changes. The studies by Fennah (1945) that involved both respiratory and oral exposure produced no detectable ill effect, as discussed above. Stammers and Whitfield (1947) reported tests in which volunteers were exposed to DDT dispersed into the air either by volatilizing units or by continuously or intermittently operated aerosol dispensers. In some instances, a slight odor and some dryness of the throat were noticed, but otherwise the results were negative.

Therapeutic Use The use of DDT for treating human body lice, head lice, and scabies has been reviewed by Simmons (1959). Obviously, these uses offered a possibility of dermal absorption, but such absorption of dry DDT is very limited. Persons who had DDT blown into their clothing as they wore it must have inhaled some of the compound, and this was especially true of persons who used hand or power equipment to apply the dust to hundreds of people per day in mass delousing stations set up to control typhus. However, the dosages absorbed cannot have been so large as in some instances in which DDT has been administered by mouth. Even smaller absorbed dosages for the general population were involved in the use of DDT for the control of other vector-borne diseases, especially malaria. These facts must not lead us to forget the tremendous contribution that DDT has made to human health through control of the vectors of typhus, malaria, plague, and several lesser diseases (Spindler, 1983; Coulston, 1985).

DDT has been used on an experimental basis at oral dosage rates varying from 0.3 to 3 mg/kg/day for periods up to 7 months in an attempt to decrease serum bilirubin levels in selected patients with jaundice. No side effects were observed. No improvement was noted in patients with jaundice based on cirrhosis who had no demonstrated liver enzyme deficiency. However, in a patient with familial, nonhemolytic, unconjugated jaundice based on a deficiency of glucuronyltransferase, treatment with DDT rapidly reduced the plasma bilirubin level to the normal range and relieved the patient of nausea and malaise from which he had suffered intermittently. The liver function tests as well as other laboratory findings remained normal. The improvement was maintained during the 6 months when DDT was administered and had persisted for 7 additional months at the time the report was written. In this case, a dosage of 1.5 mg/kg/day produced a steady rise in plasma levels of *p,p'*-DDT from an initial level of 0.005 ppm to a maximum of 1.33 ppm at the end of treatment. At this time, the concentration in body fat was 203 ppm. Plasma levels fell slowly after dosing was stopped (Thompson *et al.*, 1969). The highest daily intake in this series was six times greater than the highest level administered in earlier studies of volunteers and about 7500 times greater than the DDT intake of the general population. The highest value for *p,p'*-DDT in serum observed in the entire series was 1.330 ppm, compared to 0.996 ppm, the highest value reported by Laws *et al.* (1967) for formulation-plant workers. A lesser induction of the microsomal enzymes has been observed in workers also (Kolmodin *et al.*, 1969; Poland *et al.*, 1970).

Rappolt (1970) used a single dose of 5000 mg of DDT to promote the metabolism of phenobarbital, of which his three patients had taken an overdose. The treatment appeared useful. Neither Rappolt nor Thompson encountered any side effects of DDT. However, in addition to whatever action it may have had in promoting the metabolism of phenobarbital, the DDT administered by Rappolt must have acted largely as a pharmaceutical antidote for the barbiturate. The largest dose previously administered intentionally was 1500 mg, which caused moderate poisoning in a volunteer, who, of course, had received no barbiturate (see Table 15.8).

Accidental and Intentional Poisoning The earliest symptom of poisoning by DDT is hyperesthesia of the mouth and lower part of the face. This is followed by paresthesia of the same area and of the tongue and then by dizziness, an objective disturbance of equilibrium, paresthesia and tremor of the extremities, confusion, malaise, headache, fatigue, and delayed vomiting. The vomiting is probably of central origin and not due to local irritation. Convulsions occur only in severe poisoning.

Onset may be as soon as 30 min after ingestion of a large dose or as late as 6 hr after smaller but still toxic doses. Recovery from mild poisoning usually is essentially complete in 24 hr, but recovery from severe poisoning requires several days. In two instances, there was some residual weakness and ataxia of the hands 5 weeks after ingestion.

Involvement of the liver has been mentioned in only a small proportion of cases of accidental poisoning by DDT. In three men who ate pancakes made with DDT and who ingested 5000–6000 mg each, slight jaundice appeared after 4–5 days and lasted 3–4 days (Naevested, 1947). Hepatic involvement and convulsions were reported in an unsuccessful attempt at suicide by ingesting DDT and lindane (Eskenasy, 1972).

Cases of individual and suicidal poisoning in which effects were clearly caused by DDT are summarized in Table 15.10. All of these cases involved ingestion. The signs and symptoms of poisoning were entirely consistent with those observed in volunteers, except that the spectrum of effects was broader because some of the accidental and suicidal doses were very high. A few persons apparently have been killed by uncomplicated DDT poisoning, but none of these cases was reported in detail. Death has been caused much more frequently by the ingestion of solutions of DDT, but in most of these instances the signs and symptoms were predominantly or exclusively those of poisoning by the solvent (Hayes, 1959a). This does not mean that the toxicity of the solvent always predominates. For example, the recurrent convulsions in a case reported by Cunningham and Hill (1952), though more characteristic of poisoning by one of the cyclodienes, was certainly not typical of solvent poisoning. A 2-year-old child drank an unknown quantity of fly spray of which 5% was DDT, but the nature of the other active ingredients or the solvent was unknown. About 1 hr after taking the material, the child became unconscious and had a generalized, sustained convulsion. Convulsions were present when the child was hospitalized 2 hr after taking the poison, but the fits were controlled by barbiturates and other sedatives. Convulsions reoccurred on day 4 and again on day 21 but were stopped each time following renewal of treatment. On day 12, it was noted that the patient was deaf. Hearing began to improve about day 24 and was normal, as were other neurological and psychic findings, when the patient was seen about 2.5 months after the accident.

Clinical effects of one toxicant may be modified by

Table 15.10
Summary of the Effects of the Accidental or Suicidal Ingestion of DDT

Individual dose (mg), formulation, and number of persons	Results and reference
300–4500, in food, 1 man	onset in 1 hr; vomiting; restlessness; headache; heart weak and slow; recovery next day (Muhlens, 1946)
Unknown dose, in tarts, 25 men	onset in 2–2.5 hr; all weak and giddy; 4 vomited; 2 hospitalized; 1 confused, incoordinated, weak; one with palpitations and numbness of hands; recovery in 24–48 hr (Mackeras and West, 1946)
5000–6000, in pancakes, 3 men	onset 2–3 hr; throbbing headache; dizziness; incoordination; paresthesias of extremities; urge to defecate; wide, nonreacting pupils; reduced vision; dysarthria; facial weakness; tremor; ataxic gait; reduced sensitivity to touch; reduced reflexes; positive Romberg; slightly low blood pressure and persistent irregular heart action; partial recovery in 2–3 days, but slight jaundice appeared 4–5 days after ingestion and lasted 3–4 days; all normal 19 days after poisoning except irregular heart action in one (Naevested, 1947)
2000, in pancakes, 2 men	no illness (Naevested, 1947)
Up to 20,000, in bread, 28 men	onset in 30–60 min in those most severely affected; men first seen 2–3 hr after ingestion; in spite of severe early vomiting that reduced the effective dose, severity of illness and especially intensity of numbness and paralysis of extremities proportional to amount of DDT ingested; all but 8 men recovered in 48 hr; 5 others fully recovered in 2 weeks, but 3 men still had some weakness and ataxia of their hands 5 weeks after ingestion (Garrrett, 1947, 1950)
Unknown dose, in flour, about 100 women	onset about 3.5 hr after ingestion; total of about 85 cases of which 37 were hospitalized; symptoms mild and similar to those in earlier outbreaks except gastrointestinal disturbance in most severe cases included abdominal pain and diarrhea as well as nausea; most fully recovered in 24 hr (Jude and Girard, 1949)
Unknown dose, 14 cases	symptoms in established cases similar to those reported earlier (Francone et al., 1952)
286–1716, in meatballs, 8 cases, 11 exposed	with the exception of one man who was already sick when he received a dosage of 6 mg/kg, poisoning did not occur at dosages of 5.1–10.3 mg/kg. Ingestion of 16.3–120.5 mg/kg produced excessive perspiration, nausea, vomiting, convulsions, headache, increased salivation, tremors, tachycardia, and cyanosis of the lips. Onset varied from 2 to 6 hr, depending on dosage. Recovery required as much as 2 days (Hsieh, 1954).
Unknown dose, 1 case	death 13 hr after suicidal ingestion (Committee on Pesticides, 1951)
Unknown dose, 22 unrelated cases	22 separate cases, including 15 attempted suicides; some complicated by solvents; 3 deaths (Committee on Pesticides, 1951)

combining it with another. For example, one would not expect prolonged illness from DDT at a rate of 27 mg/kg. However, when DDT and lindane were ingested in a suicidal attempt at dosages thought to be 27 and 18 mg/kg respectively, clinical remission of convulsions and of liver involvement was delayed until day 20, and the EEG did not return to normal until day 39 (Eskenasy, 1972).

What little is known about the effect of DDT on the human heart fails to show whether cardiac arrhythmia might be a possible cause of death in acute poisoning, as is true in some species of laboratory animals. Palpitations, tachycardia, and "irregular heart action" have been noted in some but not all cases of acute poisoning (Mackerras and West, 1946; Naevested, 1947; Hsieh, 1954).

There have been no accidents or suicides involving respiratory or dermal exposure leading to recognized signs and symptoms of DDT poisoning. This is true even though sufficient respiratory exposure to acrosols or sufficient dermal exposure to solutions can cause poisoning in animals, and the difference is certainly one of dosage.

Use Experience The safety record of DDT is phenomenally good [Coulston, 1985; Food and Agriculture Organization/World Health Organization (FAO/WHO), 1985]. It has been used for mass delousing in such a way that the bodies and inner clothing of thousands of people of all ages and states of health were liberally dusted with the compound. By necessity, the applicators worked in a cloud of the material. Other applicators have sprayed the interior of hundreds of millions of homes in tropical and subtropical countries under conditions that Wolfe *et al.* (1959) showed involved extensive dermal and respiratory exposure. A smaller number of people have made or formulated DDT for many years. Extensive experience and numerous medical studies of groups of workers have been reviewed (Hayes, 1959a). Dermatitis was commonly observed among workers who used DDT solutions. The rashes were clearly due to the solvent, especially kerosene. As often happens with rashes caused by petroleum distillates, they were most severe in people when they first started work and cleared in a few days unless contamination was exceptionally severe. A smaller number of workers experienced mild narcotic effects (vertigo and nausea) from solvents when working in confined spaces. Gil and Miron (1949) reported that some persons suffered temporary irritability, fatigue, and other ill-defined symptoms after exposure in the dusty atmosphere of a delousing station, but the relation of these atypical findings to DDT was not clear. With these exceptions due largely to solvents, no illnesses clearly attributable to the formulations, much less to DDT, were revealed by the early studies.

Mild moderate poisoning by DDT itself may have occurred among a group of factory workers exposed to air concentrations of 500–4200 mg/m^3, but no measurements were made of DDT in blood, fat, or urine. The workers complained of parethesia of the extremities, headache, dizziness, and some other difficulties less clearly linked to DDT (Aleksieva *et al.*, 1959). Even higher concentrations in air have been associated with

tremor of the tongue and hands as well as with numerous subjective findings (Burkatzkaya *et al.,* 1961).

Ortelee (1958) carried out clinical and laboratory examinations of 40 workers, all of whom were exposed to a number of other pesticides. They had been employed at this work with heavy exposure for 0.4–6.5 years with slightly less exposure for as much as 8 years. Exposure was so intense that during working hours many of the men were coated with a heavy layer of concentrated DDT dust. By comparing their excretion of DDA with that of volunteers given known doses of DDT, it was possible to estimate that the average absorbed dosages of three groups of the workers with different degrees of occupational exposure were 14, 30, and 42 mg/person/day. With the exception of the excretion of DDA and the occurrence of a few cases of minor irritation of the skin and eyes, no correlation was found between any abnormality and exposure to the insecticide. Since very large doses of DDT injure the nervous system and liver of experimental animals, special attention was given to a complcte neurological examination and to laboratory tests for liver function. Although a few abnormalities were revealed, none related to DDT was detected.

Laws *et al.* (1967) studied 35 men employed from 11 to 19 years in a plant that had produced DDT continuously and exclusively since 1947 and, at the time of the study, produced 2722 metric tons per month. Findings from medical history, physical examinations, routine clinical laboratory tests, and chest x-ray films did not reveal any ill effects attributable to exposure to DDT. No case of cancer or blood dyscrasia was found among the 35 heavily exposed workers in a DDT factory, nor did the medical records of 63 men who had worked there for more than 5 years reveal these diseases. Two men were employed who had a history of successfully treated cancer before they came to work, but no employee had contracted cancer during the 19 years the plant had operated; during this period, the work force varied from 110 to 135. A study of liver function of the heavily exposed men is discussed near the end of this section.

Measurement of storage offered direct evidence of the men's heavy exposure. The overall range of storage of the sum of isomers and metabolites of DDT in the men's fat was 38–647 ppm, compared to an average of 8 ppm for the general population. Based on their storage of DDT in fat and excretion of DDA in urine, it was estimated that the average daily intake of DDT by the 20 men with high occupational exposure was 17.5–18 mg/person/day, compared to an average of 0.028 mg/person/day then found for the general population. There was significant correlation ($r = +0.64$) between the concentrations of total DDT-related material in the fat and serum of the workers. The concentration in fat averaged 338 times greater than that in serum—a factor about three times greater than that for people without occupational exposure. Compared to people in the general population, workers were found to store a smaller proportion of DDT-related material in the form of DDE; the difference was shown to be related chiefly to intensity rather than duration of exposure. DDE is relatively much less important and DDA much more important as excretory products in

Table 15.11
Average Concentration of DDT and DDE in Fat and Serum and of DDA in the Urine of Workers Engaged in the Manufacture, Formulation, or Use of DDT

Tissue	Number of workers	DDT (ppm)	DDE (ppm)	DDA (ppm)	Total as DDT (ppm)	Estimated exposure (mg/person/day)	Reference
Fat	1	648	437		1,131		Hayes *et al.* (1956)
Urine	10			0.57		14	Ortelee (1958)
Urine	16			1.7		30	Ortelee (1958)
Urine	13			2.9		42	Ortelee (1958)
Fat	3	51	44		98	3.6	Laws *et al.* (1967)
Fat	12	74	50		130	6.2	Laws *et al.* (1967)
Fat	20	161	91		263	18	Laws *et al.* (1967)
Serum	3	0.2113	0.1968		0.5412	6.3	Laws *et al.* (1967)
Serum	12	0.1420	0.1454		0.3548	8.4	Laws *et al.* (1967)
Serum	20	0.3020	0.2719		0.7371	17.5	Laws *et al.* (1967)
Urine	3			0.41			Laws *et al.* (1967)
Urine	12			0.6			Laws *et al.* (1967)
Urine	20			1.27			Laws *et al.* (1967)
Serum	18	0.573	0.506				Poland *et al.* (1970)
Serum	56	0.004[a,b]	0.052[a,b]				Morgan and Roan (1974)
Serum	32	0.002[b]	0.026[b]				Morgan and Roan (1974)
Serum	32	0.004[b]	0.047[b]				Morgan and Roan (1974)
Serum	32	0.009[b]	0.075[b]				Morgan and Roan (1974)
Serum	31	0.052[b]	0.222[b]				Morgan and Roan (1974)
Serum	5	0.004[a]	0.021[a]				Clifford and Weil (1972)
Serum	10	0.022	0.055				Clifford and Weil (1972)
Serum	4	0.087	0.072				Edmundson *et al.* (1970)
Blood	154	0.128	0.250				Edmundson *et al.* (1969a,b)
Urine				0.080			Edmundson *et al.* (1975)
Plasma	23				0.0389		Gracheva (1969)
Fat	18				5.2–45.2		
Serum	21	0.021	0.013				Keil *et al.* (1972a)
Blood	44				0.761		WHO (1973)
Blood	100				1.273		WHO (1973)
Blood	64	0.024	0.016				Violante *et al.* (1986)

[a] Control group.

[b] Approximately equal groups arranged by degree of storage.

occupationally exposed men than in men of the general population.

After Laws *et al.* (1967) had completed their study, it was found that the 36 most heavily exposed workers involved had fathered 58 children before they began working at the DDT factory and 93 children afterward (Wilcox, 1967).

By far the largest number of heavily exposed workers whose health has been investigated are those associated with malaria control in Brazil and India (WHO, 1973). In Brazil, periodic clinical examinations were made of 202 sprayers exposed to DDT for 6 or more years, 77 sprayers exposed for 13 years ending in 1959, and 406 controls. In the first examination carried out in 1971, minor differences between exposed and nonexposed groups were observed in some neurological tests, but this result was not confirmed by the second examination in the same year or by subsequent examinations. During a 3-year period, a survey of illnesses requiring medical care during the 6 months preceding each periodic medical examination failed to demonstrate any difference between exposed and control groups. A relatively small number of analyses indicated that the concentration of DDT in the blood of sprayers was about three times higher than that of controls.

In India, the blood levels of 144 sprayers were 7.5–15 times greater than those in controls and were at least as high as those reported for workers who make and formulate DDT elsewhere (see Table 15.11). When the sprayers were examined, no differences from controls were found except that knee reflexes were brisker, slight tremor was more often present, and a timed Romberg test was more poorly performed by the sprayers. The positive results led to the selection of 20 men for reexamination by a neurologist, who concluded that the differences found initially were not real or that the tests had returned to normal within the few months between the two examinations. In any event, the signs were not dosage related, since they showed no correlation with serum levels of DDT. More recently cognitive functions of Indian DDT sprayers have been tested. DDT levels were 8.5 times higher than those in controls and visuomotor functions were significantly depressed (Misra *et al.*, 1984).

Laws *et al.* (1973) made a detailed study of the liver function of 31 men who had made and formulated DDT and who had been the subjects of an earlier study already discussed. Judging from their excretion and storage, the men's exposure was equivalent to an oral intake of DDT at rates ranging from 3.6 to 18 mg/man/day for periods ranging from 16 to 25 years and averaging 21 years. All tests were in the normal range for total protein, albumin, total bilirubin, thymol turbidity, and retention of sulfobromophthalein sodium (BSP). One man had mild elevation of alkaline phosphatase (16 units) and SGPT (42 units). Another man had an alkaline phosphatase concentration of 14 units, while a third man had an SGPT level of 49 units. The α-fetoprotein test was negative for all 20 of the men for whom the test was performed.

The induction by DDT of microsomal enzymes of human liver was demonstrated first in workers, and it has been confirmed (see Section 7.4.3 and Therapeutic Use in this section). DDT may be more important than DDE in this regard, as indicated by the fact that Poland et al. (1970) observed induction in men with average serum levels of 0.573 and 0.506 ppm for DDT and DDE, respectively, while Morgan and Roan (1974) found no induction in men with corresponding values of 0.052 and 0.222 ppm.

As noted under Therapeutic Use, DDT has been used successfully to induce microsomal enzymes in order to promote metabolism of bilirubin in a case of congenital defect and to promote metabolism of phenobarbital in a case of overdose.

DDT promotes its own metabolism in some species of laboratory animals. That the same is true in humans is indicated by the fact that storage of DDT is relatively less at higher dosages (see Fig. 7.4). However, the metabolism and subsequent excretion of DDT can be promoted even more by phenobarbital and especially diphenylhydantoin (see Metabolism in Section 15.3.1.2) and to a lesser degree by some other drugs (McQueen et al., 1972). Establishment of a reduced equilibrium appeared to require about 2 months. Within this period, the regression of the level of DDT plus DDE on duration of treatment with diphenylhydantoin was highly significant ($P < 0.001$).

In addition to the studies already mentioned regarding workers with extensive storage and/or excretion of DDT as a result of truly heavy exposure to DDT, studies also have been made of a larger number of workers with lesser storage and/or excretion following lesser exposure to DDT but greater exposure to other insecticides. Continuing, meticulous study discussed by Hayes (1975) under Community Studies as well as the work of Tsutsui et al. (1974), Ouw and Shandar (1974), and Morgan and Lin (1978) has failed to reveal effects of clinical significance among workers with prolonged, moderate exposure to a wide variety of pesticides. In a review of results for 2620 persons exposed to pesticides and 1049 persons not occupationally exposed, Morgan and Lin (1978) found that, apart from serum pesticide concentrations, the only significant and consistent change associated with occupational exposure was a depression of serum bilirubin. This presumably was a reflection of a slight induction of liver microsomal enzymes. In addition, there was a tendency for serum alkaline phosphatase, serum glutamic-oxaloacetic transaminase (SGOT), serum glutamic-pyruvic transaminase (SGPT), and lactate dehydrogenase (LDH) to increase with increasing concentrations of DDT plus DDE in the serum, but the differences were small in all instances and statistically significant for SGOT and LDH only.

Wong et al. (1984) could find no significant overall cause-specific mortality excess among men potentially exposed at work to DDT from 1935 to 1976. Similarly, a population of 499 persons living downstream from a defunct DDT-manufacturing plant showed no DDT-specific illnesses or ill health despite total DDT serum levels three times the national mean (Kreiss et al., 1981). There was, however, a possible association between serum DDT and serum cholesterol, triglyceride, and γ-glutamyl transpeptidase levels.

A positive linear correlation has been reported for the concentrations of vitamin A and of DDT-related compounds in the serum of men with at least 5 years of occupational exposure to DDT. However, the workers' DDT levels were little higher than those of persons in the general population (see Table 7.15 in Hayes, 1975, and Table 15.11, herein), and their vitamin A levels were within normal limits (Keil et al., 1972b). Perhaps they were better fed than the controls.

Evidence regarding mutagenic activity of DDT and its significance in humans is uncertain. Comparing samples collected in winter and during the peak season of pesticide application, a slight increase in chromatid breaks was reported in the cultured lymphocytes of workers exposed to a wide variety of insecticides said to include DDT. A somewhat larger increase was reported for men exposed mainly to herbicides (Yoder et al., 1973). The paper failed to explain why exposure to DDT was claimed at a time when its use was banned. In another study, lymphocytes cultured from workers with an average DDT plasma level of 0.999 ppm showed significantly more chromosomal and chromatid aberrations than did cells cultured from controls with an average plasma level of 0.275 ppm. The difference was not significant in other comparisons in which the average plasma levels were 1.030 versus 0.380 ppm and 0.240 versus 0.030 ppm, respectively (Rabello et al., 1975). Examination of all of the data presented by the authors suggests that a simple dosage–effect relationship was present, with a detectable effect starting somewhere between 0.2 and 0.4 ppm and increasing at levels higher than 0.4 ppm. Some chromosomal aberrations have also been observed with human lymphocyte cultures by Preston et al. (1981), but DDT did not cause unscheduled DNA synthesis in SV40-transformed human cells (Ahmed et al., 1977).

Although there is a lot of evidence against DDT's causing liver cancer in humans in Western countries, there is still the outside possibility of it acting as a promoter of potent carcinogens. Aflatoxin is a well-known human carcinogen in areas of Southeast Asia such a Thailand, where DDT and other chlorinated insecticides are still widely used. In Denmark, Unger and Olsen (1980) have found significantly higher levels of DDE in adipose tissue from terminal cancer patients than in tissue from patients who died from other causes. In the United States, DDT and DDE levels were measured in 919 subjects in 1974 and 1975. After 10 years there was no correlation between these levels and overall mortality or cancer mortality except a slight correlation with respiratory cancer death (Austin et al., 1989). Of course, increased storage often correlates with emaciation of whatever cause (Hayes, 1975).

Atypical Cases of Various Origins It has been alleged that DDT causes or contributes to a wide variety of diseases of humans and animals not previously recognized as associated with any chemical. Such diseases included cardiovascular disease, cancer, atypical pneumonia, retrolental fibroplasia, poliomyelitis, hepatitis, and "neuropsychiatric manifestations" (Biskind, 1952, 1953; Biskind and Bieber, 1949). Without exception, the causes of these diseases were unknown or at least unproved at the time of the allegation. Needless to say, the charge that DDT predisposed to poliomyelitis was dropped after the disease was controlled through the use of vaccines. Unfortunately, there is no immediate possibility of controlling cardiovascular disease, cancer, or many of the less common conditions in humans that have been ascribed to DDT. In the meantime, such irresponsible claims could produce great harm and, if taken seriously, even interfere with scientific search for true causes and realistic means of preventing the conditions in question.

"Highly sensitive subjects" were said to experience visual disturbances, headache, perceptual abnormalities, muscular weakness, and decrease in mental and physical activity when a food oil solution containing as little as 10 ppm DDT was held beneath their nostrils. Ordinary people could not distinguish the odor of solutions containing up to 10,000 ppm from that of plain oil, and they were unaffected (Kailin and Hastings, 1966). This finding is unconfirmed; if such highly sensitive subjects exist, they are excessively rare.

There is a strong tendency to blame blood dyscrasias, other manifestations of "hypersensitivity," and, in fact, many diseases of unknown cause on any new chemical that gains widespread attention. DDT was no exception. A review of the early literature (Hayes, 1959a) indicates that blood dyscrasias and an unbelievable range of other diseases were, in fact, blamed on DDT. Only a circumstantial relationship ever was established between these diseases and exposure to DDT, and this remains true of the small number of reports of blood dyscrasias (Schüttmann, 1968; Murray et al., 1973) or angioneurotic edema (Vanat and Vanat, 1971) that appeared later. As the novelty wore off, fewer new reports appeared linking DDT to diseases of unknown cause, although the use of DDT increased greatly. It is true that available tests do not make it possible to exclude a particular compound as a cause of an isolated case of blood dyscrasia (see Section 8.1.4.1). However, it is noteworthy that the rate at which these disorders occur has remained essentially unchanged since before DDT was introduced (see Fig. 7.10 in Hayes, 1975).

Eight cases of chronic liver disease have been reported among men with prolonged occupational exposure to DDT and BHC in connection with either their manufacture or use (Schüttmann, 1968). The cases were well studied individually but not epidemiologically.

There are a few reports of acute illness among workers attributed to exposure to mixtures of DDT and other materials. Insofar as the dosage was very large, as in certain accidents that have occurred involving individuals or groups in the general population, one would expect similar results. However, in at least one instance, headache, dizziness, nausea, vomiting, pain and numbness of the limbs, and general weakness beginning 1–1.5 hr after entering a treated field (Kolyada and Mikhal'chenkova, 1973) was suggestive of food poisoning or hysteria.

Finally, there are studies of workers exposed to DDT and various other pesticides that are reported to have produced a variety of subjective and even objective medical findings. Interpretation of these reports is difficult because (a) the findings do not resemble those of poisoned animals or of persons poisoned as a result of accident or suicide and (b) the papers fail to report how the medical findings and the absenteeism of the pesticide workers compared with those of workers of comparable age, sex, and exertion who were not exposed to chemicals. The fact that the workers in question were exposed to mixtures of pesticides is not in itself an explanation because many workers, on whom careful study revealed no consistent difference from the controls, were exposed to mixtures.

The reports under discussion tend to fall into two sets, those involving general debility and those involving a single organ or system. Conditions representative of general debility include dermatitis, subtle blood changes, general weakness, palpitations, functional angiospasm, headache, dizziness, diminished appetite, vomiting, lower abdominal pain, chronic gastritis, benign chronic hepatitis, insomnia, a sympathetic vascular/asthenic syndrome, vegetative dystonia, and confusion (Jovĉiĉ and Ivanuŝ, 1968; Model', 1968; Kostiuk and Mukhtarova, 1970; Bezuglyi et al., 1973).

Organs, systems, or functions that have been studied apparently by specialists and to the complete exclusion of other organs, systems, or functions of the same workers include the respiratory system (Boiko and Krasnyuk, 1969), liver (Krasnyuk et al., 1967; Bezuglyi and Kaskevich, 1969), stomach (Krasnyuk and Platonova, 1969; Platonova, 1970), kidneys (Krasnyuk et al., 1968), labor and puerparium (Komarova, 1970; Nikitina, 1974), adrenals (Baksheyev, 1973), and skin (Karimov, 1969, 1970). An indication that the difficulties under discussion are not serious is their reversal or prophylaxis by means of diet. Leshchenko and Polonskaia (1969) described in detail two dietary supplements composed of ordinary foods plus sea kale and a selection of vitamins and trace metals. Organochlorine workers who received these diet products showed a normalization of protein metabolism manifested by an increase in total serum protein, improved lipid metabolism, and enriched vitamin and trace element supply in the organism. All of these effects led to an improvement of the detoxifying function of the liver, which was viewed as the most frequent site of adverse effects of exposure to organochlorine compounds. The frequency and degree of olfactory disorders, especially ability to detect peppermint and acetic acid in an olfactory analyzer, were reported to be greater among persons exposed to pesticides and increased with duration of exposure (Salikhodzhaev and Fershtat, 1972). Whether any of the persons exposed to pesticides experienced any clinical difficulty or social inconvenience associated with olfactory sensation is not clear.

Dosage Response The clinical effects of different dosage levels of DDT in humans are summarized in Tables 7.24 in Hayes (1975) and in Tables 15.8 and 15.10, herein. The degree of storage determined by different dosage levels of DDT has been summarized in Fig. 7.4, and details regarding higher than normal dosage rates are given in Table 15.9. A clinically useful degree of induction of microsomal enzymes was obtained with a DDT dosage of 1.5 mg/kg/day for 6 months (see paragraph on Therapeutic Use). As discussed under Use Experience and in Section 7.4.3, workers who absorbed a dosage of about 0.25 mg/kg/day showed demonstrable but only slight induction. Workers with less exposure as indicated by lower serum levels of DDT showed no detectable induction.

Storage in Fat The highest reported storage of DDT and related compounds remains that of a healthy worker whose fat contained DDT and DDE (as DDT) at concentrations of 648 and 483 ppm, respectively (Hayes *et al.*, 1956). Laws *et al.* (1967) reported considerably lower storage values among the most exposed persons in a DDT manufacturing plant (see Table 15.11). An important point evident from the table is that, whereas almost all investigations of workers are said to have been carried out on "heavily exposed" populations (or words to that effect), some of the groups studied had absorbed little more DDT than is absorbed by the general population—especially the general population of some tropical countries—as recorded in Table 15.12.

The first evidence that human beings metabolize a part of the DDT they absorb to DDE was obtained from the analysis of fat from a worker (Mattson *et al.*, 1953). The accumulation of DDE relative to total DDT-related compounds is best illustrated in humans. Of the total DDT stored in the fat of workers exposed to technical DDT (about 4% DDE) for 11–19 years, only 38% was in the form of DDE, and, of course, some of that DDE came from their diets including meat (Laws *et al.*, 1967). In India, where many people avoid meat but may consume milk, cheese, and eggs, 34–41% of total DDT stored by people without special exposure was DDE (Dale *et al.*, 1965). In the United States, during a time when DDT residues in food were decreasing, the proportion of total DDT in the form of DDE increased from about 60% in 1955 to about 80% in 1970; during the same interval the concentration of total DDT in body fat decreased from about 15 ppm to less than 10 ppm as recorded in Table 7.10 in Hayes (1975). By 1980, DDE constituted 86.7% of total DDT in one population (Kreiss *et al.*, 1981). Thus, a low proportion of DDE indicates a relatively high intake of performed DDT and relatively few years for metabolism of stored DDT to DDE.

A number of factors, especially dosage, age, sex, race, and various disease states, have been discussed in connection with the storage and excretion of DDT by people (see Section 7.2.3), but only dosage has been shown to be of practical importance.

DDT and related compounds are stored at much lower rates in the general population than in persons with occupational exposure. However, these relatively low levels of storage constitute one of the most important aspects of the measurable effects of pesticides on people. Consequently, these values have been presented and discussed in detail (see Section 7.2.2.2 and Table 15.12). Briefly, storage of total DDT in the body fat of ordinary people in the United States increased from 5.3 ppm in 1950 to about 15.6 ppm in 1955 and 1956. Thereafter, the levels decreased gradually, albeit somewhat irregularly, to about 8 ppm in 1970 and to 3 ppm in 1980 (see Fig. 7.3). In annual surveys in the United States based on 898–1920 samples per year, the geometric mean levels for total DDT in adipose tissue on a lipid basis were 7.88, 7.95, 6.88, 5.89, and 5.02 ppm for fiscal years 1970, 1971, 1972, 1973, and 1974, respectively. For each year, the values were higher for older age groups and higher for black than for white people. During fiscal year 1974, the values for persons 0–14, 15–44, and 45 years old or more were 2.15, 4.91, and 6.55 ppm, respectively, for white people and 4.02, 9.18, and 11.91 ppm, respectively, for black people (Kutz *et al.*, 1977). The values would have been somewhat lower if they had been based on wet weight.

It has been calculated that if exposure to DDT ceased it would take 10–20 years for DDT to disappear from a person but that DDE would persist throughout the life span (Morgan and Roan, 1977).

Storage in Blood No information is available on blood levels of DDT in persons poisoned by the compound. Concentrations measured in the blood or serum of workers are shown in Table 15.11. The highest value for total DDT in serum reported from several countries was 2.2017 ppm (with an average of 0.7371 ppm) based on gas chromatography (Laws *et al.*, 1967). A different situation is indicated by a report by Genina *et al.* (1969), who used a total chloride method to analyze samples of blood from controls and from persons with occupational exposure to DDT, polychloropinene, and BHC. These authors reported chloroganic compounds as high as 38.4 ppm in the blood of warehousemen. This concentration is about 20 times the highest value found by the same authors in their control group. The factor of 20 is not remarkable, but (especially in view of the fact that polychloropinene and BHC are excreted more readily than DDT and DDE) values as high as 9 ppm in the controls are completely unexpected. Whether the difference was based on massive exposure or analytical factors is unclear.

The concentrations of DDT in the blood of ordinary people are shown in Table 15.13 and are discussed in Section 7.2.2.3. It is of interest that although each person without special exposure to DDT has relatively constant serum levels of DDT and DDE, and DDE values differ more than the DDT values from person to person (Apple *et al.*, 1970). Whether this reflects differences in metabolism or differences in past exposure is unclear. Kreiss *et al.* (1981) have shown that DDE in serum samples of a community exceptionally exposed to DDT increased with age of the individual.

Surveys have demonstrated a gradual decline in the concentrations of DDT and related compounds in human fat. Presumably a similar decline has occurred in the levels of these compounds in human serum, but apparently no surveys have been carried out and, therefore, no direct evidence is available.

When storage of DDT has been found to be greater in black

Table 15.12

Concentrations of Some Chlorinated Hydrocarbon Pesticides in Body Fat of the General Population of Different Countries

Country	Year	Number of samples	Total DDT (ppm)	Total BHC (ppm)	Dieldrin (ppm)	Heptachlor epoxide (ppm)	References
North America							
Canada	1959–1960	62	4.9				Read and McKinley (1961)
	1966	47	4.39				Brown (1967)
	1966	35			0.22		Brown (1967)
	1966	42		0.07			Brown (1967)
	1966	22				0.14	Brown (1967)
	1967–1968	51	5.86				Kadis et al. (1970)
	1969	221	4.85	0.015	0.122	0.040	Ritchey et al. (1973)
	unknown				≤1.810	≤0.518	Larsen et al. (1971)
	unknown				.≤0.087	≤0.136	Larsen et al. (1971)
	unknown		5.83				Brown and Chow (1975)
	1972	168	2.57	0.65	0.069	0.043	Mes et al. (1977)
	1976	99	2.06	0.158	0.049	0.037	Mes et al. (1982)
	1979–1981	91	3.78		0.036	0.035	Williams et al. (1984)
Greenland	1974	33	3.3		0.09	0.12	Jensen and Clausen (1979)
United States	<1942	10	ND[a]				Hayes et al. (1958)
	1950	75	5.3				Laug et al. (1951)
	1955	49	19.9				Hayes et al. (1956)
	1954–1956	61	11.7				Hayes et al. (1958)
	1956	36	15.6				Hayes et al. (1971)
	1961–1962	130	12.7				Quinby et al. (1965a)
	1961–1962	28	6.7	0.20	0.15		Dale and Quinby (1963)
	1962–1963	282	11.1	0.57	0.11		Hoffman et al. (1964)
	1964	64	7.6		0.31	0.10	Zavon et al. (1965)
	1964	25	10.3	0.60	0.29	0.24	Hayes et al. (1965)
	1964–1965	18	9.0		0.002–0.8		Schafer and Campbell (1966)
	1964–1965	42	10.6				Radomski et al. (1968)
(Florida)	1964–1965	42			0.215		Fiserova-Bergerova et al. (1967)
(Chicago)	1962–1966	221–994[b]	10.4	0.48	0.14	0.16	Hoffman et al. (1967)
	1964–1965	12	11.5				Davies et al. (1968)
	1965–1967	17	5.5				Davies et al. (1968)
	1965–1967	90	8.4				Davies et al. (1968)
	1965–1967	17	7.8				Davies et al. (1968)
(Hawaii)	1965–1967	30	6.51		0.0300	0.0220	Casarett et al. (1968)
(Hawaii)	1965–1967	29	6.31		0.630	0.0320	Casarett et al. (1968)
(Hawaii)	1965–1967	30	6.17		0.0270	0.0270	Casarett et al. (1968)
	1965–1967	146			0.22		Edmundson et al. (1968)
	1965–1967	42			0.21		Radomski et al. (1968)
(11 states)	1965–1967	733	6.22	0.29	0.15	0.05	A. Yobs, personal communication (1969)
(20 states)	1965–1967	3104	7.67	0.24	0.10	0.05	A. Yobs, personal communication (1969)
(Arizona)	1966–1968	70	6.69		0.14		Morgan and Roan (1970)
	1967–1971	103	7.1				Warnick and Carter (1972)
(Idaho)	1970	200	9.9	0.3	0.2	0.1	Wyllie et al. (1972)
	1970	1412	7.87[c,d]	0.43[c,d]	0.18[c,d]	0.09[c,d]	Kutz et al. (1974b)
(Texas)	1969–1972	221	23.18	1.29	0.35		Burns (1974)
	1970	1410	7.88[d]				Kutz et al. (1977)
	1971	1612	7.95[d]				Kutz et al. (1977)
	1972	1919	6.88[d]				Kutz et al. (1977)
	1973	1092	5.89[d]				Kutz et al. (1977)
(Pennsylvania, black)	1973–1974	14	14.0[d]		0.30[d]		Domanski et al. (1977)
(Pennsylvania, white)	1973–1974	13	5.1[d]		0.24[d]		Domanski et al. (1977)
	1974	898	5.02[d]				Kutz et al. (1977)
(Louisiana)	1977	22	8.29		0.17	0.16	Greer et al. (1980)
(Florida)	unknown	10	6.71		0.15	0.06	Barquet et al. (1981)

(*continued*)

Table 15.12 (*Continued*)

Country	Year	Number of samples	Total DDT (ppm)	Total BHC (ppm)	Dieldrin (ppm)	Heptachlor epoxide (ppm)	References
Central America and Mexico							
Costa Rica	1984?	30	59.2[d]		0.16[d]	0.38[d]	Barquero and Constenla (1986)
Mexico	1975	19	21.47[d]		0.06[d]		Albert et al. (1980)
South America							
Argentina	1967	37	13.2	2.44	0.38	0.192	Wassermann et al. (1968a)
Venezuela	1964	38	10.3	0.16	0.60		W. E. Dale, personal communication (1971)
Brazil	1969–1970	38	4.1				Wassermann et al. (1972c)
Europe							
Austria	1966		6.33	1.9	0.1		Pesendorfer et al. (1973)
Belgium	1964	20	3.3				Maes and Heyndrickx (1966)
	1975	60	8.29	0.76	0.26	0.38	Djonckheere et al. (1977)
Czechoslovakia	1963–1964	229	9.6				Halacka et al. (1965)
	1975–1976	13	2.26–3.97	2.55–20.95			Dubsky et al. (1977)
Denmark	1965	18	3.3		0.20		Weihe (1966)
	1974	17	1.8		0.09	0.08	Jensen and Clausen (1979)
England	1961–1962	131	2.2		0.21		Hunter et al. (1963)
	1963–1964	66	3.3	0.42	0.26	0.1	Egan et al. (1965)
	1964	100	3.9	0.02	0.21	0.1	Robinson et al. (1965)
	1964	44	4.0		0.22		Robinson and Hunter (1966)
	1965	101	2.85	0.19	0.34		Cassidy et al. (1967)
	1965–1967	248	3.00	0.31	0.21	0.04	Abbott et al. (1968)
United Kingdom	1969–1971	201	2.5	0.29	0.16	0.03	Abbott et al. (1972)
	1976–1977	236	2.6	0.33	0.11	0.03	Abbott et al. (1981)
	1982–1983	187	1.54	0.30	0.08		Abbott et al. (1985)
Finland	1972–1974	73	2.5				Hattula et al. (1976)
	1983	65	0.33			0.002	Mussalo-Rauhama et al. (1984)
France	1961	10	5.2	1.19			Hayes et al. (1963)
Germany (East)	1966–1967	100	13.1	0.16			Engst et al. (1967)
	1958–1959	60	2.3				Maier-Bode (1960)
Germany (West)	1970	20	3.6	0.45			Acker and Schulte (1970)
			3.8	0.5	0.2		Acker and Schulte (1971)
		10	4.24	2.9	0.11	0.097	Acker and Schulte (1974)
		10	4.77	8.2	0.17	.12	Acker and Schulte (1974)
		10	5.42	5.9	0.091	0.062	Acker and Schulte (1974)
		10	8.36	4.8	0.082	0.085	Acker and Schulte (1974)
		10	7.80	6.4	0.23	0.096	Acker and Schulte (1974)
(workers)	1979?	8		54.5[d]			Baumann et al. (1980)
Hungary	1960	48	12.4				Denes (1962)
	1964	15			0.16		Denes (1966)
	1969		13.7	2.30			Berend et al. (1970)
	1970		18.9	0.76			Soos et al. (1972)
Italy	1965	9	5.0		0.594		Kanitz and Castello (1966)
	1965–1966	18	10.86	2.25	0.84	0.46	Paccagnella et al. (1967)
	1966	·22	15.48	0.08	0.68	0.23	Del Vecchio and Leoni (1967)
	1970?	31	16.75	0.02	0.10		Prati and Del Dot (1971)
	1983–1984	26	8.99[e]				Focardi et al. (1986)
Netherlands	1964	20	7.7				Wit (1964)
	1966	11	2.22	0.11	0.20	0.01	De Vlieger et al. (1968)
Norway		56	3.2				Bjerk (1972)
	1972	7	10				Kveseth et al. (1979)
	1975–1976	58	0.75–2.60				Brevik and Bjerk (1978)
	1981–1982	16	0.448				Skaare et al. (1988)

(*continued*)

Table 15.12 (*Continued*)

Country	Year	Number of samples	Total DDT (ppm)	Total BHC (ppm)	Dieldrin (ppm)	Heptachlor epoxide (ppm)	References
Poland	1965	72	13.4				Bronisz *et al.* (1967)
	1970	70	11.4	0.5	ND		Juskiewicz and Stec (1971)
	1972	15	5.23				Bojanowska *et al.* (1973)
	1977–1978	100	4.47	0.216			Syrowatka *et al.* (1979)
Romania		20		0.48–42			Mandroiu and Iordachescu (1971)
	1972–973		2.41				Ciupe (1976)
Spain	1966	41	15.7				Llinares and Wasserman (1968)
	1970s	40	4.549	0.062	0.15	0.015	Herrea-Marteache *et al.* (1978)
	1980s	55	8.95	1.38	0.27	0.16	To-Figueras *et al.* (1986)
Switzerland		12	1.9–16.3	0.3–1.8	0.07–0.57		Zimmerli and Marek (1973)
USSR		41	8.06				Vas'Kovaskaja and Komarova (1963)
		197	8.8658–15.4794	2.15			Vas'Kovskaja (1969)
Africa							
Nigeria	1967	43	8.8				Wassermann *et al.* (1968b)
	1969	41	6.5	0.19			Wassermann *et al.* (1972c)
Kenya		83	5.4		0.1	0.1	Wassermann *et al.* (1972b)
South Africa							
(Bantu)	1969	73	5.94	1.93	0.034	0.01	M. Wassermann *et al.* (1970b)
(white)	1969	41	7.16	3.27	0.047	0.01	M. Wassermann *et al.* (1970b)
Uganda		75	2.9	0.1		0.02	Wassermann *et al.* (1974a)
Asia							
Burma	unknown	43	0.3–7.0				Shure and Law (1977)
India	1964	35–67	26	1.43	0.04		Dale *et al.* (1965)
	1964	16	13				Dale *et al.* (1965)
	unknown	94	21.8				Ramachandran *et al.* (1973)
	1975–1976	100	0.45				Mukherjee *et al.* (1980)
	1981?	6	1.754	2.344			Kaphalia and Seth (1983)
	1976	14	4.7				Bhaskaran *et al.* (1979)
Iran	1974–1976	170	8.13	0.26	0.049		Hashemy-Tonkabony and Soleimani-Amin (1978)
Israel	1963–1964	254	19.2				Wassermann *et al.* (1965)
	1965–1966	71	4.6				Wassermann *et al.* (1967)
	1965–1966	133	8.2				Wassermann *et al.* (1967)
	1967–1971	63	14.4				Wassermann *et al.* (1974b)
Japan	1968–1969	241	2.4	0.12–1.28	0.13	0.02	Curley *et al.* (1970)
	1969–1970	74	6.92	12.17	0.46	0.01	Nishimoto *et al.* (1970)
	1970	21	3.69		0.33		Doguchi *et al.* (1971)
	1970		4.499	2.420	0.163		Suzuki *et al.* (1973)
	1971		2.694	3.001	0.208		Suzuki *et al.* (1973)
	1971	30	12.859	6.160	0.098		Kasai *et al.* (1972)
	1972		4.001	3.698	0.429		Suzuki *et al.* (1973)
	1972	42	5.992		0.310		Kasai *et al.* (1972)
	1973	60	6.44	2.659	0.129		Kawanishi *et al.* (1973)
	1974	17	6.87	3.0			Inoue *et al.* (1974)
	1974	30	3.59	2.36			Fukano and Doguchi (1977)
	1974	20	9.25[d]	11.90[d]			Mori *et al.* (1983)
	1976	22	4.79[d]	4.92[d]			Mori *et al.* (1983)
	1981	46	4.04[d]	3.77[d]			Mori *et al.* (1983)
Pakistan		60	25.0	0.48	0.47		Mughal and Rahman (1973)

(*continued*)

Table 15.12 (*Continued*)

Country	Year	Number of samples	Total DDT (ppm)	Total BHC (ppm)	Dieldrin (ppm)	Heptachlor epoxide (ppm)	References
Thailand	1969–1970	77	12.6	0.2	0.2		Wassermann *et al.* (1972c)
Turkey	1984–1985	48	7.12[d]	1.72[d]			Karakaya *et al.* (1987)
Oceania							
Australia	1965	53	1.81		0.05		Bick (1967)
	1965–1966	46	10.2				Wassermann *et al.* (1968a)
	1965–1966	12	10.5	0.68	0.67	0.02	Wassermann *et al.* (1968a)
	1971	75	4.94		0.21		Brady and Siyali (1972)
	1985–1986	292	3.72		0.13		Ahmad *et al.* (1988)
New Zealand	1963–1964	45		0.49			Dacre (1969)
	1966	52	5.8		0.27		Brewton and McGrath (1967)
	1965–1969	254	14.6		0.35		Copplestone *et al.* (1973)

[a] Not detected.
[b] Different numbers of samples examined for different compounds.
[c] Geometric mean.
[d] Lipid basis.
[e] Dry weight basis.

people, the difference could be accounted for by greater exposure (Hayes, 1975; D'Ercole *et al.*, 1976). However, Sandifer (1974), who found that the concentrations of DDT in the sera of blacks was two to three times greater than those in whites, also found a significant correlation between total DDT and deficiency of glucose-6-phosphate dehydrogenase, a condition much more common in blacks than whites. Thus, a genetic factor in the storage of DDT appears possible, but additional evidence would be necessary to confirm it.

Whether the high storage in blacks is strictly environmental or partly genetic, it is certain that as high or higher levels have been recorded among several groups of rural blacks in different parts of the southeastern United States than were reported by Kreiss *et al.* (1981) among blacks in Triana, Alabama, who had mean values of 0.096 and 0.062 ppm for total DDT in the serum of males and females, respectively. Other average values for rural blacks have included 0.101 ppm for women (D'Ercole *et al.*, 1976), 0.072 and 0.066 ppm for children and mothers, respectively (Keil *et al.*, 1972a,b, 1973), 0.065–0.214 ppm for blacks of different ages or rural locations (Arthur, 1976), and 0.108 and 0.105 ppm for males and females in four rural communities in the Mississippi Delta (unpublished result from CDC). Thus, there is no evidence that DDT and related compounds downstream from a former DDT factory led to greater absorption than occurred in other places.

Storage in Other Tissues With the exception of concentrations of 19–36 ppm in heart, kidney, and liver of a man who died of DDT poisoning under unstated circumstances (Luis, 1952), no information is available on tissue levels in people with heavy exposure, whether occupational or otherwise. Storage of DDT and related compounds in the organs of adults and fetuses in the general population was discussed and tabulated

by Hayes (1975). Concentrations in the viscera of adults averaged 1.0 ppm, but concentrations in lymph nodes and especially bone marrow (a fatty tissue) approached the level in adipose tissue (≤ 6.0). Concentrations in some viscera of stillborn infants were similar to those in adipose tissue of the same infants and also in adults, suggesting that there had been a mobilization of DDT from fat prior to death.

Saxena *et al.* (1987a) have reported that the levels of DDT in human leiomyomatous uterine tissue were much higher than those in normal tissue (means of 0.845 ppm and 0.103 ppm, respectively). Whether this is related to any estrogenic actions of DDT is unknown.

Secretion in Milk No information is available on the secretion of DDT in the milk of women who were occupationally exposed to the compound or who were made ill by it, regardless of circumstances. The concentrations of DDT in the milk of women in various general populations are shown in Table 15.14. As may be seen, values reported from Guatemala and early values from the USSR were much higher than those from other countries, and yet there was no indication of illness among babies fed such milk. The significance of DDT in milk and the dosages that different concentrations of it determine were discussed by Hayes (1975), Jensen (1983), Spindler (1983), and Coulston (1985).

Quinby *et al.* (1965a,b) noted that women apparently were in negative DDT balance during lactation, but no direct measurement of DDT intake of women participating in the study was made. More recently, the ingestion of DDT in food and the secretion of DDT in milk were measured in the same women, and the fact of negative balance was confirmed (Adamovic and Sokic, 1973; Adamovic *et al.*, 1978; Cocisiu *et al.*, 1976). In fact, it has been suggested that this phenomenon may be a

Table 15.13

Concentrations of Some Chlorinated Hydrocarbon Pesticides in Blood of the General Population of Different Countries

Country	Year	Number of samples	Total DDT (ppm)	Total BHC (ppm)	Dieldrin (ppm)	Heptachlor epoxide (ppm)	References
North America							
Canada			0.032				Brown and Chow (1975)
United States	1965	10	0.0418	0.0034	0.0019	0.0011	Dale et al. (1966a)
USA	1966	10, F[a]	0.0360				Dale et al. (1967)
	1966	10, M[a]	0.0746				Dale et al. (1967)
	1966–1967	53[b]	0.00501	0.00048	0.00026	0.00021	Selby et al. (1969)
	1967	64	0.01425	0.00150	0.00069	0.00000	A. Yobs, personal communication (1969)
	1968	106	0.01397	0.00000	0.00014	0.00000	A. Yobs, personal communication (1969)
	1967–1986	1000	0.0294	0.0021	0.0005	0.00007	Watson et al. (1970)
(rural black)	1968	139	0.0109		0.0002		Finklea et al. (1972)
(urban black)	1968	175	0.0125		0.0002		Finklea et al. (1972)
(rural white)	1968	210	0.0056		0.0004		Finklea et al. (1972)
(urban white)	1968	199	0.0047		0.0003		Finklea et al. (1972)
	1969	30[c,d]	0.0144	0.0030	0.0007	0.0011	Curley et al. (1969)
	1968	5[e]	0.0050	0.0012	0.0009	0.0008	Curley and Kimbrough (1969)
	1968	10[e]	0.0205	0.0034	0.0003	0.0006	Curley and Kimbrough (1969)
	1970	26	0.03169		0.00149		Radomski et al. (1971)
	1972	214[f]	0.006–0.822	0.001–0.017	0.001–0.025		Griffith and Blanke (1975)
	1970s	33, F	0–0.0782	0–0.0058	0.001		Barquet et al. (1981)
(Alaska)	1972	38[j]	0.002		0.011		Serat et al. (1977)
(urban)	1968–1970	275, M	0.0314		0.0003		Bloomer et al. (1977)
(urban)	1968–1970	205, F	0.0232		0.00015		Bloomer et al. (1977)
(rural)	1968–1970	232, M	0.0357		0.0003		Bloomer et al. (1977)
(rural)	1968–1970	243, F	0.0261		0.00011		Bloomer et al. (1977)
(black)[d]	1972–1973	209	0.007–0.292	0–0.009	0–0.003	0–0.003	D'Ercole et al. (1976)
(black)[e]	1972–1973	209	0.016–0.303	0–0.019	0–0.003	0–0.001	D'Ercole et al. (1976)
(white)[d]	1972–1973	130	0.003–0.056	0–0.009	0–0.002	0–0.002	D'Ercole et al. (1976)
(white)[e]	1972–1973	130	0.007–0.160	0–0.009	0–0.006	0–0.002	D'Ercole et al. (1976)
	1976–1980	3127	0.090	0.0002	0.0001		HANES II (1980)
(South Carolina)	1978	25			0–0.0034		Sandifer et al. (1981)
(Hawaii)	1979	200	0.004–0.152	0–0.0002	0–0.002		Takahashi and Parks (1982)
	1980	499	0.001–2.821				Kreiss et al. (1981)
South America							
Argentina	1970	20[g]	0.01934	0.02399	0.00143		Radomski et al. (1971)
	1970	18[h]	0.01327	0.00704	0.00094		Radomski et al. (1971)
	1970	19[i]	0.00869	0.00704	0.00054		Radomski et al. (1971)
Brazil	1975	32, F	0.036				Procianoy and Schvartsman (1982)
	1975?	32[d]	0.0153				Procianoy and Schvartsman (1982)
(industrial)	1980?	21	0.0219	0.0090			de Fernicola and de Azevedo (1982)
(rural)	1980?	21	0.0316	0.0087			de Fernicola and de Azevedo (1982)
Europe							
Hungary	1967–1968	120	0.034	0.019	0.001		Czegledi-Janko (1969)
Norway	1981–1982	15[e]	0.019	0.001			Skaare et al. (1988)
(immigrants)	1981–1982	5[e]	0.150	0.002			Skaare et al. (1988)
Poland			0.172, F	0.008, F			Jonczyk (1970)
	1972	15	0.030	0.084			Bojanowska et al. (1973)
	1979	100	0.0281	0.0092			Syrowatka et al. (1979)
Switzerland		13	0.0209	0.0038	0.0014		Zimmerli and Marek (1973)
Yugoslavia	1975	147	0.07478	0.00734			Reiner et al. (1977)
(urban)	1978–1979	11	0.0353				Krauthacker et al. (1980b)
(rural)	1979	41	0.0102				Krauthacker et al. (1980a)
	1980s	14, F	0.0162	0.0035			Roncevic et al. (1987)
	1978–1981	31, F	0.0215	0.0059			Bazulic et al. (1984)

(continued)

Table 15.13 (*Continued*)

Country	Year	Number of samples	Total DDT (ppm)	Total BHC (ppm)	Dieldrin (ppm)	Heptachlor epoxide (ppm)	References
Africa							
Tunisia	1980s	20	0.091	0.007			Jemma *et al.* (1986)
Asia							
India							
(Delhi)	1985?	50	0.301				Saxena *et al.* (1987b)
(Lucknow)	1981?	48, M	0.028	0.075			Kaphalia and Seth (1983)
(Lucknow)	1979–1980	29e	0.026	0.0499			Saxena *et al.* (1983)
(Lucknow)	1970s	25e	0.020	0.022			Siddiqui *et al.* (1981)
Israel	1975	19	0.0740	0.0147	0.0099	0.0136	Polishuk *et al.* (1977)
	1984–1985	14, M	0.0249		0.0027	0.0116	Pines *et al.* (1987)
Japan	1970	10	0.074	0.150			Tokutsu *et al.* (1970)
	1971		0.005	0.006	0.001		Kojima *et al.* (1971)
	1971	138	0.0183				Kasai *et al.* (1972)
	1971		0.0093	0.191	0.0030		Yamagishi *et al.* (1972a)
	1971		0.0285	0.0577			Kaku (1973)
	1972		0.001–0.078	0.030–0.067	0.003		Study Group (1972)
		37	0.0437, F	0.030–0.046	0–0.0031		Nawa (1973)
		e	0.1358	0.0326			Hara *et al.* (1973)
		d	0.0210	0.0185			Hara *et al.* (1973)
		17		0.0118			Inoue *et al.* (1974)
	1973	82	0.0179	0.0106	0.0011		Abe *et al.* (1974)
Oceania							
Australia		52	0.0172	0.0032	0.0023	0.0031	Siyali (1972)
		47	0.0167				Ouw and Shandar (1974)

a F, Female; M, male.
b Geometric mean.
c Mean of positive values only.
d Cord blood from live term infants.
e Maternal blood.
f Ages 41–60.
g Adults.
h 6–11 years old.
i 1–5 years old.
j 6–17-year-old Eskimos.

significant factor in determining the lower levels of DDT found in women than men in the general population (Adamovic and Sokic, 1973).

Johnsson *et al.* (1977) found significantly lower levels of DDT (mean of 0.008 ppm) and of DDE (mean of 0.035 ppm) than had been reported earlier for the milk of city dwellers. However, levels remained quite high (0.05–1.90 ppm) in some rural black people (Woodard *et al.*, 1976). Some evidence suggests that DDT levels are higher in milk from smokers than nonsmokers, although there may be an occupational explanation (Coulston, 1985).

Overall, despite the presence of DDT in human milk and placenta, there seems little risk to neonates in many different populations.

Excretion of DDT-Related Compounds Among workers whose DDT intake was estimated to be about 35 mg/day, Ortelee (1958) reported that the concentration of DDA in urine ranged from 0.12 to 7.56 ppm and averaged 1.71 ppm. Among workers whose exposure was about half as great, Laws *et al.*

(1967) found concentrations from 0.01 to 2.67 ppm with a mean of 0.97 ppm.

Continuous sampling of a DDT-formulating plant worker's urine showed that excretion of DDA increased promptly when exposure began on each of 5 consecutive workdays but often continued after exposure, sometimes reached a peak about midnight, and then decreased rapidly. On day 6, when there was no occupational exposure to DDT, the excretion of DDA continued until a very low level was reached. The highest concentration of DDA reported in this study was 0.68 ppm (Wolfe and Armstrong, 1971).

The urine of people in the general population contains not only DDA but also neutral compounds; the average concentrations reported by Cueto and Biros (1967) were: p,p'-DDT, 0.0007 ppm and p,p'-DDE, 0.0156 pm. Men with heavy occupational exposure to DDT excreted much more DDA but showed only a statistically insignificant increase in excretion of DDT and DDE.

The values just given for the average excretion of DDA, DDT, and DDE by different, small groups of people would

Table 15.14
Concentrations of Some Chlorinated Hydrocarbon Pesticides in Milk of the General Population of Different Countries

Country	Year	Number of samples	Total DDT (ppm)	Total BHC (ppm)	Dieldrin (ppm)	Heptachlor epoxide (ppm)	References
North America							
Canada	1967–1968	147	0.139		0.005	0.003	Ritchey et al. (1972)
	unknown	15	0.019–0.035				Musial et al. (1974)
	unknown				0.009	0.003	Larsen et al. (1971)
	unknown				0.013	0.052	Larsen et al. (1971)
	1969–1974	101					
	1970	90	0.077	0.002	0.005	0.004	Mes et al. (1977)
	1975	100	0.046	0.002	0.002	0.001	Mes and Davies (1979)
	1978–1979	154	0.039				Dillon et al. (1981)
	1982	210	0.038	0.008	0.002		Collins et al. (1982)
	1986?	18	0.016	0.006	0.0004	0.0002	Davies and Mes (1987)
United States	1950	32	0.13				Laug et al. (1951)
	1960–1961	10	0.12				Quinby et al. (1965b)
	1962	6	0.37[a]				West (1964)
	1968	unknown	0.078				Curley and Kimbrough (1969)
	1970	53	0.101			0.0066	Kroger (1972)
	1970–1971	101	0.17				Wilson et al. (1973)
	1975	55	0.114				Bradt and Herrenkohl (1976)
	1973–1974	57	0.344	0.005	0.004	0.004	Strassman and Kutz (1977)
	1971–1972	40	0.126				Savage et al. (1973)
(black)	1974	38	0.447				Woodard et al. (1976)
(white)	1974	14	0.075				Woodard et al. (1976)
(total)	1975	1436	0.070	0.003	0.002	0.001	Savage et al. (1981)
(pesticide workers)	1973–1975	34	0.719	0.022	0.006	0.003	Barnett et al. (1979)
(non-pesticide workers)	1973–1975	6	0.083	0.011	0.004	0.002	Barnett et al. (1979)
(Hawaii)	1979–1980	54	2.16[b]	0.180[b]	0.042[b]	0.036[b]	Takei et al. (1983)
(Missouri)	1977	51	0.022	0.003	0.014		Jonsson et al. (1977)
Central America and Mexico							
El Salvador	1973–1974	40	0.695	0.012	0.005	0.003	de Campos and Olszyna-Marzys (1978)
Guatemala							
(La Bomba)	1970	10	2.15	0.03	trace	0.003	Olszyna-Marzys et al. (1973)
(El Rosario)	1970	27	1.84	0.007	0.002	0.007	Olszyna-Marzys et al. (1973)
(Cerro Colorado)	1971	9	4.07	0.02		trace	Olszyna-Marzys et al. (1973)
(City)	1974	15	0.480				de Campos and Olszyna-Marzys (1978)
(Izabal)	1974	10	2.55		0.005	0.002	de Campos and Olszyna-Marzys (1978)
(Escuintla)	1974	10	3.54		0.070	0.003	de Campos and Olszyna-Marzys (1978)
Mexico	1976	15	0.266		0.030		Albert et al. (1981)
South America							
Argentina	1981	20	0.061	0.037			Landoui and Astolfi (1982)
Chile	1977	unknown	0.258				Albert (1981)
Brazil	1975–1976	26	0.090				Matuo et al. (1980)
Uruguay		10	0.230	0.057	0.032	0.002	Bauza (1975)
Europe							
Austria							
(Vienna)		22	4.725[b]	1.488[b]			Pesendorfer (1975)
(Mistelbach)		9	6.13[b]	4.013[b]			Pesendorfer (1975)
Belgium	1968	20	0.128	0.010	0.004		Heyndrickx and Maes (1969)
	1982	47	0.041	0.0567		0.0021	Rogirst et al. (1983)
Czechoslovakia	1968	unknown	0.101				Hruska (1969)
		393	0.209				Suvak (1970)
Denmark	1982	57	1.15[b]	0.08[b]	0.04[b]		Andersen and Orbaek (1982)
England	1963–1964	19	0.013	0.006			Egan et al. (1965)
United Kingdom	1979–1980	102	0.051	0.008	0.002		Collins et al. (1982)
Finland	1982	50	0.031				Wickström et al. (1983)

(continued)

Table 15.14 (*Continued*)

Country	Year	Number of samples	Total DDT (ppm)	Total BHC (ppm)	Dieldrin (ppm)	Heptachlor epoxide (ppm)	References
France		59[c]		0–0.190	0.007–0.032	0.002–0.012	Luquet *et al.* (1972)
	1971–1972		3.24[b]	2.75[b]	0.23[b]	0.28[b]	Luquet *et al.* (1974a)
	1972–1973		3.51[b]	1.77[b]		0.28[b]	Luquet *et al.* (1974b)
	1970	49		0.003–0.202	0.001	0.001	Goursaud *et al.* (1971)
	1974–1975	13	1.04[b]	0.052[b]	0.035[b]	0.08[b]	De Bellini *et al.* (1977)
Germany (West)	1970?	43	0.121				Acker and Shulte (1970)
Germany	1970?		0.569				Adamovic *et al.* (1971)
	1969	57	0.23				Engst and Knoll (1972)
	1970	18	0.16				Engst and Knoll (1972)
	1971	96	0.32				Knoll and Jayaraman (1973a,b)
	1970		4.1[b]	0.54[b]			Acker and Shulte (1971)
	1970						Acker and Shulte (1971)
	1973	184	0.23				Thielemann *et al.* (1975)
Germany (East)	1978	85	0.349				Thielemann (1979)
	1979	200	0.096		0.010		Hesse *et al.* (1981)
Germany (West)	1979–1980	unknown	2.00[b]				Acker (1981)
Hungary	1963	10	0.13–0.26[d]				Denes (1964)
Ireland	1971–1972		0.128[b]	0.001[b]	0.001[b]	0.005[b]	Downey *et al.* (1975)
Italy	1983–1985	65	0.051	0.007			Dommarco *et al.* (1987)
Netherlands	1969	50	2.7[b]				Tuinstra (1971)
	1978?	69	0.031		0.0023		Eckenhausen *et al.* (1981)
Norway	1976	45	0.050				Brevik and Bjerk (1978)
	1979	19	0.024				Skaare (1981)
	1982	34	0.024	0.002			Skaare *et al.* (1988)
(immigrants)	1982	5	0.107	0.008			Skaare *et al.* (1988)
Poland		128	0.25	0.003			Juskiewicz *et al.* (1972)
	1966	26	0.27				Bronisz and Ochynski (1968)
	1967	25	0.40				Bronisz and Ochynski (1968)
	1970?	40	0.28	0.006			Kontek *et al.* (1971)
	1979	40	0.179				Kontek *et al.* (1981)
Portugal	1972	168	0.326				Graca *et al.* (1974)
Romania	1968?	100	0.08–1.58				Unterman and Sirghie (1969)
				0.08–1.58			Mandroui and Iordachescu (1971)
Spain	1979	45	0.181	0.039	0.0005		Pozo Lora *et al.* (1979)
	1981	20	0.256	0.020	0.003	0.004	Baluja *et al.* (1982)
Sweden	1967?	unknown	0.117				Lofroth (1968)
	1967–1969	22	0.115	traces	0.001		Westoo *et al.* (1970)
	1976–1977	?	0.033		0.0007		Westoo and Noren (1978)
	1978–1979	23	0.061	0.0036	0.0008		Hofvander *et al.* (1981)
USSR	1964	16	1.22–4.88				Damaskin (1965)
	1964–1965	4505	0.1–1.0				Gracheva (1969)
	1969?	680	0.25				Gracheva (1970)
	1967	370	0.1				Komarova (1970)
	1977?	252	0.580				Gulko *et al.* (1978)
Yugoslavia	1981–1982	50	0.0743	0.011			Krauthacker *et al.* (1986)
	1977	34	0.051				Krauthacker *et al.* (1980)
Africa							
Kenya							
(nomads)	1984	13	1.69[b]	0.038[b]	2.445[b]		Kanja *et al.* (1986)
(farmers)	1985	48	9.76[b]	0.22[b]	0.310[b]		Kanja *et al.* (1986)
Nigeria	1981–1982	35	1.51[b]	0.52[b]			Atuma and Vaz (1986)
Tunisia	1980s	80	0.145	0.039	0.006		Jamma *et al.* (1986)
Asia							
India							
(Lucknow)	1970s	25	0.12	0.107			Siddiqui *et al.* (1981)
(Punjab)	1979	75	0.51	0.195			Kalra and Chawla (1981)
(Bangalore)	unknown	6	0.053	0.014			Ramakrishnan *et al.* (1985)
(Calcutta)	unknown	6	0.114	0.031			Ramakrishnan *et al.* (1985)
(Bombay)	unknown	6	0.224	0.053			Ramakrishnan *et al.* (1985)
(Ahmedabad)	1981–1982	50	0.305	0.225			Jani *et al.* (1988)
Iran	1974–1976	131	0.044	0.008	0.011		Hashemy-Tonkabony and Fateminassab (1977)

(*continued*)

Table 15.14 (*Continued*)

Country	Year	Number of samples	Total DDT (ppm)	Total BHC (ppm)	Dieldrin (ppm)	Heptachlor epoxide (ppm)	References
Iraq	1983–1984	50	0.145	0.073	0.030		Al-Omar *et al.* (1985)
Israel	1975	29	0.0717	0.0101	0.0070	0.0091	Polishuk *et al.* (1977)
	1980s	100	0.0875	0.0125			Weisenberg *et al.* (1985)
Japan	1970–1971			0.02–0.4			Narafu (1971)
	1971–1972	398	0.0562				Anonymous (1972)
	1971	43	0.179				Hidaka *et al.* (1972)
	1970	10	0.071				Tokutsu *et al.* (1970)
	1970?	5	0.160				Takeshita and Inuyama (1970)
	1970?	10	0.120				Takeshita and Inuyama (1970)
	1971?		0.04				Kojima *et al.* (1971)
	1971?	59	0.019–0.105				Kato *et al.* (1971)
	1971?	14	0.047				Sugaya *et al.* (1971)
	1971	454	0.179	0.033–0.44			Hayashi (1972a,b); Study Group, 1972
	1971–1972	398	0.056				Anonymous (1972)
	1971		0.044				Yamagishi *et al.* (1972a)
		30	2.0[b]				Mizoguchi *et al.* (1972)
		54	0.025				Taira *et al.* (1972)
	1971–1972	398	0.0626	0.105	0.0034	0.0011	Hayashi (1972a,b)
	1971–1972	5	0.027				Nagai (1972)
	1971–1972	5	0.037				Nagai (1972)
	1971–1972	5	0.016				Nagai (1972)
	1971–1972	5	0.037				Nagai (1972)
		30	0.033				Oura *et al.* (1972)
	1971–1972	123	0.105				Kawai *et al.* (1973)
	1971–1972		0.038–0.075				Kamata (1973)
	1970		3.780[b]				Suzuki *et al.* (1973)
	1971		3.592[b]				Suzuki *et al.* (1973)
	1972		3.822[b]				Suzuki *et al.* (1973)
	1973		0.0854				Kamata (1974)
	1971–1975		0.172	0.385	0.006		Matsunaga *et al.* (1975)
		26	0.061	0.067			Anonymous (1975)
	1971–1972	398	0.0626	0.1009	0.0034		Hayashi (1973, 1974)
		10	0.981		0.0051		Inuyama and Takashita (1973)
		10		0.071			
	1973	7	0.071	0.109	0.002		Shimamoto *et al.* (1973)
	1974		2.436[b]	2.313[b]			Sugaya *et al.* (1976)
			2.353[b]	2.442[b]	0.254[b]		Suzuki *et al.* (1976)
		10	0.234	0.040	not found	not found	Yamada and Sakamoto (1973)
	1977	20	1.89[b]		0.052[b]		Yakushiji *et al.* (1979)
Turkey							
(Ankara)	1984–1985	61	3.66[b]	0.97[b]			Karakaya *et al.* (1987)
(Adana-Cujurova)	1984–1985	52	10.57[b]	1.45[b]			Karakaya *et al.* (1987)
Oceania							
Australia	1970	67	0.014[e]				Newton and Greene (1972)
	1970	67	0.007[f]				Newton and Greene (1972)
	1970	67	0.066[g]				Newton and Greene (1972)
(Brisbane)	1971–1972	20	0.288				Miller and Fox (1973)
(Mareeba)	1971–1972	20	0.415				Miller and Fox (1973)
		45	0.064				Siyali (1972)
		22	0.076				Stacy and Thomas (1975)
	1980	14	0.042	0.001	0.013	0.004	Conway *et al.* (1985)
(urban)	1979–1980	45	0.046		0.009		Stacey *et al.* (1985)
(rural)	1979–1980	95	0.041		0.008		Stacey *et al.* (1985)
New Guinea	1972	16	0.004				Hornabrook *et al.* (1972)
	1972	19	0.015				Hornabrook *et al.* (1972)

[a] Maximal value.

[b] Concentration in milk fat (ppm milk fat).

[c] Not all samples tested for all compounds.

[d] Range of values for milk containing 4% fat containing 3.3–6.6 ppm.

[e] At beginning of feeding, 1.8% fat.

[f] At middle of feeding, 1.2% fat.

[g] At end of feeding, 5.1% fat.

Table 15.15
Urinary Excretion of DDA by People in the United States with Varying Degrees of Exposure to DDT[a]

Exposure	Year	Number of samples	DDA excretion (ppm)		Reference
			Range	Mean	
General population	1954	8	<0.05	—	Hayes et al. (1956)
	1957	8	<0.02–0.07	—	Hayes et al. (1971)
	1962	23	<0.02–0.18	—	Durham et al. (1965)
	1968	11	0.008–0.019	0.014	Cranmer et al. (1969)
Environmental[b]	1962	13	0.02–0.11	—	Durham et al. (1965)
Applicators	1962	11	0.02–0.17	—	Durham et al. (1965)
Formulators	1957	40	0.12–7.56	1.71	Ortelee (1958)
Makers and Formulators	1966	35	<0.01–2.67	0.97	Laws et al. (1967)
Volunteers given 3.5 mg/day orally	1953–1954	2	0.10–0.42[c]	0.21[b]	Hayes et al. (1956)
	1957–1958	6	0.06–1.98[d]	0.23[c]	Hayes et al. (1971)
Volunteers given 35 mg/day orally	1953–1954	6	0.69–9.67[c]	2.46[b]	Hayes et al. (1956)
	1957–1958	6	0.18–9.21[d]	3.09[c]	Hayes et al. (1971)

[a] Slightly modified from Hayes (1966) by permission of the National Academy of Sciences.
[b] Residents living within 500 ft of agricultural application.
[c] Based on all samples after week 35 of dosage.
[d] Based on all samples from week 35 through week 93 after dosage started.

indicate a concentration of 0.0358 ppm of DDT-related material expressed as DDT. Although the DDT intakes of these particular groups were not measured, the urinary excretion is of such an order of magnitude that it may account for the excretion of all the absorbed DDT. The excretion of DDA by people with different kinds and degrees of exposure is presented in Table 15.15.

DDT and DDE are excreted in the bile; the concentrations for five men without special exposure varied as follows: p,p'- and o,p'-DDT combined, 0.0000–0.0009 ppm and p,p'-DDE, 0.0005–0.0056 ppm. Higher levels were found in the bile of one pest-control operator (Paschal et al., 1974).

Other Laboratory Findings In the absence of occupational DDT poisoning, there has been no opportunity to explore (as has been done with the cyclodiene insecticides) the relationship between clinical and EEG findings. In fact, the only DDT workers studied in this regard were exposed also to BHC and benzilan, so the findings might have been related to one or more of the compounds or to their interaction. Electroencephalograms were obtained from 73 of these workers exposed for periods ranging from 7 months to 20 years. Just over 78% of the records were normal and 21.9% were abnormal. The most severe changes involved persons exposed to the three compounds for 1–2 years; less severe changes were seen with either shorter or longer exposure. The changes were not correlated with age; the range and mean of age for those judged abnormal were almost identical with these values for persons considered normal. Some of the records showed bitemporal sharp waves with shifting lateralization combined with low-voltage theta activity. Other records showed spike complexes, paroxysmal discharges composed of slow and sharp waves

most pronounced anteriorly, and low-voltage rhythmic spikes posteriorly. None of the persons examined showed any abnormal clinical neurological finding (Israeli and Mayersdorf, 1973; Mayersdorf and Israeli, 1974). The incidence of abnormal electroencephalograms in the general population is 9.0 or 9.2%, according to other investigators cited by Israeli and Mayersdorf. Czegledi-Janko and Avar (1970) considered that nonspecific EEG abnormalities occur in 10–20% of the general population. Under the circumstances, there is some question of whether the results are meaningful.

Clinical laboratory findings associated with DDT poisoning are not diagnostic.

Treatment of Poisoning No useful guidance regarding treatment has been gleaned from the very few cases of DDT poisoning that have occurred. Animal studies indicate that sedatives, ionic calcium, and glucose or another ready source of energy would be useful. On the basis of experience in treating people poisoned by different convulsive poisons, it seems likely that diazepam would be beneficial (see Section 15.2.5).

15.3.2 TDE

15.3.2.1 Identity, Properties, and Uses

Chemical Name TDE is 1,1-dichloro-2,2-bis(4-chlorophenyl)ethane.

Structure See Table 15.2.

Synonyms The common name TDE (ISO) is an acronym for *te*trachloro*d*iphenyl*e*thane. Except in France, it is a generally recognized name for the compound as a synthetic insecticide. This is true even though TDE is an alternative name for an unrelated compound, etoglucid, which is a chemically unrelated antineoplastic drug. For reasons that are obscure, the word DDD (an acronym for *d*ichloro*d*iphenyl*d*ichloroethane) is used very much more commonly for 1,1-dichloro-2,2-bis(chlorophenyl)ethane when viewed as a metabolite of DDT or when used as a therapeutic drug, and this distinction has been retained in this book. As it happens, the term DDD also has two meanings; it is used for 2,2′-*d*ihydroxy-6,6′-*d*inaphthyl*d*isulfide as well as for the compound under discussion. Actually, almost everything we know about the compound relevant to humans is associated with its use as a drug rather than its use as an insecticide. Nonproprietary names for the *o,p*′ isomer which is used as a drug include chlodithane (USSR) and mitotane (United States).

A proprietary name for the insecticide is Rhothane®. Code designations include D-3, ENT-4,225, ME-1,700, and NSC-38,721 (for *o,p*′ isomer only).

Physical and Chemical Properties TDE has the empirical formula $C_{14}H_{10}Cl_4$ and a molecular weight of 320.05. The pure material forms colorless crystals melting at 109–110°C. The technical material consists mainly of the *p,p*′ isomer but also contains a substantial proportion of *o,p*′ isomer and lesser proportions of related compounds. *p,p*′-TDE is more slowly dehydrochlorinated than *p,p*′-DDT, but TDE is incompatible with alkali. The solubilities are similar to those of DDT. The density of the technical material is 1.385.

History, Formulations, Uses, and Production The insecticidal properties of TDE were first described by Läuger *et al.* (1944). The formulations have included the technical material; wettable powders, 5%; emulsion concentrates, 25%; and dust, 5 and 10%.

15.3.2.2 Toxicity to Laboratory Animals

Basic Findings The effects of TDE are similar to those of DDT, but TDE is much less toxic in the rat and in humans. Gaines (1969) found the oral LD 50 in both male and female rats to be greater than 4000 mg/kg; Lehman (1951, 1952) reported 3400 mg/kg as an oral LD 50 in rats and 1200 as a dermal value in rabbits. Rabbits were killed quickly by dermal applications at the rate of 400 mg/kg/day; they were made severely ill but did not die when treated at the rate of 200 mg/kg/day for 90 days. In rats fed for 2 years, the lowest dietary level producing gross effects was 400 ppm and the lowest level fed (100 ppm, about 5 mg/kg/day) produced tissue damage. In the rat, pathology is indistinguishable from that caused by DDT (Lehman, 1951, 1952).

Absorption, Distribution, Metabolism, and Excretion The metabolism of *p,p*′-DDD has been described in Section 15.3.1.2.

Regardless of dosage form, 75% or more of *o,p*′-DDD is absorbed from the gastrointestinal tract (Korpachev, 1972a). Following repeated doses, storage of *o,p*′-DDD reached its highest point in 10–20 days and then decreased somewhat in spite of continued intake. Elimination was rapid after treatment stopped but was detectable longest in the adrenals and adipose tissues (Korpachev, 1972b). The metabolism of *o,p*′-DDD in the rat has been investigated thoroughly by Reif and Sinsheimer (1975); their major results are summarized in Figure 15.3, which also records the metabolites found in humans by Reif *et al.* (1974). More recent studies to explain the covalent binding of *o,p*′-DDD in lung and adrenals are also described in Section 15.3.1.2.

Biochemical Effects The biochemical basis for the action of *o,p*′-DDD on the adrenal is not understood fully in connection with any species. It is clear that marked species differences exist. The mechanism that leads to prompt atrophy in the dog may be quite different from the mechanisms that limit the production or increase the breakdown of corticosteroids in species in which most or all of the adrenal cells stay alive.

It is clear that a reduction of steroid production accompanies atrophy of the adrenal of the dog. A review by Kupfer (1967) considered (*a*) reduced steroid production in species other than the dog, including the possibility that such reduction is secondary to inhibition of glucose-6-phosphate dehydrogenase activity in the adrenals, and (*b*) blockage of steroid action by a steroid metabolite formed under the influence of DDD. However, the existence of these effects, much less their importance, remains obscure. Hart and Straw (1971a) showed that administration of *o,p*′-DDD to dogs for only 2–48 hr completely blocked the normal increase in steroid production in response to ACTH *in vitro* but, paradoxically, produced a marked increase in the incorporation of labeled amino acids into protein of the slices. The same authors presented evidence that the site of action is the intramitochondrial conversion of cholesterol to pregnenolone (Hart and Straw, 1971b), specifically, ACTH-activated conversion and not baseline steroid production (Hart and Straw, 1971d). A secondary site involves inhibition of intramitochondrial conversion of 11-deoxycortisol to cortisol (Hart and Straw, 1971d). Further evidence supporting the importance of the primary site was offered by Komissarenko *et al.* (1972). *o,p*′-DDD inhibited ACTH-induced steroid production by more than 97% within 2 hr, and the active principle is either *o,p*′-DDD *per se* or a derivative formed in the adrenal gland of the intact dog (Hart and Straw, 1971c). *o,p*′-DDD applied to liver slices *in vitro* is not effective in reducing ACTH-induced steroidogenesis in the slices. However, the compound did reduce the formation of corticosteroid from progesterone or deoxycorticosterone added to homogenates made from adrenal cortices from dogs, chickens, rats, and human fetuses. These results are consistent with the view that the action of *o,p*′-DDD is to block 11-β-hydroxylation (Kravchenko, 1973). Furthermore, a concentration of 16 ppm produced this effect in a monolayer culture of human fetal adrenal cells (Komissarenko *et al.*, 1971). Martz and Straw (1973) interpreted the decrease in adrenocortical heme and P-450 produced by o,p'-DDD in the dog as a suggestion that the compound is metabolized to a more active form, and this is supported by more recent *in vitro* studies with isolated adrenal mitochondria (Martz and Straw, 1980; Pohland and Counsell, 1985).

There is evidence for a peripheral action of o,p'-DDD on steroid transformation in humans also, although the site of action is different. This evidence was obtained by studying the excretion of metabolites of small injected doses of radioactive steroid both before and during administration of the drug. It was concluded that 3β-hydroxy-Δ^5-steroid dehydrogenase was inhibited (Bradlow *et al.*, 1963).

Further evidence that o,p'-DDD has some inhibitory effect on the synthesis of corticosteroids in humans was provided by *in vitro* tests on adrenal tissue removed surgically from patients, some of whom had been under treatment with the drug. Total doses prior to surgery had varied from 324 to 2280 gm and had been given over periods of 1–12 months. Compounds whose synthesis (from radioactive precursors added to incubation flasks) was inhibited in tissue from treated patients were cortisol, corticosterone, 18-hydroxycorticosterone, and aldosterone (Touitou *et al.*, 1978). Direct addition of o,p'-DDD to human adrenal tissue *in vitro* was without effect on synthesis of corticosteroids.

Following massive dosage (60 mg/kg, iv), all of the isomers of DDD inhibit ACTH-induced steroid production in the dog, but the inhibition reached 50% of control in only 27 min after dosing with the m,p' isomer compared to 87 min with the o,p' isomer and 4–18 hr with the p,p' isomer. There was a marked temporal correlation between the percentage inhibition of ACTH-induced steroid production, the disruption of normal cellular structure of the innermost zones of the adrenal cortex, and the severity of the damage to mitochondria in these zones caused by the three isomers (Hart *et al.*, 1973). The effectiveness of m,p'-DDT for treating metastatic adrenocortical carcinoma had already been demonstrated (Nichols *et al.*, 1961).

However, in humans m,p'-DDD is less effective than o,p'-DDD (de Fossey *et al.*, 1968), and Reznikov (1973) found m,p'-DDD less effective in dogs also. Administration of o,p'-DDD to dogs is followed by a decrease in plasma albumin and an increase in globulins, especially α_2-, β_1-, and γ-globulins (Vanyurykhina, 1972). The relation of these changes to the suppression of adrenal function is unknown, and their clinical significance is also unknown.

Guinea pigs receiving o,p'-DDD intraperitoneally at a rate of 100, 200, or 300 mg/kg/day for 20 days showed decreases in ascorbic acid levels corresponding to dosage (Petrun' and Nikulina, 1970). It was speculated that this might interfere with synthesis of corticosteroids.

Like other chlorinated hydrocarbon insecticides, o,p'-DDD stimulates hepatic microsomal oxygenation of both drugs and steroids and, according to a thorough review by Kupfer (1967), this may explain much of its action on corticoid metabolism in a wide range of species. Increased breakdown is evidenced by increased excretion of polar metabolites while nonpolar metabolites remain stable or even decrease—a finding encountered

in human patients (Hellman *et al.*, 1973). However, the demonstrated effect on corticoid metabolism fails to explain why o,p'- and m,p'-DDD are unique in their overall effects on the adrenal, including their ability to produce adrenocortical atrophy in the dog. Other powerful inducers of microsomal enzymes lack these effects. Furthermore, in some systems DDD is a relatively weak inducer compared, for example, to DDT and DDE (Gillett *et al.*, 1966). Whereas induction does occur in dogs, its interpretation is complex; for example, the induction caused by repeated doses can be suppressed by cortisol (Martz and Straw, 1972). Mikosha (1985) has proposed that inhibition of NADP reduction by malic enzyme in adrenals may play a role in o,p'-DDD action, perhaps by causing a decrease in steroid metabolism (Ojima *et al.*, 1985).

Effects on Organs and Tissues DDD is used to control different forms of adrenal overproduction of corticoids in humans (see Section 15.3.2.3). This therapy originally was based on the demonstration that DDD (Nelson and Woodard, 1948, 1949) and especially o,p'-DDD (Cueto and Brown, 1958; Komissarenko *et al.*, 1968) cause gross atrophy of the adrenals and degeneration of the cells of its inner cortex in dogs. This is true even though it was reported at the very first (Nelson and Woodard, 1948, 1949) that DDD produces almost no detectable damage to the adrenals of rats, mice, rabbits, and monkeys, and this finding was confirmed and extended by other investigators to other species, including humans (Zimmerman *et al.*, 1956; Komissarenko *et al.*, 1970). In the dog, o,p'-DDT produces gross atrophy of the adrenals when administered at a dosage of only 4 mg/kg/day. The dosage of technical grade DDD required to produce the same effect is 50–200 mg/kg/day (Cueto and Brown, 1958). However, in spite of its exceptional susceptibility, there is a definite threshold below which the dog does not respond. About 15% of technical DDT is o,p' isomer, much of which is gradually metabolized to o,p'-DDD. Yet dogs remained healthy and reproduced normally in a three-generation study involving dosages of technical DDT as high as 10 mg/kg/day (see Section 15.3.1.2).

DDD has been little used for Cushing's syndrome in dogs (Lubberink *et al.*, 1971), but it is effective at lower dosages than those used in humans, and side effects are less serious and less frequent (Schechter *et al.*, 1973).

It is an interesting fact that p,p'-DDE and the —OH analog of p,p'-DDD causes moderate hypertrophy of the dog adrenal and 2,2-bis(p-chlorophenyl)ethane causes moderate hyperplasia (Larson *et al.*, 1955).

The adrenal gland of the chicken, like that of the dog, undergoes some degeneration following treatment with o,p'-DDD (Komissarenko *et al.*, 1971).

The effect of DDD on thymolymphatic tissues is poorly understood. In one of the earliest studies of the compound, Lillie *et al.* (1947) reported that the spleen of all treated animals showed impressive siderosis. Much later Gawhary (1972) reported that, in rabbits, intramuscular injection of a commercial grade DDD (mainly p,p' isomer) caused acute *atrophy* of the thymus and hypertrophy of the adrenal, although the m,p'

isomer at a dosage of 100 mg/kg/day caused *hypertrophy* of the thymus and an increase in its choline acetylase activity. Decrease in the weight of the thymus and spleen as well as the adrenal glands of rats treated with *o,p'*-DDD was reported by Hamid *et al.* (1974).

Furthermore, Cueto and Moran (1968) and Cueto (1970) showed that, at a dosage of 50 mg/kg/day for 14 days, *o,p'*-DDD caused a gradually progressive hypotensive failure in dogs injected with epinephrine or norepinephrine, while leaving unchanged the cardioaccelerator and immediate pressor response of these drugs. The hypotensive failure was associated with weakening of the contractile force of the heart and with a reduction of plasma volume. The latter may have been caused by loss of fluid from the intravascular compartment and was not caused by release of histamine. The hypotensive state could be prevented to a significant degree by pretreatment with prednisolone.

The question of the hepatocarcinogenicity of chlorinated hydrocarbon insecticides is discussed in Section 15.2.3.2. In one test, no conclusion could be reached regarding either *p,p-* or *o,p'*-DDD (Innes *et al.*, 1969). In another test in mice, *p,p'*-TDE at a dietary level of 250 ppm moderately increased the incidence of liver tumors in males only and increased the incidence of lung tumors in both sexes (Tomatis *et al.*, 1974a). The *o,p'* isomer was protective in rats treated earlier with the established carcinogen dimethylbenz[*a*]anthracene (DMBA) (Kravt'sova *et al.*, 1971). Leydig cell tumors were reported in the testis of rats receiving *o,p'*-DDD at the rate of 0.6 mg/kg/day for 285–348 days (Lacassagne, 1971). This report is inconsistent with other studies (Lehman, 1951, 1952), and this may indicate that a contaminant was involved. In an NCI study (1978a) there was a possible effect of TDE in causing an increased incidence of follicular cell carcinoma or follicular cell adenoma of the thyroid in male Osborne-Mendel rats but no effects in female B6C3F1 mice.

TDE was found not to be mutagenic in *Drosophila* (Vogel, 1972). It was found mutagenic in two of three indicator organisms in host-mediated tests but not in direct tests, suggesting that a metabolite was the active agent. However, in the same series of studies, both DDT and DDA were negative (Buselmaier *et al.*, 1973).

Pathology In addition to atrophy of the zona fasciculata and zona reticularis in the dog, *o,p'*-DDD changes the ultrastructure of most cell types of the anterior pituitary of that species. The most striking feature is an increase in corticotrophocytes such as is seen following adrenalectomy, and the increase in cells is presumably associated with increased production of ACTH. The hypothalamus also is involved (Gordienko and Kozyritskii, 1970; Gordienko *et al.*, 1973). In spite of their severe nature, the changes produced in the dog adrenal are at least partially reversible (Komissarenko *et al.*, 1972). Dosage–response relationships of mitochondrial swelling and of some other details of pathology in the dog adrenal have been explored by Gordienko and Kozyritskii (1973) and by Powers *et al.* (1974), who also investigated regeneration of the gland.

Hypertrophy of the thyroid in dogs receiving 25 mg/kg and its inhibition in those receiving 50 mg/kg had been reported (Gordienko *et al.*, 1972).

15.3.2.3 Toxicity to Humans

Therapeutic Use Following the demonstration that DDD caused atrophy of a part of the adrenal cortex of dogs, the compound has been used in humans in the hope of controlling excessive cortical secretion or of reducing the size of adrenal tumors. The underlying condition may be hyperplasia or adrenocortical carcinoma. Early attempts using mixed isomers and/or dosages less than 100 mg/kg/day often were ineffective, although side effects might be produced (Sheehan *et al.*, 1953). The dosage of *o,p'*-DDD has varied from 7 to 285 mg/kg/day, but a dosage of approximately 40 or more often 100 mg/kg/day for many weeks has been necessary to produce any benefit in humans (Bergenstal *et al.*, 1960; Gallagher *et al.*, 1962; Bledsoe *et al.*, 1964; Southern *et al.*, 1966a,b; Verdon *et al.*, 1962; Wallace *et al.*, 1961; Kommissarenko and Reznikov, 1970; Gutierrez and Crooke, 1980).

The effects of idiopathic hyperplasia may be controlled; in fact, a state of adrenal insufficiency may be produced (Canlorbe *et al.*, 1971; Sizonenko *et al.*, 1974).

o,p'-DDD also may give symptomatic relief of excessive production of androgens from a virilizing adrenal carcinoma Saez *et al.*, 1971; Helson *et al.*, 1971; Korth-Schutz *et al.*, 1977) or of adrenocortical activity secondary to a tumor that produces ACTH (Carey *et al.*, 1973).

Very early attempts to use DDD for treating Cushing's syndrome often failed because the *o,p'* isomer was not used and sometimes because the dosage was small. This was true of what apparently was the first therapeutic use (Sheehan *et al.*, 1953). Using the *o,p'* isomer, a favorable response is produced in about one-fourth to one-half of patients with inoperable adrenocortical carcinoma (Hutter and Kayhoe, 1966; Canlorbe *et al.*, 1971; Hoffman and Mattox, 1972; Lubitz *et al.*, 1973; Montgomery and Struck, 1973; Gutierrez and Crooke, 1980). In fact, an occasional cure, involving complete regression of metastases, is produced by chemotherapy including *o,p'*-DDD (Schick, 1973; Perevodchikova *et al.*, 1972; Harrison *et al.*, 1973; Pellerin *et al.*, 1975; Rappaport *et al.*, 1978). Other patients may live several years (Bricaire and Luton, 1977; McKierman *et al.*, 1978). More commonly, symptoms are relieved and life is prolonged only about 7–8 months or a little longer (Hutter and Kayhoe, 1966; Canlorbe *et al.*, 1971; Hoffman and Mattox, 1972; Lubitz *et al.*, 1973) or even less (Hajjar *et al.*, 1975). The success of treatment often is indicated early by a reduction of steroid excretion (Hoffman and Mattox, 1972; Lubitz *et al.*, 1973), but steroid excretion may increase, decrease, or remain unchanged (Fukushima *et al.*, 1971). Removal of the tumor and *o,p'*-DDD treatment may be combined (Levy *et al.*, 1985). The success of treatment is greater in Cushing's syndrome due to adrenal hyperplasia (Weisenfeld and Goldner, 1962). An early example of what appeared to be complete cure was reported by Bar-Hay *et al.*

(1964). Ten of 17 patients with this condition experienced cure or remission for 12–32 months after the drug had been withdrawn (Luton et al., 1973).

The large dosage of o,p'-DDD necessary to produce clinical benefit often produces general lassitude, anorexia, nausea, vomiting, diarrhea, and/or dermatitis (Southern et al., 1961; Weisenfeld and Goldner, 1962; Danowski et al., 1964; Hutter and Kayhoe, 1966; Bochner et al., 1969; Naruse et al., 1970; Halmi and Lascari, 1971; Hoffman and Mattox, 1972; Nitschke and Link, 1972; Lubitz et al., 1973; Perevodchikova et al., 1972; Hajjar et al., 1975; Gutierrez and Crooke, 1980). Apathy may range from mild dulling of interest to profound psychotic depression (Hoffman and Mattox, 1972). Gynecomastia, hematuria, leukopenia, and thrombocytopenia have been reported more rarely (Luton et al., 1972; Perevodchikova et al., 1972). The symptoms disappear soon after administration of the drug is stopped or the dosage is reduced. Furthermore, some patients do not develop toxicity. A 10-year-old girl received 7500 mg/day for a total of 9 kg without discernible side effects (Helson et al., 1971).

Even large, therapeutic doses of o,p'-DDD cause no histological alterations of the adrenals in humans (Wallace et al., 1961). However, electron microscopy revealed degenerative changes in the mitochondria of the zona fasciculata of a patient who had received o,p'-DDD at the rate of about 3000 mg/day for 1 month (Temple et al., 1969). Dosages in the therapeutic range (specifically those between 110 and 140 mg/kg/day) produced no detectable injury to the liver, kidney, or bone marrow even though the patients exhibited the reversible symptoms listed earlier (Bergenstal et al., 1960).

Kupfer (1967) reviewed the extensive literature indicating that the effect in humans and other species except the dog is caused by stimulation of corticoid metabolism by massive doses of o,p'-DDD and not to any direct effect on the adrenal. Southern et al. (1966a,b) agreed that the effect was predominantly extra-adrenal in humans when the drug was first given but offered evidence that adrenal secretion of cortisol eventually was reduced. Even though therapeutic doses eventually have a direct effect on the adrenal, doses encountered by workers exposed to technical DDT do not (Clifford and Weil, 1972; Morgan and Roan, 1973).

Somewhat encouraging results were reported in the use of p,p'-DDD for treating diabetics with hyaline vascular changes and hyperpolysaccharidemia (Törnblom, 1959). Apparently, there has been no attempt to use o,p'-DDD for this condition.

In addition to its rather extensive use for treating Cushing's syndrome, o,p'-DDD has been used in a much lower dosage for treating spanomenorrhea associated with hypertrichosis. Menstruation was restored in 13 of 15 women with these conditions, and normal pregnancies occurred in five of them during the treatment period. The babies were normal. There was some improvement in hypertrichosis in nine and no improvement in six (Klotz et al., 1971).

At least part of the action of o,p'-DDT in controlling excessive androgens involves its action on their metabolism. It was found in a study of three patients with metastatic adrenal carcinoma and one with pernicious anemia that the compound decreased the conversion of labeled androgens to androsterone by about 76% and to etiocholanolone by about 80%. The main effect on androgen metabolism was consistent with induction of microsomal oxidase activity by the drug (Hellmann et al., 1973).

When uptake of radioactive iodine is used for diagnosis of Cushing's syndrome, [^{131}I]19-iodocholesterol is the compound usually employed. DDD labeled with ^{131}I has been used for the same purpose (Skromme-Kadlubik et al., 1972, 1973a,b, 1974). No comparative study of the duration of storage of the two compounds appears to have been made. However, it is clear that it is possible to introduce enough radiation via ^{131}I-labeled DDD either to kill rodents or to cause atrophy of their adrenal glands, depending on the schedule of administration (Skromme-Kadlubik et al., 1974). This has been viewed as an indication that ^{131}I-labeled DDD might be useful for treating human adrenal carcinoma. It certainly is an indication for caution in using the diagnostic technique in patients not already proved to have adrenal cancer.

Laboratory Findings Analytical study associated with what apparently was the first attempt to use p,p'-DDD in treating Cushing's syndrome established that the compound is concentrated in the adrenal gland. Eleven weeks after the last course of DDD, when the concentration in adipose tissue was less than half what it had been earlier, the concentration in an adrenal biopsy was 50 ppm, wet weight. On a lipid basis, the concentrations in fat and adrenal were almost identical (Sheehan et al., 1953). A patient who had received o,p'-DDD at the rate of 4000 mg/day for 58 days had a blood level of 6 ppm and excreted 8.3 mg of free and 39.7 mg of conjugated DDA in a 24-hr urine sample (Sinsheimer et al., 1972). There is evidence for two plasma pools of o,p'-DDD (Slooten et al., 1982).

Normal volunteers excreted increased concentrations of DDA within 24 hr of receiving p,p'-DDD at a rate of 5 mg/day and continued to excrete DDA at greater than predose levels for over 4 months after dosing was stopped after 81 days (Roan et al., 1971).

Treatment of appropriate cases with o,p'-DDT usually results in a decrease in urinary steroid excretion (Gutierrez and Crooke, 1980). An unusually detailed study of the individual compounds is that of Hartwig et al., (1968).

In long-term administration of o,p'-DDD (2 gm/day for 1–3 months) to patients with adrenal carcinoma or Cushing's syndrome, Ojima et al. (1984) found that plasma levels of pregnenolone, progesterone, cortisol, corticosterone, and some other C_{21} steroids were progressively decreased, as well as urinary excretion of 17-ketosteroids and 17-hydroxycorticosteroids. Touitou et al. (1985), however, have been unable to demonstrate any correlation between concentrations of o,p'-DDD in adrenals removed from patients preoperatively treated with the drug for Cushing's syndrome and inhibition of some steroid biosynthesis enzymes measured in vitro. There is a suggestion that o,p'-DDD suppresses ACTH-secreting cells in the pituitary as well as depressing steroid hormone secretion (Takamatsu *et al.*, 1981).

In some patients either *p,p'*-DDD (Törnblom, 1959) or *o,p'*-DDD (Molnar *et al.*, 1961) causes an increase in plasma cholesterol, but the opposite also may occur (Danowski *et al.*, 1964). Oddly enough, such patients are refractory to the therapeutic effects of the drug (Molnar *et al.*, 1961).

An interesting but unexplored finding is that *o,p'*-DDD has a hypouricemic effect apparently by increasing the renal clearance of uric acid (Reach *et al.*, 1978; Zumoff, 1979).

The induction of microsomal enzymes by *o,p'*-DDD (and by other drugs) may be detected by increased excretion of glucaric acid in treated patients (Sotaniemi *et al.*, 1974). Five derivatives of *o,p'*-DDD have been identified following their isolation from the urine of treated patients (Reif *et al.*, 1974).

Persons suffering from Cushing's syndrome can be distinguished from normal by their increased adrenal uptake of [^{131}I]19-iodocholesterol. In one patient under treatment with *o,p'*-DDD, uptake of radioactive iodine was reduced but not to the normal range (Morita *et al.*, 1972). DDD is commonly found in blood and tissues from the general population; for levels of it in blood, see Table 15.13.

Treatment of Poisoning   Side effects following large therapeutic doses resolve quickly if the dosage level is reduced. Therefore, it seems unlikely that a situation requiring treatment would arise. If treatment were needed, it must be symptomatic (see Section 15.2.5).

15.3.3 ETHYLAN

15.3.3.1 Identity, Properties, and Uses

Chemical Name   1,1-Dichloro-2,2-bis(4-ethylphenyl)ethane, that is, the *p,p'*-diethyl analog of DDD.

Structure   See Table 15.2.

Synonyms   Ethylan is the only common name in use, but apparently it has been approved officially only in the USSR. The trade name Perthane® often is used. Code designations for ethylan include B-63,138 and Q-137. The CAS registry number is 72-56-0.

Physical and Chemical Properties   Ethylan has the empirical formula $C_{18}H_{20}Cl_2$ and a molecular weight of 307.27. The pure compound is a crystalline solid with a melting point of 56–57°C. The technical product is a waxy solid with a melting point not below 40°C and with some decomposition above 52°C. Ethylan is practically insoluble in water but soluble in acetone, kerosene, and other organic solvents.

History, Formulations, and Uses   Ethylan was introduced in 1950. It is an insecticide used to control pear psylla, leafhoppers, various larvae on vegetables, and moths and carpet beetles on textiles. The rate of application is 1–16 kg/ha.

Perthane® as an emulsifiable concentrate contains 450 gm/liter; as a solution it contains 750 gm/liter.

15.3.3.2 Toxicity to Laboratory Animals

Basic Findings   The oral LD 50 values for ethylan were 8170 and 9.340 mg/kg in rats and mice, respectively. However, the corresponding intravenous values were only 73 and 173 mg/kg in the same species. No dermal LD 50 value could be measured; all rabbits that received a 30% solution at the rate of 3 ml/kg/day for 13 weeks survived (Finnegan *et al.*, 1955). Gaines (1960) agreed that the oral toxicity was very low (LD 50 >4000 mg/kg).

Minimal and infrequent changes were seen in the livers of rats fed dietary levels of 2500 and 5000 ppm for 2 years. There was no effect on survival, and differences in growth rate did not correspond to dosage. Thus a dietary level of 1000 ppm might be considered a no-effect level.

In contrast, the same investigators found that a dietary level of 5000 ppm was lethal to dogs within 22 weeks. Levels of 100 or 1000 ppm did not interfere with survival or growth when fed for 1 year, although the 1000 ppm level led to some atrophy of the adrenals (Finnegan *et al.*, 1955). Cortisone given at the same time as ethylan tended to block the effect of the latter on the adrenal (Bleiberg and Larson, 1957). Reznikov (1973) considered the action of *p,p'*-ethylan similar to that of *p,p'*-DDD.

Absorption, Distribution, Metabolism, and Excretion   Rats fed ethylan at a concentration of 50 ppm (about 2.5 mg/kg/day) for 6 weeks stored the compound in their fat at a concentration of 19 ppm (Finnegan *et al.*, 1955). Four generations of rats were fed a standard synthetic diet containing 20% fat to which several pesticides were added in the proportion in which they were found in the Market Basket Survey (see Section 6.1.1). The diets of the seven groups studied differed only in the kinds of fat (cottonseed oil, lard, etc.) they contained. The average concentration of added ethylan found by analysis in different samples of dietary fat varied from 2.01 to 2.71 ppm. No ethylan was detectable in the body fat or other tissues of the rats (Adams *et al.*, 1974).

After a single oral dose of [^{14}C]ethylan, rats excreted 90% of the radioactivity in their feces and 5% in their urine in 2 weeks (Bleiberg and Larson, 1957).

Biochemical Effects   Ethylan reduced excretion of 17-hydroxycorticosteroids and caused adrenal atrophy in dogs (Cobey *et al.*, 1956).

Dogs that had received ethylan for 10 or 14 days at a rate of 200 mg/kg/day slept 12–14 hr following anesthesia with sodium pentobarbital compared to only 6–7 hr following the same dosage of barbiturate before receiving ethylan. Similar studies with different DDD formulations revealed that increased sleeping time did not depend on the presence of adrenal atrophy, but they did not exclude the possibility that it depended on altered function of the adrenal. The increased sleeping time did not depend on reduced clearance of the barbiturate from the blood, which was not influenced by ethylan or DDD. Thus the cause remained obscure. Whatever the cause, the increase in sleeping time was peculiar to dogs and did not occur in rats treated with DDD (Nichols *et al.*, 1958).

In dogs, ethylan (50 mg/kg/day for 10 days) significantly increased the glutathione reductase of the adrenal cortex but not of the liver (Komissarenko *et al.*, 1978).

Effects on Organs and Tissues   Ethylan produces adrenal cortical atrophy in the dog. No such effect was noted in the rat. Presumably the effect is virtually specific for the dog, as is true of *o,p′*-DDD, which has been more extensively studied (see Section 15.3.2.2).

When ethylan was administered to mice at the highest tolerated rate for about 18 months, the results for tumorigenicity were equivocal (Innes *et al.*, 1969). Some evidence for hepatic tumor formation in female mice but not males or rats of either sex has been reported (NCI, 1979a).

Pathology   Dogs killed or rendered moribund by a dietary level of 5000 ppm (about 105 mg/kg/day) showed marked atrophy of the adrenal cortex; the medulla was unaffected. The capsule was wrinkled, the zona glomerulosa contained cells with granular and diminished cytoplasm, and there was a focal loss of these cells. The zona fasciculata was greatly narrowed, and there was extreme vacuolization among cells in the medial two-thirds. However, fat-staining material was deficient throughout the fasciculata, especially the inner part. The zona reticularis had practically disappeared, leaving only a few cells containing lipochrome pigment. There were a few focal concentrations of lymphocytes. Atrophy was present but less severe in two of three dogs that received 1000 ppm (about 21 mg/kg/day). On the contrary, severe atrophy was produced in less than 3 weeks by an oral dosage of 200 mg/kg/day (Finnegan *et al.*, 1955; Larson *et al.*, 1955).

15.3.3.3 Toxicity to Humans

Therapeutic Use   Ethylan was administered to nine men with metastatic carcinoma of the prostate and to five women with metastatic carcinoma of the breast because there were earlier reports of a favorable effect of surgical adrenalectomy on the clinical course of some patients with these diseases and because the compound had been shown to cause adrenocortical atrophy in the dog. When they received ethylan, all the patients also received ACTH either intermittently or continuously. With one exception, the dosage of ethylan varied from 50 to 150 mg/kg/day, the latter for a total of 189,000 mg within 21 days. The most intensive treatment was 200–300 mg/kg/day for a total of 96,000 mg in 6 days. The smallest dosage produced diarrhea, vomiting, and especially nausea in some patients and required cessation of treatment in some. In contrast, some patients, especially those who were less sick to begin with, tolerated the higher dosages, including 200–300 mg/kg/day, with no symptoms whatever. Marked thrombocytopenia and leukopenia were noted in one patient just after a 14-day course

of treatment. These changes, which were attributed to ethylan, resolved promptly when treatment was stopped. There was no other evidence of hematopoietic toxicity and no evidence of hepatic, renal, neural, or other toxicity. It was not considered that the relatively brief treatments influenced the clinical course in any of the cases. However, among patients receiving 150–300 mg/kg/day in divided doses, ethylan caused a marked depression of plasma 17-hydroxycorticosteroid levels, but never below the normal range. Lower dosages had no consistent effects (Taliaferro and Leone, 1957). No distinct benefit but nausea, vomiting, and skin rash were seen in four other patients with carcinoma who received ethylan at dosages of 1800–8000 mg/day for periods of 4–54 days (Weisenfeld and Goldner, 1962).

Treatment of Poisoning   In the unlikely event that treatment is required, it must be symptomatic (see Section 15.2.5).

15.3.4 METHOXYCHLOR

15.3.4.1 Identity, Properties, and Uses

Chemical Name   Methoxychlor is 1,1,1-trichloro-2,2-bis(4-methoxyphenyl)ethane or 2,2-bis(*p*-methoxyphenyl)-1,1,1-trichloroethane, that is, the *p,p′*-dimethoxy analog of *p,p′*-DDT.

Structure   See Table 15.2.

Synonyms   The common name methoxychlor (BSI, ICPC, ISO) is in general use. Other nonproprietary names have included dianisyl trichloroethane, dimethoxy-DT, DMDT (an acronym for dimethoxydiphenyltrichloroethane), and methoxy DDT. A trade name is Marlate®. Code designations include OMS-466. The CAS registry number is 72-43-5.

Physical and Chemical Properties   Methoxychlor has the empirical formula $C_{16}H_{15}Cl_3O_2$ and a molecular weight of 345.65. The pure material forms colorless crystals melting at 89°C. Technical methoxychlor is a gray flaky powder containing about 88% of the *p,p′* isomer, the remainder being mainly *o,p′* isomer, although up to 50 other contaminants have been detected (Lamoureux and Feil, 1980; West *et al.*, 1982). The density is 1.41 at 25°C. Methoxychlor is stable to heat and ultraviolet light and resistant to oxidation; it is dehydrochlorinated by alkalies and by heavy metal catalysts. The solubilities of methoxychlor are approximately the same as those of DDT. It is readily soluble in most aromatic solvents, moderately soluble in alcohols and petroleum oils, and essentially insoluble in water.

History, Formulations, Uses, and Production   Methoxychlor was first described by Läuger *et al.* (1944), and it was introduced about 1945. Formulations include wettable powder (25 and 50%), emulsifiable concentrate (24%), dusts (4–10%), and aerosols. Methoxychlor is effective against a wide range of insects affecting fruits, vegetables, forage crops, and livestock. The low toxicity of methoxychlor and its short biological half-life have been largely responsible for its greatly expanded use since the ban on DDT in many countries.

15.3.4.2 Toxicity to Laboratory Animals

Basic Findings In spite of its low toxicity, methoxychlor in sufficient dosage is capable of causing convulsions in the dog (Tegeris *et al.*, 1966). However, in the rat, the compound causes depression of the central nervous system (Lehman, 1951, 1952). Tremors have been noted but they are not a prominent symptom. In rabbits killed by a few doses, the only signs noted were diarrhea and anorexia (Smith *et al.*, 1946).

The acute toxicity of methoxychlor is very low; oral LD 50 values of 5000 mg/kg (Hodge *et al.*, 1950) and 6000 mg/kg (Lehman, 1951, 1952) have been reported for the rat and values of 1850 mg/kg (Domenjoz, 1946a) for the mouse and 2000 mg/kg for the hamster (Cabral *et al.*, 1979a).

Rats fed a dietary level of 30,000 ppm suffered a severe reduction in growth, and most of them died in less than 45 days. Those fed a dietary level of 10,000 ppm survived but gained almost no weight; paired feeding studies showed that failure of growth was due entirely to food refusal. A dietary level of 1600 ppm for 2 years caused measurable reduction of growth but produced no reduction in life span and no histological change in the tissues. Dosages of 20 mg/kg/day for 1 year or a dietary level of 200 ppm (about 10 mg/kg/day) for 2 years were both no-effect levels (Hodge *et al.*, 1950, 1952).

Rabbits are relatively susceptible to methoxychlor; a dosage of 200 mg/kg/day was fatal within 15 days (Smith *et al.*, 1946).

Dogs fed the compound in their diet in such a way that they received 1000 mg/kg/day for 6 months lost weight, and many of those that received 2000, 2500, or 4000 mg/kg/day began having convulsions within 6 weeks and died within 3 additional weeks. Strangely enough, dogs that received 2500 mg/kg/day administered by gastric tube as a suspension in 1% gum tragacanth for 5 months showed no indication of injury (Tregeris *et al.*, 1966). In an earlier study lasting 1 year, the highest dosage fed to dogs (300 mg/kg/day) produced no detectable clinical effect (Hodge *et al.*, 1952).

Swine that received methoxychlor in their diets in such a way that their dosages were 1000, 2000, and 4000 mg/kg/day lost weight for a month, but later those on the two lower dosages regained their original weight (Tegeris *et al.*, 1966).

A dietary level of 2500 ppm for 8–16 weeks produced no kill effects in chickens (Lillie *et al.*, 1973).

Absorption, Distribution, Metabolism, and Excretion In an electron microscopic study of the absorption of methoxychlor from the jejunum of the rat, material probably derived from methoxychlor was identified as intra- and intercellular densities different from those derived from the vehicles in which the compound was administered. Mixtures containing methoxychlor appeared to pass directly from the luminal border to the intercellular spaces immediately, in addition to the usual transport through the endoplasmic reticulum toward the Golgi apparatus. Furthermore, absorption of methoxychlor was accompanied by distention of vesicles and intercellular spaces (Imai and Coulston, 1968).

Storage of methoxychlor was minimal in the fat of rats that had received it for 18 weeks. In fact, no storage could be measured at a dietary level of 25 ppm, and storage decreased after the ninth week at levels of 100 and 500 ppm in spite of continued intake. No storage was detectable 2 weeks after dosing was discontinued (Kunze *et al.*, 1950).

Storage of methoxychlor in sheep reaches a steady state in 6–8 weeks or, at certain dosage levels, actually declines after that interval in spite of continued intake. Storage loss is prompt after dosing is stopped (Reynolds *et al.*, 1975, 1976).

It was recognized very early (von Oettingen and Sharpless, 1946) that methoxychlor is not excreted unchanged but as hydroxyphenyl derivatives.

Following oral administration of radioactive methoxychlor to mice, 98.3% was recovered from the excreta within 24 hr. The compound was metabolized to 2-(p-hydroxyphenyl)-2'-(methoxyphenyl)-1,1,1-trichloroethane and 2,2-bis(p-hydroxyphenyl)-1,1-trichloroethane, which were eliminated largely in conjugated form (Kapoor *et al.*, 1970). Detailed studies have also been performed with goats (Davison *et al.*, 1982, 1983). The normally low rate of storage of methoxychlor was not influenced by simutaneous feeding of DDT or dieldrin, but feeding of methoxychlor caused a small but significant reduction in dieldrin storage (Street and Blau, 1966). The metabolism of methoxychlor *in vitro* has been particularly studied in respect of the formation of estrogenic metabolites in comparison with *o,p'*-DDT (Section 15.3.1.2). For a review see Kupfer and Bulger (1987). A scheme for the probable metabolism is illustrated in Fig. 15.3. Rat liver microsomes form both the mono and dihydroxy products as well as more polar compounds (Ousterhout *et al.*, 1981; Bulger *et al.*, 1985). With (R)- and (S)-[monomethyl-$_3$H$_3$]methoxyclors, intramolecular deuterium effects and entantiotopic differentiation have been observed (Ichinose and Kurihara, 1987). Another route of metabolism is an initial dechlorination before replacement of the methoxy groups (Davison *et al.*, 1983; Kupfer and Bulger, 1987). Phenolic products from both routes appear to be converted to activated intermediates, which may bind covalently to macromolecules (Bulger *et al.*, 1983; Kupfer *et al.*, 1986; Kupfer and Bulger, 1987).

Biochemical Effects Methoxychlor induced liver microsomal enzymes in sheep, but even at a dietary level of 2500 ppm the degree of induction was less than that caused by DDT at a dietary level of 250 ppm. Methoxychlor caused no change in food consumption, body weight, liver weight, uterine weight, or estrous cycle (Cecil *et al.*, 1975). In rats, the induction is preceded by a brief inhibitory effect (Klinger *et al.*, 1973). Some increases in hepatic glucose-6-phosphatase activity have been observed in rats given methoxychlor without showing any histological damage (Morgan and Hickenbottom, 1979), and significant decreases in lactate levels occurred even at doses

<1% of the oral LD 50. Neonatal administration of methoxychlor to rats resulted in elevated levels of sex-differentiated hepatic monoamine oxidase activities in adult rats, implying changes in the brain hormone environment during development which did not become apparent until adulthood (Lamartiniere *et al.*, 1982).

Whereas massive doses of methoxychlor have an estrogenic effect in swine (Tegeris *et al.*, 1966) and perhaps other species, no such effect is detectable in chickens at a dietary level of 10 ppm (Foster, 1973) or in sheep at a dietary level of 2500 ppm (Cecil *et al.*, 1975). Even 10 ppm is a far greater residue than humans or livestock are likely to encounter.

There was no evidence that methoxychlor induced microsomal enzymes in heifers when administered at the rate of 112 mg/kg/day for 9 days, as judged by recovery of radioactivity derived from $16\alpha,17\alpha$-[^{14}C]dihydroxyprogestrone aceto-phenide (DHPA) used to synchronize estrus (Rumsey and Schrciber, 1969). However, because metabolites of DHPA were not distinguished, the study cannot be considered a critical test of induction.

Effects on Organs and Tissues Of several polycyclic aromatic compounds said to be impurities in commercial methoxychlor, only one was mutagenic and in only one strain (Grant *et al.*, 1976).

Some tumors were found in rats fed for 2 years at dietary concentrations as high as 1600 ppm, but the kind and incidence did not differ from those in controls. No tumors were found in dogs that had received dietary levels as high as 10,000 ppm (Hodge *et al.*, 1952). Negative results also were found in mice that received a single subcutaneous injection (10 mg/mouse) or in others given weekly skin applications (0.1 or 10 mg). However, it was concluded from identical study of other compounds regarded as carcinogens that the skin tests were not an adequate substitute for tests by other routes (Hodge *et al.*, 1966).

When two strains of mice were fed technical methoxychlor at a dietary level of 750 ppm for as much as 2 years, the incidence and malignancy of carcinoma of the testis were increased in one strain but not the other. The average survival of the affected group was 89.8 weeks, compared to 93.8 weeks for the controls. It was suggested that the carcinogenicity was related to the estrogenic activity of methoxychlor (Reuber, 1979a).

The occurrence of neoplasms of all sorts showed a very rough dosage response in male rats fed technical methoxychlor at dietary levels of 100 ppm or more and in females fed 10 ppm or more; tumors identified as carcinomas were found in both sexes but only in rats fed 2000 ppm for 2 years (Reuber, 1979b). The conclusion that methoxychlor is carcinogenic for the liver in C3H and BALB/c mice and Osborne–Mendel rats may be related to the covalent binding of activated metabolites (Kupfer and Bulger, 1987). However, anyone interested should consult the original reports, including NCI (1978b).

At a dietary level of 1000 ppm, the tumorigenic property of methoxychlor was less than additive when it was fed in combination with Aramite, DDT, and thiourea or Aramite, DDT, and aldrin (Deichmann *et al.*, 1967).

For other effects on organs, see the two following sections on Reproduction and Pathology.

Effects on Reproduction Because massive doses of methoxychlor have estrogenic effects, as indicated by special endocrine tests (Tullner, 1961), a comparative study was made of the effects of methoxychlor and estradiol benzoate.

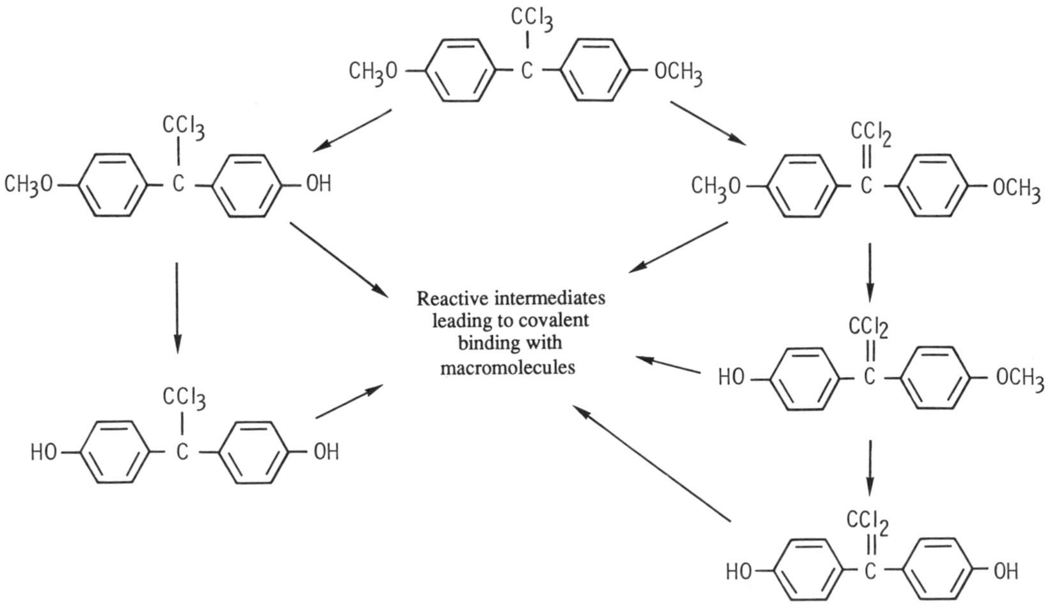

Figure 15.3 Proposed metabolic pathway and covalent binding of methoxychlor in rats.

Methoxychlor levels of 2500 and 5000 ppm reduced mating, and only one litter was produced. However, when the same rats were returned to an uncontaminated diet, they reproduced normally. A dietary level of 1000 ppm started before mating and continued throughout lactation had no effect on reproduction in that generation, but the female pups had early vaginal opening and reduced reproduction when mature, and the reproductive behavior of mature male pups was also defective (Harris *et al.*, 1974). In a recent study, male and female weanling rats were dosed with methoxychlor through puberty and gestation until day 15 of lactation in females (Gray *et al.*, 1989). Although various parameters of reproductive potential were altered in both sexes, fertility was only reduced in females when mated with untreated animals.

In vitro tests showed that pure methoxychlor is not estrogenic, although the commercial product had some activity and bishydroxy trichloroethane was quite active (Bulger and Kupfer, 1977; Bulger *et al.*, 1978a,b). The estrogenic activity of impure methoxychlor in inducing uterus growth, uterine ornithine decarboxylase activity (Bulger *et al.*, 1978a) and binding to the uterine estrogen receptor (Bulger *et al.*, 1978b) appears to be caused by the demethylated analogs (Ousterhout *et al.*, 1981; Bulger *et al.*, 1985) which are also metabolites (Fig. 15.3). By both *in vitro* and *in vivo* criteria, 1,1-dichloro-bis(4-hydroxyphenyl)ethene is the most potent agent (Bulger *et al.*, 1985; Kupfer and Bulger, 1987). More recent evidence suggests that reproductive effects of methoxychlor metabolites may be mediated, in part, by elevation of prolactin concentration and release, which in turn influences hypothalamic levels of gonadotropin-releasing hormone (Goldman *et al.*, 1986). Methoxychlor also affects the decidual cell response of the uterus (Cummings and Gray, 1987).

When mice received methoxychlor intragastrically on days 6–15 of pregnancy, dosages of 50–400 mg/kg/day reduced maternal weight gain. At 200 mg/kg/day, the compound decreased the number and weight of fetuses and caused delayed ossification, leading to wavy ribs and other bent bones. No real teratogenesis was observed (Khera *et al.*, 1978).

A predictable result of the rapid metabolism and excretion of methoxychlor is the fact that very little of it is excreted in the milk. When the compound was fed to cows at a dietary concentration of 7000 ppm, the concentration in the milk reached slightly over 2 ppm in 91 days and remained essentially constant until feeding was stopped on day 112. After dosing was stopped, the concentration in milk fell to <0.1 ppm in a week (Gannon *et al.*, 1959).

In chickens, dietary levels as high as 2500 ppm (about 145 mg/kg/day) had no effect on the health of hens or their production of hatchable eggs or on the ability of cockerels to fertilize the eggs. The hens were tested for 16 weeks and the cockerels for 8 weeks (Lillie *et al.*, 1973).

Pathology Massive doses of methoxychlor (1000, 2000, or 4000 mg/kg/day) produce dosage-dependent chronic nephritis and hypertrophy of the kidneys, mammary glands, and uteri of swine (Tegeris *et al.*, 1966). In rats, Hodge *et al.* (1950) specifically denied finding characteristic liver cell changes at any dosage level. They did find striking testicular atrophy at dietary levels of 10,000 ppm or greater, and this degree of atrophy was not present in pair-fed controls, a result later confirmed by Tullner and Edgcomb (1962). No atrophy was present in a dog that had received methoxychlor at 100 mg/kg/day for a month.

Wistar rats given methoxychlor (100 or 200 mg/kg/day) for 70 days (males) or 14 days (females) showed inhibition of spermatogenesis and folliculogenesis (Bal, 1984). There were degenerative changes in Sertoli cells and in spermatogonia and spermatocytes, with some transformed to polynucleate cells. Cytoplasmic vacuolations were observed in the epithelium of the ductus epididymis. Atresia of the ovarian follicles was evident with pyknosis and karyorrhexis of the granulosa cells.

Under certain conditions, continued massive dosage of methoxychlor produced cystic tubular nephropathy in rats (Tullner and Edgcomb, 1962).

In rats, Lehman (1951, 1952) found that the lowest dietary level producing tissue damage was 500 ppm (about 25 mg/kg/day); the effects, which were confined to the liver, consisted mainly of a slight increase in incidence of hepatic cell adenomas. In rats and monkeys the early induction of liver enzymes and the concomitant increase in hepatic endoplasmic reticulum may be temporary, disappearing in animals treated with methoxychlor for a prolonged time (Serrone *et al.*, 1965).

In dogs, a dosage of 2500 mg/kg/day caused grossly visible congestion of the intestinal mucosa. It has also caused progressive degeneration of the mitochrondria of mucosal cells of the small intestine marked in the early stages by matrical swelling and disruption of the cristae and later by disappearance of cristae and appearance of small myelin bodies. The mitochondria of these cells showed some recovery in a dog that had been returned to uncontaminated food for only 3 weeks after 12 weeks of the high dosage of methoxychlor (Tegeris *et al.*, 1968).

15.3.4.3 Toxicity to Humans

Experimental Exposure Groups of volunteers were given methoxychlor at rates of 0, 0.5, 1, and 2 mg/kg/day for 8 weeks. Even the highest dosage was without detectable effect on health, clinical chemistry, or the morphology of blood, bone marrow, liver, small intestine, or testis (Stein *et al.*, 1965; Stein, 1970). The highest dosage administered by Stein was similar to 1.4 mg/kg/day, which is considered safe for occupational intake, as reflected in the threshold limit value of 10 mg/m³.

The low sensitizing property of methoxychlor has been noted (Szarmach and Poniecka, 1973).

Use Experience There apparently has been no confirmed case of poisoning, occupational or otherwise, involving methoxychlor.

Atypical Cases of Various Origins A 21-year-old man first noticed symptoms 8–9 hr after spraying several fruit trees with a formulation diluted from a mixture containing methoxychlor (15%) and malathion (7.5%). The entire task took only 15–20 min, and afterward a shower was taken. The first symptoms were blurring of vision and gradual onset of nausea. Next morning, the man began vomiting and developed severe diarrhea. He sought medical help 24 hr after exposure and was admitted to hospital about 36 hr after exposure. He was then dehydrated and suffering severe abdominal cramps and continuing diarrhea. On day 3 after exposure, jaundice was noted and continuous, bilateral tinnitus began. On day 4 the patient was completely deaf and slightly dizzy. On day 5, rapidly progressive renal failure required hemodialysis. Soon afterward, peripheral sensory and motor neuropathy appeared, including hypoesthesias, paresthesias, persistent leg and foot pain, bilateral footdrop, and difficulty in moving the extremities. A generalized rash appeared. In spite of marked recovery, the patient still had profound, bilateral, sensorineural hearing loss, tinnitus, and moderate neuropathy of the legs and arms when he was reevaluated over 6 years later (Harell *et al.*, 1978). Clearly, the delay in onset and the character of the illness were not consistent with poisoning by methoxychlor, malathion, or a combination of them, regardless of dosage. No thought seems to have been given to other possible causes, whether toxic or otherwise.

A 49-year-old man who was exposed to a dust of methoxychlor and captan developed aplastic anemia a few weeks later and died within 6 months. He had also had light exposure to methoxychlor during the previous 2 years without symptoms (Ziem, 1982).

Laboratory Findings Most investigators have not found methoxychlor in human tissue. Apparently, the first exceptions were Griffith and Blanke (1975), who reported finding the compound infrequently and in unstated concentrations in blood taken at autopsy under the medical examiner system of Virginia. Under the circumstances of collection, the possibility of occupational exposure of the deceased could not be excluded.

The reported persistence of methoxychlor for at least 7 days on the hands of a worker (Kazen *et al.*, 1974) is interesting in view of the rapid metabolism of the compound once it is absorbed.

Treatment of Poisoning In the unlikely event that treatment is required, it must be symptomatic (see Section 15.2.5).

15.3.5 CHLOROBENZILATE

15.3.5.1 Identity, Properties, and Uses

The IUPAC name for chlorbenzilate (BS1, ISO, JMAF) is ethyl 4,4′-dichlorobenzilate. Other names are 4,4′-chlorobenzilic acid ethyl ester, ethyl 2-hydroxy-2,2-bis(3-chlorophenyl)acetate, ethyl 4,4′-dichlorodiphenyl glycollate. For the structure see Table 15.2. Proprietary names: among many have been G23992, Acaraben®, Benz O-chlor®, Benzilan®, and Kop-Mite®. The CAS registry number is 510-15-6.

Chlorobenzilate has the empirical formula $C_{16}H_{14}Cl_2O_3$ and a molecular weight of 325.20. It is a colorless solid melting at 37–37°C. It is very soluble in acetone and hexane but virtually insoluble in water. Impurities in the technical product, which is about 95% pure, can be dichlorobenzophenon, the ethyl ether of chlorobenzilate, and 4,4-dichlorobenzil.

Chlorobenzilate was introduced as a technical product in 1952. It has been used mainly as a miticide on citrus crops or to control mites in beehives. In 1978, the total usage of chlorobenzilate in the United States was estimated to have been 360,000 kg, all used on citrus crops.

15.3.5.2 Toxicity to Laboratory Animals

The acute oral LD 50 to mice, rats (Horn *et al.*, 1955), and hamsters (Cabral *et al.*, 1979b) is about 700 mg/kg. Symptoms in rats and mice include depressed motor activity and rapid, wheezing respiration. Dogs tolerated daily oral doses of 64 mg/kg for 35 weeks and rats 500 ppm in the diet for 2 years (Horn *et al.*, 1955).

After daily chlorobenzilate doses of 12.8 mg/kg to dogs, 5 days/week for 35 weeks, approximately 40% of the total dose was excreted unchanged or as urinary metabolites. No significant storage in fat of dogs or rats was reported (Horn *et al.*, 1955). Knowles and Ahmad (1971) described the conversion of chlorobenzilate by rat liver homogenates to *p,p′*-dichlorobenzilic acid, *p,p′*-dichlorobenyhydrol, *p*-chlorobenzoic acid, and *p,p′*-dichlorobenzophenone.

In carcinogenicity studies chlorobenzilate induced hepatocellular carcinomas in two strains of mice, but the evidence in rats is uncertain (NCI, 1978c). Some testicular atrophy was observed in rats.

15.3.5.3 Toxicity to Humans

A case of a pesticide sprayer poisoned by chlorobenzilate has been described (Ravindran, 1981). Symptoms included ataxia, delirium, fever, and muscle pains.

Chlorobenzilate was detected in the urine of some workers employed in Florida citrus groves. Exposed workers had levels ranging from 0.07 to 6.2 mg/liter. It should be noted that the methodology employed involved oxidation to *p,p′*-dichlorobenzophenone and would not distinguish between the parent chemical and some of its metabolites (Levy *et al.*, 1981).

15.3.6 DICOFOL

15.3.6.1 Identity, Properties, and Uses

The IUPAC name is 2,2,2-trichloro-1,1-bis(4-chlorophenyl)-ethanol. Other names include 1,1-bis(4-chlorophenyl)-2,2,2-trichloroethanol, 1,1-bis(*p*-chlorophenyl)-2,2,2-trichloroethanol, 4,4-dichloro-α-trichloro-methylbenzhydrol. For the structure see Table 15.2. Dicofol (BSI, ISO) is also called Kelthane (JMAF). Proprietary names include Acarin®, Decofol®, Hifol®, Kelthane® and Mitigan®. Dicofol has the empirical formula $C_{14}H_9Cl_5O$ and a molecular weight of 370.50.

The pure substance is colorless and melts at 78.5–79.5°C. It is soluble in most organic solvents but practically insoluble in water.

Dicofol was introduced as a commercial chemical in 1955. Like chlorobenzilate, dicofol is used mainly as a miticide for citrus fruits, nuts, cotton, and beans. Its use still appears to be widespread in many European, South American, Asian, and African countries as well as the United States.

The technical product is a brown viscous oil with a d^{25} of 1.45. The active compounds are 80% 1,1-bis(4-chlorophenyl-2,2,2-trichloroethanol and 20% 1-(2-chlorophenyl)-1-(4-chlorophenyl)-2,2,2-trichloroethanol (the o,p'-isomer). The other major impurity is 1,1,1,2-tetrachloro-2,2-bis(4-chlorophenyl)ethane (Baum *et al.*, 1976).

Dicofol is produced as water-dispersable powders, as emulsions, and in a dust.

15.3.6.2 Toxicity to Laboratory Animals

In rats and rabbits the acute oral LD 50 for technical grade dicofol seems to range from 575 to 2000 mg/kg (Smith *et al.*, 1959; Brown *et al.*, 1969; Ben-Dyke *et al.*, 1970). Dogs seem to be much less sensitive (Smith *et al.*, 1959). Rats fed dicofol for up to 2 years showed no effects on survival at levels below 1000 ppm but growth was impaired (Smith *et al.*, 1959). The maximum tolerable dose for mice in a subchronic study was 500 ppm (Sato *et al.*, 1987). Dogs fed 300 ppm showed no effect after 1 year, but some deaths occurred at 900 ppm.

Dicofol seems to be metabolized in rats to 4,4'-dichlorobenzophenone, which is stored in fat and muscle as well as being excreted in the feces (Brown *et al.*, 1969). DDE was also found, but there is doubt as to whether this was due to metabolism of dicofol or to contamination of the technical product employed. Water-soluble metabolites have been detected in the urine of mice given ^{3}H- and ^{14}C-labeled dicofol. Nearly 50% of the administered doses was excreted in the urine within 24 hr. Part may be glucuronides of 4,4'-dichlorobenzhydrol (Tabata *et al.*, 1979). More recently, Brown and Casida (1987) showed that *in vivo* mice convert dicofol to dichlorobenzophenone and dichlorobenzhydrol and that DDE originates from the impurity α-Cl-DDT.

There is little published work on the specific toxic effects of dicofol in experimental animals. Some small adverse effects associated with reproduction in rats and mice have been reported (Brown, 1972; Trifonova and Gladenko, 1980). Fed to rats for 2 weeks at 200 ppm, dicofol induced hepatic mixed-function oxidases (Den Tonkelaar and Van Esch, 1974). In a comparative study, 98% dicofol, the technical product Kelthane, and DDT were given to male rats in equimolar amounts. Dicofol produced dosage-related increases in microsomal protein, cytochrome P-450, and the specific activities of cytochrome reductase, ethoxycoumarin *O*-deethylase, aminopyrine *N*-demethylase, and glutathione *S*-transferase at a potency equivalent to that of Kelthane, DDT, or phenobarbital (Narloch *et al.*, 1987). Some evidence has been obtained for its hepato-carcinogenicity in male B6C3F1 mice but not in rats (NCI, 1978d).

15.3.6.3 Toxicity to Humans

Apparently, only one case of possible human poisoning by dicofol has been reported, and this was in combination with trichlorfon (Zolotnikova and Somov, 1978). Greenhouse workers reportedly suffered frequently from allergic dermatitis. A detailed study of the protection of workers in Florida citrus groves from contamination by dicofol has been reported (Nigg *et al.*, 1986).

Dicofol has cytokinetic and cytogenetic effects on human lymphoid cells *in vitro* (Sobti *et al.*, 1983).

15.4 BENZENE HEXACHLORIDE

15.4.1 BENZENE HEXACHLORIDE AND LINDANE

15.4.1.1 Identity, Properties, and Uses

Chemical Name "Benzene hexachloride," a term firmly established by usage, is a misnomer for 1,2,3,4,5,6-hexachlorocyclohexane. It should not be confused with hexachlorobenzene. As detailed below, the technical product is a mixture of isomers of this compound and related compounds that may vary somewhat in relative concentration.

Structure 1,2,3,4,5,6-Hexachlorocyclohexane has eight separable steric isomers, one of which (the α-isomer) exists in two enantiomorphic forms. The eight isomers are shown in Figure 15.4. Of the eight isomers, six (including the two mirror-image forms of the α isomer, plus the β, γ, δ, and ε isomers) are relatively stable, and they are the only ones commonly identified in the technical product. In addition, the crude product contains small amounts of heptachlorocyclohexane and octachlorocyclohexane. The exact composition of the crude product varies from one manufacturer to another and even from one batch to another; typical examples are shown in Table 15.16.

Synonyms The acronym for benzene hexachloride is BHC. The acronym for the proper chemical name is HCH. Both BHC and HCH are recognized as common names in ISO Recommendation R 1750. Because BHC is used more commonly in the United States, that term is used herein for the commercial mixture of isomers and related compounds.

The International Organization for Standardization reconizes as distinct common names both γ-BHC (γ-HCH) and lindane; this distinction is between the pure isomer and lindane, which is defined as not less than 99% pure γ-BHC. In the USSR, the word "lindane" is used for the pure γ isomer. Apparently, no biologically significant property of lindane has been traced to the <1% of it that is not γ-BHC.

Although BHC is the most widely used common name for the compound, other terms are used as common names in some countries: 666 in Denmark, hexaklor in Sweden, hexachloran in the USSR, and HCH in most other parts of Europe.

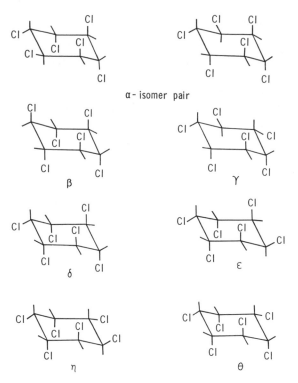

Figure 15.4 Structural isomers of BHC. The α, β, γ, and δ isomers are relatively strainless and predominate in the technical product. Unlabeled bonds represent hydrogen atoms. In the β isomer, all of the chlorine atoms are represented in the axial (*a*) position.

Proprietary names that are or have been used for BHC or its formulations include Agrocide®, Ambrocide®, Benesan®, Benexane®, Borer-Tox®, and Gamasan®.

Another common name for lindane is benhexachlor; a code designation is OMS-17. Proprietary names that are or have been used for lindane or its formulations include 666®, Ap-

Table 15.16

Composition of Five Samples of Benzene Hexachloride

Compound	Composition (%)[a]				
	A	B	C	D	E
α isomer	<70	65–70	55	55–80	61.5
β isomer	5	5–6	14	5–14	9.1
γ isomer	10–12	13	12	8–15	14.4
δ isomer	7	6	8	2–16	9.0
ε isomer	—	—	3–4	3–5	1.0
heptachlorocyclohexane	—	4	—	—	4.6
octachlorocyclohexane	—	0.6	—	—	0.4

[a] A, Slade (1945); B, Ramsey and Patterson (1946); C, Kauer *et al.* (1947); D, Riemschneider (1952); E, Hegyi and Stota (1962).

arasin®, Aphtiria®, Ben-Hex®, Borekil®, gamma-BHC®, Gammexane®, Gexane®, Jacutin®, Kwell®, Lindatox®, Lorexane®, Streunex®, Tri-6®, and Quellada®.

The CAS registry number for the mixed isomers is 608-73-1; that for lindane is 58-89-9.

Physical and Chemical Properties All isomers of BHC have the empirical formula $C_6H_6Cl_6$ and a molecular weight of 290.80. The technical mixture is an off-white to brown powder and has a persistent, musty odor. The technical mixture is stable to light, air, heat, and carbon dioxide; it is resistant to acids but susceptible to dehydrochlorination by alkali. The mixture is moderately soluble in acetone, benzene, and chlorinated hydrocarbon solvents; it is poorly soluble in kerosene, only slightly soluble in fats and oils, and almost insoluble in water.

Some physical properties of the separate isomers are shown in Table 15.17. The γ isomer is very stable to heat; it can be vaporized without appreciable decomposition by external heat

Table 15.17

Some Physical Properties of the Isomers of BHC

Property	Isomer				
	α	β	γ	δ	ε
Melting point (°C)	159–160	309–310	112–113	138–139	219–220
Vapor pressure (mm Hg at 20°C)[a]	2.5×10^{-5}	2.8×10^{-7}	9.4×10^{-6}	1.7×10^{-5}	
Solubility at 20°C (gm/100 gm)					
acetone	13.9	10.3	43.5	71.1	32.2
benzene	9.9	1.9	28.9	41.1	
chloroform	6.3	6.3	24.0	13.7	2
cyclohexanone			36.7		
ethyl ether	6.2	1.8	20.8	35.8	3
ethyl alcohol	1.8	1.1	6.4	24.2	4.2
methyl alcohol	2.3	1.6	7.4	27.3	3.7
kerosene			2.0–3.2		
xylene	8.5	3.3	24.7	42.1	
Rat fat (%)	4.05	0.66	12.55	19.10	
Water (ppm)	10	5	10	10	

[a] See text; Spencer and Cliath (1970) have calculated 3.26×10^{-5} for lindane.

or by burning a wick in which it has been incorporated. This stability, its low melting point, and its relatively high vapor pressure made it possible to use lindane as an insecticidal vapor dispensed by any of several types of vaporizers.

The values for vapor pressure given in Table 15.17 are those generally quoted. It may be that all of these values are low. Spencer and Cliath (1970), using a gas saturation technique, obtained a value of 3.26×10^{-5} mm Hg for lindane at 20°C. By measurements actually made at 20, 30, and 40°C, they obtained the equation $\log_{10} P = 13.544 - (5288/T)$, where T is the absolute temperature. They considered that lower pressures measured may have been associated with incomplete saturation of the sphere cavity in the effusion manometer method.

History, Formulations, and Uses   BHC was first made by Michael Faraday in 1825. Four of the stereoisomers were demonstrated by van der Linden (1912). During World War I, it was used as a smoke bomb. The insecticidal properties were discovered independently about 1942 by Dupire and Raucourt (1943) and by Slade (1945); it was Slade and his colleagues who showed that the γ isomer is the insecticidally effective one.

BHC is sold in relatively few formulations: concentrates (30–100%), dusts (0.5–75%), cords (63%), sprays (1.8–50%), and seed treatments (16.6%). Far more formulations of lindane occur; concentrates (99–100%), pressurized aerosols (3–11.2%), sprays (0.4–75%), dusts (0.5–1%), water-wettable powders (25%), wood preservative (75%), impregnated cords (2–20%), and seed treatments (15–25%). Lindane is sold separately or in combinations with fungicides, fertilizers, other insecticides, or wood preservatives.

Recommendations to restrict the use of lindane in continuous vaporizers were made at least as early as 1951. The recommendations were based partially on the fact that some devices overheated and dehydrochlorinated this compound, releasing highly irritating fumes of hydrochloric acid. Some authorities also objected on principle to fumigation in areas where unprotected people might be present even temporarily. The restrictions proposed by the Interdepartmental Committee on Pest Control (1951) were amplified by that organization (1953) and endorsed by others (West, 1967).

Relative to other insecticides, BHC, including lindane, has been more extensively used in some countries than in the United States and Western Europe. Furthermore, the proportion of BHC used as a crude mixture of isomers rather than as lindane has been greater in some other countries.

BHC has been of value in the control of malaria and other vector-borne diseases, but only to a small degree compared with DDT. BHC and lindane have been of value in control of grasshoppers, cotton insects, rice insects, wireworms, and other soil pests. Lindane has been used for protection of seeds, for treatment of poultry and livestock, and for control of household insects. The use of BHC on a number of crops was never practical because the technical mixture imparts to the food a marked off-flavor that is apparent at once or only after the food is cooked. The flavor has been attributed to two isomers of heptachlorocyclohexane (Scheuing and Vogelbach,

1950) and to enneachlorocyclohexane (Münchberg, 1949) in the mixture, but off-flavor is not entirely absent following the use of lindane. For humans, lindane is used as a scabicide and pediculocide, usually as lotions, creams, and shampoos.

15.4.1.2 Toxicity to Laboratory Animals

Basic Findings   Essentially nothing has been added to the description of acute poisoning by lindane given by Cameron (1945), namely increased respiratory rate, restlessness accompanied by frequency of micturition, intermittent muscular spasms of the whole body, salivation, grinding of teeth and consequent bleeding from the mouth, backward movement with loss of balance and somersaulting, retraction of the head, convulsions, gasping and biting, and collapse and death usually within a day. The few animals that survive longer but eventually die show considerable loss of weight. Symptomatology associated with other isomers is discussed under Miscellaneous Effects on Organs and Tissues in this section.

A high degree of susceptibility of rabbits to lindane applied dermally in certain formulations but not in others was reported by Lehman (1951, 1952) (Table 15.18). This susceptibility was later confirmed in connection with a formulation sold for treatment of human scabies. Some shaved weanling rabbits that received 60 mg/kg had convulsions, and some that received the same dosage following chemical depilation died after convulsions. Adult rabbits, whether depilated or not, survived the same dosage without convulsions (Hanig *et al.*, 1976).

LD 50 values for lindane administered to different species by different routes are shown in Table 15.18. For most species,

Table 15.18
Single Dose LD 50 for Lindane

Species	Route	LD 50 (mg/kg)	Reference
Rat	oral	190	Slade (1945)
		200	Cameron (1945)
		125	Lehman (1951, 1952)
		88	Gaines (1960)
		91	Gaines (1960)
	dermal	500	Cameron (1945)
		1000	Gaines (1960)
		900	Gaines (1960)
	subcutaneous	50	Coper *et al.* (1951)
Mouse	oral	86	IARC (1979)
		340–562	Miura *et al.* (1974)
	dermal	300	Cameron (1945)
Guinea pig	oral	100–127	Lehman (1948)
		100	Cameron (1945)
	dermal	400	Cameron (1945)
	subcutaneous	100	Cameron (1945)
Rabbit	oral	200	Cameron (1945)
	dermal	300	Cameron (1945)
		>4000[a]	Lehman (1951, 1952)
		>188[b]	Lehman (1951, 1952)
		50[c]	Lehman (1951, 1952)

[a] Applied in crystalline form.
[b] Applied as 2% dimethyl phthalate solution.
[c] Applied as a 1% formulation in vanishing cream.

the compound has a moderate oral toxicity not greatly different from that of DDT. It is more readily absorbed by the skin and, therefore, is more toxic than DDT by that route. The special susceptibility of calves to dermally applied BHC is remarkable. Whereas adult cattle tolerated 0.1 or 0.20% formulations, 0.05% sprays were fatal to calves (Radeleff *et al.*, 1955). In a more recent example, Frank and Braun (1984) calculated a lethal dose of 13–16 mg/kg for a calf that died in 50 hr. A calf that died in 1 hr after ingestion of lindane (about 29 mg/kg) had 15 mg/kg in its brain. Young rabbits are much more susceptible to lindane than are adults (Hanig *et al.*, 1976). Harrison *et al.* (1980) calculated that lambs poisoned by lindane had consumed only 2.5 mg/kg.

The effects of repeated oral doses of BHC and lindane may be summarized as follows. (*a*) There is no major difference between the dosages of BHC and of lindane that produce different clinical effects. (*b*) A dosage of 1.25 mg/kg/day is a no-effect level in the mouse, rat, and dog (Fitzhugh *et al.*, 1950; Mellis, 1955; Nagasaki *et al.*, 1971, 1972b; FAO/WHO, 1974). (*c*) Although dogs withstand 1.25 mg/kg/day for 2 years, some of them have convulsions and die following repeated ingestion of lindane in the range of only 2.6–5.0 mg/kg/day, and all succumb rapidly to a dosage in the range of 40–80 mg/kg/day (Woodard and Hagan, 1947; FAO/WHO, 1974). (*d*) Minor liver lesions have been reported in rats in the dosage range 2.6–5.0 mg/kg/day (Fitzhugh *et al.*, 1950; Tashkhodzhayev *et al.*, 1973). (*e*) Some investigators found that dosage at the rate of 6–10 mg/kg/day produces no effect in mice (Klimmer, 1955; Herbst *et al.*, 1975), but others found some centrilobular hypertrophic foci in the liver of mice receiving BHC at this rate (Nagasaki *et al.*, 1971, 1972b). (*f*) Dosage levels of 20 mg/kg/day or greater have produced hepatoma mainly in mice (Nagasaki *et al.*, 1971, 1972a,b, 1973; Goto *et al.*, 1972a,b; Hanada *et al.*, 1973; Thorpe and Walker, 1973; Kuwabara and Takayama, 1974), but some investigators have found no tumors, even though some did find other liver changes (Woodard and Hagan, 1947; Klimmer, 1955; Oshiba and Kawakita, 1970; Didenko *et al.*, 1973).

In rats, the acute toxicity of the isomers of BHC decreases in the order γ > α > δ > β (Woodard and Hagan, 1947). However, the toxicity of repeated doses decreases in the order β > α > γ > δ (Fitzhugh *et al.*, 1950). The long-term toxicity of the different isomers is directly related to their storage (Davidow and Frawley, 1951; Macholz *et al.*, 1986) and inversely related to their rate of metabolism.

Absorption BHC is absorbed from the gastrointestinal tract, the lungs, and the skin.

Measurement of gastrointestinal absorption is made difficult by fecal excretion. Using radioactive β-BHC, Oshiba (1972) estimated absorption of about 80%. Oshiba and Kawakita (1972c, 1973) estimated that 95% of the β isomer and 85% of the γ isomer are absorbed within 5 days. Using squalene, a compound that is completely unabsorbed by rats, as a positive control, Albro and Thomas (1974) estimated absorption of technical BHC at 95.8% within 4 days following single doses.

Variation of dosage rates from 30 to 120 mg/kg had no influence on the proportion absorbed. The overall rate of absorption of technical BHC administered in food for 14 days was essentially identical (94.9%), but average absorption of the isomers differed somewhat: α-BHC, 97.4; β-BHC, 90.7; γ-BHC, 99.4; and δ-BHC, 91.9%. These values are considered the most accurate available.

It is claimed that more rapid oral absorption of BHC occurs if it is administered with an alkyl surfactant; compared to controls, rats that received a surface-active agent had a higher concentration of BHC in the liver after 1 hr, in the blood after 24 hr, or in the kidneys after 48 hr (Litvinov and Nikonova, 1971). This increase in absorption is greater in connection with single doses than with repeated doses (Krasil'shchikov, 1972).

By autoradiography, it has been shown that all isomers of BHC are absorbed and distributed to all organs within 5 min after intraperitoneal injection (Shindo, 1972).

Transport Lindane in sheep blood is almost totally bound to serum proteins; at overall concentrations of 0.850–1.040 ppm, the proportion that was free varied from 1.29 to 1.49%. Interestingly, lindane was found almost entirely in the third fraction separated on Sephadex G200, whereas DDT eluted mainly with the first peak and dieldrin eluted mainly with the second and third peaks (Ferry *et al.*, 1972b).

Lindane may be partially displaced from blood proteins by some other compounds, and this will increase, at least temporarily, the amount that is free for toxic action or metabolism. The concentration of free lindane in the blood of sheep pretreated with lindane at the rate of 27.5 mg/kg increased slightly following intravenous injection of diphenylhydantoin, but metabolism and excretion were so rapid that total blood lindane was reduced (Ferry *et al.*, 1972a).

Distribution and Storage Davidow and Frawley (1951) showed that, although the α, β, γ, and δ isomers of BHC are stored in the fat of rats and dogs, over 30 times more β than γ is stored at equivalent dosage levels. This explains why the β isomer is more toxic when administered repeatedly even though the γ isomer is more toxic when given as a single dose. The difference in storage does not correspond to the solubility of the isomers in the fat of rats (Sedlak, 1965), nor does it depend on differences in absorption, but it must be explained by differences in metabolism. Others have confirmed the greater and more prolonged storage of the β isomer (Wakita *et al.*, 1972; Oshiba and Kawakita, 1972b,c; Srinivasan and Radhakrishnamurty, 1983a). α-Hexachlorocyclohexane also seems to accumulate more than lindane, especially in the brain, for which the β and γ isomers seem to have little affinity (Stein *et al.*, 1980; Eichler *et al.*, 1983).

In rats, lindane reaches storage equilibrium within 2–3 weeks at a dietary level of 1 or 10 ppm and in 3–7 days at a dietary level of 100 ppm. At lower dietary levels a slight decrease in storage may be observed after the third week (Oshiba and Kawakita, 1970; Oshiba, 1972). The storage of isomers of BHC is less at dietary levels of 660 and 66 ppm than at

6.6 ppm (Nagasaki, 1973). The more rapid equilibrium and relatively lesser storage at higher dosages are consistent with a dosage-related induction of microsomal enzymes.

In swine fed lindane at the high rate of 40 mg/kg/day, the highest blood level was found 13 weeks after feeding started, but the concentration in body fat did not reach maximum until weeks 27–33 (Davey and Johnson, 1974).

The time at which β-BHC reaches storage equilibrium in fat is not less than 8 weeks (Oshiba and Kawakita, 1972a; Oshiba, 1972). in mice it reaches a constant level after 12 weeks of feeding at dietary levels less than 50 ppm (Yoshimoto et al., 1972).

All isomers of BHC are preferentially stored in fat. Beyond this generalization, it appears that the adrenal (at least in the dog) has a special affinity for α-BHC unexplained by lipid content and that, because of their slow metabolism, the α and β isomers may be found in the liver in relatively high concentration (Davidow and Frawley, 1951). Strangely enough, adrenalectomized rats store more BHC in their fat than do normal rats (D. Wassermann et al., 1970).

In chickens, the concentration of lindane in fat at equilibrium is lower in relation to its concentration in the diet than is true for DDT, endrin, dieldrin, or heptachlor epoxide. By the same token, residues or lindane disappear more rapidly after dosing is discontinued (Cummings et al., 1967).

Of course, BHC is transferred via the placenta, but the rate is negligible. Hori and Kashimoto (1974) reported that only 1.6–2.2% of β-[^{14}C]BHC administered to pregnant mice was retained by the fetuses, while the dams retained 33.2–53.7%. On the other hand, a high proportion of β-[^{14}C]BHC administered to dams during lactation was secreted in their milk, so that at the end of lactation the young retained 60.0–63.8% of the total dose, while very little remained in the mothers. In another study, some uptake of [^{14}C]BHC isomers into the fetus was observed after dosage of pregnant mice. Of particular interest was the presence of radioactivity in nasal and tracheobronchial epithelia, as detected by microscopic autoradiography (Brittebo et al., 1987).

Microautoradiography after rats were fed 25 ppm lindane for 6 months followed by [^{3}H]lindane showed that radioactivity in the epithelial cells of the proximal convoluted tubules was consistent with the location and severity of granular hyaline degeneration in the kidney (Zhu et al., 1986).

Metabolism Isomers of BHC are metabolized by slightly different routes, and the biotransformation of lindane in mammals alone has become a complicated subject in drug metabolism terms. In addition, many of the products or intermediates, when given separately, are converted to other metabolites not usually detected during the metabolism of BHC isomers. A list of metabolites of lindane and related chemicals published relatively recently can be found in Macholz and Kujawa (1985). A scheme proposed for lindane metabolism by Grover and Sims (1965) laid the foundations for this field. Subsequently, new metabolites isolated from rat urine illustrated that this scheme would need revision (Chadwick and Freal, 1972a). A list of

some phenols, alcohols, and mercapturates found in excreta of animals given lindane is shown in Table 15.19.

Since the work of Grover and Sims (1965), knowledge of the metabolism of lindane has been so greatly extended that it cannot be described in full here. Metabolism involves not only phase I pathways, such as oxidation by cytochrome P-450, but also phase II pathways, such as conjugation of alcohol and phenol products to form glucuronides. The type of initial metabolism that lindane undergoes dictates the final products appearing in excreta. A recently published scheme for the metabolism of lindane by the rat is shown in Fig. 15.5. The use of microsomal systems has greatly contributed to the understanding of metabolism in vivo, although there are still unknown areas, such as the role of specific cytochrome P-450 isoenzymes. Direct hydroxylation of lindane to hexachlorocyclohexanol followed by decomposition to the pentachlorocyclohexanone and dechlorination leads to 2,4,6-trichlorophenol (Stein et al., 1977; Tanaka et al., 1977, 1979b). A related route of metabolism is initiated by dehydrogenation of lindane to γ-1,2,3,4,5,6-hexachlorocyclohexene. Subsequent hydroxylation, isomerization, and dechlorination steps result in 2,3,4,6- and 2,3,4,5-tetrachlorophenols (Chadwick et al., 1975; Stein et al., 1977; Tanaka et al., 1979a,b). Trans-dehydrochlorination of lindane can also occur, giving a 2,3,4,5,6-pentachlorocyclohexene isomer which is apparently converted to 2,4,5-trichlorophenol (Tanaka et al., 1979b). Cis-dehydrochlorination has also been reported with rat and especially human microsomes (Fitzloff et al., 1982), the resulting pentachlorocyclohexene showing little further reactivity except for undergoing epoxidation (Fitzloff and Pan, 1984). 2,3,4,5,6-Pentachloro-2-cyclohexen-1-ol and 2,4,5,6- and 2,3,4,6-tetrachloro-2-cyclohexen-1-ols, known urinary metabolites of lindane (Chadwick and Freal, 1972a; Chadwick et al., 1978a, 1981), arise by similar desaturation—hydroxylation mechanisms, perhaps involving superoxide anion (Tanaka et al., 1979a).

Under anaerobic conditions lindane undergoes dechlorination to γ-3,4,5,6-tetrachlorocyclohex-1-ene (Chadwick et al., 1978a; Kuriharu et al., 1979; Stein et al., 1980; Yamamoto et al., 1983), as well as to chlorobenzene and benzene (Baker et al., 1985) and perhaps to other chlorobenzenes (Karapally et al., 1973). Hexachlorobenzene has been proposed as another metabolite of lindane in the rat both in vivo and in vitro (Gopalaswamy and Aiyar, 1984a). Although Chadwick and Copeland (1985) have been unable to confirm these findings in in vivo studies, the persistence of HCB in the environment and tissues and the large amounts of lindane used in some countries necessitate that this aspect of metabolism be tested most rigorously.

Most of the di- and trichlorophenyl mercapturates observed in the urine of lindane-treated rats arise by conjugation of hexachlorocyclohexenes and pentachlorocyclohexenes with glutathione, followed by dechlorination (Kurihara et al., 1979; Portig et al., 1979). As with many of the later stages in lindane metabolism, it is probable that loss of the chlorines to give aromatics occurs nonenzymatically (Portig et al., 1979).

Table 15.19
Metabolites of Lindane Identified in the Urine and/or Feces of Laboratory Mammals

Metabolite[a]	Species	References
pentachlorophenol	rabbit	Karapally et al. (1973)
2,3,4,5,6-pentachloro-2-cyclohexen-1-ol	rat	Chadwick and Freal (1972a)
		Freal and Chadwick (1973)
		Chadwick et al. (1981)
	mouse	Chadwick et al. (1986)
2,3,4,6-tetrachloro-2-cyclohexen-1-ol	rat	Chadwick et al. (1978a)
		Chadwick et al. (1981)
	mouse	Chadwick et al. (1986)
2,4,5,6-tetrachloro-2-chclohexen-ol	rat	Chadwick et al. (1978a)
		Chadwick et al. (1981)
	mouse	Chadwick et al. (1986)
2,3,4,5-tetrachlorophenol	rat	Chadwick and Freal (1972a)
		Freal and Chadwick (1973)
	mouse	Chadwick et al. (1986)
	rabbit	Karapally et al. (1973)
2,3,4,6-tetrachlorophenol	rat	Chadwick and Freal (1972a)
		Freal and Chadwick (1973)
	mouse	Chadwick et al. (1986)
	rabbit	Karapally et al. (1973)
2,3,4-trichlorophenol	rabbit	Karapally et al. (1973)
2,3,5-trichlorophenol	rat	Grover and Sims (1965)
		Chadwick and Freal (1972a)
		Freal and Chadwick (1973)
	mouse	Chadwick et al. (1982)
	rabbit	Karapally et al. (1973)
2,4,5-trichlorophenol	rat	Grover and Sims (1965)
		Chadwick and Freal (1972a)
		Freal and Chadwick (1973)
	mouse	Chadwick et al. (1982)
	rabbit	Karapally et al. (1973)
2,4,6-trichlorophenol	rat	Chadwick and Freal (1972a)
		Freal and Chadwick (1973)
	mouse	Kurihara and Nakajima (1974)
		Chadwick et al. (1982)
	rabbit	Karapally et al. (1973)
2,3-dichlorophenol	rabbit	Karapally et al. (1973)
2,4-dichlorophenol	rat	Grover and Sims (1965)
	mouse	Kurihara and Nakajima (1974)
	rabbit	Karapally et al. (1973)
2,5-dichlorophenol	rabbit	Karapally et al. (1973)
2,6-dichlorophenol	rabbit	Karapally et al. (1973)
3,4-dichlorophenol	rat	Chadwick and Freal (1972a)
	rabbit	Karapally et al. (1973)
4-chlorophenol mercapturate	rat	Kurihara et al. (1979)
2,4-dichlorophenyl mercapturate	rat	Kurihara et al. (1979)
3,4-dichlorophenyl mercapturate	rat	Kurihara et al. (1979)
2,3,5-trichlorophenyl mercapturate	rat	Kurihara et al. (1979)
2,4,5-trichlorophenyl mercapturate	rat	Kurihara et al. (1979)
2,4-dichlorophenyl cysteine	rat	Macholz et al. (1985)
pentachlorobenzene	rabbit	Karapally et al. (1973)
1,2,3,4-tetrachlorobenzene	rabbit	Karapally et al. (1973)
1,2,3,5-tetrachlorobenzene	rabbit	Karapally et al. (1973)
1,2,4,5-tetrachlorobenzene	rabbit	Karapally et al. (1973)
1,2,4-trichlorobenzene	rabbit	Karapally et al. (1973)
1,2-dichlorobenzene	rabbit	Karapally et al. (1973)

[a] Cyclohexenol and phenol metabolites are often excreted as the glucuronide and sulfate conjugates.

As shown in Fig. 15.5, much of the alcohol and phenol metabolites is excreted as the glucuronides or sulfates. Proportions of these and types and quantities of alcohols and phenols can be varied in rats and mice by a number of factors *in vivo*, including age of animals (Copeland *et al.*, 1986), fiber content of diet (Chadwick *et al.*, 1978b), obesity (Chadwick *et al.*, 1986, 1987), strain (Liu and Morgan, 1986), and inducers of cytochrome P-450 (Chadwick *et al.*, 1981).

There is little evidence that lindane is converted to other

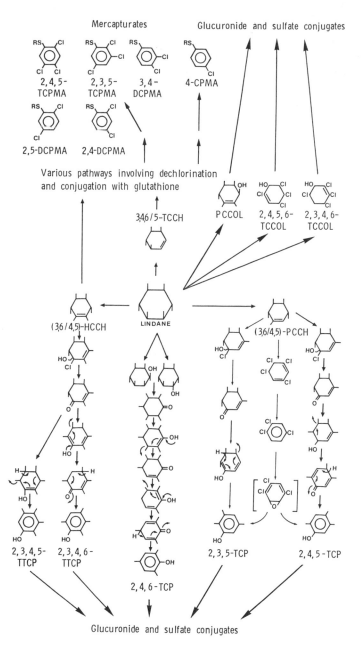

Figure 15.5 Metabolism of lindane in rats. Configurations of chlorine atoms (where known) are denoted first as above and second as below the plane of the ring. Abbreviations from top to bottom: CPMA, chlorophenyl mercapturic acid; DCPMA, dichlorophenyl mercapturic acid; TCPMA, trichlorophenyl mercapturic acid; TCCH, tetrachlorocyclohexene; PCCOL, 2,3,4,5,6-pentachloro-2-cyclohexen-1-ol; TCCOL, tetrachloro-2-cyclohexen-1-ol; HCCH, hexachlorocyclohexene; PCCH, pentachlorocyclohexene; TCP, trichlorophenol; TTP, tetrachlorophenol (adapted from Copeland *et al.*, 1986).

BHC isomers in rats (Copeland and Chadwick, 1979), although *in vitro* with reduced hematin some isomerization can occur (Saleh, 1980). Some conversion of γ-BHC to α-BHC when incubated for 1 month with either seawater and sea sediment or with the soil bacterium *Pseudomonas putida* has been reported (Benezet and Matsumura, 1973). There is also evidence for the interconversion of isomers when they are heated (Kawahara and Moku, 1972).

The metabolism of other isomers of BHC besides lindane has not been studied in as much detail as that of the γ isomer. α-BHC is converted by rats to 1,2,4-trichlorobenzene, 2,3,4-trichlorophenol, 2,4,6-trichlorophenol, 2,3,4,6-tetrachlorophenol, and other products, probably by routes very similar to those described above for lindane (Freal and Chadwick, 1973; Koransky *et al.*, 1975; Tanaka *et al.*, 1977, 1979b; Stein *et al.*, 1980; Macholz *et al.*, 1982a). A high proportion of the metabolism of α-BHC must involve conjugation with glutathione (GSH), since the level of GSH in the liver of rats is reduced by 50% 18 hr after a single dose (400 mg/kg) (Noack and Portig, 1973). The *in vitro* hepatic formation of GSH conjugates derived from α-BHC, four positional isomers of *S*-(dichlorophenyl)glutathione, has been described by Portig *et al.* (1979). GSH-mediated metabolism of radioactive α-BHC has been demonstrated in *in vitro* preparations from other tissues such as kidneys, lung, and brain (Kraus *et al.*, 1973), and the biotransformational activity of liver cytosol in this respect is inducible by pretreatment of rats with the chemical (Portig *et al.*, 1973).

Like other BHC isomers, β-BHC also gives 2,4-dichlorophenol and 2,3,4- and 2,4,6-trichlorophenol in the urine of rats, as well as 2,3,4,6-tetrachlorophenol, in both free and conjugated forms (Freal and Chadwick, 1973; Stein *et al.*, 1977; Tanaka *et al.*, 1977; Lay *et al.*, 1981; Macholz *et al.*, 1982b).

Excretion   Lindane is excreted more efficiently than the β isomer. In rats preadapted by feeding them β-BHC at a dietary level of 10 ppm for 10 days and then given a single oral dose of radioactive β-BHC, a total of 12.2–13.0% of the radioactive material was recovered in the urine and 5.4–5.8% in the feces during the first 10 days after ingestion. Comparable figures for radioactive lindane were 48.5–52.0% in urine and 20.8–22.2% in feces. The rate of urinary excretion of radioactive lindane was increased in rats fed nonradioactive compound for 49 days as compared to those fed only 10 days. There was no such increase in fecal excretion (Oshiba and Kawakita, 1972c). The results were essentially identical when either radioactive β-BHC or lindane was given first and excretion was measured while the rats continued to receive nonradioactive compounds (Oshiba and Kawakita, 1973). Dietary fiber can apparently stimulate the metabolism of lindane (Chadwick *et al.*, 1978b), and the intestinal and urinary excretion of radioactivity from labeled β-BHC is enhanced by diets containing paraffin. Whole-body elimination half-lives were reduced from 71 to 37 days in paraffin-fed rats (Richter *et al.*, 1981). Of course, many of these changes are the result of the increased metabolism described previously.

The rate at which a compound is cleared from the milk of dairy cows reflects its rate of metabolism and excretion. Under practical conditions, the times necessary for residues of different compounds to decline to nonactionable levels decreased in the following order: dieldrin > DDT and its analogs > BHC > lindane > endrin > methoxychlor (Moubry *et al.*, 1968).

Biochemical Effects   One possible basis for subtle differences in the action of different chlorinated hydrocarbon insecticides is the finding that lindane has a slightly greater inhibitory effect on Na^+,K^+-ATPase than on Mg^{2+}-ATPase, whereas chlordane and DDT behave in the opposite way. In either case, inhibition of these enzymes is thought to be related to cation transport in nerve axons, perhaps to Ca^{2+} extrusion, and therefore to the toxic action of the compounds. The inhibition of both enzymes may be observed at concentrations below 1 ppm (Koch, 1969). The inhibition of Na^+,K^+-ATPase by lindane was confirmed by Uchida *et al.* (1974), but, by comparison with other isomers and compounds, they found little correlation between the insecticidal action of lindane and either its inhibition of the enzyme or its ability to block nerve impulses in insects. In mouse synaptosomes, Na^+,K^+-ATPase activity was depressed 18 hr after lindane administration even though neither the chemical nor its metabolites were present (Magour *et al.*, 1984). *In vitro*, Na^+,K^+-ATPases in rat liver microsomes were depressed by lindane whereas the mitochondrial enzymes were stimulated. A similar depression of the microsomal enzyme was observed in *in vivo* studies (Heinevetter *et al.*, 1984, 1985). Gopalaswamy and Aiyar (1984b) have observed a depression *in vitro* of Mg^{2+}-ATPase activity of liver mitochondria caused by lindane.

Oral doses of lindane at the rate of 34 mg/kg/day for 2 days increased the urinary excretion of 5-hydroxyindoleacetic acid by 160%, indicating a change in serotonin metabolism. At a dosage of 1.7 mg/kg/day for 3 or more months, the increase was only about 105% (Khaikina and Shilina, 1971). Later studies (Shilina, 1973) indicated an unusually complex reaction; for example, brain levels of serotonin were decreased by a few doses of lindane but first increased and later uninfluenced by repeated doses. Aldegunde *et al.* (1983) also showed that an acute dose of lindane (240 mg/kg) increased brain levels of serotonin and 5-hydroxyindoleacetic acid. Although serotonin is an important neurohormone, its exact significance in connection with lindane is unknown. There have been recent studies of neurotransmitter systems (e.g., Fishman and Gianutsos, 1987b, 1988; Artigas *et al.*, 1988a; Sunol *et al.*, 1988a,b). Further discussions of the effects of lindane on brain biochemistry can be found under Effects on the Nervous System.

The induction of liver microsomal enzymes by BHC as reflected by liver morphology is discussed in Section 15.2.3.2. Of course, the induction is reflected by reduced hexobarbital sleeping time or other appropriate tests (Kolmodin *et al.*, 1969; Nadzhimutdinov *et al.*, 1973, 1974; Koransky *et al.*, 1969; Kolmodin-Hedman *et al.*, 1971; Welch *et al.*, 1971; Krampl and Hladka, 1974; Pélissier *et al.*, 1975).

In rats, the lowest dosages of lindane that shortened hexobarbital sleeping time were 150 mg/kg intraperitoneally once or about 0.05 mg/kg/day derived from a dietary level of 0.5 ppm (Kolmodin-Hedman *et al.,* 1971).

Induction of microsomal enzymes by one compound can make the difference between life and death through change in the rate of metabolism of another compound. When lindane was injected intravenously into dogs at a uniform rate, those unprotected by phenobarbital had full convulsions in 20–35 min, whereas those previously dosed with phenobarbital withstood the injection for 60 min without showing any effect except an occasional jerk. The proportion of the administered dose in the brain was significantly smaller in the phenobarbital-treated dogs (Litterst *et al.,* 1973).

Not only is lindane metabolized by the liver during life, but also breakdown of the compound continues after death. The concentration in the livers of pigeons that died after the third dose of BHC at the rate of 75 mg/kg/day fell from 153 ppm 2 hr after death to 2 ppm in 430 hr. Thus tissues must be sampled and extracted promptly (French and Jefferies, 1968).

BHC promotes not only its own metabolism but also that of parathion. When rabbits were treated with BHC for a month and then with parathion for a month and the cycle was repeated after a 4-month rest period, the rate of excretion of *p*-nitrophenol was accelerated and the degree of inhibition of plasma and erythrocyte cholinesterase was reduced compared to the action of parathion alone (Michail, 1974a).

Ascorbic acid deficiency impairs the induction of microsomal enzymes; in guinea pigs the impairment is evident after only 2 days on a deficient diet. The dietary level necessary to maintain induction is higher than that necessary to prevent scurvy (Wagstaff and Street, 1971a; Chadwick *et al.,* 1972). Deficiency of vitamin C interferes with enzyme induction in squirrel monkey also (Chadwick *et al.,* 1971b).

It is interesting that some lack of parallelism has been noted in the effects on microsomal enzyme induction, increase in cytochrome P-450, and/or change in liver morphology even in relation to the same compound (in this instance α-BHC) (Koransky *et al.,* 1969; Schulte-Hermann *et al.,* 1974; Konat and Clausen, 1973). In rats γ-BHC is apparently a more powerful inducer of the mixed-function oxidase system than β-BHC although the latter is the more potent agent in increasing liver weight (Srinivasan and Radhakrishnamurty, 1983b). At least a part of the discrepancy can be explained by inhibition of microsomal enzymes by an excess of BHC, which binds to them (Schulte-Hermann *et al.,* 1974). Furthermore, the mechanism by which lindane induces its own metabolism is different from the mechanism by which DDT stimulates lindane metabolism (Chadwick and Freal, 1972b). Metabolism of lindane is induced not only by lindane but by the α, β, or δ isomer (Chadwick *et al.,* 1971a; Freal and Chadwick, 1973), but it is unclear whether the mechanism is identical to that of induction by lindane.

Now that different cytochrome P-450 isoenzymes, which are not identical in inducibility or substrate specificity, have been demonstrated (Wolf, 1986), it seems likely that the lack of parallelism in the effects of a single inducer as well as the different effects of different inducers eventually can be ex-

plained more completely. Indeed, lindane has been shown to induce hepatic cytochrome P-450 isozymes *b*/*e* by severalfold and isozymes *c* and *d* by threefold after four ip doses to rats (25 mg/kg) (Kumar and Dwivedi, 1988).

Induction of liver microsomal enzymes is associated with an increase in DNA and in cytochrome P-450. Under ordinary conditions, the induction of DNA synthesis is greater at night and suppressed during the day. This is because this synthesis depends on food intake. If rats are adapted to an artificial feeding schedule in which eating is restricted to 5 hr in each 24, DNA synthesis begins 6–9 hr after feeding begins and independently of the schedule of lighting. The induction of DNA by BHC (α isomer) requires about 18 hr and involves two phases, the first presumably associated with action of BHC in the liver cells and the second dependent on food intake. The induction may be inhibited by actinomycin during either phase, but they differ in sensitivity by a factor of 10 (Schulte-Hermann, 1974). By controlling feeding and lighting of mice given α-BHC, DNA synthesis became synchronized in the liver (Bursch and Schulte-Hermann, 1983) and may be a model with which to study the interaction of growth stimuli with endogenous regulators of hepatic DNA replication.

Changes that may or may not be steps in the increased production of cytochrome P-450 were described by Sarkander (1974) and Sarkander *et al.* (1974). A single dose of α-BHC at the rate of 200 mg/kg leads to a significant increase in the rate at which acetate is incorporated into histones of isolated liver cell nuclei in the presence of [^{3}H]coenzyme A. There is a sharp peak of this acetylation at 1–2 hr; the process declines to control values before rising at 24 hr to a second peak about four times greater than the control value. Methylation of histones also shows two peaks but slightly later than those for acetylation. DNA-dependent RNA polymerase I activity increases promptly after dosing with α-BHC, but polymerase II activity begins to increase after 8 hr. Both reach a maximum between 36 and 42 hr after dosing when an increase in synthesis of DNA begins. An increase in histone phosphorylation was found at 42 hr.

In a similar way, Brade *et al.* (1974) demonstrated approximate doubling of the *in vivo* uptake of ^{32}P by nuclear acidic proteins during a 12-hr period after administration of α-BHC. As expected, there is an induction of ornithine decarboxylase activity and incorporation of thymidine into DNA (Murdia *et al.,* 1985).

Both CFT 1201 and SKF 525A prevent the hyperplastic but not the hypertrophic response of the rat liver to α-BHC; augmentation of DNA content, enhanced incorporation of [^{3}H]thymidine into DNA, increased mitotic rate, and increase in the number of nuclei synthesizing DNA all fail to occur, while organ weight still increases. However, CFT 1201 does not block cell proliferation in response to partial hepatectomy or the injury produced by certain drugs. Thus, CFT 1201 does not interfere with hepatocyte replication *per se* but acts at some preliminary step that is triggered by BHC and leads to replication. Because CFT 1201 and SKF 525A both inhibit reactions catalyzed by cytochrome P-450, this enzyme system may be required for the induction of liver cell proliferation by α-BHC (Schulte-Hermann et al., 1972).

An increase in lipid peroxidation has been observed following lindane treatment and probably reflects the induction of cytochrome P-450 (Junqueira et al., 1986). Induction of glutathione S-transferases after acute exposure to α-BHC and lindane has been reported and is probably associated with conjugate formation but did not seem to occur following long-term feeding experiments (Kraus et al., 1981; Wolff and Suber, 1986). The induced γ-glutamyl transpeptidase, which cleaves GSH conjugates, was isolated from BHC-induced rat liver and was identical to that in control liver but apparently slightly different from the enzyme in hepatomas (Chandar and Nagarajan, 1984). Depression of GSH in blood and long-term depression in liver of cats given 2 mg/kg of lindane have been reported (Agrawal et al., 1987).

Lindane potentiates the porphyria induced by some drugs partly by induction of δ-aminolevulinate synthetase (De Matteis, 1973). In chick embryo liver cell cultures, lindane alone causes a porphyric state by the accumulation of uroporphyrin (Sinclair and Granick, 1974) but this does not necessarily implicate an inhibition of uroporphyrinogen decarboxylase. Vila et al. (1986) have shown that although a small increase in porphyrin excretion in rats occurred after long-term treatment with lindane, there was no inhibition of the decarboxylase or even induction of aminolevulinate synthetase.

BHC or its isomers have been reported to influence the activity of a number of enzymes that have no evident relationship to the pharmacological or toxic effects of the compound. Of course, liver function tests (SGOT, serum cholinesterase, etc.) might reflect different aspects of the effect of BHC on the liver. However, when some of these tests were run on mice receiving BHC at the rate of 0.25 mg/kg/day the observed changes took the form of peaks, and the values returned to normal while dosing continued (Ito and Miyake, 1973). Changes that have been recorded after single or prolonged dosing in vivo or in vitro of lindane or BHC include inhibition of liver xanthine oxidase (Ramakrishnan et al., 1961), acid phosphatase (Gertig et al., 1971a), mitochondrial NADH oxidase (Pardini et al., 1971), ATPase (Grzycki et al., 1973; Grzycki and Zarebska, 1973), and GOT and GPT (Saigal et al., 1985). Serum lactatate dehydrogenase isoenzyme patterns are said to change with lindane treatment (Khaikina et al., 1970; Alekhina and Khaykina, 1972), and various enzymes in the small intestine can be induced initially by lindane (Zakirov et al., 1973). It is difficult to assess the meaning of some of these findings, especially when various effects on serum enzymes can be induced in vitro just by adding lindane (Gertig et al., 1971b).

An early hypothesis regarding the mode of action of γ-BHC was based on its resemblance to inositol (Slade, 1945). The history of this concept has been reviewed by van Asperen (1954). Briefly, the resemblance of lindane to inositol might explain some effects in yeasts and fungi and the partial protection of roaches by inositol against the insecticide (Srivastava, 1952). Some in vitro experiments suggest that lindane might resemble inositol in biological interactions. Hokin and Brown (1969) found that lindane was a potent inhibitor of acetylcholine-stimulated phosphatidylinositol formation in guinea pig cerebral cortex. Phosphorus turnover in phosphatidylinositol and the subsequent stimulation of RNA synthesis and initiation of DNA synthesis are inhibited by lindane in cultures of human lymphocytes stimulated by phytohemagglutinin (Fisher and Mueller, 1971).

There has been considerable interest in the turnover of inositol phospholipids after the occupation of some cell surface receptors by agonists and the involvement of Ca^{2+}. Holian et al. (1984) showed that lindane stimulated phosphatidylinositol turnover in guinea pig alveolar macrophages, calcium mobilization, and superoxide anion production. Similar studies have been conducted with human neutrophils (English et al., 1986) and neurohybridoma cells (Stark et al., 1987a). Indeed, lindane and γ-BHC have been used in a number of studies to explore the relationship between phosphatidylinositol turnover and Ca^{2+}-dependent processes (e.g., Hoffmann et al., 1980; Vu et al., 1983; Crouch and Roberts, 1985). Parries and Hokin-Neaverson (1985) have concluded that lindane does not actually act as a competitive inhibitor in enzyme systems which act on myo-inositol but that in a fairly specific manner it inhibits phosphatidylinositol synthase. Whether these effects of lindane on phosphatidylinositol metabolism are of any importance in vivo to explain toxicities remains to be determined. There is some evidence that in rats the accumulation of lindane can influence phospholipid composition, especially in the kidney, but there seems to be no evidence for a specific change in phosphatidylinositol levels (Lopez-Aparicio et al., 1988). Carrero et al. (1989) have studied the vasoactive intestinal peptide receptor/effector system in rat enterocytes for a similar involvement of Ca^{2+}.

Effects on the Nervous System The different isomers of BHC have opposite pharmacological actions. The γ isomer (lindane), which is the insecticidally active form, is a stimulant of the nervous system, causing violent epileptiform convulsions that are rapid in onset and generally followed by death or recovery within 24 hr (McNamara and Krop, 1948a,b; Coper et al., 1951; van Asperen, 1954; Joy, 1982a,b; Woolley et al., 1985). There is also evidence that lindane causes hypothermia and anorexia in rats (Aldegunde Villar et al., 1981; Woolley et al., 1985; Camon et al., 1988b).

The α, β, and δ isomers are mainly depressants of the nervous system. The β isomer produces lameness and a peculiar flaccidity of the entire musculature (Coper et al., 1951). Following subcutaneous injection of mice with α-BHC or δ-BHC, the onset of effects is delayed compared with that of the γ isomer. Poisoning by α-BHC is characterized by tremors of the extremities (especially if the animal is held up by the tail) and inability of the animals to make coordinated movements. Poisoning by the δ isomer is characterized by prostration, the animals remaining motionless for days. If death occurs, it usually is delayed. Following intravenous injection at dosages up to about 53 mg/kg, both the α and δ isomers produce hyperexcitability lasting about half a minute and followed by a state of numbness and then prompt recovery (van Asperen, 1954).

The α, β, and δ isomers counteract the effects of the γ isomer so that mortality is reduced when the same dosage of lindane is accompanied by an equal or especially a somewhat greater dosage of the α isomer (Coper *et al.*, 1951; van Asperen, 1954), β isomer (Coper *et al.*, 1951; McNamara and Krop, 1948a,b), or δ isomer (McNamara and Krop, 1948a,b; van Asperen, 1954). About 70% of technical BHC is α isomer, and in spite of the relatively low toxicity of that isomer, poisoning by the technical product is characterized by tremor and a relatively prolonged course (Coper *et al.*, 1951).

The interaction of isomers of BHC with other convulsant poisons is far from simple. The other isomers antagonize not only the convulsant action of lindane but also, in many instances, the action of other compounds or even of electrical stimulation. A reduced proportion of animals treated with pentylenetetrazole, picrotoxin, or Coramine have fits if they receive γ-BHC or β-BHC also. The δ isomer is somewhat less active in this regard, and although the α isomer antagonizes the convulsant action of coramine and pentylenetetrazole (Herken and Klempau, 1950; Herken *et al.*, 1952a; Vohland *et al.*, 1972), it is ineffective against picrotoxin (Herken *et al.*, 1952a). However, the strong inhibitory action of the γ isomer toward the convulsions caused by pentylenetetrazole is reduced by simultaneous administration of either the α or δ isomer but not by the β isomer (Coper *et al.*, 1951; Herken *et al.*, 1952a).

All of the isomers of BHC induce liver microsomal enzymes. If the action of these enzymes were sufficiently rapid in metabolizing a convulsant poison, this in itself would tend to counteract the poison. Although the α isomer does hasten and increase the inactivation of pentylenetetrazole, this action is not detectable until 60 min after the drug is administered. Therefore it cannot account for the inhibition by β-BHC of convulsions that otherwise would start 30 min after administration of pentylenetetrazole (Vohland and Koransky, 1972).

Following subcutaneous injection, either the α or δ isomer exerts an antagonistic effect against lindane long before it would exert any toxic effect if injected alone. This is considered strong evidence that the protective action of the α and δ isomers depends mainly on their lower toxicity and competition for a common receptor rather than on the difference of their pharmacological effects from those of lindane (van Asperen, 1954). The protective effect of other isomers tends to be greater if they are administered a few days before lindane (Coper *et al.*, 1951; Herken *et al.*, 1952a). Because the delay offers an opportunity for the other isomers to occupy the receptors without interference by lindane but also permits completion of the greater part of their pharmacological effects, the increased interaction suggests the importance of the blocking of critical receptors. However, the reactive site may not in-

volve exclusively a chemical "receptor" because Herken *et al.* (1952b) showed that, for many days after a single does of β-BHC, rabbits failed to have electroencephalographic seizure potentials induced by electrical stimulation of an epileptogenic area of the brain. The β isomer changed the reactivity of the thalamus.

In recent years our understanding of the mechanisms of the neurotoxic action of lindane at a molecular level has increased appreciably. Chronic administration of lindane causes a reduction in the number of muscarinic receptors in the cerebellum and diencephalon, perhaps following alterations in cholinergic transmission (Fonseca *et al.*, 1986). *In vitro,* lindane increases the calcium uptake of isolated rat brain synaptosomes (Narbonne and Lièvremont, 1983) and appears to inhibit Ca^{2+} influx at the desensitized neuromuscular junction (Lièvremont *et al.*, 1984).

The main site of action of lindane, unlike that of DDT, appears to be at the synapse with both excitatory and inhibitory effects (Joy and Albertson, 1985). The possible effect of inhibition of Na^+,K^+-ATPases on Ca^{2+} extrusion (Woolley *et al.*, 1985) has already been mentioned (see Biochemical Effects) but requires much more study at brain level. These effects occur at concentrations of lindane greater than required for antagonism of the GABA–receptor complex and among different BHC isomers are not specific for the γ-isomer (Joy and Burns, 1988; Bondy and Halsall, 1988). The actions do not appear to be a consequence of direct inhibition (Nakajima, 1983; Magour *et al.*, 1984).

Although Joy (1982b) suggested that no particular neurotransmitters or neurotransmitter systems appear to be affected by lindane, a most pertinent, more recent finding has been the demonstration that this chemical (and dieldrin) binds specifically to the picrotoxin binding site of the GABA-receptor–ionophore complex, probably in the cerebellum (Matsumura and Ghiasuddin, 1983). This may result in the effects of GABA and GABAergic transmission being disturbed (Matsumura and Ghiasuddin, 1983; Lawrence and Casida, 1984). Using t-[^{35}S]butylbicyclophosphorothionate as a specific radioligand for the picrotoxin binding site, Casida and coworkers have demonstrated that the degree of binding for lindane, other BHC isomers, dieldrin, and other chlorinated insecticides correlated with their acute toxicities and abilities to induce convulsions at similar dose levels (Lawrence and Casida, 1984; Abalis *et al.*, 1985; Casida and Lawrence, 1985; Cole and Casida, 1986). In addition, Bloomquist and Soderlund (1985) and Abalis *et al.* (1986) have shown that lindane inhibits stereospecifically the GABA-induced $^{36}Cl^-$ influx into rat brain membrane microsacs, whereas β-BHC had no effect. Diazepam will block the anorexic and hypothermic effects of lindane, and this could be taken as evidence for action at the picrotoxin receptor (Woolley *et al.*, 1985). However, the protection by lindane against the convulsant properties of pentylenetetrazole, which also acts at the GABA-receptor-linked chloride channel, after the insecticide itself has disappeared shows that the mechanism is highly complex and still far from elucidated (Vohland *et al.*, 1981; Fishman and

Gianutsos, 1987a). Although Cattabeni *et al.* (1983) and Bloomquist *et al.* (1986) have implied that impairment of the GABA-receptor–ionophore complex may not be involved in the neurotoxicity of lindane *in vivo,* more recent evidence suggests otherwise (Suñol *et al.,* 1989).

Many of the symptoms of lindane poisoning are similar to those of dysfunction of the hippocampus–limbic system (Woolley *et al.,* 1984) and measurements of glucose uptake by brain at convulsant doses of lindane show increases in the limbic regions (Camon *et al.,* 1988a). Long-term potentiation by lindane of the evoked potential elicited in the dentate gyrus after stimulation of the prepyriform cortex occurs when levels of the chemical should have greatly diminished (Woolley *et al.,* 1985). Joy and co-workers have studied the effects of lindane on kindling in some detail (Joy and Albertson, 1985). Kindling is a sequence of changes resulting from repeated stimulation of a part of the limbic system, such as the amygdala. After continual trials, progressively severe behavioral signs are observed in the rat, commencing with eye-closing or chewing and climaxing in a clonic motor seizure. Lindane at doses of 1–5 mg/kg/day, but not DDT, greatly enhances these effects (Joy *et al.,* 1982a,b, 1983; Joy, 1985; Joy and Albertson, 1985; Stark *et al.,* 1983). α-HCH also has no apparent effect, but β-HCH does result in some delayed rates of kindling acquisition (Stark *et al.,* 1986). Exposure of neonates to lindane can greatly enhance their acquisition of kindling in adulthood (Albertson *et al.,* 1985). Further studies have suggested that the granule cell population of the dentate gyrus becomes more excitable (Joy and Albertson, 1985) and by the use of this system it does now seem likely that the convulsant action of lindane is explicable by interaction with the GABA receptor (Joy and Albertson, 1987a,b, 1988). Experiments with cultured neurons from newborn rat dorsal root ganglia support the hypothesis that lindane *in vivo* inhibits the GABA receptor–channel complex but also raise the possibility of multiple receptors (Ogata *et al.,* 1988). Norepinephrine has been implicated in modulation of the spread of kindled seizures. Lindane decreases whereas β-BHC increases the number of β-adrenoceptors in cerebral cortex, a primary site of spread for seizures generated from limbic system foci (Stark *et al.,* 1987b).

Information on distribution of the isomers would be of interest in trying to understand their interaction. Autoradiographic studies failed to reveal any essential difference in the distribution of the α and γ isomers within the body as a whole (Koransky *et al.,* 1963), although minor differences do exist (Shindo, 1972). The situation is entirely different for the brain. Twenty-four hours after intraperitoneal injection of α-[^{14}C]BHC, radioactivity was found in the brain almost exclusively in the white matter, especially in the corpus callosum, anterior commissure, optic fasciculus and chiasm, lateral olfactory tract, fornix, internal capsule, corpus striatum, medullary–thalamic tract, hippocampal fimbria, cerebellar peduncle, posterior commissure, mammillotegmental tract, retroflex fasciculus, and much of the medulla oblongata (Koransky and Ullberg, 1964). Distribution of α-BHC in the brain almost

exclusively to the white matter was confirmed by Shindo (1972), who also found that accumulation of β isomer was low in the white matter but slightly higher in the gray matter, while accumulation of the γ isomer was low and uniform throughout. Furthermore, following intraperitoneal injection, the concentration of β and γ isomers in the brain began to decline gradually only 30 min after intraperitoneal injection, but the concentration of α isomer continued to increase and the isomer stayed in the brain more than 24 hr. Thus the concentration of the α isomer in the brain remains higher than that of the β isomer, even though the latter persists at a relatively very high concentration in body fat for a long period (Shindo, 1972). The long-term and selective uptake of α-BHC by the white matter of the cerebellum and cerebrum compared to the β and γ isomers has also been found in the mouse (Bergman *et al.,* 1981). Lièvremont and Potus (1981) reported that in their experiments lindane, like α-BHC, was also enriched in white matter and high-density zones of myelinated fibers. Using negative-ion chemical ionization mass spectrometry (Artigas *et al.,* 1988c), the main metabolites of BHC isomers in brain have been identified and shown to be produced at rates inversely proportional to the brain half-lives (Artigas *et al.,* 1988b).

In studies of the relationships between observable effects of lindane and the level and time course of concentrations in blood and brain, a good correlation was observed between dosages and frequency of onset of tonic seizure, intensity, and lethality (Tussell *et al.,* 1987). The incidence of response was directly proportional to the logarithm of lindane concentrations in brain and blood, and there was a high correlation between the two levels.

At dosages too low to produce clinical evidence of poisoning, electroencephalographic changes characterized by slow, high potential waves or high potential peaks may appear (Wolburg, 1973). Lindane also causes bradycardia and an increase in blood pressure in curarized dogs. The increase in pressure is blocked by yohimbine hydrochloride without any change in grand mal-type electroencephalogram. Atropine blocks the bradycardia but not the pressor effect. On the contrary, if pentobarbital is used to block the electroencephalographic changes produced by lindane, then lindane leads to a fall in blood pressure as well as to bradycardia; again, atropine prevents the bradycardia but not the change in blood pressure (McNamara and Krop, 1948b).

An unconfirmed exception to most reports of negative pathology in the nervous system is a report of a severe increased "neurophagia" and "gliophagia" in the brains of rabbits examined 12 weeks after the administration of lindane at the rate of 15 mg/kg. The liver changes in these rabbits apparently were similar to those reported by others. Brain lesions were not found in rabbits dosed at 7.5 mg/kg, although some liver change was present. Apparently, no pathology was found in rabbits dosed at 3.25 mg/kg (Ichikawa, 1972).

The effect of lindane on the uptake of α-aminobutyric acid and uridine by cultured rat C-6 glioma cells has been reported by Roux *et al.* (1980).

Mutation and Carcinogenesis In host-mediated tests in mice and in direct tests on indicator organisms, BHC was not mutagenic (Buselmaier et al., 1973; Wildemauwe et al., 1983).

Lindane applied as a seed dressing did cause polyploidy of root tip cells of wheat and other grains (Zeller and Hauser, 1974).

At concentrations of 5 and 10 ppm in the medium, lindane inhibited the division of cultured human lymphocytes, but there was no statistically significant effect of concentrations of 0.1, 0.5, or 1.0 ppm. The percentage of metaphases with structural damage to chromosomes increased with increasing concentrations of lindane, the results being statistically reliable at concentrations of 0.5 and 1.0 ppm (Tzoneva-Maneva et al., 1971). The concentrations of lindane used in these studies may be compared with 0.5 ppm, reported in the blood of people seriously poisoned by lindane.

Growth in culture of leukocytes from rats given an intraperitoneal dose of lindane (75 mg/kg) was lower than normal if the cultures were prepared up to 1 month after dosing (Friberg and Dodson, 1966). No chromosomal abnormalities were detected. Direct bone marrow preparations showed depressed mitotic rates during this time but later a rebound phenomenon. Tsushimoto et al. (1983) could find no detectable mutagenicity of lindane to Chinese hamster V79 cells, and the pesticide was less cytotoxic than DDT or chlordane.

Most, if not all, deaths following repeated dosing are also acute in the sense that they involve sudden, recent onset of convulsions. To be sure, the animals may be somewhat weakened, as evidenced by failure to grow and by abnormality of certain liver function tests. Although it is the function of the nervous system that is critical to the survival of animals that have received repeated doses of BHC or one of its isomers, it is only the visual appearance of the livers of rodents that has received much attention. This is because many investigators consider some or all of the changes in the rodent liver associated with chlorinated hydrocarbon insecticides to be neoplastic. The general aspects of this matter are discussed in Section 15.2.3.2; the sometimes conflicting details concerning technical BHC and its isomers are discussed in the following paragraphs.

Rats appear to be unsusceptible to the tumorigenic effects of lindane and BHC (IARC, 1974, 1982; NCI, 1982).

Changes described as hepatomas have been reported in mice exposed at rates in excess of 20 mg/kg/day to lindane (Goto et al., 1972a,b; Nagasaki et al., 1972a,b; Hanada et al., 1973; Thorpe and Walker, 1973), α-BHC (Goto et al., 1972a,b; Nagasaki et al., 1972a, 1973, 1974; Ito et al., 1973; Tryphonas and Iverson, 1983), β-BHC (Goto et al., 1972a,b; Thorpe and Walker, 1973), δ-BHC (Goto et al., 1972a,b), δ-BHC (Goto et al., 1972a,b), and technical BHC (Kashyap et al., 1979; Munir et al., 1983; see also IARC, 1979, 1982).

Nagasaki et al. (1972a,c; Nagasaki, 1973) gave evidence that the α isomer is more tumorigenic than the β, γ, and δ isomers; in fact, they reported no hepatomas in groups of 20 mice fed these other isomers up to dietary levels of 500 ppm (about 64 mg/kg/day), even though the incidence was 100% for mice on this dosage of α isomer. They suggested that the α isomer probably was responsible for the tumorigenic action of technical BHC, which they also reported (Nagasaki et al., 1971, 1972b; Ito et al., 1973; Ito and Miyake, 1973). Nagasaki et al. (1972c) reported that only the α isomer produced a hepatoma in rats receiving a dietary level of 1000 ppm (about 49 mg/kg/day). Thus, rats and mice showed the same reaction to different isomers, but rats were less sensitive.

Contrary to the results of Nagasaki and his colleagues, a number of authors reported liver tumors in rodents receiving high dosages of lindane; furthermore, Goto et al. (1972a,b) reported hepatomas in mice fed α, β, γ, and a mixture of δ and ε isomers, but they agreed that the α isomer or a metabolite is the most tumorigenic. Although induction of various drug-metabolizing enzymes potentially activating lindane is greater in mice than rats (Oesch et al., 1982), it has been concluded that there is little evidence for the binding of reactive metabolites to DNA as a genotoxic effect (Sagelsdorff et al., 1983; Iverson et al., 1984). In mice with a dominant mutation at the agouti locus (A^{vy}) which increases susceptibility to strain specific-spontaneous and chemically induced neoplasms, lindane appeared to act as a tumor promoter via cellular proliferation mechanism (Wolff et al., 1987).

Although the group from the Cancer Center at Nara did not find that the β isomer was carcinogenic when given alone, they did find it carcinogenic when administered in combination with a polychlorinated biphenyl (Ito and Miyake, 1973; Nagasaki et al., 1973).

On the other hand, rats fed the α isomer (which is agreed to be the most tumorigenic isomer) concomitantly with 3'-methyl-4-dimethylaminoazobenzene (3'-Me-DAB) or with ethionine developed fewer and less severe liver tumors than mice fed 3'-Me-DAB, ethionine, or even α-BHC alone. Increase in liver weight was much less in those receiving a combination of α-BHC and 3'-Me-DAB compared with 3'-Me-DAB alone. The opposite was true in connection with α-BHC and ethionine (Thamavit et al., 1974). There have been a number of studies in which lindane, α-BHC, or technical BHC was used as a promoter of rat liver tumors or foci previously initiated by carcinogens such as diethylnitrosamine (Schulte-Hermann and Parzefall, 1981; Pereira et al., 1982; Munir et al., 1984; Schulte-Hermann, 1985; Schröter et al., 1987). Lindane inhibited in vitro cell–cell communication in Chinese hamster V79 cells (Tsuchimoto et al., 1983). However, lindane protects rats against aflatoxin B_1-induced liver tumors (Angsubhakorn et al., 1989).

No abnormalities including tumors were found in mice that received dermal applications of 0.5% lindane in acetone twice a week for 15 months or in other mice observed for 10 months following subcutaneous implantation of paraffin pellets containing 3% lindane (Orr, 1948). BHC failed to promote skin tumors initiated by dimethylbenz[a]anthracene in the mouse (Munir et al., 1984).

Miscellaneous Effects on Organs and Tissues   Following sufficiently high repeated absorption of BHC or one of its isomers, degenerative changes have been observed in the kidneys (Fitzugh *et al.*, 1950; Rao *et al.*, 1972; Srinivasan *et al.*, 1984; Su and Zhou, 1986), pancreas (Watari and Torizawa, 1972), testes (Fitzugh *et al.*, 1950), and nasal mucous membrane (Sadriyeva *et al.*, 1971) of one species or another. Further discussion of antitesticular effects can be found under Effects on Reproduction. As referred to under Mutation and Carcinogenesis, lindane or BHC appears to have little or mild effects on the skin (Orr, 1948; Dikshith *et al.*, 1978a) although there is a report of more severe changes after prolonged exposure (Dikshith *et al.*, 1973). Lindane has a positive inotropic effect on guinea pig atrial tissue *in vitro* and counteracts the negative effect of varapamil (Atrakchi and West, 1985). Shivanandappa *et al.* (1982) have reported that weanling rats fed high levels of BHC (750 and 1500 ppm) for 90 days showed hypertrophy of the adrenals, reduction of steroidogenic enzymes, and accumulation of cholesterol-positive lipids. These effects, some of which are unconfirmed, have received little attention because they clearly are not neoplastic and they are produced only by dosage levels higher than those usually associated with occupational exposure.

Certain drugs, mainly alkylating agents, are used in medicine to suppress immune response and permit organ transplants. It is not known how many other compounds have some degree of immunosuppressive action, but clearly any compound that has this action to a significant degree may produce an abnormal susceptibility to infection in animals or people who absorb it. Immunosuppression has been reported in connection with a number of chlorinated hydrocarbon insecticides, and BHC is no exception (Descotes, 1986). Burkatzkaya (1963) reported a reduction of agglutination titers of cats that inhaled lindane and of rabbits that received it in their food. Rosival *et al.* (1974) reported that a 60 mg/kg dosage of lindane in rats suppressed the formation of an antibody against human serum albumin, and a dosage of 120 mg/kg inhibited both the uptake and lysis of bacteria by phagocytes. Lindane (6.25 and 25 mg/kg, equivalent to 1/20 and 1/50 of the LD 50) given to weanling rats suppressed the humoral immune response to typhoid–paratyphoid vaccine 1 or 2 weeks later (Dewan *et al.*, 1980).

There are two reasons to question these reports. First, increased susceptibility to infection is not a recognized feature of the effects of single or repeated doses of BHC in humans or animals. Second (as discussed in Section 2.4.14), it has been impossible to confirm some similar reports.

A complex action of organochlorine insecticides on the immune system has been reported by Wasserman and his colleagues. In connection with lindane, they reported a shift in the proportion of various proteins in the blood of exposed rabbits. An increase in serum albumin caused by lindane was inhibited by simultaneous administration of bacteria (*Salmonella typhi*). Furthermore, the plasma level of lindane was reduced by the bacteria. Both lindane and bacteria decreased serum protein-bound iodine (Wassermann *et al.*, 1972a). The significance of these interactions for the immune response is unknown.

The induction by BHC of antibodies against BHC might be viewed as the opposite of immunosuppression. In any event, such induction in rabbits and people has been reported. In rabbits, antibodies appeared within a week, reached maximal titer in 2 weeks, but disappeared by 12 weeks when the compound was administered by mouth. Antibodies were found in 65 of 102 persons occupationally exposed to pesticides but disappeared within 6 months after exposure was discontinued (Nikolayev and Usmanova, 1971).

Another variant on the immunological theme is the report (Omirov and Talan, 1970) that intragastric administration to rabbits of BHC—as well as one of the organic phosphorus insecticides—led to intermittent autoimmunization against liver and kidney as measured *in vitro*. Actual injury of organs associated with this mechanism apparently has not been reported.

Effects on Reproduction   The concentration of β-BHC in the fetus is low compared to the concentration in the liver of its mother. Although the level of dietary protein of the mother influences her own liver concentration of β-BHC, it does not influence the concentration in the fetus. Because of the nutritional stress, any given level of deficiency of dietary protein leads to about twice as much deposition of β-BHC in pregnant rats as in nonpregnant females. The amount of β-BHC transferred from dam to offspring is about 10 times higher during lactation than during gestation (Oshiba and Fujita, 1974).

According to one report, lindane dosages of 5 mg/kg/day were without effect on the reproduction of rats; dosage of 10 mg/kg/day for 138 days resulted in considerable reduction of fecundity and litter size (Trifonova *et al.*, 1970). In contrast, in another report, a lindane dosage of only 0.5 mg/kg/day increased the duration of diestrus and/or shortened the duration of estrus, lengthened the gestation period, decreased the number of fetuses, increased the number of dead fetuses, and decreased the growth of the young. A dosage of 0.05 was without effect (Nayshteyn and Leybovich, 1971).

In a study of teratogenesis in mice, females were given β-BHC subcutaneously at dosages of 5, 50, and 100 mg/kg/day on different days of gestation. Other females were fed a dietary level of 5 ppm, which involves an intake of about 0.66 mg/kg/day, and then were given the isomer by stomach tube at 50 and 100 mg/kg/day on days 6 and 7 of gestation. Dosages as high as 5 mg/kg/day had no statistically significant effect; dosages of 50 and 100 mg/kg/day produced some increase in the percentage of fetal immaturity and of early and late fetal death, but a clear dosage–response relationship was realized in only one of three tests (Yamagishi *et al.*, 1972a,b). Results were essentially identical when α-BHC was administered at the same dosages on days 2–6 or days 7–11 of gestation. Concentrations of BHC in the livers of the dams were five to eight times greater than those in the fetal livers (Yamagishi *et al.*, 1972c). When male Swiss mice were fed technical BHC (500 ppm) for up to 8 months and then mated, the number of dead embryos seen in females showed a significant increase (Lakkad *et al.*, 1982).

Probably related to the above effects on reproduction are the findings that (*a*) β-BHC and lindane are weakly estrogenic to female rats and mice (Raizada *et al.*, 1980; Loeber and Van Velsen, 1984; Van Velsen *et al.*, 1986) and (*b*) β-BHC, lindane, and technical BHC have adverse effects on the testes of rats and mice (Dikshith and Datta, 1972; Nigam *et al.*, 1979; Shivanandappa and Krishnakumari, 1983; Van Velsen *et al.*, 1986; Chowdhury *et al.*, 1987; Huang and Huang, 1987). Seminiferous tubules become atrophied. In rats dosed with lindane at 8 mg/kg/day for 10 days there was complete degeneration of seminiferous tubules and Leydig cells (Chowdhury *et al.*, 1987). Shivanandapp and Krishnakumari (1983) have suggested that steroid biosynthesis in the Leydig cells is inhibited. In male mice fed technical BHC (500 ppm) for 8 months meiotic division in the testes was inhibited, although this could be reversed after a return to control diet (Aravinda Babu *et al.*, 1981). The reduced sexual behavior of female rats given lindane at proestrus does not seem to be mediated through estrogenic or GABAergic actions (Uphouse, 1987); Uphouse and Williams, 1989), but by some other antiestrogenic mechanism (Cooper *et al.*, 1989).

Under conditions of practical use, lindane does not affect the reproduction of domestic animals, but there is disagreement regarding the effects of large dosages under experimental conditions. In situations in which abortion was a problem in dairy cattle, the concentrations of pesticides were no greater in aborted than in normal fetuses. Levels of lindane sufficient to keep milk off the market did not produce abortion in the herd (Macklin and Ribelin, 1971).

In one study of chickens, dietary levels of lindane as low as 0.1 ppm (about 0.0058 mg/kg) reduced egg production and hatchability, and eggshell thickness was reduced (Sauter and Steele, 1972). On the contrary, Whitehead *et al.* (1972) found that although a much higher dosage (12.5 mg/hen/day given by capsule) reduced egg production by 20–30% beginning the second or third week of feeding, production returned to its original level within 1 month after dosing was stopped. Furthermore, there was no significant decrease in eggshell thickness or in the hatchability of the eggs.

Behavioral Effects Rats receiving lindane orally at the rate of 2.5 mg/kg/day were normal in maze running but executed Skinner box tests in a way interpreted as showing increased irritability. Rats receiving dosages of 5, 10, and 50 mg/kg/day were abnormal in maze running and showed other, but irregular behavioral abnormalities. Liver function tests and histological findings were normal at all dosage levels (Desi and Major, 1972; Desi, 1974). The authors interpreted their findings as indicating the sensitivity of behavioral tests, and they recommended them for monitoring workers. It must be noted, however, that Ortega *et al.* (1957) found histological change at a dosage of 2.25 mg/kg/day; also, the exposure of workers is unlikely to be as great as the smallest dosage in any of these animal studies.

Avoidance responses in a shuttle box were decreased by administration of lindane (30 mg/kg) to rats. Pretreatment with phenobarbital and chlordiazepoxide, which may enhance GABA-mediated responses, blocked the disruptive effects of lindane (Tilson *et al.*, 1987).

Factors Influencing Toxicity Except for the obvious factor of dosage, there has been little study of factors that influence the toxicity of BHC. This toxicity is not increased appreciably when protein constitutes only 9% of the diet, but toxicity is increased by factors of 1.9 and 12.3 when protein is as low as 3.5 and 0.0%, respectively (Boyd and Chen, 1968; Boyd *et al.*, 1969). At least a part of the basis for this increased toxicity must be the increased storage of the compound at low levels of dietary protein. Rats that had received lindane at a dietary level of 10 ppm for 28 days showed average concentrations of it in liver lipid ranging from 17 to 55 ppm, depending on whether their level of protein intake had been 30% or 5%, respectively, during the same 28-day period. A similar result was obtained with β-BHC, except that storage was higher at all levels of protein even though intake of the isomer was the same. A subsample of other rats that had received β-BHC at a dietary level of 10 ppm for 28 days while receiving a regular diet had an average concentration of 47.8 ppm in liver lipid when dosage was stopped; other subsamples that were continued 6 more days without further BHC but on different levels of dietary protein showed concentrations of 2.53 ppm after 30% protein, 29.6 ppm after 20% protein, 34.3 ppm after 10% protein, and 41.2 ppm after 5% protein (Oshiba and Kawakita, 1971, 1972c,d).

Anything that causes mobilization of fat (starvation or administration of adrenalin, ACTH, or thyroid-stimulating hormone) will cause mobilization of highly fat-soluble compounds and make them more readily available for metabolism and subsequent excretion. Depending on whether the speed of metabolism is less or greater than the speed of mobilization and depending on the time of sampling, the process may result in either an increase or a decrease in the concentration of a compound in the tissues. Thus the γ isomer, which is metabolized rapidly in any case, is decreased in concentration by starvation and by fat-mobilizing hormones, whereas the concentration of β-BHC is increased in tissues other than the fat. Even the feeding of a high-fat diet produces a detectable dilution of lindane, but not of β-BHC, stored in the tissues (Oshiba and Kawakita, 1972a,b).

Different strains of mice vary greatly in susceptibility to technical BHC, the acute oral LD 50 values ranging from 411 to 1459 mg/kg (Miura *et al.*, 1973). The range of variation in susceptibility to lindane among the same five strains was less, 340–562 mg/kg. The rate at which poisoning progressed also varied, death being prompt in some and delayed in others (Miura *et al.*, 1973, 1974).

Robinson *et al.* (1975) observed a marked difference between the C57BL/6 and DBA/2 strains in mortality caused by lindane. These two strains are known to differ greatly in their responsiveness to the induction of aryl hydrocarbon hydroxylase. Nonresponsive mice (DBA/2) died when fed lindane, whereas the responsive mice (C57BL/6) did not. Although both DBA/2 and C57BL/6 mice were killed by large ip doses of lindane (50–200 mg/kg), the latter strain were completely protected by a prior dose of 3-methylcholanthrene. Liu and Morgan (1986) have demonstrated that in the uninduced C57BL/6 and DBA/2 mice the greater body fat content of the latter strain keeping up a high level of unmetabolized lindane may account partially for the strain difference.

In spite of the strain differences just mentioned, differences in susceptibility to lindane are not great among the common laboratory species. However, calves are distinctly more susceptible than rats (see Section 10.2.2).

Pathology The changes associated with fatal poisoning by one or a few doses of BHC are minor, nonspecific, and inadequate to explain death. The viscera generally are congested. Liver necrosis is neither severe nor constant. Petechial hemorrhages frequently are present as a result of convulsions. The findings are not characteristic (Cameron, 1945).

The changes associated with repeated doses occur almost entirely in the liver. They are discussed in Section 15.4.1.2 in connection with a discussion of the tumorigenicity of BHC and its isomers.

Treatment of Poisoning in Animals Abdusaidov (1972) investigated several remedies to improve liver function of rabbits receiving a combination of BHC and dimethoate orally for 90 days at rates of 3.2 and 3.8 mg/kg/day. Galascorbin (a potassium ascorbate–tannin complex) administered subcutaneously at the rate of 50 mg/kg was found best. It was reported to normalize liver function, cholinesterase activity, and the levels of cholesterol and alkaline phosphatase. The author recommended it for treatment of patients with chronic pesticide poisoning. Tilson *et al.* (1987) have used phenobarbital and chlordiazepoxide to protect rats from seizures caused by lindane. Woolley *et al.* (1985) have used diazepam to protect against the anorexic and hypothermic effects of lindane.

15.4.1.3 Toxicity to Humans

Experimental Exposure Feldmann and Maibach (1970, 1974) clearly demonstrated the absorption of lindane through human skin and estimated that within 5 days this absorption constituted 9.3% of the applied dose. Because the rate of absorption was corrected, the reported proportion represents a maximal value.

When human skin sections were bathed in lindane solutions, the outer epidermis-rich layer showed higher binding affinities than middle or inner layers and in all cases lindane was competitively extracted by a human plasma protein fraction. This seems to explain the percutaneous absorption of lindane into the body under certain circumstances (Menczel *et al.*, 1984). Washing skin samples with soap and water 3 hr after application of the insecticide resulted in an increase of it in the layer below the stratum corneum 7 hr later (Nitsche *et*

al., 1984). In an analogous study with healthy volunteers painted all over with a 0.3% lindane emulsion, absorption through the skin was reduced by taking showers with soap and water only if 8–12 hr had elapsed since application. Washing shortly after application improved absorption (Lange *et al.*, 1981). Complete baths taken 10 hr after application of lindane to dermatologic patients also enhanced absorption.

Therapeutic Use BHC has anthelmintic properties and has been explored for possible practical use in this connection. It was established that technical BHC causes a burning sensation of the tongue (Klosa, 1950; Clodi and Schnack, 1959) and causes symptoms at lower dosages than does lindane (see Table 15.20). Even for lindane, dosage levels that are dependably anthelmintic may produce serious side effects; the compound offers no advantage over available drugs and was never adopted for use.

The situation is entirely different in connection with the use of lindane to control scabies caused by the mite *Sarcoptes scabiei* or, more rarely, other species such as *Amblyseius barkeri* (Beemer *et al.*, 1970). Use against scabies is now standard and generally trouble-free (Cannon and McRae, 1948; Wooldridge, 1948; Halpern *et al.*, 1950; Panja and Choudhury,

Table 15.20
Summary of Studies of BHC as an Anthelmintic for Humans

| Formulation (% γ-isomer) | Dosage | | Effect |
	Schedule	Approximate dose/day/kg	
10–30	40 mg/day, 10 days	0.57	diarrhea after day 8[a]
	70 mg/day	1.00	dizziness, nausea, headache, pressure in temples[a]
25–60	40 mg/day, 10 days	0.57	no effect[a]
	90 mg/day	1.29	dizziness, diarrhea, pressure in temples on day 5[a]
60–85	40 mg/day, 14 days	0.57	no effect observed[a]
	110 mg/day, repeated	1.57	diarrhea after day 6[a]
100	40 mg/day, 14 days	0.57	no effect[a]
	45 mg/day, 3 days[c]	0.64	no effect, 20 patients[b]
	30–40 mg/day, 3 days[d]	0.64	6 of 15 patients poisoned, 2 with convulsions[b]
	100 mg/day	1.43	no effect[a]
	180 mg/day, repeated	2.57	dizziness and diarrhea after several days[a]

[a] Klosa (1950).
[b] Graeve and Hernnring (1951).
[c] Emulsion made by shaking.
[d] Emulsion made with a machine driven emulsifier.

1969; Soennichsen *et al.*, 1970; Hurwitz, 1973; Roed-Petersen, 1974; Herman *et al.*, 1975; Shacter, 1981; AMA, 1986). As a scabicide, lindane is applied locally, usually as a cream or ointment, but it may be formulated as an emulsion, solution, aerosol (Kleine-Natrop *et al.*, 1970), or shampoo (Elgart and Higdon, 1973). The formulation is usually 1%, but 0.3% has been recommended for babies (Hochleitner, 1973). A 0.3% solution may be used to impregnate clothing to avoid infestation (Eldridge, 1973). Formulations similar to those for mites may be used to combat human lice (Gardner, 1958; Munster *et al.*, 1962; Elgart and Higdon, 1973), but their efficiency is increased by adding an enzyme to help dislodge the nits (Gerberg, 1973) or by using chlordimeform to kill them (Makara, 1973).

A widely publicized call for reports of poisoning following the use of lindane for control of scabies revealed only a few cases, and most of them involved gross disregard of directions—specifically, application to the entire body, application for many days, and even oral administration. A single case was suggestive of hypersensitivity (Lee *et al.*, 1976; Lee and Groth, 1977). Kramer *et al.* (1980) concluded that out of 53 alleged toxicity cases due to lindane, 37 were associated with nonpharmaceutical preparations. Of the remainder, only six probable cases were associated with the 1% pharmaceutical preparations and five of these could be ascribed to inappropriate ingestion or application. It has been suggested that patients should receive better explanations of possible side effects from misuse of the insecticide, although these are rare (Rasmussen, 1981, 1984).

In a recent study, a permethrin 1% cream rinse was found to give slightly better results against head lice than lindane (98 and 76% cure rate, respectively, after 2 weeks) with possibly less dermal reactions (Bowerman *et al.*, 1987). However, lindane appears to be the better scabicide (Shacter, 1981). Because of the possible susceptibility of infants, pregnant women, and patients with highly excoriated skin, it has been suggested that other insecticides should be used in these circumstances (Pramanik and Hansen, 1979; Telch and Jarvis, 1982).

Accidental and Intentional Poisoning The clinical course of fatal poisoning clearly associated with BHC has differed significantly from the course of nonfatal poisoning only in outcome (Attygalle and Fernonda, 1959; Desbuquois *et al.*, 1963; Kay *et al.*, 1964; Paludan, 1959). Death has occurred in as little as 2 hr after ingestion (Attygalle and Fernonda, 1959) or after as long as 80 hr (Paludan, 1959).

Studies of all death certificates in appropriate categories in the United States showed that the numbers of deaths attributed to BHC including lindane were as follows: two in 1956, one in 1961, two in 1969, two in 1973, and none in 1974 (Hayes, 1977).

There are numerous reports of nonfatal illness (Osuntokun, 1964; Clodi and Schnack, 1959; Buck and Pfannenmueller, 1957; and other references cited below). In one instance in which lindane was accidentally added to dessert and thus consumed after a full meal, the average time to onset was 5 hr (Wilson, 1959). However, when lindane is taken on an empty stomach, illness may begin within 0.25 and 0.5 hr even in cases with recovery (Nicholls, 1958; Stur and Zweimüller, 1961).

Following afternoon exposure that was partly respiratory but mainly dermal, a woman became ill "the same evening." She entered hospital at 4.00 a.m. that night and responded promptly to treatment (Heilberg and Wright, 1955).

At least in the United States, a high proportion of both fatal and nonfatal poisoning by lindane has been in children who ate pellets of it intended for use in vaporizers (Joslin *et al.*, 1960; Savage *et al.*, 1971).

Nearly all of the clinical findings reported in nonfatal poisoning by BHC were encountered among a group of 11 persons who drank Nescafé accidently prepared with lindane in place of sugar in such a way that each person received approximately 0.60 gm of lindane or about 86 mg/kg. The people ranged in age from 18 to 52 years. The interval from ingestion to onset averaged about an hour but varied from 20 min (two cases) to 4 hr (one case). Initial difficulty included malaise, faintness, and dizziness followed by collapse and convulsions, sometimes preceded by screaming and accompanied by foaming at the mouth and biting of the tongue. Nausea and vomiting occurred in many cases. The patients presumably were unconscious during convulsions and certainly were unconscious afterward. Some patients had another fit following a brief return to consciousness. Loss of consciousness lasted from 0.25 to 3 hr. In nine cases there was retrograde amnesia.

On examination, the patients were found to have normal or slightly accelerated pulse and normal blood pressure. There was facial pallor in six, slight circumoral cyanosis in two, and severe cyanosis of the face and extremities in the most severely affected patients. The cyanosis apparently represented a localized vascular reaction, for the most affected person experienced no difficulty in breathing. Temperature was elevated in only one patient. The liver was slightly enlarged in two instances, but the damage persisted in only one. Most of the patients were discharged the following day; the remainder were discharged in 2 or 3 days except for one who had a residual hepatitis (Bambov *et al.*, 1966). Muscle tremors, an early finding in this group, have not been reported by other authors; conversely, ataxia was not mentioned but has been noted by others.

A moderate rise in temperature may occur in those who survive; Kay *et al.* (1964) recorded full recovery following a temperature of 38.3°C. Such a temperature may be caused by a lag in dissipating the heat associated with convulsions. A high fever may be the result of toxic action directly on the temperature control center of the brain. This phenomenon may have been involved in the deaths of children following temperatures of 39.44°C or more (Joslin *et al.*, 1960; Hayes and Vaughn, 1977).

Protracted illness caused by lindane is rare. Apparently the longest illnesses have been associated with ingestion of mixtures of DDT and lindane. The relative importance of the two compounds in prolonging symptoms is unknown. It is also unknown how much the drugs required to suppress convulsions may have served to prolong unconsciousness. At least two cases of this sort have been reported. A 2-year-old boy, who accidentally drank a mixture of unstated proportion, did not regain consciousness until the third day but then went on to complete recovery (Kluge and Olbrich, 1972). Under the conditions described, the dosage of the two active ingredients combined was about 200 mg/kg; however, it is difficult to believe that such a small child would ingest about 0.5 liter as estimated.

In an attempted suicide by ingestion of DDT and lindane at dosages of 27 and 18 mg/kg, respectively, clinical remission was delayed until day 20 and the EEG did not return to normal until day 39 (Eskenasy, 1972).

A water-wettable powder containing 7% lindane, 12% captan, 15% sulfur, and 6% malathion was clearly the cause of the unrelated deaths of two girls, one 1.9 and the other 2.5 years old. Both were in excellent condition when brought to hospital, but, within a few hours after exposure, both suffered a very sudden onset of massive pulmonary edema which was later confirmed at autopsy. There were no systemic symptoms that would implicate any of the active ingredients. Extensive study in animals showed that the powder and several of its ingredients could cause extensive pulmonary edema when insufflated into the lungs. Although it was impossible to prove, it seemed likely that the infants had aspirated the powder (McQueen et al., 1968).

In the case of probable inhalation, it was not possible to fix responsibility on any one ingredient. However, in cases in which mixtures have been ingested, the signs and symptoms may be predominantly or apparently exclusively the result of only one component. An example was the death of a 2.5-year-old boy who drank a solution containing 6% lindane and 30% malathion (Desbuquois et al., 1963); the signs were characteristic of malathion. In cases where lindane–solvent mixtures have been ingested, the pulmonary edema may be a consequence of the benzene component (Jaeger et al., 1984).

An unusual effect was associated with an attempted suicide described by Veltkamp et al. (1970). Prolongation of bleeding time to more than 15 min and reduction of factor VIII to 3% of normal clearly were the result of ingestion of a pesticide formulation. However, the relative importance of the constituents (lindane, pyrethrum, acetone, and kerosene) is entirely unknown. Fortunately, recovery was complete by day 18 and there was no relapse.

A number of the accidental cases of lindane poisoning that are reported have apparently occurred when infants or mentally disturbed patients ingested the insecticide prescribed for lice or scabies (Powell, 1980; Davies et al., 1983; Kurt et al., 1986). Sometimes misunderstandings about the use of the lindane preparations have arisen because the patient or parents did not fully understand the language in which the directions for use were written (Kurt et al., 1986).

Matsuoka (1981) described a case in which a 7-year-old was treated for scabies with lindane. The patient had a history of intractable seizures controlled by the removal of a brain glioma 5 years previously. Although he had suffered only one or two petit mal seizures a year since surgery, he had two within 12 hr of lindane administration, perhaps suggesting that he had a decreased threshold for convulsions.

In a rather interesting exposure of a population to BHC, 150 cases from 36 Indian villages were examined (Khare et al., 1977). Among these, 22 needed hospital treatment. Victims were from 7 days to 60 years of age, and there were five deaths. Domestic and wild animals and birds also died. Generally more than one person in a family was affected, but never all. Those affected came from agricultural families who, to preserve their food grains, mixed them with BHC which had been supplied as a pesticide for cane crops. Most patients exhibited classical signs of lindane poisoning including seizures and myoclonic jerks. Tremors and especially ocular defects were also observed, including defective vision, flashes of light, and water discharges. A combination of phenytoin and primidone was found to be the best treatment for controlling seizures. Laborers who had to purchase their food grains from the market were unaffected.

Use Experience Some surveys of workers have revealed a moderate number of mild, acute intoxications (Uchida et al., 1972). There have been few serious cases. A 42-year-old man who helped make lindane suffered depression, headache, vomiting, asthenia, epileptiform attacks, sleeplessness, profuse perspiration, tremor of the fingers, abnormally increased tendon and digital reflexes, oral automatism, Romberg's sign, and a number of other abnormal reflexes and neurological signs (Pernov and Kyurkchiyev, 1974). This case showed many of the elements found in occupational poisoning by dieldrin. The same similarity was noted earlier by Czegledi-Janko and Avar (1970), who studied 37 male workers exposed to lindane for as much as 2 years and, in some instances, previously exposed to aldrin. The concentration of lindane in the workers' blood varied from 0.002 to 0.340 ppm. Muscular jerking, myoclonia, and emotional changes were noted in only one man (blood level, 0.143 ppm). Minor symptoms or minor EEG changes or both were present in all workers with blood levels of 0.020 ppm or more. The clinical changes and EEG abnormalities were consistently less in association with lindane than with aldrin but the blood levels of lindane were also less. Muller et al. (1981) found abnormal EEG patterns in some workers exposed to BHC, but in a group of 60 workers producing lindane for 1–30 years no significant neurophysiological, neuromuscular or other poor health effects could be detected (Baumann et al., 1981; Brassow et al., 1981). Toxic symptoms were observed in 90% of workers engaged in the manufacture of technical BHC, some of whom showed evidence of cardiac effects (Kashyap, 1986).

Other reports of similar or milder occupational poisoning include those of Burkatzkaya et al. (1959), Wassermann et al. (1961, 1962), Shul'ga (1957), and Model and Larina (1957). Conjunctivitis and dermatitis have been reported more frequently (Wassermann et al., 1960, 1961; Behrbohm and

Brandt, 1959; da Rocha e Silva, 1961; Bruevich, 1964; Karimov, 1970) but, even so, appear to be unusual. In some instances, the exceptional findings appear to be accounted for adequately by exceptionally heavy exposure. For example, Wassermann *et al.* (1960) documented unusual conditions by striking photographs and by measured concentrations of lindane averaging from 3.2 to 48.4 mg/m^3 in the air breathed by workers carrying out various tasks. What is perhaps remarkable is that no acute intoxications were encountered under these circumstances. Even among patients being treated for various rashes, almost all of which were believed to be associated with occupational exposure in agriculture, positive skin tests to BHC were found infrequently (Szarmach and Poniecka, 1973). Furthermore, other compounds, such as DDT, may have complicated the picture (Mirakhmedov and Karimov, 1972; Yamamoto *et al.*, 1973).

Dermatitis, which occasionally is seen among workers exposed to precursors and by-products in manufacturing plants, may be of an allergic character different from that just discussed. After encountering a case so severe that the employee had to stop work for a month and after reviewing presumably similar cases reported in the literature, Hegyi and Štota (1962) explored the mixtures from which lindane was progressively removed in the process of manufacture and also explored the pure substances constituting the mixtures. They found that the worker's sensitivity to the mixtures could be accounted for almost entirely by their content of δ-heptachlorocyclohexane, to which he was extremely allergic. He was also slightly sensitive to δ-pentachlorocyclohexane, which was not originally present in the commercial product but may have been formed in the patient's environment. The δ-heptachlorocyclohexane was also tested with entirely negative results in five normal persons and in six persons with eczemas of other origins. It was concluded that the sensitivity of the one worker was specifically acquired.

The majority of effort to prevent poisoning by BHC and/or lindane has been focused on their use in vaporizing devices. The unregulated sale of these devices led to their use in thousands—probably millions—of homes and, in some instances, led to the protracted exposure of entire families to concentrations of lindane similar to those found under occupational conditions. Caution was justified by the fact that cases of acute poisoning resulted from ingestion of crystals or other solid formulations intended for use in vaporizers. A number of other illnesses in which the relationship to lindane often was circumstantial were ascribed to inhalation of fumes given off by vaporizers. Finally, it must be said that some objection to vaporizers was aesthetic in origin and based on either (*a*) doubt that constant release of any vapor into the air is an appropriate way to control insects in homes or in places where food is prepared or served or (*b*) revulsion from the unscrupulous way in which vaporizers were promoted and sold. Restrictions were recommended by the Interdepartmental Committee on Pest Control (1951, 1953). These restrictions were elaborated and supported by case reports in which poisoning was established or suspected (AMA, 1952, 1953, 1954).

The use of thermal vaporizers with lindane did cause some clear-cut instances of illness. For example, two refreshment stand operators suffered severe headache, nausea, and irritation of eyes, nose, and throat shortly after exposure to vapors from a dispenser in which lindane apparently became overheated. The symptoms abated 2 hr after the device was removed. Overheated lindane is more apt to cause respiratory distress than is lindane vaporized at lower temperatures. This is true because the greater heat releases more of the compound and, especially in the presence of some methods, also causes some splitting of the molecule into highly irritating decomposition products (AMA, 1952).

There was one case in which neurological illness followed at least 3.5 months of occupational exposure in a small room in which a vaporizer with no thermostat was kept filled with a mixture of one-third lindane and two-thirds DDT. No other person had significant exposure. The patient complained of headache, malaise, weakness, fatigue, dizziness, staggering gait, incoordination of the hands, paresthesias especially of the fingers and toes, ptosis of the right eyelid, and diplopia. The ataxia and ptosis were confirmed by medical examination, and mild inconstant nystagmus was demonstrated; however sensory findings were normal. The patient recovered to a great extent during a week in hospital without specific treatment. One month later he was almost completely recovered, although slight diplopia and nystagmus were still present (Onifer and Whisnant, 1957). Presumably, use of the vaporizer had been discontinued at the place of work, but of course some revolatilization of DDT and especially lindane would have continued from residues on surfaces. The action of lindane in this case cannot be excluded, but the signs and symptoms were essentially identical to those found after the ingestion of DDT (Hayes, 1959a).

Most other injuries attributed to vaporized lindane have involved isolated cases unexplained by dosage; they occurred in situations of which other persons did not complain. Individual sensitivity and/or sensitization may have been involved, as in the case of a family exposed for many years to a vaporizer in their basement who adopted a child who succumbed to the lindane (Morgan *et al.*, 1980). Serum levels were similar among the various members of the family. One of the more convincing of these cases concerned a 35-year-old woman who developed urticaria soon after a vaporizer was installed in her place of employment. The dermatitis improved during weekends but recurred when she returned to work. Although patch tests were negative, complete recovery followed removal of the vaporizer (AMA, 1952).

Atypical Cases of Various Origins A dramatic case involved a 35-year-old man who ate food accidentally seasoned with as much as 15–30 ml of a powder allegedly mistaken for monosodium glutamate and later identified as lindane. Grand mal seizures, vomiting, and diffuse abdominal pain began within 30 min. Taken immediately to hospital, the patient was found to be stuporous and mildly cyanotic, with accelerated pulse and respiration. He had severe acidemia. Another blood sample taken only 2 hr after the first, but when seizures had stopped, revealed a marked return of the blood pH and bicarbonate concentration to normal. During intervals of days, the patient developed marked increases in serum urea nitrogen, serum creatinine, creatine phosphokinase, lactate dehydrogenase, and glutamic-oxaloacetic transaminase, all of which returned to normal by hospital day 12–24. Clinically, the patient experienced muscle weakness and pain, myoglobinuria, acute nonoliguric renal failure, and episodic hypertension. Pancreatitis developed 13 days after ingestion; pain disappeared after 2 days, but serum amylase remained mildly elevated for an additional week. A muscle biopsy on day 15 demonstrated widespread necrosis and regeneration of individual muscle fibers. One year later, physical examination revealed normal findings including normal muscle bulk and strength (Munk and Nantel, 1977). The authors pointed out most of the unexpected findings in this case. They did not point out that the rapid cessation of convulsions and the precipitous decline of the serum level of "lindane" from 0.600 to 0.005 ppm by day 4 after ingestion were equally unexpected. The many atypical findings and the fact that the identity of the poison was inferred from gas chromatography and not confirmed by any specific test suggest that a compound other than lindane may have been involved. Rhabdomyolysis was also reported to have occurred 3 days after a 21-year-old attempted suicide by ingesting lindane (Jaeger *et al.*, 1984). Similarly, a 43-year-old woman who died 11 days after intentionally ingesting 8 oz of a 20% lindane solution had secondary renal failure and rhabdomyolysis. In addition, she presented with disseminated intravascular coagulation, which disappeared when serum lindane values fell from the initial 1.3 ppm (Sund *et al.*, 1988).

Another atypical case involved a boy who admitted having eaten about 12 chocolate biscuits he found on a dump that had been sprayed the previous night with a 4% formulation of BHC containing, it was said, only 0.5% of the γ isomer. What caused the biscuits to be discarded in the first place apparently was not explored. In any event, nausea and vomiting were delayed 3 hr after ingestion, and the boy was not hospitalized until 9.5 hr after ingestion. By that time he was stuporous; he remained so for another 9 hr, when he began to twitch, no longer to respond to painful stimuli, and to have pupils that were fixed, dilated, and diverging. It was only after this stage and after treatment with 500 ml of 10% mannitol that convulsions appeared. The boy remained in critical condition for 48 hr but recovered fully in 72 hr (MacNamara, 1970). If this illness was caused by BHC, then the CNS-depressant isomers must have predominated.

Another atypical case involved sudden onset of headache, fever, lassitude, muscular pain, and severe nausea and vomiting. After 2 days the nausea and vomiting abated somewhat, but the patient remained apathetic and even stuporous. Temperature ranged from normal to 38.3°C. On the seventh day the patient developed a stiff neck, and later diplopia, difficulty in swallowing, papilledema, abnormal reflexes, and paralysis of certain cranial nerves. There were no convulsions. A wide range of neurological diseases was considered in the differential diagnosis, but encephalitis lethargica was thought most

likely when the patient was discharged from hospital 23 days after onset. Later, at home, the patient reported that 10 hr before onset he had applied a solution of toxaphene and lindane to his sheep; final diagnosis was based on this circumstance (Pollock, 1958). There was no chemical study and no attempt to compare the case with others known to be caused by either of the compounds.

An epidemic affecting 79 persons during 1957 in the area of Carpenissi, Greece, was ascribed to BHC (Danopoulos *et al.*, 1953). In all cases the clinical picture and clinical laboratory data differed only in intensity. There were gradually appearing lassitude, weakness, stomatitis, and intestinal symptoms (colic and diarrhea), the latter lasting only a few days. Eventually there appeared an increase in muscle tone, weakness, increase in tendon reflexes, ataxia, tremor, disarthria of a slow, scanning, and undulating type, and, in some patients, delirium, athetotic movements, blindness, and convulsions. Convalescence was slow in those who survived. One boy later developed total blindness and spastic paraplegia. The entire picture suggests poisoning by a heavy metal, especially mercury. The chemical analysis available at the time was not specific for BHC; the blood levels reported (5–38 ppm) were entirely inconsistent with later results obtained by using proper methods. No search for heavy metals was attempted.

There is a report of the poisoning of four members of a family after they treated their living quarters by heating a pesticide dust on a hot plate. Presumably there was only one application. The family entered a clinic 6 months later. They showed general weakness, painful hyperesthesia, disturbed appetite, swelling of the joints, multiple exanthema, and pruritis, and they responded poorly to treatment. Although the illnesses were attributed to hexachlorocyclohexane (Rasulev *et al.*, 1965), the possibility of confusion with hexachlorobenzene is suggested by the medical findings.

In a single case, attributed to the eating of pickled peppers from a lindane-treated barrel, dizziness, ringing in the ears, nausea, vomiting, and nystagmus persisted almost 3 days (Cinotti, 1971), far longer than would be expected in connection with an even more serious illness actually caused by lindane.

The illness of 20 women 5 days after they had worked for no more than 1.5 hr in fields heavily treated with BHC, polychloropinene, and DDT (Kolyada and Mikhal'chenkova, 1973) must have been unrelated to the exposure. The same must have been true of several workers whose very complicated illness, including brief spells of unconsciousness, was attributed to lindane in the soil at a measured concentration of 0.4 ppm (Kundiev and Krasnyuk, 1965).

Dermatitis, hematuria, diarrhea, vomiting, abdominal pain, high fever, sore throat, and somnambulance in no dependable combination have been reported (Galigani and Melis, 1958; Jenkins, 1964) in instances in which the relationship between exposure and illness was circumstantial at best and even the fact of exposure was sometimes questionable.

A 9-year-old boy who had his scalp shampooed with a 1% lindane preparation developed abdominal pains and vasculitis on his lower limbs typical of Henoch-Schönlein purpura (Fagan, 1981).

A man who had suffered convulsions following trauma 14 years earlier suffered renewed convulsions that persisted intermittently for several months following heavy occupational exposure to BHC dust (Shul'ga, 1957).

Some members of two families became sick after their homes were painted with whitewash containing BHC (Mal'tseva and Savchuk, 1953), but the symptoms were not characteristic.

The nonfatal, febrile illness of a 40-year-old man involving cough, expectoration, pericarditis, and perhaps myocarditis was attributed to an "allergic reaction" to BHC and copper, mainly because the results of the spectrum of tests used to diagnose microbial disease were normal (Alix et al., 1974).

It is impossible to exclude the possibility that a particular compound is the cause of polyneuropathy in an individual case, and cases have been attributed to BHC or to BHC and DDT combined (Chakravarti, 1965; Czarski et al., 1967; Tolot et al., 1969; Rozin and Satyvaldiyev, 1970). However, it is clear that BHC causes polyneuropathy rarely, if ever. There is no case in which there is anything but circumstantial evidence for the relationship. In some instances, more than one compound was involved. Some other cases are highly suspect for other reasons. For example, it was claimed that polyneuropathy accompanied by affection of the brain was caused by a mixture of BHC and DDT and was cured within 17 days by massive treatment with cortisone, vitamins, strychnine, massage, and galvanic current (Czarski et al., 1967). Although cases of polyneuropathy may resolve spontaneously, the sad fact is that no treatment that will hasten resolution is known.

Another condition that has been attributed to BHC either alone or in combination with other compounds is aplastic anemia (Clinico-Pathologic Conference, 1955; Satieglitz et al., 1967, 1969, 1971; West, 1967; Bauer and Reisner, 1970; Best, 1963; Jedliŏka et al., 1958; Friberg and Maartensson, 1953; Marchand et al., 1956; Albahary et al., 1957; Sánchez-Medal et al., 1963; Woodliff et al., 1966a,b; West and Milby, 1965; Loge, 1965; Mendeloff and Smith, 1955; McLean, 1966; Morgan et al., 1980).

A Study Group on Blood Dyscrasias of the AMA Council on Drugs considered 1195 cases of blood disease suspected of having been caused by drugs or other chemicals between 1955 and 1962. Among the 54 compounds considered suspect to some degree were lindane, DDT, and chlordane. Some drugs are associated predominantly with specific blood disease: chloramphenicol with aplastic anemia, sulfoamides with thrombocytopenia, and phenothiazines with leukopenia. Penicillin, aspirin, and other commonly used drugs as well as the chlorinated hydrocarbon insecticides are associated with all varieties of blood diseases, but this association is coincidental and rarely present if the materials are given alone. Furthermore, in about half the cases of dyscrasia no association with any chemical can be found (Erslev and Wintrobe, 1962). Wintrobe and his colleagues (Scott et al., 1959) had reached essentially the same conclusion in connection with a very thorough review of 39 cases of aplastic anemia.

Although the causal relationship of BHC (and other compounds) in a case reported by Kotlarek-Haus et al. (1971) is no clearer than in other reports, the case itself deserves special mention. During a 2-year period, a farmer was hospitalized repeatedly for hemolytic crises. Laboratory tests were consistent with the clinical observation. Autopsy revealed a loss of erythropoietic tissue in the bone marrow. Usually an overactive bone marrow is found in hemolytic anemia. Apparently, there was an exhaustion atrophy in this case, as happens in patients who live long enough following repeated peripheral destruction of granulocytes by aminopyrine.

Although the number of reports relating BHC to aplastic anemia is considerable, one must realize that there is a great likelihood a case will be reported if a serious disease of usually undetermined cause appears to be explained by a relatively new compound. In fact, the urge to publish this kind of information is so great that one case of aplastic anemia attributed to insecticides was reported twice by separate authors, and another case was not reported a second time only because progress of the case led to a change of diagnosis (Woodliff et al., 1966b).

In a thorough review that made a plea for firmer regulations to restrict pesticides in general and BHC in particular, West concluded in 1967 that "research is urgently needed . . . to determine if there is a cause and effect relationship between exposure to lindane and adverse effects on bone marrow."

The difficulties of studying the relationship of any compound to myelogenic blood dyscrasia are very real (see Limitations of Present Tests for Hypersensitivity in Section 8.1.4.1). However, such studies as have been possible offer no support for the suspicion that lindane causes such disorders. The medical histories and physical examinations of 79 persons heavily exposed to lindane for periods of several weeks to several years revealed no illness attributable to the compound. A number of isolated hematological findings (leukopenia, leukocytosis, granulocytopenia, granulocytosis, eosinophilia, monocytosis, thrombocytopenia, and elevated blood uric acid) were found, but there was no correlation between the abnormalities and either the lindane content of the blood or the duration of exposure (Samuels and Milby, 1971). In a related study, blood samples from 40 persons employed in a lindane-processing plant were compared with samples from 40 controls; the blood lindane concentrations averaged 0.0119 and 0.0001 ppm, respectively. No evidence was found that lindane produces a hematological disorder (Milby and Samuels, 1971). In at least one other instance, careful study of heavily exposed persons failed to reveal any injury to the blood (Kleissner and Worden, 1959). One 20-year-old male is reported to have taken 4 oz of lindane per week for 18 months, yet showed no laboratory findings consistent with aplastic anemia (Purres, 1982).

Some authors of case reports have pointed out specifically that the evidence relating BHC to aplastic anemia was circumstantial. In no instance has it been possible to prove that the compound was the cause of the condition. Finally, blood dyscrasias have been found only rarely among people with heavy occupational or experimental exposure (Anonymous, 1958;

Christophers, 1969). One such report has appeared (Albahary et al., 1957), but the patient had been treated with chloramphenicol and this would seem to be a more reasonable explanation of his dyscrasia. In reporting a case of severe, but reversible, hypoplastic anemia associated with lindane exposure (Morgan et al. (1980), reviewed cases reported between 1953 and 1976. They concluded that the evidence for a link between BHC and aplastic anemia was not as good as it might be. With their own patient they were unable to explain the sudden appearance of anemia after many months of high exposure and its disappearance while BHC was still detectable in blood. Whether there is a link which originates in some of the effects of lindane on inositol metabolism in lymphocytes and so forth (Fisher and Mueller, 1971; Morgan et al., 1980; see also Section 15.4.1.2, Biochemical Effects) remains to be determined. Mead (1982) has pointed out that the cases of aplastic anemia that have been reported were associated with use of the commercial insecticide, not with the 1% pharmaceutical preparations.

A malignant otitis externa has been observed in an aplastic anemic patient who developed anemia following lindane ingestion (Schimmel et al., 1980).

There is one report (Jedliŏka et al., 1958) of paramyeloblastic leukemia appearing simultaneously in two blood cousins following their simultaneous exposure to lindane. The men, both 20 years old, had gone to school and worked together continually from the age of 14 years, and they had lived together for 4 years. For a brief period, 8 months before onset, they had been employed unloading bags of lindane at an agricultural distributing center. Other workers employed at the same time suffered no ill effect. The authors note the "constitutional, hereditary, and familial factors in the origin of the disease" and reported the cases for record without drawing any conclusion regarding cause and effect.

Far easier to explain on the basis of chance alone was a report (Klayman, 1968) by an otolaryngologist of four cases of carcinoma, one case of chronic inflammation, and one case of recurrent, spontaneous hematoma, all involving the larynx, in persons of whom one was a landscaper and most others had gardening as a hobby. There was said to have been contact with lindane in two of the cases.

In an entirely different category of atypical cases are some involving occupational exposure in the USSR and some other parts of Eastern Europe. These cases are distinct in symptomatology from certain other occupational cases in the same countries that clearly involved heavy exposure and led to signs and symptoms found in animal experiments or in accidental and intentional poisoning in people. There is not enough information to judge the degree of exposure in the atypical cases under discussion, although the authors clearly viewed it as excessive, and some authors (Husejnov, 1970) stated that intoxications have been absent when all the sanitary regulations were followed. Whatever the degree of exposure may have been, the signs and symptoms reported (mainly among groups of agricultural workers concurrently exposed to several pesticides) were not similar to those found in animals or in people whose exposure was clearly excessive. The reports under discussion tend to fall into two sets, those involving general debility and those involving a single organ or system. It was not clear, in either kind of case, whether the illness was sufficient to cause absence from work or what the sanction would be if work were missed. It also is seldom clear how often the same findings might be encountered in the general population from which the occupational sample was drawn. Conditions representative of general debility included dermatitis, subtle blood changes, general weakness, palpitations, headache, dizziness, inappetence, vomiting, lower abdominal pain, chronic gastritis, benign chronic hepatitis, insomnia, a sympathetic vascular/asthenic syndrome, vegetative dystonia, and confusion (Karimov, 1970; Khomenko and Kazakevich, 1973; Lyubchenko et al., 1973; Bezuglyi et al., 1973; Kazakevich, 1974).

Reports from the USSR sometimes speak of sensitization to pesticides without indicating whether the sensitization took the form of blood dyscrasia, dermatitis, or whatever. One such report recounts that diagnoses by degranulation of mast cells, degranulation of basophils, agglomeration of leukocytes, or blast transformation of lymphocytes were successful in a high proportion of cases (Polyak, 1974). As reviewed under Limitations of Present Tests for Hypersensitivity in Section 8.1.4.1, these tests have been available in Western Europe and the United States for many years. Their diagnostic value is unclear, and they are not generally used.

Organs or systems that have been studied apparently by specialists and to the complete exclusion of other organs or systems of the same workers include the heart (Krasnyuk, 1964a, 1969; Dunayevskiy, 1972), liver (Paramonchik, 1966; Paramonchik and Platonova, 1968; Schüttmann, 1968; Bezuglyi and Kaskevich, 1969; Katsenovich and Usmanova, 1970; Michail et al., 1972), stomach (Platonova, 1970), kidneys (Loganovskii, 1971), ovaries (Blekherman and Il'yina, 1972; Il'yina and Blekherman, 1974), adrenals (Blekherman and Il'yina, 1972), neuromuscular system (Khomenko and Kazakevich, 1973), ear (Agzamov, 1970; Muminov, 1972), nose (Salikhodzhaev and Fershtat, 1972), various internal secretory functions (Krasnyuk, 1964b), and mental disturbance (Kim et al., 1967).

Dosage Response The fatal poisoning of a 5-year-old girl weighing about 25 kg was caused by ingestion of 4.5 gm of BHC as a 30% solution in an unspecified solvent (Kwoczek, 1950); this represents a dosage of 180 mg/kg. In another fatal case, the estimated dose was 3.0 gm or approximately 200 mg/kg (Buck and Pfannenmueller, 1957). A number of deaths were caused by dosages in the order of 300 mg/kg (Joslin et al., 1960; Kay et al., 1964; Stören, 1955; Paludan, 1959), but some patients recovered in spite of about the same dosage (Clodi and Schnack, 1959; Kay et al., 1964). The difference was due at least in part to the protective effect of very prompt vomiting (Kay et al., 1964). That survival may occur after a high dosage of lindane (197 mg/kg) has been confirmed (Hayes, 1982).

It appears that BHC has caused death only when swallowed in substantial dosage. All of 11 persons who received a dosage estimated as about 86 mg/kg survived, although all had convulsions (Bambov *et al.*, 1966). On the other hand, low dosages of both the technical material and lindane may cause convulsions under certain conditions. This was illustrated most clearly when the possible use of these preparations as drugs was explored. Some children receiving lindane dermally as an emulsion at rates ranging from 50 to 100 mg/kg had convulsions (Kleine-Natrop *et al.*, 1970). Among six nonfatal cases ranging in age from 3 to 42 years, lindane ingestion was estimated as 45–247 mg/kg (Jaeger *et al.*, 1984).

Although the dosage of the few persons who have suffered occupational lindane poisoning is not known, blood levels of lindane in these workers indicate that the dosage must have been only slightly less at any one time than that which has produced acute, accidental poisoning.

Velbinger (1949) estimated that oily solutions of technical BHC administered at dosages of 16–18 mg/kg were tolerated, and he himself took 13 mg/kg without subjective or objective effect. However, much smaller dosages have produced poisoning. Studies to explore the use of BHC and lindane as anthelmintics seem to lead to two conclusions, both illustrated in Table 15.20. First, diarrhea, nausea, dizziness, headache, and a feeling of pressure in the temples are less likely following any particular dosage of lindane than of BHC and are inversely proportional to the α-isomer content of BHC. Second, an homogenized emulsion of lindane was distinctly more toxic than a less finely divided emulsion. A 26-year-old man suffered a convulsion following a single oral dose of 45 mg (about 0.6 mg/kg) in the form of a highly subdivided emulsion. Another young man, who had no side effects after two daily doses at the same rate, did have a convulsion following a third dose. Although no other fits occurred, a total of 6 of the 15 patients who received this very fine emulsion at rates of 30 or 45 mg/day experienced abdominal pain or one or more of the other symptoms mentioned above. In contrast, no side effects had been observed among 20 patients who received lindane at 45 mg/day in the form of a simple emulsion.

The threshold limit for lindane is 0.5 mg/m³, indicating that occupational absorption of about 0.07 mg/kg/day is considered safe.

Storage of BHC in Fat In one poisoning case, the concentration of lindane in fat at autopsy was 343 ppm (Joslin *et al.*, 1960). In a survey of 57 workers in a lindane factory, concentrations of β-BHC in subcutaneous adipose tissue were 300-fold higher than in serum and a significant correlation between both parameters could be established (Baumann *et al.*, 1980).

The storage of total BHC in fat of the general population of several countries is shown in Table 15.12, which indicates relatively high values for Argentina, France, Italy, India, and Japan. To this list one may add Austria (Pesendorfer *et al.*, 1973), Germany (Acker, 1974; Acker and Schulte, 1972, 1974), Hungary (Berend *et al.*, 1970), South Africa (M.

Wassermann *et al.*, 1970b), and Switzerland (Zimmerli and Marek, 1973). Investigators who reported storage of the separate isomers almost always found the β isomer predominant, and often it was the only one detected. In a few instances (Berend *et al.*, 1970; M. Wassermann *et al.*, 1970b), almost as much γ isomer as β isomer was found, undoubtedly because most of the exposure of the persons involved was to lindane rather than technical BHC. Many investigators have found traces of α isomer along with higher concentrations of other isomers, but the report of a high concentration of α isomer (1.07 ppm) in the absence of other isomers (Kadis *et al.*, 1970) is without precedent and may be incorrect.

For a time, BHC received unusually extensive use in Japan, and the highest reported values for its storage in the fat of people who were not poisoned by the compound came from that country (Nishimoto *et al.*, 1970; Doguchi *et al.*, 1971; Kasai *et al.*, 1972; Curley *et al.*, 1973; Kawanishi *et al.*, 1973; Suzuki *et al.*, 1973; Inoue *et al.*, 1974).

Storage in Blood A 41-year-old male with a history of manic-depressive disorder ingested 2 oz of Kwell. After 7 days he died from cardiopulmonary arrest. The initial blood level of lindane was 1.3 ppm, but this had declined to 0.11 ppm after 6 days and was 0.02 ppm at autopsy (Kurt *et al.*, 1986). A premature infant treated for scabies and who subsequently died had a blood level of 0.10 ppm (Pramanik and Hansen, 1979).

In an acute, nonfatal case, serum lindane concentrations of 0.84 and 0.49 ppm were found 2 and 4 hr, respectively, after ingestion (Starr and Clifford, 1972). A 2-year-old boy had convulsions and stopped breathing twice after he ate part of a vaporizer tablet. He was saved by mouth-to-mouth artificial respiration, was treated with large doses of barbiturates, and survived with sequelae. His serum lindane levels at different intervals after ingestion were: 6 hr, 0.29 ppm; 12 hr, 0.18 ppm; 25 hr, 0.20 ppm; 49 hr, 0.06 ppm; 73 hr, 0.07 ppm; and 169 hr, 0.02 ppm. Convulsions had stopped before the first blood sample was collected, but the child remained irritable for 2 days (Hayes, 1982). In a similar case, the initial blood level was 0.468 ppm. The concentration fell rapidly at first, but lindane was still somewhat above population levels 35 days later (Harris *et al.*, 1969).

In an occupational case that was described as "acute" but which had some subacute aspects, blood lindane levels were between 0.5 and 0.1 ppm. The cerebrospinal fluid contained 0.2 ppm several weeks after poisoning (Pernov and Kyurkchiyev, 1974).

In poisoning associated with a continuing high level of exposure, but without any recognized accidental gross exposure, blood levels of lindane as high as 0.340 ppm have been reported. EEG changes were observed in 15 of 17 men with blood levels greater than 0.02 ppm (Czegledi-Janko and Avar, 1970).

Children ranging in weight from 5.5 to 24 kg received near total-body application of 1% lindane lotion for either therapeutic or prophylactic treatment of scabies. The average blood level of lindane 2 hr after application was 0.013 ppm in children with active scabies, and their highest average value reached at 6 hr was 0.028 ppm. The highest value observed in one of those children was 0.048 ppm. The average blood levels of lindane during the first 12 hr were slightly lower in children with nonirritated skins who were treated only prophylactically, but the highest single value observed was in such a child. The half-lives of lindane in the blood were 17.9 and 21.4 hr, respectively, in the children with and without scabies (Ginsburg et al., 1977). Children who require retreatment may still have lindane in the blood (Ginsburg and Lowry, 1983).

Although no poisoning was involved, Milby et al. (1968) found that blood levels of lindane are a valid indicator of recent occupational or other exposure. The levels do not increase with increasing durations of exposure. The values they found for different groups overlapped considerably but the means were distinct, namely 0.0009 ppm for 21 controls employed by lindane plants but considered "unexposed"; 0.0022 ppm for eight persons who used vaporizers in the homes; 0.0046 and 0.0041 ppm, respectively, for groups of workers (37 in all) in one lindane plant that offered little opportunity for skin exposure; and 0.0306 ppm for 13 workers in another plant where skin contact was prevalent.

Baumann et al. (1980) examined workers in a factory producing lindane and compared them with an external group of clerks. The threshold limit value of 0.5 mg/m^3 was not exceeded, yet serum ranges of the exposed workers for the α, β, and γ isomers were 0.01–0.273, 0.017–0.76, and 0.005–0.188 ppm, respectively, and far above controls. A significant increase in the serum levels of β-BHC with time of employment was observed. See also Storage of BHC in Fat.

The lindane content of the blood of Argentine applicators of BHC varied from 0.0035 to 0.704 ppm (presumably depending on the quality of the technical product they used), but their levels of β-BHC were uniformly high, the averages ranging from 0.1823 to 0.2377 ppm in different provinces (Radomski et al., 1971). The highest values found in Argentine applicators were approximately equal to those reported in certain workers elsewhere who were moderately poisoned. Although the possibility of ill effect in the Argentine workers was considered, none was recognized. The difference could be due to individual variation in susceptibility or nutrition, but the possibility of differences in analytical method involving more nearly 100% detection of the Argentine residues must be considered.

Workers at a BHC manufacturing plant in India had serum levels in the range 0.143–1.152 ppm (Nigam et al., 1986). The percentage composition in the samples varied between 60 and 100% for the β-isomer. Sprayers had changes in serum residues of BHC before and after exposure (Kashyap et al., 1980).

Concentrations ranging from undetectable to 0.412 ppm BHC (but no lindane) were found in Australian workers, none of whom were ill (Siyali, 1972). Even higher levels of BHC, including lindane as high as 0.094 ppm, were found in certain pest control operators (Simpson and Shandar, 1972).

A distinctly lower average concentration of β-BHC (0.0020 ppm) was found in the blood of crop-workers in Colorado (Chase et al., 1973); in fact, it was not higher than other investigators have reported in the general population of the United States.

The storage of BHC and of other chlorinated hydrocarbon insecticides in blood of the general population of the United States has been reviewed (see Table 15.13). Concentrations of BHC in people in the United States are low. Insofar as analyses have been run on blood collected in other countries, they indicate the same distribution of the compound as is indicated by analyses of fat. Average values for β-BHC in different groups in Japan vary from 0.010 to 0.100 ppm, compared with levels of 0.003 ppm in the United States. In Japan, the concentration of β-BHC was higher in the plasma of city dwellers than in the plasma of persons living in agricultural villages but less than that in the plasma of BHC manufacturing workers (Kuwahara et al., 1972). The concentration of β-BHC in the blood of patients intoxicated by PCBs was slightly higher than in healthy persons (Abe et al., 1974).

As was true of DDT, the concentration of BHC in the blood of women gradually decreased during pregnancy and then gradually increased to approach levels found in nonpregnant controls (Curley and Kimbrough, 1969; Yamaguchi et al., 1976). Similarly, the concentrations of BHC and of some other chlorinated hydrocarbon insecticides are lower in the fat of pregnant than of nonpregnant women (Polishuk et al., 1970).

Other Storage in Adults   In one case of poisoning, the following concentrations of lindane were found at autopsy: fat, 343 ppm; liver, 88 ppm; stool, 478 ppm; and stomach contents, 105,000 ppm (Joslin et al., 1960). In another case, levels of 0.05, 0.26, 0.16, and 1.45 ppm were found at autopsy in brain, heart, liver, and fat, respectively (Kurt et al., 1986).

There have been few systematic analyses of chlorinated hydrocarbon compounds in organs. Values for a few persons in Japan (Suzuki et al., 1973) were in general agreement with those reported from Hawaii (Casarett et al., 1968; Hayes, 1975) for DDT but higher for dieldrin and BHC.

About half of 28 human gallstones (both bile pigment and mixed cholesterol types) contained α- and β-BHC in concentrations up to 0.05 ppm. No γ-BHC was found. Dieldrin and p,p'-DDT were present in most samples in concentrations up to 0.10 and 0.15, respectively (Simmons and Tatton, 1966).

Storage in the Fetus and Neonate   Although the concentrations of BHC in adult samples from Japan tend to be high, the concentrations of 0.12 ppm for β-BHC and 0.13 ppm for total BHC reported in the fat of a stillborn Japanese baby (Akasu, 1971) are somewhat low compared with values for 10 stillborns in the United States (Curley et al., 1969; Hayes, 1975). Values for β-BHC were also low in the brains, hearts, livers, and kidneys of 10 fetuses varying in age from 4 to 7 months (Shiota et al., 1974). The ratio of insecticide in the blood of newborn infants and in that of their mothers was 0.84 for α-BHC, 0.44 for β-BHC, 0.73 for lindane, 0.22 for heptachlor epoxide, 0.44 for dieldrin, 0.39 for p,p'-DDE, and 0.14 for p,p'-DDT (Radomski et al., 1971). Other authors (Polishuk et al., 1970;

Kasai *et al.*, 1972) also have reported lower concentrations in the blood of newborns than in that of their mothers.

Secretion in Milk There apparently are no data on the concentration of BHC in the milk of women with occupational exposure to it, much less in any who may have been poisoned.

In addition to reports referenced in Table 15.14, the secretion of BHC in human milk has been reported from Canada (Larsen *et al.*, 1971), France (Luquet *et al.*, 1974a,b), Germany (Adamovic *et al.*, 1971; Engst and Knoll, 1972; Knoll and Jayaraman, 1972a,b; Pfeilsticker, 1973), Japan (Takeshita and Inuyama, 1970; Tokutsu *et al.*, 1970; Kato *et al.*, 1971; Kojima *et al.*, 1971; Narafu, 1971; Sugaya *et al.*, 1971; Hayashi, 1972a,b; Mizoguchi *et al.*, 1972; Nagai, 1972; Oura *et al.*, 1972; Taira *et al.*, 1972; Yamagishi *et al.*, 1972a; Kamata, 1973, 1974; Kawai *et al.*, 1973; Suzuki *et al.*, 1973; Matsunaga *et al.*, 1975), Israel (Weisenberg *et al.*, 1985), Romania (Mandroiu and Iordachescu, 1971), and the United States (Savage *et al.*, 1973). For a review, see also Jensen (1983). Insofar as data are available, it is clear that the secretion of BHC in milk in different countries corresponds to the degree of use of the compound. Values for the United States and the United Kingdom are generally low; those for France and Japan have been relatively high. The matter has been studied most thoroughly in Japan.

Although γ-BHC may be found in milk in concentrations at least as high as 0.02 ppm soon after its absorption, it is excreted rapidly in the urine and does not persist in the body or in the milk. By contrast, β-BHC has been reported in Japanese milk at average concentrations as high as 0.23 ppm, and it persists for long periods. Occupational exposure in agriculture is of relatively little practical importance as a source of β-BHC. In fact, several groups of investigators (Takeshita and Inuyama, 1970; Kojima *et al.*, 1971; Kuroda *et al.*, 1972; Matsuda *et al.*, 1971) have found that the concentration of β-BHC is actually lower in farm women than in nonagricultural women. Although exceptions have been reported (Sugaya *et al.*, 1971; Tottori Prefectural Hygiene Research Institute, 1971), this is the usual finding, and it reflects the greater consumption of meat and dairy products in the cities, as found by a study group (1972) appointed by the Ministry of Health and Welfare and as summarized by Hayashi (1972a). Even though beef and milk are used extensively in the cities, their distribution apparently is relatively local, for human residue levels are higher in the western prefectures, where pesticide use is more extensive, than in eastern Japan (Hayashi, 1972a). Cattle acquire the isomer from rice straw. BHC formerly was used extensively for the rice crop. Although the use of BHC is now prohibited in Japan, and although human storage and excretion of other isomers have decreased, the concentration of β-BHC in human milk has shown little change. However, individual women can reduce the concentration of β-BHC in their milk to half in only a few days merely by choice of diet (Shimizu, 1972), indicating that most of the BHC in human milk is of recent dietary origin and not drawn from body stores.

By studying their diets, Shimizu (1974) estimated that

women whose milk contained β-BHC at concentrations of 0.17 and 0.60 ppm were ingesting the isomer at rates of 0.003–0.004 and 0.067 mg/day, respectively.

Because the concentration of BHC tends to be higher in human than in cow milk, it should be possible to distinguish a difference in the concentrations of the compound in groups of babies fed on the two foods. The matter was investigated by Ito and Umemura (1973), who found a significant difference in the concentration of β-BHC and DDT (but not PCBs) in the blood of groups of 3-month-old babies fed the two kinds of milk, but no difference was found in infants 1 year of age.

Discussion of Storage and Secretion Values The results for human fat, blood, and milk are in general agreement, indicating levels in different countries corresponding to their degree of use of BHC. It is clear that γ-BHC is excreted rapidly, so the finding of this isomer in any tissue or fluid is an indication of recent exposure, either occupational, accidental, or environmental. Since animals metabolize the γ isomer effectively, it is unlikely to be found in meat or eggs unless lindane was applied to livestock directly or their feed had been treated directly. On the contrary, the β isomer is metabolized slowly. It tends to become incorporated into food chains, including the rice straw–cow–human chain in Japan (Hayashi, 1973, 1974). Although less well studied, it is known that the concentration of β-BHC has been high in some fish in Japan, indicating persistence of the isomer in the aquatic environment (Hayashi, 1974).

The Japanese, who at one time had the highest human levels of BHC in general and of β-BHC in particular, have studied the matter thoroughly. Hayashi (1973), of the Department of Hygiene for Mothers and Children, National Institute of Public Health, Tokyo, stated that no case of chronic intoxication in people occurred and that detailed clinical examination of mothers and children showed no difference between groups in which the concentrations of BHC (and to a lesser extent DDT and dieldrin) in the mothers' milk were high and those in which concentrations were lower. A recent Chinese report, however, has shown a significant correlation between cerumen β-BHC levels and mortality rates from liver, colon, and lung cancer (Wang *et al.*, 1988).

Excretion in Urine and Feces In a nonfatal case the initial urine value was 0.0077 ppm. The concentration fell rapidly at first, but lindane was still detectable in the urine 35 days after ingestion. Unidentified metabolites were also detected (Harris *et al.*, 1969). The highest level of a BHC isomer reported in urine of ordinary people was 0.0009 ppm (Cueto and Biros, 1967).

Lindane in a concentration of 4870 ppm was found in the first sample of feces after ingestion of the compound (Starr and Clifford, 1972). This value, from a patient who recovered promptly, is much higher than is sometimes found at autopsy.

The urinary excretion of what was assumed to be unchanged γ-BHC at concentrations of 0.08–0.30 ppm was reported for healthy pesticide applicators (Michail, 1974b).

Five separate metabolites of lindane, either free or conjugated as ethereal sulfates, glucuronides, or mercapturic acids, were found in a sample of urine collected from a 2.5-year-old girl only 5.5 hr after she swallowed lindane. The five compounds detected were 2,4-dichlorophenol; 2,4,6-, 2,3,5-, and 2,4,5-trichlorophenols; and 2,3,4,6-tetrachlorophenol (Starr and Clifford, 1972). Only 2,3,4,6-tetrachlorophenol could be detected in the urine of an infant who died after lindane exposure (Davies *et al.*, 1983).

Metabolites of lindane were identified in the urine of 21 workers producing the insecticide (Angerer *et al.*, 1983). Fourteen mono-, di-, tri-, and -tetrachlorophenols and seven dihydroxychlorobenzenes were detected. The main metabolites present were the 2,4,6-, 2,3,5-, and 2,4,5-trichlorophenols. These trichlorophenols were also detected in the urine of forestry workers exposed to lindane (Drummond *et al.*, 1988).

In incubations of lindane with human liver microsomes, the four primary metabolites were γ-1,2,3,4,5,6-hexachlorocyclohex-l-ene, γ-1,3,4,5,6-pentachlorocyclohex-l-ene, β-1,3,4,5,6-pentachlorocyclohex-l-ene, and 2,4,6-trichlorophenol (Fitzloff *et al.*, 1982). Pentachlorobenzene and 2,3,4,6-tetrachlorophenol were also detected. Fitzloff and Pan (1984) found that β-1,3,4,5,6-pentachlorocyclohex-l-ene was further metabolized to a variety of other products including 2,4,5-trichlorophenol and the oxide derivative, which apparently is resistant to hydrolysis by microsomal epoxide hydrolase.

Other Laboratory Findings Induction of liver mixed-function oxidases by lindane has been demonstrated in humans as well as in animals. The half-life of a single (5 mg/kg) dose of phenylbutazone was 51.5 hr in men with an average plasma lindane value of 0.01840 ppm, compared to 63.9 hr in those with an average lindane concentration of 0.00002 ppm. The plasma DDE levels in these men ranged from 0.019 to 0.033 ppm but did not differ significantly between the groups (Kolmodin-Hedman, 1973a). Adult volunteers who were coated with lindane-containing cream (152–348 mg lindane/m²) showed a significant 37% increase in their ability to clear antipyrine from the plasma, although there was no correlation with plasma levels of the insecticide (Hosler *et al.*, 1980).

Storage of β-BHC, heptachlor epoxide, dieldrin, DDE, and DDT was much lower in an epileptic farmer who had been treated for 20 years with phenobarbital (21 mg five times per day) and phenytoin (90 mg four times per day) than in 391 other farmers in the same area (Schoor, 1970).

In cases of poisoning, laboratory findings (other than those involving BHC and its metabolites) are of little importance. The white cell count often is increased either as a nonspecific response to convulsions or as a response to aspiration pneumonitis. Sugar and/or albumin may be present in the urine, and blood urea nitrogen may be elevated slightly. Liver function tests may be abnormal, but they clear spontaneously.

Since liver function may be abnormal in acute poisoning, there must be some level of repeated exposure that causes liver changes. Ornithine carbamoyltransferase (OCT) was reported to be increased in workers with more than 5 years of occupational exposure to organochlorines. Less elevation was reported for BHC than for DDT (Michail *et al.*, 1972), but the degree of exposure to either compound or the presence or absence of typical signs of poisoning was not stated. A change may occur in the blood lipoproteins of healthy workers exposed mainly to lindane and DDT; 8 of 22 such exposed workers and none of 19 controls had hyper-HDL (α)-lipoproteinemia (Kolmodin-Hedman, 1973b). A significant fall in α-lipoprotein cholesterol was noted in workers who were examined 2 years after their last occupational exposure to lindane (Carlson and Kolmodin-Hedman, 1977). The significance of an observed increase in acetylcholinesterase, serum aldolase, and alkaline phosphatase in workers exposed to a variety of chlorinated hydrocarbon insecticides, including BHC, is unknown (Bogusz, 1968). Morgan and Roan (1969) found no differences in glomerular function or in tubular reabsorption of phosphate or total α-amino acid nitrogen in persons with occupational exposure to a wide variety of pesticides compared to controls. However, among pest control operators exposed to a variety of compounds including lindane, they found a significant increase in reabsorption of uric acid and a net decrease in its clearance.

A significant increase in urinary excretion of ketosteroids was reported in persons with serum β-BHC levels >0.002 ppm (Morgan and Roan, 1973), but confirmation is needed. Although liver trouble has been reported in association with a β-BHC blood level of 0.029 (Sugaya, 1972), this concentration ordinarily is not associated with any illness.

Workers manufacturing lindane had a significant rise in their luteinizing hormone levels relative to a control group (Tomczak *et al.*, 1981).

The electroencephalograms of 16 of 73 workers exposed to BHC, DDT, and benzilan were considered abnormal, even though none of the men showed any abnormal neurological finding. The abnormal EEG patterns varied. The 21.9% rate of abnormality observed among the 73 workers may be compared with abnormality rates of 9.0 and 9.2% reported by other investigators for unexposed normal populations (Israeli and Mayersdorf, 1973; Mayersdorf and Israeli, 1974). Czegledi-Janko and Avar (1970) considered that nonspecific EEG abnormalities occur in 10–20% of the general population. However, they found such changes in the EEGs of 15 of 17 workers with blood lindane levels of 0.02 ppm or more. In a group of 10 workmen who had been exposed to BHC continually, 3 showed abnormal EEG patterns and polyneuropathy (Muller *et al.*, 1981). Electromyograms of eight workers demonstrated disturbance of the peripheral motor neurons. See also Use Experience.

Pathology In the case of a 1.5-year-old boy who survived only about 12 hr after ingesting lindane with no solvent or other toxicant present, the gross findings included congestion of the lungs and kidneys, distention of the intestinal tract, and a reddish yellow appearance of the liver. Microscopically, the lungs showed edema, congestion, and bronchopneumonia. The liver exhibited fatty metamorphosis, and the kidney tubules revealed degenerative changes. There were tiny hemorrhages in the brain associated, at least in some instances, with necrosis in the walls of the small blood vessels. The change in the lung appeared to be consistent with aspiration pneumonia. The liver changes were more prominent than those seen in laboratory animals under similar conditions (Joslin *et al.*, 1960). The findings were similar in other cases in which pathology was reported (Paludan, 1959; Maresch *et al.*, 1960).

Treatment of Poisoning   Activated charcoal, liquid paraffin, and cholestyramine have been used to inhibit uptake of ingested lindane or increase its excretion (e.g., Jaeger *et al.*, 1984) with diazepam to control convulsions. Hemoperfusion over Amberlite XAD-4 has also been employed to lower serum lindane levels (Daerr *et al.*, 1985). See also Section 15.2.5.

15.5 CYCLODIENE AND RELATED COMPOUNDS

The cyclodiene insecticides discussed in this chapter are shown in Fig. 15.6. Among them are two pairs of stereoisomers: aldrin and isodrin, dieldrin and endrin. Aldrin is rapidly metabolized to its isomer, dieldrin, so that the toxicity of aldrin is essentially that of dieldrin. In a similar way, isodrin, which is little used as an insecticide, is metabolized to endrin. The difference in both toxicity and storage of the stereoisomers dieldrin and endrin is remarkable. The acute toxicity of dieldrin is less than that of endrin, but dieldrin is stored so avidly that traces of it may be found in almost everyone in the general population. On the contrary, endrin has never been detected

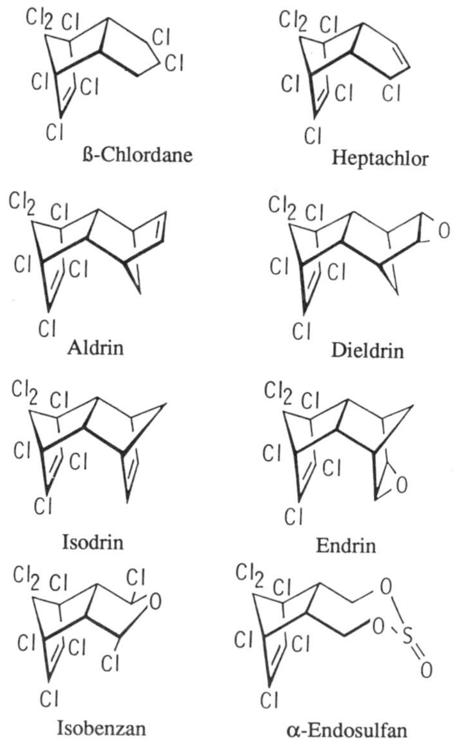

Figure 15.6 Structures of chlorinated cyclodienes and closely related insecticides.

even in healthy workers engaged in manufacturing it and has been found only in rapidly decreasing concentrations during the first few days after acute poisoning.

15.5.1 CHLORDANE

15.5.1.1 Identity, Properties, and Uses

Chemical Name   1,2,4,5,6,7,8,8-Octachloro-3a,4,7,7a-tetrahydro-4,7-methanoindan,   or   1,2,4,5,6,7,8,8-octachloro-3a,4,7,7a-hexahydro-4,7-methano-1*H*-indene.

Structure   Chlordane has two main isomers, of which the more abundant *cis*-chlordane is shown in Fig. 15.6. The *trans* isomer differs in having the chlorines at carbon atoms 1 and 2 on opposite sides of the plane of the ring. It is unfortunate that earlier sets of names used the term α-chlordane with opposite meanings and that the term γ-chlordane has been used for both the *trans* isomer and the relatively uncommon 2,2,4,5,6,7,8,8-octochloro isomer. In addition to the isomers of chlordane *per se*, technical chlordane has contained heptachlor, nonachlor, hexachlorocyclopentadiene, and other compounds. As manufacture improved, the proportion of chlordane *per se* increased and the proportion of other compounds decreased. Although chlordane is a mixture, there is no reason to assume that its composition is controlled less rigidly than the composition of other mixtures used successfully as agricultural chemicals. In fact, chlordane may be no more mixed than some technical products commonly thought of as single compounds.

Synonyms   The common name chlordane (BSI, ICPC, ISO) is in general use. The original nonproprietary name established by the Interdepartmental Committee on Pest Control was chlordan; it later was changed by ICPC to conform to the requirements for word endings in certain languages other than English. The material has been sold under the names Belt®, Corodane®, Chlortox, Niran®, Octachlor®, Octa-Klor®, Synklor®, and Toxichlor®. Code designations include ENT-9,932, M-140, and Velsicol-1,068/CD-68. The CAS registry number is 57-74-9.

Physical and Chemical Properties   Chlordane in the restricted sense has the empirical formula $C_{10}H_6Cl_8$ and a molecular weight of 409.80. The *cis* isomer melts at 106–107°C, the *trans* isomer at 104–105°C, and the 2,2,4,5,6,7,8,8-octachloro isomer at 131°C. Technical chlordane is a viscous, amber-colored liquid containing about 45 constituents (Sovocool *et al.*, 1977). It is unstable in the presence of weak alkali. Chlordane is soluble in most organic solvents including petroleum oils but is virtually insoluble in water. The vapor pressure of refined chlordane is 1×10^{-5} mm Hg at 25°C, and the density is 1.59–1.63.

History, Formulations, and Uses   Chlordane was introduced in 1945. Through 1950, the product, sometimes called "early chlordane," contained variable concentrations of an unreacted intermediate, hexachlorocyclopentadiene. From 1951 onward the concentration of this contaminant was held below 1%, with the result that the dermal and respiratory toxicities of "later chlordane" were markedly less and the oral toxicity was somewhat less. Chlordane has been available in dusts, wettable powders, granules, emulsifiable concentrates, and oil solutions. It has been used for control of insects on vegetables, small grains, maize, other oilseeds, potatoes, sugarcane, sugar beets, fruits, nuts, cotton, and jute. Chlordane has been used extensively for control of household pests and for certain wood-boring insects. The oil solution type of formulation is used almost exclusively for termite control.

15.5.1.2 Toxicity to Laboratory Animals

Basic Findings   The effects of chlordane are similar to those of other chlorinated hydrocarbon insecticides, especially the other cyclodiene compounds. Tremor is essentially absent, but convulsions are a prominent aspect of poisoning. Irritation is not an important property of later chlordane. Early chlordane was always highly irritating to the respiratory tract of animals exposed to the vapor and to the skin of those treated by this route.

The toxicity of single and repeated doses is presented in Tables 15.21 and 15.22, respectively. The no-effect levels of *cis* and *trans* isomers and of the technical product are all within the same range. Most metabolites of chlordane are far less toxic than the parent material, but oxychlordane is more toxic, having an oral LD 50 in rats of 19.1 mg/kg (FAO/WHO, 1971).

Following reports of high vapor toxicity of chlordane to pigeons (Lehman, 1950) and mice (Frings and O'Tousa, 1950), Ingle (1953) showed that the product manufactured at that time did not have this property but that, when hexachlorocyclopentadiene (Hx) was added, vapor toxicity was proportional to its concentration in the mixture. Mice kept in saturated vapor of technical chlordane for 25 days showed no symptoms. However, under otherwise identical conditions, 2.5% Hx and 97.5% chlordane in the saturation train produced symptoms in 4 days and death in 20–25 days; 5% Hx produced symptoms in 4 days and death in 10–25 days; 7.5% Hx caused 100% mortality in 48 hr; and 10% Hx caused 100% mortality within 24 hr.

Absorption, Distribution, Metabolism, and Excretion
Rats that breathed [^{14}C]chlordane vapor for 30 min retained 77% of the total inhaled (Stubblefield and Dorough, 1979). Clearance of orally dosed *cis*-[^{14}C]chlordane was faster from rats than from mice (Ewing *et al.*, 1985) and the half-life in tissues of rats tends to increase with dosage, possibly due to the accumulation of oxychlordane (Ohno *et al.*, 1986). Recent studies in mice have confirmed that unlike *cis*- and *trans*-chlordanes, nonachlors and oxychlordane readily accumulate in the body (Hirasawa and Takizawa, 1989).

Rabbits that had received four doses of α-[^{14}C]chlordane stored it in different tissues in decreasing order as follows: fat > kidney > muscle > liver > brain. The order for γ-[^{14}C]chlordane was kidney > fat > liver > muscle > brain. Oxychlordane reached higher concentrations than the parent compound, especially in fat (Balba and Saha, 1978).

In vivo and *in vitro* studies in rats have revealed two routes of biotransformation of chlordane and shown that the metabolites include *trans*-chlordane, 1,2,-dichlorochlordene, oxychlordane, 1-hydroxy-2-chlorochlordene, 1-hydroxy-2-chloro-2,3-epoxychlordene, chlordene chlorohydrin, and 1,2,-*trans*-dihydroxydihydrochlordene, as well as the metabolites of heptachlor (Tashiro and Matsumura, 1977; Brimfield and Street, 1979). *In vitro* studies showed that the livers of rat and humans have almost identical ability to degrade chlordane, except that human liver has little capacity to convert *trans*-nonachlor to *trans*-chlordane. This is consistent with the accumulation of *trans*-nonachlor in people but not in rats (Tashiro and Matsumura, 1978).

Many of the same metabolites have been identified in the urine of rabbits (Balba and Saha, 1978). When rabbits were fed radioactive isomers, they excreted, in urine and feces, 77% of the α isomer and 82% of the γ isomer (Balba and Saha, 1978).

Effects on Organs and Tissues   Altered immune competence was reported in the offspring of mice whose mothers had received chlordane at a rate of 8.0 mg/kg/day throughout gestation but not in young whose mothers received 0.16 mg/kg/day (Cranmer *et al.*, 1979; Spyker-Cranmer *et al.*, 1982; Barnett *et al.*, 1985a). This can lead to enhancement of survival to influenza type A virus infection (Menna *et al.*, 1985), perhaps by a decrease in virus-specific delayed hypersensitivity response (Barnett *et al.*, 1985b). Johnson *et al.* (1986) have recorded no enhancement of cell-mediated immunity *in vivo* after treatment of female mice with chlordane but have observed a suppression

Table 15.21
Single Dose LD 50 for Chlordane

Species	Route	LD 50 (mg/kg)	Reference
Rat, M	oral	400–500[a]	Ambrose *et al.* (1953)
Rat, F	oral	600–700[a]	Ambrose *et al.* (1953)
Rat, M	oral	600[b]	Ambrose *et al.* (1953)
Rat, F	oral	700[b]	Ambrose *et al.* (1953)
Rat, M	oral	335[c]	Gaines (1960)
Rat, F	oral	430[c]	Gaines (1960)
Rat	oral	150–225	FAO/WHO (1965)
Rat, F	dermal	530	Gaines (1960)
Mouse	oral	430	USFDA (1947)
Rabbit	oral	300[d]	Stohlman *et al.* (1950)
Rabbit	oral	100–200[e]	Stohlman *et al.* (1950)
Rabbit	oral	20–40	FAO/WHO (1965)
Goat	oral	180	Welch (1948)
Sheep	oral	500–1000	Welch (1948)

[a] Applied in cottonseed oil.
[b] Applied in ethyl alcohol.
[c] Applied in peanut oil.
[d] Applied in olive oil.
[e] Applied in Tween 20.

Table 15.22
Effect on Various Animals of Repeated Oral Doses of Chlordane

Dosage Range (mg/kg/day)	Method and concentration (ppm)	Species, number, and sex	Duration	Results	Reference
161–320	200 mg/kg/day	dog	7 days	convulsions in one	Batte and Turk (1948)
81–160	100 mg/kg/day	rat, 5	15 days	100% mortality	Ambrose *et al.* (1953)
	50 mg/kg/day	dog	37 days	100% mortality	Lehman (1951, 1952)
41–80	1000 ppm in diet	rat, 12	10 days	100% mortality	Stohlman *et al.* (1950)
	50 mg/kg/day	rat	15 days	40% mortality	Ambrose *et al.* (1953)
21–40	500 ppm in diet	rat, 12	70 days	100% mortality	Stohlman *et al.* (1950)
	25 mg/kg/day	rat, 5	15 days	no tremors or convulsions	Ambrose *et al.* (1953)
11–20	300 ppm in diet	rat, 25	100 days	25% mortality	Stohlman *et al.* (1950)
	300 ppm in diet	rat, 40	2 yr	reduced growth, liver changes obvious	Ingle (1952)
	300 ppm in diet[a]	rat, 40	2 yr	moderate toxicity	FAO/WHO (1965)
6–10	150 ppm in diet	rat, 40	2 yr	reduced growth, liver changes obvious	Ingle (1952)
	5 mg/kg/day	dog	93 wk	100% mortality	Lehman (1951, 1952)
2.6–5	75 ppm in diet	rat, 24	2 yr	moderate toxicity	Lehman (1951, 1952)
	40 ppm in diet	rat, 5	407 days	infrequent liver changes	Ambrose *et al.* (1953)
	60 ppm in diet	rat, 10 M	3 gen	symptomatology and liver change but no tumorigenesis or teratogenesis	FAO/WHO (1968)
	50 ppm in diet	rat, 40	2 yr	margination of liver cells	FAO/WHO (1965)
	75 ppm *trans* isomer in diet	rat	78 wk	no tumors	Ingle (1969)
1.26–2.5	25 ppm in diet	rat, 24	2 yr	mild toxicity	Lehman (1951, 1952)
	30 ppm in diet	rat, 40	2 yr	mild toxicity, slight liver changes	Ingle (1952)
	25 ppm[a]	rat, 40	2 yr	no liver changes	Ingle (1952)
	30 ppm in diet	rat, 10 M	3 gen	no effect on fertility	FAO/WHO (1968)
	35 ppm *cis* isomer in diet	rat	78 wk	no tumors	Ingle (1969)
0.626–1.25	no entry				
0.312–0.625	12.5 ppm in diet	rat, 12	9 mo	liver cell change in most males, no females	Ortega *et al.* (1957)
	10 ppm in diet	rat, 40	2 yr	no neurological symptoms, minimal liver cell changes	Ingle (1952)
	30 ppm in diet	dog	2 yr	increased liver weight	FAO/WHO (1968)
0.156–0.312	5 ppm in diet	rat, 40	2 yr	no effect	Ingle (1952)
	15 ppm in diet	dog	2 yr	increased liver weight	FAO/WHO (1968)
0.078–0.156	2.5 ppm in diet	rat, 24	2 yr	some liver cell changes	Lehman (1951, 1952)
	2.5 ppm in diet	rat	9 mo	cytoplasmic changes in one of five rats	Ortega *et al.* (1957)
0.039–0.078	3 ppm in diet	dog	2 yr	no effect	FAO/WHO (1968)

[a] New chlordane.

in vitro (Johnson *et al.*, 1987). Besides immune changes in offspring of mothers given chlordane, Cranmer *et al.* (1984) have shown that the plasma corticosterone levels can be elevated for much of the subsequent life. *In vitro* chlordane exhibited general stimulative effects on polymorphonuclear leukocytes from guinea-pigs (Suzaki *et al.*, 1988).

No dominant lethal changes were found when male mice received technical chlordane by gavage or intraperitoneal injection at a dosage of 50 or 100 mg/kg (Arnold *et al.*, 1977).

The incidence of hepatoma was increased in mice fed chlordane (NCI, 1977b; IARC, 1979) (see Section 15.2.3.2). However, recent studies with rats and mice fed chlordane (up to 25 ppm and 12.5 ppm respectively) have shown no significant increases in liver tumor incidence (Khasawinah & Grutsch, 1989a,b). Chlordane will promote the carcinogenic action of diethylnitrosamine (Williams and Numoto, 1984). Reactive metabolites of chlordane bind to cellular macromolecules but whether this is of any importance in the hepatocarcinogenicity is unknown (Brimfield and Street, 1981). Interestingly, chlordane at an otherwise no-effect dosage produces an increase in the number of hepatocyte nuclei with double DNA content and significant changes in chromatin distribution patterns (Nair *et al.*, 1980).

Inhalation studies with chlordane at 0–10 μg/l for 90 days, showed some alterations of liver with rats but no effects with cynomolgus monkey (Khasawinah *et al.*, 1989).

GABA turnover is apparently inhibited in the cortex and hippocampus (but less in the cerebellum) of mice given relatively high doses of chlordane (Fishman and Gianutsos, 1985). Neurotoxic effects are probably similar to those of other cyclodiene insecticides.

15.5.1.3 Toxicity to Humans

Accidental and Intentional Poisoning   Chlordane has not been a common cause of poisoning. All established cases have been associated with gross exposure. In most instances, including those with full recovery, convulsions appeared within 0.5–3 hr after ingestion (Micks, 1954; Curley and Garrettson, 1969; Aldrich and Holmes, 1969; Kutz *et al.*, 1983) or after dermal exposure involving spillage (Derbes *et al.*, 1955).

Following ingestion, some patients have experienced nausea and vomiting before signs of central nervous system overactivity appeared. However, as often as not, a convulsion was the first clear indication of illness. Convulsions often last about a minute and may recur at intervals of about 5 min. Convulsions usually are accompanied by confusion, incoordination, excitability, or, in some instances, coma. Respiratory failure may also occur (Olanoff *et al.*, 1983). In one instance, convulsions were so violent that the patient suffered compression fractures of varying severity of dorsal vertebrae four through nine, as revealed by an X-ray examination made after recovery from acute poisoning. During the acute episode, the same man experienced a brief episode of oliguria with proteinuria, hematuria, and mild hypertension, all of which returned to normal (Stranger and Kerridge, 1968). After a 21-month-old child who had a typical convulsion following ingestion of an unknown number of chlordane "pellets" was essentially recovered, she was found to have albuminuria and a positive urine culture; to what extent chlordane may have influenced the renal tract infection was unclear (Canada, 1962).

The most striking dermal case involved a woman in a formulating plant who spilled a solution of chlordane and DDT on her abdomen and thighs. About 40 min later she became confused and suddenly began having convulsions. Her associates tried to wash the poison off but left her clothes on. She was sent promptly by ambulance to a physician's office but was dead on arrival (Derbes *et al.*, 1955). Whereas the occupational origin of the woman's exposure raises the question of possible cumulative effects, there is no evidence that cumulation actually had occurred. The dose received suddenly by spillage seemed adequate to explain the rapidly fatal outcome.

One 30-year-old woman was exposed to chlordane through carelessness and overuse over a 1–4-week period. Myoclonic jerks occurred only after a delay of a month, although the patient previously suffered from circumoral numbness, anorexia, nausea, and fatigue (Garrettson *et al.*, 1985). Fatigue and anorexia became the dominant symptoms for 6 months before treatment. Of interest was metrorrhagia despite contraceptive medication. This dysfunctional bleeding was thought to be due to increased metabolism of estrogen brought on by induction of hepatic enzymes by chlordane. It ceased after the dose of estrogen was increased.

Chlordane was diluted with tap water in preparation for treating a foundation for termite control. Presumably through back siphonage, this was responsible for contamination of most of a section of a public water supply serving 42 houses and used by 105 people. The affected section of the water supply was cut off promptly and was reconnected only after replacement of the main pipes and extensive flushing of the others. Water samples collected in 35 houses downstream from the probable site of entry contained concentrations ranging from 0.0006 to 1.200 ppm. Of the inhabitants, 71 reported symptoms, and in 13 the signs and symptoms were compatible with mild acute chlordane poisoning. However, serum levels of chlordane metabolites measured soon after the incident did not correlate with the reported symptoms (Harrington *et al.*, 1978). In another episode of contamination of a public water supply by chlordane (probably intentional) many people were affected and the level in a residence near the point of intake was 6.600 ppm. Levels in other samples from residences ranged from 0 to 0.905 ppm with 44 positive households out of 70 surveyed. Although chlordane, its contaminants, or its metabolites were not detected in residents, a significant proportion reported gastrointestinal symptoms, skin and eye irritations, and headaches [Morbidity and Mortality Weekly Reports (MMWR), 1981].

Use Experience   Princi and Spurbeck (1951) were the first to study men with heavy occupational exposure to chlordane; they found no toxic effects. Entirely similar findings were reported in connection with 24 men who had made chlordane for 2 months to 5 years (Alvarez and Hyman, 1953) and in those with 15 years of exposure (Fishbein *et al.*, 1964).

One case of poisoning has been attributed to occupational exposure to chlordane in the absence of a gross accident. A man who grew trees, shrubs, and flowers commercially developed episodes of paresthesia and later twitching of the right hand and arm. Additional episodes, beginning in the same way, ended as grand mal convulsions followed by unconsciousness. The man was first studied and treated for idiopathic epilepsy but eventually remained normal, both clinically and by EEG examination, without treatment when he discontinued contact with chlordane. Almost daily for a while he had handled soil that he had treated with the compound (Barnes, 1967). The case was unusual because of the initially unilateral manifestations and because it is difficult to understand how the man's recognized exposure could have been greater than that of the factory workers just mentioned.

A survey of 1105 persons associated with pest control

showed that most of them used chlordane, but only three attributed illness to it, namely mild dizziness, headache, and weakness; the same survey revealed serious poisoning, including one death, caused by fumigants (Stein and Hayes, 1964). Epstein and Ozonoff (1987) have detailed a number of cases in which blood disorders, such as leukemias and thrombocytopenic purpura, might have been associated with chlordane or heptachlor usage, but see Peto (1980).

Retrospective mortality studies of workers employed in the manufacture of chlordane and heptachlor showed no excess of cancer 20 or more years after they entered the occupation (Wang and MacMahon, 1979a,b; Ditraglia *et al.*, 1981; Shindell *et al.*, 1981; Shindell and Ulrich, 1986). There was a significant excess of deaths from cerebrovascular disease, although previous evidence has not suggested that chlordane causes an increase in blood pressure (Princi and Spurbeck, 1951; Alvarez and Hyman, 1953; Fishbein *et al.*, 1964). It may be significant, however, that endrin has been linked to an excess of deaths due to strokes (Loevinsohn, 1987) (see Section 15.5.5.3, Use Experience).

Atypical Cases of Various Origins Typical, serious poisoning by chlordane is characterized by onset of violent convulsions within 0.5–3 hr and either death or the start of recovery within a few hours to a day. In a case ascribed to chlordane that differs from this pattern in important ways, a woman who had twice attempted to poison herself was reported to have swallowed 6 gm (104 mg/kg) of chlordane in talc. About 2.5 hr later she began to vomit, and she continued to do so for about 12 hr. She suffered chemical burns of the mouth, severe gastritis, enteritis, diffuse pneumonia, and lower nephron syndrome. She was almost completely anuric after the first few hours. The only early sign of stimulation of the central nervous system was lateral nystagmus, noted when she was hospitalized about 18 hr after the ingestion. On day 5 she did develop restlessness that gradually progressed to severe agitation; convulsions were present during the last 6 hr before death, which occurred 9.5 days after the ingestion (Derbes *et al.*, 1955). The reported dosage was adequate to cause early convulsions and death if chlordane had been the main toxicant present. The severe local irritation, the early signs of severe kidney involvement, the absence of early convulsions in a serious case, and the inconsistency of dosage response suggest that a completely different kind of poison may have been involved. The victim may not have been competent to judge, or her earnest desire for death may have led her to deceive. No chemical tests were run, but the autopsy findings of ulcers of the mouth and pharynx, severe necrotizing bronchopneumonia, and desquamation and degeneration of the renal tubular epithelium were consistent with the clinical course and suggest a heavy metal, especially mercury.

A man who developed neurological symptoms 6 months to a year after exposure to pesticides, including chlordane, had characteristic findings of multiple sclerosis in his brain and severe peripheral neuropathy at autopsy (Blisard *et al.*, 1986). These findings seemed more related to poisoning from organophosphorus chemicals than to chlordane, and there seems to be some confusion as to whether his symptoms were caused by insecticides at all. It is also difficult to explain the progressive motor neuron disease observed in a patient who was exposed to a mixture of chlordane and pyrethrin (Pall *et al.*, 1987).

The occurrence of a megaloblastic anemia accompanied by intermittent fever and followed by cholestatic hepatitis and eventual recovery (Furie and Trubowitz, 1976) was related to chlordane only circumstantially, and megaloblastic or other anemia has not been reported in established cases. The same may be said for what may have been the first illness attributed to chlordane. A 33-year-old housewife, who was a known alcoholic and had been suffering an upper respiratory infection for several days, reoccupied her apartment one evening several hours after it had been sprayed with 1 or 2% chlordane. During the night she developed severe cough and vomiting, which lasted until she was hospitalized 4 days later. She was afebrile, and the chest was clear. Signs typical of chlordane poisoning were not observed. The only remarkable physical finding was slight tenderness and enlargement of the liver. Laboratory study revealed moderate anemia and liver dysfunction. On a conservative treatment the cough and vomiting practically ceased in 3 days, and in 5 more days the liver was no longer palpable. Liver function tests improved, but the patient failed to return for recommended follow-up (Lemmon and Pierce, 1952). No similar case associated with chlordane has been reported; it does seem possible that the illness was caused by hexachloropentadiene present as a contaminant.

Chlordane has been linked to neuroblastoma, aplastic anemia, and acute leukemia but only circumstantially (Infante *et al.*, 1978).

According to the account given by a patient and her husband 3.9 years after her exposure to chlordane, that exposure consisted of spraying clothing that she moved out of a closet and then returned to the closet after the application. The clothing was sprayed while it was laid on a bed near the closet or while it was held by hand. The windows and the door of the room were open. After alternately moving and spraying clothing for about an hour, the woman cried out that she felt faint and then lost consciousness. Her husband, summoned by her call, carried her into another room and, because he thought she had no pulse or respiration, applied artificial respiration for an estimated 10 min. The woman vomited when she regained consciousness. For the next 2 days she was in a confused state. One day after exposure she suffered from headache, vomited once, and "spit up four or five tablespoons of blood." A physician consulted at this time found her extremely somnolent. Headache and lethargy continued, and within a year she lost consciousness on several occasions. During this first year, she was unable to organize her household chores including cooking. Nearly 4 years after exposure, her ability to plan and prepare meals had returned partially, but it still required considerable effort for her to organize and execute her daily routine. Neurological examination at that time disclosed an unkempt, somewhat obtunded woman, who was aware of her defects and depressed by her condition. She displayed poverty of interest and impaired memory (Stevens, 1970). If the patient's initial syncopy was causally related to her exposure, it seems more reasonable to attribute it to the solvent and propellant in the formulation, especially because there was no mention of convulsions. Because absence of respiration and pulse was reported, it seems certain that brain damage was the result of hypoxia.

An unusual case of poisoning occurred in a man with a history of schizophrenia and episodes of tremor associated with alcohol withdrawal who attempted suicide by administering 60–300 ml of a chlordane-containing solution (57–205 mg) as an enema (Marquardt, 1982). Some 4–11 hr later, when hospitalized, he was noted to be tachycardiac with fasciculations and tremors. His dose was relatively low and he survived after treatments including rectally administered activated charcoal.

Dosage Response In one patient known to be an alcoholic, death followed an oral dosage estimated at 28–56 mg/kg (Hayes, 1963). In another case, death followed failure to remove a solution of 25% chlordane and 26% DDT that soaked the victim's abdomen and thighs and, therefore, must have been at least 120 ml in volume, indicating a chlordane dosage probably in excess of 425 mg/kg (Derbes *et al.*, 1955; Hayes, 1963).

Convulsions followed by recovery occurred in infants after dosages of about 10 and 28 mg/kg, respectively (Lensky and Evans, 1952; Micks, 1954) and in an adult after 32 mg/kg (Dadey and Kammer, 1953). A man recovered after apparently consuming 216 gm of chlordane (approximately 3000 mg/kg) in a liquid pesticide formulation (Olanoff *et al.*, 1983). Whether this was the true dose or only the dose of a chlordane-containing liquid is unclear.

One poisoning by rectally administered chlordane involved a dose of 0.53–1.9 mg/kg (Marquardt, 1982). In this case symptoms were relatively mild. A dosage–response relationship has been reported for 261 people from 85 households previously treated with chlordane, in respect of sinusitis, bronchitis, and migraine symptoms, when assessed relative to indoor air levels of 1 μg/m^3 (low), 1–5 μg/m^3 (medium), and 5 μg/m^3 (high) (Menconi *et al.*, 1988).

Laboratory Findings In a fatal case of chlordane poisoning, total chlordane residues were: plasma, 4.87 ppm; liver, 59.9 ppm; brain, 23.3 ppm; and adipose tissue, 22 ppm, 2 hr after death (Kutz *et al.*, 1983).

In two cases in which violent convulsions were followed by complete recovery, the concentrations of chlordane in the earliest samples of serum taken were 3.4 and 2.71 ppm, respectively. The levels fell rapidly for 3 or 4 days and then much more slowly; easily detectable levels were still present in the last samples collected over 3 months after the accidents (Curley and Garrettson, 1969; Aldrich and Holmes, 1969). The flexure in the curve for serum is explained largely, if not entirely, by decreasing absorption. In one instance, saline purgatives were given on days 2 and 3 after ingestion, even though the child was essentially well only 16 hr after ingestion. The

resulting stools contained chlordane at concentrations of 719 and 105 ppm, respectively, showing how delayed complete evacuation may be and suggesting that the initial concentration was extremely high. In one of the cases the concentration in fat increased rapidly during the first few days after ingestion and reached an observed maximum of about 35 ppm on day 8, but no sample may have been taken at the exact crest. Three months later, the concentration had fallen only to 25.53 ppm. Somewhat higher chlordane levels might be expected in fatal cases if survival were long enough to permit distribution of the compound to the fat. A half-life of 34 days for the elimination of chlordane was calculated from kinetic studies of a patient who accidentally consumed a chlordane-containing pesticide (Olanoff *et al.*, 1983).

A dog, accidently poisoned by chlordane, had chlordane in his blood and liver at levels of 1.21 and 16 ppm, respectively (Hall, 1974).

Chlordane isomers, as such, have not usually been detected in tisues of the general population. Heptachlor epoxide is found (see Tables 15.12 and 15.13), and undoubtedly a small fraction arises from the heptachlor component of chlordane. It was not until the 1970s that a metabolite peculiar to chlordane was found in people with no special exposure. Biros and Enos (1973) found oxychlordane in 21 of 27 samples of fat obtained from routine postmortem examinations, the mean being 0.14 ppm, with a range of 0.03–0.40 ppm. Identity of the metabolite was confirmed by infrared spectroscopy and mass spectrometry. Later, *trans*-nonachlo, a minor component of both technical chlordane and technical heptachlor, was identified by mass spectometry in composites of fat samples from eight of the nine geographic regions of the United States. The concentrations were <0.1 ppm (Kutz *et al.*, 1976). Levels of *trans*-nonachlor as high as 0.00127 ppm were found in the blood of 11 of 13 persons who drank water from a municipal water system, a part of which had been contaminated by chlordane, presumably through back siphonage. One of these people had an oxychlordane blood level of 0.00037 ppm (Failing *et al.*, 1976). Oxychlordane and *trans*-nonachlor were detected in human milk at average concentrations of 0.005 and 0.001 ppm, respectively (Strassman and Kutz, 1977). *Trans*-nonachlor, oxychlordane, and heptachlor epoxide have been found in the blood of Japanese pest control operators, although at rather low levels (mean, about 0.00089 ppm total). Concentrations in the blood correlated with the number of spraying days in the 3 months prior to sampling (Saito *et al.*, 1986). Kawano and Tatsukawa (1982) also detected chlordanes in the blood of termite control operators but not in workers in other occupations. Most recently oxychlor, *trans*-nonachlor, *trans*-chlordane, *cis*-chlordane (β-chlordane), and *cis*-nonachlor have all been detected in the blood of male and female nonpesticide workers at mean levels ranging from 0.00003 to 0.00046 ppm (Wariishi *et al.*, 1986).

The EEG was normal in three nonfatal cases when it was first recorded 24 or more hours after exposure and when the patients no longer showed neurological signs (Dadey and Kammer, 1953; Curley and Garrettson, 1969; Aldrich and Holmes, 1969). The finding certainly is different from that in poisoning by dieldrin or isobenzan, in which abnormality of the EEG may persist for long periods after clinical recovery. The rapid normalization of the EEG following chlordane poisoning reflects rapid reduction of serum levels and presumably brain levels of chlordane. Whether it has any other significance is not known.

Pathology Autopsy findings in chlordane deaths were what one would expect following violent convulsions of whatever cause, namely visceral congestion, scattered petechial hemorrhages, and microscopic edema of the lungs. These findings are minimal and not diagnostic of chlordane poisoning.

Treatment of Poisoning Treatment is symptomatic (see Section 15.2.5). Heptachlor excretion after chlordane poisoning was increased 10-fold by cholestyramine treatment. Bile concentrations of heptachlor were also increased by cholecystokinin (Garrettson *et al.*, 1985).

15.5.2 HEPTACHLOR

15.5.2.1 Identity, Properties, and Uses

Chemical Name 1,4,5,6,7,8,8-Heptachloro-3a,4,7,7a-tetrahydro-4,7-methanoindane or 1,4,5,6,7,8,8-heptachloro-3a,4,7,7,7a-tetrahydro-4,7-methanol-l*H*-indene.

Structure See Fig. 15.6.

Synonyms Heptachlor (BSI, ICPC, ISO) has been sold under the trade names Drinox®, Heptagran®, and Heptamul®. Code designations include E-3,314, ENT-15,152, and Velsicol-104. The CAS registry number is 76-44-8.

Physical and Chemical Properties Heptachlor has the empirical formula $C_{10}H_5Cl_7$ and a molecular weight of 373.35. The pure material forms white crystals melting at 95–96°C. It has a mild odor similar to that of camphor. Technical heptachlor is a soft wax melting in the range 46–74°C. It contains about 72% heptachlor and 28% related compounds. Heptachlor is stable at temperatures of 150–160°C and in the presence of weak alkali, acid, light, and air. It is not compatible with strong alkali. At 27°C its solubility in grams per 100 ml is: acetone, 75; benzene, 106; carbon tetrachloride, 112; cyclohexanone, 119; xylene, 102; kerosene, 189; and alcohol, 4.5. The solubilities of heptachlor and heptachlor epoxide in water are 0.056 and 0.350 ppm, respectively (Park and Bruce, 1968). The vapor pressure is 3×10^{-4} mm Hg at 25°C, and the density is 1.57–1.59.

History, Formulations, Uses, and Production Heptachlor was first isolated from technical chlordane. Formulations have included dusts (2.5–25%), wettable powders (25%), emulsifiable concentrates (22%), and oil solutions. Heptachlor has been used for control of cotton insects, grasshoppers, soil insects, and certain crop pests. In the United States, the EPA canceled registration of heptachlor for uses other than termite control through subsurface soil treatment and the dipping of nonfood plants [*Fed. Regist.* **40**, 28850 (1975)] after July 1, 1983.

15.5.2.2 Toxicity to Laboratory Animals

Basic Findings Heptachlor causes the same kind of illness as that produced by other cyclodiene insecticides. Gaines (1960) reported oral LD 50 values of 100 and 163 mg/kg for male and female rats, respectively, and corresponding dermal values of 195 and 250 mg/kg. Other investigators have reported oral LD 50 values of 90 mg/kg (Lehman, 1951, 1952) and 55 mg/kg (Stoyanov, 1971). Heptachlor epoxide is somewhat more toxic than heptachlor administered at the same rate and under the same conditions. The fact that the toxicity of heptachlor but not that of the epoxide is increased in animals following the induction of microsomal enzymes (Sperling *et al.*, 1972) suggests that the toxicity of heptachlor is due at least in part to its biotransformation.

Unlike most cyclodiene insecticides, heptachlor is less toxic to female rats (Gaines, 1960), and this is correlated with less storage and greater excretion in females of this species (Kaul *et al.*, 1970).

Eisler (1968) reported no important difference in the toxicity of heptachlor and heptachlor epoxide to rats in 2-year studies. The no-effect level in each instance was 5 ppm (about 0.25 mg/kg/day). The same dietary level, resulting in a dosage of about 0.1 mg/kg/day, was found harmless to dogs in a 60-week study. Characteristic histological changes produced in the rat liver by dosages of 0.35 mg/kg/day for 50 weeks returned to normal during 30 additional weeks without dosing. The fact of reversibility of liver changes following feeding of heptachlor or heptachlor epoxide was confirmed by separate studies using electron microscopy. Reversion was complete within 100 days. The photoisomers of heptachlor and *cis*-chlordane produced by irradiation in acetone are more toxic to rats than the parent chemicals (Podowski *et al.*, 1979). In particular, the photoisomer of heptachlor is about 20 times more toxic to rats than heptachlor itself. Perhaps this is of relevance to the poisoning of horses and cattle kept for a week in an Australian field previously sprayed with heptachlor (Dickson *et al.*, 1984).

Absorption, Distribution, Metabolism, and Excretion Heptachlor is readily absorbed by the skin as well as by the lungs and gastrointestinal tract. In fact, it is only about twice as toxic orally as dermally. Rats retained 77% of heptachlor that they inhaled during a 30-min period (Stubblefield and Dorough, 1979).

The metabolism of heptachlor to heptachlor epoxide was reported by Davidow *et al.* (1951). Newer methods have made possible the identification of other, more easily excreted metabolites, including 1-chloro-3-hydroxychlordene, 1-hydroxychlordene, 1-hydroxy-2,3-epoxychlordene, and a dehydrogenated derivative of the latter (Brooks and Harrison, 1969; Matsumura and Nelson, 1970; Dequidt *et al.*, 1973).

Although hexadecone has no influence on the body clearance of heptachlor, unlike its effects on some other chlorinated hydrocarbons (Rozman, 1984), *trans*-stilbene oxide, an inducer of epoxide hydrolase and glutathione *S*-transferases, significantly decreased the half-life in male Sprague-Dawley rats. Radioactivity from [^{14}C]heptachlor was significantly decreased in fat, kidney, and brain but not in serum by treatment with the *trans*-stilbene oxide (Scheufler and Rozman, 1984). The effect is probably due to increased metabolism of heptachlor epoxide.

In two mares that grazed heptachlor-contaminated pasture, levels of 0.32 and 0.28 ppm heptachlor epoxide were found in blood. These mares survived; another that died had a level of 0.28 ppm in the blood and 49 ppm in the brain (Dickson *et al.*, 1984).

Biochemical Effects The ability of cyclodiene insecticides including heptachlor to induce microsomal enzymes is recorded in Table 3.6. It remains to state that no induction was detectable after feeding heptachlor or heptachlor epoxide to rats for 2 weeks at a dietary level of 1 ppm; induction did occur at 5 ppm (about 0.24 mg/kg/day) (Gillett and Chan, 1968).

Heptachlor was one-third as toxic to weanling male rats fed a 5% casein diet as to pair-fed controls receiving 20% casein, but heptachlor epoxide was equally toxic to animals on these two diets (Weatherholz *et al.*, 1969). Heptachlor was half as toxic to male weanling rats maintained on a gluten diet (10% protein) as to pair-fed rats whose diet was supplemented with casein (18% total protein) (Webb and Miranda, 1973). The differences were due to reduced ability of rats on a restricted diet to mobilize microsomal enzymes (Weatherholtz and Webb, 1971; Miranda *et al.*, 1973). This is consistent with the finding that predosing with phenobarbital increases the toxicity of heptachlor to the newborn (Harbison, 1973).

The effects of heptachlor on gluconeogenic enzymes (Kacew *et al.*, 1973) are similar to those of DDT (see Section 15.3.1.2).

Yamaguchi *et al.* (1979, 1980) have studied the effect of heptachlor epoxide, as an example of neurotoxic cyclodiene insecticides, on the synaptic regions of rat brain. As described elsewhere in this chapter for other insecticides (e.g., BHC; Section 15.4.1.2), heptachlor epoxide appears to cause an inhibition of Ca^{2+},Mg^{2+}-ATPase. This results in increased availability of Ca^{2+} to synaptic vesicles, causing an induced increase in transmitter release.

Effects on Organs and Tissues It was reported by Mestitzová (1967) that heptachlor at a dosage of 6.9 mg/kg/day increased the incidence of cataracts in rats, especially young ones born to treated mothers. The failure of others to make this observation raises a question of the identity of the pesticide used in the study. No cataract was found in any of thousands of rats and many dogs fed heptachlor or heptachlor epoxide at dietary concentrations as high as 12.5 ppm for periods as long as 2 years (Eisler, 1968). This dietary level, which is far higher than that ever encountered by people, determines dosages of approximately 0.6 and 0.26 mg/kg/day in rats and dogs, respectively.

Heptachlor was reported to cause "chromosomal mutations" as evidenced by increased resorption of fetuses and by morphological change of chromosomes (Cerey *et al.*, 1973; Sram, 1974). However, no dominant lethal changes were produced when male mice received a 1 : 3 mixture of heptachlor and heptachlor epoxide at a total dosage of 7.5 or 15 mg/kg (Arnold *et al.*, 1977).

The question of the carcinogenicity of chlorinated hydrocarbon insecticides is discussed in Section 15.2.3.2. It may be mentioned here that a few large doses of heptachlor given to suckling rats did not increase the incidence of tumors during an observation period of 106–110 weeks (Cabral *et al.*, 1972), and like other members of the chlorinated hydrocarbon insecticides, heptachlor promotes tumors initiated by diethylnitrosamine (Williams and Numoto, 1984), perhaps by inhibiting intracellular communication (Telang *et al.*, 1982). IARC Working Groups (IARC, 1976, 1982) considered the evidence inconclusive regarding the tumorigenicity of heptachlor in the rat. However, an increase in the incidence of hepatomas in the livers of male and female mice fed either heptachlor or heptachlor epoxide at a dietary level of 10 ppm has been reported (NCI, 1977c; Reuber, 1977a), and this and other studies have recently been reviewed (Reuber, 1987).

Thrombosis of the hepatic vein leading to infarcts of the liver were reported in 10.5% of male and female mice that had received heptachlor or heptachlor epoxide at a dietary level of 10 ppm. Thrombosis occurred in either the presence or absence of hepatomas (Reuber, 1977b).

Effects on Reproduction Administration of heptachlor at a rate of 10 mg/kg/day for 3 days significantly reduced the increase in weight of the ovary produced by simultaneous administration of human chorionic gonadotropin in prepubertal female rats. Heptachlor did not produce pathology or alter ovary weight when given alone (Odler, 1973).

A dosage of 6.9 mg/kg/day for 3 days significantly reduced fertility of rats and also the survival of young during the first weeks by about one-third; this effect was found more sensitive than tests of liver and kidney function (Mestizová and Beño, 1966; Mestitzová, 1967). Essentially similar results were reported for dosages of 5 and 10 mg/kg/day, and some fetal anomalies as well as resorptions were encountered. A dosage of 1 mg/kg/day apparently was harmless to reproduction (Rosival *et al.*, 1972). This negative result confirmed an earlier report of a three-generation study of rats using heptachlor at dietary levels up to 10 ppm and another using a 3 : 1 mixture of heptachlor and heptachlor epoxide at levels up to 7 ppm (about 0.35 mg/kg/day except in lactating females, in which dosage is markedly increased) (Eisler, 1968). More recently, Yamaguchi *et al.* (1987) found no increases in fetal mortality or malformation when heptachlor was administered to pregnant rats (days 7–17) at doses up to 20 mg/kg/day.

15.5.2.3 Toxicity to Humans

In January 1982, the milk supply on Oahu Island, Hawaii, was discovered to be contaminated with heptachlor (Smith, 1982).

The origin of the heptachlor was apparently foliage from pineapple plants treated with the pesticide which had been used as cattle feed. Using stored milk samples, it was possible to state that for over 2 years milk had been sold containing levels of heptachlor significantly in excess of the EPA "action level" (Smith, 1982; see also references quoted in LeMarchand *et al.,* 1986). At the time there was considerable concern that the newborn and unborn might be at risk. However, analysis of the incidence rates for 23 major congenital malformations failed to demonstrate increased incidence associated with heptachlor contamination of milk (LeMarchand *et al.,* 1986). A group of farm family members who had consumed milk contaminated with heptachlor were analyzed for serum heptachlor epoxide and oxychlordane levels. Compared to a control group, 22% of the farm family had elevated levels, but this was not accompanied by any measurable hepatic effects (Stehr-Green *et al.,* 1988).

Blood disorders (leukemias, production defects, and thrombocytopenic purpura) have been catalogued following home termite treatment with chlordane or heptachlor, but proof of a direct causal effect is lacking (Epstein and Ozonoff, 1987).

Among persons with miscellaneous occupational exposure to pesticides, heptachlor was found in blood concentrations ranging from 0.000 to 0.069 ppm, but an increase of heptachlor epoxide was small or absent (Siyali, 1972). Heptachlor generally is not detectable in tissues of the general population, but the epoxide is often found in fat (Table 15.12), blood (Table 15.13), organs, and milk. A material indistinguishable from heptachlor has been reported in the urine of ordinary people (Cueto and Biros, 1967).

The threshold limit of heptachlor (0.5 mg/m^3) indicates that occupational intake of about 0.07 mg/kg/day is considered safe.

Treatment of Poisoning   Treatment is symptomatic (see Section 15.2.5).

15.5.3 ALDRIN

Aldrin is rapidly metabolized to dieldrin by a wide range of organisms, including humans. One result is that aldrin has not been found in people of the general population or even in the body fat of people engaged in making it; only traces are found in the blood of people who make and formulate it. Persons acutely poisoned by aldrin make the conversion so rapidly that one might speculate that all the toxicity is from dieldrin. However, the toxicity of 6,7-dihydroaldrin, which is incapable of forming an epoxide, is indirect evidence that aldrin is toxic *per se* in spite of evidence that an oxygen bridge facilitates toxicity (Brooks, 1973). Aldrin and dieldrin are described separately because aldrin is a toxic compound in its own right and there is inconclusive evidence that aldrin is more likely to cause kidney or chromosomal damage. New evidence would be required to confirm these differences.

15.5.3.1 Identity, Properties, and Uses

Chemical Name   Aldrin is 1,2,3,4,10,10-hexachloro-1,4,4a,5,8,8a-hexahydro-*endo*-1,4-*exo*-5,8-dimethanonaphthalene.

Structure   See Fig. 15.6.

Synonyms   In the United States, the United Kingdom, and a number of other countries, aldrin (BSI, ISO) stands for formulations containing not less than 95% of the compound named above and not more than 5% of insecticidally active related compounds. In Canada, Denmark, and the USSR, aldrin stands for the pure compound. In France, the word is spelled aldrine. The word HHDN (ISO) also is recognized as a nonproprietary name and means, of course, the pure chemical. The word aldrin bears the same relationship to HHDN as dieldrin bears to HEOD (see Section 15.5.4). However, in this book, aldrin is used to mean the pure chemical, and technical aldrin is specified when necessary. Proprietary names include Aldrex®, Altox, Drinox, Octalene®, and Toxadrin®. Code designations for aldrin include Compound-118, ENT-15,949, and OMS-194. The CAS registry number is 309-00-2.

Physical and Chemical Properties   Aldrin has the empirical formula $C_{12}H_8Cl_6$ and a molecular weight of 364.93. The pure compound is an odorless, white, crystalline solid melting at 104–104.5°C and boiling at 145°C at 2 mm Hg.

Technical aldrin contains not less than 90% aldrin defined as a mixture, that is, not less than 85.5% of the main ingredient, not less than 4.5% of insecticidally active related compounds, and not more than 10% of other compounds. Technical aldrin is a tan to dark brown with a mild "chemical" odor and a melting point in the range 49–60°C. Aldrin is stable with alkali and alkali-oxidizing agents. It is stable with dilute acid but not with concentrated mineral acids, acid catalysts, acid-oxidizing agents, phenols, or active metals. It is not flammable. Aldrin is compatible with most pesticides and fertilizers. It is moderately soluble in paraffins, aromatics, halogenated solvents, esters, and ketones but sparingly soluble in alcohols. According to Park and Bruce (1968), the solubility of aldrin in water is 0.027 ppm. The vapor pressure is 6×10^{-6} mm Hg at 25°C, and the density is 1.70 at 20°C.

History, Formulations, and Uses   Aldrin was first described by Kearnes *et al.* (1949) and described in greater detail by Lidov *et al.* (1950). It is active against insects by contact or ingestion. It has been formulated as a seed dressing (75%), wettable powders (20–40%), dust concentrates (75%), low-percentage dusts, granules (2–25%), emulsifiable concentrates (24–48%), and mixtures (0.4–2%) with fertilizer. Aldrin has been used mainly against insects, primarily soil insects, which attack field, forage, vegetable, and fruit crops. It is not phytotoxic. It is translocated short distances in some plants, and it gives an off flavor to a few foods, notably jam made from strawberries raised in treated soil.

15.5.3.2 Toxicity to Laboratory Animals

Basic Findings The illness produced by aldrin in animals is indistinguishable from that caused by other cyclodiene insecticides. The distinction between the symptomatology associated with these compounds and that associated with DDT is discussed in Section 15.2.1.

The toxicity of single and repeated doses of aldrin in experimental animals is given in Tables 15.23 and 15.24. Technical aldrin made by the Straus process, last used in 1952, was substantially more toxic than that made by the thermal process. The chemical nature of the impurities responsible for the greater toxicity of the Straus product was not investigated (Ball *et al.*, 1953).

The dermal toxicity is only a little less than the oral toxicity. Rabbits survived no more than 10 dermal doses at the rate of 5 mg/kg/day (Lehman, 1951, 1952).

Absorption, Distribution, Metabolism, and Excretion
The conversion of aldrin to dieldrin by mammals has been demonstrated many times (Treon and Cleveland, 1955; Winteringham and Barnes, 1955; Bann *et al.*, 1956; Ivey *et al.*, 1961). The conversion occurs also in lower animals, plants, and microorganisms.

Metabolism of aldrin to dieldrin in mammals is not confined to the liver. It was detectable within the first 3 min after aldrin was added to the perfusion fluid entering isolated rabbit lung

Table 15.23
Single Dose LD 50 for Aldrin

Species	Route	LD 50 (mg/kg)	Reference
Rat	oral	67	Lehman (1951, 1952)
Rat, M	oral	54[a]	Ball *et al.* (1953)
Rat, F	oral	56[a]	Ball *et al.* (1953)
Rat, M	oral	43[b]	Ball *et al.* (1953)
Rat, F	oral	44[b]	Ball *et al.* (1953)
Rat, M	oral	14[c]	Ball *et al.* (1953)
Rat, F	oral	10[c]	Ball *et al.* (1953)
Rat, M	oral	45	Klimmer (1955)
Rat, M	oral	50	Klimmer (1955)
Rat, M	oral	49	Treon and Cleveland (1955)
Rat, F	oral	45	Treon and Cleveland (1955)
Rat, F	oral	74[b]	Treon and Cleveland (1955)
Rat, F	oral	25[c]	Treon and Cleveland (1955)
Rat, M	oral	39	Gaines (1960)
Rat, F	oral	60	Gaines (1960)
Rat, M	dermal	98[d]	Gaines (1960)
Rat, F	dermal	98[d]	Gaines (1960)
Rabbit	dermal	150[e]	Lehman (1951, 1952)
Rabbit	dermal	600–1250[f]	Treon and Cleveland (1955)

[a] Recrystallized aldrin.
[b] Aldrin made by thermal process available in 1952 and later.
[c] Aldrin made by Straus process.
[d] Applied as xylene solution.
[e] Applied as dimethyl phthalate solution.
[f] Applied as a dry powder.

preparations. Following a period of rapid uptake by the lung, the concentration of aldrin plus dieldrin reached a steady state in the perfusion fluid leaving the lung, but the ratio changed so that there was more dieldrin and less aldrin. The rate of metabolism detected did not reach a steady state during the brief period the preparation could be maintained (Mehendale *et al.*, 1974; Mehendale and El-Bassiouni, 1975).

Brandt and Hogman (1980) have examined by autoradiography the distribution of [14C]aldrin and [14C]dieldrin given to pregnant mice. Interestingly, they observed a slow but persistent uptake of both chemicals into cartilaginous tissue of both the mothers and fetuses.

Because aldrin epoxidation has been used as an assay for low-level cytochrome P-450 activity in a variety of animal tissues, cell lines, and human liver biopsies, the mechanism has been examined in some detail. Not only cytochrome P-450 induced by phenobarbital catalyzes this oxidation but also a cytochrome P-450 species induced by cyanopregnenolone. Aldrin does not, however, appear to be a substrate for the 3-methylcholanthrene-induced types of cytochrome P-450 (Wolff *et al.*, 1980; Newman and Guzelian, 1983). Most recently, Wolff and Guengerich (1987) have examined the specificities of cytochrome P-450 species for aldrin epoxidation in more detail and explored the effects of rat strain, age, sex, and physiological status. A novel aldrin metabolite, *endo*-dieldrin, was formed with one particular purified cytochrome P-450 in a sixfold excess over dieldrin (the *exo* isomer).

In extrahepatic tissues such as granuloma cells and seminal vesicles, oxidation may occur by prostaglandin endoperoxide synthase and other mechanisms involving peroxidation (Lang and Maier, 1986; Lang *et al.*, 1986).

Because aldrin is so generally metabolized to dieldrin, its further metabolism is discussed in Section 15.5.4.2.

The simultaneous administration of aldrin and DDT may alter storage of both of them, as discussed in Section 15.2.2.3.

Effects on Organs and Tissues The minimal intraperitoneal dosage of aldrin that induced chromosomal aberrations in marrow cells of both rats and mice was 9.56 mg/kg (Georgian, 1975). Usha Rani *et al.* (1980) have reported negative results at a dose of 13 mg/kg. Although some studies (see Table 15.24) have reported tumors caused by chronic administration of aldrin, Deichmann *et al.* (1978) have been unable to confirm some of these findings. Ritper has analyzed findings from six cancer studies of aldrin and dieldrin in rats and mice and failed to find reasons for discrepancies between studies (Ritper, 1979; also see NCI, 1978e).

Nephrosis has been observed in goats that were drenched with aldrin (2.5 mg/kg) every day for 21 days. Many convoluted tubules showed almost complete necrosis of the lining of the epithelial cells. Hyperplasia of the thyroid was also severe in all animals compared to controls (K. K. Singh *et al.*, 1985). Kidney damage has also been observed in dogs (Treon and Cleveland, 1955) and rats (Reuber, 1980b) after chronic administration of aldrin.

Table 15.24
Effect on Various Animals of Repeated Oral Doses of Aldrin

Dosage Range (mg/kg/day)	Method and concentration (ppm)	Species, number, and sex	Duration	Results	Reference
2.6–5	75 ppm in diet	rat, 5 M, 5 F	26 wk	survival good; increased liver weight ratio in both sexes	Treon and Cleveland (1955)
1.26–2.5	5 mg/kg/day	dog, 2		100% fatal within 24 days	Fitzhugh et al. (1964)
	50 ppm in diet	rat, 12 M, 12 F	2 yr	slight increase in mortality; increased liver weight ratio	FAO/WHO (1965)
0.626–1.25	1.5 mg/kg/day	puppy, 2 M, 1 F		fatal within 38 days	Treon and Cleveland (1955)
	2 mg/kg/day	dog, 2		100% fatal within 24 days to 1 year	Fitzhugh et al. (1964)
	20 ppm in diet	rat, 25	1 yr	increased body weight; disturbed estrus	Ball et al. (1953)
	25 ppm in diet	rat, 5 M, 5 F	26 wk	increased liver weight ratio in M	Treon and Cleveland (1955)
	25 ppm in diet	rat, 40 M, 40 F	2 yr	increased liver weight ratio; characteristic liver changes	Treon and Cleveland (1955)
	10 ppm in diet	mouse, 215	2 yr	shortening of life span; increase in benign liver tumors	Davis and Fitzhugh (1962)
	10 ppm in diet	mouse	2 yr	increased liver tumors	Reuber (1976)
	1 mg/kg/day	dog, 2		100% fatal in 1 year	Fitzhugh et al. (1964)
	1 mg/kg/day	heifer	448 days	ECG changes, no clinical effect	Rumsey and Bond (1972)
0.313–0.625	10 ppm in diet	rat, 25	1 yr	increased body weight; disturbed estrus	Ball et al. (1953)
	12.5 ppm in diet	rat, 40 M, 40 F	2 yr	increased liver weight ratio; characteristic liver changes	Treon and Cleveland (1955)
	10 ppm in diet	rat, 12M, 12F	2 yr	characteristic liver changes; increased tumors	FAO/WHO (1965)
	0.5 mg/kg/day	dog, 4	2 yr	one animal with convulsions	Fitzhugh et al. (1964)
0.156–0.313	5 ppm in diet	rat, 25	1 yr	changes not statistically significant	Ball et al. (1953)
	5 ppm in diet	rat, 5 M, 5 F	26 wk	liver changes same as control	Treon and Cleveland (1955)
	0.2 mg/kg/day	dog, 2	2 yr	no effect	Fitzhugh et al. (1964)
0.0781–0.156	2.5 ppm in diet	rat, 40 M, 40 F	2 yr	increased liver weight ratio in M, characteristic liver changes	Treon and Cleveland (1955)
	2 ppm in diet	rat, 12 M, 12 F	2 yr	characteristic liver changes; increased tumors	FAO/WHO (1965)
0.0390–0.0781	3 ppm in diet	dog, 2 M, 2 F	68 wk	increase in liver weight ratio	Treon and Cleveland (1955)
0.0193–0.0390	1 ppm in diet	dog, 2 M, 2 F	68 wk	kidney damage in F	Treon and Cleveland (1955)
0.0096–0.0193	0.5 ppm in diet	rat, 12 M, 12 F	2 yr	minimal increase in characteristic liver changes, increased tumors	FAO/WHO (1965)

Effects on Reproduction Dogs were able to reproduce when receiving oral doses at the rate of 0.2–2.0 mg/kg/day, but the pups died early, probably because of high levels of dieldrin in the milk of the dams (Kitselman, 1953).

In a three-generation test in rats, the number of pregnancies was reduced and the mortality of pups was severely increased at maternal dietary levels of 12.5 and 25 ppm (about 0.65 and 1.3 mg/kg/day except during lactation, when the dosage is much higher). At a dietary level of about 2.5 ppm (about 0.4 mg/kg/day during lactation) there was a slight to moderate increase in mortality of the pups (Treon and Cleveland, 1955).

15.5.3.3 Toxicity to Humans

Accidents and Use Experience Serious poisoning by aldrin usually involves convulsions and is entirely similar to poisoning by dieldrin (see Section 15.5.4) (Pietsch et al., 1969; Ka-zantzis et al., 1964), but a 3-year-old girl died following collapse and coma after only brief excitation and ataxia at onset (WHO, 1959). Hematuria and/or albuminuria has been noted in several cases, including some that were occupational in origin with no solvent to complicate the situation (Spiotta, 1951; Nelson, 1953).

There have been at least three outbreaks of poisoning involving a total of 53 people and caused by the consumption of seed grain treated with aldrin, sometimes in combination with other pesticides. None of the cases in Kenya involved convulsions, but five of the most severe ones there did involve unequal pupils with the smaller pupil unreactive to light and the larger reacting only sluggishly (WHO, 1958). A family outbreak in India, caused in part by BHC, occurred only after treated grain had been eaten for 6–12 months. In addition to myoclonic jerks and convulsions, the patients complained of lack of concentration, mild loss of memory, visual flashes of light and color, and of noise in their ears. EEG changes were characteristic. The most interesting finding was that diazepam was more effective than phenobarbital in controlling both the clinical and EEG features of poisoning (Gupta, 1975).

The work environment of people exposed to aldrin and related compounds can be regulated so that they remain healthy as judged by symptomatology and an impressive array of medical examinations (Princi and Spurbeck, 1951; Jager, 1970).

Acute erythematobullous dermatitis following contact with aldrin has been reported (D'Eramo and Croce, 1960), but dermatitis associated with aldrin is unusual.

Atypical Cases of Various Origins A gardener developed general malaise and giddiness 2 hr after dusting crops with 2.5% aldrin powder without observing precautions. Later he developed cyanosis, discomfort in his chest, muscular twitches about the eyelids and in the extremities, muscular weakness, incoordination, and paresthesias of the extremities. The incoordination and paresthesias lasted several months, (Frast and Poulsen, 1959). The syptoms, with the exception of paresthesias, suggest anticholinesterase poisoning, and paresthesia is not typical of aldrin poisoning. The persistence of illness is not characteristic of aldrin, or of anticholinesterases for that matter. Under the circumstances, the toxicant, if any, is open to question.

Death certainly could result from excessive exposure to aldrin. However, symptoms were not typical of aldrin in the death of a wine grower who had sprayed this compound (Symanski, 1968), and no evidence of excessive exposure was reported.

A unique case involved a 34-year-old aldrin factory worker who had had headache periodically for a year. His acute illness began at home with nausea, headache, and weakness. Although he had no further exposure, he became progressively worse and by day 4 had severe lumbar pain and albuminuria. By day 6 his face was badly swollen, and on day 13 neither kidney could be visualized when an intravenous pyelogram was attempted. It was not until day 14 that he developed epileptiform seizures with loss of consciousness. On conservative therapy for uremia and progressive renal failure, he recovered during the next 2 weeks. A renal biopsy 6 weeks after onset revealed disseminated nephrosis in a recovery stage, numerous protein casts, and multiple foci of "incipient" glomerulosclerosis (Fischer, 1966). Although some kidney injury has been observed in undoubted cases of aldrin poisoning, the relationship in the 34-year-old worker was circumstantial, and the convulsion was more likely related to azotemia than to aldrin. A distinction could have been made by analysis of serum for aldrin and dieldrin, but no analysis was reported.

Equally circumstantial was the connection between aldrin and a case of motor polyneuropathy ascribed to it by Jenkins and Toole (1964). The same applies to a case of aplastic anemia attributed to aldrin (Pick *et al.*, 1965).

Dosage Response A 3-year-old girl who was stricken 5 min after eating a cooked meal contaminated with aldrin and who died 12 hr later was thought to have consumed 120 mg of aldrin, resulting in a dosage of about 8.2 mg/kg (WHO, 1959). A 23-year-old man who intentionally drank aldrin at a dose of 25.6 mg/kg was very seriously poisoned, although eventually he recovered completely (Spiotta, 1951). One must seriously question the accuracy of the estimate of 30,000 mg as the dose taken with suicidal intent by a 17-year-old woman who lived (Phokas *et al.*, 1960).

The threshold limit value for aldrin (0.25 mg/m^3) indicates that occupational exposure at a rate of about 0.036 mg/kg/day is considered safe.

Laboratory Findings There apparently are no analytical results in connection with a fatal case. In a nonfatal case mentioned by Dale *et al.* (1966b) in which a 34-year-old man drank aldrin while drunk, the initial concentration of aldrin in the plasma was 0.036 ppm, but the concentration of dieldrin in the same sample was already 0.279 ppm. A fat sample taken 3 days after ingestion contained aldrin and dieldrin at concentrations of 5.23 and 22.26 ppm, respectively. No aldrin or metabolite was detected in any of several urine samples.

Unchanged aldrin was found at concentrations as high as 0.0039 ppm (Hayes and Curley, 1968) or even slightly over 0.1 ppm (Mick *et al.*, 1972) in the plasma of some men engaged in making or formulating the compound. No aldrin could be detected in the fat or urine of the same men.

In a case of acute aldrin poisoning with complete recovery, dieldrin was found in a concentration of 40 ppm in a fat biopsy taken 2 weeks later; no aldrin was detected. Earlier reports based on older analytical methods indicated lower concentrations in other cases (Bell, 1960). Unmetabolized aldrin is not usually found in the blood, fat, or other tissues of the general population.

As mentioned in Section 15.5.3.2, aldrin epoxidase has been used as a sensitive measurement of cytochrome P-450-mediated activities. Studies of this activity have been conducted with human liver biopsies (Williams *et al.*, 1982). It has also been used in human cytochrome P-450 polymorphism investigations (McManus *et al.*, 1984) and to study drug-metabolizing activities of tumors of human colon and rectum (Siegers *et al.*, 1984).

Treatment of Poisoning Treatment is symptomatic (see Section 15.2.5).

15.5.4 DIELDRIN

When the word dieldrin was established as a nonproprietary name by the Interdepartmental Committee on Pest Control (ICPC), it was common to define such names in terms of technical products. Specifically, dieldrin was defined as containing not less than 85% HEOD and not more than 15% of insecticidally active, related compounds. This usage was perpetuated by the International Organization for Standardization (ISO). Many authors use the term HEOD (an acronym for the chemical name) in order to specify the pure chemical. In this chapter, "dieldrin" designates the pure chemical and the term "technical dieldrin" is used when it is necessary to make a distinction.

15.5.4.1 Identity, Properties, and Uses

Chemical Name Dieldrin is 1,2,3,4,10,10-hexachloro-6,7-epoxy-1,4,4a,5,6,7,8,8a-octahydro-*endo*-1,4-*exo*-5,8-dimethanonaphthalene.

Structure See Fig. 15.6

Synonyms In most countries, the common name dieldrin (BSI, ESA, ICPC, ISO) stands for the technical product. However, in the USSR the same common name designates the pure compound. The word HEOD (BSI, ISO) also is recognized as a common name. Proprietary names include Alvit®, Octalox®, Panoram®, and Quintox®. Code designations for dieldrin have included Compound-497, ENT-16,225, and OMS-18. The CAS registry number is 60-57-1.

Physical and Chemical Properties Dieldrin has the empirical formula $C_{12}H_8Cl_6O$ and a molecular weight of 380.93. Pure dieldrin is a white, crystalline, odorless solid that melts at 176–177°C. Technical dieldrin contains not less than 95% of the 85%/15% mixture—in other words, not less than 80.75% HEOD, not less than 14.25% insecticidally active related compounds, and not over 5% of other compounds. The technical material consists of buff to light brown flakes with a mild "chemical" odor and a melting point of not less than 95°C. Dieldrin is stable to alkali, mild acids, and light. It reacts with concentrated mineral acids, acid catalysts, acid-oxidizing agents, phenols, and active metals. It is noncorrosive and nonflammable. It is slightly soluble in mineral oils, other aliphatic hydrocarbons, and alcohols; moderately soluble in acetone; and soluble in aromatic and halogenated solvents. According to Park and Bruce (1968), the solubility of dieldrin in water is 0.186 ppm at "room temperature." Whether some dieldrin dissolved in water was lost by adsorption during filtration is unclear. The vapor pressure is 1.8×10^{-7} mm Hg at 25°C. Its density is 1.70 at 20°C.

History, Formulations, and Uses The insecticidal properties of dieldrin were described first by Kearnes *et al.* (1949).

According to the experts gathered for a joint meeting (FAO/WHO, 1968), the annual world production of aldrin and dieldrin was believed to be in the order of 10,000 tons annually, of which aldrin represented the major portion. Three-quarters or more of the total production was used in agricultural fields, principally for soil treatment.

Dieldrin also was used in tropical countries as a residual spray on the inside walls and ceilings of homes for the control of vectors of diseases, mainly malaria. Zavon and Hamman (1961) stated that 9301 million pounds of dieldrin were used for public health purposes in 55 countries during the period

1952–1958. This would be 4,218,933 tons/year, a value in total disagreement with the value of 10,000 tons/year total production listed above. In temperate regions its use in homes generally was confined to cracks, crevices, and other spot treatments.

15.5.4.2 Toxicity to Laboratory Animals

Basic Findings In general, the effects of dieldrin are similar to those of other cyclodiene insecticides (see Section 15.2.1). Apparently, dieldrin is the only one of these compounds that has produced notable loss of appetite (Keane and Zavon, 1969b) or even complete refusal of food in animals (Hayes *et al.*, 1951).

The toxicity of single and repeated doses of dieldrin is shown in Tables 15.25 and 15.26. The compound is one of moderate oral toxicity. However, it is almost as toxic by the dermal as by the oral route. Its relatively high dermal toxicity does not depend on solution; very finely ground dieldrin powder is almost as poisonous as solutions of the compound (Hayes *et al.*, 1951). Undoubtedly, relatively extensive absorption by the dermal route has been an important factor leading to occupational poisoning by dieldrin.

The photoconversion isomer of dieldrin is more toxic than dieldrin to mice (Rosen and Sutherland, 1967), rats, or dogs (Walker *et al.*, 1971), but this may be of no importance under practical conditions. Although the compound is called "photodieldrin," it is formed by microorganisms (Matsumura *et al.*, 1970) as well as by light. The compound is actively metabolized to relatively water-soluble compounds by rats, rabbits, mosquito larvae, cabbages, and certain fungi. The ratio of excretion by urine and feces is opposite in rats and rabbits (Klein *et al.*, 1969a,b). In rats, the 90-day toxicity of pho-

Table 15.25
Single Dose LD 50 for Dieldrin

Species	Route	LD 50 (mg/kg)	Reference
Rat	oral	87	Lehman (1951, 1952)
Rat, M	oral	47	Treon and Cleveland (1955)
Rat, F	oral	38	Treon and Cleveland (1955)
Rat, M	oral	46	Gaines (1960)
Rat, F	oral	46	Gaines (1960)
Rat, M[a]	oral	167	Lu *et al.* (1965)
Rat, M[b]	oral	24	Lu *et al.* (1965)
Rat, M[c]	oral	37	Lu *et al.* (1965)
Rat, M	dermal	90[d]	Gaines (1960)
Rat, F	dermal	60[d]	Gaines (1960)
Rabbit	dermal	<150[e]	Lehman (1951, 1952)
Rabbit	dermal	400–450	Johnson and Eden (1953)
Rabbit	dermal	250–350[f]	Treon and Cleveland (1955)

[a] Newborn.
[b] Preweanling.
[c] Adult.
[d] Applied as xylene solution.
[e] Applied as 4% dimethyl phthalate solution.
[f] Applied as a dry powder.

Table 15.26
Effect on Various Animals of Repeated Oral Doses of Dieldrin

Dosage					
Range (mg/kg/day)	Method and concentration (ppm)	Species, number, and sex	Duration	Results	Reference
2.6–5.0	50 ppm in diet	rat 100 M, 100 F	life span	convulsions, but fewer tumors than controls	Deichman et al. (1970)
	50 ppm in diet	rat 12 M, 12 F	2 yr	some increase in mortality	Fitzhugh et al. (1964)
	5 mg/kg/day	dog, 2		both died within 35 days	Fitzhugh et al. (1964)
	2.5 mg/kg/day	sheep		toxicity in 100%; behavioral decrement within 37 days	Schnorr (1973)
	4 mg/kg/day	sheep	4 wk	fatal to 50%	Davison (1970a)
1.26–2.5	30 ppm in diet	rat 100 M, 100 F	life span	convulsions but fewer convulsions than control	Deichmann et al. (1970)
	2 mg/kg/day	dog, 2		all died within 35 days	Fitzhugh et al. (1964)
	180 ppm in diet	hamster 41 M, 38 F	life span	1 M and 1 F with liver tumors	Cabral et al. (1979b)
0.626–1.25	20 ppm in diet	rat 100 M, 100 F	life span	convulsions but fewer tumors than control	Deichmann et al. (1970)
	25 ppm in diet	rat 6 M, 6 F	2–8 mo	no illness but cytoplasmic change in liver	Ortega et al. (1957)
	25 ppm in diet	rat 20 M, 20 F	2 yr	characteristic liver changes	Treon and Cleveland (1955)
	10 ppm in diet	mouse	2 yr	shortening of life span; increase of benign liver tumors	Davis and Fitzhugh (1962)
	10 ppm in diet	mouse 30 M, 30 F		shorter lifespan, increased liver size and tumors	Walker et al. (1973) Thorpe and Walker (1973)
	10 ppm in diet	mouse 100 M, 100 F	2 yr	life span 2 yr shorter; increased tumors	Davis and Fitzhugh (1962)
	10 ppm in diet	mouse	2 yr	increased liver tumors	Reuber (1976)
	1 mg/kg/day	dog, 2	25 mo	all died within 1 yr; convulsions, fatty liver	Fitzhugh et al. (1964)
0.312–0.625	10 ppm in diet	rat 12 M, 12 F	2 yr	characteristic liver changes; increased tumors	Fitzhugh et al. (1964)
	10 ppm in diet	rat 25 M, 25 F	2 yr	animals irritable; increased liver weight ratio in F; characteristic liver changes; no increase in tumors	Walker et al. (1969) Stevenson et al. (1976)
	12.5 ppm in diet	rat 20 M, 20 F	2 yr	characteristic liver changes	Treon and Cleveland (1955)
	5 ppm in diet	mouse		no illness	Walker et al. (1973)
	25 ppm in diet	dog, 4	25 mo	all died within 33 days	Treon and Cleveland (1955)
	0.5 mg/kg/day	dog, 4	25 mo	most died within 1 yr; convulsions, fatty liver	Fitzhugh et al. (1964)
	0.5 mg/kg/day	sheep		no behavioral or other effect	Fitzhugh et al. (1964)
0.156–0.312	2.5 ppm in diet	mouse		no illness	Walker et al. (1973)
	0.2 mg/kg/day	dog, 2	25 mo	no effect	Fitzhugh et al. (1964)
0.078–0.156	2 ppm in diet	rat 12 M, 12 F	2 yr	characteristic liver changes; increased tumors	Fitzhugh et al. (1964)
	2.5 ppm in diet	rat 6 M, 6 F	2–8 mo	no illness but cytoplasmic changes in liver	Ortega et al. (1957)
	2.5 ppm in diet	rat 20 M, 20 F	2 yr	characteristic liver changes	Treon and Cleveland (1955)
	1.0 ppm in diet	mouse		no illness; no clinical enlargement of liver; no decrease of survival	Walker et al. (1973)
0.039–0.078	1.0 ppm in diet	rat 25 M, 25 F	2 yr	increased liver weight ratio in F	Walker et al. (1969) Stevenson et al. (1976)
	0.05 mg/kg/day	dog 5 M, 5 F	2 yr	increased plasma alkaline phosphatase, decreased serum protein, increased liver weight ratio in F	Walker et al. (1969)
	3 ppm	dog 2 M, 2 F	68 wk	increased liver weight ratio; kidney changes in 1 F	Treon and Cleveland (1955)
	2.5 ppm in diet	monkey	6 yr	microsomal enzyme induction only	Wright et al. (1978)

(continued)

Table 15.26   (*Continued*)

| Dosage | | | | | |
Range (mg/kg/day)	Method and concentration (ppm)	Species, number, and sex	Duration	Results	Reference
0.019–0.039	0.5 ppm in diet	rat 12 M, 12 F	2 yr	minimal liver changes	Fitzhugh *et al.* (1964)
	1.75 ppm in diet	monkey	6 yr	microsomal enzyme induction only	Weight *et al.* (1978)
0.009–0.019	1 ppm in diet	dog 2 M, 2 F	68 wk	liver enlarged but no histological changes	Treon and Cleveland (1955)
0.004–0.009	0.1 ppm in diet	rat 25 M, 25 F	2 yr	no effect	Walker *et al.* (1969) Stevenson *et al.* (1976)
	0.005 mg/kg/day	dog 5 M, 5 F	2 yr	decreased heart rate in M	Walker *et al.* (1969)

todieldrin is essentially identical to that of dieldrin, even though photodieldrin is stored to a lesser degree (Walton *et al.*, 1971).

Absorption, Distribution, Metabolism, and Excretion   Dieldrin is absorbed from the gastrointestinal tract via the hepatic portal vein rather than via the thoracic lymph duct like DDT (Heath and Vandekar, 1964; Iatropoulos *et al.*, 1975; Mueller *et al.*, 1978). The high toxicity of dieldrin when applied to the skin is evidence for the rapid absorption of the compound by that route.

Hemoglobin is largely but not entirely responsible for binding dieldrin in erythrocytes (Moss and Hathaway, 1964). Tanaka *et al.* (1981) have concluded that dieldrin is relatively slowly absorbed from the small intestine, peak blood levels occurring in rats 2.5 hr after administration. In serum, dieldrin was bound to lipoprotein and globulins and to a lesser extent albumin.

Following an oral dosage of 10 mg/kg that produced no overt illness, the concentration of dieldrin in the brain reached a maximal level in 4 hr and gradually decreased thereafter. The concentration in muscle remained essentially steady during the interval from 4 to 48 hr; there was no peak for muscle that could be interpreted as replacing a peak for the brain. The concentration of dieldrin in fat was already slightly higher than that in the brain at 1 hr, very much higher at 4 hr when the concentration in the brain was maximal, and the concentration in the fat continued to increase during the first 24 hr. Either on the basis of concentration or on the basis of the total amount in each organ, no reason was found to assign any special importance to muscle as a sink into which dieldrin is redistributed from the brain. The fat appears to be far more important in this regard. The same results were obtained in a smaller number of rats killed quickly by 150 mg/kg or more slowly by 75 mg/kg. The ratios of concentrations of dieldrin in individual tissues compared to that of the brain were essentially identical, regardless of dosage (Hayes, 1974).

The retention of dieldrin following the feeding of aldrin with the diet to four generations (P, F_1, F_2, and F_3) led to a significant increase in the concentrations of dieldrin in abdominal fat and in the lipids of the total carcass and to significantly increased retention of dieldrin in the total carcass in the second generation (F_1), with some further but statistically not significant increases in concentration and total retention of dieldrin in the F_2 and F_3 generations of mice. In the fifth (F_4) generation of experimental mice, born of parents that carried a considerable load of dieldrin but fed from weaning to age 260 days on the control diet, complete body depletion of dieldrin resulted, even though the animals had absorbed dieldrin *in utero* and via lactation. The P and F_5 generations provide "comparable" baseline data. They were essentially identical, differing only in that (*a*) the parents of the P generations, in contrast to the parents (F_4) of the F_5 generations, did not absorb pesticide *in utero* and in mothers' milk, and (*b*) the parents and grandparents of the P generation mice had no (known) exposure to aldrin or dieldrin, whereas the parents (namely F_4) of the F_5 generations were the offspring of three generations known to have ingested aldrin throughout their lifetime (Deichmann *et al.*, 1975). The experiment was complicated by an increase in total lipids per mouse in the F_1 and succeeding generations compared to the P generation, and this applied to the controls as well as the experimental animals. Pesticide storage fell to undetectable levels in mice that had received them *in utero* and from their mothers' milk. The relationship between total body lipids and concentration of pesticides in these lipids and in the entire carcass seemed inconsistent in some instances. The relation of storage to generation requires further study.

In rats, approximately 90% of excretion of dieldrin is via the feces with the remainder in the urine (Heath and Vandekar, 1964).

Rats metabolize [^{14}C]dieldrin acquired from their food to compounds excreted in both urine and feces. Some are water-soluble compounds and not recovered by ordinary extraction procedures. Details have been given by Korte and Kochen (1966), Matthews and Matsumura (1969), Matthews *et al.* (1971), McKinney *et al.* (1972), Mueller *et al.* (1975a), Bedford and Hutson (1976), Oberholser *et al.* (1977), and Chipman and Walker (1979). Similar results have been found in monkeys (Mueller *et al.*, 1975a,b) and in sheep (Hedde *et al.*, 1970; Feil *et al.*, 1970). The metabolism progresses in stages; metabolites that escape immediate excretion may undergo further biotransformation. For example, when the metabolite dihydrochlordenedicarboxylic acid marked with ^{14}C was injected intravenously into rats, it was possible to isolate nine metabolites from the urine and feces and to identify three of them, namely two isomers of dichlordihydrocarboxylic acid and the dimethyl ester of dihydrochlordenedicarboxylic acid (Lay *et al.*, 1975). The photoisomerization product of dieldrin is also metabolized by rats. In male rats, it forms ketodieldrin pentachloroketone (Klein *et al.*, 1970), which is also a metabolite of dieldrin excreted in the urine (Baldwin and Robinson, 1969; Dailey *et al.*, 1972). Other compounds found in the excreta of one or more mammalian species include the 9-hydroxy metabolite 6,7-*trans*-dihydroaldrindiol, hexachlorohexahydromethanoindenedicarboxylic acid, and two of its acylation products (Baldwin *et al.*, 1972).

The 6,7-*trans*-dihydroxyaldrin is formed by microsomes from the livers of rats, pigs, and rabbits without the addition of cofactors, but when NADPH and oxygen also are present, oxidative products are formed in some cases (Brooks *et al.*, 1970). Although Matthews and McKinney (1974) suggested that the *trans*-diol is formed by epimerization of the *cis*-diol, other workers have been unable to prove this and dieldrin is not a substrate for epoxide hydrolase (Walker *et al.*, 1986).

The greater storage of dieldrin and photodieldrin in female rats is based on their slower metabolism and lesser excretion of metabolites, compared to males (Dailey *et al.*, 1970).

There are substantial differences in the metabolism of dieldrin by rats and mice. Smaller but measurable differences in biotransformation are found between strains of mice (Hutson, 1976).

Dogs were given loading doses of dieldrin for 5 days (1.0 mg/kg/day) and then continued at 0.2 mg/kg/day for 53 days (Keane and Zavon, 1969a). Under these conditions, the concentration of dieldrin in the blood remained constant from day 7 through day 59. The concentration of dieldrin in fat was inversely proportional to the total weight of adipose tissue in different dogs. The ratio of dieldrin in fat to that in blood decreased from 216 on day 16 to 177 on day 50, and the difference was significant. It thus seems likely that a steady state of dieldrin storage in the entire body was not achieved until near the end of the experimental period, if at all. Thus, even though the level in the blood apparently was constant, the authors' conclusion that the concentration of dieldrin in fat was inversely proportional to the total body burden probably applies only to the preequilibrium state.

A steady state of storage in fat as well as in blood and liver was achieved in about 16 days in rats, and the fat-to-blood ratio was 474 (Deichmann *et al.*, 1968). Others have not explored intervals as short as 16 days but have reported achievement of storage equilibrium in rats within 6 months or less (Baron and Walton, 1971; Davison, 1973; Walker *et al.*, 1969). Chickens require 22–26 weeks to reach a steady state (Davison, 1973).

A study of the loss of dieldrin after rats had been fed a dietary level of 10 ppm (about 0.5 mg/kg/day) for 8 weeks revealed a simple exponential pattern of loss from fat and brain but an initially rapid and subsequently slower loss from blood and liver. The half-life for fat was 10.3 days and that for brain 3.0 days. The half-life for loss from liver and blood was about 1.3 days at first but later 10.2 days. Storage in the different tissues was in the following order of decreasing concentrations: fat > liver > brain > blood (Robinson *et al.*, 1969).

As far as toxicity is concerned, the metabolism of dieldrin in the rat is a true detoxication (Baldwin *et al.*, 1970a, 1972), although, on the basis of voltage clamp experiments in the squid, aldrin *trans*-diol is more active than dieldrin (Van den Bercken and Narahashi, 1974).

Dieldrin or its metabolites are excreted rapidly in the bile of rats, the rate being about three times greater in males than in females (Klevay, 1970). The dynamics of dieldrin storage in chickens is qualitatively similar to that in other vertebrates (Brown *et al.*, 1974).

Dieldrin residues of 9–11 ppm in the brains of rats were associated with convulsions (Harr *et al.*, 1970b). A wider range (1.25–26.76 ppm) was found in the brains of pheasants that died during or after dieldrin feeding; the mean was 5.75 ppm (Linder *et al.*, 1970).

Cats kept in a room that had been treated against woodworm with dieldrin developed hypersalivation, hyperesthesia, ataxia, and seizures after 4 weeks. Livers of two animals contained 10 and 8.4 ppm dieldrin and the brain contained 4 and 3.3 ppm (Gruffydd-Jones *et al.*, 1981).

The simultaneous administration of dieldrin and DDT may alter the storage of one or both, and the effect varies from one species to another as discussed in Section 15.2.2.3.

Biochemical Effects   Biochemical effects in the brain can be found under Effects on the Nervous System.

In the livers of animals that ingest dieldrin, most of the compound in the liver is in the microsomal fraction (Wright *et al.*, 1977). This is of interest because the compound induces microsomal enzymes in animals (Wright *et al.*, 1972; Virgo and Bellward, 1973a; Stevens *et al.*, 1973; Tseng and Menzer, 1974; Lacombe and Brodeur, 1974; Greene *et al.*, 1974; Chadwick *et al.*, 1975; Bellward *et al.*, 1975; Vainio and Parkki, 1976).

Induction of dieldrin metabolism by the compound itself has been demonstrated (Oberholser *et al.*, 1977), even though the results were negative in one appropriate experiment in which phenobarbital (used as a positive control) was effective (Eliason and Posner, 1971).

In rats, the dietary no-effect level for induction of metabolism of other compounds is between 1 and 5 ppm dieldrin according to Gillett and Chan (1968) or about 1 ppm (0.05 mg/kg/day) according to Kinoshita and Kempf (1970). Oral administration of dieldrin at a rate of 0.05 mg/kg/day caused a significant induction of *p*-nitroanisole-*O*-demethylase, but 1.25 mg/kg/day was the smallest dosage tested causing a significant induction of EPN-oxidase (Krampl and Hladka, 1975). In a similar way, a significant increase in the activity of the liver microsomal monooxygenase system of monkeys was observed at dietary levels of 1.75 and 5 ppm but not at 1.0 ppm or lower (Wright *et al.*, 1978).

The kinetics of the changes in rat liver microsomal and plasma enzymes caused by single and repeated administration of dieldrin has been studied in detail (Zemaitis *et al.*, 1976).

Biochemical parameters of the mouse liver returned to normal within 6 weeks after a dietary level of 20 ppm dieldrin was discontinued (Virgo and Bellward, 1975a).

In chickens no induction was observed at a dietary level of 10 ppm, but some enzymes were induced at 20 ppm (about 1.16 mg/kg/day) (Sell *et al.*, 1971).

A sufficient dosage of dieldrin causes an increase in alkaline phosphatase not only in serum but also in the liver (El-Aaser *et al.*, 1972). The same is true initially with glutaic-pyruvic transaminase and aldolase, but these enzymes promptly decrease in the liver while remaining elevated in the serum. Reversible alterations of the liver, including cell vacuolization and nuclear pyknosis, were most severe when serum enzyme levels were maximal (Krampl and Grigel, 1972). Some reports suggest that dieldrin may inhibit plasma membrane and mitochondrial Mg^{2+}-ATPases in various tissues, although aldrin may be more active in this respect (Bandyopadhyay *et al.*, 1982; Mehrotra *et al.*, 1982).

A single dieldrin dose of 20 mg/kg to rhesus monkeys elevates the uptake of glucose from the intestine and the activities of brush border sucrose, lactase, maltase, and alkaline phosphatase (Mahmood *et al.*, 1981). A similar increase in intestinal glucose transport, after *in vivo* DDT or dieldrin pretreatment, has been shown for mouse intestinal mucosal cells (Reymann *et al.*, 1983). Treatments with phenobarbital and 3-methylcholanthrene induced disaccharidase activities but failed to enhance glucose transport. In adult rats, but not perhaps in sucklings, dieldrin causes a significant rise in blood glucose levels (up to twofold) (Fox and Virgo, 1986a,b), which seems to be mediated via the central nervous system (Fox and Virgo, 1985).

A dietary level of 200 ppm, which causes decreased weight gain and other signs of toxicity, caused enlargement of the adrenals and striking changes in the production of adrenal steroids of rats (Foster, 1968). The adrenal effects appear to be a result rather than a cause of the toxicity. In a similar way, toxic levels of dieldrin reduce growth and plasma vitamin A concentration in sheep (Davison, 1970b).

A dietary level of 6.2 ppm (only 0.277 mg/kg/day), but not a level of 0.7 ppm (0.031 mg/kg/day), caused an increase in the concentration of leuteinizing hormone in the serum of both intact and castrated male rats (Blend and Lehnert, 1973).

A number of studies have demonstrated that dieldrin can depress the immune response in mice. Loose (1982) showed that isolated hepatic and splenic macrophages produced a dialyzable factor that, when added with phytohemagglutinin to splenic T-cell cultures, suppressed their stimulation. In C57BL/6 mice susceptible to mouse hepatitis virus (MHV3), sublethal doses of dieldrin will increase susceptibility and even resistant A/J mice will show increased mortality after repeated doses of the insecticide (Krzystyniak *et al.*, 1985). Again, effects seemed to be mediated by suppression of macrophage function and affecting the humoral anti-MHV3 IgG immune response (Krzystyniak *et al.*, 1986; Fournier *et al.*, 1986). Addition of dieldrin to MHV3 virus-activated macrophages *in vitro* inhibited the ability of the cells to restrict MHV3 replication. At low doses of dieldrin to a rat (5 mg/kg) the peritoneal macrophage population is increased (Kaminski *et al.*, 1982). At higher doses this response is inhibited and the phagocytic activity of the isolated cells is decreased.

Effects on the Nervous System Dieldrin has been used in many studies to typify the effects of the cyclodiene chlorinated insecticides on nerve function. As stressed many years ago, the action of dieldrin is on the central and not the peripheral system (Gowdey *et al.*, 1954; Gowdey and Stavraky, 1955). General discussions can be found in Section 15.2.3.1. Similar effects are also described under lindane in Section 15.4.1.2, Effects on the Nervous System.

Alterations in the content of biogenic amines of the brain were observed in rats following a single oral dose of dieldrin (50 mg/kg) and to a lesser extent in those receiving it in their diet at 50 ppm, that is, about 2.5 mg/kg/day (Wagner and Greene, 1978). Similar results were reported for hamsters (Willhite and Sharma, 1978). As usual with these types of study, it is difficult to known whether these changes were a cause or an effect of the basic disturbance initiated by the insecticide, and changes are not always consistent in different species (Sharma, 1976; Kohli *et al.*, 1977). Dieldrin, like other excitatory substances, increased whole-brain nucleotide levels (Joy *et al.*, 1982b). In particular, cGMP levels correlated positively with the degree of exposure of mice to dieldrin. Convulsions were not necessary to produce this effect. A variety of amino acid changes in brain have been recorded after different times following a 0.25 LD 50 dose to rats (Ahmed *et al.*, 1986).

In contrast to DDT, a major site of action of dieldrin appears to be at the synapse. Dieldrin binds to the picrotoxin binding site of the GABA-receptor–ionophore complex (Matsumura and Ghiasuddin, 1983) and this has been studied in detail using t-[^{35}S]butylbicyclophosphorothionate as a radioligand for the picrotoxin binding site (Lawrence and Casida, 1984; Abalis *et al.*, 1985; Casida and Lawrence, 1985; Eldefrawi *et al.*, 1985; Cole and Casida, 1986). The degree of binding correlates with acute toxicity and convulsions. In addition, GABA-induced $^{36}Cl^-$ flux into rat brain microsacs is inhibited (Bloomquist *et al.*, 1986). It is likely, however, that reduction in GABA-mediated inhibition is not a complete biochemical answer for the neurotoxicity of dieldrin.

At a more physiological level of dieldrin, Joy (1977) has demonstrated that in cats the convulsive action is due to the insecticide itself and not to a metabolite. Intravenous administration at dosages of 2–4 mg/kg produced fits in 2–15 min, whereas aldrin *trans*-diol at dosages up to 20 mg/kg produced no convulsions and not even a change in EEG. The effects of dieldrin on the EEG of animals have been studied many times (for instance, see Santoluchito and Morrison, 1971), without clear indications of specific changes. It has been reported that a single dose of dieldrin that produced symptoms or a series of small doses that failed to do so can change the frequency spectrum of the spontaneous EEG for as much as a year (Burchfield *et al.*, 1976).

Studies on squirrel monkeys were interpreted as showing that a dosage of 0.1 mg/kg/day interfered with acquisition of skill in a reversal behavioral task but did not impair performance after the skill had been acquired (Van Gelder and Smith, 1973; Smith *et al.*, 1976). If the results are accepted as not due to chance, then it is equally reasonable to conclude from the data presented that a dosage of 0.01 mg/kg/day improved acquisition of the skill. Whatever the interpretation, the 0.01 mg/kg/day level did cause EEG changes (Van Gelder and Cunningham, 1975), which indicates that in this connection the EEG is the more sensitive test. Carlson and Rosellini (1987) have proposed that dieldrin causes behavioral defects in rats prevented from coping with stress.

In more recent years, specific physiological lesions have become apparent. Joy (1974a) concluded that dieldrin and pentylenetetrazole share either a common mechanism of action or final common pathways responsible for electrophysiological events. This seems to be consistent with findings on the role of the GABA−receptor complex although other electrophysiological evidence does not fit entirely with the concept of antagonizing GABA-mediated inhibition (Joy and Albertson, 1985). A great many studies have been carried out by Joy to identify the exact brain region involved (for instance, see Joy, 1974a,b, 1976, 1982a,b; Joy and Albertson, 1985). The effects of lindane on kindling in rats (see Section 15.4.1.2) have been especially useful in this respect (Joy *et al.*, 1980; Joy and Albertson, 1985; Woolley *et al.*, 1985). It seems now probable that the synaptic processes of the thalamocortical relay are the synapses most severely affected by dieldrin. Perhaps the leg cocking position taken up by a beagle bitch after 2 years of treatment with dieldrin is a related phenomenon (Chambers, 1982).

Ray *et al.* (1986) have studied the effect of dieldrin on auditory evoked response and regional blood flow in four brain regions of conscious rats. Parallel increases in blood flow and evoked response amplitude were seen with especially large increases in the cerebral cortex seizures; however, there were marked but transient depressions in the auditory evoked response but more persistent depressions of blood flow.

The transient hypothermia produced by a single dose of dieldrin to rats (Wagner and Greene, 1978), together with reduction in food intake, has also been observed by Woolley *et al.* (Swanson and Woolley, 1982; Woolley *et al.*, 1985). Whether the picrotoxin-like effect of dieldrin on GABAergic pathways can account for these findings remains to be determined.

Dieldrin inhibits gap junction intercellular communication in rat glial cells at noncytotoxic concentrations. It has been proposed that such a phenomenon may contribute to the neurotoxicity of dieldrin (Suter *et al.*, 1987).

Effects on Other Organs and Tissues   Femoral bone marrow cultures from ducks that had received dieldrin at a dietary level of 30 ppm showed reduced cell division, but those from ducks at 10 ppm were normal. No significant incidence of chromosomal abnormalities was found at a dietary level of 30 ppm or less. Chromosomes were not damaged by 30 ppm or less *in vitro*, a level that would be rapidly fatal *in vivo*. Damage was produced by 100 ppm *in vitro* (Bunch and Low, 1973). A completely opposite result was reported by Majumdar *et al.* (1976) for bone marrow cells of mice dosed intraperitoneally and for human lung cell cultures. In both instances, the mitotic index varied inversely, and the percentage of cells with chromosomal abnormalities varied directly with dosage. Effects were present at the lowest dosages tested, that is, 1 mg/kg in mice and 1 ppm for human cells *in vitro*.

In a comprehensive evaluation for mutagenic activity of dieldrin, the results were negative in four mouse tests (Bidwell *et al.*, 1975). The same result was obtained in independent studies in mice, hamsters, and bacteria, and the degree of chromosome damage in short-term lymphocyte cultures from workers currently or previously employed in a dieldrin manufacturing plant did not differ significantly from that found in controls (Dean *et al.*, 1975; Bidwell *et al.*, 1975).

Pigeons fed dieldrin at rates of 4.2 and 1.0 mg/kg/day developed enlarged thyroids, loss of colloid, and hyperplastic thyroid epithelium (Jefferies and French, 1972).

Dosages of dieldrin that have produced hepatic tumors in mice are presented in Table 15.26. The implications of such tumors are discussed in Section 15.2.3.2. The dosage–effect relationship and the influence of endogenous initiation events have been considered by Tennekes *et al.* (1981, 1982, 1985). Interestingly, the logdosage–logtime curve for dieldrin is different from comparable curves for established carcinogens. This suggests that tumors in mice caused by dieldrin arise in a different manner from those caused by some other carcinogens. Perhaps the observation that Mallory bodies are found in tumors from mice treated with dieldrin but not in those caused by diethylnitrosamine is of some relevance in this context (Meierhenry *et al.*, 1983). By studying polyploidization caused by dieldrin, van Ravenzwaay *et al.* (1987, 1988; van Ravenzwaay and Kunz, 1988) have advanced the theory that such chemical promoters operate by advancing the biological age of mouse liver in the initial phases of treatment, but some evidence suggests inhibition of intercellular communication (ZhongXiang *et al.*, 1986). Hamsters are very tolerant to dieldrin. Survival at 50 weeks in those fed dietary levels as high as 180 ppm (about 14.9 mg/kg/day) was comparable to that of controls, and no significant increase in tumor incidence was noted in the treated animals (Cabral *et al.*, 1979b). Rats do not appear to develop tumors (NCI, 1978e,f). Studies of the carcinogenicities of aldrin and dieldrin have been compared by Ritper (1979).

A 10 ppm dietary concentration of dieldrin increased not only the incidence of liver tumors but also the incidence of thrombosis of the hepatic vein and consequent infarction. Tumors and thrombosis seemed unrelated (Reuber, 1977b).

Effects on Reproduction   A dietary level of 5 ppm in mice (about 0.67 mg/kg/day in adult females but much higher during lactation) did not reduce survival of adults, the percentage of pairs producing young, or the number of litters and young per producing pair. Although the reduction of the average litter size from 9.2 to 8.7 was statistically significant, it was of very questionable biological significance inasmuch as the number of young produced per day per pair by the controls (0.338) was not significantly greater than the number (0.326) produced by dieldrin-treated animals (Good and Ware, 1969). Other studies of mice showed that loss of litters was significantly increased by dietary levels of 2.5 ppm and greater but failed to show what dosage was tolerated (Virgo and Bellward, 1973b, 1975b, 1977).

Most nursing pups of rats receiving a dietary level of 2.5 ppm (about 0.396 mg/kg/day for lactating females) died in convulsions or starved. Dietary levels in excess of 0.24 ppm (about 0.014 mg/kg/day) caused a decrease in the rate of conception (Harr et al., 1970a). However, the small number of dams at each dosage level and the successful breeding of some groups at dietary levels as high as 5.0 ppm raise questions about interpretation of the results. In fact, more consistent results were reported earlier by Treon and Cleveland (1955) in a three-generation study. They found that dietary levels of 2.5 and 12.5 ppm initially reduced the number of pregnancies, but this effect tended to disappear with continued feeding. Even 2.5 ppm increased mortality among the suckling young, and at 12.5 and 25 ppm this effect was severe. In the lactating rat, a dietary level of 2.5 ppm determines a dosage of about 0.4 mg/kg/day.

Inviability of pups seems to be associated with hypoglycemia and enhanced glycogenolysis (Costella and Virgo, 1980).

Dieldrin given to rats and mice at a dosage of 3.4 mg/kg/day was reported to produce teratogenic effects, but the fewest malformations were associated with the longest duration of administration (Boucard et al., 1970). A more consistent result was reported by Chernoff et al. (1975), who found a dosage of 6 mg/kg/day nonteratogenic, although it was toxic not only to fetuses but also to the dams. A dosage of 3 mg/kg/day was toxic to fetal mice, as indicated by delayed ossification and an increase in supernumerary ribs. A dosage of 1.5 mg/kg/day was harmless to pregnant mice and their young. Dosages as high as 6 mg/kg/day were harmless in rats.

Reproduction was normal in sheep at dietary levels of dieldrin as high as 5 ppm administered over two gestation periods. However, at 25 ppm the lambs died soon after birth (FAO/WHO, 1971).

Following intravenous injection of pregnant rats with radioactive dieldrin, radioactivity in the fetus increased for 40–60 min and then decreased parallel to the simultaneous decrease in the maternal plasma (Eliason and Posner, 1971).

Factors Influencing Toxicity   Two equal doses of dieldrin within 3 weeks of each other were reported to be more toxic than the sum of the two given as a single dose (Barnes and Heath, 1964). According to Lu et al. (1965), this relationship is true only in preweanling rats; in adults divided doses are less toxic, as is usually true.

Newborn rats are less sensitive than adults to single doses of dieldrin (Lu et al., 1965).

Although there has been considerable study of the effect of protein deficiency (or excess) on the acute toxicity of pesticides (see Section 2.4.11.2), the interaction of protein with repeated doses of a pesticide has received little attention. Stoewsand and Bourke (1968) and Stoewsand et al. (1970) reported that male weanling rats maintained on a 10% casein diet died within 2 weeks after dieldrin was added to the diet at a concentration of 150 ppm. On the contrary, there were 60 and 40% survival among male rats receiving the same concentration of dieldrin but maintained on 25 and 50% casein, respectively. In fact, after initial poisoning and weight loss, the survivors stopped showing toxic signs and gained weight while still receiving dieldrin. The large dosage of dieldrin used was fatal to female rats regardless of protein intake. Investigation with [^{14}C]dieldrin showed that male rats receiving higher concentrations of protein had increased urinary and fecal excretion of metabolites and lower storage of dieldrin in the brain, liver, and fat. Similarly, Tanaka et al. (1980) demonstrated that biliary excretion of dieldrin is greater when rats are kept on a high-protein diet rather than one containing a low proportion of protein. This may explain why rats are more susceptible to dieldrin poisoning if maintained on a low-protein diet (Lee et al., 1964).

The concentrations of dieldrin in the brains of experimental animals killed by dieldrin were as follows: rat, 2.2–10.8 ppm (Hayes, 1974); cotton rat, 5.6–11.1 ppm; and cottontail rabbit, 8.5–19.1 ppm (Stickel et al., 1969).

In rats, excretion of dieldrin is approximately doubled when the compound is mobilized along with fat by starvation (Heath and Vandekar, 1964).

Pathology   Early studies found only minimal and nonspecific morphological effects of dieldrin on the nervous system. Emphasis was placed on vascular lesions (necrobiosis of the endothelium) by Harr et al. (1970b), but they considered the lesions nonspecific and so minimal that they would have been masked by conventional dietary and housing regimes or by greater genetic variability. Apparently, some statistically significant changes in the brain are the result of convulsions rather than of dieldrin per se. For example, Galasinska-Pomykol et al. (1974) reported an increase in volumes of nuclei, decrease in neurosecretory granules, and other changes in the hypothalamic neurosecretory centers of guinea pigs that had convulsions following a single oral dose of Alvit-55 but not of guinea pigs that did not have a fit before they were killed 4 hr following a dose at the same rate. On the other hand, changes were observed in some other nuclei. Some of the changes tended to regress after 8 days; changes persisted as long as 192 hr in only a few neurons of the dorsal motor nuclei (Tarmas et al., 1973).

As discussed in Section 15.2.3.2, increase in endoplasmic reticulum is the major factor leading to hypertrophy, margination, and lipospheres that together characterize the effects of tolerated dosages of chlorinated hydrocarbon insecticides on the rodent liver. A similar but less pronounced increase in smooth endoplasmic reticulum may be revealed by the electron microscope in pars recta tubules of the kidney of rats fed dieldrin at a dietary level of 5 ppm (Fowler, 1972).

15.5.4.3 Toxicity to Humans

Experimental Oral Exposure Twelve men took part in a study of HEOD (purity better than 99.9%), the compound that constitutes 85% or more of technical dieldrin. During the first 18 months, three men received a daily dose of 0.211 mg, three received 0.050 mg, three received 0.010 mg, and three served as controls. From month 18 through month 24 the six men receiving the two highest dosage levels continued to receive dieldrin at the same high levels, but the other two groups both changed to receive 0.211 mg/man/day. All dosing was stopped at the end of 24 months, but the concentration of dieldrin in the blood of all the men was followed for an additional 8 months. All the men remained in excellent health. Body weights and clinical chemistry and hematological findings, including plasma alkaline phosphatases, remained essentially unchanged throughout the 24-month exposure period and the 8-month postexposure period. There were no EEG changes related to exposure. The dosage of 0.010 mg/man/day failed to produce a detectable increase in storage above control levels. However, the other two dosage levels increased storage by factors of about 4 and 10 times. The increase was rapid at first and then more gradual. After 21 months, the data offered no evidence whatever of further increase in blood levels. The ratio of the concentration of dieldrin in adipose tissue to that in the blood was 136. The biological half-life after dosing was discontinued was 369 days (Hunter and Robinson, 1967; Hunter *et al.*, 1969; Prior and Deacon, 1969).

The corrected average for the dermal absorption of [^{14}C]dieldrin by six volunteers was 7.7% of the dose applied to a forearm. This proportion was corrected for the very small proportion (3.3%) of excretion observed within 5 days after intravenous injection of dieldrin (Feldmann and Maibach, 1974). Although such a correction is necessary and proper, the resulting estimate may lack precision.

Accidental and Intentional Poisoning Ingestion of unknown volumes of a 5% dieldrin formulation prepared from an emulsifiable concentrate killed a 2-year-old girl and poisoned her 4-year-old brother. The girl was dead before a physician arrived. Convulsions began in the boy within 15 min and became continuous for a time. The boy survived even though his temperature rose to 39.5°C (Garrettson and Curley, 1969). The fact that his temperature was reduced by means of an ice mattress and chlorpromazine hydrochloride may have contributed to his survival, and administration of large doses of barbiturates almost certainly contributed. Analytical results in the case are discussed under Laboratory Findings.

In another case the dosage was also unknown but might be supposed to be smaller, for the onset was delayed about 6 hr. The baby then suddenly lost consciousness, became dyspneic, and suffered a convulsion. Convulsions finally were controlled by treatment with phenobarbital, chloral hydrate, and chlorpromazine, but she remained unconscious. The temperature rose to 40°C; cyanosis and tachycardia increased, and the child died 20 hr after exposure (Kalushiner, quoted by AMA, 1960).

Two foodborne outbreaks are listed in Table 7.14. One of these outbreaks affecting a large number of people, of whom 79 were studied epidemiologically, was reported by WHO (1977). Illness was caused by dieldrin-contaminated rice supplied to the Public Works Department of Kayes in Mali. In most cases onset was 0.5–1.5 hr after the rice was eaten, and the delay never exceeded 6 hr. Signs and symptoms included convulsions, aching muscles, vomiting, vertigo, and fainting. Contamination of the rice was attributed to the use of dieldrin to kill rats and insects in the building where the grain had been stored.

A man who attempted suicide by drinking 9 gm (120 mg/kg) of dieldrin in toluene did not regain full consciousness until 5 days later; headache and disturbance of short-term memory persisted for several weeks, and there was evidence of mild liver damage (Black, 1974). Convulsions were so severe and persistent in spite of conventional treatment that it seems unlikely that the patient would have survived without heroic treatment, including profound muscular paralysis induced by pancuronium bromide, intermittent positive pressure ventilation, and β-sympathetic blockade.

A reduction in body temperature was described in two cases characterized by convulsions and unconsciousness; the temperature was normal and recovery well advanced 24 hr after ingestion (Fry, 1964).

Poisoning sufficiently severe to produce coma but without observed convulsions is unusual but has been reported (Barkve, 1961).

Ingestion of dieldrin by a 21-year-old man led to continuous convulsions that were controlled by conventional therapy and to two results unusual in connection with dieldrin, namely brief hematuria and total amnesia for the events leading up to and including the suicidal attempt. The hematuria began about 24 hr after ingestion and may have been due to a solvent. Renal function tests showed no residual abnormality, and liver function tests were within normal limits at all times (Jacobs and Lurie, 1967).

A 43-year-old schizophrenic who died after consuming an unknown quantity of dieldrin was found to have cerebral and pulmonary edema and large amounts of foam in the respiratory tracts (Steentoft, 1979).

Use Experience It may be that a very early report of a complete lack of injury in spite of air levels as high as 54 mg/m³ (Princi and Spurbeck, 1951) was premature. Certainly the possibility of serious poisoning was discounted in what apparently was the first report of illness among applicators (Carrillo, 1954).

Occupational poisoning has occurred among men who applied dieldrin inside houses, mainly for control of malaria, and among those who manufactured and formulated it. A few farmers have been poisoned by dieldrin; in some instances gross misuse was recognized, and unrecognized accidents may have occurred in some other instances (Paul, 1959).

Sprayers who became sick did so after they had worked for only 2 days or as much as 2 years (Hayes, 1957, 1959b; Rahman *et al.*, 1958). Among factory workers, those who developed clinical poisoning did so with decreasing frequency during their first, second, and third years of working with dieldrin. However, one was transferred to other work because of suggestive, nonincapacitating symptoms appearing as late as the ninth year of exposure (Jager, 1970).

Reported experience in the use of dieldrin involved at least 2629 sprayers (Hayes, 1957, 1959b; Zavon and Hamman, 1961) plus 826 industrial workers in a factory in the Netherlands (Jager, 1970) and 49 in a factory in the United States (Hayes and Curley, 1968). Special studies were made of all the Dutch workers who suffered poisoning and of 233 of them who were exposed for more than 4 years. It was even possible by questionnaire to trace 52 of the latter who had retired or taken other employment, and their health did not differ from that of those available for direct study (Jager, 1970; Versteeg and Jager, 1973). In general, the poisoning that occurred during early industrial experience is discussed in this section, while the detailed laboratory studies that were uniformly normal after industrial hygiene was sufficiently improved are discussed under Laboratory Findings.

Among some groups of sprayers, 2–40% were known to have developed symptoms and 47–100% of the recognized cases involved convulsions (Hayes, 1957, 1959b; Patel and Rao, 1958). Very high rates of convulsions among those recognized as ill almost certainly mean that some severe cases were missed among the entire exposed group.

Among both sprayers and factory workers, symptoms sometimes were confined to headache, nausea, vomiting, general malaise, and dizziness. In other instances, these symptoms preceded one or more epileptiform convulsions, usually followed by coma but without incontinence of urine or feces. In some instances, a fit was the first indication of illness, and there was never an aura. Patients had no memory of their fits but learned of them from their associates or inferred them when they aroused to find themselves bruised and their tongues chewed. Some persons poisoned by dieldrin have experienced sudden contraction of a major muscle, sometimes sufficient to move a part of the body or to cause the person to fall. In extreme cases, these movements were accompanied by momentary loss of consciousness (Hayes, 1957). These "jerks" or "falls," as they have been called, probably are extremely brief, incomplete fits.

Prodromal symptoms are most likely following repeated exposure, and onset with convulsions is most likely following relatively massive exposure, either with or without prior moderate exposure at a more usual rate (Jager, 1970).

Following prompt recovery from one or more convulsions, some patients seemed entirely normal. Others showed hyperexcitability and hyperactivity. A few occupational and accidental cases involved a temporary change of personality characterized by fear, weeping, difficulty in sleeping, bad dreams, mania, or other inappropriate behavior (Hayes, 1957, 1959b; Princi, 1954; Patel and Rao, 1958; Avar and Czegledi-Janko, 1970; Fry, 1964). Similar difficulties have followed prolonged eating of a mixture of aldrin and lindane or other nonoccupational exposure (Gupta, 1975; Kürsat and Türkoğlu, 1968).

The total loss of appetite and marked loss of body weight that were such striking features of some experiments with dogs and monkeys have never been reported in humans, although loss of as much as 6 kg in 4–14 days has been reported (Nelson, 1953; Glass, 1975). This difference may depend on species, but it seems more likely that it is associated with duration and intensity of dosage. People often stop exposure at the first symptom and almost always stop when it is realized that illness is serious. The animals were dosed relentlessly long after signs of illness were constant and severe.

Except for convulsions and muscular jerking, signs of poisoning are not prominent. Incoordination (especially in the Romberg and other tests), nystagmus, quivering of the outstretched fingers, sweating, dermatographia, and tachycardia may be detected in some patients.

Abnormal performance of various psychological tests administered to sprayers has been reported (Ibañez-Peterson and DeFranzetti, 1957).

With very few exceptions, persons occupationally poisoned by dieldrin recovered. No details are available concerning those who died (Hayes, 1957, 1959b), and suicide is not excluded in these instances.

Most recoveries have been prompt and permanent. Avar and Czegledi-Janko (1970) reported that three severely poisoned workers recovered within 7 months. A few sprayers and a few persons with nonoccupational exposure have had a recurrence of convulsions at intervals varying from 14 to 120 or more days after last exposure (Hayes, 1957, 1959b). Intermittent repetition of myoclonic jerking and some other symptoms (but apparently not repetition of convulsions) were observed for over a year after the eating of aldrin and BHC was discontinued (Gupta, 1975). Perhaps it is not the recurrence of myoclonic jerks or convulsions but its rarity that is remarkable. Although it is obvious that dieldrin predisposes to convulsions, it is no more clear why a person who has developed a high blood level of dieldrin has a fit at a particular moment than it is clear why an epileptic does the same thing. Fits are not continuous or even frequent in either instance, although a predisposing condition is present in each.

The initial half-life of dieldrin in the blood of workers removed from exposure is 50–150 days. However, elimination gradually becomes slower. One worker still had a blood level of 0.039 ppm 2 years after his last recognized exposure to aldrin. The half-life associated with the later, more gradual loss of dieldrin is 0.73 years (266 days) (Jager, 1970). This slow loss certainly offers a possibility for a worker to remain for some time within the threshold zone of susceptibility if the initial blood level was high.

Usually, full recovery from occupational poisoning by aldrin or dieldrin requires no more than a few weeks.

Dieldrin apparently caused a nonspecific dermatitis of the lower legs of 288 of 1209 police recruits who wore socks mothproofed with dieldrin and who were subject to extensive sweating (Ross, 1964). Evidence that dieldrin was the cause is convincing, and the rarity with which people who sweat heavily wear mothproofed fabric in direct contact with the skin seems a reasonable explanation of the rarity of such dermatitis. However, the fact that the dermatitis did not involve the recruits' feet remains unexplained.

A formulator with scleroderma had higher blood and tissue levels of dieldrin and several other organochlorine pesticides than did his fellow workers with no less exposure (Starr and Clifford, 1971). Persons with chronic skin disease may be in special danger from occupational exposure to pesticides.

Little or no progress has been made in the protection of sprayers using dieldrin in antimalarial programs because their mobility means that only personal protection can be used, and the hot, moist climates in which most of them work limit the amount of protective equipment that can be tolerated. In contrast, the industrial experience described by Jager (1970) and by Versteeg and Jager (1973) constitutes an outstanding example of the improvement of working conditions and the elimination of poisoning. This improvement was based on constantly excellent occupational medicine that was both a cause and later a result of the application of the most advanced techniques in electroencephalography and gas–liquid chromatography.

Atypical Cases of Various Origins A case resembling radiculomyelitis was attributed to dieldrin by Urbanska-Bonenberg and Langauer-Lewowicka (1966), who observed that the defect had not been described previously. It has not been reported since.

The impotence of four of five members of a team of farm workers was attributed to their exposure to four insecticides, two herbicides, and four other less toxic compounds (Espir et al., 1970). No responsibility was fixed on any particular compound, and no emphasis was given to dieldrin, which was one of the insecticides. However, this emphasis was provided by a comment (Peck, 1970), which suggested that the reported observation could be explained by a deficiency of testosterone as a direct result of stimulation of microsomal enzymes by dieldrin and other compounds to which the men were exposed. Both the paper and the comment ignored dosage relationships and epidemiological principles. If the dosages of the various pesticides encountered by farm workers were sufficient to produce impotence in some of them, then the dosages encountered by manufacturers and formulators should result in universal impotence among them. Actually, none has been observed.

Workers and their families on three Scottish farms became contaminated by dieldrin mainly by consumption of eggs from poultry which had been kept on nesting litter derived from timber treated with the insecticide (Bell and MacLeod, 1983). Eggs contained on average 0.9 mg of dieldrin. Chicken liver and meat of birds (many of which died) contained maximum levels of 142 and 17 ppm. Blood levels in humans, however, were low (see Storage in Blood and Other Tissues), and no significant clinical symptoms were reported. For these reasons a decision was taken to ignore the possibility of human poisonings resulting from the sale of some of the poultry products.

Dieldrin was the only compound mentioned specifically in connection with an alleged excess incidence of lymphomas among persons in Iowa who had consumed processed river water or water from shallow wells as compared to those whose water came from deep wells (DeKraay, 1978). No evidence was presented that any difference in the incidence of lymphoma was statistically significant or that lymphoma patients had absorbed more total dieldrin from water, food, and other sources. No consideration was given to other possible differences in the chemical content of drinking water from different sources.

A 52-year-old man, who formerly had been healthy, developed immunohemolytic anemia that was cured by splenectomy. The basis for his positive antiglobulin test was the presence of an antidieldrin IgG antibody in the serum and on the red cell membrane. The immune reaction was specific for dieldrin among seven chlorinated hydrocarbon insecticides. Neutralization of the serum antibody by prior incubation with dieldrin nullified the reaction. The spleen played a central role in cell destruction, antigen storage, and the immunopathic mechanism (Hamilton et al., 1978). In the absence of direct exposure of the patient to pesticides in his home or industrial environment, it was concluded that freshwater fish, which he ate frequently, were the source of dieldrin in his tissues. However, it was only relatively high storage of dieldrin in his spleen that may have been unusual, for the concentration of dieldrin in his body fat was identical to the average for the general population. Although there can be no doubt of the specific immune reaction in this patient involving dieldrin, one can only speculate on how many other exogenous compounds might have reacted in a similar way if they had been tested. The only thing that seems certain is that the patient developed a rare anemia at about the same time that he developed a relatively common condition, diabetes mellitus. The origin of each condition remains a mystery, just as it was before dieldrin was invented.

Dosage Response Death from dieldrin, as from most poisons, often has been associated with a massive dose as the result of accidental or especially suicidal ingestion. In one example that is worthy of mention because the compound was rigorously identified, 2 gm of dieldrin was recovered from the stomach contents alone (Weinig et al., 1966).

Two schoolboys of unstated weight drank a heaping teaspoonful of 50% dieldrin wettable powder mistaken for cocoa and made up as a drink; they vomited profusely and recovered following prolonged convulsions (Fry, 1964). The dosage ingested may have been about 29 mg/kg.

A woman in the fourth month of pregnancy survived a dose estimated as 18,000 mg even though she was unconscious for 4 days and the fetus was killed. Survival of the woman was attributed to diversion of dieldrin to the placenta and fetus (Nowak *et al.*, 1971). The concentration of dieldrin in the conceptus (discussed under Laboratory Findings) certainly indicates a high retained dosage but, in the absence of similar cases, the true dosage and the importance of pregnancy as a protective factor remain in doubt.

A dosage of 23 mg/kg led to convulsions in a child (Princi, 1954).

The average dermal dosage of antimalaria spraymen with relatively good work practices and hygiene was 1.8 mg/kg/day (Fletcher *et al.*, 1959). Judging from animal experiments, it may be assumed that a substantial part of the dosage was absorbed. Although no cases of poisoning among the sprayers had been reported at the time exposure was measured, poisoning was recognized among them later.

The measured oral dosage that volunteers tolerated was 0.21 mg/person/day or 0.0031 mg/kg/day (Hunter and Robinson, 1967). The absorbed intake tolerated by workers is clearly greater, but it must be estimated rather than measured directly. Based on the concentration of dieldrin in their fat, blood, and urine, Hayes and Curley (1968) made three estimates of the average intake of one group of workers; the results ranged from 0.72 to 1.1 mg/person/day. The plasma levels of these particular workers averaged 0.0411 ± 0.0164 ppm, far below the threshold for illness discussed under Laboratory Findings. Other estimates of the average intake of other workers fall within an only slightly wider range (0.59–1.2 mg/person/day or 0.0084–0.017 mg/kg/day) (Hunter *et al.*, 1969). According to Jager (1970), workers tolerated an intake of 0.0332 mg/kg/day for as much as 15 years without detectable effect. The estimated absorbed intake corresponding to the safe threshold (a plasma level of 0.20 ppm) is 3.6 mg/person/day.

A group of pesticide workers with elevated blood levels of dieldrin (≥0.015 ppm) showed no chronic deleterious effects as measured by extensive testing of the central nervous system (Sandifer *et al.*, 1981).

Storage in Blood and Other Tissues An attempt to relate blood levels of dieldrin to poisoning was reported by Blazques and Bianchini (1956, 1957), who used insect bioassay. Results corresponded to the degree of poisoning, but variability limited practical application of the method. Following the development of gas chromatography, it became possible to measure dieldrin in blood more accurately, and this paved the way for measuring the compound not only in persons poisoned by it but also in workers who are heavily exposed and even in the general population. Ultimately, this analytical procedure supplanted the EEG as a method for regulating the exposure of workers.

A concentration of 0.65 ppm was found in the blood of a man who successfully committed suicide with dieldrin (Hayes, 1982). Dieldrin at a level of 0.5 ppm was found in the blood of

another fatal case after oral ingestion (Steentoft, 1979). However, an initial concentration of 1.16 ppm was found in the serum of a man who had ingested dieldrin at a dosage of 120 mg/kg and who survived after treatment (Black, 1974). Maximal values in some cases, including a fatal one, may not only have been higher than the value for the earliest sample available for measurement but also higher than the initial value extrapolated pharmacokinetically. In the case described by Black (1974), the logarithm of serum values decreased as a straight line from day 3 through at least day 24, and this permitted extrapolation to a concentration of about 0.45 ppm at time zero—a value far less than the 1.16 ppm actually measured in a sample collected about 4–6 hr after ingestion. A woman who died a few minutes after injecting herself with a solution of dieldrin apparently had a blood concentration of 50 ppm (Schwär, 1965).

Concentrations of dieldrin ranging from 0.04 to 0.53 have been reported in the blood of some persons who have recovered after poisoning (Kazantzis *et al.*, 1964; Avar and Czegledi-Janko, 1970; Siyali and Simson, 1973). Brown *et al.* (1964) found blood levels of 0.13–0.37 in men who had been poisoned, and the authors estimated that the corresponding levels were 0.17–0.43 at the time of illness. In a factory where, for a time, workers were exposed to isobenzan as well as to aldrin, dieldrin, and endrin, the *blood dieldrin equivalent* (dieldrin level + 10 times the isobenzan level) associated with 20 separate episodes of intoxication ranged from 0.22 to 0.69 ppm and averaged 0.32 ppm (Jager, 1970). A follow-up covering 13 years of experience placed the average blood level in 32 cases of dieldrin intoxication at 0.28–0.29 ppm. Improved industrial hygiene had reduced the risk of poisoning to such a degree that a study of 223 workers showed no significant difference in blood and urine dieldrin levels compared to those of a control group (van Raalte, 1977).

The threshold for the concentration of dieldrin in whole blood above which illness may appear has been estimated to be 0.15–0.20 ppm (Brown *et al.*, 1964). Extensive industrial experience served to confirm 0.20 ppm as the threshold. Poisoning did not occur in men who made and formulated dieldrin when they were monitored, and anyone whose serum level reached 0.20 ppm was assigned to other duties until the level had decreased considerably (Jager, 1970; Mick *et al.*, 1972). In fact, the dieldrin equivalent actually associated with 40 instances of preventive transfer ranged from 0.21 to 0.53 ppm and averaged 0.303 ppm (Jager, 1970).

Samples collected during a 4-year-period from 233 healthy workers with long-term exposure in the same factory revealed an average blood dieldrin concentration of 0.035 ppm, which was calculated to be equivalent to a dietary intake of 0.407 mg/person/day. Among 35 men with more than 10 years of exposure, blood dieldrin averaged 0.023 ppm and ranged from <0.01 to 0.09 ppm. The corresponding values for dieldrin equivalent were 0.096 ppm and 0.02–0.21 ppm (Jager, 1970).

Poultry workers and their families exposed to dieldrin by consumption of eggs from contaminated chickens had only 0.001–0.016 ppm in their blood (Bell and MacLeod, 1983).

After a year blood levels were consistent with the view that the half-life of dieldrin in a human exposure may be about 1 year (Jager, 1970).

In a different occupational situation with no cases of poisoning, plasma levels of dieldrin ranged from 0.030 to 0.312 ppm among workers most of whose only occupational exposure was a 5-week period of formulating aldrin. Plasma levels were progressively less in warehouse workers, maintenance workers, and a supervisor (Mick *et al.*, 1972).

In a case (Black, 1974) of severe poisoning the rate of decrease of dieldrin in the serum was very rapid (1.16 to a mean of 0.45 ppm) during the period in which distribution to the tissues was undoubtedly an important factor; from day 3 forward, the half-life of dieldrin in the serum was 34 days. This may be compared to a half-life of 141–592 days (mean 369 days) reported by Hunter *et al.* (1969) for volunteers after they stopped taking small, harmless, daily doses. The much faster elimination of the large, single dose was to be expected, and it may have been accelerated by phenobarbital and other drugs used in therapy. Furthermore, consideration of the observed values kindly supplied by Dr. Black suggests that the rate of loss already had undergone some further reduction by day 54.

Persons who underwent surgical operations or complete starvation did not show an increase in the concentration of dieldrin in their blood, and the body burden was decreased by starvation (Hunter and Robinson, 1968).

Among six formulators of aldrin, the ratio of storage of dieldrin (the main compound stored) in plasma and erythrocytes varied from 1.7 : 1 to 5.8 : 1 and averaged 3.77 : 1. There was a tendency for the ratio to be higher when storage was greater (Mick *et al.*, 1971). The average ratio in 10 ordinary people was 3.8 : 1 (Dale *et al.*, 1965). Thus, the concentrations of dieldrin in the whole blood of highly exposed persons are less than those in corresponding serum samples. However, in some workers the distribution is more equal. Morgan *et al.* (1972) reported that the proportion of dieldrin in the erythrocytes was essentially the same as the hemocrit. The concentrations in the plasma and serum are indistinguishable.

In any given person, the concentration of dieldrin in β-lipoprotein usually is greater than that in α-lipoprotein (Mick *et al.*, 1971).

Unlike DDT and HCB, dieldrin was below the level of detection in cord blood even though it was present in the blood of mothers, indicating a relatively efficient placental barrier to this compound (Siyali *et al.*, 1974).

The concentration of dieldrin in fat was 89 ppm 4 days after the near-fatal ingestion of a very large dose (Black, 1974). A concentration of 60 ppm was found in the fat of a worker whose exposure was stopped 15 days earlier because of convulsions (Kazantzis *et al.*, 1964). The highest concentration found in the fat of healthy workers was 32 ppm (Hayes and Curley, 1968).

The concentration of dieldrin in the fat of pregnant women was found to average about 0.085 ppm, only about half that in nonpregnant ones (Polishuk *et al.*, 1970), but, unlike the situation for some other insecticides, the difference was not statistically significant.

Dieldrin may be found in the fat (Table 15.12), blood (Table 15.13), and in various organs of people in the general population. There are no organ values for workers or patients to compare. The top of the range for both fat and serum in the general population overlaps somewhat with the corresponding range for workers (Tables 8.1 and 8.2). The slight overlapping is explained mainly by the fact that some of the "workers," although employed at the factories or formulating plants, were actually secretaries or administrative personnel with little exposure to aldrin or dieldrin. There is also the possibility that a few persons classified as "general population" actually had an unrecognized occupational or other special exposure to one of these compounds. Perhaps the most meaningful comparison is that for samples from the general population and from workers in a factory that made aldrin, dieldrin, endrin, and certain unrelated pesticides. Analysis of the samples for dieldrin in the same laboratory gave the following means and standard errors: 0.29 ± 0.05 versus 5.67 ± 1.11 ppm for fat, 0.0019 ± 0.0003 versus 0.0185 ± 0.0019 ppm for plasma, and 0.0008 ± 0.0002 versus 0.0242 ± 0.0063 for urine (Hayes and Curley, 1968).

Ackerman (1980) has reviewed a number of studies of dieldrin levels in the population up to 1976. Although levels in the environment had declined from the mid-1960s, levels in human fat and milk fat remained constant between 0.160 and 0.220 ppm.

Excretion of Dieldrin-Related Compounds   In a child who survived poisoning by dieldrin, the concentration of the compound in urine fell very rapidly from about 0.08 ppm, and it was barely detectable when measured 7 months after ingestion. The concentration in serum fell from almost 0.3 ppm to a high population level by the seventh month and decreased only very gradually, if at all, thereafter. The initial concentration in fat was 49 ppm. This level continued to fall gradually over a period of 16 months, at the end of which time it was well within the range found in the general population (Garrettson and Curley, 1969). Incidentally, as discussed in Section 15.5.4.2, the authors' computer-assisted speculation that distribution of dieldrin to muscle constitutes an important mechanism for reducing the concentration of the compound in the brain was not confirmed when the question was studied experimentally in rats.

Dieldrin is eliminated in human urine as at least two neutral, polar metabolites. Unchanged dieldrin is not excreted, but, perhaps through thermal conversion of a conjugate, a material having the same gas chromatographic retention time can be measured in the urine of men with occupational exposure to dieldrin (Cueto and Hayes, 1962) and even in the urine of almost all men and women of the general population (Cueto and Biros, 1967). The concentrations found in the urine of spraymen in Ecuador and Panama and of workers in chemical and formulating plants in the Netherlands, Colorado, and Georgia ranged from 0.1 to 3.4 ppm expressed as dieldrin (Cueto and Hayes, 1962). This represents a minimal intake of

0.15–5.1 mg/person/day, a wider range than has been estimated from blood levels (see Dosage Response above). However, the populations under study were only partially the same, and some of the men who contributed urine may have had heavy recent exposure and may even have been poisoned. Among healthy workers, the concentration of dieldrin in urine ranged from 0.0013 to 0.0660 ppm (Hayes and Curley, 1968). The concentrations of dieldrin equivalent in the urine of five men and five women without occupational or other special exposure ranged from 0.0005 to 0.0019 ppm (Cueto and Biros, 1967). This is equivalent to an intake of 0.0007–0.0029 mg/person/day, or slightly over 10 times the range of intake estimated by Robinson and Roberts (1969) from blood levels but on average only about 0.3 times the intake as determined by residues in food.

At least one metabolite, 9-hydroxydieldrin, from human feces has been identified rigorously (Richardson and Robinson, 1971). The aldehyde of dieldrin and unidentified metabolites have been found in human bile as judged by gas chromatography. The concentration of dieldrin-related material in the bile of a pest control operator was 0.059 ppm at the time his serum level was 0.165 ppm (Paschal *et al.*, 1974).

Other Laboratory Findings   Except for analytical values related to the storage and excretion of dieldrin, the only laboratory findings of practical importance are those associated with EEG changes. EEG changes in a case of aldrin poisoning were reported at least as early as 1951 (Spiotta, 1951). As early as 1957, studies were made in workers, and the degree and kind of EEG change were found to correspond somewhat with poisoning (Winthrop and Felice, 1957; Ducharne, 1957); this was confirmed later with both aldrin and dieldrin (Kazantzis *et al.*, 1964; Avar and Czegledi-Janko, 1970). It was the EEG that was first developed to be a practical tool for monitoring workers and determining when they should be removed from exposure and when returned to work with dieldrin. Characteristic changes included bilateral synchronous spikes, spike and wave complexes, and slow theta waves (Hoogendam *et al.*, 1962, 1965; Jager, 1970). An interesting parallelism in the rate of decrease in abnormality of the EEG and the rate of decrease in the concentration of dieldrin in the serum of one patient was described by Garrettson and Curley (1969).

Workers exposed to aldrin and dieldrin and with blood levels of dieldrin as high as 0.105 ppm showed no increase in urinary excretion of 6β-hydroxycortisol, even though those with similar exposure to endrin showed a marked increase (Chamberlain, 1971; Hunter *et al.*, 1972). Thus, endrin apparently is a stronger inducer of microsomal enzymes in humans than is aldrin or dieldrin.

The failure of aldrin or dieldrin to induce microsomal enzymes in people is not unexpected. The threshold for this effect is about 0.05 mg/kg/day in rats. The dosages found ineffective in workers were approximately 0.0175 mg/kg/day (Jager, 1970). In fact, induction may have occurred in aldrin formulators with an average total-blood chlorinated hydrocarbon level of 0.349 ppm. At least, that was the interpretation of

Bonderman *et al.* (1971) based on the finding of small but statistically significant increases in erythrocyte tributyrinase and in plasma cholinesterase. Although blood levels of aldrin and/or dieldrin were not specified, the workers presumably were the same as or similar to those found to have dieldrin plasma levels as high as 0.312 ppm (Mick *et al.*, 1972).

Tests, including serum alkaline phosphatase, SGOT, SGPT, serum LDH, serum creatinine phosphokinase (CPK), and serum proteins, all reflecting liver function, have been carried out in workers with prolonged exposure to dieldrin. Only alkaline phosphatase values in men with blood dieldrin levels above 0.20 ppm differed from the average in unexposed persons, but even these values were still within the normal ranges (Jager, 1970; Bogusz, 1968). Other authors (Morgan and Roan, 1974) have found entirely normal values, but the workers whom they tested had levels less than 0.20 ppm.

If one includes induction of liver microsomal enzymes, the no-effect level demonstrated in humans for aldrin and dieldrin is above a dieldrin blood level of 0.105 ppm (Versteeg and Jager, 1973).

Treatment of Poisoning   Treatment of poisoning by dieldrin and other chlorinated hydrocarbon insecticides is discussed in Section 15.2.5.

15.5.5 ENDRIN

15.5.5.1 Identity, Properties, and Uses

Chemical Name   Endrin is 1,2,3,4,10,10-hexachloro-6,7-epoxy-1,4,4a,5,6,7,8,8a-octahydro-1,4-*endo,endo*-5,8-dimethanonaphthalene.

Structure   See Fig. 15.6.

Synonyms   The common name endrin was established by ICPC and is approved by BSI and ISO. In the Republic of South Africa, nendrin is used as a common name. Other names are Endrex® and Hexadrin. Endrin was introduced in 1951 under the code Experimental Insecticide 269. Other code designations include ENT-17,251 and OMS-197. The CAS registry number is 72-20-8.

Physical and Chemical Properties   Endrin has the empirical formula $C_{12}H_8Cl_6O$ and a molecular weight of 380.93. The technical product (85% endrin) is a light tan flowable powder with a distinct odor. The pure material is a white crystalline solid. Endrin is decomposed by heat above 200°C or by strong acids, certain metal salts, and catalytically active carriers; it is compatible with other pesticides. The compound is nonflammable. It is moderately soluble in acetone, benzene, and xylene and sparingly soluble in alcohols and petroleum distillates. Its solubility in water is reported to be 0.23 ppm. The specific gravity is 1.70 at 20°C. The vapor pressure at 25°C is 2×10^{-7} mm Hg.

History, Formulations, and Uses Endrin was introduced for experimental purposes in 1951 and registered in the United States in 1952. It is formulated as 19.2–20% emulsifiable concentrates, 50% water-wettable powders, 1–5% granules, and 1–2% dusts. Endrin has been used mainly on field crops such as cotton and grains. It has also been used for grasshoppers in noncropland and to control voles and mice in orchards.

15.5.5.2 Toxicity to Laboratory Animals

Basic Findings Convulsions produced by endrin are similar to those produced by Metrazole (pentylenetetrazole). The LT 50 associated with endrin is longer in isolated than in grouped mice, but the LD 50 is not changed (Walsh and Fink, 1970).

The acute toxicity of endrin is summarized in Table 15.27. The compound is highly toxic as compared to most commercially available chlorinated hydrocarbon insecticides. As with DDT, young rats are less susceptible than adults. The same species shows the usual difference in susceptibility of the sexes. Rats maintained on a low (3.5%) protein diet are about twice as susceptible to endrin as those receiving a normal diet (Boyd and Stefec, 1969).

The effects of repeated doses of endrin are presented in Table 15.28. Although a 90-dose LD 50 has not been done, data in the table indicate that it must be between 1 and 2 mg/kg/day. Thus, the chronicity index is approximately 7 or 8, certainly of the same order of magnitude as that of DDT.

The no-effect level in the rat is 0.05 mg/kg/day (dietary level of 1 ppm), in the mouse 0.038 mg/kg/day (dietary level of 0.3 ppm), and in the dog 0.025 mg/kg/day (dietary level of 1 ppm).

The oxidative metabolism of endrin is responsible for its relatively efficient elimination and, therefore, its relative lack of cumulative effect when administered repeatedly. However, the three known mammalian metabolites of endrin are more toxic

Table 15.27
Single Dose LD 50 for Endrin

Species	Route	LD 50 (mg/kg)	Reference
Rat, M[a]	oral	28.8	Treon et al. (1955)
Rat, F[a]	oral	16.8	Treon et al. (1955)
Rat, M[b]	oral	43.4	Treon et al. (1955)
Rat, F[b]	oral	7.3	Treon et al. (1955)
Rat[b]	oral	40	Speck and Maaske (1958)
Rat, M	oral	17.8	Gaines (1960)
Rat, F	oral	7.5	Gaines (1960)
Rat, M	oral	27	Boyd and Stefec (1969)
Rat, M[c]	oral	5.6	Bedford et al. (1975a)
Rat, F[c]	oral	5.3	Bedford et al. (1975a)
Rat, F	dermal	15	Gaines (1960)
Guinea pig, M	oral	36	Treon et al. (1955)
Guinea pig, F	oral	16	Treon et al. (1955)
Rabbit, F	oral	7–10	Treon et al. (1955)
Monkey	oral	3	Treon et al. (1955)

[a] Age, 26–31 days.
[b] Age, 6 months.
[c] Age, 12–14 weeks.

Table 15.28
Effect on Various Animals of Repeated Oral Doses of Endrin

Dosage Range (mg/kg/day)	Method and concentration (ppm)	Species, number, and sex	Duration	Results	Reference
2.6–5	100 ppm in feed	rat 20 M, 20 F	2 yr	lethal in a few weeks	Treon et al. (1955)
1.26–2.5	50 ppm in feed	rat 20 M, 20 F	2 yr	lethal in a few weeks	Treon et al. (1955)
0.626–1.25	25 ppm in feed	rat 20 M, 20 F	2 yr	increased mortality in F	Treon et al. (1955)
	5 ppm in diet	mouse		fewer pups in first litter	Good and Ware (1969)
0.312–0.625	3 ppm in diet	mouse	life span	few convulsions; no effect on mortality, weight, or food intake	FAO/WHO (1971)
0.156–0.312	5 ppm in diet	rat 20 M, 20 F	2 yr	increase in liver weight ratio in M and kidney weight ratio in F	Treon et al. (1955)
0.078–0.156	2 ppm in diet	rat	3 gen	no effect on reproduction	FAO/WHO (1971)
	2 ppm in diet	rat 50 M, 50 F	life span	few convulsions, no tumorigenesis	Deichmann et al. (1970)
	4 ppm in diet	dog 7 M, 7 F	2 yr	few convulsions, slight pathology	FAO/WHO (1971)
0.039–0.078	1 ppm in diet	rat 20 M, 20 F	2 yr	no effect	Treon et al. (1955)
	1 ppm in diet	rat	3 gen	no effect on reproduction	FAO/WHO (1971)
	0.3 ppm in diet	mouse	life span	no effect on mortality, weight or food intake	FAO/WHO (1971)
	3 ppm in diet	dog 2 M, 2 F	10 mo	increase in kidney and heart weight ratios	Treon et al. (1955)
	2 ppm in diet	dog 7 M, 7 F	2 yr	few convulsions in 1 F; slight increase in liver weight ratio	FAO/WHO (1971)
0.019–0.039	1 ppm in diet	dog 2 M, 2 F	10 mo	no effect	Treon et al. (1955)
	1 ppm in diet	dog 7 M, 7 F	2 yr	no effect	FAO/WHO (1971)

than the parent compound (Fig. 15.7). The LD 50 of 12-ketoendrin is 1.1 and 0.8 mg/kg in male and female rats, respectively, and it exerts its full effect during the first 20 hr, compared to 4–8 days for endrin. Thus, 12-ketoendrin may be responsible for much of the acute toxicity of endrin or of intermediate metabolites in the rat (Bedford *et al.*, 1975a). However, the fact that the brains of rats killed by endrin contain (in addition to endrin) substantially less 12-ketoendrin than do the brains of rats killed by 12-ketoendrin suggests that endrin is toxic *per se*. Furthermore, the production of 12-ketoendrin varies greatly from one mammalian species to another, and none has been detected in birds (Stickel *et al.*, 1979).

Absorption, Distribution, Metabolism, and Excretion Following either oral or intravenous administration of [^{14}C]endrin to rats, it is metabolized to relatively water-soluble compounds and excreted mainly in the feces (Baldwin *et al.*, 1970b; Richardson *et al.*, 1970). The half-life is 2–3 days in males and 4 days in females after a dosage of 0.2 mg/kg. With daily oral doses, rats reach maximal storage in 6 days. The concentrations in the viscera are about the same as that in fat (Klein *et al.*, 1968). In the rabbit, [^{14}C]endrin is metabolized to *anti*-12-hydroxyendrin and to a lesser extent *syn*-12-hydroxyendrin (Fig. 15.7). The hydroxylated metabolites are excreted mainly as sulfate conjugates but also as glucuronide conjugates (Bedford *et al.*, 1975b).

Over 90% of excreted activity derived from [^{14}C]endrin is found in the feces of intact rats and in the bile of those with bile fistulas. Under identical circumstances, endrin is excreted faster than dieldrin from intact rats, from bile-fistula rats (in the

bile), and from isolated, perfused rat liver preparations (Cole *et al.*, 1970).

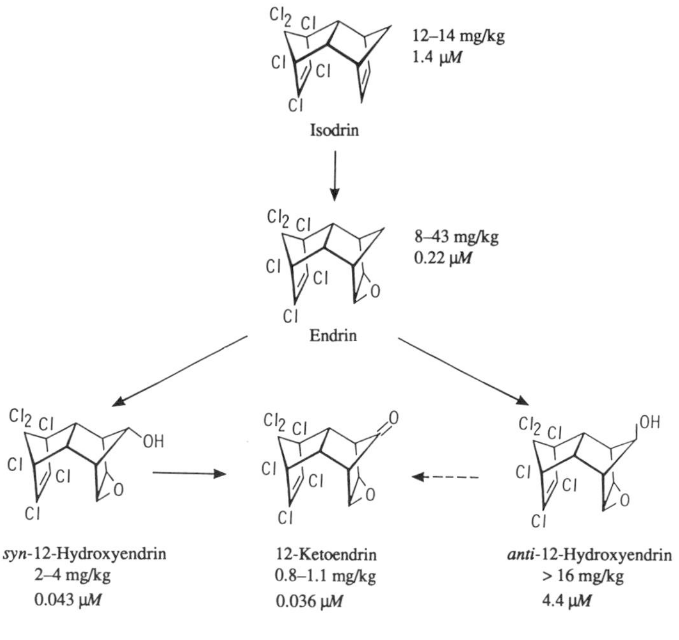

The greater susceptibility of female rats to endrin is reflected by the slower biotransformation and excretion of [^{14}C]endrin in perfused liver preparations from females (Altmeier *et al.*, 1969; Kelvay, 1970). Some evidence suggests that the difference between two strains of pine mice in their susceptibilities to endrin could be ascribed to differential metabolism (Petrella *et al.*, 1975). See also Biochemical Effects.

Biochemical Effects Increased cytochrome P-450-mediated oxidase activity has been induced in both rats and rabbits by feeding low levels of endrin (Hutson and Hoadley, 1974). In mice greater benzpyrene hydroxylase activity was found in the liver microsomes of endrin-resistant pine mice than in microsomes from susceptible ones. High levels also were found in the offspring of resistant mice, suggesting that the difference may be inherited (Webb *et al.*, 1972; Hartgrove *et al.*, 1972). The evidence for inheritance (in contrast to tolerance) is reasonable inasmuch as endrin is excreted rapidly, but final proof would require, among other things, demonstration that the young received no endrin via the placenta and milk. In nature, where the possibility of outbreeding cannot be excluded, pine mice gradually lost resistance to endrin after application of endrin as a control measure was stopped (Webb *et al.*, 1973).

The mechanism by which endrin induces mixed-function oxidase activity under practical conditions is unknown. Under some laboratory conditions, endrin inhibits this activity (Stanton and Kahn, 1972; Hundley *et al.*, 1974), whereas under other conditions it appears to be without effect of any kind (Hartgrove *et al.*, 1974). Part of the complications may involve time. Kachole and Pawar (1977) found no enzyme changes 12 hr after endrin was administered but did find induction 24 hr and more after administration. Another source of variation is excessive dosage, which may be inhibitory (Hartgrove *et al.*, 1977). In addition, species differences and the usual dosage–response relations have been demonstrated (Hartgrove *et al.*, 1977). Treatment of rats with 5 ppm endrin in their diet for 15 days reduced bile flow and phenolphthalein glucuronide excretion in males but there was a choleretic effect in females. Endrin aldehyde or endrin ketone had little influence (Young and Mehendale, 1986).

Large, single doses and small, repeated doses of endrin have largely opposite effects on the concentrations of biogenic amines in the brain (Hrdina *et al.*, 1974), but whether the changes are responsible for poisoning or secondary to it is obscure. Like lindane and some other chlorinated cyclodiene insecticides, endrin can act *in vitro* in mammalian brain preparations at sites which bind picrotoxin and which in turn block the GABA-regulated chloride ionophore (Lawrence and Casida, 1984; Eldefrawi *et al.*, 1985; Abalis *et al.*, 1986; Bloomquist *et al.*, 1986; Cole and Casida, 1986). 12-Ketoendrin seems to be particularly potent in binding and in its *in vivo* toxicity (Casida and Lawrence, 1985). As with the pairs aldrin and dieldrin, heptachlor and heptachlor epoxide (Eldefrawi *et al.*, 1985), it is the epoxide endrin which is more toxic than its

Figure 15.7 Microsomal metabolism of isodrin to endrin and then to other oxidized metabolites, showing increased acute toxicities (LD 50 values, mg/kg) and greater affinity for the picrotoxin binding site of the rat brain GABA receptor–ionophore complex as measured by the displacement of *t*-[^{35}S]butylbicyclophosphorothionate (IC 50 values, µ*M*) (data from Casida and Lawrence, 1985).

parent diene isodrin (Casida and Lawrence, 1985), a finding that can be partly ascribed to greater binding.

Effects on Organs and Tissues   A total of 1600 mice of two strains were used to explore the possible carcinogenicity of endrin. Dietary levels of 0.3 and 3.0 ppm were used, and a few convulsions were observed at the higher level. Although fibrosarcomas, hepatomas, and leukemia were observed, their incidence was not significantly higher than in the controls (FAO/WHO, 1971). Treon *et al.* (1955) mentioned an increase in the relative weight of the liver in rats receiving 5 ppm or more of endrin in the diet. Apparently, neither these authors nor others have reported, in connection with endrin, the changes that are characteristic of the effect of chlorinated hydrocarbon insecticides in rats and mice. However, in the absence of specific comparative study, it cannot be concluded that the characteristic changes are absent when relatively high but tolerated dosages are administered.

Intratesticular injection of mice with endrin caused chromosomal abnormalities (Dikshith and Datta, 1972). Studies in mice have demonstrated that endrin produces specific alterations in unmyelinated fiber bundles of peripheral nerves but does not affect myelinated fibers (Walker and Phillips, 1987).

Effects on Reproduction   Endrin is not teratogenic under practical conditions. As shown in Table 15.28, dietary levels that do not injure the parents do not injure reproduction. In fact, reproduction may continue with little change even at dosage levels that produce some convulsions. The results in wild deer mice are similar (Morris, 1968). Noda *et al.* (1972) reported increased fetal mortality and also increased fetal toxicity (primarily delayed and deviant ossification) in the offspring of rats and mice that were bred for the first time 1 week after receiving four oral doses of endrin emulsion at a rate of 0.58 mg/kg at weekly intervals. The small differences were of unstated statistical significance. Ottolenghi *et al.* (1974) found that endrin administered during pregnancy at half the LD 50 level produced a marked increase in fetal deaths of hamsters but not mice. Open eye, webbed foot, cleft palate, and especially fused ribs were seen in young hamsters and may have been related to growth retardation.

Differences in the effects of single and repeated doses administered to hamsters during pregnancy were reported by Chernoff *et al.* (1979a). A single dose as high as 10 mg/kg on day 8 did not kill the dams or young but did increase the incidence of fused ribs and meningoencephaloceles. Multiple doses as high as 3.5 mg/kg/day on days 5–14 caused maternal weight loss and mortality and fetal mortality but fewer fetal defects. Single dosages less than 5 mg/kg and repeated dosages of 1.5 mg/kg/day were ineffective. Similar but less pronounced effects were seen with rats and mice (Kavlock *et al.*, 1981).

Hamster pups from dams that had received 1.5 mg/kg/day on gestation days 5–14 were more active than controls 15 days after birth, but the difference disappeared by day 34 (Gray *et al.*, 1979).

15.5.5.3 Toxicity to Humans

Accidental and Intentional Poisoning   The most spectacular episodes of poisoning by endrin have been associated with the eating of bread made from contaminated flour. In most instances contamination occurred during shipment of the flour (Davies and Lewis, 1956; Weeks, 1967), but in some instances the way of contamination was not learned (Coble *et al.*, 1967). At least 936 persons have been made sick by eating contaminated bread, and 26 of them died. Isolated accidents often involving the ingestion of formulations are less likely to be reported, but their number has been considerable. For example, Karplus (1971) reported 13 cases, including 6 deaths in children. Reddy *et al.* (1966) reported 60 cases of which 41 were suicidal, 5 were homicidal, 13 were of unknown origin, and 1 was accidental.

The onset of poisoning may be as little as half an hour or as much as 10 hr after eating contaminated food (Davies and Lewis, 1956; Weeks, 1967). The interval usually has been 1–4 hr in cases of accidental ingestion (Weeks, 1967) and much less in cases of suicide and homicide (Reddy *et al.*, 1966).

Severe poisoning by endrin involves repeated, violent, epileptiform convulsions, each lasting several minutes and followed by semiconsciousness or coma for 15–30 min unless the next fit occurs sooner. Fits may become almost continuous. Usually, there are few or no warning symptoms in severe poisoning, and even in moderate poisoning there may be no warning before the first fit (Davies and Lewis, 1956; Reddy *et al.*, 1966). A less common but very ominous feature of serious poisoning is hyperthermia (Jedeikin *et al.*, 1979; MMWR, 1984; Runhaar *et al.*, 1985). The high fever was followed by decerebrate rigidity in 1- and 2.5-year-old children who developed temperatures of 42 and 41.7°C, respectively (Jacobziner and Raybin, 1959; Hayes, 1963). Often, lung congestion has been reported at autopsy of fatal cases (Montoya Cabrera *et al.*, 1980; MMWR, 1984; Runhaar *et al.*, 1985).

Mild illness has involved dizziness, weakness of the legs, abdominal discomfort, and nausea but usually not vomiting. Some patients were temporarily deaf and some were slightly disoriented or aggressive (Davies and Lewis, 1956).

Deaths have occurred as little as half an hour after ingestion, and most suicidal cases are dead within an hour or two (Reddy *et al.*, 1966) but it can be much longer (Runhaar *et al.*, 1985). Deaths usually have occurred in accidental cases within the first 12 hr (Weeks, 1967). In most survivors, recovery was well advanced 24 hr after poisoning, but a few complained of headache, dizziness, lethargy, weakness, and anorexia for 2–4 weeks. In one epidemic, many victims improved within the first 5 hr in the hospital, and they were promptly discharged. Except for abnormal electroencephalograms, neurological findings were normal soon after a convulsion.

The mortality rates in outbreaks involving contaminated bread have varied from 0% (Davies and Lewis, 1956; Coble *et al.*, 1967) to 9.0% (Weeks, 1967). The difference depended in part on dosage. Endrin was found in a concentration of 150 ppm in a sample of bread in an epidemic with no mortality (0/59)

(Davies and Lewis, 1956) and at concentrations of 1339–1807 in an epidemic with 9.0% (17/188) mortality (Weeks, 1967; Curley *et al.*, 1970). However, the mortality was 1.4% (7/490) in an outbreak in which a bread sample contained only 48 ppm endrin. The mortality may have been due in part to the fact that patients in the latter epidemics were treated with atropine in the belief that they were suffering from organophosphate poisoning, but see also Treatment of Poisoning.

A poisoning episode of the general population in Pakistan was reported in 1984. Altogether 192 cases of acute convulsions were reported with 19 deaths (MMWR, 1984; Rowley *et al.*, 1987). Most were male or female children, 80% being under 15 years of age. Although young children apparently had no earlier symptoms before seizures, older patients complained of headaches and/or nausea and minor muscular spasms approximately half an hour before collapsing. Interestingly, more severely ill patients did not vomit as frequently as mildly affected patients and they had higher temperatures. The evidence that endrin was the causative agent was very strong, since analyses of serum, stomach contents, and adipose tissue from convulsive patients were often positive for the insecticide. However, there was no evidence that local farmers were using endrin, nor was it available locally. So far the origin of the endrin does not appear to have been traced unequivocally but it is possible that sugar was contaminated during transport from sugarcane growers in the southern part of the Punjab. One composite sugar sample taken from the homes of three persons had an endrin level of 0.04 ppm.

Use Experience   After it became possible to measure cyclodiene compounds in blood, it was found that endrin did not accumulate, and, therefore, no endrin worker was ever transferred on this basis to a duty involving less exposure. Blood levels associated with brief, unusual occupational circumstances are discussed under Laboratory Findings.

Seven intoxications involving endrin, all characterized by one or more convulsions, were encountered in one factory. Although these illnesses were scattered over a period of 8 years, all of them occurred during the first or, sometimes, during the second year of exposure of each person involved. Recovery following occupational exposure to endrin has been essentially complete within 24 hr (Jager, 1970) and no long-term effects have been observed (Ribbens, 1985).

A study of the use of insecticides in the rural Philippines has suggested that there is a link between an increased use of insecticides and a subsequent increase in mortality in men (Loevinsohn, 1987). Increased mortality was not seen in urban men; in fact, a decrease was observed. One of the most widely used insecticides was endrin, and a significant increase in apparent strokes in younger men (15–24) was recorded. During the 1982 season, when the use of endrin was prohibited, mortality attributed to strokes decreased for all men of the rural regions in the following 2 years. Although confusion with acute endrin intoxication may be the explanation for increased mortality reported as strokes, it is interesting to compare these findings with the observations of workers employed in manufacturing chlordane and heptachlor (Wang and MacMahon, 1979b; see Section 15.5.1.3, Use Experience).

Atypical Cases of Various Origins   A case in which some symptoms persisted about 40 days (Tosa *et al.*, 1971) may not have been caused by endrin, as convulsions were not reported but signs (myofibrillar contractions and miosis) not characteristic of endrin poisoning were present.

One case of polyneuropathy following exposure to endrin and DDT has been reported (Jenkins and Toole, 1964).

A case (Kuebrich and Urban, 1973) that under other circumstances would have been diagnosed as a cerebral vascular accident was reported as endrin poisoning only because the attack came 3 hr after the patient began work in a greenhouse where endrin emulsifiable spray had been applied the day before. The progress and outcome of the case were typical of cerebral vascular accident and never were seen before or since in endrin poisoning in humans or animals.

Dosage Response   Based on a concentration of 150 ppm in the remains of a loaf of bread that had caused illness and on the amount of such bread necessary to cause different degrees of illness (Davies and Lewis, 1956), it was estimated (Hayes, 1963) that the dosage necessary to produce a single convulsion in humans is about 0.25 mg/kg, and the dosage necessary to produce repeated, nonfatal convulsions is about 1 mg/kg. In a suicide, a 49-year-old man ingested 12 gm of endrin dissolved in aromatic hydrocarbons, that is, about 100–200 mg/kg (Runhaar *et al.*, 1985).

There is no direct evidence on the repeated dosage that must be absorbed in order to produce illness. However, judging from the rapid elimination of endrin and from industrial experience, people can tolerate almost as much every day as they can tolerate for a single day.

The threshold limit value of 0.1 mg/m^3 indicates that occupational intake at a rate of 0.014 mg/kg/day is considered safe.

Laboratory Findings   In a fatal case of endrin poisoning, levels in blood were 0.450, 0.086, and 0.071 ppm at 4 hr, 6 days, and 11 days, respectively, after ingestion (Runhaar *et al.*, 1985). At the 11-day time, when the patient died, endrin levels of 89.5, 0.87, 0.89, 0.55, and 1.32 ppm were found in adipose tissue, heart, brain, kidney, and liver, respectively. Another report of tissue levels associated with fatal endrin poisoning is that of Curley *et al.* (1970), who found 0.685, 0.116, and 0.160 ppm in liver, kidney, and stomach wall, respectively; the samples were supplied separately and may have come from different persons. An earlier analysis also done by gas chromatography (Hayes, 1982) revealed the following concentrations (ppm): liver, 7.2; kidney, 0.6; brain, 0.7; lung, 0.9; and spleen, 0.4. In a second case, the values (ppm) were: liver, 10.0; kidney, 0.0; brain, 4.4; lung, 0.6; heart, 0.4; and spleen, 0.0. The first patients ate contaminated bread; the last two died after spraying endrin. Whether the 5- to 10-fold difference in results was due to more gradual absorption in the last two cases or to some other factor is unknown.

An early report (Hayes, 1963) of a concentration of 400 ppm in the fat of a man sampled 12 days after convulsions caused by endrin was based on bioassay and is entirely unconfirmed.

The endrin content of plasma from surviving patients poisoned by endrin-contaminated bread they had eaten the same day varied from <0.004 to 0.053 ppm. The plasma values tended to be inversely proportional to the interval from ingestion to onset (Coble *et al.*, 1967; Curley *et al.*, 1970). Endrin was undetectable in plasma obtained from some of the same patients 1 month later. However, a level of 0.021 ppm was found in one case 30 hr after convulsion (Coble *et al.*, 1967). Within 24 hr of poisoning in a third episode involving contaminated bread, four persons had blood levels of endrin ranging from 0.001 to 0.010 ppm, and two other persons had concentrations in the same range, although their samples were collected 72 hr after poisoning.

A man who suffered a single convulsion immediately after 4 hr of careless exposure to endrin dust he was formulating had an endrin blood level of 0.08 ppm, but he also had a dieldrin blood level of 0.11 ppm; 24 hr later his endrin level had fallen to 0.02 while the dieldrin level remained unchanged. Four days after the second sample, endrin was undetectable (<0.005 ppm). Two workers who were accidently splashed with 20% emulsifiable concentrate developed endrin blood levels of 0.09 ppm (with no other detectable cyclodiene compounds) and 0.027 ppm (with 0.01 ppm dieldrin), respectively, even though both men bathed and changed clothes promptly. Neither man became sick (Jager, 1970). In a similar way, a concentration of 0.004 ppm was found in a man who ate some contaminated bread but did not become ill (Coble *et al.*, 1967). In the outbreak of apparent endrin poisoning in Pakistan in 1984 (see under Accidental and Intentional Poisoning) serum levels in patients with convulsions ranged from 0 to 0.254 ppm (MMWR, 1984). Stomach contents from one patient whose serum was positive contained 0.307 ppm endrin.

Based on industrial experience, Jager (1970) estimated that 0.050–0.100 ppm is the concentration of endrin in the blood below which no sign or symptom is induced. The fact that people poisoned by contaminated bread had slightly lower levels suggests that the estimate of a threshold may be high or, more likely, that the highest concentrations measured in the foodborne outbreaks were slightly lower than the same patients had earlier simply because sampling often was late in accident cases. A different explanation based on a development of slight tolerance to endrin among those who make and formulate it would be logical but unsupported by available evidence.

All are agreed that blood levels drop rapidly to undetectable levels (<0.005 ppm) after heavy, accidental exposure (Curley *et al.*, 1970; Jager, 1970) and that endrin is undetectable in the blood of the general population or even the blood of endrin workers who have not experienced a very recent, gross accidental exposure (Hayes and Curley, 1968; Jager, 1970; Hunter

et al., 1972). It is even more remarkable that no endrin (<0.03 ppm) was found in the fat of healthy men employed in making and formulating it (Hayes and Curley, 1968).

In some cases of acute poisoning, endrin may be detected in urine collected within the first 24 hr at concentrations of 0.007–0.039 ppm (Coble *et al.*, 1967; Curley *et al.*, 1970).

Occupational exposure to endrin increased the excretion of 6-oxysteroid per milligram of reduced steroid from a population value of 30.7 to 91.0 μg/mg, indicating an induction of microsomal enzymes. No such effect followed exposure to aldrin and dieldrin (Chamberlain, 1971). An entirely similar conclusion was based on finding an increase in the excretion of D-glucaric acid, low blood levels of *p,p'*-DDE, and an inverse relationship between blood DDE and D-glucaric acid excretion (Jager, 1970; Hunter *et al.*, 1972).

Treatment of Poisoning   Hayden *et al.* (1965) used assisted respiration and succinylcholine at a rate of 0.5–1.0 mg/min for 24 hr to maintain effective respiration and prevent convulsions. In many instances, such heroic measures are not necessary, treatment being the same as for other chlorinated hydrocarbon insecticides (see Section 15.2.5). In a poisoning episode in Pakistan, a combination of diazepam, phenobarbital, and atropine (to control secretions) proved effective (MMWR, 1984).

15.5.6 ISOBENZAN

15.5.6.1 Identity, Properties, and Uses

Chemical Name   Isobenzan is 1,3,4,5,6,7,8,8-octachloro-1,3,3a,4,7,7a-hexahydro-4,7-methanoisobenzofuran.

Structure   The structure is shown in Fig. 15.6.

Synonyms   Isobenzan (ISO) was made and sold under the trade name Telodrin®. It had the code designations SD-4402, OMS-206, OMS-618, and ENT-25,545-X.

Physical and Chemical Properties   Isobenzan has the empirical formula $C_9H_4Cl_8O$ and a molecular weight of 411.79. The technical product (≥95% isobenzan) is a whitish to light-brown crystalline powder with a mild "chemical" odor. It is nonflammable and nonexplosive. However, it rearranges with loss of chlorine if heated above 210°C, and it also tends to rearrange in the presence of acids, certain metal salts, and catalytically active carriers. Isobenzan is soluble in acetone, benzene, toluene, xylene, heavy aromatic naphtha, and ethyl ether; slightly soluble (<1%) in kerosene and ethanol; and virtually insoluble in water. The specific gravity is 1.87 and the melting point 120°C. The vapor pressure at 25°C is 1×10^{-5} mm Hg.

History, Formulations, and Uses   Isobenzan was manufactured for Shell in Holland. Production started in 1958 and was discontinued in September 1965 (Jager, 1970). It was supplied in the form of emulsifiable concentrate, dust, and granules but never was registered for use in the United States. It has been used on alfalfa, corn, and tobacco.

15.5.6.2 Toxicity to Laboratory Animals

Basic Findings Rats become lethargic and show an elevation of their fur in about 1 hr following a dose in the LD 50 range. Soon tremors appear. The animals paw their faces, tend to carry their tails outstretched, and often gnaw the cage. Later there is frothing at the mouth, general twitching of the muscles, labored breathing, opisthotonus, and convulsions. During intervals between convulsions, the animals run around the cage. Most deaths occur within 20 hr. Recovery of survivors is rapid even in those that had violent convulsions. Symptomatology in other species differs only in degree or duration (Worden, 1969).

Isobenzan is not irritating to the skin (Worden, 1969).

The rate at which isobenzan is absorbed is strongly influenced by the formulation in which it is administered. The compound is highly toxic, as indicated by oral LD 50 values of 1.6–20 mg/kg in a number of species (see Table 15.29). Previously unpublished values within the same range were reported by Jager (1970), who also recorded a dermal LD 50 range of 20–22.5 mg/kg for xylene emulsion in the hooded rat.

There is a marked species difference in susceptibility to repeated doses of isobenzan. Rats receiving the compound orally at 2.5 mg/kg/day died within a week. However, mortality was only 20 and 0% in those that received dietary levels of 30 and 17.5 ppm (about 1.5 and 0.86 mg/kg/day), respectively, for 2 years. Both groups of rats showed immediate irritability and occasional convulsions followed by at least partial clinical recovery after several weeks of feeding (Worden, 1969). Mor-

tality was 100% within 24 or 64 days among mice on dietary levels of 10 and 5 ppm, respectively. Even at 2.5 ppm (about 0.3 mg/kg/day) isobenzan was 80% fatal to mice within 120 days (Ware and Good, 1967). Dogs survived intubation at a rate of 0.1 mg/kg/day for 2 years, but they grew slowly and showed a slight increase in serum alkaline phosphatase and increases in the relative weights of the liver, lung, and kidney (Worden, 1969). The no-effect level for rats is 0.25 mg/kg/day (Worden, 1969); that for dogs is less than 0.1 mg/kg/day but may be as high as 0.08 mg/kg/day (Brown *et al.*, 1962), a dosage not tested by Worden (1969), who reported 0.025 mg/kg/day as a no-effect level in dogs.

Absorption, Distribution, Metabolism, and Excretion
Isobenzan is absorbed by the skin as well as by the respiratory and gastrointestinal tracts.

In blood isobenzan is associated with both cellular compartments (erythrocytes) and plasma (albumin and α-globulin) (Moss and Hathway, 1964).

Brown *et al.* (1962) found that beagles developed convulsions when the concentration of isobenzan in their blood ranged from 0.042 to 0.072 ppm.

Following intravenous injection, 13 and 16% of radioactive isobenzan was excreted in 48 hr by male and female rats, respectively, in the form of a hydrophilic metabolite (Kaul *et al.*, 1970).

Biochemical Effects Isobenzan was one of the most potent cyclodiene inhibitors of beef heart mitochondrial Mg^{2+}-ATPases and rat brain synaptosome oligomycin-sensitive Mg^{2+}-ATPases (Mehrota *et al.*, 1982).

As with aldrin, dieldrin, heptachlor, and endrin, isobenzan inhibits chloride influx by mouse brain vesicles (Bloomquist *et al.*, 1986) and appears to be associated with binding to the GABA–receptor complex (Lawrence and Casida, 1984; Casida and Lawrence, 1985; Cole and Casida, 1986).

The stimulation of ammonia metabolism in brain and related amino acid metabolism were studied by Hathway and co-workers (Hathway and Mallinson, 1964; Hathway *et al.*, 1965) and is still a confusing area (Woolley *et al.*, 1985).

Effects on Organs and Tissues The maximal tolerated dosage of isobenzan failed to increase the incidence of tumors in mice treated for 18 months (Innes *et al.*, 1969).

Effects on Reproduction Although isobenzan at a dietary level of 2.5 ppm was lethal to 80% of BALB/c mice within 120 days, this strain tolerated 1 ppm (about 0.13 mg/kg/day) and reproduced normally during the same feeding interval (Ware and Good, 1967).

Pathology Although a relative increase in liver weight has been noted in rats and dogs fed high, tolerated doses, histological changes of the liver apparently have not been described and have been specifically denied (Brown *et al.*, 1962). Thyroid

Table 15.29
Single-Dose LD 50 for Isobenzan[a]

Species	Route	LD 50 (mg/kg)
Rat, M[b]	oral	11.1
Rat, F[b]	oral	8.9
Rat, M[c]	oral	6.6
Rat, F[c]	oral	6.2
Rat	subcutaneous	6–10
Mouse	oral	10.0
Mouse	subcutaneous	6–10
Guinea pig, M	oral	2.8
Guinea pig, F	oral	2.3
Hamster	oral	20.0
Hamster, M	oral	8.0
Hamster, F	oral	7.5
Rabbit	oral	4.0
Dog	oral	1.6
Cat	oral	5.0
Fowl	oral	12–14
Fowl	oral	1.8

[a] From Worden (1969).
[b] Hooded.
[c] Sprague–Dawley.

hyperplasia possibly related to isobenzan was seen in some rats fed the compound for 2 years at a dietary level of 30 ppm.

15.5.6.3 Toxicity to Humans

Accidents and Use Experience Apparently no nonoccupational accidents with isobenzan have been reported. In fact, what is known about its toxicity to people all depends on experience in a single factory complex including one unit in which isobenzan was made. The total number of persons exposed to aldrin, dieldrin, endrin, and/or isobenzan was 826. Out of an unstated proportion of these who were exposed only to isobenzan at the time, 42 were transferred to other, less hazardous work because of suggestive, nonincapacitative symptoms; an additional 30 men suffered clinical intoxication, and 16 of the 30 had one or more convulsions. In addition, among men who were exposed to both dieldrin and isobenzan at the time, 36 were transferred, and 18 were clinically intoxicated, including 8 with fits. Cases associated with isobenzan (with or without dieldrin) differed from those associated with dieldrin or endrin in that there were many complaints of headache, dizziness, drowsiness, irritability, and sometimes paresthesias, particularly in the legs. Although recovery was complete, it tended to be slow, and complaints lasted for 6 months in three cases. Intoxications with isobenzan also differed in that a high proportion of skilled workers were affected, and illness occurred among people employed for as many as 9 years and not just in people exposed for 3 or fewer years (Jager, 1970). Follow-up studies (up to a mean of 24 years) have shown no untoward effects (Versteeg and Jager, 1973; Ribbens, 1985).

Laboratory Findings The threshold blood level for isobenzan below which no signs or symptoms of intoxication occur is only 0.015 ppm. Blood levels as high as 0.030 ppm have been reported in connection with intoxications both with and without convulsions. The fatal level is not known.

The relatively prolonged course of isobenzan poisoning can be explained largely or entirely by the slow elimination of the compound; its half-life in human blood is about 2.77 years (Jager, 1970).

Typical EEG changes are found in poisoning by isobenzan. In this connection, the EEG usually recovers much quicker but has remained abnormal for more than a year (Jager, 1970).

Treatment of Poisoning Treatment is symptomatic (see Section 15.2.5).

15.5.7 ENDOSULFAN

15.5.7.1 Identity, Properties, and Uses

Chemical Name Endosulfan is a mixture of two stereoisomers of 6,7,8,9,10,10-hexachloro-1,5,5a,6,9,9a-hexahydro-6,9-methano-2,4,3-benzodioxathiepin 3-oxide. Of the two isomers, α-endosulfan (endosulfan I) has the *exo* configuration and β-endosulfan (endosulfan II) had the *endo* configuration.

Structure See Fig. 15.6.

Synonyms The common name endosulfan (ANSI, BSI, ISO) is in general use except in Iran and the USSR, where thiodan is used as a common name. Endosulfan was introduced in 1956 under code number Hoe-2671. Proprietary names include Beosit®, Cyclodan®, Malix®, Thifor®, Thimul®, and Thiodan®. Code designations for endosulfan have included FMC-5,462, Hoe-2671, OMS-204 (α-endosulfan), and OMS-205 (β-endosulfan). The CAS registry number is 115-29.7.

Physical and Chemical Properties Endosulfan has the empirical formula $C_9H_6Cl_6O_3S$ and a molecular weight of 406.95. The α isomer has a melting point of 109°C and constitutes about 70% of the pure mixture. The β isomer has a melting point of 213°C and constitutes about 30% of the mixture. Technical endosulfan contains 90–95% of the pure mixture; it is a brownish crystalline solid that smells of sulfur dioxide and melts at 70–100°C. It is stable to sunlight. Endosulfan is hydrolyzed slowly by water and acids and rapidly by bases to the alcohol and SO_2. Its decomposition is catalyzed by iron, which it corrodes. Endosulfan is moderately soluble in most organic solvents but highly insoluble in water. The vapor pressure of technical endosulfan is 9×10^{-3} mm Hg, and its density is 1.745.

History, Formulations, and Uses Endosulfan was first described in 1956 and was introduced as an experimental insecticide in the same year. It was first registered in the United States in 1960. It was formulated as emulsifiable concentrate, water-wettable powder, dust, and granules. Endosulfan has been used against a wide variety of agricultural pests but not against those of livestock, stored products, or the household.

15.5.7.2 Toxicity to Laboratory Animals

Basic Findings It has been argued (Maier-Bode, 1968) that endosulfan, as a sulfurous acid ester, differs so much from other cyclodiene insecticides that it ought to be considered separately. However, the acute illness it produces in laboratory animals or in humans is indistinguishable from that caused by other cyclodiene compounds, and its minimal storage in organisms and brief persistence in the environment are similar to these properties of endrin but different from those of dieldrin or telodrin. It is true that ataxia that progressed to complete inability to stand but never involved observed convulsions was reported in pigs and lambs that grazed in a field that had been sprayed with endosulfan (Utklev and Westbye, 1971). Although rapid recovery of surviving domestic animals is the rule, some instances of slow recovery have been reported. For example, blindness (previously unreported in connection with endosulfan but seen in connection with some other cyclodiene compounds) was observed in sheep. Onset of blindness was delayed 1 week after first exposure to pasture sprayed with endosulfan; some recovery was noted after an additional 2 weeks with full recovery at the end of the month (Doman, 1971).

The oral LD 50 values for endosulfan in male and female rats are 43 and 18 mg/kg, respectively, and the dermal values are only a little larger, 130 and 78 mg/kg, respectively (Gaines, 1969). Intraperitoneal LD 50 values in the rat varied from 22.1 to 89.4 mg/kg, depending on vehicle and sex. In the mouse, the corresponding values ranged from 6.9 to 13.5 mg/kg (Gupta, 1976). The dermal LD 50 of two lots of technical endosulfan in female rabbits was 167 and 187 mg/kg (Gupta and Chandra, 1975). α-Endosulfan is more toxic than β-endosulfan (Eldefrawi et al., 1985).

Some rats receiving repeated oral doses at a rate of 10 mg/mg/day died within 15 days. Rats survived 5 mg/kg/day for 15 days but showed liver enlargement and some other changes (Gupta and Chandra, 1977). During repeated dosing of rats (5 mg/kg for 10 days) seizures commenced 25–30 min after dosing and persisted for 60 min (Anand et al., 1980). A review by a joint committee (FAO/WHO, 1968) based largely on published reports indicated that a dietary level of 100 ppm (about 5 mg/kg/day) for 2 years reduced the growth and survival of female rats, caused enlargement and interstitial changes in the kidney of males, and produced some blood changes in both sexes. However, 50 ppm was without effect. Dogs are more susceptible than rats to poisoning by endosulfan. Dosages of only 2.5 mg/kg/day produced vomiting, tremor, and convulsions. However, dogs tolerated dosages as high as 0.75 mg/kg/day for a year.

The toxicity of endosulfan is about double in rats with moderate protein deprivation and is accentuated even more when the deprivation exceeds anything likely to occur in people (Boyd and Dobos, 1969; Krijnen and Boyd, 1971; Boyd et al., 1970).

Absorption, Distribution, Metabolism, and Excretion When given to rats by various routes, endosulfan is metabolized to the sulfate, diol, hydroxyether, ketone, and an unidentified metabolite. The ratio of the different compounds in the excreta differed not only with route but also with isomer. What is of far more importance is the fact that, when [^{14}C]endosulfan was administered to mice, only 20% of the metabolites were lipophilic (Schupan et al., 1968). The rapid production of water-soluble compounds explains the rapid excretion of endosulfan (Dorough et al., 1978). Most of the compounds formed from it by rats are produced by mice also (Deema et al., 1966). When administered in large doses endosulfan appears in the milk, largely as the sulfate (Gorbach et al., 1968).

In rabbits, the β isomer is cleared from the plasma much more rapidly than the α isomer, the terminal-slope half-lives being 5.97 and 235 hr, respectively (Gupta and Ehrnebo, 1979). The distribution of the α and β isomers in rats after administration of a mixture varies depending on the tissue. In the kidney the α isomer is the higher, whereas in seminal vesicles the β isomer predominates (Ansari et al., 1984). The sex difference in the LD 50 values in rats is probably explained by greater metabolism in the male (Dikshith et al., 1984).

Endosulfan distribution in cat brain varies with region and time after administration (Khanna et al., 1979).

Biochemical Effects Within 7 days, oral dosages of 2.5 mg/kg/day produced liver enlargement and increased pentobarbital sleeping time in female rats. These effects were not noticed in rats receiving 1.0 mg/kg/day for 15 days (Gupta and Gupta, 1977).

In vitro, endosulfan stimulates respiration of rat liver mitochondria at low concentrations but inhibits at higher levels. When state-4 respiration was stimulated, Mg^{2+}-ATPase activity was induced to a maximum 25-fold (Dubey et al., 1984). Endosulfan sulfate, endosulfan diol and endosulfan lactone were less effective.

Dorough et al. (1978) could not detect any induction of hepatic cytochrome P-450 or epoxidase activity toward aldrin after treatment of female rats with endosulfan (50 ppm of diet) for 28 days. On the other hand, Tyagi et al. (1984) have observed that multiple dosing of male rats (7.5 mg/kg body weight) did induce these parameters to a small degree. Induction appeared to be related to the quality of dietary protein.

Although there have been a number of studies on the effects of endosulfan after intratracheal administration, it is difficult to know whether the biochemical changes observed, such as lipid peroxidation (Narayan et al., 1985), are of any toxicological significance.

Endosulfan has many similar effects to lindane, dieldrin, and endrin on the GABA–receptor complex (Lawrence and Casida, 1984; Casida and Lawrence, 1985; Cole and Casida, 1986). The sulfate of endosulfan seems to be more potent than β-endosulfan (Lawrence and Casida, 1984). α-Endosulfan is more potent than β-endosulfan (Abalis et al., 1985; Eldefrawi et al., 1985). An associated inhibition of GABA-induced $^{36}Cl^-$ influx into rat brain microsacs is also observed (Abalis et al., 1986). Endosulfan appears to increase aggressive behavior and locomotor behavior in rats (Agrawal et al., 1983a; Anand et al., 1985) and this seems to involve the serotonergic system (Agrawal et al., 1983b). Young rats are often more susceptible to effects on neurotransmitter receptors than adults, and Seth et al. (1986) have reported that developing rats showed increased 5-[^{3}H]hydroxytryptamine binding and aggressive behavior when endosulfan was administered at 3 mg/kg for 30 days. Neonates receiving 1 mg/kg for 25 days showed significant changes in [^{3}H]serotonin binding and increased aggressive behavior, which persisted after cessation of treatment.

Platelet aggregation and uptake of [^{3}H]hydroxytryptamine were inhibited after rats were dosed with endosulfan (Anand et al., 1986). The administration of endosulfan to pentobarbital-anesthetized and paralyzed cats caused hypertension, capillary dilation, and increased cardiac output. Blood flow to the heart and brain occurred at the expense of that to kidneys, muscles, lung, and intestine (Anand et al., 1981). Blood flow to the brain was especially enhanced.

A single oral dose of endosulfan (5 mg/kg) to rats elevates glucose uptake by rat intestine but inhibits leucine uptake and the activity of Na^+, K^+-ATPase in the brush border (Wali *et al.*, 1982). Higher doses (40 mg/kg) are known to increase blood glucose levels (Garg *et al.*, 1980).

Both cellular and cell-mediated immune responses in rats are depressed markedly by endosulfan administration in the diet at 10 ppm for 8–22 weeks (Banerjee and Hussain, 1986).

Effects on Organs and Tissues Endosulfan was found mutagenic in a bacterial system (Dorough *et al.*, 1978) and in the micronuclear test in the bone marrow of mice (Sylianco, 1978). It also induced reverse mutations, crossovers, and mitotic gene conversions in *Saccharomyces cerevisiae* (Yadav *et al.*, 1982). However, it did not increase chromosomal changes in bone marrow and spermatogonia of rats (Dikshith *et al.*, 1978b; Dikshith and Datta, 1978). Endosulfan inhibited intercellular communication in two different *in vitro* assay systems. However, *in vivo*, oral administration of endosulfan (5 mg/kg/day) to male rats failed to enhance the incidence of γ-glutanyl transpeptidase positive foci in partially hepatectomised diethylnitrosamine-initiated animals (Flodström *et al.*, 1988).

The highest tolerated dosage of endosulfan did not increase the incidence of tumors in mice receiving it for 18 months (Innes *et al.*, 1969). In a later study no evidence was apparent for the carcinogenicity of endosulfan in rats or mice (NCI, 1978g).

Effects on Reproduction Oral dosages of 5 mg/kg/day and greater on days 6–14 of gestation increased the mortality of rat dams and increased the rates of resorption and skeletal abnormality in their fetuses (Gupta *et al.*, 1978). Oral dosage of 10 mg/kg/day for 15 days caused degeneration of many seminiferous tubules and a significant decrease in the weight of the testes (Gupta and Chandra, 1977). A dietary level of 50 ppm (about 2.5 mg/kg/day but much higher in lactating females) permitted normal reproduction in a three-generation study in rats (FAO/WHO, 1968).

15.5.7.3 Toxicity to Humans

Accidental and Intentional Poisoning Two suicides and three accidental deaths were reported by Terziev *et al.*, (1974). A 70-year-old woman died about 3 hr after she had taken only "drops" of an endosulfan formulation for stomach pains. Persons who took larger doses died quicker, some in less than an hour. The clinical picture in all cases involved gagging, vomiting, diarrhea, agitation, tonic-clonic convulsions, foaming at the mouth, dyspnea, apnea, cyanosis, and loss of consciousness. In an unsuccessful attempted suicide, three stages were observed: an acute cardiac and convulsive stage, a subacute pulmonary and convulsive stage, and finally a slow recovery (Shemesh *et al.*, 1989).

Use Experience Nine workers suffered one or more convulsions following exposure to endosulfan mainly in connection with bagging 50% water-wettable powder. Five of the men were said to have used a respirator and protective clothing; two

did not use a respirator, and the practices of the others were unknown. Six of the men had no history of a previous fit, and no history of any sort was available for the others. In the only three of these cases described in some detail, prodromal symptoms (malaise, vomiting, dizziness, weakness, or confusion) began while the man was at work and several hours before the first fit, which sometimes occurred at home or on the street. At least in one instance, a convulsion was followed by unconsciousness lasting an hour; the fit was so violent that it resulted in fractures of the fourth and fifth dorsal vertebrae. One patient remained confused for about 24 hr and then recovered rapidly (Ely *et al.*, 1967).

Three other cases were generally similar but apparently differed in detail for reasons that are not apparent. All were associated with filling bags with freshly ground endosulfan powder. Total exposure was brief in some instances. The outstanding prodromal symptom was headache, and the initial sign was fainting. The fainting was associated with or followed by "epileptoid twitching and foam at the mouth." One man bit his tongue, but apparently a full convulsion did not develop. EEG changes that promptly reverted to normal accompanied the illnesses (Israeli *et al.*, 1969).

A 23-year-old man, who had been preparing an endosulfan mixture and loading spray planes with it for about a month, stayed home for 1 day with what he thought was "flu" but may have been premonitory symptoms. He experienced dull headache, weakness, anorexia, abdominal discomfort, and a feeling of warmness. The next day he returned to work but in the afternoon, without any warning to himself or others, he suddenly "fell over backwards like a board," striking the back of his head on the concrete floor. His legs were seen to jerk mildly. His eyes were closed and he held his breath and turned blue. He was unconscious for a while and then very drowsy, recovering full consciousness about 2 hr after the fit. The only findings were a knot on his head, a chewed tongue, and complete, persisting amnesia for the period beginning about 1.75 hr before the convulsion until 1.75 hr after it. Detailed neurological examinations on days 7 and 21 were normal, but EEG records on both of these days were consistent with epilepsy (Hayes, 1982).

Atypical Cases of Various Origins A man was employed by a chemical plant where his main assignment was cleaning vats containing residues of endosulfan. The fact that he spoke only Georgian (USSR) prevented both his proper instruction and communication of his symptoms. He fainted several times and his family saw him having a convulsion during sleep. Four months after beginning his work, he had three consecutive convulsions and was admitted to a hospital. His consciousness was clouded but his vital signs were normal. The patient received diazepam and appeared to recover rapidly. However, no examination of his mental ability was possible because of the language barrier. At home, his family found him disoriented and occasionally agitated or abusive. The agitation was essentially eliminated by phenothiazine tranquilizers, but it soon became evident that the man could not converse except for answering simple questions. He could wash and feed himself but could not perform more complex activities. He was occasionally incontinent of urine. Examination at a psychiatric center 2 years later confirmed these difficulties and indicated diffuse brain damage (Aleksandrowicz, 1979). No period of apnea was observed or at least none was communicated to the medical authorities. However, it is difficult to escape the conclusion that brain damage in this case was the result of apnea during one or more convulsions.

Dosage Response   Only a small dose of endosulfan may be fatal; one victim died after swallowing only "drops" of a formulation. The absorbed dosage that affected workers is unknown. The threshold limit value of 0.1 mg/m^3 indicates that occupational intake of about 0.014 mg/kg/day is considered safe.

Laboratory Findings   In the case of a 28-year-old man who ingested 20% endosulfan powder while drunk and who was dead on arrival at hospital, α- and β-endosulfan were found in autopsy samples as follows: blood, 0.06 and 0.015 ppm; urine, 1.78 and 0.87 ppm; and liver 12.4 and 5.2 ppm, respectively. In another case, endosulfan sulfate was found in the liver at a concentration of 3.4 ppm (Demeter *et al.*, 1977; Demeter and Heyndrickx, 1978). In three other cases, the following ranges for combined isomers of endosulfan were found: blood, 4–8 ppm; liver, 0.8–1.4 ppm; kidney, 2.4–3.2 ppm; and brain, 0.25–0.30 ppm (Coutselinis *et al.*, 1978). No explanation is available for the marked difference in the ratios of blood to liver values in the two sets, but it may be pointed out that rats apparently survived plasma levels of 2.26 and 0.46 for the α- and β-isomers, respectively (Gupta, 1978). However, the synergistic effect of alcohol in the first case cannot be excluded. In a recent fatal case (Bernardelli and Gennari, 1987) endosulfan was ingested mixed with xylene. At autopsy blood contained 30 ppm, liver 20 ppm, kidney 2 ppm, and brain 0.3 ppm endosulfan. Xylene was detected only in the stomach contents (0.4 gm in a total of 50 ml), which also contained 0.5 gm of endosulfan.

In the 23-year-old man, the concentrations of endosulfan-1 and endosulfan-2 were both 0.0051 ppm in a serum sample collected 5 days after the fit; the concentrations declined gradually; they were still measurable in samples collected on day 7 but not on day 17 or 21. The concentrations of isomers 1 and 2 in subcutaneous fat were 0.28 and 0.57 ppm on day 7 and 0.13 and 0.20 ppm on day 21. Numerous other laboratory tests were normal (Hayes, 1982).

In vitro damage of human erythrocytes (membrane damage and crenation) was found at levels of 1 ppb endosulfan (Daniel *et al.*, 1986).

Treatment of Poisoning   Treatment is symptomatic (see Section 15.2.5).

15.6 TOXAPHENE

Toxaphene is a complex mixture of chemicals, many still unidentified, formed by the chlorination of technical camphene, which in turn is derived by isomerization of α-pinene, a by-product of turpentine distillation. Other products of a similar nature are made in different parts of the world, sometimes by chlorination of pinene itself. The exact compositions of these products are mostly unknown, although they can be distinguished from toxaphene (Saleh and Casida, 1977a). All will be considered under toxaphene, for which the literature is the most extensive.

15.6.1 TOXAPHENE AND ITS CONSTITUENTS

15.6.1.1 Identity, Properties, and Uses

Chemical Name   Toxaphene is chlorinated camphene containing 67–69% chlorine. Although this mixture contains more recognized compounds than most other technical pesticides, there is no evidence that toxaphene produced in the United States is any more variable in composition than other commercially available pesticides.

Analysis of technical toxaphene by gas chromatography–mass spectrometry reveals a complex of many compounds (175 and 177 reported by Casida *et al.*, 1974, and Holmstead *et al.*, 1974, respectively), mostly with 10 carbon atoms and with 6–11 chlorine atoms and 7–12 hydrogen atoms per molecule. It is important to make clear that of those identified most are chlorinated bornanes, not camphenes. During the chlorination procedure 2-*exo*,10-dichlorobornane is formed in a Wagner–Meerwein rearrangement of the camphene skeleton (Parlar *et al.*, 1977). This fact is sometimes obscured in descriptions of toxaphenes. Further chlorination causes a more or less statistical attack leading to many congeners and isomers. Three products have been identified which account significantly for the acute toxicity of toxaphene in mice, goldfish, and houseflies (Anagnostopoulos *et al.*, 1974; Casida *et al.*, 1974; Khalifa *et al.*, 1974; Nelson and Matsumura, 1975; Seiber *et al.*, 1975; Turner *et al.*, 1975, 1977; Saleh *et al.*, 1977):

2,2,5-*endo*,6-*exo*,8,9,10-Heptachlorobornane
   (known as toxicant B)
2,2,5-*endo*,6-*exo*,8,8,9,10-Octachlorobornane
2,2,5-*endo*,6-*exo*,8,9,9,10-Octachlorobornane

Other products including various nonachlorobornanes, decachlorobornanes, hexa- and heptachlorobornanes, and related chemicals can be found in the references cited.

Structure   The structures of the above chlorinated bornanes and some related congeners can be found in Fig. 15.8.

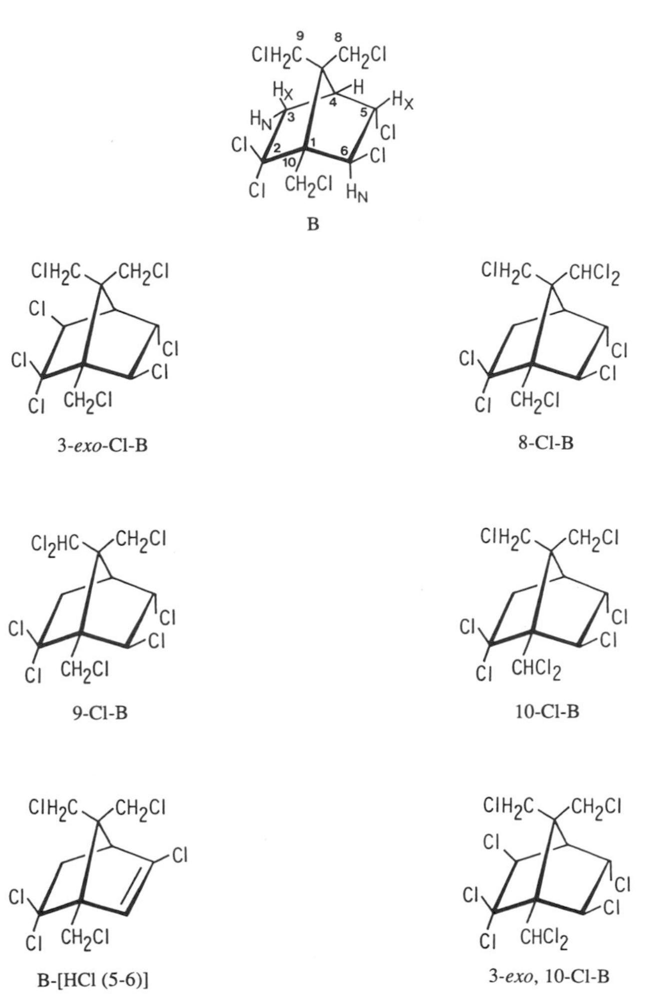

Figure 15.8 Structures of some polychlorobornane constituents of toxaphene. Abbreviated nomenclatures are shown as modified toxicant B (2,2,5-endo,6-exo,8,9,10-heptachlorobornane) (from Turner *et al.,* 1977).

Synonyms Toxaphene originally was a registered trademark of Hercules Incorporated; however, it has been dedicated to public use and is the accepted common name in the United States (ICPC) and several other countries. Other common names include camphechlor (BSI, ISO) chlorinated camphene, kamfochlor, octachloraphene, octachlorocamphene, polychlorinated camphene, toxafeen, and toxaphen. Although the terms polychlorophene and polychlorocamphene used in the USSR generally are regarded as synonyms, the material may be different, as indicated by higher toxicity associated with repeated doses in laboratory animals (see Section 15.6.1.2). The same is true of the closely related polychloropinene, which imparts an "acute piercing" odor to the organs of people killed by it. Proprietary names in addition to the former use of Toxaphene® include Agricide Maggot Killer®, Alltox®, Phenatox®, Strobane T-90®, Toxadust®, Toxakil®, Toxaspra®, and others. Code designations for toxaphene have included Compound-3,596 and Hercules-3,596. The CAS registry number is 8001-35-2. The chlorination of pinene to contain 66% chlorine produced a straw-colored liquid for-merly sold under the proprietary name Strobane®. It, or a similar product, is still in use in some countries under the name polychloropinene. Toxaphene is often combined with other insecticides.

Physical and Chemical Properties The empirical formula and molecular weight of toxicant B are $C_{10}H_{11}Cl_7$ and 379.35. Technical toxaphene is a yellow or amber, sticky wax with a slight pine odor. It is dehydrochlorinated by heat, strong sunlight, and certain catalysts, especially iron. It cannot be used with lime or other alkalies. Toxaphene is easily soluble in organic solvents including petroleum oils but is soluble in water only to the extent of about 3 ppm. The density of toxaphene is 1.66 at 20°C. It softens in the range 65–95°C. The vapor pressure is 0.2–0.4 mm Hg at 25°C.

History, Formulations, and Uses Toxaphene was first described in 1947, and it was introduced commercially the following year. It is formulated as emulsifiable concentrates, oil solutions, 40% wettable powders, 10% dust, and 10 and 20% granules.

Toxaphene is a nonsystemic contact and stomach insecticide with some action against mites. It is not toxic to plants except squash and melons. It is valued not only for its effectiveness but also because of its limited persistence in the environment and its rapid excretion by mammals. It has been used very extensively for cotton insects and to lesser degrees for a wide range of pests of beef cattle, goats, sheep, and swine and for insects attacking vegetables, small grains, and soybeans.

15.6.1.2 Toxicity to Laboratory Animals

Basic Findings The illness produced in various species by toxaphene is different from that produced by DDT, as tremor is essentially lacking, but is similar to that produced by lindane and dieldrin (see Sections 15.4.1.2 and 15.5.4.2). Whereas most animals show hyperreactivity, muscle spasms, and convulsions followed by coma, some show severe depression, drowsiness, and inappetance without any initial excitement or fit. Peculiar to toxaphene is the rapidity with which recovery sometimes occurs (Radeleff, 1964). Anorexia, oligodipsea, diuresis, glycosuria, loss of body weight, and hypothermia have been observed in rats poisoned by toxaphene. Hypothermia is most likely in animals already suffering severe protein deficiency (Boyd and Taylor, 1971).

The responses of laboratory animals to single and repeated doses of technical toxaphene are recorded in Tables 15.30 and 15.31. Toxaphene is moderately toxic by mouth but is not very poisonous when applied one time to the skin. Repeated oral doses are tolerated without any effect at levels of 0.6 mg/kg/day or slightly more by rats, dogs, and monkeys. No higher dosage was tested in monkeys. Only 4 mg/kg/day produces illness in dogs, but 75 mg/kg/day is required to produce illness in rats. Increasing dosages above about 2.2 mg/kg/day produce increasing degrees of the liver changes characteristic of stimulation of endoplasmic reticulum in rats. The fact that 43% of rats

Table 15.30
Single Dose LD 50 for Technical Toxaphene in Some Animal Species

Species	Route	LD 50 (mg/kg)	Reference
Rat, M	oral	90	Gaines (1960)
Rat, F	oral	80	Gaines (1960)
Rat	oral	69	Lehman (1951, 1952)
Rat	oral	240	Lyubenko et al. (1973a)
Rat	oral	120	USEPA (1976)
Rat	oral	270	Kuz'minskaya et al. (1980)
Rat, M	dermal	1075	Gaines (1960)
Rat, F	dermal	780	Gaines (1960)
Rat	dermal	940	Kuz'minskaya et al. (1980)
Mouse	oral	45	Lyubenko et al. (1973a)
Mouse	oral	112	USEPA (1976)
Mouse	intraperitoneal	47	Turner et al. (1977)
Mouse	intraperitoneal	33	Pollock and Kilgore (1980a)
Hamster	oral	200	Cabral et al. (1979a)
Dog	oral	49	USEPA (1976)
Cat	oral	40	USEPA (1976)
Rabbit	oral	100	USEPA (1976)
Rabbit	dermal	>4000	Lehman (1951, 1952)

were killed by polychlorophene within 6 months at a dosage of only 2.2 mg/kg/day (Lyubenko et al., 1973a,b) may indicate that the formulation tested was substantially more toxic than commercially available toxaphene. Chu et al. (1986, 1988) have concluded from a study with a Canadian toxaphene sample that the no-adverse-effect levels of the pesticide were 4 ppm (0.35 mg/kg/day) for the rat and 0.2 mg/kg/day for the dog after 13 weeks.

The acute toxicity of toxaphene can probably be ascribed to only a few of its constituents, of which the two octachlorobornanes, 2,2,5-endo,6-exo,8,8,9,10-octachlorobornane and 2,2,5-endo,6-exo,8,9,9,10-octachlorobornane, originally referred to as toxicants A-1 and A-2 respectively, are the most potent identified so far (Turner et al., 1975; Matsumura et al., 1975; Pollock and Kilgore, 1980a). Table 15.32 shows the ip LD 50 values in mice for a number of toxaphene constituents (Turner et al., 1977). Toxicity of 2,2,5-endo,6-exo,8,9,10-heptachlorobornane expecially was potentiated by the cytochrome P-450 inhibitor piperonyl butoxide (Turner et al., 1977; Saleh et al., 1977). Whether the chronic effects of toxaphene are also due to the same constituents is unknown.

Absorption, Distribution, Metabolism, and Excretion The distribution of polychlorocamphene in various lipid fractions has been investigated (Kuz'minskaya et al., 1972b), but the results are difficult to interpret because of the method of extraction. Perhaps more important is the fact that, following a single dose, residues disappeared entirely within 15 days. Combined oral and percutaneous administration enhanced toxicity (Kuz'minskaya et al., 1980).

Rats treated orally with [^{36}Cl]toxaphene and with each of several fractions of [^{36}Cl]toxaphene of equal total chlorine content excrete about 50–60% of the ^{36}Cl in the urine and 30–40% in the feces within 14 days. In each instance, about half

of the dose is excreted as chloride ion (Crowder and Dindahl, 1974; Casida et al., 1974; Ohsawa et al., 1975; Pollock and Kilgore, 1980b). Similar studies with [^{14}C]toxaphene and with [^{14}C]hepta- and [^{14}C]octachlorobornanes established that the feces contain unmetabolized compound and the metabolites include ^{14}CO$_2$ as well as acidic materials produced by partial or complete dechlorination. The tissues retain relatively low levels of ^{14}C several days after administration of [^{14}C]toxaphene or [^{14}C]Heptachlorobornane. In mice, injection iv of [^{14}C]toxaphene leads to rapid labeling of most tissues, although within 4 hr this is redistributed to adipose tissue. As with many of these types of chlorinated chemicals, persistent labeling of the adrenal cortex is observed (Mohammed et al., 1983, 1985). Most, if not all, components of toxaphene undergo extensive metabolic dechlorination in rats (Ohsawa et al., 1975; Pollock and Kilgore, 1980b). The fact that toxaphene is extensively dechlorinated by reaction with reduced hematin or reduced cytochrome P-450 in a neutral aqueous medium may help to explain its rapid metabolism (Khalifa et al., 1976).

The metabolism of 2,2,5-endo,6-exo,8,9,10-heptachlorobornane by a variety of mammalian species and chickens seems to occur partly by reductive dechlorination and dehydrochlorination at the gem-dichloro group to the respective hexachlorobornanes and hexachlorobornenes (Saleh et al., 1977, 1979). These metabolites were greatest in feces from monkeys and least in feces from chickens. In vitro experiments with rat liver preparations showed that toxaphene, as expected, can be metabolized by the microsomal mixed-function oxidases and by conjugation with glutathione and glucuronic acid, although only small amounts of mercapurates were detected in vivo (Chandurkar and Matsumura, 1979). Oxidation of 2,2,5-endo,6-exo,8,9,10-heptachlorobornane and 2-endo, 3,3,5,6-exo,8,9,10,10-nonachlorobornane was also demonstrated.

Biochemical Effects The lowest dietary level of toxaphene that produced a significant increase in any liver microsomal enzyme was 5 ppm. Enzyme activity reached an elevated steady state during the first 3 weeks of feeding (Kinoshita et al., 1966). On the other hand, Chu et al. (1986) found no significant induction of microsomal enzymes in rats 13 weeks after 100 ppm toxaphene but significant induction with 500 ppm. Another kind of evidence for the interaction of toxaphene and microsomal enzymes is the increased LD 50 of the compound in animals previously exposed to various combinations of pesticides for five or six generations (Keplinger and Deichmann, 1968). Decreased sleeping time caused by pentobarbital is also in vivo evidence for the induction of the mixed-function oxidase system (Trottman and Desaiah, 1980).

Preexposure of rats to toxaphene at a dietary level of 100 ppm for 8 days led to a reduction in the metabolism of [^{14}C]imipramine, in the production of bile, and in the biliary excretion of both endogenous and exogenous metabolites of imipramine (Mehendale, 1978).

After toxaphene administration to mice, Na$^+$,K$^+$-ATPases in liver and kidneys but not brain are inhibited (Trottman and

Table 15.31
Effect on Various Animals of Repeated Oral Doses of Technical Toxaphene

| Dosage | | | | | |
Range (mg/kg/day)	Method and concentration (ppm)	Species, number, and sex	Duration	Results	Reference
41–80	1500 ppm in feed	rat 20 M, 20 F	2 yr	occasional fits; growth retardation; moderate liver change	FAO/WHO (1969)
	1000 ppm in feed	rat 20 M, 20 F	2 yr	slight liver change	FAO/WHO (1969)
	540–1112 ppm (av) in feed	rat 50 M, 50 F		evidence of tumors in liver, thyroid, and other sites	NCI (1979b)
21–40	25 mg/kg	dog		100% mortality	Lehman (1951, 1952)
	500 ppm in feed	rat 10 M, 10 F	13 wk	no clinical effect; liver, kidney, and thyroid changes	Chu et al. (1986)
11–20	400 ppm in feed	rat	2 yr	characteristic liver change	Fitzhugh and Nelson (1951); Lehman (1951, 1952)
6–10	200 ppm in feed	rat, 6	2–6 mo	no clinical effect; many with characteristic liver change	Ortega et al. (1957)
	189 ppm in feed	rat	12 wk	no liver cell changes noted	Clapp et al. (1971)
	10 mg/kg	dog, 2		1 died in 33 days; 1 lived 3.5 yr	Lehman (1951, 1952)
2.6–5	100 ppm in feed	rat	3 gen	slight liver change; normal reproduction	Kennedy et al. (1973)
	100 ppm in feed	rat 20 M, 20 F	2 yr	no effect	FAO/WHO (1969)
	100 ppm in feed	rat	2 yr	slight characteristic liver change	Fitzhugh and Nelson (1951); Lehman (1951, 1952)
	200 ppm in feed	dog, 3		moderate liver change	FAO/WHO (1969)
	3.12–6.56 mg/kg	dog 3 M, 5 F	2 yr	no effect	FAO/WHO (1969)
	5 mg/kg	dog 6 M, 6 F	13 wk	no clinical effects; mild liver and thyroid changes	Chu et al. (1986)
	5 mg/kg	dog, 4	3+ yr	no effect	Lehman (1951, 1952)
	4 mg/kg	dog, 4	44–106 days	intermittent illness; liver and kidney damage	Lackey (1949)
1.26–2.5	50 ppm in feed	rat, 6	2–6 mo	no clinical effect; borderline liver changes	Ortega et al. (1957)
0.626–1.25	25 ppm in feed	rat	2 yr	no effect	Fitzhugh and Nelson (1951); Lehman (1951, 1952)
	25 ppm in feed	rat	3 gen	no clinical effect; normal reproduction	Kennedy et al. (1973)
	0.6–1.5 mg/kg	dog 3 M, 5 F	2 yr	no effect	FAO/WHO (1969)
	0.6–0.8 mg/kg	monkey, 2	2 yr	no effect	FAO/WHO (1969)
0.313–0.625	10 ppm in feed	rat 20 M, 20 F	2 yr	no effect	FAO/WHO (1969)
	40 ppm in feed	dog, 3		no effect	FAO/WHO (1969)
0.157–0.313	20 ppm in feed	dog 6 M, 6 F	6–24 mo	no effect	FAO/WHO (1971)

Desaiah, 1979; Fattah and Crowder, 1980). In rats, toxaphene dosing has little effect on brain synaptosome Na^+, K^+-ATPase activity or oubain and dopamine binding, although these are active in vitro (Trottman and Desaiah, 1983). Both DDT and toxaphene after acute and chronic administrations to rats depressed Na^+, K^+-ATPase activities of liver plasma membranes but, unlike DDT, toxaphene had no effect on Ca^{2+}-ATPase activity (Mourelle et al., 1985). Ca^{2+}-ATPase activity and $^{45}Ca^{2+}$ uptake by mitochondria from liver, heart, and kidney are inhibited by the addition of toxaphene in vitro (Trottman et al., 1985). In addition Ca^{2+}-ATPase activity and $^{45}Ca^{2+}$ uptake are inhibited in brain P_2 fractions from rats previously given toxaphene. Evidence obtained both in vivo and in vitro suggests that this inhibition is due to decreased levels of camodulin and it can be reversed by the addition of the calcium-binding protein (Prasado Rao et al., 1986; Moorthy et al., 1986).

Unlike DDT and chlordecone but like lindane and many of the cyclodienes, toxaphene is a sudden convulsant. In agreement with this, 2,2,5-endo,6-exo,8,9,9,10-octachlorbornane appears to be a very potent ligand for the picrotoxin binding site of mouse brain synaptosomes blocking the GABA-regulated chloride ionophore (Lawrence and Casida, 1984; Casida and Lawrence, 1985; Cole and Casida, 1986). Binding of other

Table 15.32
Single-Dose LD 50 in Mice for Some Components of Toxaphene
Administered Intraperitoneally without and with Piperonyl Butoxide[a]

Compound	LD 50 (mg/kg)	
	Without	With[b]
toxaphene	47	42
2,2,5-*endo*,6-*exo*,8,9,10-heptachlorobornane (B)	75	9.5
3-*exo*-chloro-B	>100	>100
5-*exo*-chloro-B	24	28
8-chloro-B	3.3	3.1
8-chloro-B (57%) + 9-chloro-B (43%)	2.5	1.9
10-chloro-B	>100	48
dehydrochloro(5,6)-B	65	50
dehydrochloro(5,6)-3-*exo*-chloro-B	>100	>100

[a] Data from Turner *et al.* (1977).
[b] Administered 150 mg/kg 1 hr before the insecticide.

chlorobornanes and toxaphene, together with the influence of metabolism on binding, correlates well with the LD 50 values (Table 15.32). Toxaphene caused a depression of plasma testosterone levels in male rats a few days after a single dose (120 mg/kg) but had no effect in a chronic experiment (2.4 mg/kg/day) after 3 or 6 months (Peakall, 1976). Moderate inhibition of ACTH-stimulated corticosterone synthesis was observed in adrenocortical cells isolated from female rats fed 1.2 ppm toxaphene for 5 weeks (Mohammed *et al.*, 1985). Relatively high levels of toxaphene in the diet (200 ppm) have been shown to cause changes in some aspects of the immune system of mice and their offspring (Allen *et al.*, 1983).

Mutagenesis and Carcinogenesis Toxaphene is not mutagenic at dosages of 36 and 180 mg/kg intraperitoneally or 40 mg/kg for 5 days, as judged by the dominant lethal assay in mice (Epstein *et al.*, 1972). It was mutagenic in the *Salmonella* test without requiring activation by liver homogenate (Hooper *et al.*, 1979). A number of studies suggest that toxaphene or related products are carcinogenic in mice and rats, especially for the liver and thyroid (Innes *et al.*, 1969; NCI, 1979b). See also Section 15.2.3.2. As with other chlorinated insecticides, it has been proposed that this occurs by inhibition of intercellular communication (Trosko *et al.*, 1987).

Effects on Reproduction Rats reproduced normally for five generations at a dietary level of 25 ppm (Keplinger *et al.*, 1970). A similar result was obtained at the higher dietary level of 100 ppm (about 5 mg/kg/day) for three generations (Kennedy *et al.*, 1973) or even 500 ppm (Chu *et al.*, 1988).

In studies of teratogenesis, toxaphene was administered by stomach tube to rats and mice at dosages of 15, 25, and 25 mg/kg/day on days 7–16 of gestation. In rats, the highest dosage killed one-third of the dams but reduced only slightly the fetal weight and the rate of skeletal ossification of the young of those that survived. In mice, the highest dosage killed 8% of the

dams and led to encephaloceles in 5 of 61 litters. The lower dosages did not produce any dosage-dependent effect on the young, although they did retard growth of the dams and increase the weight of their livers relative to body weight (Chernoff and Carver, 1976). Somewhat greater fetal toxicity was reported by Badayeva and Kiseleva (1976), suggesting that the preparation they studied was not identical. Mild teratogenic and gonadotoxic effects were observed when rats and hamsters were administered polychlorocamphene during pregnancy (Martson and Shepel'skaya, 1980).

Pathology Changes in the liver of rodents are typical of those produced by other chlorinated hydrocarbon insecticides (Lehman, 1951, 1952; Ortega *et al.*, 1957). See Section 15.2.3.2.

Structural and histochemical changes in the adrenal cortex, thyroid, pancreatic islets, hypophysis, and testes have been reported in rats, mice, and rabbits fed polychloropinene (Makovskaya *et al.*, 1972). Rats administered kamfochlor by stomach tube at rates of 2 mg/kg/day or higher showed circulatory disorders (hyperemia, extravasation, and hemorrhage) of the lungs and spleen and degenerative lesions (reduction of splenic follicles, disturbed spermatogenesis, and cytotoxic changes of the liver and kidney (Sosinerz *et al.*, 1972). These reports suggest that the toxaphene-like preparations available in Eastern Europe may not be identical to toxaphene.

Behavioral Effects Toxaphene, heptachlorobornane, and a mixture of the toxic octachlorobornanes were given to pregnant rats and their offspring in the diet to produce a dosage of 0.050 mg/kg/day (toxaphene) or 0.002 mg/kg/day (constituents) (Olson *et al.*, 1980). All rats were slow to learn in a swimming test at an early age in their development. In maze tests, animals given the mixture of 2,2,5-*endo*,6-*exo*-8,8,9,10- and 2,2,5-*endo*,6-*exo*-8,9,9,10-octachlorobornanes were significantly inferior in retaining knowledge than other groups, although they had no difficulty in learning test problems.

15.6.1.3 Toxicity to Humans

Experimental Exposure Twenty-five volunteers (15 men and 10 women) were exposed in a closed chamber to an aerosol of toxaphene for 30 min/day for 10 consecutive days at a maximal nominal concentration of 500 mg/m^3. After 3 weeks the same exposure was repeated for 3 days. Based on an assumed retention of 50%, the dosage was about 1 mg/kg/day. Physical (including fluoroscopic) examination and study of the blood and urine failed to reveal any toxic effect (Keplinger, 1963).

Accidental and Intentional Poisoning At least 13 persons have been killed by toxaphene (McGee *et al.*, 1952; Pollock, 1953; Hayes, 1963; Menner, 1965; Haun and Cueto, 1967; Bochkovskii and Riabov, 1970). Most of the fatal cases involved small children. One girl was only 9 months old. Ingestion of poison by the children either occurred or could not be ruled out. Even so, danger of dermal exposure cannot be considered to have been excluded. In separate accidents, two men were killed by polychloropinene, which they consumed while drunk (Bochkovskii and Riabov, 1970). The clinical course was indistinguishable from that caused by toxaphene, but the autopsy findings were unexpected, as discussed below.

Nonfatal poisoning often begins in 4 hr or less after toxaphene is ingested (McGee *et al.,* 1952). In fatal cases, severe symptoms have begun as early as half an hour after exposure (Pollock, 1953). Death was delayed 4 days in a case involving a mixture of toxaphene and DDT at a ratio of 2 : 1, but death was rapid in another case involving a similar mixture (Haun and Cueto, 1967). Death from uncomplicated toxaphene poisoning often occurs within the first 12 hr (McGee *et al.,* 1952) and occurred in one case in less than 4 hr after exposure (Pollock, 1953) On the contrary, recovery of patients who survived definite poisoning has been essentially complete in 12 hr (McGee *et al.,* 1952; Hayes, 1963).

Control of convulsions is not necessarily decisive. In one case, convulsions had been controlled for some hours, and there were hopeful signs of improvement for a time, followed by a sudden rise in temperature to 40.1°C, respiratory collapse, and death (Hayes, 1963). Nonfatal poisoning has been characterized by nausea [although this may not always occur (Wells and Milborn, 1983)], mental confusion, jerking of the arms and legs, and especially by convulsions. In some instances, convulsions have begun suddenly without any warning sign or symptom (McGee *et al.,* 1952). Fatal poisoning has been characterized by frequent, repeated, violent convulsions and by cyanosis. In some instances the cyanosis may result from mechanical interference with respiration by convulsions. However, in one carefully observed case, cyanosis appeared before convulsions (Pollock, 1953). Apparently, depression, except that seen after fits, has not been observed in human poisoning by toxaphene.

Use Experience   In spite of the acute toxicity of toxaphene, as evidenced by animal experiments and by accidental poisoning, the safety record of this insecticide under conditions of use is excellent. The good record undoubtedly is related to the rapidity with which the mixture and its most toxic constituents are metabolized and excreted.

A careful search for abnormalities of heme synthesis and sympathoadrenal activity in 45 persons occupationally exposed to toxaphene and various other pesticides failed to reveal such abnormalities or any correlation between the relevant clinical laboratory results and blood levels of pesticides (Embry *et al.,* 1972).

Exposure to dust containing 5% toxaphene and 1% lindane led to a therapeutic complication in a 53-year-old rancher, although no illness related to the formulation was involved. Much earlier, the man had been treated successfully for thrombophlebitis with warfarin sodium at a rate of 7.5 mg/day. When the condition recurred, it was found that he did not respond to warfarin at a dosage of 15 mg/day, and heparin sodium was substituted. He had recently applied the insec-

ticidal dust to sheep inside a barn. Careful monitoring demonstrated that responsiveness to warfarin returned to the normal range in about 3 months after exposure to the insecticide (Jeffrey *et al.,* 1976).

More cells with chromosomal aberrations (13.1%) were reported in women who had worked prematurely in a field sprayed with polychlorocamphene at the level of 2 kg/ha than were reported in controls (1.6%) (Samosh, 1974). Similar findings were reported for a short-term exposure of agricultural workers to polychloropinene (Samosh, 1981). In a group of 20 exposed individuals 5.6% of lymphocytes sampled had chromosome aberrations (fragmentations, coiling up, etc.), while again only 1.6% of control samples showed abnormalities. Damaged chromosomes persisted for at least 11 months after exposure.

Laboratory Findings   In a fatal case a concentration of toxaphene of 78 ppm was found in the liver and 10 ppm in postmortem blood. In another case, the concentrations were 7.85, 6.75, and 14.03 ppm in liver, kidney, and brain, respectively (Haun and Cueto, 1967).

Later it became possible to identify smaller concentrations by measuring a characteristic complex in the records of electron-capture, gas–liquid chromatography. Using this method, concentrations of 0.079 and 0.156 ppm were found in the red cells and plasma, respectively, of a man whose exposure to toxaphene presumably was occupational only. The same man had no more DDT in his red cells and plasma than people in the general population, although he was exposed to a spray containing both DDT and toxaphene. This and similar results in a fatal case (Haun and Cueto, 1967) indicate that toxaphene is absorbed more readily than DDT.

Atypical Cases of Various Origins   The illness of 3 men and 19 women has been ascribed to polychloropinene spray that was applied to a sugar beet field by aircraft while some of the people were in the field and others were close enough to inhale the fumes. The workers continued weeding for 3 hr after the spraying. No muscle twitching or convulsion was reported. Lacrimation, eye pain, headache, vertigo, nausea, abdominal pain, liquid stools, weakness, and some less defined complaints were reported (Bezuglyi and Mukhtarova, 1969). It is difficult to exclude the possibility of solvent poisoning in this instance.

Two well-described cases of respiratory disease characterized by dyspnea, mild cyanosis, rales and wheezes in the lungs, and miliary x-ray opacities of the lungs were attributed to occupational exposure to chlorinated camphene. Over a period of weeks, both cases responded to treatment with cortisone, streptomycin, and isoniazid (Warraki, 1963). Only circumstantial evidence was offered for a relationship between the illnesses and toxaphene. The same was true of a patient with a history of occupational exposure to polychlorocamphene, who was found to have liver tenderness, cholecystangiocholitis, encephalopolyneuritis, nephritis, and severe impairment of the excretory function of one kidney (Zarkevich *et al.,* 1973).

A case of alleged poisoning by a mixture of lindane and toxaphene is discussed under Lindane.

Dosage Response It was not possible to measure dosage in any fatal accident involving toxaphene. In an instance in which three of seven persons had convulsions after eating collards that had been sprayed 3 days earlier, the concentration of toxaphene on a washed sample of the food was 3126 ppm (McGee *et al.,* 1952). If one assumed that each person ate about 500 gm of the collards and absorbed half of the residue before evacuation of the food, one can estimate an absorbed dosage of about 10 mg/kg. This estimate seems reasonable in the case of persons who did not become ill but who retained their collards until evacuation was hastened by 2 oz of castor oil administered 4 hr after the food was consumed. On the contrary, the absorbed dosage may have been less than 10 mg/kg for the three persons who did have convulsions 2.5, 3.0, and 3.75 hr after eating, inasmuch as each was able to vomit a "large," "copious," or "enormous" amount of collards in response to apomorphine or other treatment shortly after her fit.

The threshold limit value (0.5 mg/m^3) indicates that occupational intake at the rate of 0.07 mg/kg/day is considered safe.

Pathology The pathology is nonspecific, involving nothing more than congestion and a few petechial hemorrhages. Polychloropinene or its formulations may be more different from toxaphene than is generally realized because an "acutely piercing" odor of the organs was noted at the autopsy of two persons killed by that mixture (Bochkovskii and Riabov, 1970). No special odor has been reported in connection with the autopsy of people killed by toxaphene although a peculiar odor was noticed during gastric aspiration and lavage of a suicide attempt (Wells and Milborn, 1983).

Treatment of Poisoning Treatment is symptomatic (see Section 15.2.5).

15.7 MIREX AND CHLORDECONE

Although structurally mirex and chlordecone may bear some resemblance to the chlorinated cyclodiene insecticides, they do not produce sudden seizures and are very slowly metabolized, often concentrating many thousandfold in food chains. In these respects they resemble DDT. There has been a tremendous increase in the literature on mirex and especially chlordecone in recent years; it has not been possible to refer to it all.

15.7.1 MIREX

15.7.1.1 Identity, Properties, and Uses

Chemical Name Mirex is 1,1a,2,2,3,3a,4,5,5,5a,5b,6-dodecachlorooctahydro-1,3,4-metheno-1*H*-cyclobuta[*cd*]-pentalene or perchloropentacyclo[5,3,0.0^{2,6}.0^{3,9}.0^{4,8}]decane.

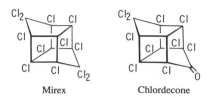

Figure 15.9 Structures of mirex and chlordecone.

Structure See Fig. 15.9.

Synonyms Mirex [ESA] was introduced under code designation GC-1283, also HRS 1276. Trade names included Dechlorane® and Ferriamicide® but products marked by the same word plus other symbols did not contain mirex. The CAS registry number is 2385-85-5.

Chemical and Physical Properties The empirical formula is $C_{10}Cl_{12}$, and the molecular weight is 545.51.

Mirex is a white crystalline solid that melts at 485°C. It is unaffected by strong acids and is nonflammable and noncorrosive. It is soluble in benzene (12.2%), carbon tetrachloride (7.2%), and xylene (14.3%) but is virtually insoluble in water.

History, Formulation, Uses, and Production Mirex was introduced in 1959 by Allied Chemical Corporation. It has been formulated mainly as fine granules made from corn cobs impregnated with vegetable oil so that they serve as bait for fire ants. The concentration of oil is about 15% and that of the active ingredient may be 0.075, 0.15, or 0.3%. The formulations of different strengths are applied at different rates in such a way that the maximal rate for the active ingredient is 10.5 gm/ha (4.25 mg/acre). Mirex is a stomach insecticide with little contact action. It was also used as a flame-retardant.

15.7.1.2 Toxicity to Laboratory Animals

Basic Findings In one study, the oral LD 50 of mirex in rats ranged from 600 to >3000 mg/kg, depending on sex and formulation. No rats were killed by dermal dosages as high as 2000 mg/kg. In a different study, the one-dose oral LD 50 of mirex in female rats was 365 mg/kg, but the 90-dose LD 50 was only 6 mg/kg/day; thus, the chronicity index was 60.8 (Gaines and Kimbrough, 1970). This value is much larger than any other chronicity index found so far for a pesticide that reached practical use. The reported failure of rats to reach a steady state of storage in 16 months (Ivie *et al.,* 1974) suggests that an even higher chronicity index might be obtained if it were based on 16-month or lifetime feeding rather than on 90-day feeding. That this speculation may not be justified is indicated by the fact that a dosage of 3.1 mg/kg/day (approximately half the 90-dose LD 50) failed to produce detectable illness in rats when administered for 90 days (Gaines and Kimbrough, 1970). The acute oral LD 50 toxicity of mirex in hamsters has been reported as 250 mg/kg for males and 125 mg/kg for females (Cabral *et al.,* 1979a). No gross changes were seen in a 9-week study on the effects of dermal application of mirex to rats (Larson *et al.,* 1979a).

Some rats died during week 3 of receiving a dietary level of 1280 ppm, and few survived a 13-week period. Poor growth, hyperexcitability, depressed hemoglobin, tremors, and convulsions were seen before death. Similar changes but no deaths were observed at 320 ppm. Significantly enlarged livers were seen in males at dietary levels of 80 ppm and higher and in females at 320 ppm. A dietary level of 20 ppm produced no effect in either sex (Larson et al., 1979a). However, as discussed under Effects on Reproduction, a dietary level of 25 ppm interfered significantly with the reproduction of rats, 5 ppm (about 0.26 mg/kg/day) being a no-effect level. Yarbrough et al. (1981) found a significant increase in liver weight after feeding male rats 5 ppm mirex for 4 weeks.

A dietary level of 5 ppm (about 0.66 mg/kg/day) produced a significant increase in mortality of one of two strains of mice (Ware and Good, 1967). Mice fed 30 ppm for 12 weeks had livers twice the size of controls (Pittz et al., 1979). Liver weight in female rabbits fed 20 ppm mirex for 8 weeks were significantly increased (Warren et al., 1978) but reproduction was unaffected.

In dogs, the oral LD 50 was estimated to be >1000 mg/kg, but a small group died within 13 weeks when fed mirex at a dietary level of 100 ppm (about 2.1 mg/kg/day). Dietary levels as high as 20 ppm for 13 weeks were without observed toxic effect (Larson et al., 1979a).

Photomirex (8-monohydromirex), which is formed in the environment from mirex, is also toxic (Hallett et al., 1978; Villeneuve et al., 1979a,b; Chu et al., 1981a). Although photomirex has been reported to be more hepatotoxic and thyrotoxic than mirex (Villeneuve et al., 1979b), this has not been confirmed by Yarbrough et al. (1981). The discrepancy between investigators may be due to different methods of preparing photomirex (Yarbrough et al., 1981).

Absorption, Distribution, Metabolism, and Excretion
Mirex is poorly absorbed from the gastrointestinal tract. After a dose of 6 mg/kg, a half-life of that absorbed was estimated as more than 100 days (Mehendale et al., 1972). At a lower dosage rate (0.2 mg/kg) an even higher proportion is excreted by rats unchanged in the feces (Gibson et al., 1972). The storage of mirex in rats is very tenacious, and no plateau of tissue levels was observed in rats fed for 16 months. Residues declined by only 40% within 10 months after rats were returned to an uncontaminated diet (Ivie et al., 1974). Of [14C]mirex inhaled by rats through cigarette smoke, 47% was exhaled and 35% remained in the lung, 11% in blood, and 1% in heart 2–4 min after inhalation (Atallah and Dorough, 1975). A free-compartment open-system model with parallel first-order elimination in the urine and feces has been developed to simulate mirex pharmacokinetics after iv and oral administration to rats (Byrd et al., 1982).

In the liver and kidney, mirex was associated mainly with the cytosol fraction (Mehendale, 1977a).

Although the conversion of mirex to Kepone in the environment has been demonstrated (Carlson et al., 1976), no evidence for this conversion was found when mirex was fed to pigs (Morgan et al., 1979). The environmentally derived pho-

tomirex is distributed and excreted in a very similar way to mirex in the rat (Hallett et al., 1978; Chu et al., 1979).

Metabolites of mirex identified in the rat include 2,8-dihydromirex and 5,10-dihydromirex (Chambers and Yarbrough, 1979). 2,8-Dihydromirex has not been shown to be further metabolized in vivo and is no more readily eliminated than mirex (Chu et al., 1980b; Chambers et al., 1982). However, cis-5,10-dihydromirex does appear to be converted to more polar metabolites, which are excreted in the urine (Yarbrough et al., 1983).

In the cow no metabolite but only unchanged mirex was found in tissues or excreta following prolonged oral dosing. Excretion of mirex in milk reached equilibrium in only about a week and then amounted to approximately 10% of the daily intake. Twenty-eight days after the last dose, the concentration of mirex was highest in fat and undetectable in muscle and brain (Dorough and Ivie, 1974). On the contrary, storage of mirex failed to reach a steady state in male goats or in one group of female goats during a period of 61 weeks when they received it orally at a rate of 1 mg/kg/day. Storage did become stable in the plasma of the same animals. Loss of stored mirex was slow in goats but not as slow as in monkeys (Smrek et al., 1977, 1978).

Using [14C]mirex, >3% of the radioactivity in the feces of monkeys was associated with a compound more polar than mirex and the radioactivity in the urine was not extracted with solvents that extract mirex. At 106 days after a single intravenous dose, radioactivity remained in all tissues but the fat contained by far the most, calculated to be about 80–97% of the dose (Kennedy et al., 1975; Wiener et al., 1976). A retention of 90% in fat also was found using gas chromatography, and a mathematical model was developed that fit available information very well and predicted an extremely long half-life in the monkey (Pittman et al., 1975, 1976). A metabolite of mirex was demonstrated chromatographically in extracts of feces collected from monkeys 2 and 5 weeks after each had received a single intravenous injection of mirex at a rate of about 1 mg/kg. The metabolite, which was not identified, was not detectable during the first few days after dosing. It was believed that the metabolite arose in the lower gut or in the feces. The feces remained positive for 14C for at least 13 months (Stein et al., 1976).

Enforced reduction of food intake to one-fourth normal failed to increase the metabolism of mirex in rats that previously had received the compound by gavage for 14 days at rates of 1.0–10 mg/kg/day. Mirex concentrations were higher in all tissues after food deprivation than after normal food intake (Villeneuve et al., 1977).

Biochemical Effects Mirex induces some microsomal enzymes in rats and mice but this induction is complex and findings are not always consistent. In both species, induction occurs at a dietary level of 1 ppm (about 0.05 and 0.12 mg/kg/day in the rat and mouse, respectively), the lowest level tested (Baker et al., 1972; Byard et al., 1974, 1975; Iverson, 1976; Villeneuve et al., 1977). At this dosage level, not all enzymes tested may be induced, and there may be no significant increase in liver weight, microsomal protein, or cytochrome P-450 (Iverson, 1976). Yarbrough et al. (1981) found that 0.5 ppm mirex or photomirex in the diet for 4 weeks significantly induced male hepatic microsomal aminopyrine N-demethylase activity but had no significant effect on aniline hydroxylase. Although higher doses (up to 75 ppm) significantly induced cytochrome P-450 levels fourfold, no greater induction of the N-demethylase activity was observed. Thus, not only is there a dosage–response relationship but also there is a qualitative difference in the cytochromes induced at different dosage levels (Baker et al., 1972). Under certain circumstances enzyme activity may be reduced (Mehendale et al., 1973). In mice fed at a dietary level of 60 ppm (about 7.44 mg/kg/day), cytochrome P-450 was elevated within 2 days, and liver weight was doubled in 2 weeks; following only 2 weeks of feeding, these and most other aspects of the induction of microsomal enzymes slowly regressed over a 4-month period, being directly related to the slow decline in the concentration of mirex in the plasma (Byard and Pittman, 1975). Mirex and chlordecone both altered the rates of aminopyrene N-demethylase activity (Chambers and Trevanthan, 1983) and p-nitrosanisole O-demethylase (Chambers and Trevanthan, 1983; Ebel, 1984) in rats, but the degree and direction depended on dose and sex. Mirex may be different from chlordecone in some respects of cytochrome P-450 induction (Crouch and Ebel, 1987), although there are differences between authors on this subject. Cis- and trans-5,10-dihydromirex are different inducers in male and female rats (Yarbrough et al., 1986a). Interestingly, the combination (1 : 1) of mirex and 3,4,5,3′,4′,5′-hexachlorobiphenyl at a total molar dose of 15 μmol/kg to mice gave significant induction of cytochrome P-450, both demethylase activities, and aniline hydroxylase, yet neither chemical at the same total dose caused significant induction (Peppriell, 1981).

Correlated with the enzyme induction, mirex causes proliferation of endoplasmic reticulum (Baker et al., 1972) and other characteristic changes in the liver (Gaines and Kimbrough, 1970; Yarbrough et al., 1981) including nodules (Byard et al., 1975). At an LD 50 level of dosage, fatty change and necrosis may overshadow more characteristic changes (Kendall, 1974a,b).

Species differences in response to mirex are marked. Ultrastructural changes associated with proliferation of the endoplasmic reticulum are more marked in mice than in other species, and at a dietary level of only 5 ppm (about 0.6 mg/kg/day) there are necrosis of hepatocytes and phagocytosis by Kupffer cells (Fulfs et al., 1975). In contrast to rats, chickens and quails did not increase liver weight or cytochrome P-450 level in response to mirex (Davison et al., 1976).

The increase in hydroxyl radical formation after dosing rats with mirex (Havkin-Frenkel et al., 1983) is probably related to some types of cytochrome P-450 induction. Whether the differences in some inducible microsomal monooxygenase activities between mirex and chlordecone (Kaminsky et al., 1978) are also seen with hydroxyl radical formation does not appear to have been studied.

In rats, the activities of liver lactate dehydrogenase, and

glutamic-oxaloacetic transaminase were reduced by dietary levels of mirex as low as 10 ppm (Abston and Yarbrough, 1974). The mirex-induced adaptive liver growth in rats is partly mediated by a hormone from the adrenals (Williams and Yarbrough, 1983) and depends on the pituitary–adrenocortical axis (Ervin and Yarbrough, 1985). In intact rats a peak of [3H]thymidine incorporation into DNA 48 hr after mirex was observed and had decreased to control values by 96 hr (Yarbrough et al., 1984). Adrenalectomy significantly reduces the liver enlargement, and the incorporation of [3H]thymidine persists for at least 96 hr. Corticosterone supplement abolishes the DNA synthesis peak altogether in adrenalectomized animals but has no effect on intact rats (Yarbrough et al., 1984). This seems to suggest that the mirex-induced liver growth has two components, a hypertrophic component mediated by corticosterone and a hyperplastic component which is independently mediated, although other evidence suggests that both are modulated by corticosterone (Wilson and Yarbrough, 1988). Thymidine kinase activity and ornithine decarboxylase activity have been used as markers for the hyperplastic and hypertrophic responses to mirex, respectively (Yarbrough et al., 1986b). Mirex may desensitize the glucocorticoid receptor-mediated response (Brown et al., 1988). The change in protein metabolism in the liver after mirex appears to be due to a decrease in catabolism rather than an increase in protein synthesized (Robinson and Yarbrough, 1980).

Ritchie and Ho (1982) found that mirex and chlordecone have different effects on the incorporation of amino acids into protein of brain and liver of mice. Chlordecone stimulated the former, mirex the latter. Mirex does not inhibit binding of t-butylbicyclophosphorothionate to the rat brain specific sites of GABA receptor as do lindane, dieldrin, and toxaphene (Lawrence and Casida, 1984), and thus it resembles DDT and chlordecone. However, DDT and mirex seem to be different from chlordecone in that they have little effect on synaptosomal Ca^{2+} uptake (Komulainen and Bondy, 1987). Leach and Charles (1987) have presented evidence that mirex may after all inhibit GABA binding but without affecting presynaptic release of GABA. Its action may be on the benzodiazepine binding sites.

Effects on Organs and Tissues Rats given mirex by oral gavage at a rate of 1.5 mg/kg/day developed hepatic centrilobular hypertrophy, and the affected cells showed a proliferation of smooth endoplasmic reticulum (Fulfs and Abraham, 1976). In fact, an increase in relative liver weight could be detected 2 days after a single oral administration, and the increase corresponded to dosage (Robinson and Yarbrough, 1978a). In some instances, the increase was 100% in 4 days after a single dose (Robinson and Yarbrough, 1978a). According to some investigators, the enlargement was without any indication of toxic effect and was almost completely reversible within 28 days (Robinson and Yarbrough, 1978b). Others have reported the degeneration of some bile canaliculi (Davison et al., 1976). In other studies, mirex- and photomirex-induced changes in the liver persisted for nearly a year after termination of treatment (Chu et al., 1981b).

Examination, especially with an electron microscope, may reveal myelin figures associated with hypertrophy of endoplasmic reticulum (Kendall, 1979).

Mirex proved negative in a dominant lethal test in rats (Khera *et al.*, 1976) and negative in the standard Ames bacterial assay (Hallett *et al.*, 1978).

The maximal tolerated dosage of mirex increased the incidence of hepatomas in two strains of mice that received it for 18 months (Innes *et al.*, 1969). In rats fed the maximal tolerated dosage and in others fed half that rate, mirex was found to be noncarcinogenic (Ulland *et al.*, 1973). However, reexamination of the data using changed criteria led to the opposite conclusion (Ulland *et al.*, 1977). Adenomas and carcinomas have been identified in livers of male rats fed mirex (100 ppm) for 13 months (Abraham *et al.*, 1983). Mirex decreased the number of tetraploid cells, especially in hepatocellular carcinomas. In 12-day-old neonates, mirex had no effect in tetraploidy or uptake of [^{3}H]thymidine into DNA, in contrast to dimethylnitrosamine (Carlson and Abraham, 1985). The binding of [^{14}C]mirex in diploid and polyploid mouse liver cells *in vitro* is total Ca^{2+}-independent and partially Na^+-dependent. Saturation of polyploid cells occurs at a threefold lower concentration of mirex than that of diploid cells and perhaps insulates them from normal regulatory signals from other cells and tissues (Charles *et al.*, 1985; Rosenbaum and Charles, 1986). Although mirex could be regarded as an epigenetic carcinogen and diethylnitrosamine and dimethylnitrosamines as genotoxic carcinogens, similar low molecular weight proteins were induced in newborn rats by all three chemicals (Timchalk *et al.*, 1985). On the other hand, whereas mirex and a phorbol ester inhibited hepatic cytosolic cyclic AMP-dependent protein kinase ratio, diethylnitrosamine had the opposite effect (Timchalk and Charles, 1986).

A different kind of effect on the liver was demonstrated by a study in which pretreatment of male rats with mirex (50 mg/kg/day orally for 3 days) caused approximately 90% suppression of biliary excretion of sulfobromophthalein, an exogenously administered polar metabolite of imipramine, and the same metabolite formed endogenously. These impairments of biliary excretion were related to neither bile flow nor rate of metabolism of imipramine. In fact, exposure to mirex increased bile flow (Mehendale, 1977c). A dosage of 5 mg/kg/day produced no discernible change. A dosage of 10 mg/kg/day inhibited Mg^{2+}-ATPase and Na^+,K^+-ATPase in the liver (Mehendale *et al.*, 1979), and the relationship probably indicates biochemical effects at the cellular membrane (Curtis and Mehendale, 1981). Mirex-induced biliary dysfunction occurs earlier than that with chlordecone and recovery is slower (Mehendale, 1981a). *In vivo*, mirex reduced the excretion of exogenous taurocholate (Curtis and Hoyt, 1984) and this is consistent with this chemical causing increased biliary tree permeability. Mirex potentiates acetaminophen hepatic toxicity in mice and to a greater extent than chlordecone (Fouse and Hodgson, 1987).

Another organ that is reproducibly affected by chronic feeding of rats with mirex and photomirex is the thyroid (Villeneuve *et al.*, 1979a,b; Yarbrough *et al.*, 1981). After 4 weeks of 75 ppm mirex or photomirex, serum triiodothyronine (T_3) and thyroxine (T_4) levels were depressed and there were changes in the thyroid structure itself (Yarbrough *et al.*, 1981). Colloid density was reduced or depleted, there was follicular atrophy, and the lining epithelial cells were hypertrophied and elongated. Similar findings were reported by A. Singh *et al.*, (1982, 1985) after feeding rats photomirex (0.05–50 mg/kg) or mirex (50 mg/kg) for 4 weeks. In addition, many deformed lysosomal bodies were observed. Effects persisted for up to and over 1 year after termination of treatment. There is some disagreement about whether photomirex is more potent than mirex in these respects (Yarbrough *et al.*, 1981). See also Effects on Reproduction.

Effects on Reproduction Administration of mirex (5 ppm of diet) to BALB/c mice for 30 days prior to mating and for 90 days after caused a reduced litter size and increased mortality of parents (Ware and Good, 1967). Wolfe *et al.* (1979) reported cessation of reproduction in a group of wild-derived mice fed 1.8 ppm for 3 months. Reduced litter sizes were also observed for rats fed 25 ppm mirex (Gaines and Kimbrough, 1970). Viability of neonates was also reduced and cataracts occurred in the surviving neonates. Cross-fostering studies showed that both cataracts and reduced viability could be partially overcome if neonates did not receive their mothers' milk. Female rats fed 5 ppm mirex produced normal litters. Similar results have been obtained with mirex and photomirex at doses of 20 and 40 ppm, respectively (Chu *et al.*, 1981c). Multiple oral doses of 0, 1.5, 3.0, 6.0, or 12.5 mg mirex/kg body weight on days 6–15 of gestation had adverse effects on the mother and offspring only at the two highest doses (Khera *et al.*, 1976). Mirex has also been shown to cause cataract formation when administered to pregnant rats at 7 mg/kg body weight daily during days 7–16 of gestation (Chernoff *et al.*, 1979b). Mirex does not seem to have a direct effect on the neonatal rat lens (Rogers, 1983). Cataract formation in fetuses seems to be associated with hypoproteinemia and edema (Grabowski, 1981; Rogers and Grabowski, 1983; Rogers *et al.*, 1984). The earliest changes observed seem to be cortical vacuoles and swelling of lens fibers with subsequent degeneration and necrosis (Scotti *et al.*, 1981; Rogers and Grabowski, 1984).

Many of the deaths among fetuses appear to be due to congestive heart failure (Grabowski and Payne, 1980, 1983a,b). The majority of edematous fetuses had abnormal ECGs, possibly due to hypovolemia.

Female goats were able to reproduce when they received oral doses of 1 mg/kg/day started at the onset of pregnancy, and the dosage was increased 61 weeks later to 10 mg/kg/day. One nanny died during delivery. No abnormalities were noted in the young (Smrek *et al.*, 1977, 1978).

Mirex inhibits ovulation induced in immature rats by pregnant mare serum (PMS) and the reaction is dosage-related in the range 5–660 mg/kg. No effect is evident at a dosage of 2.8 mg/kg. The number of ova can be increased by administering human chorionic gonadotropin 56 hr after PMS, indicating that mirex inhibits PMS-induced ovulation by means of an effect on the central nervous system controlling the release of luteinizing hormone, rather than a direct effect on the ovary (Fuller *et al.*, 1973; Fuller and Draper, 1975).

Both photomirex and mirex cause damage to rat testes with hypocellularity of the seminiferous tubules and decreased spermatogenesis (Villeneuve *et al.*, 1979a,b; Yarbrough *et al.*, 1981).

Behavioral Effects   When mirex was fed to rats at dietary concentrations of 1.78 and 17.8 ppm in one experiment and at 17.8 ppm in a second experiment, there was no detectable effect on open-field or operant behavior or on a discrimination reversal task motivated by escape from foot shock (Thorne *et al.*, 1978). However, Reiter *et al.* (1977) found that mirex produced hyporeactivity with attenuated startle response and decreased ambulation in a maze. These results were different from those with chlordecone. Other studies have also suggested briefly an influence of mirex on rat behavior (Peeler, 1976; Dietz and McMillan, 1978, 1979).

15.7.8.3 Toxicity to Humans

Apparently there has been no report of injury of a person by mirex.

Although mirex has not been used for controlling pests of domestic animals or field crops, its extensive use for control of imported fire ants in the southern United States undoubtedly has brought small amounts of it into contact with agricultural soil over wide areas. The occurrence of mirex in human fat was reported first by Kutz *et al.* (1974a) in connection with samples collected from April 1971 through April 1972 as part of the National Human Monitoring Program for Pesticides. Among about 1400 samples, mirex was found in six by gas chromatography–mass spectrometry. All six samples came from states in which the compound had been used extensively for fire ant control, and the homes of five of the persons involved were rural. However, no evidence could be found that any of the six persons had been associated directly with mirex or with the fire ant control program. Although the method used was capable of detecting a concentration of about 0.1 ppm on a lipid basis, the lowest value actually found was 0.16 ppm on the same basis. The highest value found was 5.94 ppm, and the mean was 2.49 ppm.

In a further study, 624 samples of human adipose tissue from surgical patients and cadavers were analyzed. These samples were taken from October 1975 to September 1976 in 40 sites from eight states of the southeastern United States which had some federally assisted application of the insecticide from 1965 to 1974 (Kutz *et al.*, 1985). From analysis of the data it was concluded that 10.2% of the population of this area had quantifiable levels of mirex in adipose tissue. The geometric mean of the quantifiable residues was 0.286 ppm of lipid. There appeared to be a statistical correlation between the region or location of tissue specimen collection, the presence of mirex residue, and the amount detected. The most positive state was Mississippi, with 51.1% positive samples.

Mirex was found at concentrations of 0.1–0.6 ppm in three samples of human milk collected in cities on Lake Ontario or Lake Erie (Mes *et al.*, 1978). Although mirex had been reported earlier from fish and fish-eating birds of the area, its origin remains obscure.

Treatment of Poisoning   Treatment is symptomatic (see Section 15.2.5).

15.7.2 CHLORDECONE

15.7.2.1 Identity, Properties, and Uses

Chemical Name   Chlordecone is 1,1a,3,3a,4,5,5,5a,5b,6-decachlorooctahydro-1,3,4-metheno-2*H*-cyclobuta[*cd*]pentalen-2-one.

Structure   See Fig. 15.9.

Synonyms   The common name chlordecone (BSI, ISO) is in general use. Kepone® is the trade name. The code designation is GC-1,189. The CAS registry number is 143-50-0.

Physical and Chemical Properties   Chlordecone has the empirical formula $C_{10}Cl_{10}O$ and a molecular weight of 490.61. The technical material is a solid with a purity of above 90%. It sublimes with some decomposition at about 350°C. Chlordecone is readily hydrated and can form a *gem*-diol enhancing water solubility. Chlordecone has a solubility in water of 0.4% at 100°C but is soluble in strongly alkaline aqueous solutions. It is readily soluble in acetone but less soluble in benzene and light petroleum. Its vapor pressure is $<3 \times 10^{-7}$ mm Hg at 25°C.

History, Formulations, Uses, and Production   Chlordecone was introduced in 1958 by Allied Chemical Corporation. It was used against leaf-eating insects and fly larvae. Formulations include a 50% wettable powder and 5 and 10% granules.

15.7.2.2 Toxicity to Laboratory Animals

Basic Findings   The toxicity of chlordecone to animals and possible mechanisms of action have been well described by Guzelian (1982b). Readers especially interested in discussions of the mechanisms and comparison between animal and human studies should consult this reference.

Single-dose LD 50 values for some laboratory animals are given in Table 15.33. Deaths from chlordecone are usually preceded by abnormal gait and severe tremor, which can be exacerbated by handling (Larson *et al.*, 1979a; Egle *et al.*, 1979). Oral toxicity is much greater than the toxicity induced by percutaneous absorption (Gaines, 1969). In rats given chlordecone orally (72–98 mg/kg) deaths occurred within 2–5 days. Tremor and abnormal gait developed within 4 hr, reached a peak in 2 days, and were greatly diminished by 14 days (Egle *et al.*, 1979). Interestingly, a muscle weakness developed in the second week and was still increasing by 49 days, although it had disappeared by 6 months. Weight loss also occurred. Similar

Table 15.33
Single Dose LD 50 for Chlordecone

Species	Route	LD 50 (mg/kg)	Reference
Rat, M	oral[a]	125	Gaines (1969)
Rat, F	oral[a]	125	Gaines (1969)
Rat, M	oral[a]	132	Larson et al. (1979a)
Rat, F	oral[a]	126	Larson et al. (1979a)
Rat, M	oral[b]	96	Epstein (1978)
Rat, M	dermal[c]	2000	Gaines (1969)
Rat, F	dermal[c]	2000	Gaines (1969)
Rabbit, M	oral[a]	71	Larson et al. (1979a)
Rabbit, M	oral[b]	65	Epstein (1978)
Rabbit, M	dermal[a]	410	Epstein (1978)
Rabbit, M	dermal[b]	435	Epstein (1978)
Dog, M, F	oral	250	Larson et al. (1979a)

[a] In oil.
[b] Aqueous.
[c] Xylene.

findings have been reported in the pig 48 hr after an 80 mg/kg dose of chlordecone (Soine et al., 1983). The effects of short-term and prolonged doses of chlordecone are shown in Table 15.34. In summary, as far as rats and mice are concerned, there are decreased weight gain; liver enlargement (including induction of the mixed-function oxidase system; see Biochemical Effects); ultrastructural changes in the liver, thyroid, adrenal, kidneys, and testes; and nervous symptoms including tremor; and at high doses, perhaps <50 ppm of diet, death may occur in a few months. The animals that do survive have an increased chance of developing tumors (Reuber, 1978a, 1979d). Some rats fed 25 ppm chlordecone or more showed reduced hematocrit and hemoglobin values and at higher doses sometimes had increased bleeding (Larson et al., 1979a).

Juveniles seem to be more susceptible than adults; at a level of 60 ppm, which killed young mice within 15 days, adults showed only weight loss (Huber, 1965). Mice tolerating 40 ppm for 12 months consumed 20–40% more food without an increase in body weight. At a dietary level of 30 ppm, mice developed a constant tremor by 4 weeks, but this stopped after discontinuing the treatment for a further 4 weeks. Even 5 ppm chlordecone (about 0.64 mg/kg/day) can interfere with reproduction (see Effects on Reproduction).

All of four dogs survived chlordecone at a dietary level of 25 ppm for 124 weeks. At autopsy, they showed significant increases in the weights of the liver, kidney, and heart. No other significant changes were found, and changes in organ weights were not significant in dogs receiving 1 or 5 ppm (Larson et al., 1979a).

Jager (1976), citing an unpublished report, indicated that the acute LD 50 in male rats was 132 mg/kg/day and the repeated-dose LD 50 values were 3.2 and 1.5 mg/kg/day after 3 and 6

Table 15.34
Effects on Various Animals of Repeated Oral Dosing of Chlordecone

Dose in diet (ppm)	Species and sex	Duration	Results	Reference
200	rat M	8 days	ultrastructural and biochemical liver changes	Baggett et al. (1977)
50–150	rat M, F	16 days	induction of hepatic mixed-function oxidases; decreased body weight gain and decreased biliary excretion	Mehendale et al. (1977, 1978)
1–50	mouse M	14 days	at highest levels induction of mixed-function oxidases	Fabacher and Hodgson (1976)
25	rat M, F	3 months then 4.5 months of control diet	tremors after 4 weeks; liver and adrenal hypertrophy even after recovery period	Cannon and Kimbrough (1979)
10–100	mouse M, F	up to 12 months	tremors and death at highest dose levels; liver changes; reproductive effects in females	Huber (1965)
20–40	mouse M, F	up to 90 weeks	survival reduced at high-dose level in males; hepatocellular carcinoma in both sexes	NCI (1976)
8–26	rat M, F	80 weeks then 16 weeks of control diet	increased incidence of hepatocellular carcinomas and adenomas in low-dose males	NCI (1976)
1–80	rat M, F	up to 2 years	depressed growth rate up 10 ppm; death within a few months at 50 ppm; hepatocellular carcinomas in low- or intermediate-dose groups	Reuben (1978a, 1979d); Larson et al. (1979a)
1–25	dog M, F	127 weeks	reduced weight gain at 25 ppm but no effects seen at a histological level	Larson et al. (1979a)

months of exposure, respectively. The chronicity indices for 3 and 6 months of exposure were calculated as 41 and 88. It must be recalled that it is unusual for additional exposure to produce a significant increase in the chronicity index for 3 months, and it indicates an especially persistent effect and minimal adaptation or repair. Epstein (1978) reported an LD 50 for male rats of 9.6 mg/kg when the chlordecone was administered over approximately 20 days. In rats a dietary level of 1 ppm chlordecone apparently produced no clinical or pathological effect (Larson et al., 1979a).

Absorption, Distribution, Metabolism, and Excretion Chlordecone is easily absorbed from the intestine (Boylan et al., 1978; Egle et al., 1978). Compared with other polyhalogenated chemicals such as polychlorinated biphenyls and DDT, the ratio of blood level to adipose tissue level is relatively high (Boylan et al., 1978; Egle et al., 1978). Chlordecone appears to be bound to albumin and high-density lipoproteins, whereas DDT and dieldrin are associated with β-lipoproteins mostly of low density (Skalsky et al., 1979; Soine et al., 1982). Considerable amounts may be found in the liver (Boylan et al., 1978; Egle et al., 1978).

Following a single oral dose of [^{14}C]chlordecone, tissue concentrations reached a maximum the third day and were decreasing by the fifth day. The relatively high concentration of the compound in bile, blood, and liver was noteworthy (Egle et al., 1976). The rate of clearance declined unremittingly. Half-lives in the blood were 8.5 days during the first 4 weeks, approximately 24 days during the next 8 weeks, and 45 days during the following 14 weeks. Levels in most tissues declined at a similar rate; however, the ratio of concentrations in liver and blood increased from 28 : 1 on day 1 to 126 : 1 on day 84. Total excretion of ^{14}C from radioactive chlordecone by day 84 was 65.5% in the feces and 1.6% in the urine (Egle et al., 1978).

Mice receiving chlordecone at a dietary rate of 40 ppm (about 5.1 mg/kg/day) reached a steady state of storage within 5 months. In fact, accumulation in the gonads, uterus, adrenals, spleen, heart, and muscle showed little increase in storage after the first 30 days, but storage progressed longer in the liver, brain, kidneys, and body fat. When mice were returned to a control diet, as much as 56 and 95% of the storage was lost within 24 and 150 days, respectively. Loss of storage was especially rapid from the liver and brain (Huber, 1965).

Boylan et al. (1978) presented indirect evidence for the existence of a metabolite in the feces of rats that had received [^{14}C]chlordecone. Later, chlordecone alcohol (chlordecol, decachlorooctahydro-1,3,4-metheno-2H-cyclobuta[cd]pentalen-2-ol) was identified in the feces of humans together with its glucuronide (Blanke et al., 1978; Fariss et al., 1980), but very little of these metabolites was produced by rats, mice, hamsters, or guinea pigs. However, the Mongolian gerbil is a good model for humans in this respect (Houston et al., 1981). Molowa et al. (1986a) have been able to demonstrate a cytosolic enzyme that reduces chlordecone to the alcohol in gerbil, rabbit, and human liver. The next highest activities were in kidney and intestine. The enzyme seems to be of the "aldo–keto reductase" family,

although in contrast to the aldo–keto reductase activity of cytosols toward other substrates, no chlordecone reductase activity was found in rat, hamster, mouse, and guinea pig liver. The species differences in the levels of this enzyme have been confirmed by using an antibody, raised in rabbits, to the human liver chlordecone reductase (Molowa et al., 1986b).

Following a single oral dose of [^{14}C]chlordecone at a rate of 40 mg/kg, rats excreted less than 10% of the activity in their feces during the first 24 hr and truly negligible amounts in their urine. During the next 7 days the daily rate of excretion was constant, being approximately 5% of the amount remaining to be excreted (Boylan et al., 1978). The rate reported in rats is far higher than that reported in humans. The rates are not comparable because that in the rat involved early excretion of a single dose, whereas that in humans involved late excretion after prolonged intake had stopped. Even so, the rates are so very different that it seems that excretion is inherently faster in the rat. Furthermore, relatively rapid clearance following prolonged intake has been demonstrated in mice. The contrast between the behavior of the compound in rats and mice and that in humans is striking.

The pig, like the gerbil, may be similar to humans in the metabolism of chlordecone (Soine et al., 1983). Chlordecone alcohol is found in feces; about 15% is conjugated, whereas in the bile up to 85% is in the conjugated form. Probably enterohepatic circulation occurs as in humans with conjugates hydrolyzed in the intestine or more readily being reabsorbed. Bungay et al. (1981) have described a computer-assisted model to explain chlordecone pharmacokinetics in the rat. The distribution and metabolism of chlordecone in the rat can be significantly altered by treatment with phenobarbital or SKF-525A (Aldous et al., 1983).

Besides excretion via the bile, the excretion of chlordecone occurs through the intestine wall by a process which in humans, but not rats, is inhibited by bile salts (Boylan et al., 1979). This would be similar to that process described for the excretion of other halogenated insecticides and environmental chemicals. Cholestyramine enhances chlordecone excretion in rats (Boylan et al., 1978) and humans (see Section 15.7.2.3). In rats this may be by direct binding of the insecticide, but in humans additional effects may operate, perhaps by binding bile salts which normally inhibit the nonbiliary excretion pathway (Boylan et al., 1979; Guzelian, 1982b).

In lactating animals a significant proportion (up to 52%) of a single dose of chlordecone can appear in the milk (Kavlock et al., 1980), whereas males excrete up to 33% in the feces during this time (Egle et al., 1978).

Biochemical Effects As might be expected, chlordecone induces microsomal enzymes of the liver (Fabacher and Hodgson, 1976; Mehendale et al., 1977, 1978; Kaminsky et al., 1978; Ebel, 1982; Chambers and Trevanthan, 1983). In male rats chlordecone increased the maximum rate of p-nitroanisole metabolism by rat liver microsomes by 100%, whereas mirex was less effective (Ebel, 1982, 1984). In contrast, both chemicals caused a depression of metabolism in females. It is possible that chlordecone induces constitutive forms of cytochrome P-450, although this needs further examination (Crouch and Ebel, 1987). Epoxide hydrolase is also induced by chlordecone. In mice, the no-effect level is less than a dietary level of 10 ppm (about 1.3 mg/kg/day). The compound induces enzymes in nursing mice that receive it from their mothers' milk (Fabacher and Hodgson, 1976; Mehendale *et al.*, 1977).

Lactate dehydrogenase is inhibited *in vitro* by chlordecone concentrations of 10 ppm or greater. Because this enzyme occupies a key position in the anaerobic glycolytic pathway of skeletal muscle and because similar concentrations of the insecticide may be reached in tissues, this inhibition may contribute to poisoning (Hendrickson and Bowden, 1975). The inhibition involves not only oxidation of lactate but also reduction of pyruvate and is exhibited by homologous enzymes from rabbit, beef, pig, and chicken. Changes in pH, solvents for chlordecone, and types of buffer had little effect on the degree of inhibition. Dilution experiments showed that the inhibition was fully reversible (Anderson and Noble, 1977). Chlordecone also inhibits malate dehydrogenase, an enzyme responsible for the oxidation of malate and the reduction of oxaloacetate. This inactivation, too, is reversible (Anderson *et al.*, 1977). Chlordecone, but not mirex, decreases the incorporation of amino acids into mouse brain proteins (Ritchie and Ho, 1982).

The inhibition of mitochondrial and other membrane-bound Na^+,K^+-ATPases and oligomycin-sensitive Mg^{2+}-ATPases induced by chlordecone has been extensively studied in rat and mouse liver (Desaiah *et al.*, 1977a; Curtis and Mehendale, 1979), perfused liver (Desaiah *et al.*, 1977b), heart (Desaiah, 1980), muscle (Mishra *et al.*, 1980), and especially brain (Desaiah *et al.*, 1978, 1980; Mishra *et al.*, 1980; Jordan *et al.*, 1981). The inhibition of these ATPases in brain synaptosomes is directly proportional to the degree of tremor (Jordan *et al.*, 1981). *In vitro,* addition of chlordecone also inhibited the ATPase activities of mitochondrial or synaptosomal preparations (Desaiah *et al.*, 1977a,b; 1978; End *et al.*, 1979; Mishra *et al.*, 1980; Desaiah, 1981). Compared to some tissues, brain Na^+,K^+-ATPase and heart mitochondrial Mg^{2+}-ATPase are more sensitive to chlordecone. Anti-chlordecone antibodies will reverse inhibition (Koch *et al.*, 1979).

Some theories have proposed that the net effect of chlordecone on Na^+,K^+-ATPases and oligomycin-sensitive Mg^{2+}-ATPases is interference with energy production, and certainly there is evidence which might support this theory (Desaiah *et al.*, 1977a,b; Carmines *et al.*, 1979; End *et al.*, 1979). What seems more important is that there is increasing evidence for an ATPase-linked disturbance in intracellular calcium transport (Carmines *et al.*, 1979; End *et al.*, 1979, 1981; Hoskins and Ho, 1982). A cerebrointraventricular injection of $CaCl_2$ exacerbates tremor in chlordecone-treated rats, although, interestingly, DDT-induced tremor is reduced (Herr *et al.*,% 1987). Young mice with chlordecone-induced tremors have been reported to have reduced synaptosomal calcium (Hoskins and Ho, 1982). *In vitro,* chlordecone at 5 μM inhibits basal Ca^{2+}-ATPase activity in calmodulin-depleted rat brain synaptosomes (Desaiah *et al.*, 1985). However, chlordecone decreased the calmodulin-stimu-

lated Ca^{2+}-ATPase activity at much a lower concentration (0.5 μM). Chlordecone-treated rats also show a 50% decrease in Ca^{2+}-ATPase activity in brain synaptosomes. Nuclear and cytosolic calmodulin levels were not affected, suggesting that chlordecone selectively affects membrane-bound calmodulin. Chlordecone partially depolarized synaptosomal plasma membrane *in vitro* with an increase in free synaptosomal Ca^{2+} levels in the presence of 1 mM extrasynaptosomal calcium (Komulainen and Bondy, 1987). Verapamil, a Ca^{2+} channel blocker, inhibited the increase. Although chlordecone appeared to inhibit synaptosomal K^+-stimulated uptake, this has been proposed to be due to lysis. Mirex had little effect. Komulainen and Bondy propose that chlordecone increases free intrasynaptosomal Ca^{2+} by a nonspecific leakage through the plasma membrane and by passage through voltage-sensitive Ca^{2+} channels due to membrane depolarization. This would be compatible with the theory that increased synaptosomal calcium levels cause depolarization of the membrane, promoting release of neurotransmitters (Carmines *et al.*, 1979; End *et al.*, 1979). On the other hand, it does not appear to be compatible with the proposal that chlordecone decreases synaptosomal calcium, resulting in decreased Ca-dependent release of GABA and dopamine (Hoskins and Ho, 1982).

A number of studies have been concerned with the status of neurotransmitters in chlordecone-induced neurotoxicity. Dopamine, norepinephrine, and GABA uptake into synaptosomes are all depressed (Ho *et al.*, 1981). In contrast, Fujimori *et al.* (1982b) found elevated levels of dopamine in the striatum of mice exposed to chlordecone in which the highest levels of chlordecone have been detected (Fujimori *et al.*, 1982a). However, Hong *et al.* (1984) found no changes in dopamine levels of rat striated tissue, although there was an increase in 5-hydroxyindoleacetic acid levels which was time- and dose-related to tremor. Similar findings in mice were made by Fujimori *et al* (1982b). In rats, a dosage of 25 mg/kg, which produced only slight tremor, caused a significant elevation of striatal 5-hydroxyindoleacetic acid (Hong *et al.*, 1984). 5-Hydroxytryptamine (serotonin, 5-HT) content of mouse and rat brain (Ho *et al.*, 1981; Hong *et al.*, 1984) did not significantly change, indicating that perhaps chlordecone induced the turnover of this transmitter rather than changing absolute levels. This could occur by an increase in the firing rate of the 5-HT neurons. A serotonergic receptor blocker, pizotifen, attenuates chlordecone-induced tremor, thus supporting this view (Gerhart *et al.*, 1982). A decrease in 5-HT recognition sites by 26% after 4 hr and 72% after 24 hr following an 80 mg/kg dose of chlordecone to male rats has been observed (Gandolfi *et al.*, 1984). Similar findings have been reported for females (Uphouse and Eckols, 1986). In addition, GABA turnover was inhibited in the striatum at the same time. Thus chlordecone may, through activation of 5-HT neurons, cause decreased GABAergic activity in the striatum and thereby an increase in cholinergic tone, causing tremors (Gandolfi *et al.*, 1984).

Clearly, the whole interrelationship between the effects of chlordecone on brain ATPase activities, calcium homeostasis, and neurotransmitter turnovers and releases needs considerably more careful investigation. For instance, there is also evidence that norepinephrine turnover may be involved in initial hypothermia and tremor induced by chlordecone (Chen *et al.*, 1985). Chlordecone does not bind to the picrotoxin binding site of the GABA–receptor complex as do lindane, cyclodienes, and toxaphenes (Lawrence and Casida, 1984).

Chlordecone has two effects on the liver which may be related to the inhibition of ATPases and disturbance of Ca^{2+} homeostasis that is seen in the brain. First, chlordecone, but not mirex, greatly enhances the hepatic toxicities of CCl_3 and CCl_4 (Hewitt *et al.*, 1979; Cianflone *et al.*, 1980; Curtis *et al.*, 1979, 1981; Curtis and Mehendale, 1980; Davis and Mehendale, 1980; Plaa *et al.*, 1987; Mehendale, 1989). Chlordecone is also far more potent than phenobarbital (Curtis and Mehendale, 1980; Agrawal and Mehendale, 1984a,b; Mehendale, 1989). Although there is evidence that CCl_4 is metabolized to a greater extent in chlordecone-induced animals (Klingensmith and Mehendale, 1983a), comparisons with phenobarbital demonstrate that this cannot explain the massive potentiation effect of chlordecone (Klingensmith and Mehendale, 1983a,b; Agrawal and Mehendale, 1984a,b; Mehendale and Klingensmith, 1988). In addition, CCl_4-induced lipid peroxidation is not increased and small doses of chlordecone (5 mg/kg) potentiate CCl_4 toxicity with very little induction of the hepatic monooxygenase system and increased covalent binding of CCl_4 metabolites (Davis and Mehendale, 1980). In contrast, chlordecone causes a large increase in cytosolic Ca^{2+} levels despite mitochondrial and microsomal sequestration of Ca^{2+} at elevated levels (Agrawal and Mehendale, 1984a,b). Hegarty *et al.* (1986) have reported that chlordecone potentiates the suppression of calcium sequestration by microsomes caused by CCl_4. Perfused livers from rats fed chlordecone at 10 ppm for 15 days and then given CCl_4 (100 μl/kg) progressively accumulated Ca^{2+} from perfusate, especially more than 12 hr after treatment (Agrawal and Mehendale, 1986). Partial hepatectomy protects against chlordecone-potentiated CCl_4 hepatotoxicity (Bell *et al.*, 1988; Kodavanti *et al.*, 1989; Mehendale, 1989). This supports the hypothesis that chlordecone suppresses hepatocellular regeneration after CCl_4 (although not after partial hepatectomy) (Lockard *et al.*, 1983a,b). Although chlordecone potentiates the nephrotoxicity of $CHCl_3$ (Hewitt *et al.*, 1979), it abolished the nephrotoxic effects of CBr_4 (Agrawal *et al.*, 1983b). Chlordecone and particularly mirex have been shown to increase the acute hepatotoxicity of acetaminophen in mice (Fouse and Hodgson, 1987).

The second hepatotoxic effect of chlordecone, which seems to be related to some of the biochemical effects in brain, is the impairment of biliary function (Mehendale, 1977b, 1981a,b; Curtis and Mehendale, 1979). Rats treated with chlordecone showed an impaired ability to excrete imipramine metabolite or phenolphthalein in the bile; this was not due to decreased metabolism or to cholestasis, and in fact bile flow was increased. Impairment was directly related to chlordecone content of liver, was fully reversible (Mehendale, 1981a), and seems to be due to inhibition of transfer of metabolites from hepatocyte to the bile canaliculus. Inhibition of Mg^{2+}-ATPase activity and

thus mitochondrial energy production (Desaiah *et al.*, 1977a,b) might interfere with biliary transport (Curtis and Mehendale, 1979; Mehendale, 1977a,b, 1981a,b). However, it is difficult to explain the lack of effect on endogenous organic anions such as bilirubin, and it would seem that chlordecone exerts a more subtle effect involving canalicular ATPases (Guzelian, 1982b).

Chlordecone fed to rats at 200 ppm for 8 days caused a depletion of catecholamine-containing granules of the adrenal epinephrine cells but not those of the norepinephrine cells (Baggett *et al.*, 1980). Mirex was without effect at these rates. These findings were consistent with chlordecone causing a decrease in the total catecholamine content of the gland and a small increase in norepinephrine.

Food consumption of rats tended to increase as the dietary concentration of chlordecone increased from 5 to 50 ppm for different groups. This effect was associated with a measured increase in metabolic rate (Larson *et al.*, 1979a).

Effects on Organs and Tissues   In rats and mice chlordecone causes an increased size of the liver (Huber, 1965; Baggett *et al.*, 1977; Cannon and Kimbrough, 1979; Larson *et al.*, 1979a; see also Table 15.34). This enlargement is accompanied by proliferation of the endoplasmic reticulum and associated induction of microsomal enzymes (see Table 15.34 and Biochemical Effects). Histologically, only nonspecific changes such as fatty infiltration are observed with no apparent hepatocellular necrosis.

As far as mutagenicity is concerned, there is no evidence that chlordecone is positive in the usual tests. Chlordecone was negative at a dose level of 3.6 or 11.4 mg/kg/per day for 5 days in a dominant lethal mutation study in male rats (Simon *et al.*, 1978, 1986). It was also negative when tested for enhancement of unscheduled DNA synthesis in primary cultures of adult rat hepatocytes (Williams, 1980; Prohst *et al.*, 1981).

The carcinogenic potential of chlordecone has been explored in a number of studies in rats and mice (Table 15.34). In a National Cancer Institute study with Osborne–Mendel rats and B6C3Fl mice (NCI, 1976), initial levels in the diet were too high to permit survival. After reduction in the levels, "time-weighted average" concentrations were 8 and 24 ppm (about 0.36 and 1.08 mg/kg/day) in male rats, 18 and 26 ppm (about 0.95 and 1.38 mg/kg/day) in female rats, 20 and 23 ppm (about 2.48 and 2.85 mg/kg/day) in male mice, and 20 and 40 ppm (about 2.66 and 5.32 mg/kg/day) in female mice for 80 weeks. Rats were given a normal diet for a further 32 weeks and mice for 10 weeks. At the high dose level in rats hepatocellular carcinomas were observed in 7% of males and in 22% of females, whereas none were seen in controls. Significant incidences of liver carcinomas were also observed in the mouse studies, with males more susceptible than females. No metastases to extrahepatic tissues were observed. Tumors were also recorded in other tissues, especially in female rats, and were related to dose. Animals with liver carcinomas, and many of those without, had hyperplastic nodules. Some of the other studies also showed that chlordecone is a hepatocarcinogen in rats and mice (see Epstein, 1978; Larson *et al.*, 1979a).

As with the other chlorinated insecticides (see Section 15.2.3.2), it is difficult to know the significance of the tumors caused by chlordecone and even their mechanistic origins. Chlordecone, like other chlorinated polycyclic hydrocarbons, inhibits the intercellular communication in Chinese hamster V79 cells *in vitro*, suggesting a promotive role (Tsushimoto *et al.*, 1982). Chlordecone acted as a promoter of carcinogenesis in rats following diethylnitrosamine and hepatectomy treatment. This occurred to a greater extent in females than males (Sirica *et al.*, 1989).

Chlordecone, like other chlorinated cyclic aromatic and nonaromatic chemicals, can cause changes in the adrenal (Larson *et al.*, 1979a; Cannon and Kimbrough, 1979; Baggett *et al.*, 1980; see also Biochemical Effects) with hyperplasia of the zona fasciculata and zona reticularis. Glomerulosclerosis and testicular atrophy (see Effects on Reproduction) have also been noted (Larson *et al.*, 1979a). Although mirex affects the thyroid of rats (Yarbrough *et al.*, 1981), there seems to be no clear association between chlordecone exposure and antithyroid effects (Chu *et al.*, 1980a).

Chlordecone causes a depletion of body fat in rats. Metabolic ketosis is not induced and utilization of lipids seems to be the underlying mechanism, perhaps as a consequence of altered energy balance (Klingensmith and Mehendale, 1982).

Effects on the brain can be found under Effects on the Nervous System.

In subacute studies chlordecone altered the glycogen and lipid stores of mouse muscle and caused the development of abnormal muscle mitochondria. However, muscle grip strength was unchanged (Phillips and Eroschenko, 1985a,b).

The toxic effects of chlordecone on reproductive tissues can be found under Effects on Reproduction.

No immunotoxic effects of chlordecone in male rats could be detected without first causing overt toxicity such as loss of body weight (Smialowicz *et al.*, 1985).

Effects on Reproduction   Many studies have been conducted on the effects of chlordecone on the reproduction of quails, hens, and other birds. References to some of these which are interlinked with mammalian studies can be found in Guzelian (1982b).

Two studies conducted in the 1960s showed that chlordecone fed to mice impaired their breeding. Good *et al.* (1965) found a progressive reduction in the average number of litters per pair among mice when different groups of both males and females received dietary levels of 10, 17.5, 25, 30, and 37.5 ppm. A little reproduction persisted at the highest dosage. Effects at 10 ppm were equivocal. However, when another strain of mouse was fed 10 ppm, there was a statistically significant reduction in the proportion of pairs producing litters, and the difference was more marked for second litters than for first litters. A similar result was obtained when mice were fed chlordecone at a dietary level of 5 ppm (about 0.64 mg/kg/day for nonlactating adults and higher for lactating females and for young). Finally, when the progeny of mice that had received 5 ppm were bred, the proportion of pairs producing litters was reduced compared to controls, regardless of whether the second generation received 5 ppm or control diet.

Further study showed that 14 pairs that received 40 ppm for 2 months before mating and also during the test produced no litters whatever, while 14 control pairs produced 14 first litters and 14 second litters. Reproduction resumed within 7 weeks following withdrawal of chlordecone from the females that had been sterile as a result of receiving 40 ppm for 160 days. Their initial litters were smaller and suffered greater mortality than controls; however, their second litters were slightly larger than those of controls and experienced no greater mortality. Matings between control males and females that had received 40 ppm for 2 months before mating were sterile, but control females did produce litters when mated with chlordecone-fed males. These litters were smaller than those of control females by control males, indicating that chlordecone may have affected male reproduction also, but histological examination of the testes revealed apparently normal spermatogenesis and interstitial cell content (Huber, 1965).

Rats that received chlordecone orally at a rate of 10 mg/kg/day from day 7 to day 16 of gestation suffered 19% mortality and weight loss and increased relative weight of the liver of survivors; their fetuses exhibited reduced body weight, reduced ossification, edema, undescended testes, enlarged renal pelves, and enlarged cerebral ventricles. Dosages of 6 and 12 mg/kg/day, which also produced body weight loss and relative increase in liver weight in the dams, produced only reduced body weight and reduced ossification in the fetuses. Male rats born to treated dams showed no reproductive impairment. In the mouse, toxicity to the fetus occurred at a maternal dosage of 12 mg/kg/day but not at 8 or 4 mg/kg/day, all on days 7–16 of gestation. At the highest dosage level there was increased fetal mortality and clubfoot (Chernoff and Rogers, 1976). Reproductive effects of chlordecone in rats have also been noted by Rosenstein *et al.* (1977), Cannon and Kimbrough (1979), and Chernoff *et al.* 1979b). Neuroendocrine dysfunctions can occur when rat pups are exposed to chlordecone (Cooper *et al.*, 1985).

There is now evidence to support the view that chlordecone exerts some of its reproductive effects by mimicking the effects of excessive estrogens. Vaginal smears of mice indicated that constant estrus started within 8 weeks in females after they began to receive a dietary level of 40 ppm. The same condition eventually appeared in females on 30 ppm. Examination of the ovaries of mice receiving 30 ppm showed few corpera lutea (3.8 per ovary in controls), although follicular development seemed normal. Hormone bioassay revealed that pituitary extracts from chlordecone-fed females equaled those of controls in follicle-stimulating hormone (FSH) activity but were 25% low on luteinizing hormone (LH) activity (Huber, 1965). The ability of chlordecone to cause constant estrus and other estrogen-like effects in rodents has been confirmed repeatedly (Gellert, 1978; Gellert and Wilson, 1979; Uphouse *et al.*, 1984; Sierra and Uphouse, 1986; Uphouse, 1986). Only two intraperitoneal injections of as little as 0.015 mg of chlordecone in neonatal female mice (about 0.165 mg/kg total) caused distinct morphological alterations in the epithelium lining both the vagina and the uterus. The changes showed a dosage–response relationship in the range 0.015–1.25 mg and between 2 and 10 doses. The changes appeared identical to the developmental changes induced by estradiol (Eroschenko and Mousa, 1979). However, despite the fact that in some ways the cornification of vaginal epithelial cells is similar to that seen with estradiol (Eroschenko, 1982), the effects of the two chemicals are not identical (Eroschenko and Osman, 1986).

Although chlordecone is distributed throughout male reproductive rat tissue, especially seminal vesicular fluid, it does not appear to produce dominant lethal effects (Simon et al., 1986). Chlordecone fed to male rats (up to 30 ppm for 90 days) has been reported to cause some reversible decreases in epididymal spermatazoa motility and viability and sperm reserves in the cauda epididymus (Linder et al., 1983), but other experiments have shown little effect (Cochran and Wicdow, 1984).

Chlordecone competes with estrogen for binding to nuclear and cytoplasmic estradiol receptors in target tissues (Bulger et al., 1979; Hammond et al., 1979). Incubation of rat uteri with chlordecone in vitro leads to an accumulation of estrogen receptor in the nuclear fraction and a decrease in the cytosolic fraction, indicating that translocation has occurred. Although the affinity of chlordecone for the receptor is only 0.01–0.04% that of estradiol, its estrogenic activity may be due in part to its long half-life resulting in long-term occupancy of receptors. Other investigations suggest that the effect of chlordecone may be in the hypothalamic–pituitary system (Huber, 1965; Hong and Ali, 1982; Hudson et al., 1984; Uphouse et al., 1984). However, chlordecone inhibited the effect of gonadotropin-releasing hormone on rat pituitary gonadotropes and also antagonized estradiol (Huang and Nelson, 1986). Failure of chlordecone to mimic estrogen CNS activity and perhaps even antagonize it has also been observed in vivo (Uphouse et al., 1986; Eckols et al., 1989; Williams et al., 1988, 1989). In neonatal hamsters, Gray (1982) has demonstrated that chlordecone acts like a weak estrogen in the brain so that females are masculinized and show abnormal bisexual behavior.

Unlike mirex, chlordecone was not cataractogenic in either young rats or mice (Chernoff et al., 1979b).

Effects on the Nervous System As mentioned previously, chlordecone causes a prompt onset of tremor in rats and mice (Larson et al., 1979a; Cannon and Kimbrough, 1979; Dietz and McMillan, 1979; Egle et al., 1979; Baggett et al., 1980; Huang et al., 1980; Ho et al., 1981; Jordan et al., 1981; Tilson and Mactutus, 1982; Gerhart et al., 1985). This tremor can be quantified (Gerhart et al., 1982; Tilson and Gerhart, 1982). Hyperexcitability is also characteristic of chlordecone toxicity, as is an exaggerated startle response (Reiter et al., 1977, 1982; Tilson et al., 1979). In mice the threshold for pentylenetetrazole-induced seizures was significantly reduced in chlordecone-treated animals (Huang et al., 1980). Gerhart et al. (1983) used psychopharmacological agents to determine the site of chlordecone-induced tremor of male rats. They suggested that the spinal cord and/or pontomedullary reticular formation sites are the sources of the tremor.

Some of the biochemical investigations of the brain after chlordecone treatment are considered under Biochemical Effects. Although p,p'-DDT and chlordecone both cause tremor, the mechanisms do not seem to be identical (Herr et al., 1987; Komulainen and Bondy, 1987). Pretreatment with phenytoin attenuated the tremor caused by DDT but enhanced that produced by chlordecone (Tilson et al., 1985, 1986). A number of studies suggest that endorphin levels may be altered by chlordecone treatment of adult and prepubertal mice (Hong and Ali, 1982; Ali et al., 1982; Rosencrans et al., 1982; Swanson and Woolley, 1982; Hong et al., 1985).

Chlordecone induces initial hypothermia, as do dieldrin and lindane, whereas with DDT it occurs only during severe tremor and convulsions before death (Swanson and Woolley, 1982; Hsu et al., 1986). This could be due to vasodilation mediated by an adrenergic mechanism in the brain stem rather than to decreased metabolic rate (Cook et al., 1987, 1988a,b). Investigations of ultrastructural changes induced by chlordecone have demonstrated that in mice subacute doses produced changes in peripheral unmyelinated fiber bundles including vesiculation of Schwann cell cytoplasm, dissolution of microtubules, and paracrystalline inclusion in mitochondria. In contrast, myelinated axons, myelin, and associated Schwann cells were unaffected (Phillips and Eroschenko, 1982, 1985a; also see Benet et al., 1985). Peripheral nerve conductance velocities were significantly reduced in rats given chlordecone orally at 10 mg/kg/day for 10 days (Subramony et al., 1982).

Besides tremor and irritability, chlordecone causes a number of behavioral changes. Some of these are related to the estrogenic effects of this chemical (Gray, 1982) but others seem to be defects in learning, memory, and startle responsiveness brought about by exposure to chlordecone at the neonatal stage (Squibb and Tilson, 1982a,b; Mactutus and Tilson, 1984a,b). Although mirex is more lethal than chlordecone, it does not result in the behavioral effects in weanling rats seen with the latter insecticide (Reiter and Kidd, 1978; Reiter et al., 1982).

Treatment of Poisoning in Animals Although cholestyramine is effective in increasing the fecal excretion of chlordecone and decreasing the levels in tissues (Boylan et al., 1978; see also Section 15.2.5), a definite increase in the fecal excretion of chlordecone was accomplished with light liquid paraffin added to the diet at a concentration of 8% (Richter et al., 1979).

15.7.2.3 Toxicity to Humans

Use Experience Chlordecone was manufactured in Virginia from 1965 for 8 years without reported difficulty. At that time it was decided that the factory where the compound had been made would be used exclusively for the manufacture of plastics. Very soon thereafter, a separate, small company was organized for the sole purpose of making chlordecone. Some work was begun in the autumn of 1973, and full production started in April 1974. No proper factory with exhaust ventilation, its own waste disposal system, and other hygienic equipment was available. According to Raloff (1976), the work was set up in an abandoned service station. Liquid waste was discharged directly to the community sewage system. The town's sewage digestion system began to show the effects within a month, and within another 6 months the microbiological digestors were inoperative. (There is some evidence that inactivation of the digestors was the result of the discharge into the sewer in October 1974 of an entire unsatisfactory batch of material.) In addition, no effective dust control was provided in the improvised factory. To make matters worse, personal hygiene was so poor that it was alleged that workers came home with their skin and clothes white with the powder. Some children of workers developed signs attributed to poisoning. At least one worker quit after 11 months because he had developed tremor. However, it apparently was the measurement of chlordecone in samples of urine and blood submitted by a private physician to the U.S. Public Health Service Center for Disease Control and their alerting of the Virginia State Department of Health that led to closure of the improvised plant on July 25, 1975, 4 days later. It had been in full operation for 16 months. The news report offers some detail of the environmental and liability implications that attended the closing. Absorption was probably mainly dermal (Taylor *et al.*, 1978).

Examination of 133 of the 148 present or previous employees of the chlordecone manufacturing plant revealed that 57% had symptoms of poisoning or had had them in the past. The syndrome was insidious in onset. In 23 employees with chronic intoxication, it involved weight loss, tremor especially of the upper extremities, muscle weakness, unusual eye movements spoken of as opsoclonus, ataxia and incoordination, slurred speech, mental changes, pleuritic chest pain, arthralgia, skin rash, and abnormality of routine liver function tests. It was concluded that chlordecone affects the brain as well as the peripheral nerves and muscle (Taylor *et al.*, 1978). Tremorgrams performed on three patients indicated that the usual frequency was 6–8 Hz (Taylor, 1982). Poor recent memory was reported by 13 workers, although this could not be substantiated by psychologic assessment testing. Among nine patients who complained of headache, three had a mild to moderate increase in intracranial pressure at the time of lumbar puncture (Sanborn *et al.*, 1979). Cerebrospinal fluid absorption from the subarachnoid space was impaired in all three individuals. An epidemiologic study revealed that the incidence of illness was 67% in production workers and 16% in nonproduction workers of the plant. There was no apparent association between the frequency of symptoms among community residents and the proximity of their homes to the plant. However, chlordecone blood levels as high as 0.033 ppm were found in residents of a community located within 1.6 km of the plant. The wives of two workers had had objective tremor. Both gave a history of washing their husbands' work clothing (Cannon *et al.*, 1978). Follow-up studies of 16 out of 23 patients originally examined by Taylor *et al.* (1978) were conducted between 1980 and 1982 (Taylor, 1982). Seven complained of persistent symptoms, although tremor was noted for only one worker on examination (Taylor, 1982, 1985).

Laboratory Findings   Among 32 of the men who had manufactured chlordecone and who were suffering persistent poisoning involving the nervous system, testes, and liver, whole-blood levels of the compound ranged from 0.6 to 32.0 ppm,

with an average of 5.8 ppm. The concentration in subcutaneous fat of 16 of them was only 2.2–62.0 ppm with a mean of 21.5 ppm—remarkably low in view of the blood levels. In the 10 samples that were taken, the highest concentrations were in the liver and ranged from 13.3 to 173.0 ppm with a mean of 75.9 ppm. No metabolites were identified in tissues, urine, or stool. Excretion of chlordecone was negligible in urine and sweat but occurred mainly in the feces, where it amounted to 0.019 to 0.279%/day (mean 0.075%/day) of what was estimated to be the total amount stored in the body. However, fecal excretion accounted for only 10% of biliary excretion of chlordecone estimated in six patients from samples of duodenal drainage and directly in one other from bile collected by T-tube (Cohn *et al.*, 1976, 1978; Boylan *et al.*, 1979; Guzelian, 1981). This difference suggested a therapeutic approach, which is discussed under Treatment of Poisoning.

An epidemiologic study based on a somewhat different sample revealed chlordecone in the blood of 100% of 57 workers affected in any degree, 99% of 49 unaffected workers, 94% of 32 family members of workers, 77% of 39 workers formerly employed in a different Kepone plant, 72% of 32 workers in businesses within one block of the plant where illnesses occurred, and 19% of 214 residents of the general community. The mean values were 2.53 ppm for sick workers, 0.60 ppm for healthy workers, and 0.10–0.01 ppm for the other groups (Cannon *et al.*, 1978).

In a group of workers who were associated with a plant in another city and who remained healthy, serum concentrations on the last day of exposure ranged from 0.120 to 2.109 ppm. The half-lives for disappearance of chlordecone from their sera ranged from 63 to 148 days. Half-life was not correlated with initial serum level (Adir *et al.*, 1978). The half-lives in these recently exposed healthy men were briefer than those of sick men who had been exposed longer.

An apparent threshold for disappearance of neurotoxicity was associated with a decline of blood levels of chlordecone to 0.1–1 ppm (Guzelian, 1982b).

The relatively high levels of chlordecone in blood as compared to adipose tissue, in contrast to other chlorinated lipophilic chemicals, seem to be due to specific binding to albumin and high-density lipoproteins (Skalsky *et al.*, 1979; Soine *et al.*, 1982).

Chlordecol (chlordecone alcohol) was found in the stools of patients in concentrations at least as great as those of chlordecone. The concentration of chlordecol was small in human bile and negligible in human urine and plasma (Blanke *et al.*, 1978). However, when a 46-year-old man chronically poisoned by chlordecone required cholecystectomy because of gallstones, it was found that fecal excretion of chlordecol was abolished as long as all bile was diverted through a T-tube. The concentrations of chlordecol and chlordecone in the bile were equal, and their combined excretion in the bile was four times greater than combined fecal excretion before surgery. As long as the bile was diverted, not only did fecal excretion of chlordecol stop but also fecal excretion of chlordecone increased 6–10 times over what it had been before or over what it was later when the diverted bile was continuously infused in the duodenum. This proved the presence of an extrahepatic source of decone in the stool; the intestine itself seemed the most likely source (Boylan *et al.*, 1979). These observations also strongly suggest that reabsorption of chlordecone from the intestine is largely dependent on the presence of bile.

The chlordecol found in human bile from poisoned workers was not present as the free alcohol to any great extent but mainly existed as the glucuronide (Fariss *et al.*, 1980). Another conjugate of chlordecone was also detected, possibly formed by conjugation with glutathione. Unlike rat liver, human liver and gerbil liver (see Section 15.7.2.2) formed chlordecol by the action of an aldo–keto reductase (Molowa *et al.*, 1986a). The enzyme has been purified from human liver (Molowa *et al.*, 1986b). In fact, immunoblot analyses of seven human liver samples showed the presence in four of two immunoreactive proteins whose total concentration varied over a sixfold range. Interestingly, the half-time for the disappearance of chlordecone from 22 exposed workers also varied as much as sixfold and was independent of the amount of chlordecone initially detected in the blood (Cohn *et al.*, 1978). Of 28 chlordecone-poisoned workers, only 8 patients had normal sperm counts and motility and only in one of these was chlordecone greater than 1 ppm of blood (Cohn *et al.*, 1978; Guzelian, 1981, 1982b). Arrest of sperm maturation was also observed in testicular biopsies of two patients (Guzelian, 1982b).

Pathology   Five sural nerve biopsies from workers affected by chlordecone revealed an accumulation of elongated, electron-dense, crystalloid rods and short, laminated, and parallel-membranous bodies within Schwann cell cytoplasm; redundant Schwann cell cytoplasmic folds; prominent collagen pockets, focal degradation of axon cylinders containing condensed neurofilaments, neurotubules, and dense bodies; occasional demyelinated axons; and vacuolization of nonmyelinated fibers. The predominance of involvement of nonmyelinated and smaller myelinated fibers and relative sparing of the larger myelinated fibers may explain the clinical symptomatology and electromyographic findings (Martinez *et al.*, 1978).

Six skeletal muscle biopsies from the same group of workers revealed accumulations of lipofuscin and amorphous, electron-dense structures below the sarcolemma and between myofibrils of skeletal muscle (Martinez *et al.*, 1978).

Needle liver biopsies from chlordecone-poisoned men showed minimal steatosis, focal proliferation of reticuloendothelial cells, and hypoglycogenation of nuclei. Livers were enlarged, and electron microscopic examinations showed residual bodies, branched mitochondria with paracrystalline inclusions, and proliferation of the endoplasmic reticulum (Guzelian *et al.*, 1980; Guzelian, 1985). Workers also had high levels of urinary glucaric acid, which is proposed to be derived from the hepatic endoplasmic reticulum. In addition, workers displayed an enhanced clearance of antipyrine from the blood, which usually is taken as a sign of induction of the hepatic cytochrome P-450 drug-metabolizing system.

Discussion   Whereas the acute toxicity of chlordecone is only moderate, its high degree of cumulative effect in mice (Huber, 1965) is remarkable, and it was the subject of early publication.

In fact, the protracted nature of poisoning was known to the original manufacturer before production was first started (see Gleason *et al.*, 1963, reporting brief but critical information supplied by the manufacturer).

A point that deserves more emphasis than it has received is that chlordecone is stored even more tenaciously by humans than by rodents. There was no way to predict this species difference, but routine analysis of serum samples would have detected the difference when little or no injury had occurred, and the results would have served as a warning to stop exposure. The lowest serum level eventually found associated with poisoning was one that would be alarming in connection with serum levels of other, more thoroughly studied chlorinated hydrocarbon insecticides. There seems little doubt that poisoning would have been avoided if proper attention had been given to the chemical and clinical aspects of occupational medicine and to the basic considerations of occupational hygiene.

It is interesting how much of the toxicity of chlordecone in humans can be reproduced in experimental animals, and vice versa, especially if care is taken to pick the right model for a particular effect. This includes enlargement of the liver and induction of the drug-metabolizing system, an important point for toxicological and carcinogenic considerations. Unlike many poisoning episodes, the exposure of workers to chlordecone has been used to investigate basic toxicological principles in humans with useful results such as the interindividual variability of a previously unknown aldo–keto reductase in liver (Molowa *et al.*, 1986b). Rational treatments for poisonings by these types of chemicals have also emerged (Guzelian, 1982a).

Treatment of Poisoning   The only drug that has proved useful in poisoning by chlordecone is cholestyramine. The use of this agent arose from careful consideration of data on the excretion of chlordecone by humans and animals, followed by logical experiments in rats and humans (Boylan *et al.*, 1978; Cohn *et al.*, 1978; Guzelian, 1981, 1982a, 1984, 1985). Its effects may be due not only to direct binding of chlordecone but to binding of bile salts which inhibit the nonbiliary intestinal excretion (Guzelian, 1982b). Because there is reason to think that cholestyramine might be useful for treating poisoning by some other chlorinated hydrocarbon insecticides also, it is described in Section 15.2.5.1. In spite of the importance of cholestyramine in the treatment of poisoning by chlordecone, other matters relevant to treating poisoning by chlorinated hydrocarbon insecticides ought to be considered (see Section 15.2.5).

ACKNOWLEDGMENTS

I would like to thank Miss J. Allen for help in literature searches and especially Mrs. R. Hill for arranging and typing the manuscript.

REFERENCES

Abalis, I. M., Eldefrawi, M. E., and Eldefrawi, A. T. (1985). High-affinity stereospecific binding of cyclodiene and γ-hexachlorocyclohexane to γ-aminobutyric acid receptors of rat brain. *Pestic. Biochem. Physiol.* **24,** 95–102.

Abalis, I. M., Eldefrawi, M. E., and Eldefrawi, A. T. (1986). Effect of insecticides on GABA-induced chloride influx into rat brain microsacs. *J. Toxicol. Environ. Health* **18,** 13–23.

Abbott, D. C., Goulding, R., and Tatton, J. U'G. (1968). Organochlorine pesticide residues in human fat in Great Britain. *Br. Med. J.* **3,** 146–149.

Abbott, D. C., Collins, G. B., and Goulding, R. (1972). Organochlorine pesticide residues in human fat in the United Kingdom 1969–71. *Br. Med. J.* **2,** 553–556.

Abbott, D. C., Collins, G. B., Goulding, R., and Hoodless, R. A. (1981). Organochlorine pesticide residues in human fat in the United Kingdom 1976–1977. *Br. Med. J.* **283,** 1425–1428.

Abbott, D. C., Goulding, R., Holmes, C. D., and Hoodless, R. A. (1985). Organochlorine pesticide residues in human fat in the United Kingdom 1982–1983. *Hum. Toxicol.* **4,** 435–445.

Abdusaidov, T. (1972). Effects of thiamine, ascorbic acid, galascorbin, and cocarboxylase on the functional status of the liver in combined hexachlorane and dimethoate poisoning. *Med. Zh. Uzb.* **5,** 39–41 (in Russian).

Abe, J., Inoue, Y., and Takamatsu, M. (1974). On the residual amounts of PCB and organochlorine pesticides in human blood. *Jpn. J. Hyg.* **29,** 93 (in Japanese).

Abou-Donia, M. B., and Menzel, D. B. (1968). The metabolism *in vivo* of 1,1,1-trichloro-2,2-bis(*p*-chlorophenyl)ethane (DDT), 1,1-dichloro-2,2-bis(*p*-chlorophenyl)ethylene (DDE) in the chick by embryonic injection and dietary ingestion. *Biochem. Pharmacol.* **17,** 2143–2146.

Abraham, R., Benitz, K. F., and Mankes, R. (1983). Ploidy patterns in hepatic tumors induced by mirex. *Exp. Mol. Pathol.* **38,** 271–282.

Abston, P. A., and Yarbrough, J. D. (1974). The *in vivo* effects of dietary mirex on hepatic lactic dehydrogenase and glutamic oxaloacetic transaminase levels of the rat. *J. Agric. Food Chem.* **22,** 66–68.

Acker, L. (1974). Food chemistry for the benefit of consumer protection. *Dtsch. Lebensm.-Rundsch.* **70,** 5–12 (in German).

Acker, L. (1981). Contamination of human milk with organochlorine pesticides. *Geburtshilfe Frauenheilkd.* **41,** 882–886 (in German).

Acker, L., and Schulte, E. (1970). On the presence of chlorinated biphenyls and hexachlorobenzene in addition to chlorinated insecticides in human milk and human fat tissue. *Naturwissenschaften* **57,** 497 (in German).

Acker, L., and Schulte, E. (1971). Organochlorine compounds in the human body. *Umschau* **61,** 32 (in German).

Acker, L., and Schulte, E. (1972). Occurrence of hexachlorobenzene and polychlorinated biphenyls as well as chlorinated insecticides in human adipose tissue and milk. *Nahrung* **16,** 130 (in German).

Acker, L., and Schulte, E. (1974). Organochlorine compounds in human fat. *Naturwissenschaften* **61,** 32 (in German).

Ackerman, L. B. (1980). Overview of human exposure to dieldrin residues in the environment and current trends of residue levels in tissue. *Pestic. Monit. J.* **14,** 64–69.

Adamovic, V. M., and Sokic, B. (1973). Lower level phenomena of DDT cumulation in female abdominal fatty tissue. *Arh. Hig. Rada Toksikol.* **24,** 303–306 (in Russian).

Adamovic, V. M., Sokic, B,. and Petrovic, O. (1971). On factors influencing the occurrence of organochlorine insecticides in newborns. *Ernaehrungsforschung* **16,** 579–585 (in German).

Adamovic, V. M., Sokic, B., and Jonanovic-Similganski, M. (1978). Some observations concerning the ratio of the intake of organochlorine insecticides through food and amounts excreted in the milk of breast-feeding mothers. *Bull. Environ. Contam. Toxicol.* **20,** 280–285.

Adams, M., Coon, F. B., and Poling, C. E. (1974). Insecticides in the tissues of four generations of rats fed different dietary fats containing a mixture of chlorinated hydrocarbon insecticides. *J. Agric. Food Chem.* **22,** 69–75.

Adir, J., Caplan, Y. H., and Thompson, B. C. (1978). Kepone serum half-life in humans. *Life Sci.* **22,** 699–702.

Agrawal, A. K., and Mehendale, H. H. (1984a). Perturbation of calcium homeostatis by CCl₄ in rats pretreated with chlordecone and phenobarbital. *Environ. Health Perspect.* **57,** 289–291.

Agrawal, A. K., and Mehendale, H. H. (1984b). CCl₄-induced alterations in

Ca²⁺ homeostatis by chlordecone and phenobarbital pretreated animals. *Life Sci.* **34,** 141–148.

Agrawal, A. K., and Mehendale, H. M. (1986). Effect of chlordecone on carbon tetrachloride-induced increase in calcium uptake in isolated perfused rat liver. *Toxicol. Appl. Pharmacol.* **83,** 342–348.

Agrawal, A. K., Berndt, W. O., and Mehendale, H. M. (1983a). Possible nephrotoxic effect of carbon tetrabromide and its interaction with chlordecone. *Toxicol. Lett.* **17,** 57–62.

Agrawal, A. K., Mohani, A., Zaid, N. F., and Seth, P. K. (1983b). Involvement of serotonergic receptors in endosulfan neurotoxicity. *Biochem. Pharmacol.* **32,** 3591–3593.

Agrawal, D., Khanna, R. N., Anand, M., Gupta, G. S. D., and Ray, P. K. (1987). Lindane-induced changes in glucose and glutathione levels in cats. *Toxicol. Lett.* **38,** 77–82.

Agthe, C., Garcia, H., Shubik, P., Tomatis, L., and Wenyon, E. (1970). Study of the potential carcinogenicity of DDT in the Syrian golden hamster. *Proc. Soc. Exp. Biol. Med.* **134,** 113–116.

Agzamov, S. K. (1970). Conditions of the ear in persons involved in agricultural application of chemical poisons. *Med. Zh. Uzb.* **7,** 13–15 (in Russian).

Ahmad, N., Harsas, W., Marolt, R. S., Morton, M., and Pollack, J. K. (1988). Total DDT and dieldrin content of human adipose tissue. *Bull. Environ. Contam. Toxicol.* **41,** 802–808.

Ahmed, F. E., Hart, R. W., and Lewis, N. J. (1977). Pesticide induced damage and its repair in cultured human cells. *Mutat. Res.* **42,** 161–173.

Ahmed, N. A., Rawi, J. M., and El-Behary, M. H. (1986). Effect of dieldrin injection on the level of certain amino acids and some enzymes in rat brain. *Comp. Biochem. Physiol. C* **85,** 437–442.

Akasu, F. (1971). Maternity and pollution. *J. Jpn. Obstet. Gynaecol.* **23,** 759–764. (in Japanese).

Alary, J. G., Guay, P., and Brodeur, J. (1971). Effect of phenobarbital on the metabolism of DDT in the rat and in the bovine. *Toxicol. Appl. Pharmacol.* **18,** 457–468.

Albahary, C., Dubrisay, J., and Guérin, (1957). Refractory pancytopenia due to lindane (gamma BHC). *Arch. Mal. Prof. Med. Trav. Secur. Soc.* **18,** 687–691 (in French).

Albert, L. (1981). Organochlorine pesticide residues in maternal milk and their risk to health. *Bol. Of. Sanit. Panam.* **91,** 15–29.

Albert, L., Cebrian, M. E., Mendez, F., and Portales, A. (1980). Organochlorine pesticide residues in human adipose tissue in Mexico: Results of a preliminary study in three Mexican cities. *Arch. Environ. Health* **35,** 262–269.

Albert, L., Vega, P., and Portales, A. (1981). Organochlorine pesticide residues in human milk samples from Comarca Lagunera, Mexico, 1976. *Pestic. Monit. J.* **15,** 135–138.

Albertson, T. E., Joy, R. M., and Stark, L. G. (1985). Facilitation of kindling in adult rats following neonatal exposure to lindane. *Dev. Brain Res.* **17,** 263–266.

Albro, P. W., and Thomas, R. (1974). Intestinal absorption of hexachlorobenzene and hexachlorocylohexane isomers in rats. *Bull. Environ. Contam. Toxicol.* **12,** 289–294.

Aldegunde, M., Parafita, M., and Fernandez Otero, M. P. (1983). Effect of γ-hexachlorocyclohexane on serotonin metabolism in rat brain. *Gen. Pharmacol.* **14,** 303–305.

Aldegunde Villar, M., Martin Fargueiro, I., Miguez Besada, I., and Fernandez Otero, M. P. (1981). Study of the mechanism of the hypothermic action of γ-hexachlorocyclohexane. *Acta Cient. Compostelana* **18,** 145–154.

Aldous, C. N., Chetty, C. S., and Desaiah, D. (1983). Alterations in tissue distribution of chlordecone (Kepone) in the rat following phenobarbital or SKF-S25A administration. *J. Toxicol. Environ. Health* **11,** 365–372.

Aldrich, F. D., and Holmes, J. H. (1969). Acute chlordane intoxication in a child. *Arch. Environ. Health* **19,** 129–132.

Aldridge, W. N., Clothier, B., Forshaw, P., Johnson, M. K., Parker, V. H., Price, R. J., Skilleter, D. N., Verschoyle, R. D., and Stevens, C. (1978). The effect of DDT and the pyrethroids cismethrin and decamethrin on the acetyl choline and cyclic nucleotide content of rat brain. *Biochem. Pharmacol.* **27,** 1703–1706.

Alekhina, S. M., and Khaykina, B. I. (1972). The effect of lindane on the activity of the lactate dehydrogenase and on its isoenzymatic spectrum. *Farmakol. Toksikol. (Moscow)* **35**, 734–737 (in Russian).

Aleksandrowicz, D. R. (1979). Endosulfan poisoning and chronic brain syndrome. *Arch. Toxicol.* **43**, 65–68.

Aleksieva, T., Vasilev, G., and Spasovski, M. (1959). Study of the toxic effects of DDT. *J. Hyg., Epidemiol., Microbiol. Immunol.* **5**, 8–15 (in Russian).

Ali, S. F., Hong, J. S., Wilson, W. E., Lamb, J. C., Moore, J. A., Mason, G. A., and Bonely, S. C. (1982). Subchronic dietary exposure of rats to chlordecone (Kepone) modifies levels of hypothalamic β-endorphin. *Neurotoxicology* 3(2), 119–124.

Alix, B., Courtadon, M., Jourde, M., Cassagnes, J., Chone, A. F., and Jallut, H. (1974). Acute benign pericarditis by pesticide inhalation—in relation to two cases. *Coeur Med. Interne* **13**, 165–169 (in French).

Allen, A. L., Koller, L. D., and Pollock, G. A. (1983). Effect of toxaphene exposure on immune responses in mice. *J. Toxicol. Environ. Health* **11**, 61–69.

Al-Omar, M. A., Tawfiq, S. J., and Al-Ogaily, N. (1985). Organochlorine residue levels in human milk from Baghdad. *Bull. Environ. Contam. Toxicol.* **35**, 65–67.

Altmeier, G., Klein, W., and Korte, G. (1969). Contributions to ecological chemistry. XXIV. Metabolism of 14-C-endrin in perfused rat liver. *Tetrahedron Lett.* pp. 4269–4271.

Alvarez, W. C., and Hyman, S. (1953). Absence of toxic manifestations in workers exposed to chlordane. *Arch. Ind. Hyg. Occup. Med.* **8**, 480–483.

American Medical Association (AMA) (1952). American Medical Association Council on Pharmacy and Chemistry report on: Health hazards of electric vaporizing devices for insecticides. *JAMA, J. Am. Med. Assoc.* **149**, 367–369.

American Medical Association (AMA) (1953). American Medical Association Council on Pharmacy and Chemistry report on: Health problems of vaporizing and fumigating devices for insecticides. *JAMA, J. Am. Med. Assoc.* **152**, 1232–1234.

American Medical Association (AMA) (1954). American Medical Association Council on Pharmacy and Chemistry report on: Abuse of insecticide fumigating devices. *JAMA, J. Am. Med. Assoc.* **156**, 607.

American Medical Association (AMA) (1960). American Medical Association Committee on Toxicology report on: Occupational dieldrin poisoning *JAMA, J. Am. Med. Assoc.* **172**, 2077–2080.

American Medical Association (AMA) (1986). "AMA Drug Evaluations," 3rd ed. Publishing Sciences Group, Littleton, Massachusetts.

Ambrose, A. M., Christensen, H. Robbins, D., and Rather, L. (1953). Toxicology and pharmacological studies on chlordane. *Arch. Ind. Hyg. Occup. Med.* **7**, 197–210.

Anagnostopoulos, M. L., Parlar, H., and Korte, F. (1974). Contribution to ecological chemistry LXXI: Isolation, identification and toxicology of some toxaphene components. *Chemosphere* **3**, 65–70 (in German).

Anand, M., Khanna, R. N., Gopal, K., and Gupta, G. S. (1980). Effect of endosulfan on bioelectrical activity of brain in rats. *Vet. Hum. Toxicol.* **22**, 385–387.

Anand, M., Akveld, A. C., and Saxena, P. R. (1981). Effect of a neurotoxic pesticide, endosulfan, on tissue blood flow in cats, including regional cerebral circulation. *Vet. Hum. Toxicol,* **23**, 252–258.

Anand, M., Mehrotra, S., Gopal, K., Sur, R. N., and Chandra, S. V. (1985). Role of neurotransmitter in endosulfan induced aggressive behaviour in normal and lesioned rats. *Toxicol. Lett.* **24**, 79–84.

Anand, M., Gopal, K., Agrawal, C., Chandra, S. V., Ray, P. K., Verma, M., and Shanker, K. (1986). Endosulfan induced inhibition of ^{3}H-S-hydroxytryptamine uptake in platelets. *Toxicol. Lett.* **32**, 203–208.

Andersen, J. R., and Orbaek, K. (1982). Organochlorine contaminants in human milk in Denmark, 1982. *Ambio* **13**, 266–268.

Anderson, B. M., and Noble, C., Jr. (1977). *In vitro* inhibition of lactate dehydrogenase by Kepone. *J. Agric. Food Chem.* **25**, 28–31.

Anderson, B. M., Noble, C., Jr., and Gregory, E. M. (1977). Kepone inhibition of malate dehydrogenases. *J. Agric. Food Chem.* **25**, 485–489.

Anderson, T. W. (1985). DDT: Conclusion. *IARC Sci. Publ.* **65**, 119–121.

Ando, M. (1982). Dose-dependent excretion of DDE (1,1-dichloro-2,2-bis(*p*-chlorophenyl)ethylene) in rats. *Arch. Toxicol.* **49**, 139–147.

Angerer, J., Maass, R., and Heinrich, R. (1983). Occupational exposure to hexachlorocyclohexane. VI. Metabolism of γ-hexachlorocyclohexane in man. *Int. Arch. Occup. Environ. Health* **52**, 59–67.

Angsubhakorn, S., Bhamarapravati, N., Pradesmnong, A., Im-Emgamol, N. and Sahaphong, S. (1989). Minimal dose and time protection by lindane (γ-isomer of 1,2,3,4,5,6-hexachlorocyclohexane) against liver tumors induced by aflatoxin B_1. *Int. J. Cancer,* **43**, 531–534.

Anonymous (1958). Does BHC damage the bone marrow? *Br. Med. J.* **2**, 1522–1523.

Anonymous (1972). BHC and DDT residues in human milk on the decline in Japan. *Noyaku Bijin* **56**, 458 (in Japanese).

Anonymous (1975). Results of survey of pollution of human milk by polychlorobiphenyls and organochlorine pesticides. *Annu. Rep. Kyoto Munic. Inst. Public Health* **41**, 52–53 (in Japanese).

Ansari, R. A., Siddiqui, M. K. J., and Gupta, P. K. (1984). Toxicity of endosulfan: Distribution of α- and β-isomers of racemic endosulfan following oral administration in rats. *Toxicol. Lett.* **21**, 29–33.

Apple, G., Morgan, D. P., and Roan, C. C. (1970). Determinants of serum DDT and DDE concentrations. *Bull. Environ. Contam. Toxicol.* **5**, 16–23.

Aravinda Babu, K., Nigam, S. K., Lakkad, B. C., Bhatt, D. K., Karnik, A. B., Thakora, K. N., Kashyap, S. K., and Chatterjee, S. K. (1981). Effect of hexachlorocyclohexane on somatic and meiotic divisions in mole Swiss mice. *Bull. Environ. Contam. Toxicol.* **26**, 508–512.

Arnold, D. W., Kennedy, G. L., Keplinger, M. L., and Calandra, J. C. (1977). Dominant lethal studies with technical chlordane, HCS-3260, and heptachlor: Heptachlor epoxide. *J. Toxicol. Environ. Health* **2**, 547–555.

Arthur, R. D. (1976). "The Prevalence of and Types of Pesticides in the Air of the Mississippi Delta and the Blood Serum of the General Population of Mississippi," Final Report (E-32) from the Department of Biochemistry, Mississippi State University to the Epidemiological Studies Program, Technical Services Division, U.S. Environ. Prot. Agency, Washington, D.C.

Artigas, F., Martinez, E., Canon, L., and Rodriguez-Farré, E. (1988a). Synthesis and utilization of neurotransmitters: Actions of subconvulsant doses of hexachlorocyclohexane isomers in brain monoamines. *Toxicology* **49**, 49–55.

Artigas, F., Martinez, E., Canon, L., Gelpi, E., and Rodriguez-Farré, E. (1988b). Brain metabolites of lindane and related isomers: Identification by negative ion mass spectrometry. *Toxicology* **49**, 57–63.

Artigas, F., Martinez, E., and Gelpi, E. (1988c). Organochlorine pesticides by negative ion chemical ionization. Brain metabolite of lindane. *Biomed. Mass. Spectrom.* **16**, 279–284.

Askari, E. M., and Gabliks, J. (1973). DDT and immunological responses. II. Altered histamine levels and anaphylactic shock in guinea pigs. *Arch. Environ. Health* **26**, 309–312.

Atallah, Y. H., and Dorough, H. Y. (1975). Insecticide residues in cigarette smoke, transfer and fate in rats. *J. Agric. Food Chem.* **23**, 64–71.

Atrakchi, A. H., and West, T. C. (1985). Positive inotropy, calcium dependence and arrhythmogenicity of lindane in atrial tissue from the guinea pig. *Proc. West. Pharmacol. Soc.* **28**, 65–68.

Attygalle, D. J., and Fernonda, W. D. L. (1959). Accidental poisoning with benzene hexachloride. *Ceylon Med. J.* **5**, 64–65.

Atuma, S. S., and Vaz, R. (1986). A pilot study on levels of organochlorine compounds in human milk in Nigeria. *Int. J. Environ. Anal. Chem.* **26**, 187–192.

Austin, H., Keil, J. E., and Cole, P. (1989). A prospective follow-up study of cancer mortality in relation to serum DDT. *Am. J. Public Health* **79**, 43–46.

Avar, P., and Czegledi-Janko, G. (1970). Occupational exposure to aldrin: Clinical and laboratory findings. *Br. J. Ind. Med.* **27**, 279–282.

Avrahami, M., and Gernert, I. L. (1972). Hexachlorobenzene antagonism to dieldrin storage in adipose tissue. *N. Z. J. Agric. Res.* **15**, 783–787.

Badayeva, L. N., and Kiseleva, N. I. (1976). Morphological changes in nervous structures in the body of mother and fetus during exposure to polychlorocamphene. *Vrach. Delo.* **2**, 109–113 (in Russian).

Baggett, J. McC., Klein, R. L., Mehendale, H. M., and Thureson-Klein, A. K. (1977). Acute Kepone treatment of rats: A biochemical and ultrastructural study. *Pharmacologist* **19**, 199.

Baggett, J. McC., Thureson-Klein, A., and Klein, R. L. (1980). Effects of chlordecone on the adrenal medulla of the rat. *Toxicol. Appl. Pharmacol.* **52,** 313–322.

Baker, M. T., and Van Dyke, R. A. (1984). Metabolism-dependent binding of the chlorinated insecticide DDT and its metabolite DDD to microsomal protein and lipid. *Biochem. Pharmacol.* **33,** 255–260.

Baker, M. T., Nelson, R. M., and Van Dyke, R. A. (1985). The formation of chlorobenzene and benzene by the reductive metabolism of lindane in rat liver microsomes. *Arch. Biochem. Biophys.* **236,** 506–514.

Baker, R. C., Coons, L. B., Mailman, R. B., and Hodgson, E. (1972). Induction of hepatic mixed function oxidases by the insecticide mirex. *Environ. Res.* **5,** 418–424.

Baksheyev, N. S. (1973). Prophylaxis of pathology of the fetus and newborn child (experience of the Ukrainian SSR). *Vestn. Akad. Med. Nauk SSSR* **28,** 69–75 (in Russian).

Bal, H. S. (1984). Effect of methoxychlor on reproductive systems of the rat. *Proc. Soc. Exp. Biol. Med.* **176,** 187–196.

Balba, H. M., and Saha, J. G. (1978). Studies on the distribution, excretion, and metabolism of α- and γ-isomers of ^{14}C chlordane in rabbits. *J. Environ. Sci. Health, Part B* **13,** 211–233.

Baldwin, M. K., and Robinson, J. (1969). Metabolism in the rat of the photoisomerization product of dieldrin. *Nature (London)* **224,** 283–284.

Baldwin, M. K., Robinson, J., and Carrington, R. A. G. (1970a). Metabolism of HEOD (dieldrin) in the rat: Examination of the major fecal metabolite. *Chem. Ind. (London),* pp. 595–597.

Baldwin, M. K., Robinson, J., and Parke, D. V. (1970b). Metabolism of endrin in the rat. *J. Agric. Food Chem.* **18,** 1117–1123.

Baldwin, M. K., Robinson, J., and Parke, D. V. (1972). A comparison of the metabolism of HEOD (dieldrin) in the CF1 mouse with that in the CFE rat. *Food Cosmet. Toxicol.* **10,** 333–351.

Ball, W. W., Kay, K., and Sinclair, J. W. (1953). Observations on toxicity of aldrin. I. Growth and estrus in rats. *Arch. Ind. Hyg. Occup. Med.* **7,** 292–300.

Baluja, G., Hernandez, L. M., Gonzalez, M. J., and Rico, M. C. (1982). Presence of organochlorine pesticides, polychlorinated biphenyls and mercury in Spanish milk samples. *Bull. Environ. Contam. Toxicol.* **28,** 573–577.

Bambov, C., Chomakov, M., and Dimitrova, N. (1966). Group intoxication with lindane. *Suvrem. Med.* **17,** 477–481 (in Russian).

Bandyopadhyay, S. K., Tiwari, R. K., Bhattacharyya, A., and Chatterjee, G. C. (1982). Effect of dieldrin on rat liver plasma membrane enzymes. *Toxicol. Lett.* **11,** 131–134.

Banerjee, B. D., and Hussain, Q. Z. (1986). Effect of sub-chronic endosulfan exposure on humoral and cell-mediated immune responses in albino rats. *Arch. Toxicol.* **59,** 279–284.

Bann, J. M., DeCinco, T. J., Earle, N. W., and Sun, Y. P. (1956). The fate of aldrin and dieldrin in the animal body. *J. Agric. Food Chem.* **4,** 937–941.

Bar-Hay, J., Benderly, A., and Rumney, G. (1964). Treatment of a case of nontumorous Cushing's syndrome with *o,p'*-DDD. *Pediatrics,* **33,** 239–244.

Barkve, H. (1961). Pesticides and a case of Dieldrex poisoning. *Tidsskr. Nor. Laegeforen.* **81,** 759–760 (in Norwegian).

Barnes, J. M., and Heath, D. F. (1964). Some toxic effects of dieldrin in rats. *Br. J. Ind. Med.* **21,** 280–282.

Barnes, R. (1967). Poisoning by the insecticide chlordane. *Med. J. Aust.* **1,** 972–973.

Barnett, J. B., Soderberg, L. S. F., and Menna, J. H. (1985a). The effect of prenatal chlordane exposure on the delayed hypersensitivity response of BALB/c mice. *Toxicol. Lett.* **25,** 173–183.

Barnett, J. B., Holcomb, D., Menna, J. H., and Soderberg, L. S. F. (1985b). The effect of prenatal chlordane exposure on specific anti-influenza cell-mediated immunity. *Toxicol. Lett.* **25,** 227–238.

Barnett, R. W., D'Ercole, A. J., Cain, J. D., and Arthur, R. D. (1979). Organochlorine pesticide residues in human milk samples from women living in northwest and northeast Mississippi, 1973–1975. *Pestic. Monit. J.* **13,** 47–51.

Baron, R. L., and Walton, M. S. (1971). Dynamics of HEOD (dieldrin) in adipose tissue of the rat. *Toxicol. Appl. Pharmacol.* **18,** 958–963.

Barquero, M., and Constenla, M. A. (1986). Organochlorine pesticide residues in human adipose tissue in Costa Rica. *Rev. Biol. Trop.* **34,** 7–12 (in Spanish).

Barquet, A., Morgade, C., and Pfaffenberger, C. D. (1981). Determination of organochlorine pesticides and metabolites in drinking water, human blood serum, and adipose tissue. *J. Toxicol. Environ. Health* **7,** 469–479.

Bass, S. W., Triolo, A. J., and Coon, J. M. (1972). Effect of DDT on the toxicity and metabolism of parathion in mice. *Toxicol. Appl. Pharmacol.* **22,** 684–693.

Batte, E. G., and Turk, R. D. (1948). Toxicity of some synthetic insecticides to dogs. *J. Econ. Entomol.* **41,** 102–103.

Bauer, E., and Reisner, G. (1970). Panmyelophisis after splashing with BHC in Austria. *Monatsschr. Ohrenheilkd. Laryngo-Rhinol.* **104,** 492–495 (in German).

Baum, H., Black, R. F., and Kurtz, C. P. (1976). Dicofol: Collaborative study of the hydrolysable chlorine method. *J. Assoc. Off. Anal. Chem.* **59,** 1109–1112.

Baumann, K., Angerer, J., Heinrich, R., and Lehnert, G. (1980). Occupational exposure to hexachlorocyclohexane. I. Body burdens of HCH-isomers. *Int. Arch. Occup. Environ. Health* **47,** 119–127.

Baumann, K., Behling, K., Brassow, H.-L., and Stapel, K. (1981). Occupational exposure to hexachlorocyclohexane. III. Neurophysiological findings and neuromuscular function in chronically exposed workers. *Int. Arch. Occup. Environ. Health* **48,** 165–172.

Bauza, C. F. (1975). Organochlorine pesticide residues in mothers' milk in Montevideo. *Arch. Pediatr. Urug.* **46,** 31–42.

Bazulic, D., Stampar-Plasaj, B., Bujanovic, V., Stojanovski, N., Nastev, B., Rudelic, I., Sisul, N., and Zuzek, A. (1984). Organochlorine pesticide residues in the serum of mothers and their newborns from three Yugoslav towns. *Bull. Environ. Contam. Toxicol.* **32,** 265–268.

Bedford, C. T., and Hutson, D. H. (1976). The comparative metabolism in rodents of the isomeric insecticides dieldrin and endrin. *Chem. Ind. (London),* pp. 440–447.

Bedford, C. T., Hutson, D. H., and Natoff, I. L. (1975a). The acute toxicity of endrin and its metabolites to rats. *Toxicol. Appl. Pharmacol.* **33,** 115–121.

Bedford, C. T., Harrod, R. K., Hoadley, E. G., and Hutson, D. G. (1975b). The metabolic fate of endrin in the rabbit. *Xenobiotica* **5,** 485–500.

Beemer, A. M., Kuttin, E. S., and Greenfield, S. (1970). An unusual case of dermatitis. *Harefuah* **78,** 112–113 (in Hebrew).

Behrbohm, P., and Brandt, B. (1959). On allergic and toxic skin damage during preparation and processing of hexachlorocyclohexane. *Arch. Gewerbepathol. Gewerbehyg.* **17,** 365–383 (in German).

Bell, A. (1960). Aldrin poisoning: A case report. *Med. J. Aust.* **2,** 698–700.

Bell, A. N., Young, R. A., Lockard, V. G., and Mehendale, H. M. (1988). Protection of chlordecone-potentiated carbon-tetrachloride hepatotoxicity and lethality by partial hepatectomy. *Arch Toxicol.* **61,** 392–405.

Bell, D., and MacLeod, A. F. (1983). Dieldrin pollution of a human food chain. *Hum. Toxicol.* **2,** 75–82.

Bellward, G. D., Dawson, R., and Otten, M. (1975). The effect of dieldrin-contaminated feed on rat hepatic microsomal epoxide hydrase and aryl hydrocarbon hydroxylase. *Res. Commun. Pathol. Pharmacol.* **12,** 669–684.

Ben-Dyke, R., Sanderson, D. M., and Noakes, D. N. (1970). Acute toxicity data for pesticides. *World Rev. Pestic. Control* **9,** 119–127.

Benet, H., Fujimori, K., and Ho, I. K. (1985). The basal ganglia in chlordecone-induced neurotoxicity in the mouse. *Neurotoxicology* **6**(1), 151–158.

Benezet, H. J., and Matsumura, F. (1973). Isomerization of γ-BHC to α-BHC in the environment. *Nature (London)* **243,** 480–481.

Berend, E., Kecskemeti, K., and Koppa, Gy. (1970). The level of chlorinated hydrocarbons in human tissues in Veszprem County. *Egeszsegtudomany* **14,** 388–394 (in Hungarian).

Bergenstal, D. M., Hertz, R., Lipsett, M. B., and Moy, R. H. (1960). Chemotherapy of adrenocortical cancer with *o,p'*-DDD. *Ann. Intern. Med.* **53,** 672–682.

Bergman, K., Brandt, I., Appelgren, L. E., and Slamna, P. (1981). Structure-dependent, selective localization of chlorinated xenobiotics in the cerebellum and other brain structures. *Experientia* **37,** 1184–1185.

Bernardelli, B. C., and Gennari, M. C. (1987). Death caused by ingestion of endosulfan. *J. Forensic Sci.* **32,** 1109–1112.

Best, W. R. (1963). Drug-associated blood dyscrasias. *JAMA, J. Am. Med. Assoc.* **185,** 286–290.

Bezuglyi, V. P., and Kaskevich, L. M. (1969). Some indices of the functional state of the liver in flying personnel engaged in aerial chemical operations. *Gig. Tr. Prof. Zabol.* **13,** 52–53 (in Russian).

Bezuglyi, V. P., and Mukhtarova, N. D. (1969). The clinical aspects of acute polychloropinene poisoning. *Gig. Tr. Prof. Zabol.* **13,** 53–55 (in Russian).

Bezuglyi, V. P., Odintsova, I. L., and Gorskaya, N. Z. (1973). Morphological composition of the blood in persons working with a complex of organochlorine and organophosphorus pesticides. *Vrach. Delo* **11,** 134–138.

Bhaskaran, M., Sharma, R. C., and Bhide, N. K. (1979). DDT levels in human fat samples in Delhi area. *Indian J. Exp. Biol.* **17,** 1390–1392.

Bhatia, S. C., and Venkitasubramanian, T. A. (1972). Mechanism of dieldrin-induced fat accumulation in rat liver. *J. Agric. Food Chem.* **20,** 993–996.

Bhatt, D. K., Nigam, S. K., Aravinda-Babu, K., Lakkad, B. C., Kamik, A. B., Thakore, K. N., Kashyap, S. K., and Chatterjee, S. K. (1981). Histochemical changes in ATPase distribution during hexachlorocyclohexane induced hepatocarcinogenesis in inbred Swiss mice. *Indian J. Exp. Biol.* **19,** 621–624.

Bick, M. (1967). Chlorinated hydrocarbon residues in human body fat. *Med. J. Aust.* **1,** 127–129.

Bickel, M. H. (1984). The role of adipose tissue in the distribution and storage of drugs. *Prog. Drug Res.* **28,** 273–303.

Bidwell, K., Weber, E., Nienhold, I., Connor, T., and Legator, M. S. (1975). Comprehensive evaluation for mutagenic activity of dieldrin. *Mutat. Res.* **31,** 314.

Biros, F. J., and Enos, H. F. (1973). Oxychlordane residues in human adipose tissues. *Bull. Environ. Contam. Toxicol.* **10,** 257–260.

Bishara, R. H., Born, G. S., and Christian, J. E. (1972). Radiotracer distribution and excretion study of chlorophenothane in rats. *J. Pharm. Sci.* **61,** 1912–1916.

Biskind, M. S. (1952). The new insecticides and the public health. *Harefuah* **44,** 9–13 (in Hebrew).

Biskind, M. S. (1953). Public health aspects of the new insecticides. *Am. J. Dig. Dis.* **20,** 331–341.

Biskind, M. S., and Bieber, I. (1949). DDT poisoning—a new syndrome with neuro-psychiatric manifestations. *Am. J. Psychother.* **3,** 261–270.

Bjerk, J. E. (1972). DDT and polychlorinated biphenyl residues in human material in Norway. *Tidsskr. Nor. Laegeforen.* **92,** 15–19 (in Norwegian).

Black, A. M. S. (1974). Self poisoning with dieldrin: A case report and pharmacokinetic discussion. *Anaesthesiol. Intens. Care* **2,** 369–374.

Blanke, R. V., Fariss, M. W., Guzelian, P. S., Patterson, A. R., and Smith, D. E. (1978). Identification of a reduced form of chlordecone (Kepone) in human stool. *Bull. Environ. Contam. Toxicol.* **20,** 782–785.

Blazquez, J., and Bianchini, C. (1956). Chronic occupational intoxication by dieldrin in man. *Gac. Med. Caracas* **63,** 1–39 (in Spanish).

Blazquez, J., and Bianchini, C. (1957). Study of the first cases of intoxication by dieldrin and application of xenoanalysis in people. *Bol. Of. Sanit. Panam.* **43,** 504–511 (in Spanish).

Bledsoe, T., Roland, D. P., Hey, R. L., and Liddle, G. W. (1964). An effect of *o,p'*-DDD on extra-adrenal metabolism of cortisol in man. *J. Clin. Endocrinol. Metab.* **24,** 1303–1311.

Bleiberg, M. J., and Larson, P. S. (1957). Studies on the adrenocortical effects and metabolism of 2,2 bis-(*p*-ethylphenyl)-1,1-dichloroethane (Perthane). *J. Pharmacol. Exp. Ther.* **119,** 133–134.

Blekherman, N. A., and Il'yina, V. I. (1972). Some ovarian and adrenal cortex hormonal function indexes in women working with organochlorine pesticides. *Fiziol. Zh (Kiev, 1955–1977)* **18,** 268–270 (in Ukrainian).

Blend, M. J., and Lehnert, B. E. (1973). Luteinizing hormone serum levels and body weight/organ weight ratios in male rats fed low levels of dieldrin. *Ind. Med.* **42,** 18.

Blisard, K. S., Kornfeld, M., McFeeley, P., and Smialek, J. E. (1986). The investigation of alleged insecticide toxicity: A case involving chlordane exposure, multiple sclerosis and peripheral neuropathy. *J. Forensic Sci.* **31,** 1499–1504.

Bloomer, A. W., Nash, S. I., Price, H. A., and Welch, R. L. (1977). A study of pesticide residues in Michigan's general population. *Pestic. Monit. J.* **11,** 111–115.

Bloomquist, J. R., and Soderlund, D. M. (1985). Neurotoxic insecticides inhibit GABA-dependent chloride uptake by mouse brain vesicles. *Biochem. Biophys. Res. Commun.* **133,** 37–43.

Bloomquist, J. R., Adams, P. M., and Soderlund, D. M. (1986). Inhibition of γ-aminobutyric acid stimulated chloride flux in mouse brain vesicles by polychlorocycloalkane and pyrethroid insecticides. *Neurotoxicology* **7**(3), 11–120.

Bochkovskii, F. R., and Riabov, V. G. (1970). Polychloropinene poisoning. *Sud.-Med. Ekspert.* **13,** 48–49 (in Russian).

Bochner, F., Lloyd, H. M., Roeser, H. P., and Thomas, M. J. (1969). Effects of *o,p'*-DDD and aminoglutethimide on metastatic adrenocortical carcinoma. *Med. J. Aust.* **1,** 809–812.

Bogusz, M. (1968). Influence of insecticides on the activity of some enzymes contained in human serum. *Clin. Chim. Acta* **19,** 367–369.

Boiko, V. G., and Krasnyuk, E. P. (1969). Clinical characteristics of the pathology of respiratory tracts of persons working with DDT. *Zh. Ushn., Nos. Gorl. Bolezn.* **29,** 35–38 (in Russian).

Bojanowska, A., Jonczyk, H., Rudowski, W., Traczyk, Z., and Klawe, Z. (1973). DDT and α-BHC content in blood and fatty tissue of subjects not professionally exposed to these compounds. *Pol. Tyg. Lek.* **28**(51), 1999–2001 (in Polish).

Bonderman, D. P., Mick, D. L., and Long, K. R. (1971). Occupational exposure to aldrin, 2,4-D and 2,4,5-T and its relationship to sterases. *Ind. Med. Surg.* **40,** 23–27.

Bondy, S. C., and Halsall, L. (1988). Lindane-induced modulation of calcium levels with synaptosomes. *Neurotoxicology* **9,** 645–652.

Boucard, M., Beaulaton, I. S., Mestres, R., and Allieu, M. (1970). Experimental study of teratogenesis: Influence of the period and duration of treatment. *Therapie* **25,** 907–913 (in French).

Bowerman, J. G., Gomez, M. P., Austin, R. D., and Wold, D. E. (1987). Comparative study of permethrin 1% creme rinse and lindane shampoo for the treatment of head lice. *Pediatr. Infect. Dis. J.* **6,** 252–255.

Boyd, E. M., and Chen, C. P. (1968). Lindane toxicity and protein-deficient diet. *Arch. Environ. Health* **17,** 156–163.

Boyd, E. M., and Dobos, I. (1969). Protein deficiency and tolerated oral doses of endosulfan. *Arch. Int. Pharmacodyn. Ther.* **178,** 152–165.

Boyd, E. M., and Stefec, J. (1969). Dietary protein and pesticide toxicity, with particular reference to endrin. *Can. Med. Assoc. J.* **101,** 335–339.

Boyd, E. M., and Taylor, F. I. (1971). Toxaphene toxicity in protein-deficient rats. *Toxicol. Appl. Pharmacol.* **18,** 158–167.

Boyd, E. M., Chen, C. P., and Krijen, C. J. (1969). Lindane and dietary protein. *Pharmacol. Res. Commun.* **1,** 403–412.

Boyd, E. M., Dobos, I., and Krijnen, C. J. (1970). Endosulfan toxicity and dietary protein. *Arch. Environ. Health* **21,** 15–19.

Boylan, J. J., Egle, J. L., and Guzelian, P. S. (1978). Cholestyramine: Use as a new therapeutic approach for chlordecone (Kepone) poisoning. *Science* **199,** 893–895.

Boylan, J. J., Cohn, W. J., Egle, J. L., Blanke, R. V., and Guzelian, P. S. (1979). Excretion of chlordecone by the gastrointestinal tract: Evidence for a nonbiliary mechanism. *Clin. Pharmacol. Ther.* **25,** 579–585.

Brade, W. P., Chiu, J. F., and Hnilica, L. S. (1974). Phosphorylation of rat liver nuclear acidic phosphoproteins after administration of α-1,2,3,4,5,6-hexachlorocyclohexane *in vivo*. *Mol. Pharmacol.* **10,** 398–405.

Bradlow, H. L., Fukushima, D. K., Zumoff, B., Hellman, L., and Gallagher, T. F. (1963). A peripheral action of *o,p'*-DDD on steroid biotransformation. *J. Clin. Endocrinol. Metab.* **23,** 918–922.

Bradt, P. T., and Herrenkohl, R. C. (1976). DDT in human milk: What determines the levels? *Sci. Total Environ.* **6,** 161–163.

Brady, M. N., and Siyali, D. S. (1972). Hexachlorobenzene in human fat. *Med. J. Aust.* **1,** 158–161.

Brandt, I., and Hogman, P. (1980). Selective binding of aldrin and dieldrin in cartilage. *Arch. Toxicol.* **45,** 223–226.

Brassow, H.-L., Baumann, K., and Lehnert, G. (1981). Occupational exposure to hexachlorocyclohexane. II. Health conditions of chronically exposed workers. *Int. Arch. Occup. Environ. Health* **48,** 81–87.

Bratowski, T. A., and Matsumura, F. (1972). Properties of a brain adenosine triphosphatase sensitive to DDT. *J. Econ. Entomol.* **65,** 1238–1245.

Braund, D. G., Langlois, B. E., Conner, D. J., and Moore, E. E. (1971). Feeding phenobarbital and activated carbon to accelerate dieldrin residue removal in a contaminated herd. *J. Dairy Sci.* **54,** 435–438.

Brevik, E. M., and Bjerk, J. E. (1978). Organochlorine compounds in Norwegian human fat and milk. *Acta Pharmacol. Toxicol.* **43,** 59–63.

Brewton, H. V., and McGrath, H. J. W. (1967). Insecticides in human fat in New Zealand. *N. Z. J. Sci.* **10,** 486–492.

Bricaire, H., and Luton, J. P. (1977). Does *o',p*-DDD possess antimitotic action? Reflections on its use in the treatment of suprarenal adenocarcinomas. *Nouv. Presse Med.* **6,** 3650 (in French).

Brimfield, A. A., and Street, J. C. (1979). Mammalian biotransformation of chlordane: *In vivo* and primary hepatic comparisons. *Ann. N. Y. Acad. Sci.* **320,** 247–256.

Brimfield, A. A., and Street, J. C. (1981). Microsomal activation of chlordane isomers to derivatives that irreversibly interact with cellular macromolecules. *J. Toxicol. Environ. Health* **7,** 193–206.

Brittebo, E. G., Hogman, P. G., and Brandt, I. (1987). Epithelial binding of hexachlorocyclohexanes in the respiratory and upper alimentary tracts: A comparison between α-, β-, and γ-isomers in mice. *Food Chem. Toxicol.* **25,** 773–780.

Bronisz, H., and Ochynski, J. (1968). DDT and DDE in human milk (in Polish).

Bronisz, H., Rusiecki, W., Ochynaski, J., and Bernhard, E. (1967). DDT in adipose tissue of Polish population. *Diss. Pharm. Pharmacol.* **19,** 309–314.

Brooks, G. T. (1973). The design of insecticidal chlorohydrocarbon derivatives. *In* "Drug Design" (E. J. Ariëns, ed.), Vol. 4. Academic Press, New York.

Brooks, G. T., and Harrison, A. (1969). Hydration of HEOD (dieldrin) and heptachlor epoxides by microsomes from the livers of pigs and rabbits. *Bull. Environ. Contam. Toxicol.* **4,** 352–361.

Brooks, G. T., Harrison, A., and Lewis, S. E. (1970). Cyclodiene epoxide ring hydration by microsomes from mammalian liver and houseflies. *Biochem. Pharmacol.* **19,** 255–273.

Brown, J. R. (1967). Organo-chlorine pesticides residues in human depot fat. *Can. Med. Assoc. J.* **97,** 367–373.

Brown, J. R. (1972). The effect of dietary kelthane on mouse and rat reproduction. *Pestic. Chem., Proc. Int. IUPAC Congr. Pestic. Chem., 2nd, 1971,* Vol. 6, pp. 531–548.

Brown, J. R., and Chow, L. Y. (1975). Comparative study of DDT and its derivatives in human blood samples in Norfolk County and Holland Marsh, Ontario. *Bull. Environ. Contam. Toxicol.* **13**(4), 483–488.

Brown, J. R., Hughes, H., and Viriyanondha, S. (1969). Storage, distribution and metabolism of 1,1-bis(4-chlorophenyl)-2,2,2-trichloroethanol. *Toxicol. Appl. Pharmacol.* **15,** 30–37.

Brown, L. D., Wilson, D. E., and Yarbrough, J. D. (1988). Alterations in the hepatic glycocorticoid response to mirex treatment. *Toxicol. Appl. Pharmacol.* **92,** 203–213.

Brown, M. A., and Casida, J. E. (1987). Metabolism of a dicofol impurity α-chloro-DDT, but not dicofol or dechlorodicofol, to DDE in mice and a liver microsomal system. *Xenobiotica* **17,** 1169–1174.

Brown, V. K. H., Chambers, P. L., Hunter, C. G., and Stevenson, D. E. (1962). "The Toxicity of Telodrin for Vertebrates," Tunstall Lab. Rep. R(T)-2-62 (cited by Jager, 1970).

Brown, V. K. H., Hunter, C. G., and Richardson, A. (1964). A blood test diagnostic of exposure to aldrin and dieldrin. *Br. J. Ind. Med.* **21,** 283–286.

Brown, V. K. H., Robinson, J., and Thorpe, E. (1974). The toxicity of dieldrin (HEOD) to domestic fowl. *Pestic. Sci.* **5,** 567–586.

Bruevich, T. S. (1964). Occupational dermatoses of disinfector operators provoked by hexachlorane. *Gig. Tr. Prof. Zabol.* **8,** 28–32.

Buck, R. A., and Pfannenmueller, L. (1957). Intoxications with hexachlorocyclohexane. *Arch. Toxicol.* **16,** 328–335.

Bulger, W. H., and Kupfer, D. (1977). The *in vivo* and *in vitro* estrogenic activity of methoxychlor and its bis-phenolic analog 2,2bis(BPHT) in the rat. *Pharmacologist* **19,** 199.

Bulger, W. H., Muccitelli, R. M., and Kupfer, D. (1978a). Studies on the *in vivo* and *in vitro* estrogenic activities of methoxychlor and its metabolites. Role of hepatic mono-oxygenase in methoxychlor activation. *Biochem. Pharmacol.* **27,** 2417–2423.

Bulger, W. H., Muccitelli, R. M., and Kupfer, D. (1978b). Interactions of methoxychlor, methoxychlor base-soluble contaminant, and 2,2-bis(*p*-hydroxyphenyl)-1,1,1-trichloroethane with rat uterine estrogen receptor. *J. Toxicol. Environ. Health* **4,** 881–893.

Bulger, W. H., Muccitelli, R. M., and Kupfer, D. (1979). Studies on the estrogenic activity of chlordecone (Kepone) in the rat: Effects on uterine receptor. *Mol. Pharmacol.* **15,** 515–524.

Bulger, W. H., Temple, J. E., and Kupfer, D. (1983). Covalent binding of [^{14}C]methoxychlor metabolite(s) to rat liver microsomal components. *Toxicol. Appl. Pharmacol.* **63,** 367–374.

Bulger, W. H., Feil, V., and Kupfer, D. (1985). Role of hepatic monooxygenases in generating estrogenic metabolites from methoxychlor and from identified contaminants. *Mol. Pharmacol.* **27,** 115–124.

Bunch, T. D., and Low, J. B. (1973). Effects of dieldrin on chromosomes of semi-domestic mallard ducks. *J. Wildl. Manage.* **37,** 51–57.

Bungay, P. M., Dedrick, R. C., and Mathews, H. B. (1981). Enteric transport of chlordecone (Kepone) in the rat. *J. Pharmacokinet. Biopharm.* **9,** 309–341.

Bunyan, P. J., Townshend, M. G., and Taylor, A. (1972). Pesticide induced changes in hepatic microsomal enzyme systems: Some effects of 1,1-di(*p*-chlorophenyl)-2,2,2-trichloroethane (DDT) and 1,1-di(*P*-chlorophenyl)-2,2-dichloroethylene (DDE) in the rat and Japanese quail. *Chem.-Biol. Interact.* **5,** 13–26.

Burchfield, J. L., Duffy, F. H., and Sim, V. M. (1976). Persistent effects of sarin and dieldrin upon the primate electroencephalogram. *Toxicol. Appl. Pharmacol,* **35,** 365–379.

Burkatzkaya, E. N. (1963). The effect of hexachlorocyclohexane γ-isomer on the immunobiological reactivity of the body. *Gig. Sanit.* **28,** 29–33 (in Russian).

Burkatzkaya, E. N., Ivanova, E. V., and Krasniuk, E. P. (1959). Working hygiene and the state of health of workers producing insecticides containing BHC. *Gig. Sanit.* **24,** 17–22 (in Russian).

Burkatzkaya, E. N., Voitenko, G. A., and Krasniuk, E. P. (1961). Working conditions and health status of workers at DDT production plants. *Gig. Sanit.* **26,** 24–29 (in Russian).

Burlington, H., and Linderman, V. F. (1950). Effect of DDT on testes and secondary sex characteristics of White Leghorn cockerels. *Proc. Soc. Exp. Biol. Med.* **74,** 48–51.

Burns, E. C., Dahm, P. A., and Lindquist, D. A. (1957). Secretion of DDT metabolites in the bile of rats. *J. Pharmacol. Exp. Ther.* **121,** 55–62.

Burns, J. E. (1974). Organochlorine pesticide and polychlorinated biphenyl residues in biopsied human adipose tissue—Texas 1969–72. *Pestic. Monit. J.* **7,** 122–126.

Bursch, W., and Schulte-Hermann, R. (1983). Synchronization of hepatic DNA synthesis by scheduled feeding and lighting in mice treated with the chemical inducer of liver growth α-hexachlorocyclohexane. *Cell Tissue Kinet.* **16,** 125–134.

Buselmaier, W., Röhrborn, G., and Propping, P. (1973). Comparative investigations on the mutagenicity of pesticides in mammalian test systems. *Mutat. Res.* **21,** 25–26.

Byard, J. L., and Pittman, K. A. (1975). Early liver changes produced by mirex and their reversibility. *Toxicol. Appl. Pharmacol.* **33,** 130.

Byard, J. L., Koepke, U. C., Abraham, R., Goldberg, L., and Coulston, F. (1974). Biochemical changes produced in the liver by mirex. *Toxicol. Appl. Pharmacol.* **29,** 126–127.

Byard, J. L., Koepke, U. C., Abraham, R., Goldberg, L., and Coulston, F. (1975). Biochemical changes in the liver of mice fed mirex. *Toxicol. Appl. Pharmacol.* **33,** 70–77.

Byrd, R. A., Young, J. F., Kimmel, C. A., Morris, M. D., and Holson, J. F. (1982). Computer simulation of mirex pharmacokinetics in the rat. *Toxicol. Appl. Pharmacol.* **66,** 182–192.

Cabral, J. R. P. (1985). DDT: Laboratory evidence. *IARC Sci. Publ.* **65,** 101–105.

Cabral, J. R. P., Testa, M. C., and Terracini, B. (1972). Lack of long-term effects from heptachlor administration to suckling rats. *Tumori* **58**, 49–53.

Cabral, J. R. P., Raitano, F., Mollner, T., Bronczyk, S., and Shubik, P. (1979a). Acute toxicity of pesticides in hamsters. *Toxicol. Appl. Pharmacol.* **48**, A192.

Cabral, J. R. P., Hall, R. K., Bronczyk, S. A., and Shubik, P. (1979b). A carcinogenicity study of the pesticide dieldrin in hamsters. *Cancer Lett.* **6**, 241–246.

Cabral, J. R. P., Hall, R. K., Rossi, L., Bronczyk, S. A., and Shubik, P. (1982a). Lack of carcinogenicity of DDT in hamsters. *Tumori* **68**, 5–10.

Cabral, J. R. P., Hall, R. K., Rossi, L., Bronczyk, S. A., and Shubik, P. (1982b). Effects of long-term intake of DDT in rats. *Tumori* **68**, 11–17.

Cameron, G. R. (1945). Risks to man and animals from the use of 2,2-bis(*p*-chlorophenyl)-1,1,1-trichlorethane (DDT): With a note on the toxicity of γ-benzene hexachloride (666, Gammexane). *Br. Med. Bull.* **3**, 233–235.

Cameron, G. R., and Burgess, F. (1945). The toxicity of 2,2-bis(*p*-chlorophenyl)-1,1,1-trichloroethane (DDT). *Br. Med. J.* **1**, 865–871.

Camon, L., Sola, C., Martinez, E., Sanfeliu, C., and Rodriguez-Farré, E. (1988a). Cerebral glucose uptake in lindane-treated rats. *Toxicology*, **49**, 381–387.

Camon, L., Martinez, E., Artigas, F., Sola, C., and Rodriguez-Farré, E. (1988b). The effect of nonconvulsant doses of lindane on temperature and body weight. *Toxicology*, **49**, 389–394.

Campos, H. A., and Jurupe, H. (1970a). A histamine-dependent increase of 5-hydroxytryptamine in the rat brain *in vivo. Experientia,* **26**, 613–614.

Canada (1962). "Chlordane Poisoning. Information Release to Poison Control Centers," Release No. 2. Reprinted in: "World Health Organization Information Circular on Toxicity of Pesticides to Man," No. 11, p. 10. World Health Organ., Geneva, 1963.

Canlorbe, P., Bader, J. C., and Job, J. C. (1971). Diagnostic problems arising from a virilizing tumor of the adrenal cortex. (Case report—literature review.) *Sem. Hop.* **47**, 2255–2270 (in French).

Cannon, A. B., and McRae, M. R. (1948). Treatment of scabies. *JAMA, J. Am. Med. Assoc.* **138**, 557–560.

Cannon, S. B., and Kimbrough, R. D. (1979). Short-term chlordecone toxicity in rat including effects on reproduction, pathological organ changes and their reversibility. *Toxicol. Appl. Pharmacol.* **47**, 469–476.

Cannon, S. B., Veazey, J. M., Jackson, R. S., Burse, V. W., Hayes, C., Straub, W. E., Landrigan, P. J., and Liddle, J. A. (1978). Epidemic Kepone poisoning in chemical workers. *Am. J. Epidemiol.* **107**, 529–537.

Carey, R. M., Orth, D. N., and Hartmann, W. H. (1973). Malignant melanoma with ectopic production of adrenocorticotrophic hormone: Palliative treatment with inhibitors of adrenal steroid biosynthesis. *J. Clin. Endocrinol. Metab.* **36**, 482–487.

Carlson, D. A., Konyha, K. D., Wheeler, W. B., Marshall, G. P., and Zaylshie, R. G. (1976). Mirex in the environment: Its degradation to Kepone and related compounds. *Science* **194**, 939–941.

Carlson, J., and Abraham, R. (1985). Nuclear ploidy of neonatal rat livers: Effects of two hepatic carcinogens (mirex and diethylnitrosamine). *J. Toxicol. Environ. Health* **15**, 551–559.

Carlson, J. N., and Rosellini, R. A. (1987). Exposure to low doses of the environmental chemical dieldrin causes behavioural deficit in animals prevented from coping with stress. *Psychopharmacology* **91**, 122–126.

Carlson, L. A., and Kolomodin-Hedman, B. (1977). Decrease in α-lipoprotein cholesterol in men after cessation of exposure to chlorinate hydrocarbon pesticides. *Acta Med. Scand.* **201**, 375–376.

Carmines, E. L., Carchman, R. A., and Borzelleca, J. F. (1979). Kepone: Cellular sites of action. *Toxicol. Appl. Pharmacol.* **49**, 543–550.

Carrero, I., Fernandez-Moreno, M. D., Pérez-Albarsanz, M. A., and Prieto, J. C. (1989). Lindane effect upon the vasoactive intestinal peptide receptor/effector system in rat enterocytes. *Biochem. Biophys. Res. Commun.* **159**, 1391–1396.

Carrillo, S. J. (1954). The use of dieldrin in Venezuela. *Bol. Of. Sanit. Panam.* **37**, 76–81 (in Spanish).

Casarett, L. J., Fryer, G. C., Yauger, W. L., and Klemmer, H. W. (1968). Organochlorine pesticide residues in human tissue—Hawaii. *Arch. Environ. Health* **17**, 306–311.

Case, R. A. M. (1945). Toxic effects of 2,2-bis(*p*-chlorophenyl)-1,1,1-trichlorethane (DDT) in man. *Br. Med. J.* **2**, 842–845.

Casida, J. E., and Lawrence, L. J. (1985). Structure–activity correlations for interactions of bicyclophosphorus esters and some polychlorocycloalkane and pyrethroid insecticides with brain-specific *t*-butylbicyclophosphorothionate receptor. *Environ. Health Perspect.* **61**, 123–132.

Casida, J. E., Holmstead, R. L., Khalifa, S., Knox, J. R., Ohsawa, T., Palmer, K. J., and Wong, R. Y. (1974). Toxaphene insecticide: A complex biodegradable mixture. *Science* **183**. 520–521.

Cassidy, W., Fisher, A. J., Peden, J. D., and Parry-Jones, A. (1967). Organochlorine pesticide residues in human fats from Somerset. *Mon. Bull. Minist. Health Public Health Lab. Serv. (G.B.)* **26**, 2–6.

Cattabeni, F., Pastorello, M. C., and Eli, M. (1983). Convulsions induced by lindane and the involvement of the GABAergic system. *Arch. Toxicol., Suppl.* **6**, 244–249.

Cecil, H. C., Harris, S. J., Bitman, J., and Reynolds, P. (1975). Estrogenic effects and liver microsomal enzyme activity of technical methoxychlor and technical 1,1-trichloro-2,2-bis(*p*-chlorophenyl)ethane in sheep. *J. Agric. Food Chem.* **23**, 401–403.

Cerey, K., Izakovic, V., and Ruttkay-Nedecka, J. (1973). Effect of heptachlor on dominant lethality and bone marrow in rats. *Mutat. Res.* **21**, 26.

Chadwick, R. W., and Copeland, M. F. (1985). Investigation of HCB as a metabolite from female rats treated daily for 6 days with lindane. *J. Anal. Toxicol.* **9**, 262–266.

Chadwick, R. W., and Freal, J. J. (1972a). The identification of five unreported lindane metabolites recovered from rat urine. *Bull. Environ. Contam. Toxicol.* **7**, 137–146.

Chadwick, R. W., and Freal, J. J. (1972b). Comparative acceleration of lindane metabolism to chlorophenols by pretreatment of rats with lindane or with DDT and lindane. *Food Cosmet. Toxicol.* **10**, 789–795.

Chadwick, R. W., Cranmer, F. L., and Peoples, A. J. (1971a). Comparative stimulation of γ-HCH metabolism by pretreatment of rats with γ-HCH, DDT, and DDT + γ-HCH. *Toxicol. Appl. Pharmacol.* **18**, 685–695.

Chadwick, R. W., Cranmer, M. F., and Peoples, A. J. (1971b). Metabolic alterations in the squirrel monkey induced by DDT administration and ascorbic acid deficiency. *Toxicol. Appl. Pharmacol.* **20**, 308–318.

Chadwick, R. W., Peoples, A. J., and Cranmer, M. F. (1972). The effect of ascorbic acid deficiency and protein quality on stimulation of hepatic microsomal enzymes in guinea pigs. *Toxicol. Appl. Pharmacol.* **22**, 308–309.

Chadwick, R. W., Linko, R. S., Freal, J. J., and Robbins, A. L. (1975). The effect of age and long-term low-level DDT exposure on the response to enzyme induction in the rat. *Toxicol. Appl. Pharmacol.* **31**, 469–480.

Chadwick, R. W., Freal, J. J., Sovocool, G. W., Bryden, C. C., and Copeland, M. F. (1978a). The identification of three previously unreported lindane metabolites from mammals. *Chemosphere* **7**, 633–640.

Chadwick, R. W., Copeland, M. F., and Chadwick, C. J. (1978b). Enhanced pesticide metabolism, a previously unreported effect of dietary fibre in mammals. *Food Cosmet. Toxicol.* **16**, 217–225.

Chadwick, R. W., Copeland, M. F., Mole, M. L., Nesnow, S., and Cook, N. (1981). Comparative effect of pretreatment with phenobarbital, Aroclor 1254 and β-naphthoflavone on the metabolism of lindane. *Pestic. Biochem. Physiol.* **15**, 120–136.

Chadwick, R. W., Chuong, L. T., and Williams, K. (1985). Dehydrogenation: A previously unreported pathway of lindane metabolism in mammals. *Pestic. Biochem. Physiol.* **5**, 575–586.

Chadwick, R. W., Copeland, M. F., Wolff, G. L., Cook, N., Whitehouse, D. A., and Mole, M. L. (1986). Effects of age and obesity on the metabolism of lindane by black *a/a*, yellow A^{vy}/*a* and pseudoagouti A^{vy}/*a* phenotypes of (YS × VY)F$_1$ hybrid mice. *J. Toxicol. Environ. Health* **16**, 771–796.

Chadwick, R. W., Copeland, M. F., Wolff, G. L., Stead, A. G., Mole, M. L., and Whitehouse, D. A. (1987). Saturation of lindane metabolism in chronically treated (YS × VY)F$_1$ hybrid mice. *J. Toxicol. Environ. Health* **20**, 411–434.

Chakravarti, H. S. (1965). Polyneuritis due to DDT. *J. Indian Med. Assoc.* **45**, 598–599.

Chamberlain, J. (1971). The determination of urinary 6-oxygenated cortisol in evaluating liver function. *Clin. Chim. Acta* **34**, 269–271.

Chambers, J. E., and Trevanthan, C. A. (1983). Effect of mirex, dechlorinated mirex derivatives and chlordecone on microsomal mixed-function oxidase activity and other hepatic parameters. *Toxicol. Lett.* **16**, 109–115.

Chambers, J. E., and Yarbrough, J. D. (1979). Disposition and excretion of mirex, 2,8-dihydromirex and 5,10-dihydromirex by adult rats. *Fed. Proc., Fed. Am. Soc. Exp. Biol.* **38**, 266.

Chambers, J. E., Case, R. S., Alley, E. G., and Yarbrough, J. D. (1982). Short-term fate of mirex and 2,8-dihydromirex in rats. *J. Agric. Food Chem.* **30**, 378–382.

Chambers, P. L. (1982). A possible site of action of dieldrin in the brain. *Arch. Toxicol. Suppl.* **5**, 112–115.

Chandar, N., and Nagarajan, B. (1984). Induction of γ-glutamyltranspeptidase by hexachlorocyclohexane. *Biochem. Int.* **8**, 41–48.

Chandurkar, P. S., and Matsumura, F. (1979). Metabolism of toxaphene components in rats. *Arch. Environ. Contam. Toxicol.* **8**, 1–24.

Charles, A. K., Rosenbaum, D. P., Ashok, L., and Abraham, R. (1985). Uptake and disposition of mirex in hepatocytes and subcellular fractions in CD1 mouse liver. *J. Toxicol. Environ. Health* **15**, 395–403.

Chase, H. P., Barnett, S. E., Welch, N. N., Briese, F. W., and Krassner, M. L. (1973). Pesticides and US farm labor families. *Rocky Mt. Med. J.* **70**, 27–31.

Chen, P. H., Tilson, H. A., Marbury, G. D., Karoum, F., and Hong, J. J. (1985). Effect of chlordecone (Kepone) on the rat brain concentrations of 3-methoxy-4-hydroxyphenylglycol: Evidence for a possible involvement of the norepinephrine system in chlordecone-induced tremor. *Toxicol. Appl. Pharmacol.* **77**, 158–164.

Chernoff, N., and Carver, B. D. (1976). Fetal toxicity of toxaphene in rats and mice. *Bull. Environ. Contam. Toxicol.* **15**, 660–664.

Chernoff, N., and Rogers, E. H. (1976). Fetal toxicity of Kepone in rats and mice. *Toxicol. Appl. Pharmacol.* **38**, 189–194.

Chernoff, N., Kavlock, R. J., Kathrein, J. R., Dunn, J. M., and Haseman, J. K. (1975). Prenatal effects of dieldrin and photodieldrin in mice and rats. *Toxicol. Appl. Pharmacol.* **31**, 302–308.

Chernoff, N., Kavlock, R. J., Hanisch, R. C., Whitehouse, D. A., Gray, J. A., Gray, L. E., and Sovocool, G. W. (1979a). Perinatal toxicity of endrin in rodents. I. Fetotoxic effects of prenatal exposure in hamsters. *Toxicology* **13**, 155–165.

Chernoff, N., Linder, R. E., Scott, T. M., Rogers, E. H., Carver, B. D., and Kavlock, R. J. (1979b). Fetotoxicity and cataractogenicity of mirex in rats and mice with notes on Kepone. *Environ. Res.* **18**, 257–269.

Chhabra, R. S., and Fouts, J. R. (1974). Stimulation of hepatic drug metabolizing enzymes by DDT, polycyclic hydrocarbons or phenobarbital in adrenalectomized or castrated mice. *Toxicol. Appl. Pharmacol.* **28**, 465–476.

Chin, Y., and T'Ant, C. (1946). The effect of DDT on cutaneous sensation in man. *Science* **103**, 654.

Chipman, J. K., and Walker, C. H. (1979). The metabolism of dieldrin and two of its analogues. The relationship between rates of microsomal metabolism and rates of excretion of metabolites in the male rat. *Biochem. Pharmacol.* **28**, 1337–1345.

Chowdhury, A. R., Venkatakrishna-Bhatt, H., and Gautam, A. K. (1987). Testicular changes of rats under lindane treatment. *Bull. Environ. Contam. Toxicol.* **38**, 154–156.

Christophers, A. J. (1969). Hematological effects of pesticides. *Ann. N.Y. Acad. Sci.* **160**, 352–355.

Chu, I., Villeneuve, D. C., Secours, V., Becking, G. C., Viau, A., and Benoit, F. (1979). The absorption, distribution and excretion of photomirex in the rat. *Drug. Metab. Dispos.* **7**, 24–27.

Chu, I., Villeneuve, D. C., Becking, G. C., Iverson, F., Ritter, L., Valli, V. E., and Reynolds, L. M. (1980a). Short-term study of the combined effects of mirex, photomirex, and Kepone with halogenated biphenyls in rats. *J. Toxicol. Environ. Health* **6**, 421–432.

Chu, I., Villeneuve, D. C., Becking, G. C., and Viau, A. (1980b). Tissue distribution and elimination of 2,8-dihydromirex in the rat. *J. Toxicol. Environ. Health* **6**, 713–721.

Chu, I., Villeneuve, D. C., Valli, V. E., Secours, V. E., and Becking, G. C. (1981a). Chronic toxicity of photomirex in the rat. *Toxicol. Appl. Pharmacol.* **59**, 268–278.

Chu, I., Villeneuve, D. C., MacDonald, B. L., Secours, V. E., and Valli, V. E. (1981b). Reversibility of the toxicological changes induced by photomirex and mirex. *Toxicology* **21**, 235–250.

Chu, I., Villeneuve, D. C., Secours, V. E., Valli, V. E., and Becking, G. C. (1981c). Effects of photomirex and mirex on reproduction in the rat. *Toxicol. Appl. Pharmacol.* **60**, 549–556.

Chu, I., Villeneuve, D. C., Sun, C.-W., Secours, V., Procter, B., Arnold, E., Clegg, D., Reynolds, L., and Valli, V. E. (1986). Toxicity of toxaphene in the rat and beagle dog. *Fundam. Appl. Toxicol.* **7**, 408–418.

Chu, I., Secours, V., Villeneuve, D. C., Valli, V. E., Nakamura, A., Colin, D., Clegg, D. J., and Arnold, E. P. (1988). Reproduction study of toxaphene in the rat. *J. Environ. Sci. Health, Part B* **23**, 101–126.

Chung Hwang, E., and Van Woert, M. H. (1981). p,p'-DDT-induced alterations in brain serotonin metabolism. *Neurotoxicology* **2**, 649–657.

Cianflone, D. J., Hewitt, W. R., Villeneuve, D. C., and Plaa, G. L. (1980). Role of biotransformation in the alterations of chloroform hepatotoxicity produced by Kepone and mirex. *Toxicol. Appl. Pharmacol.* **53**, 140–149.

Cinotti, V. (1971). Poisoning with Radosan and Gamacid caused vertiginous disorders. *Srp. Arh. Celok. Lek.* **98**, 1213–1217 (in Serbian).

Ciupe, R. (1976). Determination of BHC, p,p'-DDT, and p,p'-DDE in food and adipose tissue. *Igiena* **15**(2), 113–117 (in Romanian).

Clapp, K. L., Nelson, D. M., Bell, J. T., and Rousek, E. J. (1971). A study of the effects of toxaphene on the hepatic cells of rats. *Proc. Annu. Meet.— Am. Soc. Anim. Sci., West. Sect.* **22**, 313–323.

Clark, D. E., Ivie, G. W., and Camp, B. J. (1981). Effects of dietary hexachlorobenzene or *in vivo* biotransformation, residue deposition, and elimination of certain xenobiotics by rats. *J. Agric. Food Chem.* **29**, 600–608.

Clemmesen, J., Fugelsang-Fredericksen, V., and Plum, C. M. (1974). Are anticonvulsants oncogenic? *Lancet* **1**, 705–707.

Clifford, N. J., and Weil, J. (1972). Cortisol metabolism in persons occupationally exposed to DDT. *Arch. Environ. Health* **24**, 145–147.

Clinico-Pathologic Conference (1955). Exposure to insecticides, bone marrow failure, gastrointestinal bleeding, and uncontrolled infections. *Am. J. Med.* **19**, 274–284.

Clodi, P. H., and Schnack, H. (1959). An attempted suicide with gamma-hexachlorcyclohexane (Inexid). *Wien. Z. Inn. Med. Ihre Grenzgeb.* **40**, 414–417 (in German).

Cobey, F. A., Taliaferro, I., and Haag, H. B. (1956). Effect of DDD and some of its derivatives on plasma 17-OH-corticosteroids in the dog. *Science* **123**, 140–141.

Coble, Y., Hildebrandt, P., Davis, J., Raasch, F., and Curley, A. (1967). Acute endrin poisoning. *JAMA, J. Am. Med. Assoc.* **202**, 489–493.

Cochran, R. C., and Wiedow, M. A. (1984). Chordecone lacks estrogenic properties in the male rat. *Toxicol. Appl. Pharmacol.* **76**, 519–525.

Cocisiu, M., Aizicovici, H., Nistor, C., Unterman, H. W., Barbuta, R., and Gugles, E. (1976). Variation of the DDT and HCH contents of maternal milk in connection with food intake. *Igiena* **25**, 105–108 (in Romanian).

Cohn, W. J., Blanke, R. V., Griffith, F. D., and Guzelian, P. S. (1976). Distribution and excretion of Kepone (KP) in humans. *Gastroenterology* **71**, A-8/901.

Cohn, W. J., Boylan, J. J., Blanke, R. V., Fariss, B. S., Howell, J. R., and Guzelian, P. S. (1978). Treatment of chlordecone (Kepone) toxicity with cholestyramine. Results of a controlled trial. *N. Engl. J. Med.* **298**, 243–248.

Cole, J. F., Klevay, L. M., and Zavon, M. R. (1970). Endrin and dieldrin: A comparison of hepatic excretion in the rat. *Toxicol. Appl. Pharmacol.* **16**, 547–555.

Cole, L. M., and Casida, J. E. (1986). Polychlorocycloalkane insecticide-induced convulsions in mice in relation to disruption of the GABA-regulated chloride ionophore. *Life Sci.* **39**, 1855–1862.

Collins, G. B., Holmes, D. C., and Hoodless, R. A. (1982). Organochlorine pesticide residues in human milk in Great Britain 1979–80. *Hum. Toxicol.* **1**, 425–431.

Committee on Pesticides (1951). American Medical Association Council on Pharmacy and Chemistry report on pharmacologic and toxicologic aspects of DDT (chlorphenothane U.S.P.). *JAMA, J. Am. Med. Assoc.* **145**, 728–733.

Cook, L. L., Gordon, C. J., Tilson, H. A., and Edens, F. W. (1987). Chlordecone-induced effects on thermoregulatory processes in the rat. *Toxicol. Appl. Pharmacol.* **90**, 126–134.

Cook, L. L., Edens, F. W., and Tilson, H. A. (1988a). Possible brainstem involvement in the modification of thermoregulatory processes by chlordecone in rats. *Neuropharmacology*, **27**, 871–879.

Cook, L. L., Edens, F. W., and Tilson, H. A. (1988b). Pharmacological evaluation of central adrenergic involvement in chlordecone-induced hypothermia. *Neuropharmacology*, **27**, 881–887.

Cooper, J. R., Vodicnik, M. J., and Gordon, J. H. (1985). Effects of perinatal Kepone exposure on sexual differentiation of the rat brain. *Neurotoxicology* **6**(1), 183–190.

Cooper, R. L., Chadwick, R. W., Rehnberg, G. C., Goldman, J. M., Booth, K. C., Hein, J. F., and McElroy, W. K. (1989). Effect of lindane on hormonal control of reproductive function in the female rat. *Toxicol. Appl. Pharmacol.* **99**, 384–394.

Copeland, M. F., and Chadwick, R. W. (1979). Bioisomerization of lindane in rats. *J. Environ. Pathol. Toxicol.* **2**, 737–749.

Copeland, M. F., and Cranmer, M. F. (1974). Effects of *o,p'*-DDT on the adrenal gland and hepatic microsomal enzyme system of the beagle dog. *Toxicol. Appl. Pharmacol.* **27**, 1–10.

Copeland, M. F., Chadwick, R. W., Cooke, N., Whitehouse, D. A., Hill, D. M. (1986). Use of γ-hexachlorocyclohexane (lindane) to determine the ontogeny of metabolism in the developing rat. *J. Toxicol. Environ. Health* **18**, 527–542.

Coper, H., Herken, H., and Klempau, I. (1951). On the pharmacology and toxicology of chlorinated cyclohexane. *Naunyn-Schmiedebergs Arch. Exp. Pathol. Pharmakol.* **212**, 463–479 (in German).

Copplestone, J. F., Hunnego, J. N., and Harrison, D. L. (1973). Insecticides in adult New Zealanders—a five year study. *N.Z. J. Sci.* **16**, 27–39.

Costella, J. C., and Virgo, B. B. (1980). Is dieldrin-induced congenital inviability mediated by central nervous system hyperstimulation or by altered carbohydrate metabolism. *Can. J. Physiol. Pharmacol.* **58**, 633–637.

Coulston, F. (1985). Reconsideration of the dilemma of DDT for the establishment of an acceptable daily intake. *Regul. Toxicol. Pharmacol.* **5**, 332–383.

Coutselinis, A., Kentarchou, P., and Boukis, D. (1978). Concentration levels of endosulfan in biological material (report of three cases). *Forensic Sci.* **11**, 75.

Cranmer, J. M., Cranmer, M. F., and Goad, P. T. (1984). Prenatal chlordane exposure: Effects on plasma corticosterone concentrations over the lifespan of mice. *Environ. Res.* **35**, 204–210.

Cranmer, J. S., Avery, D. L., and Barnett, J. B. (1979). Altered immune competence of offspring exposed during development to the chlorinated hydrocarbon pesticide chlordane. *Teratology* **19**, 23A.

Cranmer, M. F. (1970). Effect of diphenylhydantoin on storage of DDT in the rat. *Toxicol. Appl. Pharmacol.* **17**, 315.

Cranmer, M. F. (1972). Absence of conversion of *o,p'*-DDT to *p,p'*-DDT in the rat. *Bull. Environ. Contam. Toxicol.* **7**, 121–124.

Cranmer, M. F., Carroll, J. J., and Copeland, M. F. (1969). Determination of DDT and metabolites, including DDA, in human urine by gas chromatography. *Bull. Environ. Contam. Toxicol.* **4**, 214–223.

Cranmer, M. F., Peoples, A., and Chadwick, R. (1972). Biochemical effects of repeated administration of *p,p'*-DDT on the squirrel monkey. *Toxicol. Appl. Pharmacol.* **21**, 98–101.

Crouch, L. S., and Ebel, R. E. (1987). Influence of chlordecone and mirex exposure on benzo[*a*]pyrene metabolism of rat liver microsomes. *Xenobiotica* **17**, 25–34.

Crouch, M. F., and Roberts, M. L. (1985). The effects of γ-hexachlorocyclohexane on amylase secretion and inositol phospholipid metabolism in mouse pancreatic acini. *Biochim. Biophys. Acta* **844**, 149–157.

Crowder, L. A., and Dindal, E. F. (1974). Fate of ³⁶Cl-toxaphene in rats. *Bull. Environ. Contam. Toxicol.* **12**, 320–327.

Cueto, C., Jr. (1970). Cardiovascular effects of *o,p'*-DDD. *Ind. Med. Surg.* **39**, 31–32.

Cueto, C., Jr., and Biros, F. J. (1967). Chlorinated insecticides and related materials in human urine. *Toxicol. Appl. Pharmacol.* **10**, 261–269.

Cueto, C., Jr., and Brown, J. H. U. (1958). Biological studies on an adrenocorticolytic agent and the isolation of the active components. *Endocrinology (Baltimore)* **62**, 334–339.

Cueto, C., Jr., and Hayes, W. J., Jr. (1962). The detection of dieldrin metabolites in human urine. *J. Agric. Food Chem.* **10**, 366–369.

Cueto, C., Jr., and Moran, N. C. (1968). The circulatory effects of catecholamines and ouabain in glucocorticoid-deficient animals. *J. Pharmacol. Exp. Ther.* **164**, 31–44.

Cummings, A. M., and Gray, L. E. (1987). Methoxychlor affects the decidual cell response of the uterus but not other progestational parameters in female rats. *Toxicol. Appl. Pharmacol.* **90**, 330–336.

Cummings, J. G., Eidelman, M., Turner, V., Reed, D., Zee, K. T., and Cook, R. E. (1967). Residues in poultry tissues from low level feeding of five chlorinated hydrocarbon insecticides to hens. *J. Assoc. Off. Anal. Chem.* **50**, 418–425.

Cunningham, R. E., and Hill, F. S. (1952). Convulsions and deafness following ingestion of DDT. *Pediatrics* **9**, 745–747.

Curley, A., and Garretson, L. K. (1969). Acute chlordane poisoning. *Arch. Environ. Health* **18**, 211–215.

Curley, A., and Kimbrough, R. (1969). Chlorinated hydrocarbon insecticides in plasma and milk of pregnant and lactating women. *Arch. Environ. Health* **18**, 156–164.

Curley, A., Copeland, M. F., and Kimbrough, R. D. (1969). Chlorinated hydrocarbon insecticides in organs of stillborn and blood of newborn babies. *Arch. Environ. Health* **19**, 628–632.

Curley, A., Jennings, R. W., Mann, H. T., and Sedlak, V. (1970). Measurement of endrin following epidemics of poisoning. *Bull. Environ. Contam. Toxicol.* **5**, 24–29.

Curley, A., Burse, V. W., Jennings, R. W., Villanueva, E. C., Tomatis, L., and Akazaki, K. (1973). Chlorinated hydrocarbon pesticides and related compounds in adipose tissue from people of Japan. *Nature (London)* **242**, 338–340.

Curtis, L. R., and Hoyt, D. (1984). Impaired biliary excretion of taurocholate associated with increased biliary tree permeability in mirex- or chlordecone-pretreated rats. *J. Pharmacol. Exp. Ther.* **231**, 495–501.

Curtis, L. R., and Mehendale, H. M. (1979). The effects of Kepone treatment on biliary excretion of xenobiotics in the male rat. *Toxicol. Appl. Pharmacol.* **47**, 295–303.

Curtis, L. R., and Mehendale, H. M. (1980). Specificity of chlordecone-induced potentiation of carbon tetrachloride hepatotoxicity. *Drug Metab. Dispos.* **8**, 23–27.

Curtis, L. R., and Mehendale, H. M. (1981). Hepatobiliary dysfunction and inhibition of adenosine triphosphatase activity of bile canaliculi-enriched fractions following *in vivo* mirex, photomirex, and chlordecone exposures. *Toxicol. Appl. Pharmacol.* **61**, 429–440.

Curtis, L. R., Williams, W. L., and Mehendale, H. M. (1979). Potentiation of the hepatotoxicity of carbon tetrachloride following preexposure to chlordecone (Kepone) in the male rat. *Toxicol. Appl. Pharmacol.* **51**, 283–293.

Curtis, L. R., Thureson-Klein, A. K., and Mehendale, H. M. (1981). Ultrastructural and biochemical correlates of the specificity of chlordecone-potentiated carbon tetrachloride hepatotoxicity. *J. Toxicol. Environ. Health* **7**, 499–517.

Czarski, Z., Checinski, S., and Berbec, W. (1967). A case of poisoning with chlorinated hydrocarbons from the insecticide Ditox. *Pol. Tyg. Lek.* **22**, 27–29 (in Polish).

Czegledi-Janko, G. (1969). Residues of chlorinated hydrocarbons in the blood of inhabitants of Budapest in 1967–1968 with particular reference to lindane. *Z. Gesamte Hyg. Ihre Grenzgeb.* **15**, 766–761.

Czegledi-Janko, G., and Avar, P. (1970). Occupational exposure to lindane: Clinical and laboratory findings. *Br. J. Ind. Med.* **27**, 283–286.

Dacre, J. C. (1969). Residual metabolites of hexachlorocyclohexane in human adipose tissues. *Proc. Univ. Otago Med. Sch.* **47**(3), 74–76.

Dadey, J. L., and Kammer, A. G. (1953). Chlordane intoxication: A report of a case. *JAMA, J. Am. Med. Assoc.* **153**, 723–725.

Daerr, W., Kaukel, E., and Schmoldt, A. (1985). Hemoperfusion—a therapeutic alternative for early treatment of acute lindane poisoning. *Dtsch. Med. Wochenschr.* **110**, 1253–1255 (in German).

Dailey, R. E., Walton, M. S., Beck, V., Leavens, C. L., and Klein, A. K. (1970). Excretion, distribution, and tissue storage of a ^{14}C-labelled photoconversion product of ^{14}C-dieldrin. *J. Agric. Food Chem.* **18,** 443–445.

Dailey, R. E., Klein, A. K., Brouwer, E., Link, J. D., and Braunberg, R. C. (1972). Effect of testosterone on metabolism of ^{14}C-photodieldrin in normal, castrated and oophorectomized rats. *J. Agric. Food Chem.* **20,** 371–376.

Dale, W. E., and Quinby, G. E. (1963). Chlorinated insecticides in the body fat of people in the United States. *Science* **142,** 593–595.

Dale, W. E., Gaines, T. B., Hayes, W. J., Jr., and Pearce, G. W. (1963). Poisoning by DDT: Relation between clinical signs and concentration in rat brain. *Science* **142,** 1474–1476.

Dale, W. E., Copeland, M. F., and Hayes, W. J., Jr. (1965). Chlorinated insecticides in the body fat of people in India. *Bull. W. H. O.* **33,** 471–477.

Dale, W. E., Copeland, M. F., Pearce, G. W., and Miles, J. W. (1966a). Concentration of o,p'-DDT in rat brain at various intervals after dosing. *Arch. Int. Pharmacodyn. Ther.* **162,** 40–43.

Dale, W. E., Curley, A., and Cueto, C., Jr. (1966b). Hexane extractable chlorinated pesticides in human blood. *Life Sci.* **5,** 47–54.

Dale, W. E., Curley, A., and Hayes, W. J., Jr. (1967). Determination of chlorinated insecticides in human blood. *Ind. Med. Surg.* **36,** 275–280.

Damaskin, V. I. (1965). The extent of the accumulation of DDT in the human body in connection with its assimilation and food, and its toxic effect. *Gig. Sanit.* **30,** 109–111.

Dangerfield, W. G. (1946). Toxicity of DDT to man. *Br. Med. J.* **1,** 27.

Daniel, C. S., Agarwal, S., and Agarwel, S. S. (1986). Human red blood cell membrane damage by endosulfan. *Toxicol. Lett.* **32,** 113–118.

Danopoulos, E., Melissinos, K., and Katsas, G. (1953). Serious poisoning by hexachlorocyclohexane. Clinical and laboratory observations on five cases. *Arch. Ind. Hyg. Occup. Med.* **8,** 582–587.

Danowski, T. S., Sarver, H. E., Moses, C., and Boness, J. V. (1964). o,p'-DDD therapy in Cushing's syndrome and in obesity with cushingoid changes. *Am. J. Med.* **37,** 235–250.

da Rocha e Silca, E. O. (1961). A case of hypersensitivity to chlorinated insecticides (DDT and BHC). *Arq. Hig. Saude Publica* **26,** 51–55 (in Portuguese).

Datta, P. R. (1970). *In vitro* detoxication of p,p'-DDT via p,p'-DDE to p,p'-DDA in rats. *Ind. Med. Surg.* **39,** 190–194.

Datta, P. R., and Nelson, M. F. (1970). p,p'-DDT detoxication by isolated perfused rat liver and kidney. *Ind. Med. Surg.* **39,** 195–198.

Davey, R. J., and Johnson, L. A. (1974). Tissue residues, blood chemistry and physiological response of lindane-treated swine. *J. Anim. Sci.* **38,** 318–324.

Davidow, B., and Frawley, J. P. (1951). Tissue distribution, accumulation, and elimination of the isomers of benzene hexachloride. *Proc. Soc. Exp. Biol. Med.* **76,** 780–783.

Davidow, B., Hagan, E. C., and Radomski, J. L. (1951). A metabolite of chlordane in tissues of animals. *Fed. Proc., Fed. Am. Soc. Exp. Biol.* **10,** 291.

Davies, D., and Mes, J. (1987). Comparison of the residue levels of some organochlorine compounds in breast milk of the general and indigenous Canadian populations. *Bull. Environ. Contam. Toxicol.* **39,** 743–749.

Davies, G. M., and Lewis, I. (1956). Outbreak of food poisoning from bread made from chemically contaminated flour. *Br. Med. J.* **2,** 393–398.

Davies, J. E., Edmundson, W. F., Schneider, N. J., and Cassidy, J. D. (1968). Problems of prevalence of pesticide residues in humans. *Pestic. Monit. J.* **2**(2), 80–85.

Davies, J. E., Edmundson, W. F., Carter, C. H., and Barquet, A. (1969). Effect of anticonvulsant drugs on dichophane (D.D.T.) residues in man. *Lancet* **2,** 7–9.

Davies, J. E., Didhia, H. V., Morgade, C., Barquet, A., and Maibach, H. I. (1983). Lindane poisonings. *Arch. Dermatol.* **119,** 142–144.

Davis, K. J., and Fitzhugh, O. G. (1962). Tumorigenic potential of aldrin and dieldrin for mice. *Toxicol. Appl. Pharmacol.* **4,** 187–189.

Davis, M. E., and Mehendale, H. M. (1980). Functional and biochemical correlates of chlordecone exposure and its enhancement of CCl_4 hepatotoxicity. *Toxicology* **15,** 91–103.

Davison, K. L. (1970a). Dieldrin accumulation in tissues of sheep. *J. Agric. Food Chem.* **18,** 1156–1160.

Davison, K. L. (1970b). Growth, hemoglobin, body composition and vitamin A in sheep fed dieldrin. *J. Anim. Sci.* **31,** 567–575.

Davison, K. L. (1973). Dieldrin ^{14}C balance in rats, sheep and chickens. *Bull. Environ. Contam. Toxicol,* **10,** 16–24.

Davison, K. L., Mollenhauer, H. H., and Younger, R. L. (1976). Mirex-induced hepatic changes in chickens, Japanese quail, and rats. *Arch. Environ. Contam. Toxicol.* **4,** 469–482.

Davison, K. L., Feil, V. J., and Lamoureux, C. H. (1982). Methoxychlor metabolism in goats. *J. Agric. Food Chem.* **30,** 130–137.

Davison, K. L., Lamoureux, C. H., and Feil, V. J. (1983). Methoxychlor metabolism in goats. 2. Metabolites in bile and movement through skin. *J. Agric. Food Chem.* **312,** 164–166.

Dean, B. J., Doak, S. M. A., and Somerville, H. (1975). The potential mutagenicity of dieldrin (HEOD) in mammals. *Food Cosmet. Toxicol.* **13,** 317–323.

Dean, M. E., Smeaton, T. C., and Stock, B. H. (1980). The influence of fetal and neonatal exposure to dichlorodiphenyltrichloroethane (DDT) on the testosterone status of neonatal male rat. *Toxicol. Appl. Pharmacol.* **53,** 315–322.

de Bellini, Y., Cressely, J., Deluzarche, A., and Hazemann, A. (1977). Organochlorine pesticides in women's milk. *Ann. Falsif. Exp. Chim.* **70,** 567.

de Campos, M., and Olszyna-Marzys, A. E. (1978). Contamination of human milk with chlorinated pesticides in Guatemala and in El Salvador. *Arch. Environ. Contam. Toxicol.* **8,** 43–58.

Dedek, W., and Schmidt, R. (1972). Studies on transplacental transport and metabolism of ^{3}H- and ^{14}C-labelled DDT in pregnant mice under hunger stress. *Pharmazie* **27,** 294–297.

Deema, P., Thompson, E., and Ware, G. W. (1966). Metabolism, storage and excretion of C^{14}-endosulfan in the mouse. *J. Econ. Entomol.* **59,** 546–550.

de Fernicola, N. A. G. G., and de Azevedo, F. A. (1982). Serum levels of organochlorine insecticides in humans in São Paulo, Brazil. *Vet. Hum. Toxicol.* **24,** 91–93.

de Fossey, B. M., Luton, S. P., and Bricaire, H. (1968). Our experience of o,p'-DDD in the treatment of hypercorticisms. *Ann. Endocrinol.* **29,** 93–102 (in French).

Deichmann, W. B., and Keplinger, M. L. (1970). Protection against the acute effects of certain pesticides by pretreatment with aldrin, dieldrin, and DDT. *In* "Pesticides Symposia" (W. B. Deichman, J. L. Radomski, and R. A. Penalver, eds.), pp. 121–123. Halos and Associates, Miami, Florida.

Deichmann, W. B., and MacDonald, W. E. (1976). Liver cancer deaths in the continental USA from 1930 to 1972. *Am. Ind. Hyg. Assoc. J.* **37,** 495–498.

Deichmann, W. B., and MacDonald, W. E. (1977). Organochlorine pesticides and liver cancer deaths in the United States, 1930–1972. *Ecotoxicol. Environ. Saf.* **1,** 89–110.

Deichmann, W. B., Witherup, S., and Kitzmiller, K. V. (1950). "The Toxicity of DDT. I. Experimental Observations." Kettering Lab., Cincinnati, Ohio.

Deichmann, W. B., Keplinger, M. L., Sala, F., and Glass, E. (1967). Synergism among oral carcinogens. IV. The simultaneous feeding of four tumorigens to rats. *Toxicol. Appl. Pharmacol.* **11,** 88–103.

Deichmann, W. B., Dressler, I., Keplinger, M., and McDonald, W. E. (1968). Retention of dieldrin in blood, liver and fat of rats fed dieldrin for six months. *Ind. Med. Surg.* **37,** 837–839.

Deichmann, W. B., Keplinger, M. L., Dressler, I., and Sala, F. (1969). Retention of dieldrin and DDT in the tissues of dogs fed aldrin and DDT individually and as a mixture. *Toxicol. Appl. Pharmacol.* **14,** 205–213.

Deichmann, W. B., MacDonald, W. E., Blum, E., Bevilacqua, M., Radomski, J., Keplinger, M. L., and Balkus, M. (1970). Tumorigenicity of aldrin, dieldrin, and endrin in the albino rat. *Ind. Med. Surg.* **39,** 426–434.

Deichmann, W. B., MacDonald, W. E., and Cubit, D. A. (1971a). DDT tissue retention: Sudden rise induced by the addition of aldrin to a fixed DDT intake. *Science,* **172,** 275–276.

Deichmann, W. B., MacDonald, W. E., Beasley, A. G., and Cubit, D.

(1971b). Subnormal reproduction in beagle dogs induced by DDT and aldrin. *Ind. Med. Surg.* **40,** 10–20.

Deichmann, W. B., MacDonald, W. E., and Cubit, D. A. (1975). Dieldrin and DDT in the tissues of mice fed aldrin and DDT for seven generations. *Arch. Toxicol.* **34,** 173–182.

Deichmann, W. B., MacDonald, W. E., and Lu, F. C. (1978). Effects of chronic aldrin feeding in two strains of female rats and a discussion on the risks of carcinogens in man. *Dev. Toxicol. Environ. Sci.* **4,** 407–413.

DeKraay, W. H. (1978). Pesticides and lymphoma in Iowa. *J. Iowa Med. Soc.* **68,** 50–53.

Del Vecchio, V., and Leoni, V. (1967). Research on levels of chlorinated insecticides in biological material. Note II. CI: Chlorinated insecticides in adipose tissue of some groups of the Italian population. *Nuovi Ann. Ig. Microbiol.* **18,** 107–128 (in Italian).

De Matteis, F. (1973). Drug interactions in experimental hepatic porphyria. A model for the exacerbation by drugs of human variegate porphyria. *Enzyme* **16,** 266–275.

Demeter, J., and Heyndrickx, A. (1978). Two lethal endosulfan poisonings in man. *J. Anal. Toxicol.* **2,** 68–74.

Demeter, J., Heyndrickx, A., Timperman, J., Lefevere, M., and DeBeer, J. (1977). Toxicological analysis in a case of endosulfan suicide. *Bull. Environ. Contam. Toxicol.* **18,** 110–114.

Denes, A. (1962). Food chemistry problems of chlorinated hydrocarbon residues. *Nahrung* **6,** 48–56 (in German).

Denes, A. (1964). Investigation of chlorinated hydrocarbon residues in animal and vegetable fats. *In* "1963 Year Book." Institute of Nutrition, Budapest, Hungary (in Hungarian).

Denes, A. (1966). Dieldrin residues in foodstuffs and biological material. *In* "1965 Year Book," pp. 47–49. Institute of Nutrition, Budapest, Hungary (in Hungarian).

Den Tonkelaar, E. M., and Van Esch, G. J. (1974). No-effect levels of organochlorine pesticides based on induction of microsomal liver enzymes in short-term toxicity experiments. *Toxicology* **2,** 371–380.

Dequidt, J., Erb, F., Brice, A., and Van Aerde, C. (1973). Accumulation and transformation of heptachlor by the rat. *Bull. Soc. Pharm. Lille* **4,** 153–163 (in French).

D'Eramo, N., and Croce, E. (1960). Acute erythematic-bullous dermatitis caused by contact with aldrin. *Riv. Infort. Mal. Prof.* **47,** 534–537 (in Italian).

Derbes, V. J., Dent, J. H., Forrest, W. W., and Johnson, M. F. (1955). Fatal chlordane poisoning. *JAMA, J. Am. Med. Assoc.* **158,** 1367–1369.

D'Ercole, A. J., Arthur, R. D., Cain, J. D., and Barrentine, B. F. (1976). Insecticide exposure of mothers and newborns in a rural agricultural area. *Pediatrics* **57,** 869–874.

Desaiah, D. (1980). Comparative effects of chlordecone and mirex on rat cardiac ATPases and binding of [^{3}H]-catecholamines. *J. Environ Pathol. Toxicol.* **4,** 237–248.

Desaiah, D. (1981). Interaction of chlordecone with biological membranes. *J. Toxicol. Environ. Health* **8,** 719–730.

Desaiah, D., Ho, I. K., and Mehendale, H. M. (1977a). Effects of Kepone and mirex on mitochondrial Mg^{2+}ATPase activity in rat liver. *Toxicol. Appl. Pharmacol.* **39,** 219–228.

Desaiah, D., Ho, I. K., and Mehendale, H. M. (1977b). Inhibition of mitochondrial Mg^{2+}ATPase activity in isolated perfused rat liver by Kepone. *Biochem. Pharmacol.* **26,** 1155–1159.

Desaiah, D., Mehendale, H. M., and Ho, I. K. (1978). Kepone inhibition of mouse brain synaptosomal ATPase activities. *Toxicol. Appl. Pharmacol,* **45,** 268–269.

Desaiah, D., Gilliland, I. K., Ho, I. K., and Mehendale, H. M. (1980). Inhibition of mouse brain synaptosomal ATPases and ouabain binding by chlordecone. *Toxicol. Lett.* **6,** 275–285.

Desaiah, D., Chetty, C. S., and Prasada Rao, K. S. (1985). Chlordecone inhibition of calmodulin activated calcium APTase in rat brain synaptosomes. *J. Toxicol. Environ. Health* **16,** 189–195.

Desbuquois, G., Lutier, J., and Lebrettevillois, G. (1963). Acute fatal intoxication by ingestion of lindane and malathion by an infant. *Arch. Mal. Prof. Med. Trav. Secur. Soc.* **24,** 409–411.

Descotes, J. (1986). "Immunotoxicology of Drugs and Chemicals." Elsevier, Amsterdam.

Desi, I. (1974). Neurotoxicological effect of small quantities of lindane. *Int. Arch. Arbeitsmed.* **33,** 153–162 (in German).

Desi, I., and Major, M. (1972). Neurotoxic effect of small lindane doses in animal experiments. *Egeszsegtudomany* **38,** 98–99 (in Hungarian).

de Vlieger, M., Robinson, J., Baldwin, M. K., Crabtree, A. N., and van Dijk, M. C. (1968). The organochlorine insecticide content of human tissue. *Arch. Environ. Health,* **17,** 759–767.

Dewan, A., Gupta, S. K., Jani, J. P., and Kashyap, S. K. (1980). Effect of lindane on antibody response to typhoid vaccine in weanling rats. *J. Environ. Sci. Health, Part B* **B15,** 395–402.

Dickson, J., Peet, R. L., Duffy, R. J., Bolton, J., Hilbert, B., and McGill, C. (1984). Heptachlor poisoning in horses and cattle. *Aust. Vet. J.* **61,** 331.

Didenko, G. G., Chernov, O. V., and Gupalovich, T. D. (1973). Study of possible blastomogenic effects of gammon-BHCB (lindane). *Gig. Sanit.* **38,** 98–99 (in Russian).

Dietz, D. D., and McMillan, D. E. (1978). Effects of mirex and Kepone on schedule controlled responding. *Pharmacologist* **20,** 225.

Dietz, D. D., and McMillan, D. E. (1979). Comparative effects of mirex and Kepone on schedule-controlled behaviour in the rat. I. Multiple fixed-ratio 12-fixed interval 2 min schedule. *Neurotoxicology* **1,** 369–385.

Dikshith, T. S. S., and Datta, K. K. (1972). Effect of intratesticular injection of lindane and endrin on the testes of rats. *Acta Pharmacol. Toxicol.* **31,** 1–10.

Dikshith, T. S. S., and Datta, K. K. (1978). Endosulfan: Lack of cytogenetic effects in male rats. *Bull. Environ. Contam. Toxicol,* **20,** 826–833.

Dikshith, T. S. S., Chandra, P., and Datta, K. K. (1973). Effect of lindane on the skin of albino rats. *Experientia* **29,** 684–685.

Dikshith, T. S. S., Datta, K. K., Kushwah, H. S., and Raizada, R. B. (1978a). Histopathological and biochemical changes in guinea pigs after repeated dermal exposure to benzene hexachloride. *Toxicology* **10,** 55–66.

Dikshith, T. S. S., Nath, G., and Datta, K. K. (1978b). Combined cytogenic effects of endosulfan and metepa in male rats. *Indian J. Exp. Biol.* **16,** 1000–1002.

Dikshith, T. S. S., Raizada, R. B., Shivastava, M. K., and Kaphalia, B. S. (1984). Response of rats to repeated oral administration of endosulfan. *Ind. Health* **22,** 295–304.

Dillon, J. C., Martin, G. B., and O'Brien, H. T. (1981). Pesticide residues in human milk. *Food Cosmet. Toxicol.* **19,** 437–442.

Ditraglia, D., Brown, D. P., Namekata, T., and Iverson, N. (1981). Mortality study of workers employed at organochlorine pesticide manufacturing plants. *Scand. J. Work Environ. Health* **7,** Suppl. 4, 140–146.

Djonckheere, W., Steurbaxt, W., Verstraeten, R., and Kips, R. H. (1977). Residues of organochlorine pesticides in human fat in Belgium. *Meded. Fac. Lanbouwwet. Rijksuniv. Gent* **42,** 1839–1847.

Dobson, R. C., Fahey, J. E., Ballee, D. C., and Baugh, E. R. (1971). Reduction of chlorinated hydrocarbon residues in swine. *Bull. Environ. Contam. Toxicol.* **6,** 391–400.

Doguchi, M., Wshio, F., Niwayama, K., and Nishida, K. (1971). Pesticide content of human female fat in a metropolitan area. *Annu. Rep. Tokyo Metrop. Res. Lab. Public Health* **22,** 131–133 (in Japanese).

Doman, I. (1971). Thiodan poisoning in sheep. *Magy. Allatorv. Lapja,* **26,** 342–343 (in Hungarian).

Domanski, J. J., Nelson, L. A., Guthrie, F. E., Domanski, R. E., Mark, R., and Postlethwaite, R. W. (1977). Relation between smoking and levels of DDT and dieldrin in human fat. *Arch. Environ. Health* **32,** 196–199.

Domenjoz, R. (1944). Experimental investigation with a new insecticide (Neocide Geigy): A contribution to the theory of of action of contact poison. *Schweiz. Med. Wochenschr.* **74,** 952–958 (in German).

Domenjoz, R. (1946a). On the biological action of a DDT-derivative. *Arch. Int. Pharmacodyn.* **73,** 128–146 (in German).

Domenjoz, R. (1946b). Biological action of a few derivatives of DDT. *Helv. Chim. Acta* **29,** 1317–1322 (in French).

Dommarco, R., Muccio, A. D., Camoni, I., and Gigli, B. (1987). Organochlorine pesticide and polychlorinated biphenyl residues in human milk from Rome (Italy) and surroundings. *Bull. Environ. Contamin. Toxicol.* **39**, 919–925.

Dorough, H. W., and Ivie, G. W. (1974). Fate of mirex-^{14}C during and after a 28-day feeding period to a lactating cow. *J. Environ. Qual.* **3**, 65–67.

Dorough, H. W., Huhtaren, K., Marshall, T. C., and Bryant, H. E. (1978). Fate of endosulfan in rats and toxicological considerations of apolar metabolites. *Pestic. Biochem. Physiol.* **8**, 241–252.

Downey, W. K., Flynn, M. P., and Aherne, S. A. (1975). Organochlorine content of milks, dairy products and animal feed ingredients: Ireland 1971–1972. *J. Dairy Res.* **42**, 21–29.

Draize, J. G., Nelson, A. A., and Calvery, H. O. (1944). The percutaneous absorption of DDT (2,2-bis-(*p*-chlorophenyl)-1,1,1-trichloroethane) in laboratory animals. *J. Pharmacol. Exp. Ther.* **82**, 159–166.

Drummond, L., Gillanders, E. M., and Wilson, H. K. (1988). Plasma γ-hexachlorocyclohexane concentrations in forestry workers exposed to lindane. *Br. J. Ind. Med.* **45**, 493–497.

Dubey, R. K., Beg, M. U., and Singh, J. (1984). Effects of endosulfan and its metabolites on rat liver mitochondrial respiration and enzyme activities *in vitro*. *Biochem. Pharmacol.* **33**, 3405–3410.

Dubois, J. M., and Bergman, C. (1977). Asymmetrical currents and sodium currents in Ranvier nodes exposed to DDT. *Nature (London)* **266**, 741–742.

Dubsky, H., Rittich, B., Sommerova, H., Marek, V., Hana, K., and Janoušek, S. (1977). Determination of chlorinated pesticides in food and human fat tissues. *Vet. Med. (Prague)* **22**, 629–633 (in Czech).

Ducharne, P. L. P. (1957). "Electroencephalographic Study of Dieldrin," Symp. Acerca de Ciertos Aspectos del uso del dieldrin en Venezuela. Division de Malariologia, Direccion de Salud Publica, Ministerio de Sanidad y Asistencia Social (in Spanish).

Duggan, R. E. (1968). Residues in food and feed. Pesticide residue levels in food in the United States from July 1, 1963 to June 30, 1967. *Pestic. Monit. J.* **2**, 2–46.

Dunayevskiy, G. A. (1972). The functional condition of the circulatory organs in workers involved in organochlorine compounds' manufacturing. *Gig. Tr. Prof. Zabol.* **16**, 48–50 (in Russian).

Dupire, A., and Raucourt, M. (1943). A new insecticide: The hexachloride of benzene. *C. R. Seances Acad. Agric. Fr.* **29**, 470–472 (in French).

Durham, W. F., Ortega, P., and Hayes, W. J., Jr. (1963). The effect of various dietary levels of DDT on liver function, cell morphology, and DDT storage in the rhesus monkey. *Arch. Int. Pharmacodyn. Ther.* **141**, 111–129.

Durham, W. F., Armstrong, J. F., and Quinby, G. E. (1965). DDA excretion levels. *Arch. Environ. Health* **11**, 76–79.

Ebel, R. E. (1982). Alterations in microsomal cytochrome P-450 catalysed reactions as a function of chlordecone (Kepone) induction. *Pestic. Biochem. Physiol.* **18**, 113–121.

Ebel, R. E. (1984). Hepatic microsomal *p*-nitroanisole *O*-demethylase. Effects of chlordecone or mirex induction in male and female rats. *Biochem. Pharmacol.* **33**, 559–564.

Eckenhausen, F. W., Bennett, D., Beynon, K. I., and Elgar, K. E. (1981). Organochlorine pesticide concentration in perinatal samples from mother and babies. *Arch. Environ. Health* **36**, 81–92.

Eckols, K., Williams, J., and Uphouse L. (1989). Effects of chlordecone on progesterone receptors in immature and adult rats. *Toxicol. Appl. Pharmacol.* **100**, 506–516.

Edmundson, W. F., Davies, J. E., and Hull, W. (1968). Dieldrin storage levels in necropsy adipose tissue from a South Florida population. *Pestic. Monit. J.* **2**, 86–89.

Edmundson, W. F., Davies, J. E., Nachman, G. A., and Roeth, R. L. (1969a). *p,p'*-DDT and *p,p'*-DDE in blood samples of occupationally exposed workers. *Public Health Rep.* **84**, 53–58.

Edmundson, W. F., Davies, J. E., Cranmer, M., and Nachman, G. A. (1969b). Levels of DDT and DDE in blood and DDA in urine of pesticide formulators following a single intensive exposure. *Ind. Med. Surg.* **38**, 145–150.

Edmundson, W. F., Davies, J. E., and Cranmer, M. (1970). DDT and DDE in blood and urine of men exposed to 3 percent DDT aerosol. *Public Health Rep.* **85**, 457–463.

Egan, H., Goulding, R., Ropburn, J., and Tatton, J. O'G. (1965). Organochlorine pesticide residues in human fat and human milk. *Br. Med. J.* **2**, 66–69.

Egle, J. L., Jr., Gochberg, B. J., and Borzelleca, J. F. (1976). The distribution of ^{14}C-Kepone in the rat. *Pharmacologist* **18**, 195.

Egle, J. L., Jr., Fernandez, S. B., Guzelian, P. S., and Borzelleca, J. F. (1978). Distribution and excretion of chlordecone (Kepone) in the rat. *Drug. Metat. Dispos.* **6**, 91–95.

Egle, J. L., Jr., Guzelian, P. S., and Borzelleca, J. F. (1979). Time course of the acute toxic effects of sublethal doses of chlordecone (Kepone). *Toxicol. Appl. Pharmacol.* **48**, 533–536.

Eichler, D., Heupt, W., and Paul, W. (1983). Comparative study on the distribution of α- and γ-hexachlorocyclohexane in the rat with particular reference to the problem of isomerization. *Xenobiotica* **13**, 639–647.

Eisler, M. (1968). Heptachlor: Toxicology and safety evaluation. *Ind. Med. Surg.* **37**, 840–844.

El-Aaser, A.-B. A., Reid, E., and Stevenson, D. E. (1972). Alkaline phosphatase patterns in dieldrin-treated dogs. *Hoppe-Seyler's Z. Physiol. Chem.* **353**, 667–673.

Eldefrawi, M. E., Sherby, S. M., Abalis, I. M., and Eldefrawi, A. T. (1985). Interactions of pyrethroid and cyclodiene insecticides with nicotinic acetylcholine and GABA receptors. *Neurotoxicology* **6**(2), 47–62.

Eldridge, B. F. (1973). Repellents and impregnants for the control of body lice. *Sci. Publ.—Pan Am. Health Organ.* **263**,177–178.

Elgart, M. L., and Higdon, R. S. (1973). Pediculosis pubis of the scalp. *Arch. Dermatol.* **107**, 916–917.

Eliason, B. C., and Posner, H. S. (1971). Reduced passage of carbon-14-dieldrin to the fetal rat by phenobarbital but not by eight other drugs or dieldrin. *Am. J. Obstet. Gynecol.* **110**, 943–947.

Ely, T. D., MacFarlane, J. W., Galen, W. P., and Hine, C. H. (1967). Convulsions in Thiodan workers: A preliminary report. *J. Occup. Med.* **9**, 35–37.

Embry, T. L., Morgan, D. P., and Roan, C. C. (1972). Search for abnormalities of heme synthesis and sympathoadrenal activity. *J. Occup. Med.* **14**, 918–921.

End, D. W., Carchman, R. A., Ameen, R., and Dewey, W. L. (1979). Inhibition of rat brain mitochondrial calcium transport by chlordecone. *Toxicol. Appl. Pharmacol.* **51**, 189–196.

End, D. W., Carchman, R. A., and Dewey, W. L. (1981). Neurochemical correlates of chlordecone neurotoxicity. *J. Toxicol. Environ. Health,* **8**, 707–718.

Engebretson, K. A., and Davison, K. L. (1971). Dieldrin accumulation and excretion by rats fed phenobarbital and carbon. *Bull. Environ. Contam. Toxicol.* **6**, 391–400.

English, D., Schell, M., Siakotos, A., and Gabig, T. G. (1986). Reversible activation of the neutrophil superoxide generating system by hexachlorocyclohexane: Correlation with effects on a sub-cellular superoxide-generating fraction. *J. Immunol.* **137**, 283–290.

Engst, R., and Knoll, R. (1972). Organochlorine pesticide residues in human milk. *Pharmazie* **27**, 526–531 (in German).

Engst, R., Knoll, R., and Nickel, B. (1967). Concentration of chlorinated hydrocarbons especially DDT and its metabolic DDE in human fat. *Pharmazie* **22**, 654–661 (in German).

Epstein, S. S. (1978). Kepone—hazard evaluation. *Sci. Total Environ.* **9**, 1–62.

Epstein, S. S., and Ozonoff, D. (1987). Leukemias and blood dyscrasias following exposure to chlordane and heptachlor. *Teratogen, Carcinogen. Mutagen.* **7**, 527–540.

Epstein, S. S., and Shafner, H. (1968). Chemical mutagens in the human environment. *Nature (London)* **219**, 385–387.

Epstein, S. S., Arnold, E., Andrea, J., Bass, W., and Bishop, Y. (1972). Detection of chemical mutagens by the dominant lethal assay in the mouse. *Toxicol. Appl. Pharmacol.* **23**, 288–325.

Eriksson, P., and Nordberg, A. (1986). The effects of DDT, DDOH-palmitic acid, and a chlorinated paraffin on muscarinic receptors and the sodium-dependent choline uptake in the central nervous system of immature mice. *Toxicol. Appl. Pharmacol.* **85**, 121–127.

Eriksson, P., Flakeborn, Y., Nordberg, A., and Slanina, P. (1984). Effects of

DDT on muscanine and nicotine-like binding sites in CNS of immature and adult mice. *Toxicol. Lett.* **22**, 329–334.

Eroschenko, V. P. (1982). Surface changes in oviduct, uterus and vaginal cells of neonatal mice after estradiol-17β and the insecticide chlordecone (Kepone) treatment: A scanning electron microscopic study. *Biol. Reprod.* **26**, 707–720.

Eroschenko, V. P., and Mousa, M. A. (1979). Neonatal administration of insecticide chlordecone and its effects on the development of the reproductive tract in the female mouse. *Toxicol. Appl. Pharmacol.* **49**, 151–159.

Eroschenko, V. P., and Osman, F. (1986). Scanning electron microscopic changes in vaginal epithelium of suckling neonatal mice in response to estradiol or insecticide chlordecone (Kepone) passage in milk. *Toxicology* **38**, 175–185.

Erslev, A. J., and Wintrobe, M. M. (1962). Detection and prevention of drug-induced blood dyscrasias. *JAMA, J. Am. Med. Assoc.* **181**, 116–119.

Ervin, M. G., and Yarbrough, J. D. (1985). Mirex-induced liver enlargement in rats is dependent upon an intact pituitary–adrenalcortical axis. *Life Sci.* **36**, 139–145.

Esaac, E. G., and Matsumura, F. (1980). Mechanisms of reductive dechlorination of DDT by rat liver microsomes. *Pestic. Biochem. Physiol.* **10**, 81–93.

Eskenasy, J. J. (1972). Status epilepticus by dichlorodiphenyltrichloroethane and hexachlorcyclohexane poisoning. *Rev. Roum. Neurol.* **9**, 435–442 (in Romanian).

Espinosa-Gonzalez, J., and Thiel, R. (1987). Insecticide residues in the milk of Panamanian mothers. *Rev. Med. Panama* **12**, 139–143 (in Spanish).

Espir, M. L. E., Hall, J. W., Shirreffs, J. G., and Stevens, D. L. (1970). Impotence in farm workers using toxic chemicals. *Br. Med. J.* **1**, 423–425.

Ewing, A. D., Kadry, A. M., and Dorough, H. W. (1985). Comparative disposition and elimination of chlordane in rats and mice. *Toxicol. Lett* **26**, 233–239.

Eyzaguirre, C., and Lilienthal, J. L., Jr. (1949). Veratrinic effects of pentamethylenetetrazol (Metraxol) and 2,2-bis(p-chlorophenyl)-1,1,1-trichloroethane (DDT) on mammalian neuromuscular function. *Proc. Soc. Exp. Biol. Med.* **70**, 272–275.

Fabacher, D. L., and Hodgson, E. (1976). Induction of hepatic mixed-function oxidase enzymes in adult and neonatal mice by Kepone and mirex. *Toxicol. Appl. Pharmacol.* **38**, 71–77.

Fagan, J. E. (1981). Henoch-Schönlein purpura and (γ)-benzene hexachloride. *Pediatrics* **67**, 310–311.

Failing, F., Rimer, C., Wooley, R., Sandifer, S. H., Hutcheson, R. H. J., Saucier, J. W., Ward, C., and Kutz, F. W. (1976). Chlordane contamination of a municipal water system—Tennessee. *Morbid. Moral. Wkly. Rep.* **25**, 117.

Fariss, M. W., Blanke, R. V., Boylan, J. J., King, S. T., and Guzelian, P. S. (1978). Reductive biotransformation of chlordecone in man and rat. *Toxicol. Appl. Pharmacol.* **45**, 337.

Fariss, M. W., Blanke, R. V., Saady, J. J., and Guzelian, P. S. (1980). Demonstration of major metabolic pathways for chlordecone (Kepone) in humans. *Drug. Metab. Dispos.* **8**, 434–438.

Farkas, I., Desi, I., and Klemeny, T. (1968). The effect of DDT in the diet on the resting and loading electrocorticogram record. *Toxicol. Appl. Pharmacol.* **12**, 518–525.

Farkas, I., Desi, I., and Kemeny, T. (1969). Effect of orally consumed DDT on the rest and load EEG curves. *Egeszsegtudomany* **13**, 195–201 (in Hungarian).

Fattah, K. M. A., and Crowder, L. A. (1980). Plasma membrane ATPases from various tissues of the cockroach (*Periplaneta americana*) and mouse influenced by toxaphene. *Bull. Environ. Contam. Toxicol.* **24**, 356–363.

Fawcett, S. C., Bunyan, P. J., Huson, L. W., King, L. J., and Stanley, P. I. (1981). Excretion of radioactivity following the intraperitoneal administration of ^{14}C-DDT, ^{14}C-DDD, ^{14}C-DDE and ^{14}C-DDMU to the rat and Japanese quail. *Bull. Environ. Contam. Toxicol.* **27**, 386–392.

Fawcett, S. C., King, L. F., Bunyan, P. J., and Stanley, P. I. (1987). The metabolism of ^{14}C-DDT, ^{14}C-DDD, ^{14}C-DDE and ^{14}C-DDMU in rats and Japanese quail. *Xenobiotica* **17**, 525–538.

Feil, V. J., Hedde, R. D., Zaylskie, R. G., and Zachrison, C. H. (1970). Dieldrin-^{14}C metabolism in sheep: Identification of *trans*-6,7-dihydroxydihydroaldrin and hydro-1,4-*endo*-5,8-*exo*-dimethanonaphthalene. *J. Agric. Food Chem.* **18**, 120–124.

Feil, V. J., Lamoureux, C. H., Styrvoky, E., Zaylskie, R. G., Thacker, E. J., and Holman, G. M. (1973). Metabolism of *o,p'*-DDT in rats. *J. Agric. Food Chem.* **21**, 1072–1078.

Feil, V. J., Lamoureux, C. H., and Zaylskie, R. G. (1975). Metabolism of *o,p'*-DDT in chickens. *J. Agric. Food Chem.* **23**, 382–388.

Feldman, R. J., and Maibach, H. I. (1970). Pesticide percutaneous penetration in man. *J. Invest. Dermatol.* **54**, 435–436.

Feldmann, R. J., and Maibach, H. I. (1974). Percutaneous penetration of some pesticides and herbicides in man. *Toxicol. Appl. Pharmacol.* **28**, 126–132.

Fennah, R. G. (1945). Preliminary tests with DDT against insect pests of food-crops in the Lesser Antilles. *Trop. Agric.* **22**, 126–132.

Ferrigan, L. W., Hunter, C. G., and Stevenson, D. E. (1965). Observations on the effects of continued oral exposure of rats to dieldrin. *Food Cosmet. Toxicol,* **3**, 149–151.

Ferry, D. G., Owen, D., and McQueen, E. G. (1972a). The effect of phenytoin on the binding of pesticides to serum proteins. *Proc. Univ. Otago Med. Sch.* **50**, 8–9.

Ferry, D. G., Owen, D., Ballard, D. L., and McQueen, E. G. (1972b). Pesticides and serum proteins. *Proc. Univ. Otago Med. Sch.* **50**, 10–11.

Finklea, J., Priester, L. E., Creason, J. P., Hauser, T., Hinners, T., and Hammer, D. I. (1972). Polychlorinated biphenyl residues in human plasma expose a major urban pollution problem. *Am. J. Public Health* **62**, 645–651.

Finnegan, J. K., Hennigar, G. R., Smith, R. B., Jr., Larson, P. S., and Haag, H. B. (1955). Acute and chronic toxicity studies on 2,2-bis-*p*-ethylphenyl-1,1-dichloroethane (Perthane). *Arch. Int. Pharmacodyn. Ther.* **103**, 404–418.

Fischer, R. (1966). Toxic renal failure induced by the pesticide aldrin. *Muench. Med. Wochenschr.* **108**, 1379–1381 (in German).

Fiserova-Bergerova, V., Radomski, J. L., Davies, J. E., and Davies, J. H. (1967). Levels of chlorinated hydrocarbon pesticides in human tissues. *Ind. Med. Surg.* **36**, 65–70.

Fishbein, L. F. (1974). Chromatographic and biological aspects of DDT and its metabolites. *J. Chromatogr.* **98**, 177–251.

Fishbein, W. I., White, J. V., and Isaacs, H. J. (1964). Survey of workers exposed to chlordane. *Ind. Med. Surg.* **33**, 726–727.

Fisher, D. B., and Mueller, G. C. (1971). Gamma-hexachlorocyclohexane inhibits the initiation of lymphocyte growth by phytohemagglutinin. *Biochem. Pharmacol.* **20**, 2515–2518.

Fishman, B. E., and Gianutsos, G. (1985). Inhibition of 4-aminobutyric acid (GABA) turnover by chlordane. *Toxicol. Lett.* **26**, 219–223.

Fishman, B. E., and Gianutsos, G. (1987a). Differential effects of gamma-hexachlorocyclohexane (lindane) on pharmacologically-induced seizures. *Arch. Toxicol.* **59**, 397–401.

Fishman, B. E., and Gianutsos, G. (1987b). Opposite effects of hexachlorocyclohexane (lindane) isomers on cerebellar cyclic GMP: Relation of cyclic GMP accumulation to seizure activity. *Life Sci.* **41**, 1703–1709.

Fishman, B. E., and Gianutsos, G. (1988). CNS biochemical and pharmacological effects of the isomers of hexachlorocyclohexane (lindane) in the mouse. *Toxicol. Appl. Pharmacol.* **93**, 146–153.

Fitzhugh, O. G. (1948). Use of DDT insecticides on food products. *Ind. Eng. Chem.* **40**, 704–705.

Fitzhugh, O. G. (1970). A summary of a carcinogenic study of DDT in mice from Food and Drug Administration, USA. *In* "FAO/WHO 1969 Evaluations of Some Pesticide Residues in Foods," pp. 61–64. World Health Organ., Geneva.

Fitzhugh, O. G., and Nelson, A. A. (1947). The chronic oral toxicity of DDT (2,2-bis-*p*-chlorophenyl-1,1,1-trichloroethane). *J. Pharmacol. Exp. Ther.* **89**, 18–30.

Fitzhugh, O. G., and Nelson, A. A. (1951). Comparison of chronic effects produced in rats by several chlorinated hydrocarbon insecticides. *Fed. Proc., Fed. Am. Soc. Exp. Biol.* **10**, 295.

Fitzhugh, O. G., Nelson, A. A., and Frawley, J. P. (1950). The chronic toxicities of technical benzene hexachloride and its alpha, beta, and gamma isomers. *J. Pharmacol. Exp. Ther.* **100**, 59–66.

Fitzhugh, O. G., Nelson, A. A., and Quaife, M. L. (1964). Chronic oral toxicity of aldrin and dieldrin in rats and dogs. *Food Cosmet. Toxicol.* **2**, 551–562.

Fitzloff, J. F., and Pan, J. C. (1984). Epoxidation of the lindane metabolite, beta-PCCH, by human- and rat-liver microsomes. *Xenobiotica* **14**, 599–604.

Fitzloff, J. F., Portig, J., and Stein, K. (1982). Lindane metabolism by human and rat liver microsomes. *Xenobiotica* **12**, 197–202.

Fletcher, T. E., Press, J. M., and Wilson, D. B. (1959). Exposure of spraymen to dieldrin in residual spraying. *Bull. W. H. O.* **20**, 15–25.

Flodström, S., Wärngård, L., Hemming, H., Fransson, R., and Ahlborg, U. G. (1988). Tumour promotion related effects by the cyclodiene insecticide endosulfan studied in vitro and in vivo. *Pharmacol. Toxicol.* **62**, 230–235.

Focardi, S., Fossi, C., Leonzio, C., and Romei, R. (1986). PCB congeners, hexachlorobenzene, and organochlorine insecticides in human fat in Italy. *Bull. Environ. Contamin. Toxicol.* **36**, 644–650.

Fonseca, M. I., Aguilar, J. S., Lopez. C., Garcia Fernandez, J. C., and De Robertis, E. (1986). Regional effect of organochlorine insecticides on cholinergic muscarine receptors of rat brain. *Toxicol. Appl. Pharmacol.* **84**, 192–195.

Food and Agriculture Organization (FAO). (1972). "Production Yearbook—1971," Vol. 25, pp. 499–537. Food Agric. Organ., Rome.

Food and Agriculture Organization/World Health Organization (FAO/WHO) (1965). "Evaluation of the Toxicity of Pesticide Residues in Food," Monograph prepared by the Joint Meeting of the FAO Committee on Pesticides in Agriculture and the WHO Expert Committee on Pesticide Residues, which met in Rome, 15–22 March 1965, WHO/Food Add./27.65. Food Agric. Organ./World Health Organ., Rome.

Food and Agriculture Organization/World Health Organization (FAO/WHO) (1968). "1967 Evaluations of Some Pesticide Residues in Food," Monograph prepared by the Joint Meeting of the FAO Working Party of Experts on Pesticide Residues and the WHO Expert Committee on Pesticide Residues, which met in Rome, 4–11 December 1967, WHO/Food Add./68.30. Food Agric. Organ./World Health Organ., Rome.

Food and Agriculture Organization/World Health Organization (FAO/WHO) (1969). "1968 Evaluations of Some Pesticide Residues in Food," Monograph prepared by the Joint Meeting of the FAO Working Party of Experts on Pesticide Residues and the WHO Expert Committee on Pesticide Residues which met in Geneva, 9–16 December 1968, WHO/Food Add./69.35. Food Agric. Organ./World Health Organ., Geneva.

Food and Agriculture Organization/World Health Organization (FAO/WHO) (1971). "1970 Evaluations of Some Pesticide Residues in Food," Monograph prepared by the Joint Meeting of the FAO Working Party of Experts and the WHO Expert Group on Pesticide Residues which met in Rome, 9–16 November 1970, WHO/Food Add./71.42. Food Agric. Organ./World Health Organ., Rome.

Food and Agriculture Organization/World Health Organization (FAO/WHO) (1974). "1973 Evaluations of Some Pesticide Residues in Food," Monograph prepared by the Joint Meeting of the FAO Working Party of Experts on Pesticide Residues and the WHO Expert Committee on Pesticide Residues that met in Geneva from 26 November to 5 December 1973, WHO Pestic. Residues Ser., No. 3. Food Agric. Organ./World Health Organ., Geneva.

Food and Agriculture Organization/World Health Organization (FAO/WHO) (1985). "Pesticide Residues in Food —1984: Report of the Joint Meeting on Pesticide Residues, Rome, 24 September–30 October 1984," FAO Plant Prod. Prot. Pap. No. 62. Food Agric. Organ./World Health Organ., Rome.

Foster, T. S. (1968). Effect of some pesticides on the adrenal glands in the rat. *J. Biochem. (Tokyo)* **46**, 1115–1120.

Foster, T. S. (1973). Evaluation of the possible estrogenic activity of methoxychlor in the chicken by means of feeding trials. *Bull. Environ. Contamin. Toxicol.* **9**, 234–242.

Fournier, M., Bernier, J., Flipo, D., and Krzystyniak, K. (1986). Evaluation of pesticide effect on humoral response to sheep erythrocytes and mouse

hepatitis virus 3 by immunosorbent analysis. *Pestic. Biochem. Physiol.* **26**, 353–364.

Fouse, B. L., and Hodgson, E. (1987). Effects of chlordecone and mirex on the acute hepatotoxicity of acetaminophen in mice. *Gen. Pharmacol.* **18**, 623–630.

Fowler, B. A. (1972). The morphologic effects of dieldrin and methyl mercuric chloride on pars recta segment of rat kidney proximal tubules. *Am. J. Pathol.* **69**, 163–178.

Fox, G. R., and Virgo, B. B. (1985). The effects of phenobarbital, atropine, L-α-methyldopa, and DL-propranolol on dieldrin-induced hyperglycemia in the adult rat. *Toxicol Appl. Pharmacol.* **78**, 342–350.

Fox, G. R., and Virgo, B. B. (1986a). Relevance of hyperglycemia to dieldrin toxicity in suckling and adult rats. *Toxicology* **38**, 315–326.

Fox, G. R., and Birgo, B. B. (1986b). Effects of dieldrin on hepatic carbohydrate metabolism in the suckling and adult rat. *Can. J. Physiol. Pharmacol.* **64**, 694–698.

Francone, M. P., Mariani, F. H., and Demare, C. (1952). Clinical picture of intoxication by DDT. *Rev. Asoc. Med. Argent.* **6**, 56–59 (in Spanish).

Frank, R., and Braun, H. E. (1984). Lindane toxicity to four-month-old calves. *Bull. Environ. Contam. Toxicol.* **32**, 533–536.

Freal, J. J., and Chadwick, R. W. (1973). Metabolism of hexachlorocyclohexane to chlorophenols and effect of isomer pretreatment on lindane metabolism in rat. *J. Agric. Food Chem.* **21**, 424–427.

French, M. C., and Jefferies, D. J. (1968). Disappearance of gamma BHC from avian liver after death. *Nature (London)* **219**, 164–166.

French, M. C., and Jefferies, D. J. (1969). Degradation and disappearance of ortho, para isomer of technical DDT in living and dead avian tissues. *Science* **165**, 914–916.

Friberg, L., and Maartensson, J. (1953). Case of panmyelophthisis after exposure to cholorophenothane and benzene hexachloride. *Arch. Ind. Hyg. Occup. Med.* **8**, 166–169.

Friberg, R. D., and Dodson, V. N. (1966). Cytogenetic studies of rats injected with lindane. *Toxicol. Appl. Pharmacol.* **8**, 341.

Fries, G. F., Marrow, G. S., Jr., Gordon, C. H., Dryden, L. P., and Hartman, A. M. (1970). Effect of activated carbon on elimination of organochlorine pesticides from rats and cows. *J. Dairy Sci.* **53**, 1632–1637.

Fries, G. F., Marrow, G. S., Jr., Lester, J. W., and Gordon, C. H. (1971). Effects of microsomal enzyme inducing drugs on DDT and dieldrin elimination from cows. *J. Dairy Sci.* **54**, 364–368.

Frings, H., and O'Tousa, J. E. (1950). Toxicity to mice of chlordane vapor and solutions administered cutaneously. *Science* **111**, 658–660.

Frost, I., and Poulsen, E. (1959). Aldrin poisoning. *Ugeskr. Laeg.* **121**, 1406 (in Danish).

Fry, D. R. (1964). Human dieldrin poisoning. *Lancet* **1**, 764.

Fujimori, K., Benet, H., Mehendale, H. M., and Ho, I. K. (1982a). Comparison of brain discrete areas distributions of chlordecone and mirex in the mouse. *Neurotoxicology* **3** (2), 125–130.

Fujimori, K., Nabeshima, T., Ho, I. K., and Mehendale, H. M. (1982b). Effect of oral administration of chlordecone and mirex on brain biogenic amines in mice. *Neurotoxicology* **3** (2), 143–148.

Fukano, S., and Doguchi, M. (1977). PCT, BPC, and pesticide residues in human fat and blood. *Bull. Environ. Contam. Toxicol.* **17**, 613–617.

Fukushima, D. K., Bradlow, H. L., and Hellman, L. (1971). Effects of o,p'-DDD on cortisol and 6 beta-hydroxycortisol secretion and metabolism in man. *J. Clin. Endocrinol. Metab.* **32**, 192–200.

Fulfs, J. C., and Abraham, R. (1976). Effects of mirex and chloroquine on PCB-induced hepatic porphyria in the rat. *Toxicol. Appl. Pharmacol.* **37**, 119–120.

Fulfs, J. C., Abraham, R., and Coulston, F. (1975). Comparative ultrastructural and cytochemical studies in livers of mice, rats, and monkeys fed various levels of mirex. *Toxicol. Appl. Pharmacol.* **33**, 130–131.

Fuller, G. B., and Draper, S. W. (1975). Effect of mirex on induced ovulation in immature rats. *Proc. Soc. Exp. Biol. Med.* **148**, 414–417.

Fuller, G. B., Draper, S. W., and Gowdy, W. P. (1973). Effect of mirex on induced ovulation in immature rats. *J. Anim. Sci.* **36**, 211.

Furie, B., and Trubowitz, S. (1976). Insecticides and blood dyscrasias: Chlordane exposure and self-limited refractory megaloblastic anemia. *JAMA, J. Am. Med. Assoc.* **235**, 1720–1722.

Gabliks, J., Askari, E. M., and Yolen, N. (1973). DDT and immunological responses. I. Serum antibodies and anaphylactic shock in guinea pigs. *Arch. Environ. Health* **26**, 305–308.

Gabliks, J., Al-Zubaidy, T., and Askari, E. (1975). DDT and immunological responses. 3. Reduced anaphylaxis and mast cell populations in rats fed DDT. *Arch. Environ. Health* **30**, 81–84.

Gaines, T. B. (1960). The acute toxicity of pesticides to rats. *Toxicol. Appl. Pharmacol.* **2**, 88–99.

Gaines, T. B. (1969). Acute toxicity of pesticides. *Toxicol. Appl. Pharmacol.* **14**, 515–534.

Gaines, T. B., and Kimbrough, R. D. (1970). Oral toxicity of mirex in adult and suckling rats, with notes on the ultrastructure of liver changes. *Arch. Environ. Health* **21**, 7–14.

Galand, P., Mairesse, N., Degraef, C., and Rooryck, J. (1987). o,p'-DDT(1,1,1-trichloro-2(p-chlorophenyl)-2-(o-chlorophenyl)ethane is a purely estrogenic agonist in the rat uterus *in vivo* and *in vitro*. *Biochem. Pharmacol.* **36**, 397–400.

Galasinska-Pomykol, I., and Stefanska-Sulik, E. (1974). Morphological analysis of cells of the subthalamic nuclcus of guinea pigs treated with the pesticide "Alvit-55." *Med. Pr.* **25**, 27–37 (in Polish).

Galasinska-Pomykol, I., Tarmas, J., and Stefanska-Sulik, E. (1974). Morphological pattern of hypothalamic neurosecretory centers during convulsive state induced by pesticides. *Endokrynol. Pol.* **25**, 193–204 (in Polish).

Galigani, D., and Melis, R. (1958). Poisoning by synthetic insecticides. *Minerva Med.* **48**, 3753–3763 (in French).

Gallagher, T. F., Fukushima, D. K., and Hellmann, L. (1962). The effect of ortho, para' DDD on steroid hormone metabolites in adrenocortical carcinoma. *Metab., Clin. Exp.* **11**, 1155–1161.

Gandolfi, O., Cheney, D. C., Hong, J., and Costa, E. (1984). On the neurotoxicity of chlordecone: A role for γ-aminobutyric acid and serotonin. *Brain Res.* **303**, 117–123.

Gannon, N., Link, R. R., and Decker, G. C. (1959). Insecticide residues in the milk of dairy cows fed insecticides in their daily ration. *J. Agric. Food Chem.* **7**, 829–832.

Gardner, J. (1958). Pediculosis capitis in preschool and school children: Control with a shampoo containing gamma benzene hexachloride. *J. Pediatr.* **52**, 448–450.

Garg, A., Kunwar, K., Das, N., and Gupta, P. K. (1980). Endosulfan intoxication: Blood glucose, electrolytes, Ca levels, ascorbic acid and glutathione in rats. *Toxicol. Lett.* **5**, 119–123.

Garrett, R. M. (1947). Toxicity of DDT for man. *J. Med. Assoc. State Ala.* **17**, 74–76.

Garrettson, L. K., and Curley, A. (1969). Dieldrin: Studies in a poisoned child. *Arch. Environ. Health* **19**, 814–822.

Garrettson, L. K., Guzelian, P. S., and Blanke, R. V. (1985). Subacute chlordane poisoning. *J. Toxicol. Clin. Toxicol.* **22**, 565–571.

Gawhary, A. S. (1972). The effects of 2,2-bis(para-chloro-phenyl) 1,1-dichloroethane (DDD) on choline acetylase of the thymus gland. *Biochem. Pharmacol.* **21**, 887–890.

Gellert, R. J. (1978). Kepone, mirex, dieldrin, and aldrin: Estrogenic activity and the induction of persistent vaginal estrus and anovulation in rats following neonatal treatment. *Environ. Res.* **16**, 131–138.

Gellert, R. J., and Wilson, C. (1979). Reproductive function in rats exposed prenatally to pesticides and polychlorinated biphenyls (PCB). *Environ. Res.* **18**, 437–443.

Gellert, R. J., Heinrichs, W. L., and Swerdloff, R. S. (1972). DDT homologues: Estrogen-like effects on the vagina, uterus, and pituitary of the rat. *Endocrinology (Baltimore)* **91**, 1095–1100.

Genina, S. A., Svetlaja, E. N., and Komarova, L. I. (1969). Blood levels of organic chlorine pesticides and some hematological indicators in people employed in applying pesticides from the air. *In* "The Hygiene of Application and the Toxicology of Pesticides and the Clinical Features of Pesticide Poisoning. A Collection of Papers," Issue No. 7, pp. 492–496. Vniigintoks, Kiev (in Russian).

Georgian, I. (1975). The comparative cytogenic effects of aldrin and phosphamidon. *Mutat. Res.* **31**, 103–108.

Gerberg, E. J. (1973). Head lice: Control and nit removal. *Sci. Publ.—Pan Am. Health Organ.* **263**, 196–198.

Gerhart, J. M., Hong, J. L., Uphouse, L. L., and Tilson, H. A. (1982). Chordecone-induced tremor: Quantification and pharmacological analysis. *Toxicol Appl. Pharmacol.* **66**, 234–243.

Gerhart, J. M., Hong, J. L., and Tilson, H. A. (1983). Studies on the possible sites of chlordecone-induced tremor in rats. *Toxicol Appl. Pharmacol.* **70**, 382–389.

Gerhart, J. M., Hong, J. S., and Tilson, H. A. (1985). Studies on the mechanism of chordecone-induced tremor in rats. *Neurotoxicology* **61** (1),211–229.

Gertig, H., Nowaczyk, W., and Sawicka, B. (1971a). The effect of aldrin, dieldrin, lindane, DDT, DDD, and DDE on the activity of alkaline and acid phosphatase. *Diss. Pharm. Pharmacol.* **23**, 541–543.

Gertig, H., Nowaczyk, W., and Sierznat, M. (1971b). The effect of aldrin, dieldrin, lindane, DDT, DDD, and DDE on the activity of aspartate and alanine aminotransferase. *Diss. Pharm. Pharmacol.* **23**, 545–548.

Ghiasuddin, S. M., and Matsumura, F. (1979). DDT inhibition of Ca-ATPase of the peripheral nerves of the American lobster. *Pestic. Biochem. Physiol.* **10**, 151–161.

Gibson, J. R., Ivie, G. W., and Dorough, H. W. (1972). Fate of mirex and its major photodecomposition product in rats. *J. Agric. Food Chem.* **20**, 1246–1248.

Gil, G. P., and Miron, B. F. (1949). Investigations of intoxication by DDT in man. *Med. Colon.* **14**, 459–470 (in French).

Gillett, J. W. (1968). No effect level of DDT in induction of microsomal epoxidation. *J. Agric. Food Chem.* **16**, 295–297.

Gillett, J. W., and Chan, T. M. (1968). Cyclodiene insecticides as inducers, substrates and inhibitors of microsomal epoxidation. *J. Agric. Food Chem.* **16**, 590–593.

Gillett, J. W., Chan, T. M., and Terriere, L. C. (1966). Interactions between DDT analogs and microsomal epoxidase systems. *J. Agric. Food Chem.* **14**, 540–545.

Gingell, R., and Wallcave, L. (1974). Species differences in the acute toxicity and tissue distribution of DDT in mice and hamsters. *Toxicol. Appl. Pharmacol.* **28**, 385–394.

Ginsburg, C. M., and Lowry, W. (1983). Absorption of gamma benzene hexachloride following application of Karell shampoo. *Pediatr. Dermatol.* **1**, 74–76.

Ginsburg, C. M., Lowry, W., and Reisch, J. S. (1977). Absorption of lindane (gamma benzene hexachloride) in infants and children. *J. Pediatr.* **91**, 998–1000.

Glass, W. I. (1975). Dieldrin poisoning: Case report. *N. Z. Med. J.* **81**, 202–203.

Gleason, M. N., Gosselin, R. E., and Hodge, H. C. (1963). "Clinical Toxicology of Commercial Products: Acute Poisoning (Home and Farm)." Williams & Wilkins, Baltimore, Maryland.

Gold, B., and Brunk, G. (1982). Metabolism of 1,1,1-trichloro-2,2-bis(p-chlorophenyl)ethane and 1,1-dichloro-2,2-bis(p-chlorophenyl)ethane in the mouse. *Chem.-Biol. Interact.* **41**, 327–339.

Gold, B., and Brunk, G. (1983). Metabolism of 1,1,1-trichloro-2,2-bis(p-chlorophenyl)ethane (DDT), 1,1-dichloro-2,2-bis(p-chlorophenyl)ethane, and 1-chloro-2,2-bis(p-chlorophenyl)ethane in the hamster. *Cancer Res.* **43**, 2644–2647/

Gold, B., and Brunk, G. (1984). A mechanistic study of the metabolism of 1,1-dichloro-2,2-bis(p-chlorophenyl)ethane (DDD) to 2,2-bis(p-chlorophenyl)acetic acid (DDA). *Biochem. Pharmacol.* **33**, 979–982.

Gold, B., and Brunk, G. (1986). The effect of subchronic feeding of 1,1-dichloro-2,2-bis(4'-chlorophenyl)ethane (DDE) on its metabolism in mice. *Carcinogenesis (London)* **7**, 1149–1153.

Gold, B., Leuschen, T., Brunk, G., and Gingell, R. (1981). Metabolism of a DDT metabolite via chloroepoxide. *Chem.-Biol. Interact.* **35**, 159–176.

Goldman, J. M., Cooper, R. L., Rehnberg, G. L., Hein, J. F., McElroy, W. K., and Gray, L. E. (1986). Effect of low subchronic doses of methoxychlor on the rat hypothalamic–pituitary reproductive axis. *Toxicol. Appl. Pharmacol.* **86**, 474–483.

Goldman, M. (1981). The effect of a single dose of DDT on thyroid function in male rats. *Arch. Int. Pharmacodyn. Ther.* **252**, 327–334.

Good, E. E., and Ware, G. W. (1969). Effects of insecticides on reproduction in the laboratory mouse. IV. Endrin and dieldrin. *Toxicol. Appl. Pharmacol.* **14**, 201–203.

Good, E. E., Ware, G. W., and Miller, D. F. (1965). Effects of insecticides on reproduction in the laboratory mouse: Kepone. *J. Econ. Entomol.* **58**, 754–757.

Gopalaswamy, U. V., and Aiyar, A. S. (1984a). Biotransformation of lindane in the rat. *Bull. Environ. Contamin. Toxicol.* **32**, 148–156.

Gopalaswamy, U. V., and Aiyar, A. S. (1984b). Effects of lindane on liver mitochondrial funtion in the rat. *Bull. Environ. Contamin. Toxicol.* **33**, 106–113.

Gorbach, S. G., Christ, O. E., Kellner, H. M., Kloss, G., and Boerner, E. (1968). Metabolism of endosulfan in milk sheep. *J. Agric. Food Chem.* **16**, 950–953.

Gordienko, V. M., and Kozyritskiĭ, V. G. (1970). The effect of o,p'-dichlorodiphenyldichloroethane on the ultrastructure of cells of the anterior lobe of the hypophysis in dogs. *Arkh. Anat., Gistol. Embriol.* **58**, 49–57 (in Russian).

Gordienko, V. M., and Kozyritskiĭ, V. G. (1973). Alterations in the ultrastructure of the adrenal cortex of the dog after short-term and long-term administration of o,p'-DDD. *Arkh. Anat. Gistol. Embriol.* **65**, 90–95 (in Russian).

Gordienko, V. M., Bogomolets, Y. O., and Kozyritskiĭ, V. G. (1972). Electron microscopic study of the dog thyroid gland following administration of different doses of o,p'-dichlorodiphenyldichloroethane (o,p'-DDD). *Tsitol. Genet.* **6**, 392–394 (in Russian).

Gordienko, V. M., Kozyritskiĭ, V. G., and Drozdovich, I. I. (1973). Response of the hypothalamo-hypophyseal system in the development of hypocorticism. *Arkh. Anat. Gistol Embriol.* **65**, 62–68 (in Russian).

Gordon, H. T., and Welsh, J. H. (1948). The role of ions in axon surface reactions to toxic organic compounds. *J. Cell. Comp. Physiol.* **31**, 395–420.

Goto, M., Hattori, M., and Miyagama, T. (1972a). Contribution on ecological chemistry. Toxicity of alpha-BHC in mice. *Chemosphere* **1**, 153–154 (in German).

Goto, M., Hattori, M., Miyagama, T., and Enomoto, M. (1972b). Contribution on ecological chemistry. II. Hepatoma-formation in mice after administration of HCH-isomers in high doses. *Chemosphere* **1**, 279–282 (in German).

Goursaud, J., Luquet, F. M., and Casalis, J. (1971). Pesticide residue contamination of human milk in the northern province of France and Pas-de-Calais. *Lait* **51**, 559–567 (in French).

Gowdey, C. W., and Stavraky, G. W. (1955). A study of the autonomic manifestations seen in acute aldrin and dieldrin poisoning. *Can. J. Biochem. Physiol.* **33**, 272–282.

Gowdey, C. W., Graham, A. R., Seguin, J. J., and Stavraky, G. W. (1954). The pharmacological properties of the insecticide dieldrin. *Can. J. Biochem. Physiol.* **32**, 498–503.

Graboswki, C. T. (1981). The plasma proteins and colloid osmotic pressure of blood of rat fetuses prenatally exposed to mirex. *J. Toxicol. Environ. Health* **7**, 705–714.

Grabowski, C. T., and Payne, D. B. (1980). An electrocardiographic study of cardiovascular problems in mirex-fed rat fetuses. *Teratology* **22**, 167–177.

Grabowski, C. T., and Payne, D. B. (1983a). The causes of perinatal exposure of rats to the pesticide mirex. Part 1. Pre-parturition observations of the cardiovascular system. *Teratology* **27**, 7–11.

Grabowski, C. T., and Payne, D. B. (1983b). The causes of perinatal death induced by prenatal exposure of rats to the pesticide mirex. Part II. Postnatal observations. *J. Toxicol. Environ. Health* **11**, 301–315.

Graca, I., Silva Fernandes, A. M. S., and Maurao, H. C. (1974). Organochlorine insecticide residues in human milk in Portugal. *Pestic. Monit. J.* **8**, 148–156.

Gracheva, G. V. (1969). The possibility of DDT accumulation in the organism of persons not having occupational contact with it. *Faktory Vneshn. Sred. Ikh Znach. Zdorov'ya Naseleniya* **1**, 125–129 (in Russian).

Gracheva, G. V. (1970). DDT excretion with the milk of nursing mothers occupationally unexposed to the effect of this insecticide. *Vopr. Pitan.* **29**, 75–78 (in Russian).

Graeve, K., and Herrnring, G. (1951). On the toxicity of gamma-hexachlorocyclohexane. *Arch. Int. Pharmacodyn. Ther.* **85**, 64–72 (in German).

Graillot, C., Gak, J.-C., Lancret, C., and Truhaut, R. (1975). Investigations on the states and mechanisms of toxic action of organochlorine insecticides. II. Study on the long-term toxic effects of DDT in the hamster. *Eur. J. Toxicol.* **8**, 353–359 (in French).

Grant, E. L., Mitchell, R. H., West, P. R., Mazuch, L., and Ashwood-Smith, M. J. (1976). Mutagenicity and putative carcinogenicity tests of several polycyclic aromatic compounds associated with impurities of the insecticide methoxychlor. *Mutat. Res.* **40**, 225–228.

Gray, L. E. (1982). Neonatal chlordecone exposure alters behavioural sex differentiation in female hamsters. *Neurotoxicology* **3** (2),67–80.

Gray, L. E., Jr., Kavlock, R., Chernoff, N., Lawton, D., and Gray, J. (1979). The effects of endrin administration during gestation on the behavior of the golden hamster. *Toxicol. Appl. Pharmacol.* **48**, A200.

Gray, L. E., Ostby, J., Ferrell, J., Rehnberg, G., Linder, R., Cooper, R., Goldman, J., Slott, V., and Laskey, J. (1989). A dose response analysis of methoxychlor-induced alterations of reproductive development and function in the rat. *Fundam. Appl. Toxicol.,* **12**, 92–108.

Greene, F. E., Stevens, J. T., Soliman, M. R. I., and Oberholser, K. A. (1974). Effects of perinatal dieldrin exposure on hepatic microsomal enzymes of immature and adult rats. *Toxicol. Appl. Pharmacol.* **29**, 128.

Greer, E. S., Miller, D. J., Bruscato, F. N., and Holt, R. L. (1980). Investigation of pesticide residues in human adipose tissue in the northeast Louisiana area. *J. Agric. Food Chem.* **28**, 76–78.

Griffith, F. D., Jr., and Blanke, R. V. (1975). Pesticides in people. Blood organochlorine pesticide levels in Virginia residents. *Pestic. Monit. J.* **8**, 219–224.

Grover, P. L., and Sims, P. (1965). The metabolism of α-2,3,4,5,6-pentachlorocyclohex-1-ene and γ-hexachlorocyclohexane in rats. *Biochem. J.* **96**, 521–525.

Gruffydd-Jones, T. J., Evans, R. J., Brown, P., and Sullivan, K. (1981). Dieldrin poisoning of cats after woodworm treatment. *Vet. Rec.* **108**, 540.

Grzycki, S., and Zarebska, A. (1973). Histoenzymatic studies on the liver cell after the administration of gamma-benzene hexachloride (lindane). *Z. Mikrosk.-Anat. Forsch.* **87**, 470–476 (in German).

Grzycki, S., Czerny, K., and Zarebska, A. (1973). Studies on the functional topography of the hydrolytic enzymes in the epithelium of the convoluted renal tubules. *Acta Histochem.* **47**, 350–357 (in German).

Gulko, A. G., Zimnitsa, N. I., Diskalenko, A. P., Chernokan, V. F., and Bubucha, V. F. (1978). Pesticide carriers among certain population groups of Moldavia. *Gig. Sanit.* **43**, 36–41 (in Russian).

Gupta, P. C. (1975). Neurotoxicity of chronic chlorinated hydrocarbon insecticide poisoning—a clinical and electro-encephalographic study in man. *Indian J. Med. Res.* **63**, 601–605.

Gupta, P. K. (1976). Endosulfan-induced neurotoxicity in rats and mice. *Bull. Environ. Contam. Toxicol.* **15**, 708–713.

Gupta, P. K. (1978). Distribution of endosulfan in plasma and brain after repeated oral administration to rats. *Toxicology* **9**, 371–377.

Gupta, P. K., and Chandra, S. V. (1975). The toxicity of endosulfan in rabbits. *Bull. Environ. Contam. Toxicol.* **14**, 513–519.

Gupta, P. K., and Chandra, S. V. (1977). Toxicity of endosulfan after repeated oral administration to rats. *Bull. Environ. Contam. Toxicol.* **18**, 378–384.

Gupta, P. K., and Ehrnebo, M. (1979). Pharmacokinetics of α- and β-isomers of racemic endosulfan following intravenous administration in rabbits. *Drug Metab. Dispos.* **7**, 7–10.

Gupta, P. K., and Gupta, R. C. (1977). Effect of endosulfan pretreatment on organ weights and on pentobarbital hypnosis in rats. *Toxicology* **7**, 283–288.

Gupta, P. K., Chandra, S. V., and Saxena, D. K. (1978). Teratogenic and embryotoxic effects of endosulfan in rats. *Acta Pharmacol. Toxicol.* **42**, 150–152.

Gutierrez, M. L., and Crooke, S. T. (1980). Mitotane (o,p'-DDD) *Cancer Treat. Rev.* **7**, 49–55.

Guzelian, P. S. (1981). Therapeutic approaches for chlordecone poisoning in humans. *J. Toxicol. Environ. Health* **8**, 757–766.

Guzelian, P. S. (1982a). Chlordecone poisoning: A case study in approaches for the detoxification of humans exposed to environmental chemicals. *Drug Metab. Rev.* **13**, 663–679.

Guzelian, P. S. (1982b). Comparative toxicology of chlordecone (Kepone) in humans and experimental animals. *Annu. Rev. Pharmacol. Toxicol.* **22**, 89–113.

Guzelian, P. S. (1984). New approaches for treatment of humans exposed to a slowly excreted environmental chemical (chlordecone). *Z. Gastroenterol.* **22**, 16–20 (in German).

Guzelian, P. S. (1985). Clinical evaluation of liver structure and function in humans exposed to halogenated hydrocarbons. *Environ. Health Perspect.* **60**, 159–164.

Guzelian, P. S., Vranian, G., Boylan, J. J., Cohn, W. J., and Blanke, R. V. (1980). Liver structure and function in patients poisoned with chlordecone (Kepone). *Gastroenterology* **78**, 206–213.

Haag, H. B., Finnegan, J. K., Larson, P. S., Dreyfuss, M. L., Main, R. J., and Riese, W. (1948). Comparative chronic toxicity for warm-blooded animals of 2,2-bis-(p-chlorophenyl)-1,1,1-trichloroethane (DDT) and 2,2-bis-(p-chlorophenyl)-1,1-dichloroethane (DDD). *Ind. Med. Surg.* **17**, 477–484.

Hajjar, R. A., Hickey, R. C., and Samoan, N. A. (1975). Adrenal cortical carcinoma: A study of 32 patients. *Cancer (Philadelphia)* **35**, 549–554.

Halacka, K., Kaki, J., and Vymetal, F. (1965). A reflection in human fat tissue of the extensive use of DDT. *Czech. Hyg.* **10**, 188–192 (in Czech).

Hall, E. T. (1974). An apparent case of chlordane poisoning. *Bull. Environ. Contamin. Toxicol.* **12**, 555–561.

Hallett, D. J., Khera, K. S., Stoltz, D. R., Chu, I., Villeneuve, D. C., and Trivett, G. (1978). Photomirex: Synthesis and assessment of acute toxicity, tissue distribution, and mutagenicity. *J. Agric. Food Chem.* **26**, 288–291.

Halmi, K. A., and Lascari, A. D. (1971). Conversion of virilization to feminization in a young girl with adrenal cortical carcinoma. *Cancer (Philadelphia)* **27**, 931–935.

Halpern, L. K., Woolridge, W. E., and Weiss, R. S. (1950). Appraisal of the toxicity of the gamma isomer of hexachlorocyclohexane in clinical usage. *Arch. Dermatol. Syphilol.* **62**, 648–650.

Hamid, J., Sayeed, A., and McFarlane, H. (1974). The effect of 1-(0-chlorophenyl)-1-(p-chlorophenyl)-2,2-dichloroethane (o,p'-DDD) on the immune response in malnutrition. *Bri. J. Exp. Pathol.* **55**, 94–100.

Hamilton, H. E., Morgan, D. P., and Simmons, A. (1978). A pesticide (dieldrin)-induced immunohemolytic anemia. *Environ. Res.* **17**, 155–164.

Hammond, B., Bahr, J., Dial, O., McConnel, J., and Metcalf, R. (1978). Reproductive toxicology of mirex and Kepone. *Fed. Proc., Fed. Am. Soc. Exp. Biol.* **37**, 501.

Hammond, B., Katyzenellenbogen, B. S., Krauthammer, N., and McConnell, J. (1979). Estrogenic activity of the insecticide chlordecone (Kepone) and interaction with uterine estrogen receptors. *Proc. Natl. Acad. Sci. U.S.A.* **76**, 6641–6645.

Hanada, M., Yutani, C., and Miyaji, T. (1973). Induction of hepatoma in mice by benzene hexachloride. *Gann* **64**, 511–513.

HANES II (1980). "Health and Nutrition Examination Survey II: Laboratory Findings of Pesticide Residues, National Survey." U.S. Environ. Prot. Agency. Washington, D.C.

Hanig, J. P., Yoder, P. D., and Krop, S. (1976). Convulsions in weanling rabbits after a single topical application of 1% lindane. *Toxicol. Appl. Pharmacol.* **38**, 463–469.

Hansell, M. M., and Ecobichon, D. J. (1975). The morphological effects of maternally administered phenobarbital and DDT on hepatic cell structure in young rats. *Toxicol. Appl. Pharmacol.* **33**, 144.

Hara, A., Iwasaki, I., Nawa, H., Yoshioka, Y., and Yokoo, S. (1973). Organochlorine insecticide residues in the blood of pregnant women and in umbilical cord blood. *Igaku no Ayumi* **84**, 79–80 (in Japanese).

Harbison, R. B. (1973). DDT, heptachlor, chlordane, and parathion toxicity in adult, newborn, and phenobarbital-treated newborn rats. *Toxicol. Appl. Pharmacol.* **25**, 472–473.

Harell, M., Shea, J. J., and Emmett, J. R. (1978). Bilateral sudden deafness following combined insecticide poisoning. *Laryngoscope* **88**, 1348–1351.

Harr, J. R., Claeys, R. R., Bone, J. R., and McCorde, T. W. (1970a). Dieldrin toxicosis: Rat production. *Am. J. Vet. Res.* **31**, 181–189.

Harr, J. R., Claeys, R. R., and Benedict, N. (1970b). Dieldrin toxicosis in rats: Long-term study of brain and vascular effects. *Am. J. Vet. Res.* **31**, 1853–1862.

Harrington, J. M., Baker, E. L., Jr., Folland, D. S., Saucier, J. W., and Sandifer, S. H. (1978). Chlordane contamination of a municipal water system. *Environ. Res.* **15**, 155–159.

Harris, C. J., Williford, E. A., Kemberling, S. R., and Morgan, D. P. (1969). Pesticide intoxications in Arizona. *Ariz. Med.* **26**, 872–876.

Harris, S. J., Cecil, H. C., and Bitman, J. (1974). Effect of several dietary levels of technical methoxychlor on reproduction in rats. *J. Agric. Food Chem.* **22**, 969–973.

Harrison, J. H., Mahoney, E. M., and Bennett, A. H. (1973). Tumors of the adrenal cortex. *Cancer (Philadelphia)* **32**, 1227–1235.

Harrison, M. A., Nicholls, T. J., and Rousseaux, C. G. (1980). Lindane toxicity in lambs. *Aust. Vet. J.* **56**, 42.

Harrison, R. D. (1975). Comparative toxicity of some selected pesticides in neonatal and adult rats. *Toxicol. Appl. Pharmacol.* **32**, 443–446.

Hart, M. M., and Straw, J. A. (1971a). Effects of 1-(o-chlorophenyl)-1-(p-chlorophenyl)-2,2-dichloroethane and puromycin on adrenocorticotropic hormone-induced steroidogenesis and on amino acid incorporation in slices of dog adrenal cortex. *Biochem. Pharmacol.* **20**, 257–263.

Hart, M. M., and Straw, J. A. (1971b). Studies on the site of action of o,p'-DDD in the dog adrenal cortex. I. Inhibition of ACTH-mediated pregnenolone synthesis. *Steroids* **17**, 559–574.

Hart, M. M., and Straw, J. A. (1971c). Effect of 1-(o-chlorophenyl)-1-(p-chlorophenyl)-2,2-dichloroethane. *Biochem. Pharmacol.* **20**, 1679–1688.

Hart, M. M., and Straw, J. A. (1971d). Effect of 1-(o-chlorophenyl)-1-(p-chlorophenyl)-2,2-dichloroethane *in vivo* on baseline and adrenocorticotrophic hormone-induced steroid production in dog adrenal slices. *Biochem. Pharmacol.* **20**, 1689–1691.

Hart, M. M., Regan. R. L., and Adamson, R. H. (1973). The effect of isomers of DDD on the ACTH-induced steroid output, histology, and ultrastructure of the dog adrenal cortex. *Toxicol. Appl. Pharmacol.* **24**, 101–113.

Hartgrove, R. W., Jr., Petrella, V. J., and Webb, R. E. (1972). Microsomal activity in endrin susceptible and resistant pine mice. *Toxicol. Appl. Pharmacol.* **22**, 298.

Hartgrove, R. W., Jr., Hundley, S. G., and Webb, R. E. (1974). Comparative inductive effects of phenobarbital and endrin on liver microsomal activity in endrin-resistant and susceptible pine voles. *Toxicol. Appl. Pharmacol.* **29**, 92.

Hartgrove, R. W., Jr., Hundley, S. G., and Webb, R. E. (1977). Characterization of the hepatic mixed function oxidase system in endrin-resistant and -susceptible pine voles. *Pestic. Biochem. Physiol.* **7**, 146–153.

Hartwig, W., Massalski, W., Kasperlik-Zaluska, A., Migdalska, B., Szamatowics, M., and Jakowicki, J. (1968). Hormonally active carcinoma of the adrenal cortex treated with o,p'-DDD. *Endokrynol. Pol.* **19**, 57–69 (in Polish).

Hashemy-Tonkabony, S. E., and Fateminassab, F. (1977). Chlorinated pesticide residues in milk of Iranian nursing mothers. *J. Dairy Sci.* **60**, 1858–1860.

Hashemy-Tonkabony, S. E., and Soleimani-Amin, M. J. (1978). Chlorinated pesticide residues in the bodyfat of people of Iran. *Environ. Res.* **16**, 419–422.

Hassall, K. A. (1971). Reductive dechlorination of DDT: The effect of some physical and chemical agents on DDD production by pigeon liver preparations. *Pestic. Biochem. Physiol.* **1**, 259–266.

Hathway, D. E., and Mallinson, A. (1964). Chemical studies in relation to convulsive conditions. Effect of Telodrin on the liberation and utilization of ammonia in rat brain. *Biochem. J.* **90**, 51–60.

Hathway, D. E., Mallinson, A., and Akintonwa, D. A. A. (1965). Effects of dieldrin, picrotoxin and Telodrin on the metabolism of ammonia in brain. *Biochem. J.* **94**, 676–686.

Hattula, M. L., Ikkala, J., Isomaki, M., Maatta, K., and Arstila, A. U. (1976). Chlorinated hydrocarbon residues (PCB and DDT) in human liver, adipose tissue, and brain in Finland. *Acta Pharmacol. Toxicol.* **39**, 545–554.

Haun, E. C., and Cueto, C., Jr. (1967). Fatal toxaphene poisoning in a 9-month-old child. *Am. J. Dis. Child.* **113**, 616–618.

Havkin-Frenkel, D., Rosen, J. D., and Gallo, M. A. (1983). Enhancement of hydroxyradical formation in rat liver microsomes by mirex. *Toxicol. Lett.* **15**, 219–223.

Hayashi, M. (1972a). Pollution of mothers' milk by organochlorine pesticides. *Jpn. J. Public Health* **19**, 437–441 (in Japanese).

Hayashi, M. (1972b). Pesticide pollution of mother's milk. *J. Jpn. Med. Assoc.* **68**, 1281–1286 (in Japanese).

Hayashi, M. (1973). Pollution of mothers' milk by organochlorine compounds. *Pediatrics* **14**, 527–531.

Hayashyi, M. (1974). Mothers' milk and environmental pollution. *J. Pediatr. Pract.* **37**, 1113–1119.

Hayden, M. J., Muelling, R. J., Noonan, J. A., and Bosomworth, P. P. (1965). A report of endrin poisoning. *J. Ky. Med. Assoc.* **63**, 33–34.

Hayes, W. J., Jr. (1957). Dieldrin poisoning in man. *Public Health Rep.* **72**, 1087–1091.

Hayes, W. J., Jr. (1959a). Pharmacology and toxicology of DDT. *In* "DDT: The Insecticide Dichlorodiphenyl-Trichloroethane and Its Significance" (P. Müller, ed.), Vol. 2, pp. 9–247. Birkhaeuser, Basel.

Hayes, W. J., Jr. (1959b). The toxicity of dieldrin to man. *Bull. W. H. O.* **20**, 891–912.

Hayes, W. J., Jr. (1963). "Clinical Handbook on Economic Poisons: Emergency Information for Treating Poisoning," Public Health Serv. Publ. No. 476. U.S. Gov. Printing Office, Washington, D.C.

Hayes, W. J., Jr. (1965). Review of the metabolism of chlorinated hydrocarbon insecticides especially in mammals. *Annu. Rev. Pharmacol.* **5**, 27–52.

Hayes, W. J., Jr. (1969). Sweden bans DDT. *Arch. Environ. Health* **18**, 872.

Hayes, W. J., Jr. (1974). Distribution of dieldrin following a single oral dose. *Toxicol. Appl. Pharmacol.* **28**, 485–492.

Hayes, W. J., Jr. (1975). "Toxicology of Pesticides." Williams & Wilkins, Baltimore, Maryland.

Hayes, W. J., Jr. (1976a). Mortality in 1969 from pesticides, including aerosols. *Arch. Environ. Health* **31**, 61–72.

Hayes, W. J., Jr. (1976b). Dosage relationships associated with DDT in milk. *Toxicol. Appl. Pharmacol.* **38**, 19–28.

Hayes, W. J., Jr., and Curley, A. (1968). Storage and excretion of dieldrin and related compounds. *Arch. Environ. Health* **16**, 155–162.

Hayes, W. J., Jr., and Vaughn, W. K. (1977). Mortality from pesticides in the United States in 1973 and 1974. *Toxicol. Appl. Pharmacol.* **42**, 235–252.

Hayes, W. J., Jr., Ferguson, F. F., and Cass, J. S. (1951). The toxicology of dieldrin and its bearing on field use of the compound. *J. Trop. Med.* **31**, 519–522.

Hayes, W. J., Jr., Durham, W. F., and Cueto, C., Jr. (1956). The effect of known repeated oral doses of chlorophenothane (DDT) in man. *JAMA, J. Am. Med. Assoc.* **162**, 890–897.

Hayes, W. J., Jr., Quinby, G. E., Walker, K. C., Elliott, J. W., and Upholt, W. M. (1958). Storage of DDT and DDE in people with different degrees of exposure to DDT. *AMA Arch. Ind. Health* **18**, 398–406.

Hayes, W. J., Jr., Dale, W. E., and LeBreton, R. (1963). Storage of insecticides in French people. *Nature (London)* **199**, 1189–1191.

Hayes, W. J., Jr., Dale, W. E., and Burse, V. W. (1965). Chlorinated hydrocarbon pesticides in the fat of people in New Orleans. *Life Sci.* **4**, 1611–1615.

Hayes, W. J., Jr., Dale, W. E., and Pirkle, C. I. (1971). Evidence of safety of long-term, high, oral doses of DDT for man. *Arch. Environ. Health* **22**, 119–135.

Heath, D. F., and Vandekar, M. (1964). Toxicity and metabolism of dieldrin in rats. *Br. J. Ind. Med.* **21**, 269–279.

Hedde, R. D., Davison, K. L., and Robbins, J. D. (1970). Dieldrin-14-C metabolism in sheep: Distribution and isolation of urinary metabolites. *J. Agric. Food Chem.* **18**, 116–119.

Hegarty, J. M., Glende, F. A., and Recknagel, R. O. (1986). Potentiation by chlordecone of the defect in hepatic microsomal calcium sequestration induced by carbon tetrachloride. *J. Biochem. Toxicol.* **1** (2),73–78.

Hegyi, E., and Stota, Z. (1962). The nature of the allergen in the manufacture of hexachlorocyclohexane. *J. Invest. Dermatol.* **38**, 111–113.

Heiberg, O. M., and Wright, H. N. (1955). Benzene hexachloride poisoning. *AMA Arch. Ind. Health* **11**, 457–458.

Heinevetter, D., Lewerenz, H. J., Plass, R., and Macholz, R. (1984). Comparative studies on the effect of hexachlorocyclohexane (HCH) and HCH metabolites on ATPases in rats and mice. *Z. Gesamte Hyg. Ihre Grenzgeb.* **30**, 576–579 (in German).

Heinevetter, D., Lewerenz, H. J., Plass, R., and Macholz, R. (1985). Effect of lindane and lindane metabolites on microsomal and mitochondrial ATPases in vitro. *J. Environ. Sci. Health, Part B* **20**, 539–558.

Heinricks, W. J., Gellert, R. J., Bakke, J. L., and Lawrence, N. L. (1971). DDT administered to neonatal rats induces persistent estrus syndrome. *Science* **173**, 642–643.

Hellman, L., Bradlow, H. L., and Zumoff, B. (1973). Decreased conversion of androgens to normal 17-ketosteroid metabolites as a result of treatment with *o,p'*-DDD. *J. Clin. Endocrinol. Metab.* **36**, 801–803.

Helson, L., Wollner, N., Murphy, L., and Schwartz, M. K. (1971). Metastatic adrenal cortical carcinoma: Biochemical changes accompanying clinical regression during therapy with *o,p'*-DDD. *Clin. Chem. (Winston-Salem, N.C.)* **17**, 1191–1193.

Henderson, G. L., and Woolley, D. E. (1969). Tissue concentrations of DDT: Correlation with neurotoxicity in young and adult rats. *Proc. West. Pharmacol. Soc.* **12**, 58–62.

Henderson, G. L., and Woolley, D. E. (1970). Mechanisms of neurotoxic action of 1,1,1-trichloro-2,2-bis-(*p*-chlorophenyl)-ethane (DDT) in immature and adult rats. *J. Pharmacol. Exp. Ther.* **175**, 60–68.

Hendrickson, C. M., and Bowden, J. A. (1975). The *in vitro* inhibition of rabbit muscle lactate dehydrogenase by mirex and Kepone. *J. Agric. Food Chem.* **23**, 407–409.

Herbst, M., Weisse, I., and Koellmer, H. (1975). A contribution to the question of the possible hepatocarcinogenic effects of lindane. *Toxicology* **4**, 91–96.

Herken, H., and Klempau, I. (1950). Neurotropic effects of some hexachlorocyclohexanes. *Naturwissenschaften* **37**, 493–494 (in German).

Herken, H., Kewitz, H., and Klempau, I. (1952a). Loss of effect of poison-induced seizures by hexachlorocyclohexane. *Naunyn-Schmiedebergs Arch. Exp. Pathol. Pharmakol.* **215**, 217–230 (in German).

Herken, H., Monnier, M., Coper, H., and Laue, H. (1952b). Inhibition of subcortical seizure potential caused by β-hexachlorocyclohexane. *Experientia* **8**, 432–434 (in German).

Herman, P., Jacobs, M., Hughes, G., Smith, B., McClintock, B., Farrar, W., and Holder, W. (1975). Scabies—Florida, New Mexico. *Morbid. Mortal. Wkly. Rep.* **24**, 118–123.

Herr, D. W. and Tilson, H. A. (1987). Modulation of p,p'-DDT-induced tremor by catecholaminergic agents. *Toxicol. Appl. Pharmacol.* **91**, 149–158.

Herr, D. W., Hong, J. S., and Tilson, H. A. (1985). DDT-induced tremor in rats: Effects of pharmacological agents. *Psychopharmacology* **86**, 426–431.

Herr, D. W., Hong, J. S., Chen, P., Tilson, H., and Harry, G. J. (1986). Pharmacological modification of DDT-induced tremor and hyperthermia in rat: Distributional factors. *Psychopharmacology* **89**, 278–283.

Herr, D. W., Gallus, J. A., and Tilson, H. A. (1987). Pharmacological modification of tremor and enhanced acoustic startle by chlordecone and p,p'-DDT. *Psycopharmacology* **91**, 320–325.

Herr, D. W., Mailman, R. B., and Tilson, H. A. (1989). Blockade of only spinal α-adrenoceptors is insufficient to attenuate DDT-induced alterations in motor function. *Toxicol. Appl. Pharmacol.* **101**, 11–26.

Herrera-Marteache, A, Polo Villar, L. M., Jodral Villarejo, M., Pollo Villar, G., Mallor, J., and Pozo Lora, R. (1978). Organochlorine pesticides residues in human fat in Spain. *Rev. Sanid. Hig. Publica* **52**, 1125–1144 (in Spanish).

Hesse, V., Gabrio, T., Kirst, E., and Plenert, W. (1981). Investigation of the contamination of women's milk, cow milk and butter in the DDR with chlorinated hydrocarbons. *Koinderarzth. Prax.* **49**, 292 (in German).

Hewitt, W. R., Miyajima, H., Cote, M., and Plaa, G. L. (1979). Acute alteration of chloroform-induced hepato- and nephrotoxicity by mirex and Kepone. *Toxicol. Appl. Pharmacol.* **48**, 509–527.

Heyndrickx, A., and Maes, R. (1969). The excretion of chlorinated hydrocarbon insecticides in human mother milk. *J. Pharm. Belg.* **9–10**, 459–463.

Hidaka, K., Ohe, T., and Fujiwara, K. (1972). PCB and organochlorine pesticides in mother's milk. *Igaku no Ayumi* **82**, 519–520 (in Japanese).

Higginson, J. (1985). DDT: Epidemiological evidence. *IARC Sci. Publ.* **65**, 101–105.

Hirasawa, F. and Takizawa, Y. (1989). Accumulation and declination of chlordane congeners in mice. *Toxicol Lett.* **47**, 109–117.

Ho, I. K., Fujimori, K., Huang, T. P., and Chang-Tusi, H. (1981). Neurochemical evaluation of chlordecone toxicity in the mouse. *J. Toxicol. Environ. Health* **8**, 701–706.

Hochleitner, H. (1973). The epidemiology, clinics and treatment of scabies. *Wien. Klin. Wochenschr.* **85**, 197–202 (in German).

Hodge, H. C., Maynard, E. A., Thomas, J. F., Blanchet, H. J., Jr., Wilt, W. G., Jr., and Mason, K. E. (1950). Short-term oral toxicity tests of methoxychlor (2,2-di(*p*-methoxyphenyl)-1,1,1-trichloroethane) in rats and dogs. *J. Pharmacol. Exp. Ther.* **99**, 140–148.

Hodge, H. C., Maynard, E. A., and Blanchet, H. J., Jr. (1952). Chronic oral toxicity tests of methoxychlor (2,2-di-(*p*-methoxyphenyl)-1,1,1-trichloroethane) in rats and dogs. *J. Pharmacol. Exp. Ther.* **104**, 60–66.

Hodge, H. C., Maynard, E. A., Downs, W. L., Ashton, J. K., and Salerno, L. L. (1966). Tests on mice for evaluating carcinogenicity. *Toxicol. Appl. Pharmacol.* **9**, 583–596.

Hoffman, D. G., Worth, H. M., Emmerson, J. L., and Anderson, R. C. (1970). Stimulation of hepatic drug-metabolizing enzymes by chlorophenothane (DDT): The relationship to liver enlargement and hepatotoxicity in the rat. *Toxicol Appl. Pharmacol.* **16**, 171–178.

Hoffman, D. L., and Mattox, V. R. (1972). Treatment of adrenocortical carcinoma with *o,p'*-DDD. *Med. Clin. North Am.* **56**, 999–1012.

Hoffman, I., and Lendle, L. (1948). The mode of action of a new insecticide. *Naunyn-Sohmiedebergs Arch. Exp. Pathol. Pharmakol.* **205**, 223–242 (in German).

Hoffman, W. S., Fishbein, W. I., and Andelman, M. B. (1964). The pesticide content of human fat tissue. *Arch. Environ. Health* **9**, 387–394.

Hoffman, W. S., Adler, H., Fishbein, W. I., and Bauer, F. C. (1967). Relation of pesticide concentration in fat to pathological changes in tissues. *Arch. Environ. Health* **15**, 758–765.

Hoffman, R., Erzberger, P., Frank, W., and Ristow, H. (1980). Increased phosphatidylinositol synthesis in rat embryo fibroblasts after growth stimulation and its inhibition by δ-hexachlorocyclohexane. *Biochim. Biophys. Acta* **618**, 282–292.

Hofvander, Y., Hagman, U., Linder, C. E., Vaz, R., and Slorach, S. A. (1981). WHO collaborative breast feeding study. I. Organochlorine contaminants in individual samples of Swedish human milk, 1978–1979. *Acta Paediatr. Scand.* **70**, 3–8.

Hokin, M. R., and Brown, D. F. (1969). Inhibition by gamma-hexachlorocyclohexane of acetylcholine-stimulated phosphatidylinositol synthesis in cerebral cortex slices and of phosphatidic acid–inositol transferase in cerebral cortex particulate fractions. *J. Neurochem.* **16**, 475–483.

Holian, A., Marchiarullo, M. A., and Stickle, D. F. (1984). γ-Hexachlorocyclohexane activation of alveolar macrophage phosphatidylinositol cycle, calcium mobilization and O_2^- production. *FEBS Lett.* **176**, 151–154.

Holmstead, R. L., Khalifa, S., and Casida, J. E. (1974). Toxaphene composition analyzed by combined gas chromatography–chemical-ionization mass spectrometry. *J. Agric. Food Chem.* **22**, 939–944.

Hong, J. S., and Ali, S. F. (1982). Chlordecone (Kepone®) exposure in the neonate selectively alters brain and pituitary endorphin levels in prepubertal and adult rats. *Neurotoxicology* **3** (2),111–117.

Hong, J. S., Tilson, H. A., Uphouse, L. L., Gerhart, J., and Wilson, W. E. (1984). Effects of chlordecone exposure on brain neurotransmitters: Possible involvement of the serotonin system in chlordecone-elicited tremor. *Toxicol. Appl. Pharmacol.* **73**, 336–344.

Hong, J. S., Hudson, P. M., Yoshikawa, K., Ali, S. F., and Mason, G. A. (1985). Effect of chlordecone administration on brain and pituitary peptide systems. *Neurotoxicology* **6** (1),167–182.

Hong, J. S., Herr, D. W., Hudson, P. M., and Tilson, H. A. (1986). Neurochemical effects of DDT in rat brain in vivo. *Arch. Toxicol., Suppl.* **9**, 14–26.

Hoogendam, I., Versteeg, J. P. J., and de Vlieger, M. (1962). Electroencephalograms in insecticide toxicity. *Arch. Environ. Health* **40**, 86–94.

Hoogendam, I., Versteeg, J. P. J., and de Vlieger, M. (1965). Nine years' toxicity control in insecticide plants. *Arch. Environ. Health* **10**, 441–448.

Hooper, N. K., Ames, B. N., Saleh, M. A., and Casida, J. E. (1979). Toxaphene, a complex mixture of polychloroterpenes and a major insecticide, is mutagenic. *Science* **205**, 591–593.

Hori, S., and Kashimoto, T. (1974). Transfer of beta-BHC from mother to suckling mouse. *J. Food Hyg. Soc. Jpn.* **15**, 446–450 (in Japanese).

Horn, H. J., Bruce, R. B., and Paynter, O. E. (1955). Toxicology of chlorobenzilate. *J. Agric. Food Chem.* **3**, 752–756.

Hornabrook, R. W., Dyment, P. G., Gomes, E. D., and Wiseman, J. S. (1972). DDT residues in human milk from New Guinea natives. *Med. J. Aust.* **1**, 1297–1300.

Hoskins, B., and Ho, I. K. (1982). Chlordecone-induced alterations in content and subcellular distribution of calcium in mouse brain. *J. Toxicol. Environ. Health* **9**, 535–544.

Hosler, J., Tschanz, C., Hignite, C. E., and Azarnoff, D. C. (1980). Topical application of lindane cream (Kwell) and antipyrine metabolism. *J. Invest. Dermatol.* **74**, 51–53.

Houston, J. E., Mutter, L. C., Blanke, R. V., and Guzelian, P. S. (1981). Chlordecone alcohol formation in the Mongolian gerbil (*Meriones unguiculatus*): A model for human metabolism of chlordecone (Kepone). *Fundam. Appl. Toxicol.* **1**, 293–298.

Hrdina, P. D., Singhal, R. L., Peters, D. A. V., and Ling, G. M. (1973). Some neurochemical alterations during acute DDT poisoning. *Toxicol Appl. Pharmacol.* **25**, 276–288.

Hrdina, P. D., Singhal, R. L., and Peters, D. A. V. (1974). Changes in brain biogenic amines and body temperature after cyclodiene insecticides. *Toxicol. Appl. Pharmacol.* **29**, 119.

Hrdina, P. D., Singhal, R. L., and Ling, G. M. (1975). DDT and related hydrocarbon insecticides: Pharmacological basis of their toxicity in mammals. *Adv. Pharmacol. Chemother.* **12**, 31–88.

Hruska, J. (1969). DDT residues in the milk, butter, and fat of cattle, *Veterinarstvi* **19**, 493–498 (in Czech).

Hsieh, H. C. (1954). DDT intoxication in a family in southern Taiwan. *Arch. Ind. Hyg. Occup. Med.* **10**, 334–346.

Hsu, Y. N., Lin, M. T., Hong, J. S., and Tsai, M. C. (1986). Effect of chlordecone exposure on thermoregulation in the rat. *Pharmacology* **32**, 292–300.

Huang, E. S., and Nelson, F. R. (1986). Anti-estrogenic action of chlordecone in rat pituitary gonadotrophs *in vitro*. *Toxicol. Appl. Pharmacol.* **82**, 62–69.

Huang, Q., and Huang, X. (1987). The effect of benzene hexachloride on mouse sperm. *Zhejiang Yike Daxue Xuebao* **16**, 9–12.

Huang, T. P., Ho, I. K., and Henendale, H. M. (1980). Assessment of neurotoxicity induced by oral administration of chlordecone (Kepone) in the mouse. *Neurotoxicology* **2**, 113–124.

Huber, J. J. (1965). Some physiological effects of the insecticide Kepone in the laboratory mouse. *Toxicol. Appl. Pharmacol.* **7**, 516–524.

Hudson, P. M., Yoshikawa, K., Ali, S. F., Lamb, J. C., Peel, J. R., and Hong, J. S. (1984). Estrogen-like activity of chlordecone (Kepone) on the hypothalamo–pituitary axis—effects on the pituitary enkephalin system. *Toxicol. Appl. Pharmacol.* **74**, 383–389.

Hudson, P. M., Chen, P. H., Tilson, H. A., and Hong, J. S. (1985). Effects of *p,p*-DDT on the rat brain concentrations of biogenic amine and amino acid neurotransmitters and their association with *p,p'*-DDT-induced tremor and hyperthermia. *J. Neurochem.* **45**, 1349–1355.

Hueper, W. C. (1942). "Occupational Tumors and Allied Diseases." Thomas, Springfield, Illinois.

Hundley, S. G., Hartgrove, R. W., Jr., and Webb, R. E. (1974). Transfer of endrin via milk in endrin-susceptible and resistant pine mice and the resultant effects on liver microsomal activity in the neonate. *Toxicol. Appl. Pharmacol.* **29**, 127–128.

Hunter, C. G., and Robinson, J. (1967). Pharmacodynamics of dieldrin (HEOD). I. Ingestion by human subjects for 18 months. *Arch. Environ. Health* **15**, 614–626.

Hunter, C. G., and Robinson, J. (1968). Aldrin, dieldrin, and man. *Food Cosmet. Toxicol.* **6**, 253–260.

Hunter, C. G., Robinson, J., and Richardson, A. (1963). Chlorinated insecticide content in human body fat in southern England. *Br. Med. J.* **1,** 221–224.

Hunter, C. G., Robinson, J., and Roberts, M. (1969). Pharmacodynamics of dieldrin (HEOD). Ingestion by humans subjects for 18 to 24 months and postexposure for eight months. *Arch. Environ. Health* **18,** 12–21.

Hunter, J., Maxwell, J. D., Stewart, D. A., Williams, R., Robinson, J., and Richardson, A. (1972). Increased hepatic microsomal enzyme activity from occupational exposure to certain organochlorine pesticides. *Nature (London)* **237,** 399–401.

Hurwitz, S. (1973). Scabies in babies. *Am. J. Dis. Child.* **126,** 226–228.

Husejnov, M. K. (1970). The prevention of agricultural chemicals intoxication among collective farm workers. *Azerb. Med. Zh.* **47,** 27–30 (in Russian).

Hutson, D. H. (1976). Comparative metabolism of dieldrin in two strains of mouse (FC1 and LACG). *Food Cosmet. Toxicol.* **14,** 577–591.

Hutson, D. H., and Hoadley, E. C. (1974). The oxidation of a cyclic alcohol (12-hydroxyendrin) to a ketone (12-keto-endrin) by microsomal monooxygenation. *Chemosphere* **3,** 205–210.

Hutter, A. M., and Kayhoe, D. E. (1966). Adrenal cortical carcinoma. II. Results of treatment with *o,p'*-DDD in 138 patients. *Am. J. Med.* **41,** 581–592.

Hwang, E. C., and van Woert, M. H. (1978). *p,p'*-DDT-induced neurotoxic syndrome: Experimental myoclonus. *Neurology* **28,** 1020–1025.

Iatropoulos, M. J., Milling, A., Mueller, W. F., Nohynek, G., Rozman, K., Coulston, F., and Korte, F. (1975). Absorption, transport and organotropism of dichlorobiphenyl (DCB), dieldrin, and hexachlorobenzene (HCB) in rats. *Environ. Res.* **10,** 384–389.

Ibañez-Petersen, E. H., and DeFranzetti, R. P. (1957). Psychometric studies and their clinical value in dieldrin spraymen. *Bol. Of. Sanit. Panam.* **43,** 531–533 (in Spanish).

Ichikawa, H. (1972). Pathology of BHC poisoning. *Biotechnol Bioeng. Symp.* **3,** 111–116.

Ichinose, R., and Kurihara, N. (1987). Intramolecular deuterium isotope effect and crantiotopic differentiation in oxidative demethylation of chiral (monomethyl-d3)methoxychlor in rat liver microsomes. *Biochem. Pharmacol.* **36,** 3761–3756.

Il'yina, V. I., and Blekherman, N. A. (1974). Data on the status of the specific female functions of the organism in female workers exposed to hexachlorocyclohexane. *Pediatr., Akush. Ginekol.* **36,** 46–49 (in Russian).

Imai, H., and Coulston, F. (1968). Ultrastructural studies of absorption of methoxychlor in the jejunal mucosa of the rat. *Toxicol. Appl. Pharmacol.* **8,** 135–158.

Infante, P. F., Epstein, S. S., and Newton, W. A. (1978). Blood dyscrasias and childhood tumors and exposure to chlordane and heptachlor. *Scand. J. Work. Environ. Health* **4,** 137–150.

Ingle, L. (1952). Chronic oral toxicity of chlordane to rats. *Arch. Ind. Hyg. Occup. Med.* **6,** 357–367.

Ingle, L. (1953). The toxicity of chlordane vapors. *Science* **118,** 213–214.

Innes, J. R., Ulland, B. M., Vallerio, M. G., Petricelli, L., Fishbein, L., Hart, E. R., Pallotta, A. J., Bates, R. R., Falk, H. L., Gart, J. J., Klein, M., Mitchell, I., and Peters, J. (1969). Bioassay of pesticides and industrial chemicals for tumorigenicity in mice: A preliminary note. *J. Natl. Cancer Inst. (U.S.)* **42,** 1101–1114.

Inoue, Y., Abe, J., Takamatsu, M., and Aoki, N. (1974). A study on the qualitative and quantitative ratio of PCB and organochlorine pesticide residues in the blood and the adipose tissue. *Jpn. J. Hyg.* **29,** 92 (in Japanese).

Interdepartmental Committee on Pest Control (1951). A statement on the health hazards of thermal generators as used for the control of flying insects. *J. Econ. Entomol.* **44,** 1027.

Interdepartmental Committee on Pest Control (1953). A revised statement of the health hazards of insecticide vaporizers as used for the control of flying insects. *J. Econ. Entomol.* **46,** 181.

International Agency for Research on Cancer (IARC) (1974). World Health Organization, International Agency for Research on Cancer. Some organochlorine pesticides. *IARC Monogr. Eval. Carcinog. Risk Chem. Man* **5.**

International Agency for Research on Cancer (IARC) (1979). World Health Organization, International Agency for Research on Cancer. Some halogenated hydrocarbons. *IARC Mongr. Eval. Carcinog. Risk Chem. Man,* **20.**

International Agency for Research on Cancer (IARC) (1982). World Health Organization, International Agency for Research on Cancer. Chemicals, Industrial Processes and Industries Associated with Cancer in Humans. *IARC Monogr. Eval. Carcinog. Risk Chem. Man, Suppl.* **4.**

International Agency for Research on Cancer (IARC) (1983). World Health Organization, International Agency for Research on Cancer. Miscellaneous Pesticides. *IARC Mongr. Eval. Carcinog. Risk Chem. Man,* **30.**

(IARC) International Agency for Research on Cancer (1987). "World Health Organization, International Agency for Research on Cancer. Overall Evaluations of Carcinogenicity: An Update of IARC Monographs 1–42," Suppl. 7. Int. Agency Res. Cancer, Lyon.

Inuyama, Y., and Takashita, T. (1973). Survey of pesticide residues and PCB in mother's milk and human adipose tissue. *Annu. Rep. Shimane Prefect. Inst. Public Health Environ. Pollut.* **15,** 37–39 (in Japanese).

Ireland, J. S., Mukku, V. R., Robison, A. K., and Stancel, G. M. (1980). Stimulation of uterine deoxyribonucleic acid synthesis by 1,1,1-trichloro-2-(*p*-chlorophenyl)-2-)*o*-chlorophenyl)ethane (*o,p'*-DDT). *Biochem. Pharmacol.* **29,** 1469–1474.

Ishikawa, Y., Charalambous, P., and Matsumura, F. (1989). Modification by pyrethroids and DDT of phosphorylation activities of rat brain sodium channel. *Biochem. Pharmacol.* **38,** 2449–2457.

Israeli, R., and Mayersdorf, A. (1973). Pathological changes in the EEG during work with halogen-containing insecticides. *Zentralbl. Arbeitsmed. Arbeitsschutz* **23,** 340–343 (in German).

Israeli, R., Kristal, N., and Tiberin, P. (1969). Endosulfan poisoning: A preliminary report on three cases. *Zentralbl. Arbeitsmed. Arbeitsschutz* **19,** 1–3 (in German).

Ito, K., and Umemura, N. (1973). Environmental pollution and preservation of health of mothers and their children—on the pollution by organochlorine pesticides. *Jpn. J. Public Health* **20,** 406 (in Japanese).

Ito, K., Nagasaki, H., Arai, M., Sugihara, S., and Makiura, S. (1973). Histological and ultrastructural studies on the hepatocarcinogenicity of benzene hexachloride in mice. *JNCI, J. Natl. Cancer Inst.* **51,** 817–826.

Ito, N., Hananouchi, M., Sugihara, S., Shirai, T., Tsuda, H., Fukushima, S., and Nagasaki, H. (1976). Reversibility and irreversibility of liver tumours in mice induced by the α-isomer of 1,2,3,4,5,6-hexachlorocyclohexane. *Cancer Res.* **36,** 2227–2234.

Ito, T., and Miyake, Y. (1973). Influence of pesticides on enzymes in living bodies. *Annu. Rep. Res. Inst. Environ. Pollut., Kinki Univ.* **1,** 5–8 (in Japanese).

Iverson, F. (1976). Induction of paraoxon dealkylation by hexachlorobenzene (HCB) and mirex. *J. Agric. Food Chem.* **24,** 1238–1246.

Iverson, F., Ryan, J. J., Lizotte, R., and Hierlihy, S. T. (1984). *In vivo* and *in vitro* binding of α- and γ-hexachlorocyclohexane to mouse liver macromolecules. *Toxicol. Lett.* **20,** 331–335.

Ivey, M. C., Claborn, H. U., Mann, H. D., Radeleff, R. D., and Woodward, G. T. (1961). Aldrin and dieldrin content of body tissues of livestock receiving aldrin in their diet. *J. Agric. Food Chem.* **9,** 374–376.

Ivie, G. W., Gibson, J. R., Bryant, H. E., Begin, J. J., Barnett, J. R., and Dorough, H. W. (1974). Accumulation, distribution, and excretion of mirex-^{14}C in animals exposed for long periods to the insecticide in the diet. *J. Agric. Food Chem.* **22,** 646–653.

Jacobs, P., and Lurie, J. B. (1967). Acute toxicity of the chlorinated hydrocarbon insecticides. *S. Afr. Med. J.* **41,** 1147–1150.

Jacobziner, H., and Raybin, H. W. (1959). Briefs on accidental chemical poisonings in New York City. *N.Y. State J. Med.* **59,** 2017–2022.

Jaeger, U., Podczeck, A., Haubenstock, A., Pirich, K., Donner, A., and Hruby, K. (1984). Acute oral poisoning with lindane–solvent mixtures. *Vet. Hum. Toxicol.* **26,** 11–14.

Jager, K. W. (1970). "Aldrin, Dieldrin, Endrin and Telodrin." Am. Elsevier, New York.

Jager, R. J. (1976). Kepone chronology. *Science* **193,** 95–96.

Jandacek, R. J. (1982). The effect of nonabsorbable lipids on the intestinal absorpiton of lipophiles. *Drug Metab. Rev.* **13,** 695–714.

Jani, J. P., Patel, J. S., Shah, M. P., Gupta, S. K., and Kashyap, S. K. (1988). Levels of organochlorine pesticides in human milk in Ahmedabad, India. *Int. Arch. Occup. Environ. Health* **60**, 111–113.

Jansson, B., Jensen, S., Olsson, M., Renberg, L., Sundström, G., and Vaz, R. (1975). Identification by GC-MS of phenolic metabolites of PCB and *p,p'*-DDE isolated from Baltic guillemot and seal. *Ambio* **4**, 93–97.

Jedeikin, R., Kaplan, R., Shapira, A., Radwan, H., and Hoffman, S. (1979). The successful use of "high level" PEEP in near fatal endrin poisoning. *CRC Crit. Care Med.* **7**, 168–170.

Jedliŏka, V., Heřmanska, Z., Šmida, I., and Kouba, A. (1958). Paramyeloblastic leukaemia appearing simultaneously in two blood cousins after simultaneous contact with Gammexane (hexachlorocyclohexane). *Acta Med. Scand.* **161**, 447–451.

Jefferies, D. J., and French, M. C. (1972). Changes induced in the pigeon thyroid by *p,p'*-DDE and dieldrin. *J. Wildl. Manage.* **36**, 24–30.

Jeffery, W. H., Ahlin, T. A., Goren, C., and Hardy, W. R. (1976). Loss of warfarin effect after occupational insecticide exposure. *JAMA, J. Am. Med. Assoc.* **236**, 2881–2882.

Jemma, Z., Sabbah, S., Driss, M. R., and Bouguerra, M. L. (1986). Hexachlorobenzene in Tunisian mothers' milk, cord blood and foodstuffs. *IARC Publ.* **77**, 139–142.

Jenkins, M. Q. (1964). Poisoning of the month. *J. S. C. Med. Assoc.* **60**, 17–18.

Jenkins, R. B., and Toole, J. F. (1964). Polyneuropathy following exposure to insecticides. Two cases of polyneuropathy with albuminocytologic dissociation in the spinal fluid following exposure to DDD and aldrin and DDT and endrin. *Arch. Intern. Med.* **113**, 691–695.

Jensen, A. A. (1983). Chemical contaminants in human milk. *Residue Rev.* **89**, 1–128.

Jensen, G. E., and Clausen, J. (1979). Organochlorine compounds in adipose tissue of Greenlanders and southern Danes. *J. Toxicol. Environ. Health* **5**, 617–629.

Jensen, J. A., Cueto, C., Dale, W. E., Rothe, C. F., Pearce, G. W., and Mattson, A. M. (1957). Metabolism of insecticides. DDT metabolites in feces and bile of rats. *J. Agric. Food Chem.* **5**, 919–925.

Jensen, S., and Jansson, B. (1976). Anthropogenic substances in seal from the Baltic: Methyl sulfone metabolites of PCB and DDE. *Ambio* **5**, 257–260.

Jeyaratnam, J., and Forshaw, J. (1974). A study of the cardiac effects of DDT in laboratory animals. *Bull. W.H.O.* **51**, 531–535.

Johnson, B. L., and Eden, W. G. (1953). The toxicity of aldrin, dieldrin, and toxaphene to rabbits by skin absorption. *J. Econ. Entomol.* **46**, 702–703.

Johnson, K. W., Holsapple, M. P., and Munson, A. E. (1986). An immunotoxicological evaluation of gamma-chlordane. *Fundam. Appl. Toxicol.* **6**, 317–326.

Johnson, K. W., Kaminski, N., and Munson, A. E. (1987). Direct suppression of cultured spleen cell responses by chlordane and the basis for differential effects on *in vivo* and *in vitro* immunocompetence. *J. Toxicol. Environ. Health* **22**, 497–515.

Jonczyk, H. (1970). The content of organochlorine insecticides in the blood of healthy persons. *Rocz. Panstw. Zakl. Hig.* **21**, 589–593 (in Polish).

Jonsson, V., Liu, G. J. K., Armbruster, J., Kettlehut, L. L., and Drucker, B. (1977). Chlorohydrocarbon pesticide residues in human milk in Greater St. Louis, Missouri, 1977. *Am. J. Clin. Nutr.* **30**, 1106–1109.

Jordan, J. E., Grice, T., Mishra, S. K., and Desaiah, D. (1981). Acute chlordecone toxicity in rats: A relationship between tremor and ATPase activities. *Neurotoxicology* **2**, 355–364.

Joslin, E. F., Forney, R. L., Huntington, R. W., Jr., and Hayes, W. J., Jr. (1960). A fatal case of lindane poisoning. *In* "Proceedings of the National Association of Coroners Seminars, 1958, 1959," pp. 53–57. S. R. Gerber, Cleveland, Ohio.

Jovčic, B., and Ivanuŝ, J. (1968). Variations in the electroencephalogram in workers exposed to insecticides. *Zentralbl. Arbeitsmed. Arbeitsschutz.* **18**, 270–272 (in German).

Joy, R. M. (1973). Electrical correlates of preconvulsive and convulsive doses of chlorinated hydrocarbon insecticides in the CNS. *Neuropharmacology* **12**, 63–76.

Joy, R. M. (1974a). Alteration of sensory and motor evoked responses by dieldrin. *Neuropharmacology* **13**, 93–110.

Joy, R. M. (1974b). Temporal sequencing of dieldrin induced epileptiform spikes in the cat. *Proc. West. Pharmacol. Soc.* **17**, 82–96.

Joy, R. M. (1976). The alteration by dieldrin of cortical excitability conditioned by sensory stimuli. *Toxicol. Appl. Pharmacol.* **38**, 357–368.

Joy, R. M. (1977). Contrasting actions of dieldrin and aldrin-transdiol, its metabolite, on cat CNS function. *Toxicol. Appl. Pharmacol.* **42**, 137–148.

Joy, R. M. (1982a). Chlorinated hydrocarcon insecticides. *In* "Pesticides and Neurological Diseases" (D. Ecobicon and R. M. Joy, eds.), pp. 91–150. CRC Press, Boca Raton, Florida.

Joy, R. M. (1982b). Mode of action of lindane, dieldrin and related insecticides in the central nervous system. *Neurobehav. Toxicol. Teratol.* **4**, 813–823.

Joy, R. M. (1985). The effects of neurotoxicants on kindling and kindled seizures. *Fundam. Appl. Toxicol.* **5**, 41–65.

Joy, R. M., and Albertson, T. E. (1985). Lindane and limbic system excitability. *Neurotoxicology* **6** (2),193–214.

Joy, R. M., and Albertson, T. E. (1987a). Factors responsible for increased excitability of dentate gyrus granule cells during exposure to lindane. *Neurotoxicology* **8**, 517–527.

Joy, R. M., and Albertson, T. E. (1987b). Interactions of lindane with synaptically mediated inhibition and facilitation in the dentate gyrus. *Neurotoxicology* **8**, 529–542.

Joy, R. M., and Albertson, T. E. (1988). Convulsant-induced changes in perforant path–dentate gyrus excitability in urethane anaesthetized rats. *J. Pharmacol. Exp. Ther.* **246**, 887–895.

Joy, R. M., and Burns, V. W. (1988). Exposure to lindane and two other hexachlorocyclohexane isomers increases free intracellular calcium levels in neurohybridoma cells. *Neurotoxicology* **9**, 637–644.

Joy, R. M., Stark, L. G., Peterson, S. L., Bowyer, J. F., and Albertson, T. E. (1980). The kindled seizures: Production of and modification by dieldrin in rats. *Neurobehav. Toxicol.* **2**, 117–124.

Joy, R. M., Stark, L. G., and Albertson, T. E. (1982a). Proconvulsant effects of lindane: Enhancement of amygdaloid kindling in the rat. *Neurobehav. Toxicol. Teratol.* **4**, 347–354.

Joy, R. M., Giri, S. N., and Schiedt, M. J. (1982b). Elevation of brain cyclic nucleotides during acute dieldrin exposure. *Bull. Environ. Contam. Toxicol.* **28**, 611–616.

Joy, R. M., Stark, L. G., and Albertson, T. E. (1983). Proconvulsant action of lindane compared at two different kindling sites in the rat—amygdala and hippocampus. *Neurobehav. Toxicol. Teratol.* **5**, 461–465.

Judah, J. D. (1949). Studies on the metabolism and mode of action of DDT. *Br. J. Pharmacol. Chemother.* **4**, 120–131.

Jude, A., and Girard, P. (1949). Toxicity of DDT intoxication by accidental ingestion. *Ann. Med. Leg.* **29**, 209–213 (in French).

Junqueira, V. B. C., Simizu, K., Videla, L. A., and Barros, S. B. DeM. (1986). Dose-dependent study of the effects of acute lindane administration on rat liver superoxide anion production, antioxidant enzyme activities and lipid peroxidation. *Toxicology* **41**, 193–204.

Juszkiewicz, T., and Stec, J. (1971). Polychlorinated insecticide residues in adipose tissue of farmers in the Lublin Province (Poland). *Pol. Tyg. Lek.* **26**, 462 (in Polish).

Juskiewicz, T., Stec, J., Radomanski, T., and Trebicka-Kwiatkowska, B. (1972). Residues of chlorinated hydrocarbon insecticides in human milk. *Pol. Tyg. Lek.* **27**, 616–619 (in Polish).

Kacew, S., and Singhal, R. L. (1972). Role of adrenals in acute effects of *p,p'*-DDT renal glucose metabolism. *Fed. Proc., Fed. Am. Soc. Exp. Biol.* **31**, 1727.

Kacew, S., and Singhal, R. L. (1973). Adaptive response of hepatic carbohydrate metabolism to oral administration of *p,p'*-1,1,1-trichloro-2,2-bis-(*p*-chlorophenyl)ethane in rats. *Biochem. Pharmacol.* **22**, 47–57.

Kacew, S., Sutherland, D. J. B., and Singhal, R. L. (1973). Biochemical changes following chronic administration of heptachlor epoxide and endrin to male rats. *Environ. Physiol. Biochem.* **3**, 221–229.

Kachole, M. S., and Pawar, S. S. (1977). Effect of endrin on microsomal electron transport reactions. Part I. Sleeping time, electron transport components and protection by pretreatment. *Indian J. Biochem. Biophys.* **14**, 45.

Kadis, V. W., Breitkreitz, W. E., and Johasson, O. J. (1970). Insecticide levels in human tissues of Alberta residents. *Can. J. Public Health* **61**, 413–416.

Kagan, Y. S., Rodionov, G. A., Woronina, L. Y., Velichko, L. S., Kulagin, O. M., and Peremitina, A. D. (1969). Effect of DDT on the functional and morphological condition of the liver. *Vrach. Delo* **12**, 101–105 (in Russian).

Kailin, E. W., and Hastings, A. (1966). Electromyographic evidence of DDT-induced myasthenia. *Med. Ann. D.C.* **35**, 237–244.

Kaku, S. (1973). An epidemiological study on organochlorine pesticide contamination. On the pesticide residues in the plasma of so-called healthy Japanese in 1971. *Kurume Igakkai Zasshi* **36**, 307–326.

Kalra, R. L., and Chawla, R. P. (1981). Occurrence of DDT and BHC residues in human milk. *Experientia* **37**, 404–405.

Kamata, T. (1973). On the present status of environmental pollution by organochlorine pesticide residues. *Jpn. J. Pub. Health* **20**, 405 (in Japanese).

Kamata, T. (1974). Hygienic studies on pesticide residues. Part 4. Environmental contamination by organochlorine pesticides. *Med. J. Hiroshima Univ.* **22**, 315–325 (in Japanese).

Kaminski, N. E., Robert, J. F., and Guthrie, F. E. (1982). The effects of DDT and dieldrin on rat peritoneal macrophages. *Pestic. Biochem. Physiol.* **17**, 191–195.

Kaminsky, L. S., Piper, L. J., McMartin, D. N., and Fasco, M. J. (1978). Induction of microsomal cytochrome P-450 by mirex and Kepone. *Toxicol. Appl. Pharmacol.* **43**, 327–338.

Kanitz, S., and Castello, G. (1966). On the presence of residues of some pesticides in human adipose tissue and in some foods. *G. Ig. Med. Prev.* **7**, 1–19 (in Italian).

Kanja, L., Skare, J. U., Nafstad, I., Maitai, C. K., and Lokken, P. (1986). Organochlorine pesticide in human milk from different areas of Kenya 1983–1985. *J. Toxicol. Environ. Health* **19**, 449–464.

Kaphalia, B. S., and Seth, T. D. (1983). Chlorinated pesticide residues in blood plasma and adipose tissue of normal and exposed human population. *Indian J. Med. Res.* **77**, 245–247.

Kapoor, I. P., Metcalf, R. L., Nystrom, R. F., and Sangha, G. K. (1970). Comparative metabolism of methoxychlor, methiochlor, and DDT in mouse, insects, and in a model ecosystem. *J. Agric. Food Chem.* **18**, 1145–1152.

Karakaya, A. E., and Ozalp, S. (1987). Organochlorine pesticides in human adipose tissue collected in Ankara (Turkey) 1984–1985. *Bull. Environ. Contamin. Toxicol.* **38**, 941–945.

Karakaya, A. E., Burgaz, S., and Kanzik, I. (1987). Organochlorine pesticide contaminants in human milk from different regions of Turkey. *Bull. Environ. Contam. Toxicol.* **39**, 506–510.

Karapally, J. C., Saha, J. G., and Lee, Y. W. (1973). Metabolism of lindane^{14}C in the rabbit: Ether soluble urinary metabolites. *J. Agric. Food Chem.* **21**, 811–818.

Karimov, A. M. (1969). Skin sensitivity to organochlorine insecticides. *Med. Zh. Uzb.* **9**, 58–60 (in Russian).

Karimov, A. M. (1970). Occupational skin diseases in cotton growers caused by chemical poisons and measures for their prevention. *Gig. Tr. Prof. Zabol.* **14**, 35–37 (in Russian).

Karnik, A. B., Thakore, K. N., Nigam, S. K., Babu, K. A., Lakkad, B. C., Bhatt, D. K., Kashyap, S. K., and Chatterjee, S. K. (1981). Studies on glucose-6-phosphatase, fructose-1,6-diphosphatase activity, glycogen and endoplasmic reticulum changes during hexachlorocyclohexane induced hepatocarcinogenesis in pure inbred Swiss mice. *Neoplasma* **28**, 575–584.

Karplus, M. (1971). Endrin poisoning in children. *Harefuah* **81**, 113–116 (in Hebrew).

Kasai, A., Asanuma, S., and Nakamura, S. (1972). Studies on organochlorine pesticide residues in human organs. Part II. *J. Jpn. Assoc. Rural Med.* **21**, 296–297 (in Japanese).

Kashyap, S. K. (1986). Health surveillance and biological monitoring of pesticide formulators in India. *Toxicol. Lett.* **33**, 107–114.

Kashyap, S. K., Nigam, S. K., Karnik, A. B., Gupta, R. C., and Chatterjee, S. K. (1977). Carcinogenicity of DDT (dichlorodiphenyltrichloroethane) in pure inbred Swiss mice. *Int. J. Cancer* **19**, 725–729.

Kashyap, S. K., Nigam, S. K., Gupta, R. C., Karnik, A. B., and Chatterjee, S. K. (1979). Carcinogenicity of hexachlorocyclohexane (BHC) in pure inbred Swiss mice. *J. Environ. Sci. Health, Part B* **14**, 305–318.

Kashyap, S. K., Gupta, S. K., Karnik, A. B., Parikh, J. R., and Chatterjee, S. K. (1980). Scope and need of toxicological evaluation of pesticides under field conditions—medical surveillance of malaria spraymen exposed to HCH (hexachlorocyclohexane) in India. *Stud. Environ. Sci.* **7**, 53–61.

Kato, K., Yamada, T., Watanabe, S., Wada, Y., Fukuda, M., Kuroda, M., Nakaoka, S., Takahashi, T., Miyashiro, K., Masuda, J., and Yasukata, S. (1971). Analyses of residual pesticides in vegetables, cows' milk and mothers' milk. *Annu. Rep. Kanazawa Prefect. Inst. Public Health* **21**, 85–92 (in Japanese).

Katsenovich, R. A., and Usmanova, I. Y. (1970). On the appearance of liver autoantibodies in persons in contact with pesticides. *Med. Zh. Uzb.* **7**, 6–8 (in Russian).

Kauer, K., DuVall, R., and Alquist, F. (1947). Epsilon isomer of 1,2,3,4,5,6-hexachlorocyclohexane. *Ind. Eng. Chem.* **39**, 1335–1338.

Kaul, R., Klein, W., and Korte, F. (1970). Contributions to ecological chemistry. XX. Distribution, excretion and metabolism of Telodrin and heptachlor in rats and male rabbits. The end product of heptachlor metabolism in warm-blooded animals. *Tetrahedron* **26**, 331–337.

Kavlock, R. J., Chernoff, N., Rogers, E., and Whitehouse, D. (1980). Comparative tissue distribution of mirex and chlordecone in fetal and neonatal rats. *Pestic. Biochem. Physiol.* **14**, 227–235.

Kavlock, R. J., Chernoff, N., Hanisch, R. C., Gray, J., Rogers, E., and Gray, L. E. (1981). Perinatal toxicity of endrin in rodents. II. Fetotoxic effects of prenatal exposure in rats and mice. *Toxicology* **21**, 141–150.

Kawahara, T., and Moku, M. (1972). Studies on organochlorine pesticide residues in crops and soils. Report XVI. Degradation and isomerization of BHC isomers by heating. *Bull. Agric. Chem. Insp. Stn. (Jpn.)* **12**, 35–37.

Kawai, Y., Hori, Y., Nigawa, Y., Yamamoto, I., Tsuzuki, T., Kitayama, M., and Mori, K. (1973). On the pollution of mothers' milk by pesticides and PCB in Hokkaido. *J. Food Hyg. Soc. Jpn.* **14**, 302–303 (in Japanese).

Kawanishi, A., Asanuma, S., and Nakamura, S. (1973). Studies on the organochlorine pesticide residues in humans. Report 4. *J. Jpn. Assoc. Rural Med.* **22**, 278–279 (in Japanese).

Kawano, M., and Tatsukawa, R. (1982). Chlordanes and related compounds in blood of pest control operators (PCOs). *Nippon Nogei Kagaku Kaishi* **56**, 923–929 (in Japanese).

Kay, R. W. W., Kuder, G. G., Sessler, W. A., and Lewis, R. (1964). Fatal poisoning from ingestion of benzene hexachloride. *Ghana Med. J.* **3**, 72–74.

Kazakevich, R. L. (1974). State of the nervous system in persons with a prlonged professional contact with hexachlorocyclohexane and products of its synthesis. *Vrach. Delo.* **2**, 129–133 (in Russian).

Kazantzis, G., McLaughlin, A. I. G., and Prior, P. F. (1964). Poisoning in industrial workers by the insecticide aldrin. *Br. J. Ind. Med.* **21**, 46–51.

Kazen, C., Bloomer, A., Welch, R., Oudbier, A., and Price, H. (1974). Persistence of pesticides on the hands of some occupationally exposed people. *Arch. Environ. Health* **29**, 315–318.

Keane, W. T., and Zavon, M. R. (1969a). The total body burden of dieldrin. *Bull. Environ. Contam. Toxicol.* **4**, 1–16.

Keane, W. T., and Zavon, M. R. (1969b). Dieldrin poisoning in dogs: Relation to obesity and treatment. *Br. J. Ind. Med.* **26**, 338–341.

Kearnes, C. W., Weinman, C. G., and Decker, G. C. (1949). Insecticidal properties of some new chlorinated organic compounds. *J. Econ. Entomol.* **42**, 127–134.

Keil, J. E., Weston, W., III, Loadholt, C. B., Sandifer, S. H., and Colcolough, J. J. (1972a). DDT and DDE residues in blood from children, South Carolina—1970. *Pestic. Monit. J.* **6**, 1–3.

Keil, J. E., Sandifer, S. H., Finklea, J. H., and Priester, L. E. (1972b). Serum vitamin A elevation in DDT exposed volunteers. *Bull Environ. Contam. Toxicol.* **8**, 317–320.

Keil, J. E., Loadholt, C. B., Sandifer, S. H., Weston, W., III, Gadsden, R.

H., and Hames, C. G. (1973). Sera DDT elevation in black components of two southeastern communities: Genetics or environment? *In* "Pesticides and the Environment: A Continuing Controversy" (W. B. Diechman ed.), pp. 203–213. Intercontinental Medical Book Corp., New York.

Keller, W. C., and Yeary, R. A. (1980). A comparison of the effects of mineral oil, vegetable oil and sodium sulfate on the intestinal absorption of DDT in rodents. *Clin. Toxicol.* **16**, 223–231.

Kelner, M. J., McLenithan, J. C., and Anders, M. W. (1986). Thiol stimulation of the cytochrome P-450-dependent reduction of 1,1,1-trichloro-2,2-bis(*p*-chlorophenyl)ethane (DDT) to 1,1,1,-dichloro-2,2-bis(*p*-chlorophenyl)ethane (DDD). *Biochem. Pharmacol.* **35**, 1805–1807.

Kelvay, L. M. (1970). Endrin excretion by the isolated perfused liver: A sexual difference. *Proc. Soc. Exp. Biol. Med.* **136**, 878–879.

Kendall, M. W. (1974a). Acute histopathologic alterations induced in livers of rat, mouse, and quail by the fire-ant poison, mirex. *Anat. Rec.* **178**, 388.

Kendall, M. W. (1974b). Acute hepatotoxic effects of mirex in the rat. *Bull. Environ. Contam. Toxicol.* **12**, 617–621.

Kendall, M. W. (1979). Light and electron microscopic observations of the acute sublethal hepatotoxic effects of mirex in the rat. *Arch. Environ. Contam. Toxicol.* **8**, 25–41.

Kennedy, G. L., Jr., Frawley, J. P., and Calendra, J. C. (1973). Multigeneration reproductive effects of three pesticides in rats. *Toxicol. Appl. Pharmacol.* **25**, 589–596.

Kennedy, M. W., Pittman, K. A., and Stein, V. M. (1975). Fate of ^{14}C mirex in the female rhesus monkey. *Toxicol. Appl. Pharmacol.* **33**, 161–162.

Keplinger, M. L. (1963). Use of humans to evaluate safety of chemicals. *Arch. Environ. Health* **6**, 342–349.

Keplinger, M. L., and Diechmann, W. B. (1968). Susceptibility of offspring of mice fed pesticides to single oral doses of pesticides. *Am. Ind. Hyg. Assoc. J.* **29**, Suppl. 2, 111–112.

Keplinger, M. L., Diechmann, W. B., and Sala, F. (1970). Effect of combinations of pesticides on reproduction in mice. *In* "Pesticides Symposia" (W. B. Deichmann, J. L. Radomski, and R. A. Penalver, eds.), pp. 125–138. Halos and Associates, Miami, Florida.

Khaikina, B. I., and Shilina, V. F. (1971). The effect on serotonin metabolism of some organochlorine pesticides. *Farmakol. Toksikol. (Moscow)* **34**, 357–359 (in Russian).

Khaikina, B. I., Kuz'minskaia, U. A., and Alakhina, S. M. (1970). The effect of some pesticides on the isoenzymatic activity of serum lactic dehydrogenase. *Byull. Eksp. Biol. Med.* **70**, 39–41 (in Russian).

Khairy, M. (1959). Changes in behaviour associated with a nervous system poison (DDT). *Q. J. Exp. Physiol.* **11**, 91–94.

Khalifa, S., Mon, T. R., Engel, J. L., and Casida, J. E. (1974). Isolation of 2,2,5-*endo*,6-*exo*,3,9,10-heptachlorobornane and an octachloro toxicant from technical toxaphene. *J. Agric. Food Chem.* **22**, 653–657.

Khalifa, S., Holmstead, R. L., and Casida, J. E. (1976). Toxaphene degradation by iron(II) protoporphyrin system. *J. Agric. Food Chem.* **24**, 277–282.

Khanna, R. N., Misra, D., Anand, M., and Sharma, H. K. (1979). Distribution of endosulfan in cat brain. *Bull. Environ. Contam. Toxicol.* **22**, 72–79.

Khare, S. B., Rizvi, A. G., Shukla, O. P., Singh, R. R. P., Perkash, O., Misra, V. D., Gupta, J. P., and Sethi, P. K. (1977). Epidemic outbreak of neuro-ocular manifestations due to chronic BHC poisoning. *J. Assoc. Physicians India* **25**, 215–222.

Khasawinah, A. M., and Grutsch, J. F. (1989a). Chlordane: thirty-month tumorgenicity and chronic toxicity test in rats. *Reg. Toxicol. Pharmacol.* **10**, 95–109.

Khasawinah, A. M., and Grutsch, J. F. (1989b). Chlordane: a 24-month tumorgenicity and chronic test in mice. *Regul. Toxicol Pharmacol.* **10**, 244–254.

Khasawinah, A. M., Hardy, C. J., and Clark, G. C. (1989). Comparative inhalation toxicity of technical chlordane in rats and monkeys. *J. Toxicol. Environ. Health,* **28**, 327–347.

Khera, K. S., Villeneuve, D. C., Terry, G., Panopio, L., Nash, L., and Trivett, G. (1976). Mirex: A teratogenicity, dominant lethal and tissue distribution study in rats. *Food Cosmet. Toxicol.* **14**, 25–29.

Khera, K. S., Whalen, C., and Trivett, G. (1978). Teratogenicity studies on linuron, malathion, and methoxychlor in rats. *Toxicol. Appl. Pharmacol.* **45**, 435–444.

Khomenko, N. R., and Kazakevich, R. L. (1973). Abnormalities of the knee reflex in chronic BHC and thiram poisoning. *Gig. Tr. Prof. Zabol.* **17**, 56–57 (in Russian).

Kim, A. S., Aminov, K. A., and Zaitsev, A. A. (1967). Psychosis with poisoning by fenthion and hexachlorane. *Nauchn. Tr., Samark. Med. Inst.* **37**, 282–287 (in Russian).

Kimbrough, R. D., Gaines, T. B., and Hayes, W. J., Jr. (1968). Combined effect of DDT, pyrethrum, and piperonyl butoxide on rat liver. *Arch. Environ. Health* **16**, 333–341.

Kinoshita, F. K., and Kempf, C. K. (1970). Quantitative measurements of hepatic microsomal enzyme induction after dietary intake of chlorinated hydrocarbon insecticides. *Toxicol Appl. Pharmacol.* **17**, 288.

Kinoshita, F. K., Frawley, J. P., and DuBois, K. P. (1966). Quantitative measurement of induction of hepatic mocrosomal enzymes by various dietary levels of DDT and toxaphene in rats. *Toxicol. Appl. Pharmacol.* **9**, 505–513.

Kitselman, C. H. (1953). Long term studies on dogs fed aldrin and dieldrin in sublethal dosages, with references to the histopathological findings and reproduction. *J. Am. Vet. Med. Assoc.* **123**, 28.

Klayman, M. B. (1968). Exposure to insecticides. *Arch. Otolaryngol.* **88**, 116–117.

Klein, A. K., Laug, E. P., Datta, P. R., and Mendel, J. L. (1965). Evidence for the conversion of *o,p'*-DDT (1,1,1-trichloro-2-*o*-chlorophenyl-2-*p*-chlorophenylethane) to *p,p'*-DDT (1,1,1-trichloro-2,2-bis(*p*-chlorophenyl)ethane) in rats. *J. Am. Chem. Soc.* **87**, 2520–2522.

Klein, A. K., Laug, E. P., Datta, P. R., Watts, J. O., and Chen, J. T. (1969a). Metabolites: Reductive dechlorination of DDT to DDD and isomeric transformation of *o,p'*-DDT to *p,p'*-DDD *in vitro. J. Assoc. Off. Anal. Chem.* **47**, 1129–1145.

Klein, A. K., Kaul, R., Parlar, Z., Zimmer, M., and Korte, F. (1969b). Contributions to ecological chemistry. XIX. Metabolism of photodieldrin-14-C in warm-blooded animals, insects, and plants. *Tetrahedron Lett.,* pp. 3197–3199.

Klein, A. K., Dailey, R. E., Walton, M. S., Beck, V., and Link, J. D. (1970). Metabolites isolated from urine of rats fed ^{14}C-photodieldrin. *J. Agric. Food Chem.* **18**, 705–708.

Klein, W., and Korte, F. (1970). Metabolism of chlorinated hydrocarbons. *In* "Chemistry of Plant Protection and Pest Control Agents" (R. Wegler, ed.). Vol. 1, pp. 199–218. Springer-Verlag, Berlin (in German).

Klein, W., Mueller, W., and Korte, F. (1968). Insecticides in metabolism. 16. Excretion, distribution and metabolism of C-14 endrin rats. *Ann. Chim. (Paris)* **7**, [13], 180–185.

Kleine-Natrop, H. E., Roder, H., and Kadner, H. (1970). Note on timely scabies treatment. *Dtsch. Gesundheitswes.* **25**, 2082–2084 (in German).

Kleinfeld, M. (1967). Cancer of urinary bladder in a dye plant: A medical environmental study. *In:* "Bladder Cancer: A Symposium" (W. B. Diechmann, ed.). Aesculapius, Birmingham, Alabama.

Kleissner, M., and Worden, A. N. (1959). BHC and bone marrow. *Br. Med. J.* **1**, 971.

Klevay, L. M. (1970). Dieldrin excretion by the isolated perfused rat liver: A sexual difference. *Toxicol. Appl. Pharmacol.* **17**, 813–815.

Klimmer, O. R. (1955). Experimental investigations of the toxicology of chlorinated hydrocarbon insecticides. *Nauyn-Schmiedebergs Arch. Exp. Pathol. Pharmakol.* **227**, 183–195 (in German).

Klingensmith, J. S., and Mehendale, H. M. (1982). Chlordecone-induced fat depletion in the male rat. *J. Toxicol. Environ. Health* **10**, 121–129.

Klingensmith, J. S., and Mehendale, H. M. (1983a). Hepatic microsomal metabolism of CCl$_4$ after pretreatment with chlordecone, mirex or phenobarbital in male rats. *Drug Metab. Dispos.* **11**, 329–334.

Klingensmith, J. S., and Mehendale, H. M. (1983b). Destruction of hepatic mixed-function oxygenase parameters by CCl$_4$ in rats following acute treatment with chlordecone, mirex and phenobarbital. *Life Sci.* **33**, 2339–2348.

Klinger, W., Gmyrek, D., and Gruebner, I. (1973). Investigation of different substances and classes of substances. III. Chlorinated insecticides. *Arch. Int. Pharmacodyn. Ther.* **202**, 270–280 (in German).

Klosa, J. (1950). On the toxicology of hexachlorocyclohexane. *Pharmazie* **5**, 615–616 (in German).

Klotz, H. P., Thibaut, E., and Russo, F. (1971). Weak doses of *o,p'*-DDD in the spanomenorrhea with hypertrichosis. *Ann. Endocrinol.* **32**,763–767 (in French).

Kluge, W., and Olbrich, H. (1972). Poisoning by a DDT–lindane combination. *Z. Aerzt. Fortbild.* **66**, 980–982 (in German).

Knoll, W., and Jayaraman, S. (1972a). Organochlorine pesticide residues in human milk. *Z. Gesamte Hyg. Ihre Grenzgeb.* **19**, 43–45 (in German).

Knoll, W., and Jayaraman, S. (1972b). On the contamination of human milk with chlorinated hydrocarbons. *Nahrung* **17**, 599–615 (in German).

Knoll, W., and Jayaraman, S. (1973). Organochlorine pesticide residues in human milk. *Z. Gesamte Hyg. Ihre Grenzgeb.* **19**, 43–45 (in German).

Knoll, W., and Jayaraman, S. (1973). On the contamination of human milk with chlorinated hydrocarbons. *Nahrung* **17**, 599–615 (in German).

Knowles, C. O., and Ahmad, S. (1971). Comparative metabolism of chlorobenzilate, chloropropylate and bromopropylate acaricides by rat hepatic enzymes. *Can. J. Physiol. Pharmacol.* **49**, 590–597.

Koch, R. B. (1969). Chlorinated hydrocarbon insecticides. Inhibition of rabbit brain ATPase activities. *J. Neurochem.* **16**, 269–271.

Koch, R. B., Patel, T. N., Glick, B., Stinson, R. J., and Lewis, E. A. (1979). Properties of an antibody to kelevan isolated by affinity chromatography: Antibody reactivation of ATPase activities inhibited by pesticides. *Pestic. Biochem. Physiol.* **12**, 130–140.

Kodavanti, P. R. S., Joshi, U. M., Young, R. A., Bell, A. N., and Mehendale, H. M. (1989). Role of hepatocellular regeneration in chlordecone potentiated hepatotoxicity of carbon tetrachloride. *Arch. Toxicol.,* **63**, 367–375.

Kohli, K. K., Chandrasekaran, V. P., and Venkitasubramanian, T. A. (1977). Stimulation of serotonin metabolism by dieldrin. *J. Neurochem.* **28**, 1397–1399.

Kojima, S., Saito, M., Konno, H., and Ozawa, K. (1971). Results of investigation of organochlorine pesticide residues in mothers' milk and in the blood of the mothers. *Annu. Rep. Akita Prefect. Inst. Public Health* **16**, 65–68 (in Japanese).

Kolmodin, B., Azarnoff, D. L., and Sjöqvist, F. (1969). Effect of environmental factors on drug metabolism: Decreased plasma half-life of antipyrine in workers exposed to chlorinated hydrocarbon insecticides. *Clin. Pharmacol. Ther.* **10**, 638–642.

Kolmodin-Hedman, B. (1973a). Decreased plasma half-life of phenylbutazone in workers exposed to chlorinated pesticides. *Eur. J. Clin. Pharmacol.* **5**, 195–198.

Kolmodin-Hedman, B. (1973b). Changes in drug metabolism and lipoproteins in workers occupationally exposed to DDT and lindane. *Arch. Hig. Rada Toksikol.* **24**, 289–296.

Kolmodin-Hedman, B., Alexanderson, B., and Sjöqvist, F. (1971). Effect of exposure to lindane on drug metabolism. Decreased hexobarbital sleeping times and increased antipyrine disappearance rate in rats. *Toxicol. Appl. Pharmacol.* **20**, 299–307.

Kolyada, I. S., and Mikhal'chenkova, O. F. (1973). Acute organochlorine pesticide poisoning. *Gig. Tr. Prof. Zabol.* **17**, 43 (in Russian).

Komarova, L. I. (1970). The excretion of DDT in mothers' milk and its effect on the organism of mother and child. *Pediatr., Akush. Ginekol.* **1**, 19–20 (in Russian).

Komissarenko, V. P., and Reznikov, A. G. (1970). Chlodithane (*o,p'*-DDD) treatment in Itsenko-Cushing's disease. *Vrach. Delo* **8**, 107–112 (in Russian).

Komissarenko, V. P., Reznikov, A. G., Gordienko, V. M., and Zak, K. P. (1968). Effect of *o,p'*-DDD on the morphology and function of adrenal cortex in dogs. *Endocrinol. Exp.* **2**, 21–28 (in Russian).

Komissarenko, V. P., Rezinikov, A. G., and Gordienko, V. M. (1970). An experimental study of the action of *o,p'*-DDD on the functioning and structure of the adrenal cortex. *Vopr. Endokrinol. Obmena Veschestv. Sb.* **1**, 5–10 (in Russian).

Komissarenko, V. P., Karvchenko, V. O., Tron'ko, M. D., and Turchin, I. S. (1971). Effect of *o,p'*-DDD (clodithane) on secretion and metabolism of

corticosteroids in chickens. *Fiziol. Zh. (Kiev, 1955–1957)* **17**, 435–441 (in Russian).

Komissarenko, V. P., Gordiyenko, V. M., and Reznikov, A. G. (1972). Restorative processes in the adrenal cortex of dogs following administration of TDE. *Probl. Endokrinol.* **18**, 74–81 (in Russian).

Komissarenko, V. P., Chelnakova, I. S., and Mikosha, A. S. (1978). The activity of glutathione reductase in the adrenal glands and the liver of dogs following the administration of *o,p'*-DDD, Perthane and ACTH. *Probl. Endokrinol.* **24**, 95–98 (in Russian).

Komulainen, H., and Bondy, S. C. (1987). Modulation of levels of free calcium within synaptosomes by organochlorine insecticides. *J. Pharmacol. Exp. Ther.* **241**, 575–581.

Konat, G., and Clausen, J. (1973). The cytochrome P-450 complex and esterase of the liver and brain in lindane, Aroclor 1254, and DDT-induced intoxication of the mouse. *Environ. Physiol. Biochem.* **3**, 139–147.

Kontek, M., Kubachi, S., Paradowski, S., and Wierzchowiecka, B. (1971). Chlorinated insecticides in human milk. *Pediatr. Pol.* **46**, 183–188.

Kontek, M., Banaszak, S., Didowicz-Parzycka, J., Kubacki, S., and Kossowski, A. (1981). Comparative investigations of organic chloride pesticides in human milk before and after withdrawal of these agents from chemical plant protection. *Pol. Tyg. Lek.* **36**, 9–11 (in Polish).

Koransky, W., and Ullberg, S. (1964). Distribution in the brain of ^{14}C-benzenehexachloride. Autoradiographic study. *Biochem. Pharmacol.* **13**, 1537–1538 (plus plates).

Koransky, W., Portig, J., and Münch, G. (1963). Absorption, distribution and metabolism of α- and γ-hexachlorocyclohexane. *Naunyn-Schmiedebergs Arch. Exp. Pathol. Pharmakol.* **244**, 564–575 (in German).

Koransky, W., Magour, S., Noack, G., and Schulte Hermann, R. (1969). The influence of inducing substances on drug-oxidases and other redox enzymes of the liver. *Naunyn Schmiederberg's Arch. Exp. Pathol. Pharmakil.* **263**, 281–296 (in German).

Koransky, W., Munch, G., Noack, G., Portig, J., Sodomann, S., and Wirsching, M. (1975). Biodegradation of α-hexachlorocyclohexane. V. Characterization of the major urinary metabolites. *Naunyn Schmiedeberg's Arch. Pharmacol.* **288**, 65–78 (in German).

Korpachev, V. U. (1972a). Dependence of *o,p'*-DDD absorption on dose and drug form. *Farm Zh.* **27**, 64–66 (in Russian).

Korpachev, V. U. (1972b). Accumulation and elimination of *o,p'*-DDD in organs and tissues of guinea pigs and dogs. *Fiziol. Zh.* **18**, 585–590 (in Russian).

Korte, F. (1979). Transformation of *p,p'*-DDT in the environment. *In* "Environmental Health Criteria 9. DDT and Its Derivatives." United Nations Environmental Programme and the World Health Organization, Geneva.

Korte, F., and Kochen, W. (1966). Metabolism of insecticides. XII. Isolation and identification of metabolites of ^{14}aldrin from the urine of rabbit. *Med. Pharmacol. Exp.* **15**, 409–414 (in German).

Korth-Schutz, S., Levine, L. S., Roth, J. A., Saenger, P., and New, M. I. (1977). Virilizing adrenal tumor in a child suppressed with dexamethasone for three years. Effect of *o,p'*-DDD on serum and urinary androgens. *J. Clin. Endocrinol. Metab.* **44**, 433–439.

Koschier, F. J., Gigliotti, P. J., and Hong, S. K. (1980). The effect of bis(*p*-chlorophenyl)acetic acid on the renal function of the rat. *J. Environ. Pathol. Toxicol.* **4**, 209–217.

Koster, R. (1947). Differentiation of gluconate, glucose, calcium, insulin effect on DDT poisoning in cats. *Fed. Proc., Fed. Am. Soc. Exp. Biol.* **6**, 346.

Kostiuk, O. T., and Mukhtarova, N. D. (1970). Catecholamines and the functional state of the hypothalamus under the action of a complex of organochlorine and organophosphorus pesticides. *Gig. Tr. Prof. Zabol.* **14**, 35–38 (in Russian).

Kotlarek-Haus, S., Dzierzkowa-Borodej, W., and Lawinska, B. (1971). Autoimmune hemolytic anemia after handling insecticides and herbicides, with simultaneous detection of the Australia antigen (Au 1) in the serum. *Folia Haematol. (Leipzig)* **95**, 249–253 (in German).

Kramer, M. S., Hutchinson, T. A., Rudnick, S. A., Leventhal, J. M., and Feinstein, A. R. (1980). Operational criteria for adverse drug reactions in evaluating suspected toxicity of a popular scabicide. *Clin. Pharmacol. Ther.* **27**, 149–155.

Krampl, V., and Grigel, M. (1972). Relationships between serum enzymes and morphological changes occurring in the rat liver after administration of chlorinated cyclodiene insecticides. *Prak. Lek.* **24**, 121–125 (in Czech).

Krampl, V., and Hladka, A. (1974). The effect of simultaneous administration of lindane and phenobarbital upon stimulation of microsomal liver enzymes. *Prak. Lek.* **26**, 169–172 (in Czech).

Krampl, V., and Hladka, A. (1975). Dose-dependent extent of microsomal enzyme induction by aldrin and dieldrin in rats. *Bull. Environ. Contam. Toxicol.* **14**, 571–578.

Krasil'shchikov, D. G. (1972). The penetration of hexachlorane into white rat liver and adipose tissue as affected by the presence of determents in water. *Gig. Sanit.* **37**, 96–97.

Krasnyuk, E. P. (1964a). Electrocardiographic changes in persons working with organic chlorine insecticides. *Sov. Med.* **28**, 134–137 (in Russian).

Krasnyuk, E. P. (1964b). The internal secretory function in persons working with organochlorine insecticides. *In* "Labor Hygiene," pp. 186–190. Zdorov'ya, Kiev (in Russian).

Krasnyuk, E. P. (1969). Ballistocardiographic changes in those working with organochlorine compounds. *Gig. Tr.* **5** (1),203–207 (in Russian).

Krasnyuk, E. P., and Platonova, V. I. (1969). Functional disorders of the stomach under the prolonged effects of organochlorine chemical poisons. *Vrach. Delo.* **9**, 99–101 (in Russian).

Krasnyuk, E. P., Onikiyenko, F. A., and Osknskaya, L. S. (1967). Pathology of the liver in persons working with DDT. *Vrach. Delo* **1**, 92–95 (in Russian).

Krasnyuk, E. P., Loganovskii, N. G., Makovskaya, E. I., and Rappoport, M. B. (1968). Functional and morphological changes in the kidneys during the effects of DDT on the body. *Sov. Med.* **31**, 38–42 (in Russian).

Kraus, P., Noack, G., and Portig, J. (1973). Biodegradation of alpha-hexachlorocyclohexane. II. Glutathione-mediated conversion to hydrophilic substance by particulate fractions of rat liver and by homogenates of various rat organs. *Naunyn-Schmiedeberg's Arch. Pharmacol.* **279**, 199–202 (in German).

Kraus, P., Gross, B., and Kloft, H. D. (1981). The elevation of rat liver glutathione-*S*-transferase activity by alpha-hexachlorocyclohexane. *Biochem. Pharmacol.* **30**, 355–361.

Krauthacker, B., Alebic-Kolbah, T., Buntic, A., Tkalčević, B., and Reiner, E. (1980a). Organochlorine pesticides in blood serum of the general Yugoslav population and in occupationally exposed workers. *Int. Arch. Occup. Environ. Health* **45**, 217–220.

Krauthacker, B., Alebic-Kolbah, T., Kralj, M., Tkalčević, B., and Reiner, E. (1980b). DDT residues in samples of human milk, and in mothers' and cord blood serum in a continental town in Croatia (Yugoslavia). *Int. Arch. Occup. Environ. Health* **46**, 267–273.

Krauthacker, B., Kralj, M., Tkalčević, B., and Reiner, E. (1986). Levels of β-HCH, HCB, *p,p'*-DDE, *p,p'*-DDT and PCBs in human milk from a continental town in Croatia, Yugoslavia. *Int. Arch. Occup. Environ. Health* **58**, 69–74.

Kravchenko, V. I. (1973). The effect of *o,p'*-DDD on the formulation of corticosteroids by the adrenal tissue *in vitro*. *Probl. Endokrinol.* **19**, 76–79 (in Russian).

Kravt'sova, O. L., Korenevs'kyy, L. I., and Reznikov, O. H. (1971). The influence of *o,p'*-DDD on the development of DMBA-induced mammary gland tumors and adrenal cortex function in rats. *Dopov. Akad. Nauk. Ukr. RSR, Ser. B: Geol., Geofiz., Khim. Biol.* **30** (3),943–945 (in Russian).

Kreiss, K., Zack, M. M., Kimbrough, R. D., and Needham, L. C. (1981). Cross-sectional study of a community with exceptional exposure to DDT. *JAMA, J. Am. Med. Assoc.* **245**, 1926–1930.

Krijnen, C. J., and Boyd, E. M. (1971). The influence of diets containing from 0 to 81 per cent of protein on tolerated doses of pesticides. *Comp. Gen. Pharmacol.* **2**, 373–376.

Kroger, M. (1972). Insecticide residues in human milk. *J. Pediatr.* **80**, 401–405.

Krzystyniak, K., Hugo, P., Flipo, D., and Fournier, M. (1985). Increased susceptibility to mouse hepatitis virus 3 of peritoneal macrophages exposed to dieldrin. *Toxicol. Appl. Pharmacol.* **80**, 397–408.

Krzystyniak, K., Bernier, J., Hugo, P., and Fournier, M. (1986). Suppression of MHV3 virus-activated macrophages by dieldrin. *Biochem. Pharmacol.* **35**, 2577–2586.

Kuebrich, W., and Urban, I. (1973). Endrin poisoning—a contribution to the neurophysiology of epileptic attacks. *Z. Aerztl. Fortbild.* **67**, 1076–1078.

Kujawa, M., Macholz, R., and Knoll, R. (1985). Enzymic degradation of DDT. Part 5. Direct transformation of DDD (dichlorodiphenyldichloroethane) to an aldehyde. *Nahrung* **29**, 517–522.

Kumar, A., and Dwivedi, P. O. (1988). Relative induction of molecular forms of cytochrome P-450 in γ-hexachlorocyclohexane exposed rat liver microsomes. *Arch. Toxicol.* **62**, 479–481.

Kundiev, Yu. I., and Krasnyuk, E. P. (1965). Possible consequences of the introduction of hexachloran into the soil. *Hyg. Sanit. (USSR)* **30**, 116–119 (in Russian).

Kunz, W., Schaude, G., Schmid, W., and Siess, M. (1966). Liver hypertrophy caused by foreign agents. *Naunyn-Schmiedebergs Arch. Pharmakol. Exp. Pathol.* **254**, 470–488 (in German).

Kunze, F. M., Laug, E. P., and Prickett, C. S. (1950). The storage of methoxychlor in the fat of the rat. *Proc. Soc. Exp. Biol. Med.* **75**, 415–416.

Kupfer, D. (1967). Effects of some pesticides and related compounds on steroid function and metabolism. *Residue Rev.* **19**, 11–30.

Kupfer, D., and Bulger, W. H. (1979). A novel *in vitro* method for demonstrating proestrogens. Metabolism of methoxychlor and *o,p'*-DDT by liver microsomes in the presence of uteri and effects on intracellular distribution of estrogen receptors. *Life Sci.* **25**, 975–984.

Kupfer, D., and Bulger, W. H. (1987). Biochemical toxicology of methoxychlor and related chlorinated hydrocarbons. *Rev. Biochem. Toxicol.* **8**, 183–215.

Kupfer, D., Bulger, W. H., and Nanni, F. (1986). Characteristics of the active oxygen in covalent binding of the pesticide methoxychlor to hepatic microsomal proteins. *Biochem. Pharmacol.* **35**, 2775–2780.

Kurihara, N., and Nakajima, M. (1974). Studies on BHC isomers and related compounds. VIII. Urinary metabolites produced from γ- and β-BHC in the mouse: Chlorophenyl conjugates. *Pestic. Biochem. Physiol.* **4**, 220–231.

Kurihara, N., Tanaka, K., and Nakajima, M. (1979). Mercapturic acid formation from lindane in rats. *Pestic. Biochem. Physiol.* **10**, 137–150.

Kuroda, H., Yano, T., Kagawa, K., and Mitsumune, M. (1972). On the residual organochlorine pesticides in mothers' milk. *J. Shikoku Public Health Soc.* **17**, 79–80 (in Japanese).

Kürsat, A., and Türkoğlu, N. (1968). Interesting poisoning cases with dieldrin and other insecticides. *Saglik Derg.* **42**, 3–20 (in Turkish).

Kurt, T. L., Bost, R., Gilliland, M., Reed, G., and Petty, C. (1986). Accidental Kwell (lindane) ingestions. *Vet. Hum. Toxicol.* **28**, 569–571. *Note:* the wrong title and authors were printed in the original. See *Index Medicus* Vol. 28.

Kutz, F. W., Yobs, A. R., Johnson, W. G., and Wiersma, G. B. (1974a). Mirex residues in human adipose tissue. *Environ. Entomol.* **3**, 882–884.

Kutz, F. W., Yobs, A. R., Johnson, W. G., and Wiersma, G. B. (1974b). Pesticide residues in adipose tissue of the general population of the United States, FY 1970 survey. *Bull. Soc. Pharmacol. Environ. Pathol.* **2**, 4–10.

Kutz, F. W., Sovocool, W., Strassman, S., and Lewis, R. G. (1976). *trans*-Nonachlor residues in human adipose tissue. *Bull. Environ. Contam. Toxicol.* **16**, 9–14.

Kutz, F. W., Yobs, A. R., Strassman, S. C., and Viar, J. F., Jr. (1977). Effects of reducing DDT usage on total DDT storage in humans. *Pestic. Monit. J.* **11**, 61–63.

Kutz, F. W., Strassman, S. C., Sperling, J. F., Cook, B. T., Sunshine, I., and Tessari, J. (1983). A fatal chlordane poisoning. *J. Toxicol. Clin. Toxicol.* **20**, 167–174.

Kutz, F. W., Strassman, S. C., Stroup, C. R., Carra, J. S., Leininger, C. C., Watts, D. C., and Sparacino, C. M. (1985). The human body burden of mirex in the south eastern United States. *J. Toxicol. Environ. Health* **15**, 385–394.

Kuwabara, N., and Takayama, S. (1974). Comparison of histogenesis of liver in mice administered respectively BHC, DDT, and 2,7-FAA. *Proc. Jpn. Cancer Assoc.* **33**, 50 (in Japanese).

Kuwahara, Y., Koga, Y., Yamaguchi, S., Matsumoto, H., Matsuo, S., Kaku, S., Tateishi, M., Shiramizu, M., Ide, I., Goto, K., Karatsu, M., and Hinagata, K. (1972). Epidemiological study of pesticide pollution. I. Organochlorine pollution. *Jpn. J. Hyg.* **27**, 103 (in Japanese).

Kuz'minskaya, U. A., Klisenko, M. A., and Khaykina, B. I. (1972a). Peculiarities of the distribution of some pesticides in the lipid fractions of the liver. *Vopr. Pitan.* **31**, 48–52 (in Russian).

Kuz'minskaya, U. A., Novachik, V., and Klisenko, M. A. (1972b). Distribution of polychlorocamphene in lipid fractions of tissues. *Gig. Sanit.* **37**, 96–97 (in Russian).

Kuz'minskaya, U. A., Yakushko, V. E., Bersan, L. V., and Vercmenko, L. M. (1980). Study of the complex action of poly(chlorocamphene) using the orthogonal experimental design method. *Gig. Sanit.* 82–83 (in Russian).

Kveseth, N. J., Bjerk, J. E., Fimreite, N., and Stenersen, J. (1979). Residues of DDT in a Norwegian fruitgrowing district two and four years after the termination of DDT usage. *Arch. Environ. Contam. Toxicol.* **8**, 201–212.

Kwano, M., and Tatsukawa, R. (1982). Chlordanes and related compounds in blood of pest control operators. *Nippon Nogei Kagaku Kaishi* **56**, 923–929 (in Japanese).

Kwoczek, J. (1950). Toxicity of DDT and hexachlorocyclohexane preparations. *Med. Monatsschr.* **4**, 25–28 (in German).

Lacassagne, A. (1971). Critical review of experimental tumours of Leydig cells, more particularly in the rat. *Bull. Cancer* **58**, 235–276 (in French).

Lackey, R. W. (1949). Observations on the acute and chronic toxicity of toxaphene in the dog. *J. Ind. Hyg. Toxicol.* **31**, 117–120.

Lacombe, R., and Brodeur, J. (1974). The effect of pretreatment with dieldrin on certain *in vivo* parameters of enzyme induction in mice. *Toxicol. Appl. Pharmacol.* **27**, 70–85.

Lakkad, B. C., Nigam, S. K., Karnik, A. B., Thakora, K. N., Aravindra Babu, K., Blatt, D. K., and Kashyap, S. K. (1982). Dominant-lethal study of technical-grade hexachlorocyclohexane in Swiss mice. *Mutat. Res.* **101**, 315–320.

Lamartiniere, C. A., Luther, M. A., Lucier, G. W., and Illsley, N. P. (1982). Altered imprinting of rat liver monoamine oxidase by *o,p'*-DDT and methoxychlor. *Biochem. Pharmacol.* **31**, 647–651.

Lamoureux, C. H., and Feil, V. J. (1980). Gas chromatographic and mass spectrometric characterization of impurities in technical methoxychlor. *J. Assoc. Off. Anal. Chem.* **63**, 1007–1037.

Landoui, J. H., and Astolfi, E. A. (1982). Organochlorinated pesticides residues in human milk—Rep. Argentina—10 years monitoring. *Pap. Int. Symp., Chem. Environ., Copenhagen, 1982.*

Lang, B., and Maier, P. (1986). Lipid peroxidation dependent aldrin epoxidation in liver microsomes, hepatocytes and granulation tissue cells. *Biochem. Biophys. Res. Commun.* **138**, 24–32.

Lang, B., Frei, K., and Maier, P. (1986). Prostaglandin synthase dependent aldrin epoxidation in hepatic and extrahepatic tissue of rats. *Biochem. Pharmacol.* **35**, 3643–3645.

Lange, M., Nitzsche, K., and Zesch, A. (1981). Percutaneous absorption of lindane in healthy volunteers and scabies patients. *Arch. Dermatol. Res.* **271**, 387–399.

Larsen, A. A., Robinson, J. M., Schmitt, N., and Hole, L. (1971). Pesticide residues in mother's milk and human fat from intensive use of soil insecticides. *HSMHA Health Rep.* **86**, 477–481.

Larson, P. S., Hennigar, G. R., Finnegan, J. K., Smith, R. B., Jr., and Haag, H. B. (1955). Observations on the relation of chemical structure to the production of adrenal cortical atrophy or hypertrophy in the dog by derivatives of 2,2-bis(*p*-chlorophenyl)-1,1-dichloroethane (DDD, TDE). *J. Pharmacol. Exp. Ther.* **115**, 408–412.

Larson, P. S., Egle, J. L., Jr., Hennigar, G. R., Lane, R. W., and Borzelleca, J. F. (1979a). Acute, subchronic, and chronic toxicity of chlordecone. *Toxicol. Appl. Pharmacol.* **48**, 29–41.

Larson, P. S., Egle, J. L., Jr., Hennigar, G. R., and Borzelleca, J. F. (1979b). Acute and subchronic toxicity of mirex in the rat, dog, and rabbit. *Toxicol. Appl. Pharmacol.* **49**, 271–277.

Laug, E. P., Nelson, A. A., Fitzhugh, O. G., and Kunze, F. M. (1950). Liver-cell alteration and DDT storage in the fat of the rat induced by dietary levels of 1 to 50 ppm of DDT. *J. Pharmacol. Exp. Ther.* **98**, 268–273.

Laug, E. P., Kunze, F. M., and Prickett, C. S. (1951). Occurrence of DDT in human fat and milk. *Arch. Ind. Hyg. Occup. Med.* **3**, 245–246.

Laüger, P., Martin, H., and Müller, P. (1944). Constitution and toxic effects of natural and synthetic insecticides. *Helv. Chim. Acta.* **27**, 892–928 (in German).

Laüger, P., Pulver, R., and Montigel, C. (1945a). Mode of action of 4,4'-dichlorodiphenyl-trichloromethyl-methane (DDT-Geigy) in warm-blooded organisms. *Experientia* **1**, 120–121 (in German).

Laüger, P., Pulver, R., and Montigel, C. (1945b). Mode of action of 4,4'-dichlorodiphenyl-trichlor-methylmethane (DDT-Geigy) in warm-blooded animals. *Helv. Physiol. Pharmacol. Acta* **3**, 405–415 (in German).

Lawrence, L. J., and Casida, J. E. (1984). Interactions of lindane, toxaphene and cyclodienes with brain specific *t*-butylcyclophosphorothionate receptor. *Life Sci.* **35**, 171–178.

Laws, E. R., Jr. (1971). Evidence of antitumorigenic effects of DDT. *Arch. Environ. Health* **23**, 181–183.

Laws, E. R., Jr., Curley, A., and Biros, F. J. (1967). Men with intensive occupational exposure to DDT. A clinical and chemical study. *Arch. Environ. Health* **15**, 766–775.

Laws, E. R., Maddrey, W. D., Curley, A., and Burse, V. W. (1973). Long-term occupational exposure to DDT. *Arch. Environ. Health* **27**, 318–321.

Lay, J. P., Weisgerber, I., and Klein, W. (1975). Conversion of the aldrin/dieldrin metabolite dihydrochlordene dicarboxylic acid-^{14}C in rats. *Pestic. Biochem. Physiol.* **5**, 226–232.

Lay, J. P., Klein, W., Korte, F., and Richter, E. (1981). Metabolism of β-hexachlorocyclohexane-^{14}C in rats following low dosing in the diet. *J. Environ. Sci. Health, Part B* **16**, 227–238.

Leach, J. F., and Charles, A. K. (1987). Regional mirex distribution and its effects on γ-aminobutyric acid and flunitrazepam binding in mouse strains. *J. Toxicol. Environ. Health* **21**, 423–433.

Lee, B., and Groth, P. (1977). Scabies: Transcutaneous poisoning during treatment. *Pediatrics* **59**, 643.

Lee, B., Groth, P., and Turner, W. (1976). Suspected reactions to benzene hexachloride. *JAMA, J. Am. Med. Assoc.* **236**, 2846.

Lee, M., Harris, K., and Trowbridge, H. (1964). Effect of the level of dietary protein on the toxicity of dieldrin for the laboratory rat. *J. Nutr.* **84**, 136–144.

Lehman, A. J. (1948). The toxicology of the new agricultural chemicals. *Q. Bull.— Assoc. Food Drug Off.* **12**, 82.

Lehman, A. J. (1950). Some toxicological reasons why certain chemicals may or may not be permitted as food additives. *Q. Bull.—Assoc. Food Drug Off.* **14**, 82–98.

Lehman, A. J. (1951). Chemicals in foods: A report to the Association of Food and Drug Officials on current developments. Part II. Pesticides. Section I: Introduction. *Q. Bull.—Assoc. Food Drug Off.* **15** (I),122–125 Lehman, A. J. (1952). Chemicals in foods: A report to the Association of Food and Drug officials on current developments. Part II. Pesticides. Section II. Dermal toxicity. Section III. Subacute and chronic toxicity. Section IV. Biochemistry. Section V. Pathology. *Q. Bull.—Assoc. Food Drug Off.* **16** (II), 3–9; (III), 47–53; (IV), 85–91; (V), 126–132.

Lehman, A. J. (1965). "Summaries of Pesticide Toxicity." Assoc. Food Drug Off. U.S., Topeka, Kansas.

Leighty, E. G. (1981). Decreased retention of fatty acid conjugated DDT metabolites in rats given injections of heparin, bile salts or leirthin. *Res. Commun. Chem. Pathol. Pharmacol.* **31**, 69–76.

Leighty, E. G., Fentiman, A. F., and Thompson, R. M. (1980). Conjugation of fatty acids to DDT in the rat: Possible mechanism for retention. *Toxicology* **15**, 77–82.

LeMarchand, L., Kolonel, L. N., Siegel, B., and Dendle, W. H. (1986). Trends in birth defects for a Hawaiian population exposed to heptachlor and for the United States. *Arch. Environ. Health* **41**, 145–148.

Lemmon, G. B., and Pierce, W. F. (1952). Intoxication due to chlordane. Report of a case. *JAMA, J. Am. Med. Assoc.* **149**, 1314–1316.

Lensky, G. B., and Pierce, W. F. (1952). Human poisoning by chlordane. Report of a case. *JAMA, J. Am. Med. Assoc.* **149**, 1394–1395.

Leshchenko, P. D., and Polonskaia, M. N. (1969). New products in the prophylactic nutrition of workers in the organochlorine industry. *Vrach. Delo* **8**, 106–110 (in French).

Levy, J. M., Lutz, P., Wagner, C., Sauer, P., Seiller, F., Fischbach, M., Segura, N., and Sauvage, P. (1985). Favorable outcome of a recurring malignant adrenocortical tumor under *o,p'*-DDD therapy. *Ann. Pediatr.* **32**, 541–544 (in French).

Levy, K. A., Brady, S. E., and Pfaffenberger, C. D. (1981). Chlorobenzilate residues in citrus-workers. *Bull. Environ. Contam. Toxicol.* **27**, 235–238.

Lewis, W. H., and Richards, A. G., Jr. (1945). Non-toxicity of DDT on cells in cultures. *Science* **102**, 330–331.

Lidov, R. E., Bluestone, H., and Soloway, S. B. (1950). Alkali-stable poly-chloro-organic insect toxicants, aldrin and dieldrin. *Adv. Chem.* **1**, 175–183.

Lièvremont, M., and Potus, J. (1981). Intracerebral distribution of lindane in the rat; observations a short time after single dose administration. *C.R. Seances Acad. Sci., Ser. 3* **292**, 1163–1168 (in French).

Lièvremont, M., Barnier, J. V., and Potus, J. (1984). γ-Hexachlorocyclohex-ane inhibition of the calcium fluxes at the desensitized mouse neu-romuscular junction. *Toxicol. Appl. Pharmacol.* **76**, 280–287.

Lillie, R. D., and Smith, M. I. (1944). Pathology of experimental poisoning in cats, rabbits, and rats with 2,2-bis-(*para*-chlorphenyl)-1,1,1-trichloreth-ane. *Public Health Rep.* **59**, 979–984.

Lillie, R. D., Smith, M. I., and Stohlman, E. F. (1947). Pathologic action of DDT and certain of its analogs and derivatives. *Arch. Pathol.* **43**, 127–142.

Lillie, R. J., Cecil, H. C., and Bitman, J. (1973). Methoxychlor in chicken breeder diets. *Poult. Sci.* **52**, 1134–1138.

Linder, R. E., Scotti, T. M., McElroy, W. K., Laskey, J. W., Stracler, L. F., and Powell, K. (1983). Spermotoxicity and tissue accumulation of chlor-decone (Kepone) in male rats. *J. Toxicol. Environ. Health* **12**, 183–192.

Linder, R. L., Dahlgren, R. B., and Greichus, Y. A. (1970). Residues in the brain of adult pheasants given dieldrin. *J. Wildl. Manage.* **34**, 954–956.

Litterst, C. L., Miller, E., Michel, T., Olivito, V., and Van Loon, E. J. (1973). Distribution and penetration of lindane into brains of normal and phenobar-bital pretreated dogs. *Toxicol. Appl. Pharmacol.* **25**, 484–485.

Litvinov, N. N., and Nikonova, A. G. (1971). The action of alkyl sulfate on the resorption of pesticides and on their content in animal organs. *Gig. Sanit.* **36**, 21–25 (in Russian).

Liu, P. T., and Morgan, D. P. (1986). Comparative toxicity and biotransfor-mation of lindane in C57BL/6 and DBA/2 mice. *Life Sci.* **39**, 1237–1244.

Llinares. V. M., and Wasserman, M. (1968). Storage of DDT in the body fat of the people of Spain. Unpublished data (cited by Wassermann *et al.,* 1968b).

Lockard, V. G., Mehendale, H. M., and O'Neal, R. M. (1983a). Chlor-decone-induced potentiation of carbon tetrachloride hepatotoxicity: A light and electron microscopic study. *Exp. Mol. Pathol.* **39**, 230–245.

Lockard, V. G., Mehendale, H. M., and O'Neal, R. M. (1983b). Chlor-decone-induced potentiation of carbon tetrachloride hepatotoxicity: A mor-phometric and biochemical study. *Exp. Mol. Pathol.* **39**, 246–255.

Loeber, J. G., and Van Velsen, F. L. (1984). Uterotropic effect of beta-HCH, a food chain contaminant. *Food Addit. Contam.* **1**, 63–66.

Loevinsohn, M. E. (1987). Insecticide use and increased mortality in rural central Luzon, Philippines. *Lancet* **1**, 1359–1362.

Lofroth, G. (1968). Pesticides and catastrophe. *New Sci.* **40**, 567–568.

Loganovskii, N. G. (1971). The effect of hexachlorane on the functional state of the kidneys. *Gig. Tr. Prof. Zabol.* **15**, 46–48.

Loge, J. P. (1965). Aplastic anemia following exposure to benezene hex-acholoride (lindane). *JAMA, J. Am. Med. Assoc.* **193**, 110–114.

Loose, L. D. (1982). Macrophage induction of 7-suppressor cells in pesticide-exposed and protozoan-infected mice. *Environ. Health Perspect.* **43**, 89–97.

Lopez-Aparicio, P., Del Hoyo, N., and Perez-Albarsanz, M. A. (1988). Lin-dane distribution and phospholipid alterations in rat tissues after admin-istration of lindane-containing diet. *Pestic. Biochem. Physiol.* **31**, 109–119.

Lu, F. C., Jessup, D. C., and Lavalle, A. (1965). Toxicity of pesticides in young versus adult rats. *Food Cosmet. Toxicol.* **3**, 591–596.

Lubberink, A. A. M. E., Rijnberk, A., Der Kinderen, P. J., and Thijssen, J. H. H. (1971). Hyperfunction of the adrenal cortex: A review. *Aust. Vet. J.* **47**, 504–509.

Lubitz, J. A., Feeman, L., and Okum, R. (1973). Mitotane use in inoperable adrenal cortical carcinoma. *JAMA, J. Am. Med. Assoc.* **233**, 1109–1112.

Ludke, J. L. (1974). Interaction of dieldrin and DDE residues in Japanese quail (*Coturnix coturnix japonica*). *Bull. Environ. Contam. Toxicol.* **11**, 297–302.

Luis, P. (1952). A case of detection of DDT in viscera. *Rev. Asoc. Bioquim. Argent.* **17**, 334–338 (in Spanish).

Lund, B., Klasson-Wehler, F., and Brandt, I. (1986). *o,p'*-DDD in the mouse lung: Selective uptake, covalent binding and effect on drug metabolism. *Chem.-Biol. Interact.* **60**, 129–141.

Lund, B., Bergman, A., and Brandt, I. (1988). Metabolic activation of a DDT-metabolite,3-methylsulfonyl-DDE, in the adrenal *zona fasciculata* in mice. *Chem.-Biol. Interact.* **65**, 24–40.

Lund, B. O., Ghantous, H., Bergman, A., and Brandt, I. (1989). Covalent binding of four DDD isomers in the mouse lung: Lack of structure specific-ity. *Pharmacol. Toxicity.*, **65**, 282–286.

Luquet, F. M., Goursaud, J., and Gaudier, B. (1972). Study of the pollution of human milk by residual pesticides. *Pathol. Biol.* **20**, 137–143 (in French).

Luquet, F. M., Goursand, J. G., and Casalis, J. (1974a). Residues of organochlorine pesticides in the milk of animals and humans. *Ann. Falsif. Expert. Chim.* **67**, 217–239 (in French).

Luquet, F. M., Goursand, J. G., and Casalis, J. (1974b). Residues of organochlorine pesticides in the milk of animals and humans. *Lait* **54**, 269–301 (in French).

Luton, J. P., Valcke, J. C., Remy, J. M., Mathieu de Fossey, B., and Bricaire, H. (1972). Gynecomastia after long-term treatment of Cushing's disease with *o,p'*-DDT. *Ann. Endocrinol.* **33**, 290–293 (in French).

Luton, J. P., Remy, J. M., Valcke, J. C., Laudat, P., and Bricaire, H. (1973). Cure or remission of Cushing's disease by prolonged therapeutic use of *o,p'*-DDD (with reference to 17 observations). *Ann. Endocrinol.* **34**, 351–376 (in French).

Lyubchenko, P. N., Chemnyy, A. B., Boyarchuk, Z. I., Ginzburg, D. A., and Sukova, V. M. (1973). Effects of a BHC–thiram combination in humans. *Gig. Tr. Prof. Zabol.* **17**, 50–52 (in Russian).

Lyubenko, P. K., Stefanskiy, K. S., and Rosenfel'd, A. A. (1973a). Procedure in using polychlorocamphene in agriculture and its content in soil and plants. *Khim. Sel'sk. Khoz.* **11**, 28–29 (in Russian).

Lyubenko, P. K., Stefanskiy, K. S., and Rozenfel'd, A. A. (1973b). Regula-tions for polychlorocamphene use in agriculture and content of it in soil and plants. *Khim. Sel'sk. Khoz.* **11**, 908–909 (in Russian).

MacCormack, J. D. (1945). Infestation and DDT. *Ir. J. Med. Sci.* **6**, 627–634.

Macek, K. J., Rodgers, C. R., Stalling, D. L., and Korn, S. (1970). The uptake, distribution, and elimination of dietary 14-C-DDT and 14-C-di-eldrin in rainbow trout. *Trans. Am. Fish. Soc.* **99**, 689–695.

Macholz, R. M., and Kujawa, M. (1985). Recent state of lindane metabolism. Part III. *Residue Rev.* **94**, 119–149.

Macholz, R. M., Knoll, R., Lewerenz, H. J., Petrzika, M., and Engst, R. (1982a). Metabolism of α-hexachlorocyclohexane. Free metabolites in urine and organs of rats. *Xenobiotica* **12**, 227–231.

Macholz, R. M., Knoll, R., Lewerenz, H. J., and Plass, R. (1982b). Bio-degradation of beta-hexahlorocyclohexane. Free metabolites in rat urine and organs. *Arch. Toxicol.* **50**, 85–88.

Macholz, R. M., Seidler, H., Petrzika, M., and Kujawa, J. (1985). Identification of an amino acid conjugate in the urine following administration of lindane to rats. *Z. Gesamte Hyg. Ihre Grenzgeb.* **31**, 177–178 (in German).

Macholz, R. M., Bleyl, D. W. R., Klepel, H., Knoll, R., Kujawa, M., Lewerenz, H. J., Mueller, D., and Plass, R. (1986). Comparison of dis-tribution and toxicity of α-, β- and γ-hexachlorocyclohexane (HCH) after application to rats for 30 days. *Nahrung* **30**, 701–708 (in German).

Mackeras, I. M., and West, R. F. K. (1946). "DDT" poisoning in man. *Med. J. Aust.* **1**, 400–401.

Macklin, A. W., and Ribelin, W. E. (1971). The relation of pesticides to abortion in dairy cattle. *J. Am. Vet. Med. Assoc.* **159**, 1743–1748.

MacMahon, B. (1985). Phenobarbital: Epidemiological evidence. *IARC Sci. Publ.* **65**, 101–105.

MacNamara, B. G. P. (1970). Benzene hexacholoride poisoning. *Br. Med. J.* **3**, 585.

Mactutus, C. F., and Tilson, H. A. (1984a). Evaluation of neonatal chlordecone neurotoxicity during early development. *Neurobehav. Toxicol. Teratol.* **6**, 67–73.

Mactutus, C. F., and Tilson, H. A. (1984b). Neonatal chlordecone exposure impairs early learning and retention of active avoidance in the rat. *Neurobehav. Toxicol. Teratol.* **6**, 75–83.

Maes, R., and Heyndrickx, A. (1966). Distribution of organic chlorinated insecticides in human tissues. *Meded. Rijksfac. Landbouw wet. Gent* **31**, 1021–1025.

Magour, S. Mäser, H., and Steffen, I. (1984). Effect of lindane on synaptosomal Na$^+$/K$^+$-ATPase in relation to its subcellular distribution in the brain. *Acta Pharmacol. Toxicol.* **54**, 299–303.

Mahmood, A., Agarwel, N., Sanyal, S., Dudeja, P. K., and Subrahmanyam, D. (1981). Acute dieldrin toxicity effect on the uptake of glucose and leucine on brush border enzymes in monkey intestine. *Chem.-Biol. Interact.* **37**, 165–170.

Maier-Bode, H. (1960). DDT in body fat of people. *Med. Exp.* **1**, 146–152 (in German).

Maier-Bode, H. (1968). Properties, effect, residues and analytics of the insecticide endosulfan. *Residue Rev.* **22**, 1–44.

Majumdar, S. K., Kopleman, H. A., and Schnitman, M. J. (1976). Dieldrin-induced chromosome damage in mouse bone-marrow and WI-38 human lung cells. *J. Hered.* **67**, 303–307.

Makara, G. (1973). Chlorphenamidine as an ovicide and the efficiency of heat in killing lice and nits. *Sci. Publ.—Pan. Am. Health Organ.* **263**, 198–200.

Makovskaya, Y. I., Shamray, P. F., and Grigor'yeva, N. N. (1972). Structural and histochemical changes in internal secretion glands during polychloropinene poisoning. *Vrach. Delo* **2**, 128–131 (in Russian).

Mal'tseva, Z. I., and Savchuk, T. F. (1953). The possibility of chronic poisoning with the use of BHC for disinfection of habitable dwellings. *Gig. Sanit.* **12**, 43–45 (in Russian).

Mandroiu, V., and Iordachescu, M. (1971). Determination of the BHC content in the human organism. *Igiena* **20**, 363–364 (in Romanian).

Marchand, M., Dubrulle, P., and Goudemand, M. (1956). Agranulocytosis in a subject exposed to vapor of hexochlorocyclohexane. *Arch. Mal. Prof. Med. Trav. Secur. Soc.* **17**, 256–258 (in French).

Maresch, W., Lembeck, F., and Lipp, W. (1960). Poisonings in infancy. *Wien Klin. Wochenschr.* **72**, 411–416 (in German).

Markarian, D. S. (1966). Cytogenetic effect of some chlorine-containing organic insecticides on mouse bone-marrow cell nuclei. *Genetika* **1**, 132–137.

Marquardt, E. D. (1982). Suicide attempt with rectally administered chlordane. *Drug Intell. Clin. Pharm.* **16**.

Martinez. A. J., Taylor, J. R., Dyck, P. J., Jouff, S. A., and Isaacs, E. (1978). Chlordecone intoxication in man. II. Ultrastructure of peripheral nerves and skeletal muscle. *Neurology* **28**, 631–635.

Martson, L. V., and Shepel'skaya, N. R. (1980). Study of the reproductive function in animals exposed to polychlorocamphene. *Gig. Sanit.*, pp. 14–16 (in Russian).

Martz, F., and Straw, J. A. (1972). Effects of mitotane (*o,p'*-DDD) on hepatic drug metabolism in dogs. *Fed. Proc., Fed. Am. Soc. Exp. Biol.* **31**, 581.

Martz, F., and Straw, J. A. (1973). Mitotane decreases adrenal cortical heme and P450. *Fed. Proc., Fed. Am. Soc. Exp. Biol.* **32**, 734.

Martz, F., and Straw, J. A. (1977). The *in vitro* metabolism of 1-(o-chlorophenyl)-1-(p-chlorophenyl)-2,2-dichloroethane (*o,p*-DDD) by dog adrenal mitochondria and metabolite covalent binding to mitochondrial macromolecules. A possible mechanism for the adrenocorticolytic effect. *Drug. Metabl. Dispos.* **5**, 482–486.

Martz, F., and Straw, J. A. (1980). Metabolism and covalent binding of 1-(o-chlorophenyl)-1-(p-chlorophenyl)-2,2-dichloroethane (*o,p*-DDD). Correlation between adrenocorticolytic activity and metabolic activation by adrenocortical mitochondria. *Drug Metab. Dispos.* **8**, 127–130.

Maslansky, C. J., and Williams, G. M. (1981). Evidence for an epigenetic mode of action in organochlorine pesticide hepatocarcinogenicity: A lack of genotoxicity in rat, mouse, and hamster hepatocytes. *J. Toxicol. Environ. Health* **8**, 121–130.

Mason, T. J., McKay, F. W., Hoover, F., Blot, W. J., and Fraumeni, J. F., Jr. (1975). "Atlas of Cancer Mortality for U. S. Counties: 1950–1969," Publ. No. (NIH) 75-780. U.S. Department of Health, Education and Welfare, Public Health Service, Washington, D. C.

Matsuda, H., Shimamoto, T., Ito, T., and Ogida, K. (1971). On the analytical results of organochlorine pesticide residues in mothers' milk. *Annu. Rep. Ehime Prefect. Hyg. Lab.* **33**, 43–48 (in Japanese).

Matsumura, F., and Ghiasuddin, S. M. (1983). Evidence for similarities between cyclodiene type insecticides and picrotoxin in their action mechanisms. *J. Environ. Sci. Health, Part B*, **B18**, 1–14.

Matsumura, F., and Patil, K. C. (1969). Adenosine triphosphatase sensitive to DDT in synapses of rat brain. *Science* **166**, 121–122.

Matsumura, F., and Nelson, J. O. (1970). Identification of the major metabolic product of heptachlor epoxide in rat feces. *Bull. Environ. Contam. Toxicol.* **5**, 489–492.

Matsumura, F., Patil, K. C., and Bousch, G. M. (1970). Formation of "photodieldrin" by microorganisms. *Science* **170**, 1206–1207.

Matsumura, F., Howard, R. W., and Nelson, J. O. (1975). Structure of the toxic fraction A of toxaphene. *Chemosphere* **5**, 271–276.

Matsunaga, K., Ogino, Y., Morita, K., Sueiishi, T., Imanaka, M., Mukada, K., Namba, S., Tada, Y., and Takata, M. (1975). Hygienic studies on pesticide residues. Part 3. Organochlorine pesticide residues in human milk. *Annu. Rep. Hyg. Lab. Okayama Prefect.* **22**, 35–38 (in Japanese).

Matsuoka, L. Y. (1981). Convulsions following application of gamma benzene hexachloride. *J. Am. Acad. Dermatol.* **5**, 98–99.

Matthews, H. B., and Matsumura, F. (1969). Metabolic fate of dieldrin in the rat. *J. Agric. Food Chem.* **17**, 845–852.

Matthews, H. B., and McKinney, J. D. (1974). Dieldrin metabolism to *cis*-dihydroaldrindiol and epimerization of *cis*- to *trans*-dihydroaldrindiol by rat liver microsomes. *Drug Metab. Dispos.* **2**, 333–340.

Matthews, H. B., McKinney, J. D., and Lucier, G. W. (1971). Dieldrin metabolism, excretion, and storage in male and female rats. *J. Agric. Food Chem.* **19**, 1244–1248.

Matthews, H. B., Domanski, J. J., and Guthrie, F. E. (1976). Hair and its associated lipids as an excretory pathway for chlorinated hydrocarbons. *Xenobiotica* **6**, 425–429.

Mattson, A. M., Spillane, J. T., Baker, C., and Pearce, G. W. (1953). Determination of DDT and related substances in human fat. *Anal. Chem.* **25**, 1065–1070.

Matuo, Y. K., Lopes, J. N., and Lopes, J. L. (1980). DDT levels in human milk from Ribeirao Preto (Brazil). *Rev. Bras. Biol.* **40**, 293–296 (in Portuguese).

Mayer, F. L., Street, J. C., and Neubold, J. M. (1970). Organochlorine insecticide interactions affecting residue storage in rainbow trout. *Bull. Environ. Contam. Toxicol.* **5**, 300–310.

Mayer, R. T., and Himel, C. M. (1972). Dynamics of fluorescent probe–cholinesterase reactions. *Biochemistry* **11**, 2082–2090.

Mayersdorf, A., and Israeli, R. (1974). Toxic effects of chlorinated hydrocarbon insecticides on the human electroencephalogram. *Arch. Environ. Health* **28**, 159–163.

McBlain, W. A. (1987). The levo enantimer of *o,p'*-DDT inhibits the binding of 17β-estradiol to the estrogen receptor. *Life Sci.* **40**, 215–221.

McCann, J., and Ames, B. N. (1976). Detection of carcinogens as mutagens in the *Salmonella*/microsome test: Assay of 300 chemicals: Discussion. *Proc. Natl. Acad. Sci. U.S.A.* **73**, 950–954.

McCann, J., Chol, E., Yamasaki, E., and Ames, B. N. (1975). Detection of carcinogens as mutagens in the *Salmonella*/microsome test: Assay of 300 chemicals. *Proc. Natl. Acad. Sci. U.S.A.* **72**, 5135–5139.

McGee, L. C., Reed, H. L., and Fleming, J. P. (1952). Accidental poisoning by toxaphene. Review of toxicology and case reports. *JAMA, J. Am. Med. Assoc.* **149**, 1124–1126.

McKiernan, P., Doyle, D. A., Duffy, G. J., Towers, R. P., Duff, F. A., and O'Donovan, D. K. (1978). Brief report. *o,p'*-DDD and adrenal carcinoma. *Ir. J. Med. Sci.* **147**, 437–440.

McKinney, J. D., Boozier, E. L., Hopkins, H. P., and Suggs, J. E. (1969). Synthesis and reactions of a proposed DDT metabolite, 2,2'-bis-(p-chlorophenyl)-acetaldehyde. *Experientia* **25**, 897–898.

McKinney, J. D., Matthews, H. B., and Fishbein, L. (1972). Major fecal metabolite of dieldrin in rat. Structure and chemistry. *J. Agric. Food Chem.* **20**, 597–602.

McLachlan, J. A., and Dixon, R. L. (1972). Gonadal function in mice exposed prenatally to p,p'-DDT. *Toxicol. Appl. Pharmacol.* **22**, 327.

McLean, J. A. (1966). Aplastic anaemia associated with insecticides. *Med. J. Aust.* **1**, 996.

McManus, M. E., Boobis, A. R., Minchin, R. F., Schwartz, D. M., Murray, S., Davies, D. S., and Thorgeirsson, S. S. (1984). Relationship between oxidative metabolism of 2-acetylaminofluorene, debrisoquine, bifuralol, and aldrin in human liver microsomes. *Cancer Res.* **44**, 5692–5697.

McNamara, B. P., and Krop, S. (1948a). Observations on the pharmacology of the isomers of hexachlorocyclohexane. *J. Pharmacol. Exp. Ther.* **92**, 140–146.

McNamara, B. P., and Krop, S. (1948b). The treatment of acute poisoning produced by gamma hexachlorocyclohexane. *J. Pharmacol. Exp. Ther.* **92**, 147–152.

McQueen, E. G., Brosnan, C., and Ferry, D. G. (1968). Poisoning from a rose spray containing lindane and malathion. *N. Z. Med. J.* **67**, 533–537.

McQueen, E. G., Owen, D., and Ferry, D. G. (1972). Effect of phenytoin and other drugs in reducing serum DDT levels. *N. Z. Med. J.* **75**, 208–211.

Mead, R. J. (1982). Lindane, Kwell and aplastic anemia. *Postgrad. Med.* **72**, 28.

Medley, J. G., Bond, C. A., and Woodham, D. W. (1974). The cumulation and disappearance of mirex residues. I. In tissues of roosters fed four concentrations of mirex in their feed. *Bull. Environ. Contam. Toxicol.* **11**, 217–223.

Mehendale, H. M. (1977a). Chemical reactivity–absorption, retention, metabolism, and elimination of hexachlorocyclopentadiene. *Environ. Health Perspect.* **21**, 275–278.

Mehendale, H. M. (1977b). Effect of preexposure to Kepone on the biliary excretion of imipramine and sulfobromophthalein. *Toxicol. Appl. Pharmacol.* **40**, 247–259.

Mehendale, H. M. (1977c). Mirex-induced impairment of hepatobiliary function. Suppressed biliary excretion of imipramine and sulfobromophthalein. *Drug Metab. Dispos.* **5**, 56–62.

Mehendale, H. M. (1978). Pesticide-induced modification of hepatobiliary function: Hexachlorobenzene, DDT and toxaphene. *Food Cosmet. Toxicol.* **16**, 19–25.

Mehendale, H. M. (1981b). Chlordecone-induced hepatic dysfunction. *J. Toxicol. Environ. Health* **8**, 743–755.

Mehendale, H. M. (1989). Mechanism of the lethal interaction of chlordecone and CCl₄ at non-toxic doses. *Toxicol. Lett.* **49**, 215–241.

Mehendale, H. M., and El-Bassiouni, E. A. (1975). Uptake and disposition of aldrin and dieldrin by isolated perfused rabbit lung. *Drug. Metab. Dispos.*, **3**, 543–556.

Mehendale, H. M., and Klingensmith, J. C. (1988). *In vivo* metabolism of CCl₄ by rats pretreated with chlordecone, mirex, or phenobarbital. *Toxicol. Appl. Pharmacol.* **93**, 247–256.

Mehendale, H. M., Fishbein, L., Fields, M., and Matthews, H. B. (1972). Fate of mirex-¹⁴C in the rat and plants. *Bull. Environ. Contam. Toxicol.*, **8**, 200–207.

Mehendale, H. M., Chen, P. F., Fishbein, L., and Matthews, H. B. (1973). Effect of mirex on the activities of various rat hepatic mixed-function oxidases. *Arch. Environ. Contam. Toxicol.*, **1**, 245–254.

Mehendale, H. M., El-Bassiouni, E. A., and McKinney, J. D. (1974). Disposition of aldrin by isolated perfused rabbit lung preparations. *Fed. Proc., Fed. Am. Soc. Exp. Biol.* **33**, 534.

Mehendale, H. M., Takanaka, A., Desaiah, D., and Ho, I. K. (1977). Kepone induction of hepatic mixed function oxidases. *Life Sci.*, **20**, 991–998.

Mehendale, H. M., Takanaka, A., Desaiah, D., and Ho, I. K. (1978). Effect of preexposure to kepone on hepatic mixed function oxidases in the female rat. *Toxicol. Appl. Pharmacol.*, **44**, 171–180.

Mehendale, H. M., Ho, I. K., and Desaiah, D. (1979). Possible molecular mechanism of mirex-induced hepatobiliary dysfunction. *Drug Metab. Dispos.*, **7**, 28–33.

Mehendale, H. M., Purushotham, K. R., and Lockard, V. G. (1989). The time course of liver injury and [³H]thymidine incorporation in chlordecone-potentiated CHCl₃ hepatotoxicity. *Exp. Mol. Pathol.*, **51**, 31–47.

Mehrota, B. D., Bansal, S. K., and Desaiah, D. (1982). Comparative effects of structurally related cyclodiene pesticides on ATPases. *J. Appl. Toxicol.* **2**, 278–283.

Meierhenry, E. F., Reubner, B. H., Gershwin, M. E., Hsieh, L. S., and French, S. W. (1983). Dieldrin-induced Mallory bodies in hepatic tumors of mice of different strains. *Hepatology* **3**, 90–95.

Mellis, R. (1955). Tolerability of small doses of lindane by warm-blooded animals. *Nuovi Ann. Ig. Microbiol.* **6**, 90.

Menconi, S., Clark, J. M., Langenberg, P., and Hryhorczyk, D. (1988). A preliminary study of potential human health effects in private residences following chlordane applications for termite control. *Arch. Environ. Health* **43**, 349–352.

Menczel, E., Bucks, D., Maibach, H., and Wester, R. (1984). Lindane binding to sections of human skin: Skin capacity and isotherm determinations. *Arch. Dermatol. Res.* **276**, 326–329.

Mendeloff, A. I., and Smith, D. E. (1955). Exposure to insecticides, bone marrow failure, gastrointestinal bleeding, and uncontrollable infections. *Am. J. Med.* **19**, 274–284.

Menna, J. H., Barnett, J. B., and Soderberg, L. S. (1985). Influenza type A infection of mice exposed in utero to chlordane; survival and antibody studies. *Toxicol. Lett.* **24**, 45–52.

Menner, K. (1965). Experiences of poisonings of infants. *Med. Welt* **13**, 634–638 (in German).

Menzie, C. M. (1969). "Metabolism of Pesticides," Spec. Sci. Rep., Wildl. No. 127. U. S. Govt. Printing Office, Washington, D.C.

Mes, J., and Davies, D. J. (1979). Presence of polychlorinated biphenyl and organochlorine pesticide residues and the absence of polychlorinated terphenyls in Canadian human milk samples. *Bull. Environ. Contam. Toxicol.* **21**, 381–387.

Mes, J., Campbell, D., Robinson, R., and Davis, D. (1977). Polychlorinated biphenyls and organochlorine residues in adipose tissue of Canadians. *Bull. Environ. Contam. Toxicol.* **17**, 196–203.

Mes, J., Davies, D. J., and Miles, W. (1978). Traces of mirex in some Canadian human milk samples. *Bull. Environ. Contam. Toxicol.* **19**, 564–570.

Mes, J., Davis, D. J., and Turton, D. (1982). Polychlorinated biphenyl and other chlorinated hydrocarbon residues in adipose tissue of Canadians. *Bull. Environ. Contam. Toxicol.* **28**, 97–104.

Mes, J., Davies, D. J., Turton, D., and Sun, W. (1986). Levels and trends of chlorinated hydrocarbon contaminants in the breast milk of Canadian women. *Food Addit. Contam.* **3**, 313–322.

Mestitzová, M. (1967). On reproduction studies and the occurrence of cataracts in rats after long-term feeding of the insecticide heptachlor. *Experientia* **23**, 42–43.

Mestitzová, M., and Beño, M. (1966). Toxicologic characteristics of small repeated doses of heptachlor. *Prac. Lek.* **18**, 153–157 (in Slovakian).

Mestitzová, M., Kovac, J., and Durcek, K. (1970a). Heptachlor induced changes in fenitrothion metabolism. *Bull. Environ. Contam. Toxicol.* **5**, 195–201.

Mestitzová, M., Kovac, J., Durcek, K., and Hladka, A. (1970b). Toxicity of an organophosphate (fenitrothion) in rats chronically poisoned with an organochlorine (heptachlor). *Prac. Lek.* **22**, 361–365.

Mestitzová, M., Kovac, J., and Durcek, K. (1971). Metabolic studies of combinations of pesticides. *Int. Arch. Arbeitsmed.* **22**, 223–238 (in German).

Metcalf, R. L. (1973). A century of DDT. *J. Agric. Chem.* **21**, 511–519.

Michail, G. (1974a). Experimental studies on toxic effects of BHC and parathion administered jointly. *J. Jpn. Assoc. Rural Med.* **22**, 772–773 (in Japanese).

Michail, G. (1974b). On the preliminary study of occupational chronic exposure in plant protection. *J. Jpn. Assoc. Rural Med.* **22**, 773 (in Japanese).

Michail, G., Zlavog, A., Anghelache, V., and Bodnar, J. (1972). Serum ornithine carbamoyltransferase, test for evaluating hepatic alterations caused by some industrial toxic substances. *Igiena* **21,** 267–276 (in Romanian).

Mick, D. L., Long, K. R., Dretchen, J. S., and Bonderman, D. P. (1971). Aldrin and dieldrin in human blood components. *Arch. Environ. Health* **23,** 177–180.

Mick, D. L., Long, K. R., and Bonderman, D. P. (1972). Aldrin and dieldrin in the blood of pesticide formulators. *Am. Ind. Hyg. Assoc. J.* **33,** 94–99.

Micks, D. W. (1954). Potential health hazards of organic insecticides. *Tex. State J. Med.* **50,** 148–153.

Mikosha, A. S. (1985). Effect of chloditan on activity of malate enzymes in adrenal gland. *Vopr. Med. Khim.* **31,** 61–64.

Milby, T. H., and Samuels, A. J. (1971). Human exposure to lindane: Comparison of an exposed and unexposed population. *J. Occup. Med.* **13,** 256–258.

Milby, T. H., Samuels, A. J., and Ottoboni, F. (1968). Human exposure to lindane: Blood lindane levels as a function of exposure. *J. Occup. Med.* **10,** 584–587.

Miller, G. J., and Fox, J. A. (1973). Chlorinated hydrocarbon pesticide residues in Queensland human milks. *Med. J. Aust.* **2,** 261–264.

Miller, P. E., and Fink, G. B. (1973). Brain serotonin level and pentylenetetrazol seizure threshold in dieldrin and endrin treated mice. *Proc. West. Pharmacol. Soc.* **16,** 195–197.

Mirakhmedov, U. M., and Karimov, A. M. (1972). The effect of pesticides on the skin of agricultural workers. *Vestn. Dermatol. Venerol.* **46,** 50–52 (in Russian).

Miranda, C. L., Webb, R. E., and Ritchey, S. J. (1973). Effect of dietary protein quality, phenobarbital and SKF 525-A on heptachlor metabolism in the rat. *Pestic. Biochem. Physiol.* **3,** 456–461.

Mishra, S. K., Koury, M., and Desaiah, D. (1980). Inhibition of calcium ATPase activity in rat brain and mucle by chlordecone. *Bull. Environ. Contamin. Toxicol.* **25,** 262–268.

Misra, U. K., Nag, D., and Murti, C. R. (1984). A study of cognitive functions in DDT sprayers. *Indian Health* **22,** 199–206.

Mitjavila, S., Carrera, G., Boigegrain, R.-A., and Derache, R. (1981a). I. Evaluation of the toxic risk of DDt in the rat: During accumulation. *Arch. Environ. Contam. Toxicol.* **10,** 459–469.

Mitjavila, S., Carrera, G., and Fernandez, Y. (1981b). II. Evaluation of the toxic risk of accumulated DDT in the rat: During fat mobilization. *Arch. Environ. Contam. Toxicol.* **10,** 471–481.

Miura, K., Ino, T., and Iizuka, M. (1973). Comparison of susceptibility of various strains of mice to acute toxicity of BHC. *Med. Biol.* **86,** 391–396.

Miura, K., Ino, T., and Iizuka, S. (1974). Comparison of susceptibilities to the acute toxicity of BHC in strains of experimental mice. *Exp. Anim.* **23,** 198 (in Japanese).

Mizoguchi, M., Yamagishi, T., Ushio, F., Fujimoto, C., Takeba, K., Kani, T., Haruta, M., Yasuhara, K., and Kubota, H. (1972). On the residual amount of organochlorine pesticides in human milk in Tokyo metropolitan area. *Jpn. J. Public Health* **19,** 541–544 (in Japanese).

Model', A. A. (1968). Peculiarities of neurological symptoms in chronic DDT poisoning. *Sov. Med.* **31,** 110–114 (in Russian).

Model', A. A., and Larina, M. B. (1957). On BHC poisoning. *Zh. Nevropatol. Psikhiatr. Im. S. S. Korsakova* **57,** 20–21 (in Russian).

Mohammed, A., Andersson, O., Biessmann, A., and Slanina, P. (1983). Fate and specific tissue retention of toxaphene in mice. *Arch. Toxicol.* **54,** 311–321.

Mohammed, A., Hallberg, E., Rydström, J., and Slanina, P. (1985). Toxaphene: Accumulation in the adrenal cortex and effect on ACTH-stimulated corticosteroid synthesis in the rat. *Toxicol. Lett.* **24,** 134–143.

Molnar, G. D., Nunn, S. L., and Tauxe, W. N. (1961). The effect of *o,p'*-DDD therapy on plasma cholesterol in adrenal carcinoma. *Proc. Staff Meet. Mayo Clin.* **36,** 618–620.

Molowa, D. T., Wrighton, S. A., Blanke, R. V., and Guzelian, P. S. (1986a). Characterization of a unique aldo-keto reductase responsible for the reduction of chlordecone in the liver of the gerbil and man. *J. Toxicol. Environ. Health* **17,** 375–384.

Molowa, D. T., Shayne, A. G., and Guzelian, P. S. (1986b). Purification and characterization of chlordecone reductase from human liver. *J. Biol. Chem.* **261,** 12624–12627.

Montgomery, J. A., and Struck, R. F. (1973). The relation of the metabolism of anticancer agents to their activity. *Fortschr. Arzneimittelforsch.* **17,** 32–304 (in German).

Montoya-Cabrera, M. A., de Aquino, Jaso-M. E., Reynoso Garcia, M., Vargas de la Rosa, R., and Hernandez-Zamora, A. (1980). Fatal endrin poisoning. *Bol. Med. Hosp. Infant. Mex. (Span. Ed.)* **37,** 417–423 (in Spanish).

Moorthy, K. S., Trottman, C. H., Spann, C. H., and Desaiah, D. (1986). *In vivo* effects of toxaphene on canodulin-regulated calcium-pump activity in rat brain. *J. Toxicol. Environ. Health* **20,** 249–259.

Morbidity and Mortality Weekly Reports (MMWR) (1981). Chlordane contamination of a public water supply—Pittsburgh, Pennsylvania. *Morbid. Mortal. Wkly. Rep.* **30,** 571–578.

Morbidity and Mortality Weekly Reports. (MMWR) (1984). Acute convulsions associated with endrin poisoning—Pakistan. *Morbid. Mortal. Wkly. Rep.* **33,** 687–693.

Morgan, D. P., and Lin, I. L. (1978). Blood organochlorine pesticide concentrations, clinical hematology and biochemistry in workers occupationally exposed to pesticides. *Arch. Environ. Contam. Toxicol.* **7,** 423–447.

Morgan, D. P., and Roan, C. C. (1969). Renal function in persons occupationally exposed to pesticides. *Arch. Environ. Health* **19,** 633–636.

Morgan, D. P., and Roan, C. C. (1970). Chlorinated hydrocarbon pesticide residue in human tissues. *Arch. Environ. Health* **20,** 452–457.

Morgan, D. P., and Roan, C. C. (1971). Absorption, storage, and metabolic conversion of ingested DDT and metabolites in man. *Arch. Environ. Health* **22,** 301–308.

Morgan, D. P., and Roan, C. C. (1972). Loss of DDT from storage in human body fat. *Nature (London)* **238,** 221–223.

Morgan, D. P., and Roan, C. C. (1973). Adrenocortical function in persons occupationally exposed to pesticides. *J. Occup. Med.* **15,** 26–28.

Morgan, D. P., and Roan, C. C. (1974). Liver function in workers having high tissue stores of chlorinated hydrocarbon pesticides. *Arch. Environ. Health* **29,** 14–17.

Morgan, D. P., and Roan, C. C. (1977). The metabolism of DDT in man. *Essays Toxicol.* **5,** 39.

Morgan, D. P., Roan, C. C., and Paschal, E. H. (1972). Transport of DDT, DDE and dieldrin in human blood. *Bull. Environ. Contam. Toxicol.* **8,** 321–326.

Morgan, D. P., Sandifer, S. H., Hetzler, H. L., Slach, E. F., Brady, C. D., and Colcolough, J. (1979). Test for *in vivo* conversions of mirex to Kepone. *Bull. Environ. Contam. Toxicol.* **22,** 238–244.

Morgan, D. P., Roberts, R. J., Walter, A. W., and Stockdale, E. M. (1980). Anemia associated with exposure to lindane. *Arch. Environ. Health* **35,** 307–310.

Morgan, J. M., and Hickenbottom, J. P. (1979). Comparison of selected parameters for monitoring methoxychlor hepatotoxicity. *Bull. Environ. Contam. Toxicol.* **23,** 275–280.

Mori, Y., Kikuta, M., Okinaga, E., and Okura, T. (1983). Levels of PCBs and organochlorine pesticides in human adipose tissue collected in Ehime prefecture. *Bull. Environ. Contam. Toxicol.* **30,** 74–79.

Morita, R., Lieberman, L. M., Beierwaltes, W. H., Conn, J. W., Ansari, A. N., and Nishiyama, H. (1972). Percent uptake of ^{131}I radioactivity in the adrenal from radioiodinated cholesterol. *J. Clin. Endocrinol. Metab.* **34,** 36–43.

Morohashi, K., Yoshioka, H., Sogawa, K., Fujii-Kuriyama, Y., and Omura, T. (1984). Induction of mRNA coding for phenobarbital-inducible form of microsomal cytochrome P-450 in rat liver by administration of 1,1-di(*p*-chlorophenyl)-2,2-dichloroethylene and phenobarbital. *J. Biochem. (Tokyo)* **95,** 949–957.

Morris, R. D. (1968). Effects of endrin feeding on survival and reproduction in the deer mouse, *Peromyscus maniculatus. Can. J. Zool.* **46,** 951–958.

Moss, J. A., and Hathway, D. E. (1964). Transport of organic compounds in the mammal—partition of dieldrin and Telodrin between the cellular components and soluble proteins of blood. *Biochem. J.* **91,** 384–393.

Moubry, R. J., Myrdal, G. R., and Sturges, A. (1968). Residues in food and feed. Rate of decline of chlorinated hydrocarbon pesticides in dairy milk. *Pestic. Monit. J.* **2**, 72–79.

Mourelle, M., Garcia, M., and Aguilar, C. (1985). Adenosine triphosphatase activities in plasma liver membranes of rats treated with DDT and toxaphene. *J. Appl. Toxicol.* **5**, 39–43.

Mueller, W. F., Nohynek, G., Woods, G., Korte, F., and Coulston, F. (1975a). Comparative metabolism of dieldrin-^{14}C in mouse, rat, rabbit, rhesus monkey and chimpanzee. *Chemosphere* **4**, 89–92.

Mueller, W. F., Woods, G., Korte, F., and Coulston, F. (1975b). Metabolism and organ distribution of dieldrin C in rhesus monkeys after single oral and intravenous administration. *Chemosphere* **4**, 93–98.

Mueller, W. F., Iatropoulos, M. J., Rozman, K., Korte, F., and Coulston, F. (1978). Comparative kinetic, metabolic, and histopathologic effects of chlorinated hydrocarbon pesticides in rhesus monkeys. *Toxicol. Appl. Pharmacol.* **45**, 283–284.

Mughal, H. A., and Rahman, A. (1973). Organochlorine pesticide content of human adipose tissue in Karachi. *Arch. Environ. Health* **27**, 396–398.

Muhlens, K. (1946). Significance of dichlor-diphenyl-trichlor methylmethane peparations as an arthropod poison in plagues, with regard to one experience. *Dtsch. Med. Wochenschr.* **71**, 164–169 (in German).

Mukkherjee, D., Ghosh, B. N., Chakraborty, J., and Roy, B. R. (1980). Pesticide residues in human tissues in Calcutta. *Indian J. Med. Res.* **72**, 583–587.

Muller, D., Klepel, H., Macholz, R., and Knoll, R. (1981). Electroneurographic and electroencephalographic finding in patients exposed to hexachlorocyclohexane. *Psychiatr. Neurol. Med. Psychol.* **33**, 468–472.

Muminov, A. I. (1972). Functional condition of the hearing organ in persons with pesticide intoxication. *Vestn. Otorinolaringol.* **34**, 33–35 (in Russian).

Münchberg, P. (1949). On the chemistry of impurities of hexachlorocyclohexanes. *Anz. Schaedlingskd.* **22**, 116–119.

Munir, K. M., Soman, C. S., and Bhide, S. V. (1983). Hexachlorocyclohexane-induced tumorigenicity in mice under different experimental conditions. *Tumori* **69**, 383–386.

Munir, K. M., Rao, K. V. K., and Bhide, S. V. (1984). Effect of hexachlorocyclohexane on diethylnitrosamine-induced hepatocarcinogenesis in rat and its failure to promote skin tumors on dimethylbenz[a]anthracene initiation in mouse. *Carcinogenesis (London)* **5**, 479–481.

Munk, Z. M., and Nantel, A. (1977). Acute lindane poisoning with development of muscle necrosis. *Can. Med. Assoc. J.* **117**, 1050–1054.

Munster, A. J., Bollman, H., and Saunders, J. C. (1962). Hexachlorocyclohexane in the treatment of pediculosis. *Arch. Pediatr.* **79**, 94–95.

Murdia, U. K., Munir, K. M., and Bhide, S. V. (1985). Induction of early biochemical events on hexachlorocyclohexane treatment on mouse liver. *Indian J. Biochem. Biophys.* **22**, 223–225.

Murray, C. P. F. V., Sauceda, F. M., and Navarez, G. M. (1973). Environmental contamination and the health of children. *Salud. Publ. Mex.* **15**, 91–100 (in Spanish).

Musial, C. J., Hutzinger, O., Zitko, V., and Crocker, J. (1974). Presence of PCB, DDE and DDT in human milk in the provinces of New Brunswick and Nova Scotia, Canada. *Bull. Environ. Contam. Toxicol.* **12**, 258–267.

Mussalo-Rauhamaa, H., Pyysalo, H., and Moilanen, R. (1984). Influence of diet and other factors on the levels of organochlorine compounds in human adipose tissue in Finland. *J. Toxicol. Environ. Health.* **13**, 689–704.

Mutter, L. C., Blanke, R. V., Jandacek, R. J., and Guzelian, P. S. (1988). Reduction in the body content of DDE in the Mongolian gerbil treated with sucrose polyester and caloric restriction. *Toxicol. Appl. Pharmacol.* **92**, 428–435.

Nadzhimutdinov, K. N., Muzrabekov, S. M., and Kamilov, I. K. (1973). Effect of hexachlorocyclohexane on the action of Hexenal and Corazol. *Med. Zh. Uzb.* **4**, 54–57 (in Russian).

Nadzhimutdinov, K. N., Kamilov, I. K., and Muzrabekov, S. M. (1974). Influence of pesticides on the duration of hexobarbital-induced sleep. *Farmakol. Toksikol. (Moscow)* **37**, 533–537 (in Russian).

Naevested, R. (1947). Poisoning by DDT powder as well as other poisons. *Tidsskr. Nor. Laegeforen.* **67**, 261–263 (in Norwegian).

Nagai, I. (1972). Residues of organochlorine pesticides in mothers' milk in Yamaguchi Prefecture. *Annu. Rep. Yamaguchi Prefect. Res. Inst. Public Health* **14**, 93–94 (in Japanese).

Nagasaki, H. (1973). Experimental studies on chronic toxicity of benzene hexachloride (BHC). *J. Nara Med. Assoc.* **24**, 1–26 (in Japanese).

Nagasaki, H., Tomii, S., Mega, T., Marugami, M., and Ito, N. (1971). Development of hepatomas in mice treated with benzene hexachloride. *Gann* **62**, 431.

Nagasaki, H., Tomii, S., Mega, T., Marugami, M., and Ito, N. (1972a). Hepatocarcinogenic effect of α-, β-, γ-, and δ-isomers of benzene hexachloride in mice. *Gann* **63**, 393.

Nagasaki, H., Tomii, S., Mega, T., Marugami, M., and Ito, N. (1972b). Carcinogenicity of benzene hexachloride. *In* "Topics in Chemical Carcinogenesis" (W. Nakahara, ed.), pp. 343–353. University Park Press, Baltimore, Maryland.

Nagasaki, H., Tomii, S., Tsumashika, T., Marusami, M., Arai, M., and Ito, N. (1972c). On the experimental tumorigenesis of the liver of mice and rats by the induction of BHC isomers, α-, β-, γ-, δ. *Proc. Jpn. Cancer Assoc.* **31**, 33.

Nagasaki, H., Arai, M., Makjura, S., Sugihara, S., Hirao, K., Matsumura, K., and Ito, N. (1973). Studies on interactions of HCB isomers and PCBs in the induction of liver tumors in the mouse. *Collect. Lect. Abstr. United Soc. Cancer Jpn., p. 160.*

Nagasaki, H., Aoi, H., Makiura, S., Aoki, Z., Arai, M., Konishi, Y. and Ito, N. (1974). Characteristic features of hepatoma of mice due to α-BHC and several factors of carcinogenesis. *Proc. Jpn. Cancer Assoc.* **33**, 78 (in Japanese).

Nair, K. K., Bartels, P. H., Mahon, D. C., Olson, G. B., and Oloffs, P. C. (1980). Image analysis of hepatocyte nuclei from chlordane-treated rats. *Anal. Quant. Cytol.* **2**, 285–289.

Nakajima, M. (1983). Biochemical toxicology of lindane and its analogs. *J. Environ. Sci. Health, Part B*, **B18**, 147–172.

Narafu, T. (1971). Pollution of cows' milk and human milk by BHC. *J. Clin. Nutr.* **39**, 26–34.

Narayan, S., Bajpai, A., Chauhan, S. S., and Misra, U. K. (1985). Lipid peroxidation in lung and liver of rats given DDT and endosulfan intratracheally. *Bull. Environ. Contam. Toxicol.* **34**, 63–67.

Narbonne, P., and Lièvremont, M. (1983). *In vitro* demonstration of the effect of lindane on isolated synaptomsoma preparations. *C. R. Seances Acad. Sci., Ser. 3* **296**, 811–814.

Narloch, B. A., Lawton, M. P., Moody, D. E., Hammock, B. D., and Shull, L. R. (1987). The effects of dicofol on induction of hepatic microsomal metabolism in rats. *Pestic. Biochem. Physiol.* **28**, 362–370.

Naruse, R., Sasaki, T., Yamoka, T., Matsuoka, K., Negoro, Y., Itasaka, Y., Urushibata, K., Chin, T., Kaot, K., Kako, K., Goto, Y., Eguchi, Y., Yogo, H., Tomita, A., and Asai, M. (1970). Clinical use of o,p'-DDD in adrenal cortex cancer. *Horumon to Rinsho* **18**, 241–244 (in Japanese).

National Cancer Institute (NCI) (1976). "Report on Carcinogenesis Bioassay of Technical Grade Chlordecone (Kepone)." Carcinog. Program, Div. Cancer Cause and Prev., U.S. Govt. Printing Office, Washington, D.C.

National Cancer Institute (NCI) (1977a). "Bioassay of Lindane for Possible Carcinogenicity," Techn. Rep. Ser. No. 14, DHEW Publ. No. (NIH) 77-814. U.S. Govt. Printing Office, Washington, D.C.

National Cancer Institute (NCI) (1977b). "Bioassay of Chlordane for Possible Carcinogenicity," Tech. Rep. Ser. No. 8, DHEW Publ. No. (NIH) 77-808. U.S. Govt. Printing Office, Washington, D.C.

National Cancer Institute (NCI) (1977c). "Bioassay of Heptachlor for Possible Carcinogenicity," Tech. Rep. Ser. No. 9, DHEW Publ. No. (NIH) 77-809. U.S. Govt. Printing Office, Washington, D.C.

National Cancer Institute (NCI) (1978a). "Bioassay of DDT, TDE, and p,p'-DDE for Possible Carcinogenicity," Carcinogenesis Tech. Rep. Ser. No. 131, DHEW Publ. No. (NIH) 78-1325. U.S. Govt. Printing Office, Washington, D.C.

National Cancer Institute (NCI) (1978b). "Bioassay of Methoxychlor for Possible Carcinogenicity," Tech. Rep. Ser. No. 35, DHEW Publ. No. (NIH) 78-835. U. S. Govt. Printing Office, Washington, D.C.

National Cancer Institute (NCI) (1978c). "Bioassay of Chlorobenzilate for

Possible Carcinogenicity," Tech. Rep. Ser. No. 75, DHEW Publ. No. (NIH) 78-1325. U.S. Govt. Printing Office, Washington, D.C.

National Cancer Institute (NCI) (1978d). "Bioassay of Dicofol for Possible Carcinogenicity," Tech. Rep. Ser. No. 90, DHEW Publ. No. (NIH) 78-1340. U.S. Govt. Printing Office, Washington, D.C.

National Cancer Institute (NCI) (1978e). "Bioassay of Aldrin and Dieldrin for Possible Carcinogenicity," Tech. Rep. Ser. No. 21, DHEW Publ. No. (NIH) 78-821. U.S. Govt. Printing Office, Washington, D.C.

National Cancer Institute (NCI) (1978f). "Bioassay of Dieldrin for Possible Carcinogenicity in Rats," Carcinogenesis Tech. Rep. Ser. No. 22, DHEW Publ. No. (NIH) 78-822. U.S. Govt. Printing Office, Washington, D.C.

National Cancer Institute (NCI) (1978g). "Bioassay of Endosulfan for Possible Carcinogenicity," Tech. Rep. Ser. No. 621, DHEW Publ. No. (NIH) 78-1312. U.S. Govt. Printing Office, Washington, D.C.

National Cancer Institute (NCI) (1979a). "Bioassay of p,p'-Ethyl-DDD for Possible Carcinogenicity," Carcinogenesis Tech. Rep. Ser., DHEW Publ. No. (NIH) 79-1712. U.S. Govt. Printing Office, Washington, D.C.

National Cancer Institute (NCI) (1979b). "Bioassay of Toxaphene for Possible Carcinogenesis," Carcinogenesis Tech. Rep. Ser. No. 37, DHEW Publ. No. (NIH) 79-837. U.S. Govt. Printing Office, Washington, D.C.

Nawa, H. (1973). Studies on intoxication by organochlorine pesticides for agricultural use. Part 2. Examination of concentration of organochlorine pesticides in sera of healthy people and of patients with various diseases. *J. Okayama Med. Soc.* **85**, 47–58 (in Japanese).

Nayshteyn, S. Y., and Leybovich, D. L. (1971). Low doses of DDT, γ-HCCH and mixtures of these: Effect on sexual function and embryogenesis in rats. *Gig. Sanit.* **36**, 19–22 (in Russian).

Neal, P. A., von Oettingen, W. F., Smith, W. W., Malmo, R. B., Dunn, R. C., Moran, H. E., Sweeney, T. R., Armstrong, D. W., and White, W. C. (1944). Toxicity and potential dangers of aerosols, mists, and dusting powders containing DDT. *Public Health Rep, Suppl.* **177**, 1–32.

Neal, P. A., Sweeney, T. R., Spicer, S. S., and von Oettingen, W. F. (1946). The excretion of DDT (2,2-bis-(p-chlorophenyl)-1,1,1-trichloroethane) in man, together with clinical observations. *Public Health Rep.* **61**, 403–409.

Nelson, A. A., and Woodard, G. (1948). Adrenal cortical atrophy and liver damage produced in dogs by feeding 2,2-bis-(parachlorophenyl)-1,1-dichlorethane (DDD). *Fed. Proc., Fed. Am. Soc. Exp. Biol.* **7**, 277.

Nelson, A. A., and Woodard, G. (1949). Severe adrenal cortical atrophy (cytotoxic and hepatic damage produced in dogs by feeding 2,2-bis-(parachlorophenyl)-1,1-dichlorethane (DDD or TDE). *Arch. Pathol.* **48**, 387–394.

Nelson, A. A., Draize, J. H., Woodard, G., Fitzhugh, O. G., Smith, R. B., Jr., and Calvery, H. O. (1944). Histopathological changes following administration of DDT in several species of animals. *Public Health Rep.* **59**, 1009–1020.

Nelson, E. (1953). Aldrin poisoning. *Rocky Mt. Med. J.* **50**, 483–486.

Nelson, J. A. (1973). Effects of DDT analogs and polychlorinated biphenyls (PCB) mixtures on ³H-estradiol binding to rat uterine receptor. *Fed. Proc., Fed. Am. Soc. Exp. Biol.* **32**, 236.

Nelson, J. O., and Matsumura, F. (1975). A simplified approach to studies of toxic toxaphene components. *Bull. Environ. Contam. Toxicol.* **13**, 464–470.

Newman, S. L., and Guzelian, P. S. (1983). Identification of the cyanopregnenolone-inducible form of hepatic cytochrome P-450 as a catalyst of aldrin epoxidation. *Biochem. Pharmacol.* **32**, 1529–1531.

Newton, K. G., and Greene, N. C. (1972). Organochlorine pesticide residue levels in human milk—Victoria, Australia—1970. *Pestic. Monit. J.* **6**, 4–8.

Nicholls, R. W. (1958). A case of acute poisoning by BHC. *Med. J. Aust.* **1**, 42–43.

Nichols, J., Kaye, S., and Larson, P. S. (1958). Barbiturate potentiating action of DDD and Perthane. *Proc. Soc. Exp. Biol. Med.* **98**, 239–242.

Nichols, J., Prestley, W. E., and Nichols, F. (1961). Effects of m,p-DDT in a case of adrenal cortical carcinoma. *Curr. Ther. Res.* **3**, 266–271.

Nigam, S. K., Lakkad, B. C., Karnik, A. B., Thakore, K. N., Bhatt, D. K., Aravindra Babu, K., and Kashyap, S. K. (1979). Effect of hexachlorocy-

clohexane feeding on testicular tissue of pure inbred Swiss mice. *Bull. Environ. Contam. Toxicl.* **23**, 431–437.

Nigam, S. K., Bhatt, D. K., Karnik, A. B., Thakore, K. N., Babu, K. A., Lakkad, B. C., Kashyap, S. K., and Chatterjee, S. K. (1981). Experimental studies on insecticides commonly used in India. *J. Cancer Res. Clin. Oncol.* **99**, 143–152.

Nigam, S. K., Thakore, K. N., Karnik, A. B., and Lakkad, B. C. (1984). Hepatic glycogen, iron distribution and histopathological alterations in mice exposed to hexachlorocyclohexane. *Indian J. Med. Res.* **79**, 571–579.

Nigam, S. K., Karnik, A. B., Majumder, S. K., Visweswariah, K., Suryanarayana Raju, G., Muktha Bai, K., Lakkad, B. C., Thakore, K. N., and Chatterjee, B. B. (1986). Serum hexachlorocyclohexane residues in workers engaged at a HCH manufacturing plant. *Int. Arch. Occup. Environ. Health* **57**, 315–320.

Nigg, H. N., Stamper, J. H., and Queen, R. M. (1986). Dicofol exposure to Florida citrus applicators: Effects of protective clothing. *Arch. Environ. Contam. Toxicol.* **15**, 121–134.

Nikitina, Y. I. (1974). Course of labor and puerperium in vineyard workers and milkmaids in the Crimea. *Gig. Tr. Prof. Zabol.* **18**, 17–20 (in Russian).

Nikolayev, A. I., and Usmanova, I. Y. (1971). Production of antibodies to pesticides. *Lab. Delo* **11**, 676–678 (in Russian).

Nishimoto, T., Uyeta, M., and Taue, S. (1970). The accumulation of organ ochlorine pesticides in human adipose tissue. *Prog. Med.* **73**, 275–277.

Nitsche, K., Lange, M., Bauer, E., and Zesch, A. (1984). Quantitative distribution of locally applied lindane in human skin and subcutaneous fat *in vitro*. Dependence of penetration on the applied concentration, skin state, duration of action and nature and time of washing. *Dermatosen. Beruf. Umwelt* **32**, 161–165 (in German).

Nitschke, U., and Link, K. (1972). Clinical and biochemical aspects of hormone-producing adrenal carcinomas. *Z. Gesamte Inn. Med. Ihre Grenzgeb.* **27**, 896–905 (in German).

Noack, G., and Portig, J. (1973). Biodegradation of alpha-hexachlorocyclohexane. III. Decrease in liver non-protein thiol after intragastric application of the drug. *Naunyn-Schmiedeberg's Arch. Pharmacol.* **280**, 183–189.

Noda, K., Hirabayashi, M., Yonemura, I., Maruyama, M., and Endo, I. (1972). Influence of pesticides on embryos. II. On the influence of organochlorine pesticides. *Pharmacometrics* **6**, 673–679.

North, H. H., and Menzer, R. E. (1973). Metabolism of DDT in human embryonic lung cell cultures. *J. Agric. Food Chem.* **21**, 509–510.

Nowak, W., Lotocki, W., Szrzedzinski, J., Stasiewicsz, A., and Badusrki, J. (1971). Dieldrin poisoning during pregnancy. *Pol. Tyg. Lek.* **25**, 958–959 (in Polish).

Oberholser, K. M., Wagner, S. R., and Greene, F. E. (1977). Factors affecting dieldrin metabolism by rat liver microsomes. *Drug. Metab. Dispos.* **5**, 302–309.

Obuchowska, D., and Pawlowska-Tochman, A. (1973). The effect of the gamma-isomer of HCH (lindane) on the ultrastructure of the liver cell. *Medicine (Baltimore)* **28**, 63–66.

Odler, M. (1973). The effect of some chlorinated insecticides on the activity of chorionic gonadotrophin in rats. *Comp. Gen. Pharmacol.* **4**, 293–295.

Oesch, F., Freidberg, T., Herbst, M., Paul, W., Wilhelm, N., and Bentley, P. (1982). Effects of lindane treatment on drug metabolizing enzymes and liver weight of CF1 mice in which it evoked hepatomas and in nonsusceptible rodents. *Chem.-Biol. Interact.* **40**, 1–14.

Offner, H., Konat, G., and Clausen, J. (1973). The effect of DDT, lindane and Aroclor 1254 on brain cell culture. *Environ. Physiol. Biochem.* **3**, 204–211.

Ofner, R. R., and Calvery, H. O. (1945). Determination of DDT (2,2-bis-(p-chlorophenyl)-1,1,1-trichloroethane) and its metabolite in biological materials by use of the Schecter-Haller method. *J. Pharmacol. Exp. Ther.* **85**, 363–370.

Ogata, N., Vogel, S. M., and Narahashi, T. (1988). Lindane but not deltamethrin blocks a component of GABA-activated chloride channels. *FASEB J.* **2**, 2895–2900.

Ohno, Y., Kawanishi, T., Takahashi, A., Nakaura, S., Kawashima, K., Tanaka, S., Takanaka, A., Omori, Y., Sekita, H., and Uchiyama, M. (1986). *J. Toxicol. Sci.* **11**, 111–123.

Ohsawa, T., Knox, J. R., Khalifa, S., and Casida, J. E. (1975). Metabolic dechlorination of toxaphene in rats. *J. Agric. Food Chem.* **23**, 98–106.

Ohyama, T., Takahashi, T., and Ogawa, H. (1982). Effects of dichlorodiphenyltrichloroethane and its analogues on rat liver mitochondria. *Biochem. Pharmacol.* **31**, 397–404.

Ojima, M., Saito, M., and Fukushima, S. (1984). Effect of an insecticide (*o,p'*-DDD) on human adrenal synthesis. *Nippon Naibunpi Gakkai Zasshi* **60**, 852–871 (in Japanese).

Ojima, M., Saitoh, M., Itoh, N., Kusano, Y., Fukuchi, S., and Naganuma, H. (1985). Effect of *o,p'*-DDD on adrenal steroidogenesis and hepatic steroid metabolism. *Nippon Naibunpi Gakkai Zasshi* **61**, 168–178 (in Japanese).

Olanoff, L. S., Bristow, W. J., Colcolough, J., and Reigart, J. R. (1983). Acute chlordane intoxication. *J. Toxicol. Clin. Toxicol.* **20**, 291–306.

O'Leary, J. A., Davies, J. E., and Feldman, M. (1970). Spontaneous abortion and human pesticide residues of DDT and DDE. *Am. J. Obstet. Gynecol.* **108**, 1291–1292.

Olson, K. L., Matsumura, F., and Boush, G. M. (1980). Behavioural effects on juvenile rats from perinatal exposure to low levels of toxaphene, and its toxic components; toxicant A, and toxicant B. *Arch. Environ. Contam. Toxicol.* **9**, 247–257.

Olszyna-Marzys, A. E., de Campos, M., Farvar, M. T., and Thomas, M. (1973). Residues of chlorinated pesticides in human milk in Guatemala. *Bol. Of. Sanit. Panam.* **74**, 93–107 (in Spanish).

Omirov, P. Y., and Talan, K. A. (1970). Rabbit autoimmunization under conditions of chronic poisoning with hexachlorane (BHC) and methyl mercaptophos. *Med. Zh. Uzb.* **7**, 11–12 (in Russian).

Onifer, T. M., and Whisnant, J. P. (1957). Cerebellar ataxis and neuronitis after exposure to DDT and lindane. *Proc. Staff Meet. Mayo Clin.* **32**, 67–72.

Orr, J. W. (1948). Absence of carcinogenic activity of benzene hexachloride ('Gammexane'). *Nature (London)* **162**, 189.

Ortega, P. (1966). Light and electron microscopy of dichlorodiphenyltrichloroethane (DDT) poisoning in the rat liver. *Lab. Invest.* **15**, 657–679.

Ortega, P., Hayes, W. J., Jr., Durham, W. F., and Mattson, A. (1956). "DDT in the Diet of the Rat," Public Health Monogr. No. 43, Public Health Serv. Publ. No. 484. U.S. Govt. Printing Office, Washington, D.C.

Ortega, P., Hayes, W. J., Jr., and Durham, W. F. (1957). Pathologic changes in the liver of rats after feeding low levels of various insecticides. *Arch. Pathol.* **64**, 614–622.

Ortelee, M. F. (1958). Study of men with prolonged intensive occupational exposure to DDT. *Arch. Ind. Health* **18**, 433–440.

Oshiba, K. (1972). Experimental studies on the fate of β- and γ-BHC *in vivo* following daily administration. *J. Osaka City Med. Cent.* **21**, 1–9 (in Japanese).

Oshiba, K., and Fujita, T. (1974). Interaction between toxicant and nutrition. Part 7. Effects of dietary protein levels on the β-BHC deposition in dam and offspring of rats during gestation and lactation. *J. Food Hyg. Soc. Jpn.* **15**, 342–348 (in Japanese).

Oshiba, K., and Kawakita, H. (1970). Interaction between toxicant and nutrition. II. Relationship between concentrations of γ-BHC in diet and deposition of the chemical in animal tissues. *J. Food Hyg. Soc. Jpn.* **11**, 445–448 (in Japanese).

Oshiba, K., and Kawakita, H. (1971). The relationship between toxic substances and nutrition. Part 5. Effects of dietary protein and fat starvation on excretion of accumulated BHC. *Rep. Osaka Munic. Inst. Public Health* **34**, 158 (in Japanese).

Oshiba, K., and Kawakita, H. (1972a). Interaction between toxicants and nutrition. III. Distribution and deposition of β-BHC in rat tissues. *J. Food Hyg. Soc. Jpn.* **13**, 184–188 (in Japanese).

Oshiba, K., and Kawakita, H. (1972b). Interaction between toxicants and nutrition. IV. Effect of lipid metabolism on reduction of BHC deposition in rat tissues. *J. Food Hyg. Soc. Jpn.* **13**, 189–194 (in Japanese).

Oshiba, K., and Kawakita, H. (1972c). Relationship between toxic substances

and nutrition. VI. Absorption and excretion of benzene hexachloride. *J. Food Hyg. Soc. Jpn.* **13**, 244–245 (in Japanese).

Oshiba, K., and Kawakita, H. (1972d). Interaction between toxicant and nutrition. V. The fate of β- and γ-BHC *in vivo* following dietary protein levels. *J. Food Hyg. Soc. Jpn.* **13**, 383–387 (in Japanese).

Oshiba, K., and Kawakita, H. (1973). Interactions between toxicants and nutrition. Part 6. Studies on absorption and excretion of BHC in rats. *J. Food Hyg. Soc. Jpn.* **14**, 452–456 (in Japanese).

Osuntokun, B. O. (1964). "Gammelin 20" poisoning: A report of two cases. *West Afr. Med. J.* **13**, 207–210.

Ottoboni, A. (1969). Effect of DDT on reproduction in the rat. *Toxicol. Appl. Pharmacol.* **14**, 74–81.

Ottoboni, A. (1972). Effect of DDT on the reproductive lifespan in the female rat. *Toxicol. Appl. Pharmacol.* **22**, 497–502.

Ottoboni, A., Bissell, G. D., and Hexter, A. C. (1977). Effects of DDT on reproduction in multiple generations of beagle dogs. *Arch. Environ. Contam. Toxicol.* **6**, 83–101.

Ottolenghi, A. D., Haseman, J. K., and Suggs, F. (1974). Teratogenic effects of aldrin, dieldrin, and endrin in hamsters and mice. *Teratology* **9**, 11–16.

Oura, H., Kobayashi, H., Oura, T., Senda, I., and Kubota, K. (1972). On the pollution of human milk by PCB and organochlorine pesticides. *J. Jpn. Assoc. Rural Med.* **21**, 300–301 (in Japanese).

Ousterhaut, J., Struck, R. F., and Nelson, J. A. (1981). Estrogenic activities of methoxychlor metabolites. *Biochem. Pharmacol.* **30**, 2869–2871.

Ouw, K. H., and Shandar, A. G. (1974). A health survey of Wee Waa residents during 1973 aerial spraying season. *Med. J. Aust.* **2**, 871–873.

Paccagnella, B., Prati, L., and Cavazzini, G. (1967). Organochlorine insecticides in the adipose tissue of persons living in the province of Ferrara. *Nuovi Ann. Ig. Microbiol.* **18**, 17–26 (in Italian).

Palin, K. J., Wilson, C. G., Davis, S. S., and Phillips, A. J. (1982). The effects of oils on the lymphatic absorption of DDT. *J. Pharm. Pharmacol.* **34**, 707–710.

Pall, H. S., Williams, A. C., Waring, R., and Elias, E. (1987). Motorneurone disease as manifestation of pesticide toxicity. *Lancet* **2**, 685.

Palmer, K. A., Green, S., and Legator, M. S. (1972). Cytogenic effects of DDT and derivatives of DDT in a cultured mammalian cell line. *Toxicol. Appl. Pharmacol.* **22**, 355–364.

Paludan, J. (1959). Poisoning with gamma-hexachlorocyclohexane. *Ugeskr. Laeg.* **121**, 2023–2028 (in Danish).

Panja, R. K., and Choudhury, S. (1969). A clinical trial with gamma benzene hexachloride in scabies. *Indian J. Dermatol.* **14**, 136–137.

Paramonchik, V. M. (1966). State of the protein forming function of the liver in persons working with chlororganic chemical poisons. *Vrach. Delo* **11**, 85–88 (in Russian).

Paramonchik, V. M., and Platonova, V. I. (1968). The functional state of the liver and stomach in persons exposed to the action of organochlorine chemical poisons. *Gig. Tr. Prof. Zabol.* **12**, 27–31 (in Russian).

Pardini, R. S., Heidker, J. C., and Payne, B. (1971). The effect of some cyclodiene pesticides, benzenehexachloride and toxaphene on mitochondrial electron transport. *Bull. Environ. Contam. Toxicol.* **6**, 436–444.

Park, K. S., and Bruce, W. N. (1968). The determination of the water solubility of aldrin, dieldrin, heptachlor, and heptachlor epoxide. *J. Econ. Entomol.* **61**, 770–774.

Parlar, H., Nitz, S., Gäb, S., and Korte, F. (1977). A contribution to the structure of the toxaphene components. Spectroscopic studies on chlorinated bornane derivatives. *J. Agric. Food Chem.* **25**, 68–72.

Parries, G. S., and Hokin-Neaverson, M. (1985). Inhibition of phosphatidylinositol synthase and other membrane-associated enzymes by steroisomers of hexachlorocyclohexane. *J. Biol. Chem.* **260**, 2687–2693.

Paschal, E. H., Roan, C. C., and Morgan, D. P. (1974). Evidence of excretion of chlorinated hydrocarbon pesticides by the human liver. *Bull. Environ. Contam. Toxicol.* **12**, 547–554.

Patel, T. B., and Rao, V. N. (1958). Dieldrin poisoning in man. A report of 20 cases in Bombay State. *Br. Med. J.* **1**, 919–921.

Paul, A. H. (1959). Dieldrin poisoning. *N. Z. Med. J.* **58**, 393.

Peakall, D. B. (1976). Effects of toxaphene on hepatic enzyme induction and circulating steroid levels in the rat. *Environ. Health Perspect.* **13,** 117–120.

Pearce, G. W., Mattson, A. M., and Hayes, W. J., Jr. (1952). Examination of human fat for presence of DDT. *Science* **116,** 254–256.

Pearl, W., and Kupfer, D. (1972). Stimulation of dieldrin elimination by a thiouracil derivative and DDT in the rat: Enhancement of dieldrin oxidative metabolism? *Chem.-Biol. Interact.* **4,** 91–96.

Peck, A. W. (1970). Impotence in farm workers. *Br. Med. J.* **1,** 690.

Peeler, D. F. (1976). Open field activity as a function of preweaning or generational exposure to mirex. *J. Miss. Acad. Sci.* **21,** 58.

Pélissier, M. A., Manchon, P., Atteba, S., and Albrecht, R. (1975). Some effects of treatment with lindane on the microsomal enzymes of rat liver. *Food Cosmet. Toxicol.* **13,** 437–440 (in French).

Pellerin, D., Harouchi, A., and Soulier, Y. (1975). Corticosuprarenal tumors of children. Concerning 10 cases. *Ann. Chir. Infant.* **16,** 155–179 (in French).

Peppriell, J. (1981). The induction of hepatic microsomal mixed-function oxidase activities in the mouse by mirex, 3,4,5,3′,4′,5′-hexachlorobiphenyl, and equimolar dosages of both. *Environ. Res.* **26,** 402–408.

Peraino, C., Fry, R. J. M., Staffeldt, E., and Christopher, J. P. (1975). Comparative enhancing effects of phenobarbital, amobarbital, diphenylhydantoin, and dichlorodiphenyltrichloroethane on 2-acetylaminofluorene-induced hepatic tumorigenesis in the rat. *Cancer Res.* **35,** 2884–2890.

Pereira, M. A., Herren, S. L., Britt, A. L., and Khoury, M. M. (1982). Sex difference in enhancement of GGTase-positive foci by hexachlorobenzene and lindane in rat liver. *Cancer Lett.* **15,** 95–101.

Perevodchikova, N. I., Platinskiy, L. V., and Kerstsman, V. I. (1972). The treatment of inoperable forms of malignant tumors of the adrenal cortex with *o,p′*-DDD. *Vopr. Onkol.* **18,** 24–29 (in Russian).

Pernov, K., and Kyurkchiyev, S. (1974). Acute occupational poisoning by lindane. *Gig. Tr. Prof. Zabol.* **12,** 46–47 (in Russian).

Pesendorfer, H. (1975). Organochlorine pesticide (DDT, etc.) and polychlorinated biphenyl (PCB) compound residues in human milk (from the area of Vienna and lower Austria). *Wien. Klin. Wochenschr.* **87,** 732–736 (in German).

Pesendorfer, H., Eichler, I., and Glofke, E. (1973). Informative analyses of organochlorine pesticide and PCB residues in human adipose tissue (from the area of Vienna). *Wien. Klin. Wochenschr.* **85,** 218–222 (in German).

Peterson, J. E., and Robinson, W. H. (1964). Metabolic products of *p,p′*-DDT in the rat. *Toxicol. Appl. Pharmacol.* **6,** 321–327.

Peto, R. (1980). Distorting the epidemiology of cancer: The need for a more balanced overview. *Nature (London)* **284,** 297–300.

Petrella, V. J., Fox, J. P., and Webb, R. E. (1975). Endrin metabolism in endrin-susceptible and -resistant strains of pine mice. *Toxicol. Appl. Pharmacol.* **34,** 283–291.

Petrun', N. M., and Nikulina, G. G. (1970). The effect of chronic administration of different doses of *o,p′*-DDD on the ratio of ascorbic and dehydroascorbic acid in the adrenals and some other organs of guinea-pigs. *Vopr. Endokrinol. Obmenu Veschestv* **1,** 19–22 (in Russian).

Pfeilsticker, K. (1973). Pesticides in baby food. *Monatsschr. Kinderheilkd.* **121,** 551–553 (in German).

Philips, F. S., and Gilman, A. (1946). Studies on the pharmacology of DDT (2,2-bis-(parachlorophenyl)-1,1,1-trichloroethane). I. The acute toxicity of DDT following intravenous injection in mammals with observations on the treatment of acute DDT poisoning. *J. Pharmacol. Exp. Ther.* **86,** 213–221.

Philips, F. S., Gilman, A., and Crescitelli, F. N. (1946). Studies on the pharmacology of DDT (2,2-bis-parachlorophenyl)-1,1,1-trichloroethane). II. The sensitization of the myocardium to sympathetic stimulation during acute DDT intoxication. *J. Pharmacol. Exp. Ther.* **86,** 222–228.

Phillips, D. E., and Eroschenko, V. P. (1982). An electron microscopic study of chlordecone (Kepone) induced peripheral nerve damage in adult mice. *Neurotoxicology* **3** (2), 155–162.

Phillips, D. E., and Eroschenko, V. P. (1985a). An electron microscopic study of alterations in mouse peripheral nerve and skeletal muscle after chlordecone exposure. *Neurotoxicology* **6** (1),141–150.

Phillips, D. E., and Eroschenko, V. P. (1985b). Effect of the insecticide chlordecone on the ultrastructure of mouse skeletal muscle. *Neurotoxicology* **6,** (3),45–52.

Phokas, E., Andriotakis, K. N., and Kaklamanis, P. M. (1960). On two cases of poisoning by aldrin. *Hellen. Iatr.* **29,** 910–916 (in Greek).

Pick, I. A., Josha, H., Leffkowitz, M., and Gutman, A. (1965). Aplastic anemia following exposure to aldrin. *Harefuah* **68,** 164–167 (in Hebrew).

Pietsch, R. L., Finklea, J. F., and Ecotr, W. L. (1969). Stolen pesticides. *J. S. C. Med. Assoc.* **65,** 237–238.

Pines, A., Cucos, S., Pnina, E., and Ron, M. (1987). Some organochlorine insecticide and polychlorinated biphenyl blood residues in infertile males in the general Israeli population of the middle 1980's. *Arch. Environ. Contam. Toxicol.* **16,** 587–597.

Pittman, K. A., Kennedy, M. W., and Treble, D. H. (1975). Mirex kinetics in the rhesus monkey. *Toxicol. Appl. Pharmacol.* **33,** 196–197.

Pittman, K. A., Wiener, M., and Treble, D. H. (1976). Mirex kinetics in the rhesus monkey. II. Pharmacokinetic model. *Drug. Metab. Dispos.* **4,** 288–295.

Pittz, E. P., Rourke, D., Abraham, R., and Coulston, F. (1979). Alterations in hepatic microsomal proteins of mice administered mirex orally. *Bull. Environ. Contam. Toxicol.* **21,** 344–351.

Plaa, G. L., Caille, G., Vezina, M., Moritake, I., and Cote, M. G. (1987). Chloroform interaction with chlordecone and mirex: Correlation between biochemical and histological indexes of toxicity and quantitative tissue levels. *Fundam. Appl. Toxicol.* **9,** 198–207.

Planche, G., Croisy, A., Malaveille, C., Tomatis, L., and Bartsch, H. (1979). Metabolic and mutagenicity studies on DDT and 15 derivatives. Detection of 1,1-bis(*p*-chlorophenyl)-2,2-dichloroethane and 1,1-bis(*p*-chlorophenyl)-2,2,2-trichloroethyl acetate (Kelthane acetate) as mutagens in *Salmonella typhimurium* and of 1,1-bis(*p*-chlorophenyl) ethylene oxide, a likely metabolite, as an alkylating agent. *Chem.-Biol. Interact.* **25,** 157–175.

Platonova, V. I. (1970). Disturbances of the functional conditions of the stomach with the prolonged effect on the body of some organochlorine pesticides. *Gig. Tr.* **6,** 142–147 (in Russian).

Pocock, D. E., and Vost, A. (1974). DDT absorption and chylomicron transport in rat. *Lipids* **9,** 374–381.

Podowski, A. A., Banerjee, B. C., Feroz, M., Dudek, M. A., Willey, R. C., and Khan, M. A. Q. (1979). Photolysis of heptachlor and *cis*-chlordane and toxicity of their photoisomers to animals. *Arch. Environ. Contam. Toxicol.* **8,** 509–518.

Pohland, R. C., and Counsell, R. E. (1985). *In vitro* and *in vivo* metabolism of a radioiodinated analog of 1-(2-chlorophenyl)-1-(4-chlorophenyl)-2,2-dichloroethane. *Drug. Metab. Dispos.* **13,** 113–115.

Poland, A., Smith, D., Kuntzman, R., Jacobson, M., and Conney, A. H. (1970). Effect of intensive occupational exposure to DDT on phenylbutazone and cortisol metabolism in human subjects. *Clin. Pharmacol. Ther.* **11,** 724–732.

Polishuk, Z. W., Wasserman, M., Wasserman, D., Groner, Y., Luzarovici, S., and Tomatis, L. (1970). Effects of pregnancy on storage of organochlorine insecticides. *Arch. Environ. Health* **20,** 215–217.

Polishuk, Z. W., Ron, M., Wassermann, M., Cucos, S., Wassermann, D., and Lemesch, C. (1977). Organochlorine compounds in human blood plasma and milk. *Pestic. Monit. J.* **10,** 121–129.

Pollock, G. A., and Kilgore, W. W. (1980a). Toxicities and descriptions of some toxaphene fractions: Isolation and identification of a highly toxic component. *J. Toxicol. Environ. Health* **6,** 115–125.

Pollock, G. A., and Kilgore, W. W. (1980b). Excretion and storage of [^{14}C]toxaphene and two isolated [^{14}C]toxaphene fractions. *J. Toxicol. Environ. Health* **6,** 127–140.

Pollock, R. W. (1953). Toxaphene poisoning—report of a fatal case. *Northwest Med.* **52,** 293–294.

Pollock, R. W. (1958). Toxaphene–lindane poisoning by cutaneous absorption: Report of a case with recovery. *Northwest Med.* **57,** 325–326.

Polyak, N. R. (1974). Immunoserological and immunocytological reactions in response to sensitization with some pesticides. *Gig. Tr. Prof. Zabol.* **5,** 14–17 (in Russian).

Popp, J. A., Scortichini, B. H., and Garvey, L. K. (1985). Quantitative evaluation of hepatic foci of cellular alteration occurring spontaneously in Fischer-344 rats. *Fundam. Appl. Toxicol.* **5,** 314–319.

Portig, J., Kraus, P., Sodomann, S., and Noack, G. (1973). Biodegradation of alpha-hexachlorohexane. I. Glutathione-dependent conversion to a hydrophilic metabolite by rat liver cytosol. *Naunyn-Schmiedeberg's Arch. Pharmacol.* **279,** 185–198.

Portig, J., Kraus, P., Stein, K., Koransky, W., Noack, G., Gross, B., and Sodomann, S. (1979). Glutathione conjugate formation from hexachlorocyclohexane and pentachlorocyclohexane by rat liver *in vitro. Xenobiotica* **9,** 353–378.

Pott, P. (1775). "Chirurgical Observations Relative to the Cataract, the Polypus of the Nose, the Cancer of the Scrotum, etc." T. F. Carnegy, London.

Pott, P. (1790). "The Chirurgical Works of Percival Pott, FRS, Surgeon to St. Bartholomew's Hospital, A New Edition with his Last Corrections." L. Johnson, London.

Powell, G. M. (1980). Toxicity of lindane. *Cent. Afr. J. Med.* **26,** 170.

Powers, J. M., Hennigar, G. R., Grooms, G., and Nichols, J. (1974). Adrenal cortical degeneration and regeneration following administration of DDT. *Am. J. Pathol.* **75,** 181–194.

Pozo Lora, R., Marteache, A. H., Villar, L. M. P., Gimenez, R. L., Villarejo, M. J., and Perez, J. I. (1979). Plaquicidas organoclorados en leches humanas espanolas. *Rev. Esp. Pediatr.* **35,** 93–110 (in Spanish).

Pramanik, A. K., and Hansen, R. C. (1979). Transcutaneous gamma benzene hexachloride absorption and toxicity in infants and children. *Arch. Dermatol.* **15,** 1224–1225.

Prasado Rao, K. S., Trottman, C. H., Morrow, W., and Desaiah, D. (1986). Toxaphene inhibition of calmodulin dependent calcium ATPase in rat brain synaptosomes. *Fundam. Appl. Toxicol.* **6,** 642–653.

Prati, L., and Del Dot, M. (1971). Studies on synthetic organochlorine pesticide accumulation levels in human adipose tissues in the province of Trento. *Ig. Mod.* **64,** 36–44 (in Italian).

Preston, R. J., Au, W., Bender, M. A., Brewen, J. G., Carrano, A. V., Heddle, J. A., McFee, A. F., Wolff, S., and Wassom, J. S. (1981). Mammalian *in vivo* and *in vitro* cytogenic assays: A report of the U.S. EPA Gene-Tox Program. *Mutat. Res.* **87,** 143–188.

Princi, F. (1954). Toxicity of the chlorinated hydrocarbon insecticides. *Atti Congr. Int. Med. Lav., 11th,* pp. 253–272 (in Italian).

Princi, F., and Spurbeck, G. H. (1951). A study of workers exposed to insecticides chlordan, aldrin, dieldrin. *Arch. Ind. Hyg. Occup. Med.* **3,** 64–72.

Prior, P. F., and Deacon, P. A. (1969). Spontaneous sleep in healthy subjects in long-term serial electroencephalographic recordings. *Electroencephalogr. Clin. Neurophysiol.* **27,** 422–424.

Procianoy, R. S., and Schvartsman, S. (1982). Serum DDT levels in an nonoccupationally exposed pediatric population (São Paulo, Brazil). *J. Trop. Pediatr.* **28,** 308–309.

Prohst, G. S., McMahon, R. E., Hill, L. E., Thompson, C. Z., Epp, J. K., and Neal, S. B. (1981). Chemically-induced unscheduled DNA synthesis in primary rat hepatocyte cultures: A comparison with bacterial mutagenicity using 218 compounds. *Environ. Mutat.* **3,** 11–32.

Purres, J. (1982). Safety of gamma benzene hexachloride. *J. Am. Acad. Dermatol.* **7,** 407–408.

Quinby, G. E., Hayes, W. J., Jr., Armstrong, J. F., and Durham, W. F. (1965a). DDT storage in the US population. *JAMA, J. Am. Med. Assoc.* **191,** 109–113.

Quinby, G. E., Armstrong, J. F., and Durham, W. F. (1965b). DDT in human milk. *Nature (London)* **207,** 726–728.

Rabello, M. N., Becak, W., Almeida, W. F., Pigati, P., Ungaro, M. T., Murata, T., and Pereira, C. A. B. (1975). Cytogenic study on individuals occupationally exposed to DDT. *Mutat. Res.* **28,** 449–454.

Radeleff, R. D. (1964). "Veterinary Toxicology." Lea & Febiger, Philadelphia, Pennsylvania.

Radeleff, R. D., Woodard, G. T., Nickerson, W. J., and Bushland, R. C. (1955). The acute toxicity of chlorinated hydrocarbon and organic phosphorus insecticides to livestock. *U.S., Dep. Agric., Tech. Bull.* **1122.**

Radomski, J. L., Deichmann, W. B., MacDonald, W. E., and Glass, E. M. (1965). Synergism among oral carcinogens. I. Results of simultaneous feeding of four tumorigens to rats. *Toxicol. Appl. Pharmacol.* **7,** 652–656.

Radomski, J. L., Deichmann, W. B., and Clizer, E. E. (1968). Pesticide concentrations in the liver, brain, and adipose tissue of terminal hospital patients. *Food Cosmet. Toxicol.* **6,** 209–220.

Radomski, J. L., Astolfi, E., Deichmann, W. B., and Rey, A. A. (1971). Blood levels of organochlorine pesticides in Argentina: Occupationally and nonoccupationally exposed adults, children, and newborn infants. *Toxicol. Appl. Pharmacol.* **20,** 186–193.

Rahman, J., Singh, M. V., and Datia, S. P. (1958). Toxicity of dieldrin to human beings. *Bull. Natl. Soc. Ind. Mal. Mosq. Dis.* **6,** 107–111.

Raizada, R. B., Misra, P., Saxena, I., Datta, K. K., and Dikshith, T. S. S. (1980). Weak estrogenic activity of lindane in rats. *J. Toxicol. Environ. Health* **6,** 483–492.

Raloff, J. (1976). The Kepone episode. *Chemistry* **49,** 20–21.

Ramachandran, M., Sharma, M. I. D., Sharma, S. C., Mathur, P. S., Aravindakshan, A., and Edward, G. J. (1973). DDT and its metabolites in human body fat in India. *Bull. W.H.O.* **49,** 637–638

Ramachandran, M., Zaidi, S. S. A., Banerjee, B. D., and Hussain, Q. Z. (1984). Urinary excretion of DDA: 2,2-bis(4-chlorophenyl) acetic acid as an index of DDT exposure in men. *Indian J. Med. Res.* **80,** 483–486.

Ramakrishnan, N., Kaphalia, B. S., Seth, T. D., and Roy, N. K. (1985). Organochlorine pesticide residues in mother's milk: A source of toxic chemicals in suckling infants. *Hum. Toxicol.* **4,** 7–12.

Ramakrishnan, S., Srinivasan, V., and Nedungadi, T. M. B. (1961). Effect of gammexane on flavoprotein enzymes of rat liver. *Curr. Sci.* **30,** 416–417.

Ramsey, L. L., and Patterson, W. I. (1946). Separation and purification of some constituents of commercial hexachlorocyclohexane. *J. Assoc. Off. Agric. Chem.* **29,** 337–346.

Rao, P. P., Rao, M. R., Visweswariah, K., and Majumder, S. K. (1972). Comparative toxicological study of the new isolate X-factor and other components of BHC on albino rats. *Bull. Grain Technol.* **10,** 89–96.

Rappaport, R., Schweisguth, O., Cachin, O., and Pellerin, D. (1978). Malignant suprarenaloma with metastases. Extraction and treatment by o,p'-DDD following recovery. *Arch. Fr. Pediatr.* **35,** 551–554.

Rappolt, R. T. (1970). Use of oral DDT in three human barbiturate intoxications: CNS arousal and/or hepatic enzyme induction by reciprocal detoxicants. *Ind. Med. Surg.* **39,** 319.

Rasmussen, J. E. (1981). The problem of lindane. *J. Am. Acad. Dermatol.* **15,** 507–516.

Rasmussen, J. E. (1984). Pediculosis and the pediatrician. *Pediatr. Dermatol.* **2,** 74–79.

Rasulev, I. A., Salikhov, K. K., and Barabash, Z. E. (1965). The clinical picture of hexachlorocyclohexane poisoning. *Med. Zh. Uzb.* **1,** 14–16 (in Russian).

Ravindran, M. (1978). Toxic encephalopathy from chlorobenzilate poisoning: Report of a case. *Clin. Encephalogr.* **9,** 170–172.

Ray, D. E., Lister, T., and Joy, R. M. (1986). The action of dieldrin on regional brain blood flow in the rat. *Pestic. Biochem. Physiol.* **25,** 205–210.

Reach, G., Elki, F., Parry, C., Corrol, P., and Milliez, P. (1978). Increased urate excretion after o,p'-DDD. *Lancet* **1,** 1269.

Read, S. T., and McKinley, W. P. (1961). DDT and DDE content of human fat. A survey. *Arch. Environ. Health* **3,** 209–211.

Reddy, D. B., Edward, V. D., and Rao, K. V. (1966). Fatal endrin poisoning. A detailed autopsy, histopathological and experimental study. *J. Indian Med. Assoc.* **46,** 121–124.

Reif, V. D., and Sinsheimer, J. E. (1975). Metabolism of 1-(o-chlorophenyl)-1-(p-chlorophenyl)-2,2-dichloro-ethane (o,p'-DDD) in rats. *Drug Metab. Dispos.* **3,** 15–25.

Reif, V. D., Sinsheimer, J. E., Ward, J. C., and Schteingart, D. E. (1974). Aromatic hydroxylation and alkyl oxidation in metabolism of mitotane (o,p'-DDD) in humans. *J. Pharm. Sci.* **63,** 1730–1736.

Reiner, E., Krauthacker, B., Stipceuvic, M., and Stefanac, Z. (1977). Blood levels of chlorinated hydrocarbon residues in the population of a continental town in Croatia (Yugoslavia). *Pestic. Monit. J.* **11,** 54–55.

Reiter, L. W., and Kidd, K. (1978). The behavioral effects of subacute exposre to Kepone or mirex on the weanling rat. *Toxicol. Appl. Pharmacol.* **45**, 357.

Reiter, L. W., Kidd, K., Ledbetter, G., Chernoff, N., and Gray, L. E. (1977). Comparative behavioral toxicology of mirex and Kepone in the rat. *Toxicol. Appl. Pharmacol.* **41**, 143.

Reiter, L. W., Kidd, K., Ledbetter, G., Gray, L. E., and Chernoff, N. (1982). Comparative behavioral toxicology of mirex and Kepone in the rat. *Toxicol. Appl. Pharmacol.* **41**, 143.

Reuber, M. D. (1976). Histopathology of carcinomas of the liver in mice ingesting dieldrin or aldrin. *Tumori* **62**, 463–472.

Reuber, M. D. (1977a). Histopathology of carcinomas of the liver in mice ingesting heptachlor or heptachlor epoxide. *Exp. Cell Biol.* **45**, 147–157.

Reuber, M. D. (1977b). Hepatic vein thrombosis in mice ingesting chlorinated hydrocarbons. *Arch. Toxicol.* **38**, 163–168.

Reuber, M. D. (1978a). Carcinogenicity of Kepone. *J. Toxicol. Environ. Health* **4**, 895–911.·

Reuber, M. D. (1978b). Carcinomas of the liver in Osborne-Mendel rats ingesting DDT. *Tumori* **64**, 571–577.

Reuber, M. D. (1979a). Interstitial cell carcinomas of the testis in Balb/c male mice ingesting methoxychlor. *J. Cancer Res. Clin. Oncol.* **93**, 173–179.

Reuber, M. D. (1979b). Carcinomas of the liver in Osborne-Mendel rats ingesting methoxychlor. *Life Sci.* **24**, 1367–1371.

Reuber, M. D. (1979c). Carcinogenicity of toxaphene: A review. *J. Toxicol. Environ. Health* **5**, 729–748.

Reuber, M. D. (1979d). Carcinomas of the liver in rat ingesting Kepone. *Neoplasma* **26**, 231–235.

Reuber, M. D. (1980a). Carcinogenicity and toxicity of methoxychlor. *Environ. Health Perspect.* **36**, 205–219.

Reuber, M. D. (1980b). Carcinogenicity of chlorobenzilate in mice, rats and dogs. *Clin. Toxicol.* **16**, 67–98.

Reuber, M. D. (1980c). Significance of acute and chronic renal disease in Osborne-Mendel rats ingesting dieldrin or aldrin. *Clin. Toxicol.* **17**, 159–170.

Reuber, M. D. (1987). Carcinogenicity of heptachlor and heptachlor epoxide. *J. Environ. Pathol. Toxicol. Oncol.* **7**, 85–114.

Reymann, A., Brown, W., and Drager, J. (1983). Effects of DDT and dieldrin on intestinal glucose transport and brush border hydrolases. A comparison with phenobarbital and methylcholanthrene. *Biochem. Pharmacol.* **32**, 1759–1763.

Reynolds, P. J., Lindahl, I. L., Cecil, H. C., and Bitman, J. (1975). DDT and methoxychlor accumulation and depletion in sheep. *J. Anim. Sci.* **41**, 274.

Reynolds, P. J., Lindahl, I. L., Cecil, H. C., and Bitman, J. (1976). A comparison of DDT and methoxychlor accumulation and depletion in sheep. *Bull. Environ. Contam. Toxicol.* **16**, 240–247.

Reznikov, A. G. (1973). Experimental data on adrenocorticolytic activity of *m,p'*-DDD and *p,p'*-Perthane. *Probl. Endokrinol.* **19**, 71–74 (in Russian).

Ribbens, P. H. (1985). Mortality studies of industrial workers exposed to aldrin, dieldrin and endrin. *Int. Arch. Occup. Environ. Health* **56**, 75–79.

Richardson, A., and Robinson, J. (1971). The identification of a major metabolite of HEOD (dieldrin) in human feces. *Xenobiotica* **1**, 213–219.

Richardson, A., Robinson, J., and Baldwin, M. K. (1970). Metabolism of endrin in the rat. *Chem. Ind. (London)*, pp. 502–503.

Richardson, J. A., Keil, J. E., and Sandifer, S. H. (1975). Catecholamine metabolism in humans exposed to pesticides. *Environ. Res.* **9**, 290–294.

Richter, E., Lay, J. P., Klein, W., and Korte, F. (1979). Enhanced elimination of Kepone-^{14}C in rats fed liquid paraffin. *J. Agric. Food Chem.* **27**, 187–189.

Richter, E., Luger, W., Klein, W., Korte, F., and Weger, N. (1981). Excretion of β-hexachlorocyclohexane by the rat as influenced by oral paraffin, squalane and Lutrol E 400. *Ecotoxicol. Environ. Saf.* **5**, 270–280.

Riemschneider, R. (1952). Contact insecticides based on halogenated hydrocarbons. III. Further development of insecticides of the chlorinated-hydrocarbon class. *Euclides* **12**, 35–41, 91–105.

Ritchey, W. R., Savary, G., and McCully, J. A. (1972). Organochlorine insecticide residues in human milk, evaporated milk, and some milk substitutes in Canada. *Can. J. Public Health* **63**, 125–132.

Ritchey, W. R., Savary, G., and McCully, K. A. (1973). Organochlorine insecticide residues in human adipose tissue of Canadians. *Can. J. Public Health* **64**, 380–383.

Ritchie, G. P., and Ho, I. K. (1982). Effects of chlordecone and mirex on amino acids incorporation into brain and liver proteins in the mouse. *Neurotoxicology* **3** (4),243–248.

Ritper, D. L. (1979). Comparison of carcinogenicity studies with aldrin and dieldrin. *J. Assoc. Off. Anal. Chem.* **62**, 900–903.

Roan, C., Morgan, D., and Paschal, E. H. (1971). Urinary excretion of DDA following ingestion of DDT and DDT metabolites in man. *Arch. Environ. Health* **22**, 309–315.

Robinson, J., and Hunter, C. G. (1966). Organochlorine insecticides: Concentrations in human blood and adipose tissue. *Arch. Environ. Health* **13**, 558–563.

Robinson, J., and Roberts, M. (1969). Estimation of the exposure of the general population to dieldrin (HEOD). *Food Cosmet. Toxicol.* **7**, 501–514.

Robinson, J., Richardson, A., Hunter, C. G., Crabtree, A. N., and Rees, H. J. (1965). Organochlorine insecticide content of human adipose tissue in southeastern England. *Br. J. Ind. Med.* **22**, 220–229.

Robinson, J., Roberts, M., Baldwin, M., and Walker, A. I. T. (1969). The pharmacokinetics of HEOD (dieldrin) in the rat. *Food Cosmet. Toxicol.* **7**, 317–332.

Robinson, J. R., Felton, J. S., Levitt, R. C., Thorgeirsson, S. S., and Nebert, D. W. (1975). Relationship between "aromatic hydrocarbon responsiveness" and the survival times in mice treated with various drugs and environmental compounds. *Mol. Pharmacol.* **11**, 850–865.

Robinson, K. M., and Yarbrough, J. D. (1978a). Liver response to oral administration of mirex in rats. *Pestic. Biochem. Physiol.* **8**, 65–72.

Robinson, K. M., and Yarbrough, J. D. (1978b). A study of mirex induced changes in liver metabolism and function with emphasis on liver enlargement. *Fed. Proc., Fed. Am. Soc. Exp. Biol.* **37**, 699.

Robinson, K. M., and Yarbrough, J. D. (1980). Liver protein synthesis and catabolism in mirex-pretreated rats with enlarging livers. *J. Pharmacol. Exp. Ther.* **215**, 82–85.

Robison, A. K., Mukku, V. R., Spalding, D. M., and Stancel, G. M. (1984). The estrogenic activity of DDT: The *in vitro* induction of an estrogenic-inducible protein by *o,p'*-DDT. *Toxicol. Appl. Pharmacol.* **76**, 537–543.

Robison, A. K., Sirbasku, D. A., and Stancel, G. M. (1985a). DDT supports the growth of an estrogen-responsive tumor. *Toxicol. Lett.* **27**, 109–113.

Robison, A. K., Schmidt, W. A., and Stancel, G. M. (1985b). Estrogenic activity of DDT: Estrogen-receptor profiles and the responses of individual uterine cell types following *o,p'*-DDT administration. *J. Toxicol. Environ. Health* **16**, 493–508.

Roed-Petersen, J. (1974). The course of scabies during system and local steroid therapy. *Ugeskr. Laeg.* **136**, 262–263 (in Danish).

Rogers, J. M. (1983). The effects of mirex on the neonatal rat lens *in vitro*, with a comparison to Kepone. *Toxicol. Lett.* **18**, 241–244.

Rogers, J. M., and Grabowski, C. T. (1983). Mirex-induced fetal cataracts: Lens growth, histology and cation balance, and relationship to edema. *Teratology* **27**, 343–349.

Rogers, J. M., and Grabowski, C. T. (1984). Postnatal mirex cataractogenesis in rats: Lens cation balance, growth and histology. *Exp. Eye Res.* **39**, 563–573.

Rogers, J. M., Morelli, L., and Grabowski, C. T. (1984). Plasma glucose and protein concentrations in rat fetuses and neonates exposed to cataractogenic doses of mirex. *Environ. Res.* **34**, 155–161.

Rogirst, A., Vandexande, A., Gordts, L., and Beernaert, H. (1983). Organochlorine pesticide residues and PCB in maternal milk. *Arch. Belg. Med. Soc., Hyg., Med. Trav. Med. Leg.* **41**, 424–432.

Rojanapo, W., Tepsuwan, A., Kupradinum, P., and Chutimataewin, S. (1987). Modulation of hepatocarcinogenicity of aflatoxin B₁ by the chlorinated insecticide, DDT. In 'Eicosanoids, Lipid Peroxidation and Cancer.' (S. K. Nigam, D. C. H. McBrien and T. F. Slater, eds.) pp. 327–338, Springer-Verlag, Berlin.

Roncevic, N., Parkov, S., Galetin-Smith, R., Vukavic, T., Vojinovic, M., and

Djordjevic, M. (1987). Serum concentrations of organochlorine compounds during pregnancy and the newborn. *Bull. Environ. Contam. Toxicol.* **38**, 117–124.

Rosen, J. D., and Sutherland, D. J. (1967). The nature and toxicity of the photoconversion products of aldrin. *Bull. Environ. Contam. Toxicol.* **2**, 1–9.

Rosenbaum, D. P., and Charles, A. K. (1986). In vitro binding of mirex by mouse hepatocytes. *J. Toxicol. Environ. Health* **17**, 385–393.

Rosencrans, J. A., Hong, J. S., Squibb, R. E., Johnson, J. H., Wilson, W. E., and Tilson, H. A. (1982). Effects of perinatal exposure to chlordecone (Kepone) on neuroendocrine and neurochemical responsiveness of rats to environmental challenges. *Neurotoxicology* **3** (2),131–142.

Rosenstein, L., Brica, A., Rogers, N., and Lawrence, S. (1977). Neurotoxicity of Kepone in perinatal rats following *in utero* exposure. *Toxicol. Appl. Pharmacol.* **41**, 142–143.

Rosival, L., Cerey, K., Ruttkayova, J., Vargova, M., and Tildyova, K. (1972). Recent achievements in pesticide toxicology studies. *Egeszsegtudomany* **16**, 63–69 (in Hungarian).

Rosival, L., Barlogova, S., and Grunt, Yu. (1974). Effect of lindane on certain immunological reactions in rats. *Gig. Tr. Prof. Zabol.* **6**, 53–55 (in Russian).

Ross, C. M. (1964). Sock dermatitis from dieldrin. *Br. J. Dermatol.* **76**, 494–495.

Rossi, L., Ravera, M., Repetti, G., and Santi, L. (1977). Long-term administration of DDT or phenobarbital-Na in Wistar rats. *Int. J. Cancer* **19**, 179–185.

Rossi, L., Barbieri, O., Sanguineti, M., Cabral, J. R. P., Bruzzi, P., and Santi, L. (1983). Carcinogenicity study with technical-grade dichlorophenyltrichloroethane and 1,1-dichloro-2,2-bis(*p*-chlorophenyl)ethylene in hamsters. *Cancer Res.* **43**, 776–781.

Rothe, C. F., Mattson, A. M., Nueslein, R. M., and Hayes, W. J., Jr. (1957). Metabolism of chlorophenothane (DDT): Intestinal lymphatic absorption. *Arch. Ind. Health* **16**, 82–86.

Roux, F., Treich, I., and Fournier, F. (1980). Different levels of changes induced by the insecticide lindane in cultured C-6 glioma cells. *Toxicology* **17**, 261–264.

Rowley, D. L., Rab, M. A., Hardjotanojo, W., Liddle, J., Bur, V. W., Saleem, M., Sokal, D., Falk, H., and Head, S. L. (1987). Convulsions caused by endrin poisoning in Pakistan. *Pediatrics* **79**, 928–934.

Rozin, D. G., and Satyvaldiyev, A. S. (1970). A case of acute poisoning with BHC. *Med. Zh. Uzb.* **7**, 74 (in Russian).

Rozman, K. K. (1984). Phase II enzyme induction reduces body burden of heptachlor in rats. *Toxicol. Lett.* **20**, 5–12.

Rumsey, T. S., and Bond, J. (1972). Effect of aldrin, urea and DES on the physiology of beef heifers fed a concentrate or roughage diet. *J. Anim. Sci.* **35**, 978–985.

Rumsey, T. S., and Schreiber, E. C. (1969). Excretion of radiocarbon of C-14-labeled 16-*alpha*-dihydroxyprogesterone acetophenide (DHPA) by beef heifers. *J. Agric. Food Chem.* **17**, 1210–1212.

Runhaar, E. A., Sangster, B., Greve, P. A., and Voortman, M. (1985). A case of fetal endrin poisoning. *Hum. Toxicol.* **4**, 241–247.

Rybakova, M. N. (1968). The effect of certain pesticides on the hypophysis and its gonadotrophic function. *Gig. Sanit.* **33**, 27–31 (in Russian).

Sadriyeva, R. V., Absalyamov, I. F., and Flebkashanskaya, N. V. (1971). The dynamics of morphological changes in the nasal mucous membrane in prolonged peroral administration of small doses of hexachlorane. *Vestn. Otorinolaringo.* **33**, 92–95 (in Russian).

Saez, J. M., Loras, B., Morera, A. M., and Bertrand, J. (1971). Studies of androgens and their precursors in adrenocortical virilizing carcinoma. *J. Clin. Endocrinol. Metab.* **32**, 462–469.

Sagelsdorff, P., Lutz, W. K., and Schlatter, C. (1983). The relevance of covalent binding to mouse liver DNA to the carcinogenic action of hexachlorocyclohexane isomers. *Carcinogenesis (London)* **4**, 1267–1273.

Saigal, S., Bhatnagar, V. K., and Singh, V. S. (1985). Effects of lindane and Diazinon on transaminases in rats. *Environ. Ecol.* **3**, 408–410.

Saito, I., Kawamura, N., Uno, K., Hisanaga, N., Takeucki, Y., Ono, Y., Iwata, M., Gotoh, M., Okutani, H., Matsumoto, T., Fukaya, Y., Yoshitomi, S., and Ohno, Y. (1986). Relationship between chlordane and its metabolites in blood of pest control operators and spraymen. *Int. Arch. Occup. Environ. Health* **58**, 91–97.

Saitoh, K., Shaw, S., and Tilson, H. A. (1986). Noradrenergic influence on the prepulse inhibition of acoustic startle. *Toxicol. Lett.* **34**, 209–216.

Saleh, M. A. (1980). Isomerization of lindane by reduced hematin. *Bull. Environ. Contam. Toxicol.* **25**, 833–836.

Saleh, M. A., and Casida, J. E. (1977a). Consistency of toxaphene composition analysed by open tubular column gas–liquid chromatography. *J. Agric. Food Chem.* **25**, 63–68.

Saleh, M. A., Turner, W. V., and Casida, J. E. (1977). Polychlorobornane components of toxaphene: Structure toxicity relations and metabolic reductive dechlorination. *Science* **198**, 1256–1258.

Saleh, M. A., Skinner, R. F., and Casida, J. E. (1979). Comparative metabolism of 2,2,5-*endo*,6-*exo*,8,9,10-heptachlorobornane and toxaphene in six mammalian species and chickens. *J. Agric. Food Chem.* **27**, 731–737.

Salikhodzhaev, S. S., and Fershtat, V. N. (1972). Condition of the olfactory analyzer under the effect of organochlorine and organophosphorus pesticides. *Gig. Sanit.* **37**, 95–96 (in Russian).

Samosh, L. V. (1974). Chromosome aberrations and the character of satellite associations following accidental exposure of the human body to polychlorocamphene. *Tsitol. Genet.* **8**, 24–27 (in Russian).

Samosh, L. V. (1981). Chromosomal aberrations in the lymphocytes of workers during the use of polychloropinene in agriculture. *Tsitol. Genet.* **15**, 62–67 (in Russian).

Sampson, D. A., Pitas, R. E., and Jensen, R. G. (1980). Effect of chronic ingestion of DDT on physiological and biochemical aspects of fatty acid deficiency. *Lipids* **15**, 815–822.

Samuels, A. J., and Milby, T. H. (1971). Human exposure to lindane: Clinical, hematological and biochemical effects. *J. Occup. Med.* **13**, 147–151.

Sanborn, G. E., Selhorst, J. B., Calabrese, V. P., and Taylor, J. R. (1979). Pseudotumor cerebri and insecticide intoxication. *Neurology* **29**, 1222–1227.

Sánchez-Medal, L., Castanedo, J. P., and Garcia-Rojas, F. (1963). Insecticides and aplastic anemia. *N. Engl. J. Med.* **269**, 1365–1367.

Sandifer, S. H. (1974). Industrial and agricultural chemicals. *Pediatrics* **53**, 843–844.

Sandifer, S. H., Cupp, C. M., Wilkins, R. T., Loadholt, B., and Schuman, S. H. (1981). A case-control study of persons with elevated blood levels of dieldrin. *Arch. Environ. Contam. Toxicol.* **10**, 35–45.

Santolucito, J. A., and Morrison, G. (1971). EEG of rhesus monkeys following prolonged low-level feeding of pesticides. *Toxicol. Appl. Pharmacol.* **19**, 147–154.

Sanyal, S., Agarwal, N. J., and Subrahmanyam, D. (1986). Effect of acute sublethal and chronic administration of DDT (chlorophenotane) on brain lipid metabolism of rhesus monkeys. *Toxicol. Lett.* **34**, 47–54.

Sarett, H. P., and Jandorf, B. J. (1947). Effect of chronic DDT intoxication in rats on lipids and other constituents of the liver. *J. Pharmacol. Exp. Ther.* **91**, 340–344.

Sarkander, H. I. (1974). Temporal relationship between rat liver histone acetylation and nuclear RNA polymerase activities after α-hexachlorocyclohexane application. *Naunyn-Schmiedeberg's Arch. Pharmacol.* **282**, R83.

Sarkander, H. I., Kemmerle, M., and Brade, W. (1974). Rat liver histone modifications and their relationship to DNA-dependent RNA polymerase activities during α-hexachlorocyclohexane induced liver proliferation. *Naunyn-Schmiedeberg's Arch. Pharmacol.* **284**, 39–53.

Sato, H., Toyoda, K., Furukawa, F., Hasegawa, R., Takahashi, M., and Hayashi, Y. (1987). Subchronic oral toxicity test of dicofol (1,1-bis(*p*-chlorophenyl)-2,2,2-trichloroethanol) as the basis for the design of a long-term carcinogenicity study in B6C3F1 mice. *Eisei Shikensho Hokoku* **(105)**, 42–45 (in Japanese).

Sauter, E. A., and Steele, E. E. (1972). The effect of low level pesticide feeding on the fertility and hatchability of chicken eggs. *Poult. Sci.* **51**, 71–76.

Savage, E. P., Bagby, J. R., Jr., Mounce, L., Williams, L. P., Jr., Cholas, P. H., and Cholas, G. (1971). Pesticide poisonings in rural Colorado. *Rocky Mt. Med. J.* **68**, 29–33.

Savage, E. P., Tessari, J. D., Malberg, J. W., Wheeler, H. W., and Bagby, J.

R. (1973). Organochlorine pesticide residues and polychlorinated biphenyls in human milk. *Pestic. Monit. J.* **7,** 1–5.

Savage, E. P., Keefe, T. J., Tessari, J. D., Wheeler, H. W., Applehans, F. M., Goes, E. A., and Ford, S. A. (1981). National study of chlorinated hydrocarbon insecticide residues in human milk, U.S.A. I. Geographic distribution of dieldrin, heptachlor, heptachlor epoxide, chlordane, oxychlordane, and mirex. *Am. J. Epidemiol.* **113,** 413–422.

Saxena, M. C., Siddiqui, M. K. J., Agarwal, V., and Kuuty, D. (1983). A comparison of organochlorine insecticide contents in specimens of maternal blood, placenta and umbilical-cord blood from stillborn and liveborn cases. *J. Toxicol. Environ. Health* **11,** 71–79.

Saxena, S. P., Khare, C., Farooq, A., Murugesan, K., Buckshee, K., and Chandra, J. (1987a). DDT and its metabolites in leiomyomatous and normal human uterine tissue. *Arch. Toxicol.* **59,** 453–455.

Saxena, S. P., Share, C., Farooq, A., Murugesan, K., and Chandra, J. (1987b). DDT residues in blood of residents of areas surrounding a DDT manufacturing factory in Delhi. *Bull. Environ. Contam. Toxicol.* **38,** 392–395.

Schafer, M. L., and Campbell, J. E. (1966). Distribution of pesticide residues in human body tissues from Montgomery County, Ohio. *Adv. Chem. Ser.* **60,** 89–98.

Schechter, R. D., Stabenfeldt, G. H., Gribble, D. H., and Ling, G. V. (1973). Treatment of Cushing's syndrome in the dog with adrenocorticolytic agent (*o,p'*-DDD). *J. Am. Vet. Med. Assoc.* **162,** 629–639.

Scheufler, E., and Rozman, K. (1984). Enhanced total body clearance of heptachlor from rats by stilbeneoxide. *Toxicology* **32,** 93–104.

Scheuing, G., and Vogelbach, G. (1950). γ- and δ-Hexachlorocyclohexane. Odor components of technical hexachlorocyclohexanes. *Naturwissenschaften* **37,** 211–212 (in German).

Schick, M. (1973). Survival with adrenal carcinoma. *JAMA, J. Am. Med. Assoc.* **224,** 1763.

Schimmel, M., Abrahamov, A., and Brama, I. (1980). A rare complication of aplastic anemia due to lindane intoxication. *Harefuah* **98,** 355–356 (in Hebrew).

Schmidt, R. (1973). Effect of 1,1,1-trichloro-2,2-bis(*p*-chlorophenyl)ethane (DDT) on the prenatal development of the mouse (under consideration of distribution of tritium-labeled and carbon-14-labeled DDT in pregnant mice). *Biol. Rundsch.* **11,** 316–317 (in German).

Schnorr, J. K. (1973). Effects of dieldrin on learning and retention of a visual discrimination task in sheep. *Diss. Abstr. Int. B* **33,** 3995B.

Schoor, W. P. (1970). Effect of anticonvulsant drugs on insecticide residues. *Lancet* **2,** 520–521.

Schroeder, G., and Dorozalska, A. (1975). Degradation of DDT and its analogues. *Wiad. Chem.* **29,** 553–565.

Schröter, C., Parzefall, W., Schröter, H., and Schulte-Hermann, R. (1987). Dose–response studies on the effects of α-, β-, and γ-hexachlorocyclohexane on putative preneoplastic foci monooxygenases, and growth in rat livers. *Cancer Res.* **47,** 80–88.

Schulte-Hermann, R. (1974). Control by feeding habits of the induction of hepatic DNA synthesis by α-hexachlorocyclohexane. *Naunyn-Schmiedeberg's Arch. Pharmacol.* **282,** R88.

Schulte-Hermann, R. (1985). Tumor promotion in liver. *Arch. Toxicol.* **57,** 147–158.

Schulte-Hermann, R., and Parzefall, W. (1981). Failure to discriminate initiation from promotion of liver tumours in a long-term study with the phenobarbital-type inducer α-hexachlorocyclohexane and the role of sustained stimulation of hepatic growth and monooxygenases. *Cancer Res.* **41,** 4140–4146.

Schulte-Hermann, R., Koransky, W., Leberl, C., and Noack, G. (1971). Hyperplasia and hypertrophy of rat liver induced by α-hexachlorocyclohexane and butylhydroxytoluene. Retention of the hyperplasia during involution of the enlarged organ. *Virchows Arch. B.* **9,** 125–134.

Schulte-Hermann, R., Schlicht, I., Koransky, W., Leberl, C., Eulenstedt, C., and Zimek, M. (1972). Selective inhibition of liver-cell proliferation by CFT 1201 and SKF 525 A. Studies on growth processes induced by drugs and by partial hepatectomy. *Naunyn-Schmiedeberg's Arch. Pharmacol.* **273,** 109–122.

Schulte-Hermann, R., Leberl, C., Langgraf, H., and Koransky, W. (1974).

Liver growth and mixed-function oxidase activity: Dose-dependent stimulatory and inhibitory effects of α-hexachlorocyclohexane. *Naunyn-Schmiedeberg's Arch. Pharmacol.* **285,** 355–366.

Schupan, I., Ballschmiter, K., and Tolo, G. (1968). Some metabolites of endosulfans in rats and mice. *Z. Naturforsch., C: Biochem., Biophys., Biol., Virol.* **23c,** 701–707 (in German).

Schüttmann, W. (1968). Chronic liver damage after occupational exposure to dichlorodiphenyltrichloroethane (DDT) and hexachlorocyclohexane (HCH). *Int. Arch. Gewerbepathol. Gewerbehgy.* **24,** 193–210 (in German).

Schwabe, U., and Wendling, I. (1967). Increased metabolism of drugs by small doses of DDT and other chlorinated hydrocarbon insecticides. *Arzneim.-Forsch.* **17,** 614–618 (in German).

Schwär, T. G. (1965). Intravenous dieldrin solution administration. *J. Forensic Med.* **12,** 142–145.

Scott, J. L., Cartwright, G. E., and Wintrobe, N. M. (1959). Acquired aplastic anemia: An analysis of thirty-nine cases and a review of the pertinent literature. *Medicine (Baltimore)* **38,** 119–172.

Scotti, T. M., Chernoff, N., Linder, R., and McElroy, W. K. (1981). Histopathologic lens changes in mirex-exposed rats. *Toxicol. Lett.* **9,** 289–294.

Sedlak, V. A. (1965). Solubility of benzene hexachloride isomers in rat fat. *Toxicol. Appl. Pharmacol.* **7,** 79–83.

Seiber, J. N., Landrum, P. F., Madden, S. C., Nugent, K. D., and Winterlin, W. L. (1975). Isolation and gas chromatographic characterization of some toxaphene components. *J. Chromatogr.* **114,** 361–368.

Selby, L. A., Newell, K. W., Hauser, G. A., and Junker, G. (1969). Comparison of chlorinated hydrocarbon pesticides in maternal blood and placental tissues. *Environ. Res.* **2,** 247–255.

Sell, J. L., Davison, K. L., and Puyear, R. L. (1971). Aniline hydroxylase, *N*-demethylase and cytochrome P_{450} in liver microsomes of hens fed DDT and dieldrin. *J. Agric. Food Chem.* **19,** 58–60.

Serat, W. F., Lee, M. K., Van Loon, A. J., Mengle, D. C., Ferguson, J., Burks, J. M., and Bender, T. R. (1977). DDT and DDE in the blood and diet of Eskimo children from Hooper Bay, Alaska. *Pestic. Monit. J.* **11,** 1–4.

Serrone, D. M., Stein, A. A., and Coulston, F. (1965). Biochemical and electron microscopic changes observed in rats and monkeys medicated orally with methoxychlor. *Toxicol. Appl. Pharmacol.* **7,** 497.

Seth, P. K., Saidi, N. F., Agrawal, A. K., and Anand, M. (1986). Neurotoxicity of endosulfan in young and adult rats. *Neurotoxicology* **7** (2),623–635.

Shabad, L. M., Kolesnichenko, T. S., and Nikonova, T. V. (1972). On a possible blastomogenicity of DDT. *Vopr. Pitan.* **30,** 63–66 (in Russian).

Shacter, B. (1981). Treatment of scabies and pediculosis with lindane preparations: An evaluation. *J. Am. Acad. Dermatol.* **5,** 517–527.

Shah, P. V., Monroe, R. J., and Guthrie, F. E. (1981). Comparative rates of dermal penetration of insecticides in mice. *Toxicol. Appl. Pharmacol.* **59,** 414–423.

Shankland, D. L. (1982). Neurotoxic action of chlorinated hydrocarbon insecticides. *Neurobehav. Toxicol. Teratol.* **4,** 805–811.

Sharma, R. P. (1976). Influence of dieldrin on serotonin turnover and 5-hydroxyindole acid efflux in mouse brain. *Life Sci.* **19,** 537–542.

Sheehan, H. L., Summers, V. K., and Nichols, J. (1953). DDD therapy in Cushing's syndrome. *Lancet* **1,** 312–314.

Shemesh, Y., Bourvine, A., Gold, D., and Bracha, P. (1989). Survival after acute endolsulfan intoxication. *J. Toxicol. Clin. Toxicol.* **26,** 265–268.

Shilina, V. F. (1973). Effect of lindane on the serotonin level in the blood and tissues of rats. *Farmakol. Toksikol. (Moscow)* **36,** 687–688 (in Russian).

Shimamoto, T., Matsueda, H., Yoshinouchi, M., Okinaga, E., Mori, K., Yamatake, S., Nakajima, S., and Aihara, M. (1973). Results of a survey on PCB and organochlorine pesticide residues in mothers' milk. *Annu. Rep. Ehime Prefect. Inst. Hyg. Sci.* **35,** 71–73 (in Japanese).

Shimizu, S. (1972). β-BHC residues in human milk and an attempt to reduce the residue by serving diets low in β-BHC content. *Jpn. J. Public Health* **19,** 376–382 (in Japanese).

Shimizu, S. (1974). Results of pursuing investigation on pesticide residues in Saga Prefecture. *Jpn. J. Public Health* **21,** 239–245.

Shindell, S., and Ulrich, S. (1986). Mortality of workers employed in the manufacture of chlordane: An update. *J. Occup. Med.* **28,** 497–501.

Shindell, S., Ulrich, I. S., and Geifer, E. E. (1981). Epidemiology of chlorinated hydrocarbon insecticides. In "Toxicology of Halogenated Hydrocarbons: Health and Ecological Effects" (M. A. Q. Kahn and R. H. Stanton, eds.). Pergamon, New York.

Shindo, H. (1972). Applications of whole body autoradiography to the studies of drug metabolism and disposition. *Annu. Rep. Sankyo Res. Lab.* **24**, 1–72 (in Japanese).

Shiota, K., Tanimura, T., Nishimura, H., Mizutani, T., and Matsumoto, M. (1974). Polychlorinated biphenyls, BHC, and DDE in human fetal tissues. *Congenital Anom.* **13**, 179.

Shirasu, Y., Moriya, M., Kato, K., Furuhashi, A., and Kada, T. (1976). Mutagenicity screening of pesticides in the microbial system. *Mutat. Res.* **40**, 19–30.

Shirasu, Y., Moriya, M., Kato, K., Lienard, F., Tezuka, H., Teramoto, S., and Kada, T. (1977). Mutagenicity screening of pesticides and modification products: A basis of carcinogenicity evaluation. *Cold Spring Harbor Conf. Cell Proliferation* **4**.

Shivanandappa, T., and Krishnakumari, M. K. (1983): Hexachlorocyclohexane-induced testicular dysfunction in rats. *Acta Pharmacol. Toxicol.* **52**, 12–17.

Shivanandappa, T., Krishnakumari, M. K., and Majumder, S. K. (1982). Inhibition of steroidogenic activity in the adrenal cortex of rats fed benzene hexachloride (hexachlorocyclohexane). *Experientia* **38**, 1251–1253.

Shul'ga, A. I. (1957). On the problem of BHC poisoning. *Klin. Med. (Moscow)* **5**, 139–142 (in Russian).

Shure, K. A., and Law, A. (1977). DDT residues in adipose tissue of people in Rangoon area. *Southeast Asian J. Trop. Med. Public Health* **8**, 71–73.

Siddiqui, M. K. J., Saxena, M. C., Bhargava, A. K., Seth, T. D., Krishna Murti, C. R., and Kutty, D. (1981). Agrochemicals in the maternal blood, milk and cord blood: A source of toxicants for prenates and neonates. *Environ. Res.* **24**, 24–32.

Sieber, S. M. (1976). The lymphatic absorption of *p,p'*-DDT and some structurally-related compounds in the rat. *Pharmacology* **14**, 443–454.

Sieber, S. M., Cohn, V. H., and Wynn, W. T. (1974). The entry of foreign compounds into the thoracic duct lymph of rat. *Xenobiotica* **4**, 265–284.

Siegers, C. P., Schumann, S., Thies, E., Böse-Younes, H., and Younes, M. (1984). Aldrin epoxidase and dimethylhydrazine demethylase activities in tumorous and non-tumorous tissue of the human colon and rectum. *Cancer Lett.* **23**, 39–43.

Sierra, V., and Uphouse, L. (1986). Long-term consequences of neonatal exposure to chlordecone. *Neurotoxicology* **7** (2), 609–622.

Simmons, J. H., and Tatton, J. O. (1966). Organochlorine pesticides in gallstones. *Clin. Chem. (Winston-Salem, N.C.)* **12**, 697–700.

Simmons, S. W. (1959). The use of DDT insecticides in human medicine. In "DDT: The Insecticide Dichlorodiphenyl-trichloroethane and Its Significance" (P. Müller, ed.), Vol. 2, pp. 251–502. Birkhaeuser, Basel.

Simon, G. S, Kipps, B. R., Tarcliff, R. G., and Borzelleca, J. F. (1978). Failure of Kepone and hexachlorobenzene to induce dominant lethal mutations in the rat. *Toxicol. Appl. Pharmacol.* **45**, 330–331.

Simon, G. S., Egle, J. L., Dougherty, R. W., and Borzelleca, J. F. (1986). Dominant lethal assay of chlordecone and its distribution in the male reproductive tissues of the rat. *Toxicol. Lett.* **30**, 237–245.

Simpson, G. R., and Shandar, A. (1972). Exposure to chlorinated hydrocarbon pesticides by pest control operators. *Med. J. Aust.* **2**, 1060–1063.

Sinclair, P. R., and Granick, S. (1974). Uroporphyrin formulation induced by chlorinated hydrocarbons (lindane, polychlorinated biphenyls, tetrachloro-dibenzo-*p*-dioxin). Requirements for endogenous iron, protein synthesis and drug-metabolizing activity. *Biochem. Biophys. Res. Commun.* **61**, 124–133.

Singh, A., Villeneuve, D. C., Bhatnagar, M. K., and Valli, V. E. O. (1982). Ultrastructure of the thyroid glands of rats fed photomirex: An 18 month recovery study. *Toxicology* **23**, 309–319.

Singh, A., Bhatnagar, M. K., Villeneuve, D. C., and Valli, V. E. (1985). Ultrastructure of the thyroid glands of rats fed photomirex: A 48-week recovery study. *J. Environ. Pathol. Toxicol. Oncol.* **6**, 115–126.

Singh, K. K., Jha, G. J., Chauhan, H. V. S., and Singh, P. N. (1985).

Pathology of chronic aldrin intoxication in goats. *Zentralbl. Veterinaermed.* **32**, 437–444.

Singhal, R. L., and Kacew, S. (1976). The role of cyclic AMP in chlorinated hydrocarbon-induced toxicity. *Fed. Proc., Fed. Am. Soc. Exp. Biol.* **35**, 2618–2623.

Sinsheimer, J. E., Guilford, J., Bobrin, L. D., and Schteingart, D. E. (1972). Identification of *o,p'*-dichloro-diphenylacetic acid as a urinary metabolite of 1-(*o*-chlorophenyl)-1-(*p*-chlorophenyl)-2,2-dichloroethane. *J. Pharm. Sci.* **61**, 314–316.

Sirica, A. E., Wilkerson, C. S., Wu, L. L., Fitzgerald, R., Blanke, R. V., and Guzelian, P. S. (1989). Evaluation of chlordecone in a two-stage model of hepatocarcinogenesis: A significant sex difference in the hapatocellular carcinoma incidence. *Carcinogenesis (London)* **10**, 1047–1054.

Siyali, D. S. (1972). Hexachlorobenzene and other organochlorine pesticides in human blood. *Med. J. Aust.* **2**, 1063–10-66.

Siyali, D. S., and Simon, R. E. (1973). Chlorinated hydrocarbon pesticides in human blood and fat. *Med. J. Aust.* **1**, 212–213.

Siyali, D. S., Stricker, P., and Tischler, E. 1974). Placental barrier reduced pesticide intake to fetus. *Med. J. Aust.* **1**, 285.

Sizonenko, P. C., Doret, A. M., Riondel, A. M., and Paunier, L. (1974). Cushing's syndrome due to bilateral adrenal cortical hyperplasia in a 13-year-old girl: Successful treatment with *o,p'*-DDD. *Helv. Paediatr. Acta* **29**, 195–202.

Skaare, J. U. (1981). Persistent organochlorinated compounds in Norwegian human milk in 1979. *Acta Pharmacol. Toxicol.* **49**, 384–3898.

Skaare, J. U., Tuveng, J. M., and Sande, H. A. (1988). Organochlorine pesticides and polychlorinated biphenyls in maternal adipose tissue, blood, milk and cord blood from mothers and their infants living in Norway. *Arch. Environ. Contam. Toxicol.* **17**, 55–63.

Skalsky, H. L., Fariss, M. W., Blanke, R. V., and Guzelian, P. S. (1979). The role of plasma proteins in the transport and distribution of chlordecone (Kepone) and other polyhalogenated hydrocarbons. *Ann. N.Y. Acad. Sci.* **320**, 231–237.

Skromme-Kadlubik, G., Alvarez-Cervera, J., and Cortes-Marmolejo, F. (1972). Studies of suprarenal scintigraphy in humans using ^{131}I-DDD. *J. Nucl. Med.* **13**, 282–284.

Skromme-Kadlubik, G., Alvarez-Cervera, J., and Cortes-Marmolejo, F. (1973a). Human suprarenal gammagrams using DDD labeled with I-131. *Arch. Inst. Cardiol. Mex.* **43**, 245–248.

Skromme-Kadlubik, G., Alvarez-Cervera, J., and Cortes-Marmolejo, F. (1973b). Adrenal scanning with dichloro-diphenyl-dichloro-ethane-[131]I(DDD-^{131}I)—a clinical report on 100 subjects. *Int. J. Nucl. Med. Biol.* **2** -83–96.

Skromme-Kadlubik, G., Ferez, A., and Celis, C. (1974). Selective atrophy of adrenal cortex by dichloro-diphenyl dichloroethane I-131 (DDD-I-131). *Arch. Inst. Cardiol. Mex.* **44**, 869–873.

Slade, R. E. (1945). The γ-isomer of hexachlorocyclohexane (Gammexane). An insecticide with outstanding properties. *Chem. Ind. (London)*, pp. 314–319.

Slooten, H. V., Seters, A. P. V., Smeenk, D., and Moolengar, A. J. (1982). *o,p'*-DDD (mitotane) levels in plasma and tissues during chemotherapy and at autopsy. *Cancer Chemother. Pharmacol.* **9**, 85–88.

Smialowicz, R. J., Luebka, R. W., Riddle, M. M., Rogers, R. R., and Rowe, D. G. (1985). Evaluation of the immunotoxic potential of chlordecone with comparison to cyclophosphamide. *J. Toxicol. Environ. Health* **15**, 561–574.

Smith, M. I., and Stohlman, E. F. (1944). The pharmacologic action of 2,2-bis-(*p*-chlorophenyl)-1,1,l-trichloroethane and its estimation in the tissues and body fluids. *Public Health Rep.* **59**, 984–993.

Smith, M. I., and Stohlman, E. F. (1945). Further studies on the pharmacologic action of 2,2-bis-(*p*-chlorophenyl)-1,1,1-trichloroethane (DDT). *Public Health Rep.* **60**, 289–301.

Smith, M. I., Bauer, H., Stohlman, E. F., and Lillie, R. D. (1946). The pharmacologic action of certain analogues and derivatives of DDT. *J. Pharmacol.* **88**, 359–365.

Smith, R. B., Larson, P. S., Finnegan, J. K., Haag, H. B., Hennigar, R. G., and Cobey, F. (1959). Toxicological studies on 2,2-bis(chlorophenyl)-2,2,2-trichloroethanol (Kelthane). *Toxicol. Appl. Pharmacol.* **1**, 119–134.

Smith, R. J. (1982). Hawaiian milk contamination creates alarm. *Science* **217**, 137–140.

Smith, R. M., Cunningham, W. L., Van Gelder, G. A., and Karas, G. G. (1976). Dieldrin toxicity and successive discrimination reversal in squirrel monkeys (*Saimiri sciureus*). *J. Toxicol. Environ. Health* **1**, 737–747.

Smrek, A. L., Adams, S. R., Liddle, J. A., and Kimbrough, R. D. (1977). Pharmacokinetics of mirex in goats. 1. Effect of reproduction and lactation. *J. Agric. Food Chem.* **25**, 1321–1325.

Smrek, A. L., Adams, S. R., Liddle, J. A., and Kimbrough, R. D. (1978). Pharmacokinetics of mirex in goats. 2. Residue tissue levels, trans-placental passage during recovery. *J. Agric. Food Chem.* **26**, 945–947.

Sobti, R. C., Krishan, A., and Davies, J. (1983). Cytokinetic and cytogenetic effects of agricultural chemicals on human lymphoid cells *in vitro*. II. Organochlorine pesticides. *Arch. Toxicol.* **52**, 221–231.

Soennichsen, N., Barthelmes, R., and Barthelmes, H. (1970). Studies on the currently increased occurrence and clinical and therapeutic aspects of scabies. *Dtsch. Gesundheitswes.* **28**, 1178–1183 (in German).

Soine, P. J., Blanke, R. V., Guzelian, P. S., and Schwartz, C. C. (1982). Preferential binding of chlordecone to the protein and high density lipoprotein fractions of plasma from humans and other species. *J. Toxicol. Environ. Health* **9**, 107–118.

Soine, P. J., Blanke, R. V., and Schwartz, C. C. (1983). Chlordecone metabolism in the pig. *Toxicol. Lett.* **17**, 35–41.

Soos, K., Cieleszky, V., and Tarjan, R. (1972). The development of the level of chlorinated hydrocarbons in the adipose tissue of the population of Budapest in 1970. *Egeszsegtudomany* **16**, 70–76 (in Hungarian).

Sosinerz, M., Szczurek, Z., Knapek, R., and Kolodziejczyk, A. (1972). Morphologic studies on short-term subacute toxicity of Kamfochlor. *Patol. Pol.* **23**, 199–202 (in Polish).

Sotaniemi, E. A., Medzihradsky, F., and Eliasson, G. (1974). Glucaric acid as an indicator of use of enzyme-inducing drugs. *Clin. Pharmacol. Ther.* **15**, 417–423.

Southern, A. L., Weisenfield, S., Laufer, A., and Goldner, M. G. (1961). Effect of *o,p'*-DDD in a patient with Cushing's syndrome. *J. Clin. Endocrinol. Metab.* **21**, 201–208.

Southern, A. L., Tochimoto, S., Isurugi, K., Gorcher, G. G., Krikun, E., and Stypulkowski, W. (1966a). The effect of 2,2-bis-(2-chlorophenyl-4-chlorophenyl)-1,1,1-dichloroethane (*o,p'*-DDD) on the metabolism of infused cortisol-7-H. *Steroids* **7**, 11–29.

Southern, A. L., Tochimoto, S., Strom, L., Ratuschni, A., Rass, H., and Gorcher, G. (1966b). Remission in Cushing's syndrome with *o,p'*-DDD. *J. Clin. Endocrinol. Metab.* **26**, 268–278.

Sovocool, G. W., Lewis, R. G., Harless, R. L., Wilson, N. K., and Zehr, R. D. (1977). Analysis of technical chlordane by gas chromatography mass spectrometry. *Anal. Chem.* **49**, 734–740.

Speck, L. B., and Maaske, C. A. (1958). The effects of chronic and acute exposure of rats to endrin. *AMA Arch. Ind. Health* **18**, 268–272.

Spencer, W. F., and Cliath, M. M. (1970). Vapor density and apparent vapor pressure of lindane (gamma-BHC). *J. Agric. Food Chem.* **18**, 529–530.

Sperling, F., Ewenike, H. K. U., and Farber, T. (1972). Changes in LD 50 of parathion and heptachlor following turpentine pretreatment. *Environ. Res.* **5**, 164–171.

Spicer, S. S., Sweeney, T. R., von Oettingen, W. F., Lillie, R. D., and Neal, P. A. (1947). Toxicological observations on goats fed large doses of DDT. *Vet. Med. (Prague)* **42**, 289–293.

Spindler, M. (1983). DDT: Health aspects in relation to man and risk/benefit assessment based thereupon. *Residue Rev.* **90**, 1–34.

Spiotta, E. J. (1951). Aldrin poisoning in man. Report of a case. *Arch. Ind. Hyg. Occup. Med.* **4**, 560–566.

Spyker-Cranmer, J. M., Barnett, J. B., Avery, D. L., and Cranmer, M. F. (1982). Immunoteratology of chlordane: Cell-mediated and humoral immune responses in adult mice exposed *in utero*. *Toxicol. Appl. Pharmacol.* **62**, 402–408.

Squibb, R. E., and Tilson, H. A. (1982a). Effects of gestational and perinatal exposure to chlordecone (Kepone) on the neurobehavioral development of Fischer-344 rats. *Neurotoxicology* **3** (2),17–26.

Squibb, R. E., and Tilson, H. A. (1982b). Neurobehavioral changes in adult Fischer-344 rats exposed to dietary levels of chlordecone (Kepone): A 90 day chronic dosing study. *Neurotoxicology* **3** (2),59–65.

Sram, R. (1974). Evaluation of the genetic danger of chemical substances. *Gig. Sanit.* **4**, 80–83 (in Russian).

Srinivasan, K., and Radhakrishnamurty, R. (1983a). Studies on the distribution of the β- and γ-isomers of hexachlorocyclohexane. *J. Environ. Sci. Health, Part B.* **18**, 401–418.

Srinivasan, K., and Radhakrishnamurty, R. (1983b). Induction of liver mixed function oxygenase system by β- and γ-hexachlorocyclohexane. *Indian J. Biochem. Biophys.* **20**, 84–91.

Srinivasan, K., Ramesh, H. P., and Radhakrishnamurty, R. (1984). Renal tubular dysfunction caused by dietary hexachlorocyclohexane (HCH) isomers. *J. Environ. Sci. Health, Part B* **19**, 453–466.

Srivastava, A. S. (1952). Metabolic relationship between *meso*-inositol and lindane. *Science* **115**, 403–404.

Stacey, C. I., and Tatum, T. (1985). House treatment with organochlorine pesticides and their levels in human milk—Perth, Western Australia. *Bull. Environ. Contam. Toxicol.* **35**, 202–208.

Stacey, C. I., and Thomas, B. W. (1975). Organochlorine pesticide residues in human milk, Western Australia 1970–71. *Pestic. Monit. J.* **9**, 64–66.

Stacey, C. I., Perriman, W. S., and Whitney, S. (1985). Organochlorine pesticide residue levels in human milk: Western Australia, 1979–1980. *Arch. Environ. Health* **40**, 102–108.

Stammers, F. M. G., and Whitfield, F. G. S. (1947). Toxicity of DDT to man and animals. *Bull. Entomol. Res.* **38**, 1–73.

Stanton, R. H., and Khan, M. A. Q. (1972). Oxidation of cyclodiene insecticides by sunfish, mouse and rat liver mixed-function oxidase. *Am. Zool.* **12**, 38.

Stark, L. G., Joy, R. M., and Albertson, T. E. (1983). The persistence of kindled amygdaloid seizures in rats exposed to lindane. *Neurobehav. Toxicol. Teratol.* **4**, 221–226.

Stark, L. G., Albertson, T. E., and Joy, R. M. (1986). Effects of hexachlorocyclohexane isomers on the acquisition of kindled seizures. *Neurobehav. Toxicol. Teratol.* **8**, 487–491.

Stark, L. G., Chuang, R. Y., and Joy, R. M. (1987a). Biochemical markers of exposure to proconvulsant and anticonvulsant chlorinated hydrocarbons. *Epilepsia* **8**, 44.

Stark, L. G., Joy, R. M., and Hollinges, M. A. (1987b). Effects of two isomers of hexachlorocyclohexane (HCH) on cortical beta-adrenoceptors in rat brain. *Exp. Neurol.* **98**, 276–284.

Starr, H. G., Jr., and Clifford, N. J. (1971). Absorption of pesticides in a chronic skin disease. *Arch. Environ. Health* **22**, 396–400.

Starr, H. G., Jr., and Clifford, N. J. (1972). Acute lindane intoxication. A case study. *Arch. Environ. Health* **25**, 374–375.

Steentoft, A. (1979). A case of fatal dieldrin poisoning. *Med. Sci. Law* **19**, 268–269.

Stehr-Green, P. A., Wohlleb, J. C., Royce, W., and Head, S. L. (1988). An evaluation of serum pesticide residue levels and liver function in persons exposed to dairy products contaminated with heptachlor. *JAMA, J. Am. Med. Assoc.* **259**, 374–377.

Stein, A. A. (1970). Comparative toxicology of methoxychlor. *In* "Pesticides Symposia" (W. B. Diechmann, J. L. Radomski, and R. A. Penalver, eds.). Halos and Associates, Miami, Florida.

Stein, A. A., Serrone, D. M., and Coulston, F. (1965). Safety evaluation of methoxychlor in human volunteers. *Toxicol. Appl. Pharmacol.* **7**, 499.

Stein, K., Portig, J., and Koransky, W. (1977). Oxidative transformation of hexachlorocyclohexane in rats and with rat liver microsomes. *Naunyn-Schmiederberg's Arch. Pharmacol.* **298**, 115–128.

Stein, K., Portig, J., Fuhrmann, H., Koransky, W., and Noack, G. (1980). Steric factors in the pharmacokinetics of lindane and α-hexachlorocyclohexane in rats. *Xenobiotica* **10**, 65–77.

Stein, V. B., Pittman, K. A., and Kennedy, M. W. (1976). Characterization of a mirex metabolite from monkeys. *Bull. Environ. Contam. Toxicol.* **15**, 140–146.

Stein, W. J., and Hayes, W. J., Jr. (1964). Health survey of pest control operators. *Ind. Med. Surg.* **33**, 549–555.

Stevens, H. (1970). Neurotoxicity of some common halogenated hydrocarbons. *In* "Laboratory Diagnosis of Diseases Caused by Toxic Agents" (F. W. Sunderman and F. W. Sunderman, Jr., eds.). Warren H. Green, St. Louis, Missouri.

Stevens, J. T., Wagner, S. R., Zemaitis, M. A., and Greene, F. E. (1973). Effect of chronic dieldrin exposure on the hepatic microsomal mixed function oxidase system from male and female rats. *Toxicol. Appl. Pharmacol.* **25**, 484.

Stevens, J. T., Oberholser, K. M., Wagner, S. R., and Greene, F. E. (1977). Content and activities of microsomal electron transport components during the development of dieldrin-inducer hypertrophic hypoactive endoplasmic transport. *Toxicol. Appl. Pharmacol.* **39**, 411–421.

Stevenson, D. E., and Walker, A. I. T. (1969). Hepatic lesions produced in mice by dieldrin and other hepatic enzyme inducing components. *Eur. J. Toxicol.* **2**, 83–84.

Stevenson, D. E., Thorpe, E., Hunt, P. F., and Walker, A. I. T. (1976). The toxic effects of dieldrin in rats: A reevaluation of data obtained in a two-year feeding study. *Toxicol. Appl. Pharmacol.* **36**, 247–254.

Stickel, W. H., Stickel, L. F., and Spann, J. W. (1969). Tissue residues of dieldrin in relation to mortality in birds and mammals. *In* "Chemical Fallout" (M. W. Miller and G. G. Berg, eds.), pp. 174–204. Thomas, Springfield, Illinois.

Stickel, W. H., Kaiser, T. E., and Reichel, W. L. (1979). Endrin versus 12-keto-endrin in birds and rodents. *ASTM Spec. Tech. Publ.* **STP 693**, 61–68.

Stieglitz, R., Stobbe, H., and Schüttmann, W. (1967). Bone marrow damages after occupational exposure to the insecticide gammahexachlorocyclohexane (lindane). *Acta Haematol.* **38**, 337–350.

Stieglitz, R., Stobbe, H., Schüttmann, W., Herrmann, H., and Schmidt, U. (1969). On the pathomechanism of panmyelophthises induced by the insecticide lindane. *Folia Haematol. (Leipzig)* **91**, 293–301 (in German).

Stieglitz, R., Schüttmann, W., and Stobbe, H. (1971). Panmyelophthisis from occupational exposure to toxicants. *Dtsch. Gesundheitswes.* **26**, 910–916 (in German).

Stijve, T., and Cardinale, E. (1972). On the residues associated with the use of technical grade BHC with special reference to the occurrence and determination of three pentachlorocyclohex-1-ene isomers. *Mitt. Geb. Lebensmittelunters. Hyg.* **63**, 142–152 (in German).

Stoewsand, G. S., and Bourke, J. B. (1968). The influence of dietary protein on the resistance to dieldrin toxicity in the rat. *Ind. Med. Surg.* **37**, 526.

Stoewsand, G. S., Broderick, E. J., and Bourke, J. B. (1970). Dietary protein and dieldrin toxicity. *Ind. Med. Surg.* **39**, 356–360.

Stohlman, E. F., and Lillie, R. D. (1948). The effect of DDT on the blood sugar and of glucose administration on the acute and chronic poisoning of DDT in rabbits. *J. Pharmacol. Exp. Ther.* **93**, 351–361.

Stohlman, E. F., Throp, W. T. S., and Smith, M. I. (1950). Toxic action of chlordan. *Arch. Ind. Hyg. Tidskr.* **36**, 77–81.

Stören, G. (1955). A fatal case of poisoning by Jacutin (lindane) insecticide and moth-proofing agent. *Nord. Hyg. Tidskr.* **36**, 77–81 (in Swedish).

Stoyanov, K. (1971). Biochemical alterations occurring in rats and sheep after acute poisoning with heptachlor. *Vet. Med. Nauki* **8**, 65–70 (in Russian).

Stranger, J., and Kerridge, G. (1968). Multiple fractures of the dorsal part of the spine following chlordane poisoning. *Med. J. Aust.* **1**, 267–268.

Strassman, S. C., and Kutz, F. W. (1977). Insecticide residues in human milk from Arkansas and Mississippi, 1973–1974. *Pestic. Monit. J.* **10**, 130–133.

Street, J. C. (1964). DDT antagonism to dieldrin storage in adipose tissue of rats. *Science* **146**, 1580–1581.

Street, J. C., and Blau, A. D. (1966). Insecticide interactions affecting residue accumulation in animal tissues. *Toxicol. Appl. Pharmacol.* **8**, 497–504.

Street, J. C., and Chadwick, R. W. (1967). Stimulation of dieldrin metabolism by DDT. *Toxicol. Appl. Pharmacol.* **11**, 68–71.

Street, J. C., Wang, M., and Blau, A. D. (1966a). Drug effects on dieldrin storage in rat tissue. *Bull. Environ. Contam. Toxicol.* **1**, 6–15.

Street, J. C., Chadwick, R. W., Wang, M., and Phillips, R. L. (1966b).

Insecticide interactions affecting residue storage in animal tissues. *J. Agric. Food Chem.* **14**, 545–549.

Street, J. C., Mayer, F. L., and Wagstaff, D. J. (1969). Ecological significance of pesticide interactions. *Ind. Med. Surg.* **38**, 409–414.

Stubblefield, W. A., and Dorough, H. W. (1979). Quantitative administration of insecticide vapors to rats. *Toxicol. Appl. Pharmacol.* **48**, A138.

Study Group Ministry of Health and Welfare for Organochlorine Pesticide Residues in Mothers' Milk (1972). Studies on the analysis of pesticide residues in foods. VII. Organochlorine pesticide residues in mothers' milk. *J. Food Hyg. Soc. Jpn.* **13**, 422–437 (in Japanese).

Stur, O., and Zweimüller, E. (1961). Diagnosis and therapy of acute gamma-hexachlorocyclohexane poisoning in infants. *Dtsch. Med. Wochenschr.* **86**, 1474–1476 (in German).

Su, Y., and Zhou, Y. (1986). Histopathological effects of technical benzene hexachloride and lindane on rat liver and kidney. *Zhonghua Yufangyixue Zazhi* **20**, 356–358 (in Chinese).

Subramony, S. H., Reddy, R. V., and Desaiah, D. (1982). Effects of chlordecone on nerve conductance in rats. *Fed. Proc., Fed. Am. Soc. Exp. Biol.* **41**, 1578.

Sugaya, A. (1972). On the chronic cases of disturbance due to organochlorine pesticides. *J. Jpn. Assoc. Rural Med.* **21**, 362–363 (in Japanese).

Sugaya, A., Hayashi, S., Meguro, Y., Minagawa, N., Sasaki, S., Suzuki, Y., and Watabe, K. (1976). Amount of organochlorine pesticide residues in human body. *J. Jpn. Soc. Rural Med.* **1–2**, 43–47 (in Japanese).

Sugaya, T. *et al.* (1971). Organochlorine pesticide residues in human milk. *J. Jpn. Assoc. Rural Med.* **19**, 379–380 (in Japanese).

Sund, R. R. C. V., Shreenivas, R., Singh, V., Perez, A. A., and Wolf, A. (1988). Disseminated intravascular coagulation in a case of fatal lindane poisoning. *Vet. Hum. Toxicol.* **30**, 132–134.

Sundström, G. (1977). Metabolic hydroxylation of the aromatic rings of 1,1-dichloro-2,2-bis(4-chlorophenyl)ethylene (p,p'-DDE) by the rat. *J. Agric. Food Chem.* **25**, 18–21.

Sundström, G., Jansson, B., and Jenson, S. (1975). Structure of phenolic metabolites of p,p'-DDE in rat, wild seal and guillemot. *Nature (London)* **255**, 627–628.

Suñol, C., Tusell, J. M., Gelpi, E., and Rodriguez-Farré, E. (1988a). Convulsant effect of lindane and regional brain concentration of GABA and dopamine. *Toxicology* **49**, 247–252.

Suñol, C., Tusell, J. M., Gelpi, E., and Rodriguez-Farré, E. (1988b). Regional concentrations of GABA, serotonin and noradrenaline in brain at onset of seizures induced by lindane (γ-hexachlorocyclohexane). *Neuropharmacology* **27**, 677–681.

Sunōl, C., Tusell, J. M., Gelpí, E., and Rodríguez-Farré, E. (1989). GABA-ergic modulation of lindane (γ-hexachlorocyclohexane)-induced seizures. *Toxicol. Appl. Pharmacol.*, **100**, 1–8.

Suter, S., Trosko, J. E., Fouly, M. H., Lockwood, L. R., and Koestner, A. (1987). Dieldrin inhibition of gap junctional intercellular communication in rat glial cells as measured by the fluorescence photobleaching and scrape loading/dye transfer assays. *Fundam. Appl. Toxicol.* **9**, 785–794.

Suvak, L. N. (1970). DDT in mothers' milk. *Zdravooch. Kosinev* **13**, 19–21 (in Russian).

Suzaki, E., Inoue, B., Okimasu, E., Ogata, M., and Utsumi, K. (1988). Stimulative effect of chlordane on the various functions of guinea-pigs leukocyte. *Toxicol. Appl. Pharmacol.* **93**, 137–145.

Suzuki, Y., Sugaya, H., and Sasaki, S. (1973). Results of 3 years' tracing investigation of organochlorine pesticide residues in humans. *J. Jpn. Assoc. Rural Med.* **22**, 276–277 (in Japanese).

Suzuki, Y., Sugaya, H., and Sasaki, S. (1976). Organochlorine pesticide residues in humans 1975. *J. Jpn. Assoc. Rural Med.* **25**, 498–499 (in Japanese).

Swanson, K., and Woolley, D. (1978). Neurotoxic effects of dieldrin. *Toxicol. Appl. Pharmacol.* **45**, 339.

Swanson, K., and Woolley, D. E. (1982). Comparison of the neurotoxic effects of chlordecone and dieldrin in the rat. *Neurotoxicology* **3** (2), 81–102.

Sylianco, C. Y. L. (1978). Some interactions affecting the mutagenicity potential of dipyrone, hexachlorophene, Thiodan and malathion. *Mutat. Res.* **53**, 272–272.

Symanski, H. J. (1968). A case of fatal occupational aldrin intoxication. *Ind. Med. Surg.* **37,** 551.

Syrowatka, T., Palut, D., Gorski, T., and Tulczynski, A. (1979). Residues of chloro-organic pesticides in adipose tissue of the population of Warsaw and environs. *Rocz. Panstw. Zakl. Hig.* **40,** 505–509 (in Polish).

Syrowatka, T., Gorski, T., and Palut, D. (1981). Residues of organic chlorine pesticides in the blood of the population of Warsaw and environs in the fourth trimester of 1979. *Rocz. Panstw. Zakl. Hig.* 267–269 (in Polish).

Szarmach, H., and Poniecka, H. (1973). Contact allergy in agriculture. *Przegl. Dermatol.* **60,** 479–484 (in Polish).

Tabata, K., Mijata, T., and Saito, T. (1979). Water soluble metabolites of dicofol in mouse urine. *Appl. Entomol. Zool.* **14,** 490–493.

Taira, M., Hashimoto, S., and Shimohira, I. (1972). Organochlorine pesticide residues in human breast milk. *Bull. Hyogo Prefect. Public Health Lab.* **7,** 19–23 (in Japanese).

Takahashi, W., and Parks, L. H. (1982). Organochlorine pesticide residues in human tissues, Hawaii, 1968–1980. *Hawaii Med. J.* **41,** 250–251.

Takamatsu, J., Kitazawa, A., Nakata, K., and Furukawa, K. (1981). Does mitotane reduce endogenous ACTH secretion? *N. Engl. J. Med.* **305,** 957.

Takei, G. H., Kauahikaua, S. M., and Leong, G. H. (1983). Analyses of human milk samples collected in Hawaii for residues of organochlorine pesticides and polychlorobiphenyls. *Bull. Environ. Contam. Toxicol.* **30,** 606–613.

Takeshita, T., and Inuyama, Y. (1970). Organochlorine residues in mothers' milk and blood. *Annu. Rep. Shimane Prefect. Inst. Public Health* **12,** 27–28 (in Japanese).

Taliaferro, I., and Leone, L. (1957). Inhibitory effect of Perthane (2,2-bis-[paraethylphenyl]-1,1-dichloroethane) on adrenocortical function in human subjects. *N. Engl. J. Med.* **257,** 855–860.

Tanaka, K., Kurihara, N., and Nakajima, M. (1977). Pathways of chlorophenol formation in oxidative biodegradation of BHC. *Agric. Biol. Chem.* **41,** 723–725.

Tanaka, K., Kurihara, N., and Nakajima, M. (1979a). Oxidative metabolism of tetrachlorocyclohexenes, pentachlorocyclohexenes, and hexachlorocyclohexenes with microsomes from rat liver and house fly abdomen. *Pestic. Biochem. Physiol.* **10,** 79–95.

Tanaka, K., Kurihara, N., and Nakajima, M. (1979b). Oxidative metabolism of lindane and its isomers with microsomes from rat liver and house fly abdomen. *Pestic. Biochem. Physiol.* **10,** 96–103.

Tanaka, R., Fujisawa, S., Nakai, K., and Minagawa, K. (1980). Distribution and biliary excretion of carbaryl, dieldrin and paraquat in rats: Effect of diets. *J. Toxicol. Sci.* **5,** 151–162.

Tanaka, R., Fujisawa, S., and Nakai, K. (1981). Study on the absorption and protein binding of carbaryl, dieldrin and paraquat in rats fed on protein diet. *J. Toxicol. Sci.* **6,** 1–11.

Tarján, R., and Kemény, T. (1969). Multigeneration studies on DDT in mice. *Food Cosmet. Toxicol.* **7,** 215–222.

Tarmas, J., Stefanska-Sulik, E., and Pieczko-Kuduk, I. (1973). Morphologic changes in the central nervous system in guinea pigs under the influence of the pesticide Alvit 55. *Patol. Pol.* **24,** 295–302 (in Polish).

Tashiro, S., and Matsumura, F. (1977). Metabolic routes of *cis-* and *trans-*chlordane in rats. *J. Agric. Food Chem.* **25,** 872–880.

Tashiro, S., and Matsumura, F. (1978). Metabolism of *trans-*nonachlor and related chlordane components in rat and man. *Arch. Environ. Contam. Toxicol.* **7,** 113–127.

Tashkhodzhayev, P. I., Nadzhimutdinov, K. N., and Sharipova, N. M. (1973). Effect of hexachlorocyclohexane on the general morphology and ultrastructure of the liver. *Med. Zh. Uzb.* **12,** 23–27 (in Russian).

Taylor, J. R. (1982). Neurological manifestations in humans exposed to chlordecone and follow-up results. *Neurotoxicology* **3** (2),9–16.

Taylor, J. R. (1985). Neurological manifestations in humans exposed to chlordecone: Follow-up results. *Neurotoxicology* **6** (1),231–236.

Taylor, J. R., Selhorst, J. B., Houff, S. A., and Martinez, A. J. (1978). Chlordecone intoxication in man. I. Chemical observations. *Neurology* **28,** 626–630.

Tegeris, A. S., Earl, F. L., Smalley, H. E., and Curtis, J. M. (1966). Methoxychlor toxicity. Comparative studies in the dog and swine. *Arch. Environ. Health* **13,** 776–787.

Tegeris, A. S., VanderWeide, G. C., and Curtis, J. M. (1968). Progressive ultrastructural changes in the mucosal epithelium of the small intestine of beagle dogs fed methoxychlor. *Exp. Mol. Pathol.* **8,** 243–257.

Telang, S., Tong, C., and Williams, G. M. (1982). Epigenetic membrane effects of a possible tumor promoter type on cultured liver cells by the nongenotoxic organochlorine pesticides chlordane and heptachlor. *Carcinogenesis (London)* **3,** 1175–1178.

Telch, J., and Jarvis, A. (1982). Acute intoxication with lindane. *Can. Med. Assoc. J.* **126,** 662–663.

Telford, H. S., and Guthrie, J. E. (1945). Transmission of the toxicity of DDT through the milk of white rats and goats. *Science* **102,** 647.

Temple, T. E., Jones, D. J., Liddle, G. W., and Dexter, R. N. (1969). Treatment of Cushing's disease: Correction of hypercortisolism by *o,p'*-DDD without induction of aldosterone deficiency. *N. Engl. J. Med.* **281,** 801–805.

Tennekes, H. A., Wright, A. S., Dix, K. M., and Koeman, J. H. (1981). Effects of dieldrin, diet, and bedding on enzyme function and tumor incidence in livers of male CF-1 mice. *Cancer Res.* **41,** 3615–3620.

Tennekes, H. A., Edler, L., and Kunze, H. W. (1982). Dose–response analysis of the enhancement of liver tumor formation in CF-1 mice by dieldrin. *Carcinogenesis (London)* **3,** 941–945.

Tennekes, H. A., van Ravenzwaay, B., and Kunz, H. W. (1985). Quantitative aspects of enhanced liver tumour formation in CF-1 mice by dieldrin. *Carcinogenesis (London)* **6,** 1457–1462.

Terracini, B., Testa, M. C., Cabral, J. R., and Day, N. (1973). The effects of long-term feeding of DDT to BALB/c mice. *Int. J. Cancer* **11,** 747–764.

Terziev, G., Dimitrova, N., and Rusev, P. (1974). Forensic medical and forensic chemical study of acute lethal poisonings with Thiodan. *Folia Med. (Plovdiv)* **16,** 325–329.

Thamavit, W., Hiasa, Y., Ito, N., and Bhamarapravati, N. (1974). The inhibitory effects of α-benzene hexachloride on 3′-methyl-4-dimethylaminoazobenzene and DL-ethionine carcinogenesis in rats. *Cancer Res.* **34,** 337–340.

Thielemann, H. (1979). Results from experimental studies on the question of the contamination of human milk by total DDT (DDT + DDE) in the urban district of Halle (Saale) in 1978. *Pharmazie* **34,** 665–666 (in German).

Thielemann, H., Grahneis, H., and Haase, H. H. (1975). Studies concerning contamination of human milk with DDT within the city limits of Halle (Saale). *Z. Gesamte Hyg. Ihre Grenzgeb.* **21,** 685–687 (in German).

Thompson, R. P. H., Pilcher, C. W. T., Robinson, J., Stathers, G. M., McLean, A. E. M., and Williams, R. (1969). Treatment of unconjugated jaundice with dicophane. *Lancet* **2,** 4–6.

Thorne, B. M., Taylor, E., and Wallace, T. (1978). Mirex and behavior in the Long-Evans rat. *Bull. Environ. Contam. Toxicol.* **19,** 351–359.

Thorpe, E., and Walker, A. I. T. (1973). The toxicology of dieldrin (HEOD). II. Comparative long-term oral toxicity studies in mice with dieldrin, DDT, phenobarbitone, β-BHC and γ-BHC. *Food Cosmet. Toxicol.* **11,** 433–442.

Tilson, H. A., and Gerhart, J. G. (1982). Time course and dose response assessment of chlordecone (C)-induced tremors in rats. **2,** 114.

Tilson, H. A., and Mactutus, C. F. (1982). Chlordecone neurotoxicity: A brief overview. *Neurotoxicology* **3** (2),1–8.

Tilson, H. A., Byrd, N., and Riley, M. (1979). Neurobehavioral effects of exposing rats to Kepone via the diet. *Environ. Health Perspect.* **33,** 321.

Tilson, H. A., Hong, J. S., and Mactutus, C. F. (1985). Effects of 5,5-diphenylhydantoin (phenytoin) on neurobehavioral toxicity of organochlorine insecticides and permethrin. *J. Pharmacol. Exp. Ther.* **233,** 285–289.

Tilson, H. A., Hudson, P. M., and Hong, J. S. (1986). 5,5-Diphenylhydantoin antagonizes neurochemical and behaviour effects of *p,p'*-DDT but not of chlordecone. *J. Neurochem.* **47,** 1870–1878.

Tilson, H. A., Shaw, S., and McLamb, R. L. (1987). The effects of lindane, DDT, and chlordecone avoidance responding and seizure activity. *Toxicol. Appl. Pharmacol.* **88,** 57–65.

Timchalk, C., and Charles, A. K. (1986). Differential effects of carcinogens on hepatic cytosolic cyclic AMP-dependent protein kinase activity. *J. Am. Coll. Toxicol.* **5,** 267–273.

Timchalk, C., Charles, A. K., and Abraham, R. (1985). Comparative changes in rat liver cytosolic proteins by mirex, diethylnitrosamine and dimethylnitrosamine exposure. *Proc. Soc. Exp. Biol. Med.* **180,** 214–223.

Tinsley, I. J., and Lowry, R. R. (1972). An interaction of DDT in the metabolism of essential fatty acids. *Lipids* **7,** 182–185.

To-Figueras, J., Rodamilans, M., Goméz, J., and Corbella, J. (1986). Hexachlorobenzene residues in the general population of Barcelona (Spain). *IARC Sci. Publ.* **77,** 147–148.

Tokutsu, K., Koyama, T., and Yokoyama, T. (1970). Pesticide residue in mother's milk and plasma in Wakayama Prefecture. *Annu. Rep. Wakayama Prefect. Inst. Public Health* **19,** 59–62 (in Japanese).

Tolot, F., Lenglet, J. P., Prost, G., and Bertholon, J. (1969). Polyneuritis due to lindane. *J. Med. Lyon* **50,** 747–748.

Tomatis, L., and Turusov, V. (1975). Studies on the carcinogenicity of DDT. *Gann Monogr. Cancer Res.* **17,** 219–241.

Tomatis, L., Turusov, V., Day, N., and Charles, R. T. (1972). The effect of long-term exposure to DDT on CF-1 mice. *Int. J. Cancer* **10,** 489–506.

Tomatis, L., Partensky, C., and Montesano, R. (1973). The predictive value of mouse liver tumor induction in carcinogenicity testing—a literature survey. *Int. J. Cancer* **12,** 1–20.

Tomatis, L., Turusov, V., Charles, R. T., and Boicchi, M. (1974a). Effect of long-term exposure to 1,1-dichloro-2,2-bis(*p*-chlorophenyl)ethylene, to 1,1-dichloro-2,2-bis(*p*-chlorophenyl)ethane, and to the two chemicals combined on CF-1 mice. *J. Natl. Cancer Inst. (U.S.)* **52,** 883–891.

Tomatis, L., Turusov, V., Charles, R. T., Boicchi, M., and Gati, F. (1974b). Liver tumors in CF-1 mice exposed for limited periods to technical DDT. *Z. Krebsforsch.* **82,** 25–35.

Tomczak, S., Baumann, K., and Lehnert, G. (1981). Occupational exposure to hexachlorocyclohexane. IV. Sex hormone alterations in HCH-exposed workers. *Int. Arch. Occup. Environ. Health* **48,** 283–287.

Tomii, S., Nagasaki, H., and Mega, Y. (1972). Studies on BHC as a carcinogen. *Jpn. J. Hyg.* **27,** 113 (in Japanese).

Torda, C., and Wolff, H. G. (1949). Effect of convulsant and anticonvulsant agents on the activity of carbonic anhydrase. *J. Pharmacol. Exp. Ther.* **95,** 444–447.

Törnblom, N. (1959). Administration of DDD (2,2-bis(parachlorophenyl)-1,1-dichloroethane) to diabetics with hyaline vascular changes and hyperpolysaccharidemia. *Acta. Med. Scand.* **16,** 23–27.

Tosa, Y., Yasugi, N., Okada, N., Nagami, H., and Seki, R. (1971). A case of survival in endrin poisoning. *J. Jpn. Assoc. Rural Med.* **19,** 370–371 (in Japanese).

Tottori Prefectural Hygiene Research Institute (1971). Tests and investigations on pesticide residues in mothers' milk and blood. *Rep. Tottori Prefect. Hyg. Res. Inst.* **11,** 19 (in Japanese).

Touitou, Y., Bogdan, A., and Luton, J. P. (1978). Changes in corticosteroid synthesis of the human adrenal cortex *in vitro,* induced by treatment with *o,p'*-DDD for Cushing's syndrome: Evidence for the sites of action of the drug. *J. Steroid Biochem.* **9,** 1217–1224.

Touitou, Y., Moolenaar, A. J., Bogdan, A., Auzeby, A., and Luton, J. P. (1985). *o,p'*-DDD (mitotane) treatment for Cushing's syndrome: Adrenal drug concentration and inhibition *in vitro* of steroid synthesis. *Eur. J. Clin. Pharmacol.* **29,** 483–487.

Tovari, G. (1971). Acute poisoning by Thiodan in cattle. *Magy. Allatorv. Lapja* **26,** 343–345 (in Hungarian).

Treinen, K. A., and Kulkarni, A. P. (1986). Human placental calcium ATPase: *In vitro* inhibition by DDT homologues. *Toxicol. Lett.* **30,** 223–229.

Treon, J. F., and Cleveland, F. P. (1955). Toxicity of certain chlorinated hydrocarbon insecticides for laboratory animals with special reference to aldrin and dieldrin. *J. Agric. Food Chem.* **3,** 402–408.

Treon, J. F., Cleveland, F. P., and Cappel, J. (1955). Toxicity of endrin for laboratory animals. *J. Agric. Food Chem.* **3,** 842–848.

Trifonova, T. K., and Gladenko, I. N. (1980). Determination of gonado- and embryotoxicity of pesticides. *Veterinariya (Kiev)* **6,** 58–59 (in Russian).

Trifonova, T. K., Gladenko, In. N., and Shulyak, V. D. (1970). Effect of gamma-BHC and Sevin on reproduction. *Veterinariya (Kiev)* **47,** 91–93 (in Russian).

Triolo, A. J., and Coon, J. M. (1966a). Toxicologic interactions of chlorinated hydrocarbon and organophosphate insecticides. *J. Agric. Food Chem.* **14,** 549–555.

Triolo, A. J., and Coon, J. M. (1966b). The protective effect of aldrin against the toxicity of organo-phosphate anticholinesterases. *J. Pharmacol. Exp. Ther.* **154,** 613–623.

Trosko, J. E., Jone, C., and Chang, C. C. (1987). Inhibition of gap junctional-mediated intercellular communication *in vitro* by aldrin, dieldrin, and toxaphene: A possible cellular mechanism for their tumor-promoting and neurotoxic effects. *Mol. Toxicol.* **1,** 83–93.

Trottman, C. H., and Desaiah, D. (1979). Adenosine triphosphatase activities in brain, kidney and liver of mice treated with toxaphene. *J. Environ. Sci. Health, Part B* **14,** 393–404.

Trottman, C. H., and Desaiah, D. (1980). Induction of rat hepatic microsomal enzymes by toxaphene pretreatment. *J. Environ. Sci. Health, Part B* **B15,** 121–134.

Trottman, C. H., and Desaiah, D. (1983). Effect of toxaphene on the binding of ³H-labelled ouabain and dopamine to rat brain synaptosomes. *Toxicol. Lett.* **18,** 323–330.

Trottman, C. H., Prasada Rao, K. S., Morrow, W., Uzodinman, J. E., and Desaiah, D. (1985). *In vitro* effects of toxaphene or mitochondrial calcium uptake in selected rat tissues. *Life Sci.* **36,** 427–433.

Tryphonas, L., and Iverson, F. (1983). Sequential histopathic analysis of alpha-hexachlorocyclohexane-induced hepatic megalocytosis and adenoma formation in the HPBD mouse. *JNCI, J. Natl. Cancer Inst.* **71,** 1307–1318.

Tseng, Y. C. L., and Menzer, R. E. (1974). Effect of hepatic enzyme inducers on the *in vivo* and *in vitro* metabolism of dicrotophos, dimethoate, and phosphamidon in mice. *Pestic. Biochem. Physiol.* **4,** 425–437.

Tsushimoto, G., Trosko, J. E., Chang, C. C., and Matsumura, F. (1982). Inhibition of intercellular communication by chlordecone (Kepone) and mirex in Chinese hamster v 79 cells *in vitro. Toxicol. Appl. Pharmacol.* **64,** 550–556.

Tsushimoto, G., Chang, C. C., Trosko, J. E., and Matsumura, F. (1983). Cytotoxic, mutagenic, and cell–cell communication inhibitory properties of DDT, lindane, and chlordane on Chinese hamster cells *in vitro. Arch. Environ. Contam. Toxicol.* **12,** 721–730.

Tsutsui, J., Kato, T., and Nishikawa, T. (1974). Results of health survey on persons engaging in pesticide application in Suzuka area, Mie Prefecture. *J. Jpn. Assoc. Rural Med.* **23,** 518–521 (in Japanese).

Tuinstra, L. G. M. T. (1971). Organochlorine insecticide residues in human milk in the Leiden region. *Ned. Melk Zuiveltijdschr.* **25,** 24–32 (in Dutch).

Tullner, W. W. (1961). Uterotrophic action of the insecticide methoxychlor. *Science* **133,** 647–648.

Tullner, W. W., and Edgcomb, J. H. (1962). Cystic tubular nephropathy and decrease in testicular weight in rats following oral methoxychlor treatment. *J. Pharmacol. Exp. Ther.* **138,** 126–130.

Turner, W. V., Khalifa, S., and Casida, J. E. (1975). Toxaphene toxicant A. Mixture of 2,2,5-*endo*,6-*exo*,8,8,9,10-octachlorobornane and 2,2,5-*endo*,6-*exo*,8,9,9,10-octachlorobornane. *J. Agric. Food Chem.* **23,** 991–994.

Turner, W. V., Engel, J. L., and Casida, J. E. (1977). Toxaphene components and related compounds: Preparation and toxicity of some hepta-, octa-, and nonachlorobornanes, hexa- and heptachlorobornenes, and a hexachlorobornadiene. *J. Agric. Food Chem.* **25,** 1394–1401.

Tussell, J. M., Sunol, C., Gelpi, E., and Rodriguez-Farré, E. (1987). Relationship between lindane concentration in blood and brain and convulsant response in rats after oral or intraperitoneal administration. *Arch. Toxicol.* **60,** 432–437.

Tyagi, S. R., Singh, Y., Srivastava, P. K., and Misra, U. K. (1984). Induction of hepatic mixed function oxidase system by endosulfan in rats. *Bull. Environ. Contam. Toxicol.* **32,** 550–556.

Tzoneva-Maneva, M. T., Kalianova, F., and Georgieva, V. (1971). Influence of Diazinon and lindane on the mitotic activity and the caryotype of human lymphocytes, cultivated *in vitro. Bibl. Haematol. (Basel)* **38,** 344–347.

Uchida, A., Ishige, T., Saito, M., and Oikawa, K. (1972). Results of the status of acute pesticide intoxications. *J. Jpn. Assoc. Rural Med.* **21,** 235–235 (in Japanese).

Uchida, M., Kurihara, N., Fujita, T., and Nakajima, M. (1974). Inhibitory effects of BHC isomers on Na$^+$-K$^+$-ATPase, yeast growth, and nerve conduction. *Pestic. Biochem. Physiol.* **4,** 260–265.

Ulland, B. M., Weisburger, E. K., and Weisburger, J. H. (1973). Chronic toxicity and carcinogenicity of industrial chemicals and pesticides. *Toxicol. Appl. Pharmacol.* **25,** 446.

Ulland, B. M., Page, N. P., Squire, R. A., Weisburger, E. K., and Cypher, R. L. (1977). A carcinogenicity assay of mirex in Charles River CD rats. *J. Natl. Cancer Inst. (U.S.)* **58,** 133–140.

Unger, M., and Olsen, J. (1980). Organochlorine compounds in the adipose tissue of diseased people with and without cancer. *Environ. Res.* **23,** 257–263.

Unterman, H. W., and Sirghie, E. (1969). Storage of organochlorine in the human organism. *Igiena* **18,** 221–226 (in Romanian).

Uphouse, L. (1986). Single injection with chlordecone reduces behavioral receptivity and fertility of adult rats. *Neurobehav. Toxicol. Teratol.* **8,** 121–126.

Uphouse, L. (1987). Decreased rodent sexual receptivity after lindane. *Toxicol. Lett.* **39,** 7–14.

Uphouse, L., and Eckols, K. (1986). Serotonin receptors in striatum after chlordecone treatment of adult female rats. *Neurotoxicology* **7** (1),25–32.

Uphouse, L., and Williams, J. (1989). Diestrous treatment with lindane disrupts the female rat reproductive cycle. *Toxicol. Lett.,* **48,** 21–28.

Uphouse, L., Mason, G., and Hunter, V. (1984). Persistent vaginal estrus and serum hormones after chlordecone (Kepone) treatment of adult female rats. *Toxicol. Appl. Pharmacol.* **72,** 177–186.

Uphouse, L., Eckols, K., Sierra, V., Kolodziej, M., and Brown, H. (1986). Failure of chlordecone (Kepone) to induce behavioral estrus in adult ovariectomized female rats. *Neurotoxicology* **7** (1),127–142.

Urbanska-Bonenberg, L., and Langauer-Lewowicka, H. (1966). Polyorganic toxic action of dieldrin. *Med. Pr.* **17,** 336–339.

U.S. Department of Agriculture (1945a). Release of February 13, 1945. Bureau of Entomology and Plant Quarantine, U.S. Dept. Agric., Washington, D.C.

U.S. Department of Agriculture (1945b). "Outlook for Supplies of DDT Insecticides," Release of August 6, 1945. Bureau of Entomology and Plant Quarantine, U.S. Dept. Agric., Washington, D. C.

U.S. Department of Agriculture (1949). "USDA Entomologists Recommend Substitute Insecticide for DDT to Control Insects on Dairy Cattle and in Dairy Barns," New Release, March 24, 1949. Agricultural Research Administration, U.S. Dept. Agric. Washington, D. C.

U.S. Food and Drug Administration (1947). "Quarterly Report No. 3." U. S. Food Drug Admin., Washington, D. C.

U.S. Environmental Protection Agency (USEPA) (1976). "Criteria Document for Toxaphene," EPA-440/9-76/014, Office of Water Planning and Standards, Washington, D.C.

Usha Rani, M. V., Reddi, O. S., and Reddy, P. P. (1980). Mutagenicity studies involving aldrin, endosulfan, dimethoate, phosphamidon, carbaryl and Ceresan. *Bull. Environ. Contam. Toxicol.* **25,** 277–282.

Utklev, H. E., and Westbye, C. (1971). Endosulfan poisoning. *Nor. Veterinaertidsskr.* **83,** 31 (in Swedish).

Vaarama, A. (1947). The influence of DDT pesticides upon plant mitosis. *Hereditas* **33,** 191–219.

Vainio, H. (1975). Stimulation of microsomal drug-metabolizing enzymes in rat liver by 1,1,1-trichloro-2,2-bis(*p*-chlorophenyl)ethane (DDT), pregnenolone-16α-carbonitrile (PCN), and polychlorinated biphenyls (PCBs). *Environ. Qual. Saf.* **3,** 486–490.

Vaino, H., and Parkki, M. G. (1976). Enhancement of microsomal monooxygenase, epoxide hydrase and UDP-glucuronyltransferase by aldrin, dieldrin and isosafrole administrations in rat liver. *Toxicology* **5,** 279–286.

van Asperen, K. (1954). Interaction of the isomers of benzene hexachloride in mice. *Arch. Int. Pharmacodyn. Ther.* **99,** 368–377.

Vanat, S. V., and Vanat, I. M. (1971). Contribution to the toxic–allergic reaction induced by DDT. *Klin. Med. (Moscow)* **49,** 126–127 (in Russian).

Van den Bercken, J., and Narahashi, T. (1974). Effects of aldrin-transdiol—a metabolite of the insecticides dieldrin—on nerve membrane. *Eur. J. Pharmacol.* **27,** 255–258.

van der Linden, T. (1912). Decomposition of benzene hexachloride in trichlorobenzene. *Ber. Dtsch. Chem. Ges.* **45,** 231–247 (in German).

Van Gelder, G. A., and Cunningham, W. L. (1975). The effect of low-level dieldrin exposure on the EEG and learning ability of the squirrel monkey. *Toxicol. Appl. Pharmacol.* **33,** 142.

Van Gelder, G. A., and Smith, R. M. (1973). Delayed acquisition of a successive reversal behavioral task in dieldrin-dosed squirrel monkeys. *Toxicol. Appl. Pharmacol.* **25,** 485.

van Raalte, H. G. S. (1977). Human experience with dieldrin in perspective. *Ecotoxicol. Environ. Saf.* **1,** 203–210.

van Ravenswaay, B., and Kunz, W. (1988). Quantitative aspects of accelerated nuclear polyploidization and tumour formation in dieldrin treated CF-1 mouse liver. *Br. J. Cancer* **58,** 52–56.

van Ravenzwaay, B., Tennekes, H., Stoehr, M., and Kunz, W. (1987). The kinetics of nuclear polyploidization and tumor formation in livers of CF-1 mice exposed to dieldrin. *Carcinogenesis (London)* **8,** 265–269.

van Ravenswaay, B., Toussaint, H. J. M., and Schmitt, R. L. (1988). Dieldrin-induced changes in isozyme composition in the livers of CF-1 mice. *Int. J. Cancer* **41,** 305–308.

Van Velsen, F. L., Danse, L. H. J. C., Van Leluwen, F. X. R., Dormans, J. A. M. A., and Van Logten, M. J. (1986). The subchronic oral toxicity of the β-isomer of hexachlorocyclohexane in rats. *Fundam. Appl. Toxicol.* **6,** 697–712.

Vanyurykhina, L. T. (1972). Effect of adrenal cortex function inhibitor clodithane (*o,p'*-DDD) on blood serum proteins. *Fiziol. Zh. (Kiev, 1955–1977)***18,** 591–595 (in Russian).

Vas'Kovskaja, L. F. (1969). Accumulation of certain chloroorganic insecticides in the bodies of experimental animals and humans. *Kiev, Vniggintox* **7,** 503–796 (in Russian).

Vas'Kovskaja, L. F., and Komarova, L. I. (1963). Quoted by Y.S. Kagan *et al., Residue Rev.* **27,** 43–79 (in Russian).

Vaz, A., Pereira, R. S., and Malheiro, D. M. (1945). Calcium in prevention and treatment of experimental DDT poisoning. *Science* **101,** 434–436.

Velbinger, H. H. (1947a). Question of "DDT"—toxicity for humans. *Dtsch. Gesundheitswes.* **2,** 355–358 (in German).

Velbinger, H. H. (1947b). Contribution on the toxicology of "DDT"—active substances of dichlorodiphenyltrichloromethylmethane. *Pharmazie* **2,** 268–274 (in German).

Velbinger, H. H. (1949). Different effects of the new insecticides "DDT," Gammexan and E605. *Pharmazie* **4,** 165–176 (in German).

Veltkamp, J. J., Stevens, P., von der Plas, M., and Loeliger, E. A. (1970). Production site of bleeding factor (acquired morbus von Willebrand). *Thromb. Diath. Haemorrh.* **23,** 412.

Verdon, T. A., Bruton, J., Herman, R. H., and Beisel, W. R. (1962). Clinical and chemical response of functioning adrenal cortical carcinoma to *ortho,para*-DDD. *Metab., Clin. Exp.* **11,** 226–234.

Versteeg, J. P. J., and Jager, K. W. (1973). Long-term exposure to the insecticide aldrin, dieldrin, endrin, and Telodrin. *Br. J. Ind. Med.* **30,** 201–202.

Vila, M. C., Aldonatti, C., and San Martin de Viale, L. C. (1986). Evaluation of porphyrinogenic effect of lindane in rats. *Acta Physiol. Latinoam.* **36,** 69–76.

Villeneuve, D. C., Yagminas, A. P., Marino, I. A., Chu, I., and Reynolds, L. M. (1977). Effects of food deprivation in rats previously exposed to mirex. *Bull. Environ. Contam. Toxicol.* **18,** 278–284.

Villeneuve, D. C., Ritter, L., Felsky, G., Norström, R. J., Marion, I. A., Valli, V. E., Chu, I., and Becking, G. C. (1979a). Short-term toxicity of photomirex in the rat. *Toxicol. Appl. Pharmacol.* **47,** 105–114.

Villeneuve, D. C., Valli, V. E., Chu, I., Secours, V., Ritter, L., and Becking, G. C. (1979b). 90-Day toxicity of photomirex in the male rat. *Toxicology* **12,** 235–250.

Violante, F. S., Gennari, P., Raffi, G. B., Coltelli, E., Lev, D., Minak, G., and Tiraferri, S. (1986). Study of DDT blood level in a group of workers exposed to pesticides. *Arch. Environ. Health* **41,** 117–119.

Virgo, B. B., and Bellward, G. D. (1973a). Effect of dietary dieldrin on the liver and drug metabolism in the SWV mouse. *Proc. Can. Fed. Biol. Soc.* **16,** 69.

Virgo, B. B., and Bellward, G. D. (1973b). Effect of dieldrin on mouse reproduction. *Proc. Can. Fed. Biol. Soc.* **16**, 103.

Virgo, B. B., and Bellward, G. D. (1975a). Effects of dietary dieldrin on the liver and drug metabolism in the female Swiss-Vancouver mouse. *Can. J. Physiol. Pharmacol.* **53**, 903–911.

Virgo, B. B., and Bellward, G. D. (1975b). Effects of dietary dieldrin on reproduction in the Swiss-Vancouver (SMV) mouse. *Environ. Physiol. Biochem.* **5**, 440–450.

Virgo, B. B., and Bellward, G. D. (1977). Effects of dietary dieldrin on offspring viability, maternal behavior, and milk production in the mouse. *Res. Commun. Chem. Pathol. Pharmacol.* **17**, 399–409.

Vogel, E. (1972). Mutagenicity studies with DDT and its metabolites DDE, DDD, DDOM and DDA in *Drosophila melanogaster*. *Mutat. Res.* **16**, 157–164.

Vohland, H. W., and Koransky, W. (1972). Effect of α-hexachlorocyclohexane on metabolism and excretion of pentetrazol (Cardiazol) in the rat. *Naunyn-Schmiedeberg's Arch. Pharmacol.* **273**, 99–108.

Vohland, H. W., Koransky, W., and Zufelde, H. (1972). Effect of α-hexachlorocyclohexane on the convulsive activity of pentetrazol (Cardiazol) in the rat. *Naunyn-Schmiedeberg's Arch. Pharmacol.* **275**, 289–298.

Vohland, H. W., Portig, J., and Stein, K. (1981). Neuropharmacological effects of isomers of hexachlorocyclohexane. 1. Protection against pentylenetetrazol-induced convulsions. *Toxicol. Appl. Pharmacol.* **57**, 425–438.

von Oettingen, W. F., and Sharpless, N. E. (1946). The toxicity and toxic manifestations of 2,2-bis-(*p*-chlorophenyl)-1,1,1-trichloroethane (DDT) as influenced by chemical changes in the molecule. A contribution to the relation between chemical constitution and toxicological action. *J. Pharmacol. Exp. Ther.* **88**, 400–413.

Vu, N., Chepko, G., and Zelenka, P. (1983). Decreased turnover of phosphatidylinositol accompanies *in vitro* differentiation of embryonic chicken lens epithelial cells into lens fibres. *Biochim. Biophys. Acta* **750**, 105–111.

Wagner, S. R., and Greene, F. E. (1974). Effects of acute and chronic dieldrin exposure on brain biogenic amines of male and female rats. *Toxicol. Appl. Pharmacol.* **29**, 119.

Wagner, S. R., and Greene, F. E. (1978). Dieldrin-induced alterations in biogenic amine content of rat brain. *Toxicol. Appl. Pharmacol.* **43**, 45–55.

Wagstaff, D. J., and Street, J. C. (1971a). Ascorbic acid deficiency and induction of hepatic microsomal hydroxylative enzymes by organochlorine pesticides. *Toxicol. Appl. Pharmacol.* **19**, 10–19.

Wagstaff, D. J., and Street, J. C. (1971b). Antagonism of DDT storage in guinea pigs by dietary dieldrin. *Bull. Environ. Contam. Toxicol.* **6**, 273–278.

Wakita, M., Hoshino, S., Morimoto, K., Yamada, K., Miyata, K., and Tsubota, H. (1972). BHC (1,2,3,4,5,6-hexachlorocyclohexane) residues in sheep. *Jpn. J. Zootech. Sci.* **43**, 620–624 (in Japanese).

Wali, R. K., Singh, R., Dudeja, P. K., and Mahmood, A. (1982). Effect of a single oral dose of endosulfan on intestinal uptake of nutrients and on brush-border enzymes in rats. *Toxicol. Lett.* **12**, 7–12.

Walker, A. I. T., Stevenson, D. E., Robinson, J., Thorpe, E., and Roberts, M. (1969). The toxicology and pharmacodynamics of dieldrin (HEOD): Two-year oral exposures of rats and dogs. *Toxicol. Appl. Pharmacol.* **15**, 345–373.

Walker, A. I. T., Thorpe, E., Robinson, J., and Baldwin, M. K. (1971). Toxicity studies on the photo-isomerisation product of dieldrin. *Meded. Fac. Landbouwwet. Rijksuniv. Gent* **36**, 398–409.

Walker, A. I. T., Thorpe, E., and Stevenson, D. E. (1973). The toxicology of dieldrin (HEOD). I. Long-term oral toxicity studies in mice. *Food Cosmet. Toxicol.* **11**, 415–432.

Walker, C. H., Timms, C. W., Wolf, C. R., and Oesch, F. (1986). The hydration of sterically hindered epoxides by epoxide hydrolase of the rat and rabbit. *Biochem. Pharmacol.* **35**, 499–503.

Walker, J. F., and Phillips, D. E. (1987). An electron microscopic study of endrin induced alterations in unmyelinated fibers of mouse sciatic nerve. *Neurotoxicology* **8** (1),55–64.

Wallace, Z. E., Silverstein, J. N., Villadolid, L. S., and Weisenfeld, S. (1961). Cushing's syndrome due to adrenocortical hyperplasia. *N. Engl. J. Med.* **265**, 1088–1093.

Walsh, G. M., and Fink, G. B. (1970). Temporal aspects of acute endrin toxicity in mice. *Proc. West. Pharmacol. Soc.* **13**, 81–83.

Walton, M. S., Bastone, V. B., and Baron, R. L. (1971). Subchronic toxicity of photodieldrin, a photodecomposition product of dieldrin. *Toxicol. Appl. Pharmacol.* **20**, 82–88.

Wang, C. M., and Matsumura, F. (1969). Dieldrin effect on the ion transport activities in liver tissues. *Bull. Environ. Contam. Toxicol.* **41**, 144–151.

Wang, H. H., and MacMahon, B. (1979a). Mortality of pesticide applicators. *J. Occup. Med.* **221**, 741–744.

Wang, H. H., and MacMahon, B. (1979b). Mortality of workers employed in the manufacture of chlordane and heptachlor. *J. Occup. Med.* **21**, 745–748.

Wang, X. Q., Gao, P. Y., Lin, Y. Z., and Chen, C. M. (1988). Studies on hexachlorocyclohexane and DDT contents in human cerumen and their relationship to cancer mortality. *Biomed. Environ. Sci.* **1**, 138–151.

Ware, G. W., and Good, E. E. (1967). Effects of insecticides on reproduction in the laboratory mouse. II. Mirex, Telodrin and DDT. *Toxicol. Appl. Pharmacol.* **10**, 54–61.

Wariishi, M., Suzuki, Y., and Nishiyama, K. (1986). Chlordane residues in normal human blood. *Bull. Environ. Contam. Toxicol.* **36**, 635–643.

Wärngård, L., Flodström, S., Ljungquist, S., and Ahlborg, U. G. (1985). Inhibition of metabolic cooperation in Chinese hamster lung fibroblast cells (V79) in culture by various DDT-analogs. *Arch. Environ. Contam. Toxicol.* **14**, 541–546.

Wärngård, L., Flodström, S., Ljungquist, S., and Ahlborg, U. G. (1987). Interaction between quercetin, TPA and DDT in the V79 metabolic cooperation assay. *Carcinogenesis (London)* **8**, 1201–1205.

Wärngård, L., Fransson, R., Flodström, S., Drakenberg, T.-B., and Ahlborg, U. G. (1988). Calmodulin involvement in TPA and DDT induced inhibition of intercellular communication. *Chem.-Biol. Interact.* **65**, 41–49.

Wärngård, L., Hemming, H. J., Flodström, S., Duddy, S. K., and Kass, G. E. N. (1989). Mechanistic studies on the DDT-induced inhibition of intercellular communication. *Carcinogenesis (London)* **10**, 471–476.

Warnick, S. L., and Carter, J. E. (1972). Some findings in a study of workers occupationally exposed to pesticides. *Arch. Environ. Health* **25**, 265–270.

Warraki, S. (1963). Respiratory hazards of chlorinated camphene. *Arch. Environ. Health* **7**, 253–256.

Warren, R. J., Kirkpatrick, R. L., and Young, R. W. (1978). Barbiturate-induced sleeping times, liver weights, and reproduction of cottontail rabbits after mirex ingestion. *Bull. Environ. Contamin. Toxicol.* **19**, 223–228.

Wasicky, R., and Unti, O. (1944). Dichloro-diphenyl trichloroethane (DDT) does not control culicine larvae. *Arch. Hig.* **9**, 87–102.

Wasicky, R., and Unti, O. (1945). Dichloro-diphenyl-trichloroethane (DDT). Recent investigations on its properties and uses. *Arch. Hig.* **10**, 49–64.

Wassermann, D., Wassermann, M., and Lazarovici, S. (1970). Effects of adrenalectomy on the storage of organochlorine insecticides. *Bull. Environ. Contam. Toxicol.* **5**, 373–378.

Wassermann, M., Iliescu, S., Mandric, G., and Horvath, P. (1960). Toxic hazards during DDT- and BHC-spraying of forests against *Lymantria monacha*. *AMA Arch. Ind. Health* **21**, 503–508.

Wassermann, M., Pebdefunda, G., Merling, M., Mihail, G., Sandulescu, G., and Vancea, G. (1961). Research on environmental conditions and on occupational pathology of *Anopheles* eradicators. Chronic poisoning by hexachlorocyclohexane (HCH). II. Clinical modifications caused by the action of HCH on *Anopheles* eradicators. *Arch. Mal. Prof. Med. Trav. Secur. Soc.* **22**, 308–317 (in French).

Wassermann, M., Mihail, G., Vancea, G., Mandric, G., Iliescu, S., Raileanu, D. B., Losubas, I. S., and Nestor, L. (1962). Research on environmental conditions and on the occupational pathology of *Anopheles* eradicators. Chronic poisoning by hexachlorocyclohexane (HCH). Correlation between clinical, chronaximetric and biochemical disorders. *Arch. Mal. Prof. Med. Trav. Secur. Soc.* **23**, 18–31 (in French).

Wassermann, M., Gon, M., Wassermann, D., and Zellermayer, L. (1965). DDT and DDE in the body fat of people in Israel. *Arch. Environ. Health* **11**, 375–379.

Wassermann, M., Wassermann, D., Zellermayer, L., and Gon, M. (1967).

Pesticides in people. Storage of DDT in the people of Israel. *Pestic. Monit. J.* **1**, 14–20.

Wassermann, M., Curnow, D. H., Forte, P. N., and Groner, Y. (1968a). Storage of organochlorine pesticides in the body fat of people in Western Australia. *Ind. Med. Surg.* **37**, 295–300.

Wassermann, M., Sofuluwe, G. I., Wassermann, D., Groner, Y., and Lazarovitch, S. (1968b). Storage of organochlorine insecticides in the body fat of people in Nigeria. *In* "Proceedings of the Largos International Seminar on Occupational Health for Developing Countries, Lagos, Nigeria, April 1–6."

Wassermann, M., Wassermann, D., and Ivriani, I. (1970a). Organochlorine insecticides in the plasma of occupationally exposed workers. *In* "Pesticides Symposia" (W. B. Diechmann, J. L. Radomski, and R. A. Penalver, eds.), Halos and Associates, Miami, Florida.

Wassermann, M., Wassermann, D., Lazarovici, S., Coetzee, A. M., and Tomatis, L. (1970b). Present state of the storage of the organochlorine insecticides in the general population of South Africa. *S. Afr. Med. J.* **44**, 646–648.

Wassermann, M., Wassermann, D., Kedar, E., and Djavaherian, M. (1971). Immunological and detoxication interactions in *p,p'*-DDT fed rabbits. *Bull. Environ. Contam. Toxicol.* **6**, 426–534.

Wassermann, M., Wassermann, D., Kedar, E., Djavaherian, M., and Cucos, S. (1972a). Effects of dieldrin and gamma BHC on serum proteins and PBI. *Bull. Environ. Contam. Toxicol.* **8**, 177–185.

Wassermann, M., Rogoff, M. G., Tomatis, L., Day, N. E., Wassermann, D., Djavaherian, M., and Guttel, C. (1972b). Storage of organochlorine insecticides in the adipose tissue of people of Kenya. *Ann. Soc. Belge Med. Trop.* **52**, 509–514.

Wassermann, M., Nogueira, D. P., Tomatis, L., Athie, E., Wassermann, D., Djavaherian, M., and Guttel, C. (1972c). Storage of organochlorine insecticides in people of São Paulo, Brazil. *Ind. Med. Surg.* **41**, 22–25.

Wassermann, M., Trishnanada, M., Tomatis, L., Day, N. E., Wassermann, D., Rungpitarangsi, V., Chiamsakol, V., and Cucos, S. (1972d). Storage of organochlorine insecticides in the adipose tissue of people in Thailand. *Southeast Asian J. Trop. Med. Public Health* **3**, 280–285.

Wassermann, M., Sofoluwe, G. O., Tomatis, L., Day, N. E., Wassermann, D., and Lazarovici, S. (1972e). Storage of organochlorine insecticides in people in Nigeria. *Environ. Physiol. Biochem.* **2**, 59–67.

Wassermann, M., Tomatis, L., Wassermann, D., Day, N. E., and Djavaherian, M. (1974a). Storage of organochlorine insecticides in adipose tissue of Ugandans. *Bull. Environ. Contam. Toxicol.* **12**, 501–508.

Wassermann, M., Tomatis, L., Wassermann, D., Day, N. E., Groner, Y., Lazarovici, S., and Rosenfeld, D. (1974b). Epidemiology of organochlorine insecticides in the adipose tissue of Israelis. *Pestic. Monit. J.* **8**, 1–7.

Watari, N. (1973). Ultrastructural alterations of the mouse liver after the prolonged administration of BHC. *J. Clin. Electron Microsc.* **5**, 1410–1420, 1449–1456.

Watari, N., and Torizawa, K. (1972). Ultrastructural alterations of the mouse pancreas after prolonged administration of BHC. *J. Electron Microsc.* **21**, 334 (in Japanese).

Watson, M., Benson, W. W., and Gabica, J. (1970). Serum organochlorine pesticide levels in people in southern Idaho. *Pestic. Monit. J.* **4**, 47–50.

Weatherholz, W. M., and Webb, R. E. (1971). Influence of dietary protein on the activity of microsomal epoxidase in the growing rat. *J. Nutr.* **101**, 9–12.

Weatherholz, W. M., Campbell, T. C., and Webb, R. E. (1969). Effect of dietary protein levels on toxicity and metabolism of heptachlor. *J. Nutr.* **98**, 90–94.

Webb, R. E., and Miranda, C. L. (1973). Effect of the quality of dietary protein on heptachlor toxicity. *Food, Cosmet. Toxicol.* **11**, 63–67.

Webb, R. E., Randolph, W. C., and Horsfall, F. (1972). Hepatic benzpyrene hydrolase activity in endrin susceptible and resistant pine mice. *Life Sci.* **11**, (Part 2), 477–483.

Webb, R. E., Hartgrove, R. W., Randoolph, W. C., Petrella, V. J., and Hortsfall, F., Jr. (1973). Toxicity studies in endrin-susceptible and resistant strains of pine mice. *Toxicol. Appl. Pharmacol.* **25**, 42–47.

Weeks, D. E. (1967). Endrin food-poisoning. A report on four outbreaks caused by two separate shipments of endrin contaminated flour. *Bull. W.H.O.* **37**, 499–512.

Weihe, M. (1966). Chlorinated insecticides in the body fat of people in Denmark. *Ugeskr. Laeg.* **128**, 881–882.

Weinig, E., Machbert, G., and Zink, P. (1966). Proof of dieldrin in dieldrin poisoning. *Arch. Toxikol.* **22**, 115–124.

Weisenberg, E., Arad, I., Grauer, F., and Sahm, Z. (1985). Polychlorinated biphenyls and organochlorine insecticides in human milk in Israel. *Arch. Environ. Contam. Toxicol.* **14**, 517–521.

Weisenfeld, S., and Goldner, M. G. (1962). Treatment of advanced malignancy and Cushing's syndrome with DDD. *Cancer Chemother. Rep.* **16**, 335–339.

Welch, H. (1948). Tests of the toxicity to sheep and cattle of certain of the newer insecticides. *J. Econ. Entomol.* **41**, 36–39.

Welch, R. M., Levin, W., and Conney, A. H. (1969). Estrogenic action of DDT and its analogs. *Toxicol. Appl. Pharmacol.* **14**, 358–367.

Welch, R. M., Levin, W., Kuntzman, R., Jacobson, M., and Conney, A. H. (1971). Effect of halogenated hydrocarbon insecticides on the metabolism and uterotrophic action of estrogens in rats and mice. *Toxicol. Appl. Pharmacol.* **19**, 234–246.

Wells, W. L., and Milborn, H. T. (1983). Suicide attempt by toxaphene ingestion: A case report. *J. Miss. State Med. Assoc.* **24**, 329–330.

Welsh, J. H., and Gordon, H. T. (1946). The mode of action of DDT. *Fed. Proc., Fed. Am. Soc. Exp. Biol.* **5**, 1.

West, I. (1964). Pesticides as contaminants. *Arch. Environ. Health* **9**, 626–631.

West, I. (1967). Lindane and hematologic reactions. *Arch. Environ. Health* **15**, 97–101.

West, I., and Milby, T. H. (1965). Public health problems arising from the use of pesticides. *Residue Rev.* **11**, 140–159.

West, P. R., Chaudhary, S. K., Branton, G. R., and Mitchell, R. H. (1982). High-performance liquid chromatographic analysis of impurities and degradation products of methoxychlor. *J. Assoc. Off. Anal. Chem.* **65**, 1457–1470.

Westoo, G., and Noren, K. (1978). Organochlorine contaminants in human milk, Stockholm, 1967–1977. *Ambio* **7**, 62–64.

Westoo, G., Noren, K., and Andersson, M. (1970). Levels of organochlorine pesticides and polychlorinated biphenyls in margarine, vegetable oils, and some foods of animal origin on the Swedish market in 1967–69. *Var. Foeda* **22**, 9–31.

White, W. C., and Sweeney, T. R. (1945). The metabolism of 2,2-bis(*p*-chlorophenyl)-1,1,1-tricholorethane (DDT). I. A metabolite from rabbit urine di-(*p*-chlorophenyl)-acetic acid; its isolation, identification, and synthesis. *Public Health Rep.* **60**, 66–71.

Whitehead, C. C., Downing, A. G., and Pettigrew, R. J. (1972). The effects of lindane on laying hens. *Br. Poult. Sci.* **13**, 293–299.

Wickström, K., Pyysalo, H., and Siimes, M. A. (1983). Levels of chlordane, hexachlorobenzene, PCB and DDT compounds in Finnish milk in 1982. *Bull. Environ. Contam. Toxicol.* **31**, 251–256.

Wiener, M., Pittman, K. A., and Stein, V. (1976). Mirex kinetics in rhesus monkey. I. Disposition and excretion. *Drug Metab. Dispos.* **4**, 281–287.

Wigglesworth, V. B. (1945). A case of DDT poisoning in man. *Br. Med. J.* **1**, 517.

Wilcox, A. R. (1967). "USPH Investigation—DDT Health Effects," Interoffice ccorrespondence to M. V. Anthony. Stauffer Chemical Co.

Wildemauwe, C., Lontie, J.-F., Schoofs, L., and van Larebeke, N. (1983). The mutagenicity in procaryocytes of insecticides, acaricides, and nematicides. *Residue Rev.* **89**, 129–178.

Willhite, C., and Sharma, R. P. (1978). Acute dieldrin exposure in relation to brain monoamine oxidase activity and concentration of brain serotonin and 5-hydroxyindoleacetic acid. *Toxicol. Lett.* **2**, 71–75.

Williams, C. H., and Casterline, J. L. (1970). Effects on toxicity and on enzyme activity of the interactions between aldrin, chlordane, piperonyl butoxide and Banol in rats. *Proc. Soc. Exp. Biol. Med.* **135**, 46–50.

Williams, D. J., and Rabin, B. R. (1971). Disruption by carcinogens of the hormone dependent association of membranes with polysomes. *Nature (London)* **232**, 102–105.

Williams, D. T., LeBel, G. L., and Jenkins, E. (1984). A comparison of organochlorine residues in human adipose tissue autopsy samples from two Ontario municipalities. *J. Toxicol. Environ. Health* **13**, 19–29.

Williams, F. M., Woodhouse, K. W., Middleton, D., Wright, P., James, O., and Rawlins, M. D. (1982). Aldrin epoxidation in small samples of human liver. *Biochem. Pharmacol.* **31**, 3701–3703.

Williams, G. M. (1980). Classification of genotoxic and epigenetic hepatocarcinogens using liver culture assays. *Ann. N.Y. Acad. Sci.* **349**, 273–282.

Williams, G. M., and Numoto, S. (1984). Promotion of mouse liver neoplasms by the organochlorine pesticides chlordane and heptachlor in comparison to dichlorodiphenyltrichloroethane. *Carcinogenesis (London)* **5**, 1689–1696.

Williams, G. M., Telang, S., and Tong, C. (1981). Inhibition of intercellular communication between liver cells by the liver tumor promoter 1,1,1-trichloro-2,2-bis(p-chlorophenyl)ethane. *Cancer Lett.* **11**, 339–344.

Williams, J., Eckols, K., Stewart, G., and Uphouse, L. (1988). Proestrous effects of chlordecone on the serotonin system. *Neurotoxicology* **9**, 597–610.

Williams, J., Eckols, K., and Uphouse, L. (1989). Estradiol and chlordecone interactions with the estradiol receptor. *Toxicol. Appl. Pharmacol.*, **98**, 413–421.

Williams, J. D., and Yarbrough, J. D. (1983). The relationship between mirex-induced liver enlargement and the adrenal glands. *Pestic. Biochem. Physiol.* **19**, 15–22.

Wilson, D. J., Locker, D. J., Ritzen, C. A., Watson, J. T., and Schaffner, W. (1973). DDT concentrations in human milk. *Am. J. Dis. Child.* **125**, 814–817.

Wilson, D., and Yarbrough, J. D. (1988). Autoradiographic analysis of hepatocytes in mirex-induced adaptive liver growth. *Am. J. Physiol.* **255**, G132–G139.

Wilson, H. F., Allen, N. N., Bohstedt, G., Betheil, J., and Lardy, H. A. (1946). Feeding experiments with DDT-treated pea vine silage with special reference to dairy cows, sheep, and laboratory animals. *J. Econ. Entomol.* **39**, 801–806.

Wilson, J. S. (1959). Lindane poisoning in a family. *Med. J. Aust.* **2**, 684.

Wilson, K. A., and Cook, R. M. (1970). Metabolism of xenobiotics in ruminants: Use of activated carbon as an antidote for pesticide poisoning in ruminants. *J. Agric. Food Chem.* **18**, 437–440.

Winteringham, F. P. W., and Barnes, J. M. (1955). Comparative response of insects and mammals to certain halogenated hydrocarbons used as insecticides. *Physiol. Rev.* **35**, 701–739.

Winthrop, G. J., and Felice, J. F. (1957). A clinical toxicological study of spraymen of a chlorinated hydrocarbon insecticide. *Bol. Of. Sanit. Panam.* **43**, 512–517.

Wit, S. L. (1964). Aspects of toxicology and chemical analysis of insecticide residues. *Voeding* **25**, 609–628.

Wolburg, I. (1973). The use of electroencephelography in industrial toxicology. *Act. Nerv. Super.* **15**, 226–235 (in German).

Wolf, C. R. (1986). Cytochrome P-450s: Polymorphic multigene families involved in carcinogen activation. *Trends Genet.* **2**, 209–214.

Wolfe, H. R., and Armstrong, J. F. (1971). Exposure of formulating plant workers to DDT. *Arch. Environ. Health* **23**, 169–176.

Wolfe, H. R., Walker, K. C., Elliott, J. W., and Durham, W. F. (1959). Evaluation of the health hazards involved in house spraying with DDT. *Bull. W.H.O.* **20**, 1–14.

Wolfe, J. L., Esher, R. J., Robinson, K. M., and Yarbrough, J. D. (1979). Lethal and reproductive effects of dietary mirex and DDT on old-field mice, *Peromyscus polionotus. Bull. Environ. Contam. Toxicol.* **21**, 397–402.

Wolff, G. L., and Suber, R. L. (1986). Hepatic glutathione S-transferase activity in mice. Effects of A^{vy}/-genotype, obesity, lindane treatment, and sex. *Proc. Soc. Exp. Biol. Med.* **181**, 535–541.

Wolff, G. L., Roberts, D. W., Morrissey, R. L., Greenman, D. L., Allen, R. R., Campbell, W. L., Bergman, H., Nesnow, S., and Frith, C. H. (1987). Tumourigenic responses to lindane in mice: Potentiation by a dominant mutation. *Carcinogenesis (London)* **8**, 1889–1897.

Wolff, T., and Guengerich, F. P. (1987). Rat liver cytochrome P-450 isozymes as catalysts of aldrin epoxidation in reconstituted monooxygenase systems and microsomes. *Biochem. Pharmacol.* **36**, 2581–2588.

Wolff, T., Greim, H., Huang, M., Miwa, G., and Lu, A. Y. H. (1980). Aldrin epoxidation catalysed by purified rat-liver cytochromes P-450 and P-448. *Eur. J. Biochem.* **111**, 545–551.

Wong, O., Brocker, W., Davis, H. V., and Nagle, G. S. (1984). Mortality of workers potentially exposed to organic and inorganic brominated chemicals, DBCP, TRIS, PBB and DDT. *Br. J. Ind. Med.* **41**, 15–24.

Woodard, B. T., Ferguson, B. B., and Wilson, D. J. (1976). DDT levels in milk of rural indigent blacks. *Am. J. Dis. Child.* **130**, 400–403.

Woodard, G., and Hagan, E. C. (1947). Toxicological studies on the isomers and mixtures of isomers of benzene hexachloride. *Fed. Proc., Fed. Am. Soc. Exp. Biol.* **6**, 386.

Woodard, G., Ofner, R. R., and Montgomery, C. M. (1945). Accumulation of DDT in body fat and its appearance in the milk of dogs. *Science* **102**, 177–178.

Woodliff, H. J., Connor, P. M., and Scopa, J. (1966a). Aplastic anaemia associated with insecticides. *Med. J. Aust.* **1**, 628–629.

Woodliff, H. J., Connor, P. M., and Scopa, J. (1966b). Aplastic anaemia associated with insecticides (letter). *Med. J. Aust.* **1**, 915–916.

Wooldridge, W. E. (1948). The gamma isomer of hexachlorocyclohexane in the treatment of scabies. *J. Invest. Dermatol.* **10–11**, 363–366.

Woolley, D. E. (1982). Neurotoxicity of DDT and possible mechanisms of action. In "Mechanisms of Action of Neurotoxic Substances" (K. Pradad and A. Vernadakis, eds.), pp. 95–141. Raven Press, New York.

Woolley, D. E. (1985). Application of neurophysiological techniques to toxicological problems: An overview. *Fundam. Appl. Toxicol.* **5**, 1–8.

Woolley, D., Zimmer, L., Hasson, Z., and Swanson, K. (1984). Do some insecticides and heavy metals produce long-term potentiation in the limbic system? In "Cellular and Molecular Toxicology" (T. Narahashi, ed.), pp. 45–69. Raven Press, New York.

Woolley, D., Zimmer, L., Dodge, D., and Swanson, K. (1985). Effects of lindane-type insecticides in mammals: Unsolved problems. *Neurotoxicology* **6** (2), 165–192.

Worden, A. N. (1969). Toxicity of Telodrin. *Toxicol. Appl. Pharmacol.* **14**, 556–573.

World Health Organization (WHO) (1958). "Note by Secretariat on Aldrin Poisoning in Kenya," Inf. Circ. Toxic. Pestic. Man, No. 1, p. 3. World Health Organ., Geneva.

World Health Organization (WHO) (1959). "Report of Fatal Case of Aldrin Poisoning in an African Child (personal communication)," Inf. Circ. Toxic. Pestic. Man, No. 3, p. 1. World Health Organ., Geneva.

World Health Organization (WHO) (1971). The place of DDT in operations against malaria and other vector-borne diseases. In "Official Records of the World Health Organization, No. 190," Executive Board Forty-Seventh Session. Part II. Report on the Proposed Program and Budget Estimates for 1972. Appendix 14, pp. 176–182. World Health Organ., Geneva.

World Health Organization (WHO) (1973). "Safe Use of Pesticides. Twentieth Report of the WHO Expert Committee on Insecticides," Tech. Rep. Ser. No. 513. World Health Organ., Geneva.

World Health Organization (WHO) (1974). Some organochlorine pesticides. *IARC Monogr. Eval. Carcinog. Risk Chem. Man* **5**.

World Health Organization (WHO) (1977). Outbreak of food poisoning of chemical origin. *Wkly. Epidemiol. Rec.* **52**, 217.

World Health Organization (WHO) (1979). "Environmental Health Criteria 9. DDT and Its Derivatives." United National Environment Programme and the World Health Organization, Geneva.

Wrenn, T. R., Weyant, J. R., Fries, G. F., and Bitman, J. (1971a). Effect of several dietary levels of o,p'-DDT on reproduction and lactation in the rat. *Bull. Environ. Contam. Toxicol.* **6**, 471–479.

Wrenn, T. R., Randall, J., Weyant, R., Fries, G. F., and Bitman, J. (1971b). Influence of dietary o,p'-DDT on reproduction and lactation of ewes. *J. Anim. Sci.* **33**, 1288–1292.

Wright, A. S., Potter, D., Wooder, M. F., Donninger, C., and Greenland, R. D. (1972). The effects of dieldrin on the subcellular structure and function of mammalian liver cells. *Food Cosmet. Toxicol.* **10**, 311–322.

Wright, A. S., Akintonwa, D. A. A., and Wooder, M. F. (1977). Studies on the interactions of dieldrin with mammalian liver cells at the subcellular level. *Ecotoxicol. Environ. Saf.* **1**, 7–16.

Wright, A. S., Donninger, C., Greeland, R. D., Stemmer, K. L., and Zavon,

M. R. (1978). The effect of prolonged ingestion of dieldrin on the livers of male rhesus monkeys. *Ecotoxicol. Environ. Saf.* **1**, 477–502.

Wyllie, J., Gabica, J., and Benson, W. W. (1972). Comparative organochlorine pesticide residues in serum and biopsied lipoid tissue: A survey of 200 persons in southern Idaho—1970. *Pestic. Monit. J.* **6**, 84–88.

Yadav, A. S., Vashishat, R. K., and Kakar, S. N. (1982). Testing of endosulfan and fenitrothion for genotoxicity in *Saccharomyces cerevisiae*. *Mutat. Res.* **105**, 403–407.

Yakushiji, T., Watanabe, I., Kuwabara, K., Yoshida, S., Koyana, K., and Kunita, N. (1979). Levels of polychlorinated biphenyls (PCBs) and organochlorine pesticides in human milk and blood collected in Osaka Prefecture from 1972 to 1977. *Int. Arch. Occup. Environ. Health* **43**, 1–15.

Yamada, T., and Sakamoto, Y. (1973). Results of survey of pesticide residues in mother's milk and soil. *Annu. Rep. Hiroshima Prefect. Inst. Prevent. Environ. Pollut.* **3**, 57–58 (in Japanese).

Yamagishi, T., Takeba, K., Fujimoto, C., Morimoto, K., and Haruta, M. (1972a). On the organochlorine pesticide residues in mother's body and her fetus' body. *Rep. Tokyo Public Health Stud.* **50**, 44–45 (in Japanese).

Yamagishi, T., Fugimoto, C., Takeba, K., Morimoto, K., and Haruta, M. (1972b). Effects of β-BHC on the mouse fetus. *Rep. Tokyo Public Health Stud.* **50**, 46–47 (in Japanese).

Yamagishi, T., Takeba, K., Fujimoto, C., Morimoto, K., and Haruta, M. (1972c). On the effects of β-BHC on the fetus of mouse. IV. *J. Clin. Nutr.* **41**, 599–604.

Yamaguchi, I., Matsumura, F., and Kadous, A. A. (1979). Inhibition of synaptic ATPases by heptachlorepoxide in rat brain. *Pestic. Biochem. Physiol.* **11**, 285–293.

Yamaguchi, I., Matsumura, F., and Kadous, A. A. (1980). Heptachlor epoxide: Effects on calcium-mediated transmitter release from brain synaptosomes in rat. *Biochem. Pharmacol.* **29**, 1815–1823.

Yamaguchi, M., Tanaka, S., Kawashima, K., Nakaura, S., and Tananaka, A. (1987). Effects of heptachlor on fetal developments of rats. *Eisei Shikensho Hokoku* **105**, 33–36 (in Japanese).

Yamaguchi, S., Kaku, S., Kuwahara, Y., and Yamada, A. (1976). Epidemiological findings and evaluation of the amount of organochlorine pesticides in human blood plasma in Japan. (1976). *Arch. Environ. Contam. Toxicol.* **3**, 448–460.

Yamamoto, K., Konoshita, K., and Uchihira, T. (1973). A case of secondary erythroderma possibly due to BHC. *Case Hist.* **6**, 61–62.

Yamamoto, T., Egashira, T., Yamanaka, Y., Takerni, Y., and Kuroiwa, Y. (1983). Initial metabolism of gamma-hexachlorocyclohexane (γ-HCH) by rat liver microsomes. *J. Pharmacobio-Dyn.* **6**, 721–728.

Yarbrough, J. D., Chambers, J. E., Grimley, J. M., Alley, E. G., Fang, M. M., Morrow, J. T., Ward, B. C., and Conroy, J. D. (1981). Comparative study of 8-monohydromirex and mirex toxicity in male rats. *Toxicol. Appl. Pharmacol.* **58**, 105–117.

Yarbrough, J. D., Grimley, J. M., Karl, P. I., Chambers, J. E., Case, R. S., and Alley, E. G. (1983). Tissue disposition, metabolism, and excretion of *cis*- and *trans*-5,10-dihydrogen mirex. *Drug Metab. Dispos.* **11**, 611–614.

Yarbrough, J. D., Brown, L. D., and Grimley, J. O. (1984). Mirex-induced adaptive liver growth: A corticosterone-mediated response. *Cell Tissue Kinet.* **17**, 465–473.

Yarbrough, J. D., Grimley, J. M., and Alley, E. G. (1986a). Induction of the hepatic cytochrome P-450 dependent monooxygenase system by *cis*- and *trans*-5,10-dihydrogen mirex. *Toxicol. Lett.* **32**, 65–71.

Yarbrough, J. D., Grimley, J. M., and Karl, P. I. (1986b). Relationship of ornithine decarboxylase and thymidine kinase to mirex-induced liver growth. *Am. J. Physiol.* **251**, G859–G865.

Yoder, J. M., Watson, M., and Benson, W. W. (1973). Lymphocyte chromosome analysis of agricultural workers during extensive occupational exposure to pesticides. *Mutat. Res.* **21**, 335–340.

Yoshimoto, H., Kaneko, T., Horiuchi, S., Yonemaru, H., and Ideda, Y. (1972). Long-term toxicity of beta-BHC. *Folia Pharmacol. Jpn.* **68**, 243 (in Japanese).

Young, R. A., and Mehendale, H. M. (1986). Effect of endrin and endrin derivatives on hepatobiliary function and carbon tetrachloride-induced hepatotoxicity in male and female rats. *Food Chem. Toxicol.* **34**, 863–868.

Zaidi, S. S. A. (1987). Possible role of rat liver NADPH cytochrome P-450 reductase in the detoxication of DDT to DDD. *Bull. Environ. Contamin. Toxicol.* **39**, 327–333.

Zakirov, U. B., Volokhvyanskiy, Y. A., and Kadyrov, U. Z. (1973). Effect of small doses of hexachlorocyclohexane after a lengthy period of administration on the activity of small intestine enzymes. *Med. Zh. Uzb.* **12**, 28–31 (in Russian).

Zarkevich, N. F., Brusilovskiy, Y. S., and Orlov, N. S. (1973). Evaluation of the functional state of the kidneys using radioisotope renography in nephropathies of chemical etiology. *Gig. Tr. Prof. Zabol.* **17**, 28–32 (in Russian).

Zavon, M. R., and Hamman, R. E. (1961). Human experience with dieldrin in malaria control programs. *Am. J. Public Health* **51**, 1026–1034.

Zavon, M. R., Hine, C. H., and Parker, K. D. (1965). Chlorinated hydrocarbon insecticides in human body fat in the United States. *JAMA, J. Am. Med. Assoc.* **193**, 837–839.

Zeidler, O. (1874). Compounds of chloral with bromo- and chlorobenzene. *Ber. Dtsch. Chem. Ges.* **7**, 1180–1181 (in German).

Zein-el-Dine, K. (1946). The insecticide DDT. *J. Egypt. Med. Assoc.* **29**, 38–54.

Zeller, F. J., and Hauser, H. (1974). Induction of polyploidy in cereal grains in lindane-based seed dressings. *Experientia* **30**, 345–348.

Zemaitis, M. A., Oberholser, K. M., and Greene, E. E. (1976). Effects of acute and chronic dieldrin administration on liver and plasma esterases of the rat. *Toxicol. Appl. Pharmacol.* **37**, 29–37.

Zhong-Xiang, L., Kavanagh, T., Trosko, J. E., and Chang, C. C. (1986). Inhibition of gap junctional intercellular communication in human teratocarcinoma cells by organochlorine pesticides. *Toxicol. Appl. Pharmacol.* **83**, 10–19.

Zhu, J., Feng, Z., and Chen, J. (1986). Studies on the distribution and fate of [γ-^{3}H]hexachlorocyclohexane in rats. *Pestic. Biochem. Physiol.* **25**, 414–419.

Ziem, G. (1982). Aplastic anaemia after methoxychlor exposure. *Lancet* **2**, 1349.

Zimmerli, B., and Marck, B. (1973). The pesticide burden of the Swiss population (analyses of prepared meals, human fat, human serum, cigarettes, and cosmetics). *Mitt. Geb. Lebensmittelunters. Hyg.* **64**, 459–479 (in German).

Zimmerman, B., Bloch, H. S., Williams, W. L., Hitchcock, C. R., and Hoeischer, B. (1956). Effects of DDT (1,1,-dichloro-2,2-his(p-chloro-phenyl)-ethane) on human adrenal. Attempt to use adrenal destructive agent in treatment of disseminated mammary and prostatic cancer. *Cancer (Philadelphia)* **9**, 940–948.

Zolotnikova, G. P., and Somov, B. A. (1978). On the role of pesticides in the occurrence of occupational dermatitis in workers of hothouses. *Vestn. Dermatol. Venerol.* **4**, 76–79 (in Russian).

Zumoff, B. (1979). The hypouricemic effect of o,p-DDD. *Am. J. Med. Sci.* **278**, 145–147.

Organic Phosphorus Pesticides

Michael A. Gallo and Nicholas J. Lawryk
University of Medicine and Dentistry of New Jersey

16.1 CLASSIFICATION OF ORGANIC PHOSPHORUS COMPOUNDS

Organic phosphorus compounds share a common chemical structure, but they differ greatly in the details of their structure, in their physical and pharmacological properties, and consequently in the uses to which they have been put or for which they have been proposed. No chemical classification has been proposed that will divide this wide variety of compounds into pharmacologically and toxicologically homogeneous groups with no overlapping. The scheme adopted in this book is based on that of Holmstedt (1959). Two main changes have been made. The distinction between P=O and P=S substitutions was dropped to avoid placing the metabolites of many insecticides in a group different from that of the parent compound. The subheadings under the main groups have been changed so that pesticides fall mainly into two groups and so that compounds with similar pharmacologic properties fall into as few groups as possible.

Although this book is concerned with pesticides, it is necessary to examine the historical significance and briefly compare the properties of some other organic phosphorus compounds.

In 1820, Lassaigne first synthesized esters of phosphorus. Later in that century, the German chemist Michaelis developed a much more comprehensive understanding of the chemistry of organic phosphorus compounds, particularly those involving the phosphorus–nitrogen bond. Later in the career of Michaelis, A. E. Arbuznov in Russia conducted research on trivalent phosphorus compounds, including the Michaelis–Arbuznov reaction to form the phosphorus–carbon bond. This work was continued by his son, B. A. Arbuznov (Eto, 1979).

Although a number of organic phosphorus compounds were synthesized or discovered prior to the early part of this century, knowledge of their adverse effects on living organisms was not documented until 1932, when Lang and Kreuger observed toxic effects on rats in their quest to discover new organic pesticides. This discovery resulted in a number of new potential uses for organic phosphorus compounds, including their employment as nerve gases in World War II.

Saunders in England and Schrader in Germany worked on toxic organic phosphorus compounds during World War II. Saunders, in his attempts to develop nerve gases, synthesized diisopropyl fluorophosphate (DFP). In 1937, Schrader discovered the insecticidal properties of organic phosphorus compounds leading to the development of the systemic insecticide OMPA (presently known as schradan) in 1941. Schrader is also credited with the 1944 discovery of the first marketed organic phosphorus pesticide, Bladan, which contained TEPP as its active ingredient.

Most environmentally persistent organic chlorine pesticides have been used with decreasing frequency since 1957, as they were replaced by compounds more capable of biodegradation to less harmful products. Since integrated pest control management involves the use of these less persistent and more specific pesticides, organic phosphorus pesticides were the first compounds of choice for these applications, and they were later replaced by carbamate pesticides. However, the rapid biodegradation of carbamate pesticides has resulted in the present utilization of both carbamate and organic phosphorus pesticides for these purposes, with the use of organic chlorine pesticides reserved in the event of special problems [U.S. Department of Health, Education, and Welfare (USDHEW), 1969].

According to Holmstedt (1959), Schrader noted as early as 1937 that the general formula for anticholinesterase organic phosphorus compound is in which X is the leaving group. All

$$\begin{array}{c} R_1 \diagdown \quad \diagup O \text{ (or S)} \\ P \\ R_2 \diagup \quad \diagdown X \end{array}$$

the compounds may be placed in four main categories, depending on the character of the X constituent, as follows:

   I. X contains a quaternary nitrogen
  II. X = F
 III. X = CN, OCN, SCN, or a halogen other than F
 IV. X = other moieties (see below)

Examples are given in Table 16.1.

The first of these categories is small. Although categories II and III are somewhat larger, only a very few compounds in one of them (II) have been used or even considered as pesticides. There seems to be no need to subdivide these categories at this time. On the other hand, category IV may be subdivided usefully into at least eight groups on the basis of their R_1 and R_2 constituents. Several of these groups differ either quantitatively or qualitatively in toxicity, and in some instances the basis for the difference is known. For example, the basis for the quantitative difference in the toxicities of dimethoxy and diethoxy compounds is known and is discussed in Section 16.2.1.4. Some, but not necessarily all, compounds in four of the groups produce delayed paralysis in hens and undoubtedly would do the same in humans if absorbed in sufficient quantity (see Section 16.4.1). The eight groups and an example of each are as follows:

1. Dimethoxy — Section 16.6
2. Diethoxy — Section 16.7
3. Other dialkoxy — Section 16.8
4. Diamino — Section 16.9
5. Chlorinated and other substituted dialkoxy — Tables 16.14 and 16.46
6. Trithioalkyl — Section 16.10
7. Triphenyl and substituted triphenyl — Tables 16.14 and 16.46
8. Mixed substituent — Section 16.11

In each of the first seven groups, it is understood that R_1 and R_2 are identical, with the exception that thio isomers formed by rearrangement of certain compounds are still classified as belonging to the parent group. For example, isomalathion, the *S*-methyl isomer, which is formed from malathion during tropical storage of some formulations, is classified as a dimethoxy compound (see Use Experience in Section 16.6.1.3). Most, but not all, dithioalkyl and diphenyl compounds, substituted or otherwise, are in fact trithioalkyl and triphenyl compounds. In the last group (mixed constituent compounds), R_1 and R_2 are different. In fact, in many compounds of this group, all four substitutions on the phosphorus are different, and the compound is optically active. However, there are exceptions, such as edifenphos (see Section 16.10.4), in which the X group or leaving group is identical to one of the R groups and the compound is not optically active.

16.1.1 CHARACTERISTICS OF THE MAIN CATEGORIES

Organic phosphorus compounds containing a quaternary nitrogen are called phosphorylcholines. They not only are powerful inhibitors of cholinesterase, they also are directly cholinergic. This combination of properties helps to explain why some of them are among the most toxic synthetic compounds known. They are valuable investigative tools. One of them, ecothio-

Table 16.1

Examples of the Four Main Categories of Organic Phosphorus Compounds

Group	X constituents	Example
I	substituted quaternary nitrogen	Ecothiopate isodide
II	F	Sarin $(iC_3H_7O)_2 P(O) \!-\! F$ DFP
III	CN, OCN, SCN, or halogen other than F	Tabun Parathion
IV	alkyl; alkoxy or alkylthio; aryl or heterocyclic; aryloxy, arylthio, or one of their heterocyclic analogs; nitrogen; or disubstituted phosphoryl groups	Triorthocresyl phosphate

pate iodide, is used in the management of glaucoma. Their use as war gases has been discussed.

Although less toxic on the average than the phosphorylcholines, the fluorophosphates are, nonetheless, highly toxic. This property and their relatively great volatility make some of them suitable for war gases. Those proposed for this use have been called *nerve gases* because their effect is predominantly on the nervous system. Much of what is known about organic phosphorus compounds in general was derived from the study of these fluorophosphates. A very few (dimefox and mipafox) have been used or proposed as pesticides.

Organic phosphorus compounds containing some combination of cyanide or a halogen other than fluorine are generally intermediate in toxicity between the fluorophosphates and the broad category containing the majority of pesticides. A few of these compounds have been proposed for use as war gases.

The fourth category of organic phosphorus compounds is a

broad one. Unlike phosphocholines, the X group in category IV contains no quaternary nitrogen, but like phosphocholines, the group usually is attached by a P—O or P—S bond. A few of the compounds involve a P—N or P—C bond. The X group may be alkoxy, alkylthio, aryloxy, arylthio, or a heterocyclic analog. The nonring compounds include esters, thioesters, and vinyl esters. A number are disubstituted phosphoryl compounds. Category IV compounds with a P—N bond include azides and amines. Category IV compounds with a P—C linkage include chloroalkyl and heterocyclic moieties. The toxicity of representatives of category IV ranges from that of the nerve gases to less than that of table salt. Most organic phosphorus pesticides belong to this category; in fact, the vast majority are either dimethoxy or diethoxy compounds and thus fall into one of its first two groups, based on the configuration of the R_1 and R_2 substituents.

Considering only compounds of category IV that have been used or considered as pesticides, a higher proportion of the dimethoxy and diethoxy compounds are insecticides and/or acaricides, and a higher proportion of the other groups have other uses. Thus merphos (Section 16.10.1) is a defoliant, trimiphos is a fungicide, crufomate is a veterinary anthelmintic, and gophacide is a rodenticide. The fact that one is used to kill ground squirrels and another is used as a drug emphasizes their wide range of toxicity. The toxicity of some of the compounds to flowering plants, fungi, and other organisms almost certainly reflects different modes of action. However, in mammals, the only recognized modes of action involve inhibition of cholinesterase leading to acute poisoning or, in a few instances, inhibition of what is now called neuropathy target esterase (NTE) leading to paralysis.

Category IV also contains some other compounds that are useful, although they have no known pesticidal action. An example is tri-o-cresyl phosphate (TOCP), which is a valuable additive for gasoline and special lubricants.

16.1.2 POSSIBLE SUBDIVISIONS WITHIN CATEGORIES OR INDEPENDENT OF THEM

Based on use, chemistry, or other diverse characteristics, several subdivisions of the organic phosphorus compounds may be recognized; among them are those discussed under the following subheadings.

Systemic Antiparasitics   The astonishing fact that some pesticides are both effective and safe when administered systemically to mammals for control of parasites in the gastrointestinal tract or in the tissues is reviewed in Section 2.4.7.1. Examples include crufomate, trichlorfon, dichlorvos, ronnel, diphacinone, and coumaphos, all of which have been used in animals. The one that has received the greatest use by human patients is trichlorfon (see Section 16.6.6.3).

Other Systemic Drugs Used in Human Medicine   Paraoxon, schradan, and TEPP (see Sections 16.7.5.3 and 16.9.1.3)

are well as some other highly toxic organic phosphorus compounds, including DFP (see Section 16.5.3.3), have been used in treating patients with glaucoma and myasthenia gravis with the objective of producing prolonged inhibition of cholinesterase.

Antiparasitics for Dermal Application   Organic phosphorus compounds applied to human skin, hair, or clothing for control of lice or mites include malathion and temephos.

Plant Systemics   A combination of properties permits some compounds or their transformation products to be absorbed by one portion of a plant and to be translocated to other parts in sufficient concentration to kill insects that feed on them, especially by sucking the plant juices. Such compounds are called *systemics* or *plant systemics*. Under practical conditions, they may be applied to the leaves and translocated to other parts of the plant, or they may be applied to the soil, absorbed by the roots, and translocated to all the structures above ground. Examples of systemic organic phosphorus insecticides include demeton, demeton-S-methyl, demephion, crufomate, dicrotophos, dimefox, dimethoate, disulfoton, endothion, ethoate-methyl, pyrazophos, fenchlorphos, formothion, heptenophos, menazon, mephosfolan, methamidophos, mevinphos, monocrotophos, omethoate, oxydemeton-methyl, oxydisulfoton, phorate, phosfolan, phosphamidon, prothoate, schradan, thiometon, and vamidothion.

16.1.3 NOMENCLATURE OF ISOMERS

Some of the organic phosphorus insecticides contain two asymmetrically substituted, nonterminal atoms joined by a double bond and, therefore, occur in two stereoisomeric forms. It sometimes has occurred that the isomers of a compound were at least partially separated, characterized entomologically or in some other way, and designated α and β before the orientation of their moieties had been defined. When the orientation was learned, it was long customary to designate the two forms by the prefixes *cis-* and *trans-*, meaning "on this side" and "across," respectively. In considering the orientation of similar moieties in space across the double bond, emphasis generally was placed on carbon chains, but the rules were not precise or failed to cover some situations. This became a source of confusion in organic chemistry. The problem was not restricted to phosphorus compounds and had no special implications for toxicology. A rigid set of rules was developed for determining which moiety on one side of a plane is to be compared to which moiety on the other side. Rather than imposing the new rules on the old terms, new terms were used, presumably on the basis that new wine ought to be put into new bottles. The new terms are Z (from the German *zusammen,* meaning together), and E (from *entgegen,* meaning opposite). The entire matter has been discussed in great detail by the International Union for Pure and Applied Chemistry (IUPAC, 1970). Unfortunately, the new rules for defining the precedence of moieties sometimes are opposite to earlier custom. The result is that some isomers formerly designated *cis* are now correctly designated *E*, even though the terms themselves have opposite meanings. Examples include the isomers of monocrotophos, dicrotophos, mevinphos, and phosphamidon.

16.2 TOXICOLOGY

The toxic signs and symptoms that characterize poisoning by nearly all organic phosphorus compounds are thought to depend on the inhibition of acetylcholinesterase or (in the case of the phosphorylcholines) on this action plus direct cholinergic activity, which produces the same end result. This distinctive illness and the closely related pharmacological actions leading to it are the subject of this section. For convenience, the phenomena of potentiation and neurotoxicity, which are other aspects of the toxicology of organic phosphorus compounds, are covered in separate sections. This separation is justified by the fact that the pharmacological basis of each phenomenon is different.

16.2.1 PHARMACOLOGICAL BASIS

The chief pharmacologic basis of the toxic effect characteristic of all the organic phosphorus compounds under discussion at this point is inhibition of acetylcholinesterase leading to an abnormal accumulation of acetylcholine in the tissues. An understanding of this simple statement requires some explanation.

16.2.1.1 Acetylcholine

Only a bare outline of cholinergic mechanisms can be offered in this book. Those interested in details should consult books devoted exclusively to these mechanisms such as those edited by Koelle (1963), Waser (1975), and Goldberg and Hanin (1976).

Anatomy of Cholinergic Function Acetylcholine is the chemical mediator responsible for physiological transmission of nerve impulses from (*a*) preganglionic to postganglionic neurons of both the parasympathetic and sympathetic nervous systems, (*b*) postganglionic parasympathetic fibers to effector organs and postganglionic sympathetic fibers to sweat glands, (*c*) motor nerves to skeletal muscle, and (*d*) some nerve endings within the central nervous system.

The fibers listed under *a* and *b* are parts of the autonomic nervous system. Their anatomy and that of nerves to skeletal muscles are well understood. The situation is less clear for the central nervous system. Although it has been clear for a long time that some activities of the central nervous system depend on acetylcholine, the anatomical relationships have remained obscure. A discussion of this matter is beyond the scope of this book. However, it is of interest that organic phosphorus compounds have been important in its investigation. It is unlikely that acetylcholine is without function at any point at which it is released. On this basis, the accumulation of acetylcholine in different parts of the brain has been charted in animals poisoned by these compounds. A single example of such research is that of Stavinoha *et al.* (1976).

Autonomic Nervous System Table 16.2 outlines certain anatomical and pharmacological features of the autonomic nervous system that are basic to an understanding of the action of

Table 16.2

Summary of the Anatomy, Physiology, and Pharmacology of the Autonomic Nervous System

	Parasympathetic	Sympathetic
Location of cell body of		
preganglionic fiber	brain stem and sacral cord (S_2–S_4)	cord (T_1–L_2)
postganglionic fiber	ciliary, spenopalatil, submandibular, and otic ganglia associated with cranial nerves III, VII, and IX and in or near organ innervated by cranial nerves X and XI and the pelvic nerve	ganglia in three locations: paravertebral (e.g., sympathetic chain ganglia), prevertebral (e.g., ciliac, aorticorenal, superior mesenteric, and inferior mesenteric ganglia), and peripheral (e.g., hypogastric and pelvic plexi)
Chemical mediation of transmission from		
preganglionic fiber	acetylcholine	acetylcholine
postganglionic fiber	acetylcholine (relaxation of cardiac sphincter due to adrenergic fibers)	norepinephrine (except cholinergic, sympathetic nerves to sweat glands)
Chemicals that mimic effect of stimulation of		
preganglionic fiber on ganglia	nicotine	nicotine
postganglionic fiber on effector organs	muscarine (also produces sweating)	—
Chemicals that block action of nerves or drugs on		
ganglia	hexamethonium	hexamethonium
effector organs	atropine	ergot blocks receptors that are stimulated (α-adrenotropic receptors); DCI[a] blocks receptors in the heart and those that are inhibited (β-adrenotropic receptors)

[a] DCI, Dichloroisoprotenol.

acetylcholine. For a detailed description of the physiology of this system, the reader may consult Hillarp (1960). Briefly, the autonomic nervous system is a visceral, efferent system concerned with the innervation of smooth muscle, heart muscle, and glands. It is composed of two portions, the parasympathetic and the sympathetic nervous systems. Both involve cell bodies located in the central nervous system (CNS) and other cells located outside the CNS. However, the two systems differ in function, anatomy, and chemistry. The parasympathetic system is concerned with normal function and is necessary to life. Its central cell bodies are located in the brain stem and the sacral cord; the peripheral cell bodies in the head are located in small ganglia close to the innervated organs, while the peripheral cells of the remainder of the parasympathetic system are located somewhat diffusely near or in the organs they serve. The sympathetic nervous system is concerned with response to emergencies; it is not necessary to life, except perhaps under conditions of stress. The central nervous system cell bodies of the sympathetic system lie in the thoracic and upper lumbar spinal cord; its peripheral cell bodies lie chiefly in the chain ganglia near the cord or in relatively large ganglia within the abdominal cavity.

The central cells of both systems contain acetylcholine, and this ester mediates transmission of the nerve impulse across the synapse, separating the preganglionic fibers from the peripheral neurons. Transmission from postganglionic parasympathetic fibers is also mediated by acetylcholine, but (with the exception of nerves to sweat glands) impulses from postganglionic sympathetic fibers are transmitted by noradrenaline. In addition, the transmission of impulses from motor nerves to skeletal muscle is mediated by acetylcholine.

Thus, the pre- and postganglionic fibers of the parasympathetic systems and the somatic motor nerves may be classified chemically as well as anatomically and physiologically. Fibers releasing acetylcholine are called cholinergic; those releasing noradrenaline are called adrenergic.

In general, the effects of stimulation of the two parts of the autonomic system are opposite (see Table 16.3). The contrast in response may involve the same structure, e.g., contraction (parasympathetic) and relaxation (sympathetic) of the muscles of the fundus of the urinary bladder. Contrast in response may involve opposing structures, e.g., contraction of the circular muscle of the iris (parasympathetic), which constricts the pupil of the eye, or contraction of the radial muscle (sympathetic), which dilates the pupil. In some instances, the two systems have parallel functions. For example, stimulation of both kinds of nerves to the salivary glands causes secretion, but of a somewhat different form of saliva.

Function of Acetylcholine   According to present concepts, acetylcholine is released from the endings of cholinergic fibers in response to the conduction of an action potential along the fiber. The acetylcholine is produced under the influence of choline acetylase within vesicles that occur throughout the cell but are numerous at the axonal endings. The release of acetylcholine at the junction between pre- and postganglionic

Table 16.3

Effect of Stimulation of Autonomic Nerves on Organs and Tissues of Humans

Organ or tissue	Parasympathetic	Sympathetic
Eye		
radial muscle of iris	—	contraction
circular muscle of iris	contraction	—
ciliary muscle	contraction	—
Glands		
sweat	—	secretion[a]
salivary	secretion	secretion
lacrimal	secretion	—
respiratory tract	secretion	—
gastrointestinal tract	secretion	—
adrenal medulla	—	secretion[b]
Heart		
sinus nodal rhythm	slowing	acceleration
refractory period, AV node	increased	reduced
atrial conduction rate	increased	increased
atrial contraction force	decreased	increased
ventricular contraction force	unknown	increased
Blood vessels to		
muscles	—	dilatation
heart	constriction	dilatation
skin	—	constriction
viscera	—	constriction
salivary glands	dilatation	constriction
erectile tissue	dilatation	constriction
Muscles of		
hair	—	contraction
intestinal wall	contraction	relaxation
cardiac sphincter	relaxation[a]	
spleen	—	contraction
fundus of urinary bladder	contraction	relaxation
trigone and sphincter of same	relaxation	contraction
uterus	—	contraction
Liver	—	glycogenolysis

[a] See note on chemical mediation in Table 16.2.

[b] The stimulation is preganglionic; the adrenal medulla is analogous to a ganglion.

fibers (synapse) or between a nerve fiber and an effector cell (neuroeffector junction) and contact of the neurohumor with cholinergic receptors in the surface of the target cell accomplish transmission of the impulse. Under normal circumstances, the acetylcholine released at any junction is hydrolyzed by acetylcholinesterase almost instantly. There is no accumulation of the ester. The rapid destruction accounts for the brevity and unity of each normal propagated impulse. Thus, the normal function of acetylcholine depends on its rapid destruction by acetylcholinesterase.

If anything interferes with this destruction, acetylcholine tends to accumulate at the junctions where it is produced. A small excess of neurohormone produces abnormally great stimulation, but a further excess may have the opposite effect. For example, a small increase in acetylcholine at the neuromuscular junction of skeletal muscles produces fasciculations, but a further increase produces profound weakness and, eventually, flaccid paralysis. The cholinergic nerve endings on smooth muscle and glands are less susceptible than those on skeletal muscle to blocking by an excess of acetylcholine. Therefore, in poisoning, bronchospasm, cramping of the intestinal muscles, and excessive secretions often persist after weakness of the voluntary muscles has become severe.

It is interesting that by use of ^{32}P-labeled DFP, it was possible to estimate that the number of sites phosphorylated at each striated muscle end plate of the mouse was about 90,000,000 for the sternomastoid and about 30,000,000 for the diaphragm. By using three methods that are relatively specific for acetylcholinesterase, it was found that about 35% of DFP-reactive sites at muscle end plates are acetylcholinesterase. Thus, the mean value for the number of acetylcholinesterase molecules per endplate of the sternomastoid and diaphragm were 31,000,000 and 11,000,000 respectively (Rogers *et al.*, 1969). Of course, the proportion of reactive sites that are acetylcholinesterase must be far less than 35% in non-specialized portions of striated muscles. Reactive sites are widely distributed in the liver and kidney cytoplasma and in kidney nuclei, but the proportion of cholinesterase was small (Barnard *et al.*, 1970). The same is likely to be true of most tissues.

Hydrolysis of Acetylcholine   The hydrolysis of acetylcholine is thought to be facilitated by its attachment to special reactive sites on the surface of the protein constituting the enzyme acetylcholinesterase, as illustrated in Fig. 16.1A. The strong positive charge on the quaternary nitrogen of the choline moiety forms an electrostatic linkage with the anionic site of the enzyme. This ionic bond is reinforced by auxiliary binding forces between two of the methyl groups on the nitrogen and the surface of the protein. It is thought that the attachment of the choline moiety is a necessary prerequisite to the formation of a covalent bond between the carbonyl atom of the acetate moiety and the esteratic site of the enzyme. Acetylation of the enzyme is rapidly followed by breakage of the ester linkage and the elimination of choline. The acetylated enzyme then reacts with water to regenerate the enzyme and release acetic acid.

16.2.1.2 Compounds That Mimic Acetylcholine or Block Its Action

Much of what is known about the anatomy and function of the autonomic nervous system was learned from experiments with compounds that were found to mimic or block the effects of stimulation of specific nerves. See Table 16.2.

Cholinomimetic Compounds   Compounds that mimic one or more of the actions of acetylcholine are said to be cholinomimetic. This property is shared by (*a*) compounds that act on cholinergic receptors and produce an effect similar to that of acetylcholine and (*b*) compounds that potentiate or preserve acetylcholine so that its own action is increased. The only known mechanism for "potentiating or preserving" the neurohormone is through inhibition of the enzyme that normally hydrolyzes it. The most important inhibitors of this enzyme are

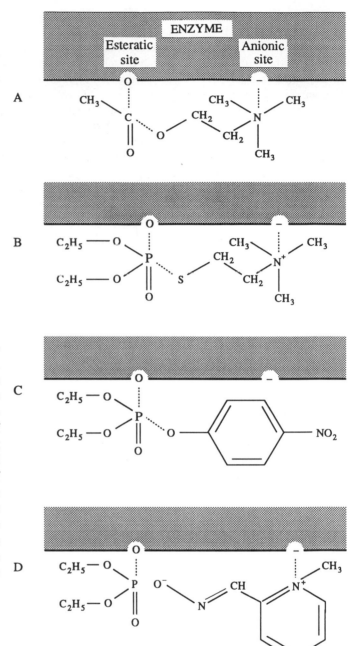

Figure 16.1   Reaction of acetylcholine (A), ecothiophate (B), and paraoxon (C) with acetylcholinesterase and positioning of 2-PAM for reactivation of the enzyme inhibited by diethoxy phosphate (D) derived from either of the two inhibitors.

the organic phosphorus compounds considered in this chapter and certain carbamates considered in the next chapter.

Compounds that mimic acetylcholine by direct action on cholinergic sites include nicotine and muscarine (Table 16.4). These compounds have been used to demonstrate that cholinergic receptors are not not identical. As summarized in Table 16.2, very dilute solutions of nicotine stimulate parasympathetic and sympathetic ganglia and (not shown in the table) the neuromuscular junction of skeletal muscle. Nicotine

Table 16.4
Comparison of Acetylcholine and Some Other Compounds That Affect the
Autonomic Nervous System

Action	Compound
Transmission of all cholinergic nerve impulses	Acetylcholine chloride
Direct stimulation of parasympathetic postganglionic fibers and sympathetic fibers to sweat glands	Muscarine
Direct stimulation of autonomic ganglia and neuromuscular junctions followed by paralysis at higher concentrations	Nicotine
Blocking of muscarinic receptors	Atropine
Blocking of nicotinic receptors in autonomic ganglia	Hexamethonium chloride

has little or no effect on cholinergic receptors innervated by postganglionic parasympathetic fibers, but muscarine acts on them in a way essentially identical to that of the normal neurohormone. In view of these facts, it is customary to distinguish "nicotinic" and "muscarinic" effects of the organic phosphorus compounds and certain carbamates that inhibit cholinesterase and, therefore, produce abnormally high concentrations of acetylcholine at receptor sites.

Blocking of Cholinergic Receptors   Blocking agents include nicotine (at all but the weakest concentration), hexamethonium and related compounds, and atropine and analogs of atropine (Table 16.4). Although very weak concentrations of nicotine are cholinomimetic, stronger solutions are inhibitory, so that nicotine is a powerful ganglionic blocking agent. Hexamethonium has a similar but more easily regulated action, adapting it to medical use. In contrast to these ganglionic blocking agents, atropine and its analogs block the action of acetylcholine or muscarine on cholinergic effectors innervated by postganglionic, parasympathetic fibers. Atropine has little or no effect on the neuromuscular junction. Succinylcholine chloride, a molecule quite similar to hexamethonium chloride, blocks nerve impulses at the neuromuscular junction and is used in medicine as a muscle relaxant. Finally, curare and related compounds block the action of acetylcholine or nicotine at the neuromuscular junctions of skeletal muscle. Like hexamethonium chloride and succinylcholine chloride, tubocurarine chloride, an active principle of curare, contains two quarternary nitrogens.

Thus, the actions of these blocking agents, as well as the stimulatory actions of nicotine and muscarine, demonstrate inherent differences in cholinergic receptors. At high concentrations, even inorganic phosphorus compounds act as inhibitors of the acetylcholine receptor, but this effect is rapidly reversible (Bartels and Nachmansohn, 1969).

16.2.1.3 Reaction of Enzymes with Organic Phosphorus Compounds

Classes of Esterases   Organic phosphorus compounds are esters. From the standpoint of their interaction with these compounds, esterases are divided into three classes designated by the letters A, B, and C. With the exception of acetylcholinesterase, the normal substrates and normal functions of A- and B-esterases are unknown. For a far more detailed discussion of the different kind of esterases than can be given below, see Heath (1961) and Walker and Mackness (1987).

A-esterases hydrolyze organic phosphorus compounds to products that are entirely inactive as cholinesterase inhibitors and, in most instances, of low toxicity in other ways. Thus, the poisons under discussion serve as substrates of A-esterases and are detoxified by them. The acidic group of the organic phosphorus compound is the one most subject to hydrolysis. However, all ability to phosphorylate enzymes disappears if any side chain is hydrolyzed, leaving an —OH group attached to the phosphorus atom (Heath, 1961). Humans and other mammalian species possess A-esterase in the liver and the high-density lipoprotein fraction of plasma. Contrasting elution profiles using organic phosphates and pyrethroids as substrates implies the existence of several forms of A-esterases. Human A-esterase provides some protection against Diazinon, pirimiphos-methyl, and other pesticides in which the active oxon is a good substrate for the enzyme. However, a bimodal distribution of paraoxonase activity suggests a variation in human susceptibility to organic phosphorus compounds. Likewise, the greater susceptibility of birds to the effects of organic phosphorus compounds may be due to much lower A-esterase activities (Walker and Mackness, 1987). Phosphorylphosphatase is an alternative term for A-esterase. A-esterases must not be confused with aliesterases, which are enzymes that hydrolyze simple esters such as phenyl acetate, the natural substrates of which are also unknown. Aliesterases may be A-, B-, or C-esterases (Heath, 1961).

B-esterases, including cholinesterases, react with organic phosphorus compounds but become firmly—in some instances, irreversibly—phosphorylated and, therefore, inhibited in the process. This inhibition is discussed in more detail below. These two forms of esterase, A and B, differ in their reaction with organic phosphorus compounds only in the rate at which the phosphorylated enzyme is hydrolyzed by water in the tissues to release the enzyme and the phosphorus acid. No one knows why the two groups do not grade into one another, but they are distinct. Most direct inhibitors react with A-esterases fast enough that, 1 hr after intravenous injection, they are nearly completely decomposed and further inhibition of cholinesterase stops.

C-esterases do not react with organic phosphorus compounds and are, therefore, of no known interest in connection with pesticides.

Inhibition of Cholinesterase   As discussed in Section 16.2.1.1, the function of acetylcholinesterase is to hydrolyze acetylcholine. The initial reversible complex formed between acetylcholinesterase and the drug ecothiopate is entirely analogous to that between the enzyme and its normal substrate (see Fig. 16.1B). Most organic phosphorus pesticides lack a positive charge in the acidic group; these compounds react with the esteratic site on the acetylcholinesterase molecule but not with the anionic site (see Fig. 16.1.C). Whether or not the anionic site is involved, the splitting off of the acidic group of the organic phosphorus compound is entirely analogous to the splitting off of choline from acetylcholine. However, the bond between the phosphorus atom and the esteratic site of the enzyme is more stable than the bond between the carbonyl carbon of acetate and the same enzyme site. Breaking of the phosphorus–enzyme bond requires an hour to weeks (1 to >1000 hr), depending on the compound involved (see Section 16.2.1.4). Breaking of the carbon–enzyme bond from acetylcholine is complete in a few microseconds (Wilson, 1951). Thus, the phosphorylated enzyme is inhibited because its active site is occupied and, therefore, incapable of carrying out its normal function.

The reactive group of the esteratic site is the hydroxyl group of serine. If the enzyme is phosphorylated by a ^{32}P-tagged inhibitor and then hydrolyzed either by hydrochloric acid or by the brief action of trypsin at 37°C, the ^{32}P is found to be attached to serine (Schaffer *et al.*, 1954). The reaction of the serine hydroxyl with phosphorus is aided by acidic and basic moieties present in the esteratic site.

Not all cholinesterases with both an esteratic and anionic site are identical. There is evidence that the distance between these two sites in bovine erythrocyte cholinesterase is between 4.3 and 4.7Å whereas in housefly cholinesterase it is between 5.0 and 5.5Å (Hollingworth *et al.*, 1967a). Advantage may be taken of this and other differences to design insecticides that are effective but safe (Metcalf and Metcalf, 1973).

Pseudocholinesterase, including the cholinesterase found in plasma, is a less specialized enzyme than acetylcholinesterase. Unlike acetylcholinesterase, it lacks an anionic site in a position that specially adapts it to react with acetylcholine. It does, however, react slowly with acetylcholine. It also reacts with a wide range of other esters. There is marked species variation in the activity and specificity of pseudocholinesterases (Ecobichon and Comeau, 1973).

Accumulation of Acetylcholine   As a result of the continuing and perhaps increased production of acetylcholine at cholinergic nerve endings during poisoning and because of the inhibition of cholinesterase, there is a measurable increase in the concentration of acetylcholine. For example, its concentration in the brain of control rats was 2.78 ppm, but its concentration in the brain of rats at different intervals after subcutaneous injection with Diazinon at the rate of 45 mg/kg was 4.75 in 1 hr, 4.89 in 24 hr, 3.15 in 72 hr, and 2.74 in 96 hr (Kar and Matin, 1971).

The accumulation of acetylcholine begins, of course, with its release from the synaptic vesicles. A reduction in the number of these vesicles together with other changes has been demonstrated by electron microscopy in poisoned rats. The same study revealed a relative absence of these changes in rats protected by an oxime (Dishovski and Kotev, 1972).

Inhibition of Other Enzymes Organic phosphorus anticholinesterases phosphorylate a number of other enzymes, including acid phosphatase, aliesterases, lipases, trypsin, chymotrypsin, succinoxidase, ascorbic acid oxidase, dehydrogenase, sulfhydryl enzymes, and others. The reaction with these enzymes is generally slower than that with cholinesterases. So far as is known, none of these other reactions has any clinical consequence. The potentiation of certain organic phosphorus compounds by others depends at least in part on inhibition of aliesterases. Although potentiation is rarely of clinical importance, it is of great theoretical interest, and it is discussed in general terms in Section 2.4.3 and in connection with organic phosphorus insecticides in Section 16.3.1.

β-Glucuronidase activity is decreased in the liver and increased in the serum of rats receiving parathion at dosages as low as 0.25 mg/day, but the action is indirect; paraoxon and several other anticholinesterase inhibitors were ineffective when tested *in vivo* (Williams, 1970).

Rats receiving acute intraperitoneal doses of 500 mg/kg malathion or 40 mg/kg Diazinon showed increased activities of cerebral glycogen phosphorylase, phosphoglucomutase, and hexokinase, as well as decreased cerebral glycogen and cholinesterase activity. The alterations in enzymes associated with cerebral glycolysis and glycogenolysis are probably in response to increased energy demands in tissues following organic phosphorus pesticide exposure, as exemplified by increased blood lactate and glucose levels (Husain and Matin, 1986a,b; Matin and Husain, 1987).

Another enzyme inhibited by parathion is choline acetyltransferase (ChAc) responsible for synthesis of acetylcholine. Using preparations from the brains of treated mice, it was found that activity decreased as follows: synthesis of acetylcholine > choline uptake = inhibition of ChAc > inhibition of cholinesterase. DFP failed to influence choline uptake or synthesis of acetylcholine (Muramatsu and Kuriyama, 1976), emphasizing the different spectrum of effects of different compounds.

Relation to Microsomal Enzymes The relation of organic phosphorus compounds to microsomal enzymes has been most thoroughly explored in connection with parathion. Even here, the relationship is complex and incompletely understood. It has

been shown clearly that the conversion of parathion to paraoxon (toxication) and to O,O-diethylthiophosphate (detoxication) depends on these enzymes (Neal, 1967a; Nakatsugawa and Dahm, 1967). The net effect of microsomal enzymes on the toxicity of organic phosphorus compounds represents a balance of at least two oxidative reactions. However, the net effect of biotransformation involves not only the microsomal reactions but also those associated with A-esterases. Experiments involving injection of a preparation by way of the hepatic portal vein in some animals and a systemic vein in others serve to isolate the effects of biotransformation from other factors such as sequestration in relatively nonsusceptible tissues that can influence observed toxicity. In any event, the net effect of the passage of organic phosphorus compounds through the liver is opposite for different compounds. In animals that have received only enough barbiturate to permit cannulation of a vein, the liver increases the toxicity of parathion but decreases the toxicity of dichlorvos (Gaines *et al.*, 1966). The same conclusion about the toxicity of parathion had been reached earlier by comparing toxicities by the intraperitoneal and intramuscular routes (Holtz and Westermann, 1959), and it has been reached from other evidence (Hollwich and Diekhues, 1974). Only 2.5% of [^{14}C]parathion was recovered as paraoxon following perfusion of isolated rat liver (Fuhremann *et al.*, 1974) and, therefore, it is strange that the net effect of the liver on parathion is toxication.

Experiments that tend to isolate metabolite effects in the intact animal rarely have been carried out in animals pretreated with classical stimulators or inhibitors of microsomal enzymes. However, in many instances, chlorinated hydrocarbon insecticides, which are inducers of microsomal enzymes, are protective against single doses of many organic phosphorus compounds (see Section 16.2.2.3). DDT or DDE protected mice against parathion but not paraoxon. The effect probably involved increased production of a nontoxic metabolite rather than decreased production of paraoxon (Bass *et al.*, 1972). The patterns of induction and of clinical protection vary from species to species (Chapman and Leibman, 1971). The same often is true of the classical inducers, phenobarbital and benzpyrene (Alary and Brodeur, 1969; Villeneuve *et al.*, 1970; Harbison, 1975a,b) and of 4-aminobutyric acid. The classical inhibitor SKF 525A has little effect on the brain cholinesterase activity of rats intoxicated by parathion, but carbon tetrachloride reduced this activity, presumably by increasing the conversion of parathion to paraoxon (Orzel and Weiss, 1966). The effects of carbon tetrachloride are difficult to interpret because they are different for different organic phosphorus compounds (Szutowski, 1975).

Many investigators have found that anticholinesterase insecticides given alone inhibit a wide range of microsomal enzymes (Gundu Rao and Anders, 1973; Stevens, 1973, 1974; Weber *et al.*, 1974; Stevens and Greene, 1974) but, under certain circumstances, negative results are obtained (Thomas and Schien, 1974; Thomas and Mawhinney, 1974). When given in combination with various chlorinated hydrocarbon insecticides, parathion increases the induction of some of these same enzymes and decreased the induction of others (Mac-Donald *et al.*, 1970).

At least in connection with the toxication of indirect inhibitors, it may be that extrahepatic microsomal biotransformation may be of greater importance than hepatic metabolism in determining toxicity. In any event, it has been found that, in terms of protein content, the microsomal fraction of rat brain is about 3% as effective as the same fraction from liver in converting parathion to paraoxon (Norman and Neal, 1974).

Relation to Transferases   Organic phosphorus molecules can be split not only by A-esterases and mixed-function oxygenases, but also by certain transferases. These include glutathione *S*-alkyltransferase (Dauterman, 1971) and glutathione *S*-aryltransferase (Hollingworth *et al.*, 1973). The latter enzyme is soluble and occurs in the postmitochondrial supernatant of rat and mouse liver. It converts parathion and related compounds to *S-p*-nitrophenylglutathione and the corresponding dialkyl phosphothioic or phosphoric acid.

Relation of Cholinesterase Inhibition to Illness   Reasons for believing that phosphorylation of acetylcholinesterase is the biochemical lesion in typical poisoning by organic phosphorus compounds in mammals include the following:

1. The character of illness produced is what would be predicted to result from inhibition of acetylcholinesterase and the consequent accumulation of acetylcholine in the tissues. Carbamates that inhibit cholinesterase produce the same kind of illness, even though the compounds are dissimilar in other ways. Many, if not all, differences between the effects of various dosing schedules, routes of administration, and compounds (whether organic phosphorus or carbamate) can be explained by differences in the absorption, distribution, and metabolism of the inhibitors.

2. The degree and duration of illness are related to the inhibition of acetylcholinesterase. Compounds that produce typical poisoning inhibit the enzyme or are converted in the body to compounds that do. For direct inhibitors, there is a fairly good correlation between toxicity *in vivo* and ability to inhibit acetylcholinesterase *in vitro*. This is discussed in Section 16.2.1.4 in connection with Fig. 16.2. Failure of the degree of illness resulting from repeated doses to correspond well with the degree of inhibition of acetylcholinesterase can be explained, at least in part, by the ability of the body to adapt to increased concentration of acetylcholine. This matter is discussed in greater detail below.

   Recovery from illness parallels recovery of activity of acetylcholinesterase. In acute poisoning by either direct or indirect inhibitors, the duration of illness is related to the stability of the phosphorylated enzyme. Thus, acetylcholinesterase inhibited by a dimethoxy compound is reactivated faster by water in the tissues than enzyme inhibited by a diethoxy or especially a diisopropoxy

compound; illness caused by dimethoxy compounds tends to run the shortest course. The relationship between clinical recovery and reactivation of acetylcholinesterase activity is most dramatic in both humans and animals when reactivation is actively promoted by a nucleophilic drug. The facts that only certain oximes are active and that the enzyme cannot be reactivated after inhibition by certain compounds or after aging lend proof to the belief that inhibition of acetylcholinesterase is the biochemical lesion.

3. Neither the kind nor degree of illness observed in poisoning by organic phosphorus compounds corresponds with the inhibition of other enzymes, although such inhibition is known to occur.

4. Illness may be lessened and shortened in experimental animals by prophylactic use of compounds (e.g., eserine) that temporarily occupy the active site of acetylcholinesterase and thus prevent phosphorylation of the enzyme until there has been time for destruction of the organic phosphorus compound by A-esterases.

5. Specific aspects of illness may be lessened and shortened in experimental animals by the prophylactic use of compounds that block the action of acetylcholine by covering its receptor surfaces at parasympathetic nerve endings (atropine), ganglia (hexamethonium), and myoneural junctions (D-tubocurarine). Of these drugs, atropine has distinct therapeutic value in both humans and animals.

The clearly established fact that the most important effects of organic phosphorus compounds are due to inhibition of acetylcholinesterase does not exclude the logical possibility that some of them or their metabolites may have other modes of action. For example, paranitrophenol causes headache and irritation of the urinary tract. It is difficult to exclude the possibility that paranitrophenol derived from parathion contributes to the clinical picture of poisoning by the insecticide. On the other hand, there is no objective evidence for this relationship, and none may exist because parathion is so much more toxic than its metabolite.

It has been reported that kymographic records of the movement of rats' jaws following oral administration of fenitrothion tended to correspond to the degree of inhibition of blood cholinesterase. However, at a dosage 0.5 mg/kg, change in the amplitude of movement of the jaw was more sensitive than change in blood cholinesterase activity (13 and 0% change, respectively) (Nishimura *et al.*, 1978). Although the finding is fascinating, it does not exclude a change in the activity of acetylcholinesterase in the nervous system or even a change in enzyme activity in the blood under other conditions of measurement.

Practical application of the relation of cholinesterase to illness is discussed under Abnormal Cholinesterase Values and Their Interpretation in Section 16.2.2.3. The section considers the possibility that in very rare instances organic phosphorus insecticides may cause death without significantly lowering the cholinesterase levels.

Cumulation of Effect versus Tolerance   It is not uncommon for organisms to exhibit both cumulative effects and tolerance in response to different dosages of the same compound. It often happens that one phenomenon is predominant and the other receives little or no attention. However, in connection with several organic phosphorus compounds that have been studied, rather minute differences in experimental design determined whether cumulation of effect or tolerance, or some elements of both, became evident.

Poisoning is partly cumulative in connection with dosages sufficiently large that they produce marked inhibition of blood cholinesterase within a few days. In tests in which guinea pigs and rabbits were subjected to LD 50 tests with either sarin or tetraethylpyrophosphate after one to nine nonlethal doses of the same compound, it was concluded that susceptibility (compared to controls that received no predosing) was increased about 1.5 times when blood cholinesterase was reduced by half (Callaway and Davies, 1957).

Recovery is apparently complete if a poisoned animal or human has time to re-form the critical quota of cholinesterase. Experiments with rats show that gradual depression of the blood cholinesterase by repeated, small, tolerated doses does not make the animals significantly more susceptible to a challenge dose. Field experience suggests that the same is true of humans. Thus, there may be a physiological adjustment to the stress of repeated, small, tolerated doses that is at least partially independent of the blood cholinesterase *per se*. On the contrary, repeated doses that produce only detectable clinical injury in rats tend not only to reduce cholinesterase levels progressively but also to produce cumulative clinical injury. Thus, if a small second dose of poison is administered before physiological adjustment is complete, the effect is partially additive.

One of the most striking examples of tolerance is that involving schradan. Whereas all rats died after six to seven subcutaneous doses at the rate of 1 mg/kg/day, all survived 0.5 mg/kg/day for 56 days followed by 1 mg/kg/day for 26 days. However, the tolerance was limited; the rats that had survived 26 days at 1 mg/kg/day all died after only two doses at 2 mg/kg/day (Rider *et al.*, 1952). In a similar way, tolerance to schradan was induced in rats started at 0.5 mg/kg/day and gradually increased to 2.5 mg/kg/day; of the experimental animals, 80% survived the entire procedure, including those receiving the drug for 10 days at 2.5 mg/kg/day, but only 6.25% of the controls survived 7 days when started at this dosage. The adaptation was related to the rate at which cholinesterase was depressed. Rats survived when diaphragm cholinesterase was lowered to 20% of normal gradually over a period of 20 days, but others died when the enzyme level was lowered to the same extent in 6 days. In rats adapted to schradan, interruption of daily injections was followed after 12 days by recovery of normal sensitivity to the compound. Recovery of normal sensitivity was paralleled by recovery of diaphragm cholinesterase activity to near-normal levels (McPhillips and Coon, 1966).

Chlorfenvinphos produces in rats a far more prompt tolerance, probably depending on a different mechanism. Oral pretreatment of rats with the compound at 15 mg/kg (one-half the usual oral LD 50 value) increased the LD 50 of a second dose given 24 hr later by only 1.4-fold when the second dose was intravenous but by 3-fold when the second dose was oral. In comparison with controls, pretreatment reduced the concentration of the compound in the plasma (as judged by the area under the curve) following the second oral dose. Pretreatment also reduced the rate of inhibition of red cell and brain cholinesterase so that the activities of these enzymes were actually higher in the experimental rats following the second dose than they were in control rats following a single dose at the same rate (Tsuda *et al.*, 1989).

The development of tolerance may be implied by response to a single dose or by response to repeated doses at the same rate. Clinical improvement following a single dose often occurs before cholinesterase activity returns to normal, and effects correlate much more poorly with the degree of cholinesterase inhibition following repeated dosing than after a single dose. It was shown long ago that electrical discharges, reflex activity, and neuromuscular activity return spontaneously toward normal following irreversible inhibition of cholinesterase in spite of the persistence of high concentrations of acetylcholine in the structures under study (Barnes, 1953; McNamara *et al.*, 1954; Robinson *et al.*, 1954; Meeter and Wolthuis, 1968a). Such findings suggest that there may be adaptation to persistent high levels of acetylcholine. That this is in fact true in relation to brain acetylcholine was shown by Smith *et al.* (1968).

In experimental animals, it sometimes happens that tolerance for continuing inhibition of cholinesterase becomes progressively evident during continuing intake of one of its inhibitors. Animals may recover from initial illness while receiving the same or an even greater dosage of a poison. For example, Barnes and Denz (1954) found that female rats became severely ill after receiving demeton for 3–4 weeks at a dietary level of 50 ppm, but recovered completely while continuing to eat the same feed. Furthermore, their actual intake of the insecticide increased as they recovered. During the second week, their feed intake was reduced to about 62 gm/kg/day, determining a demeton intake of 3.1 mg/kg/day, which made them sick; intake reached its highest rate (145 gm/kg/day) during the 13th week, determining a demeton intake of 7.25 mg/kg/day, on which they thrived. Hayes (1982) reported a similar phenomenon with parathion. Dosages high enough to cause illness inhibit food intake, but the appetite of survivors recovers so that it at least approaches that of normal animals.

Loss of appetite leading to weight loss has not been reported in people with daily exposure to an organic phosphorus compound. However, it is common to find groups of workers who remain well in spite of substantial continuing reduction of plasma and red cell cholinesterase levels.

Clinical recovery and recovery of blood cholinesterase activity or improvement in enzyme activity only has been observed in animal experiments with other compounds; examples and the sections in which they are discussed include oxydemeton-methyl (Section 16.6.4.2), formothion (Section 16.6.17.2), phosphamidon (Section 16.6.22.2), Diazinon (Section 16.7.2.2.), and chlorfenvinphos (Section 16.7.7.2).

It is interesting that adaptation is evident in behavioral as well as in other toxicological effects. Learning of a one-trial, passive-avoidance task was blocked in mice by a single dose of parathion but not by repeated smaller doses that also produced marked inhibition of cholinesterase (Reiter *et al.*, 1973b). In a study in which rats were trained in Skinner operant boxes before receiving daily doses of DFP, tolerance was evident by the ninth injection. From other details of the study it was concluded that the biochemical process of tolerance had a major central nervous system component (Russell *et al.*, 1971). Whereas the sensitivity of both muscarine and nicotine receptors to acetylcholine may be reduced by repeated doses of DFP, the muscarine receptors may be of greater importance in behavioral response (Overstreet *et al.*, 1974; Russell *et al.*, 1975). Changes in the sensitivity of muscarinic acetylcholine receptor can be demonstrated biochemically and are associated with tolerance to low levels of acetylcholinesterase (Schiller and Overstreet, 1979).

Rats adapted to some organic phosphorus compounds showed cross-tolerance to some but not all other organic phosphorus compounds. Animals adapted to schradan were more sensitive than normal animals to a single large dose of schradan or of acetylcholine (McPhillips and Coon, 1966).

Whether cumulative effects or tolerance will follow repeated exposure may be complicated by potentiation (see Section 16.3.1) if pretreatment with one compound is followed by challenge with a second. Thus increased susceptibility to acutely injected trichlorfon and physostigmine was observed in rats prefed either schradan or parathion at a dietary level of 50 ppm for 40 days (Hagan *et al.*, 1971).

Tolerance to both single and repeated doses of cholinesterase inhibitors might be explained, at least in part, by tolerance to acetylcholine. In addition, increased production of acetylcholinesterase at nerve endings would help to explain tolerance to repeated doses of inhibitors, although it would not, of course, explain the tolerance often observed in connection with gradual reduction of enzyme activities to low levels.

Tolerance to Increased Acetylcholine That this tolerance can develop was demonstrated by Krivoy and Wills (1956), who found that sympathetic ganglia exposed to constant concentrations of acetylcholine undergo fairly rapid adaptation to their altered environment, so that the evoked postganglionic action potential returns to normal magnitude after a period of depression. The ultimate desensitization reached in the unpoisoned phrenic nerve–diaphragm preparation was found to be linearly related to the log of the concentration of acetylcholine between 0.07 and 1.1 m*M* (Meeter, 1969).

Increased Cholinesterase Production in Response to Inhibition It is technically difficult to demonstrate increased production of an enzyme while inhibition of its activity continues. However, it is clear that if increased production occurred, it would tend to limit the net rate of inhibition. That increased production of red cell and plasma enzymes does occur in some instances is indicated by the fact that their levels sometimes become more normal while dosing continues. Another indication that a new norm for production has been achieved is that the plasma cholinesterase activity sometimes overshoots the normal level for a time after dosing is stopped (Hayes and Durham, 1954; Frawley and Fuyat, 1957). This was observed in dogs during the period of recovery following inhibition by parathion at oral dosage rates in the range of 0.021 to 4 mg/kg/day (Hayes and Durham, 1954; Frawley and Fuyat, 1957). Similar observations were made in rats in connection with several compounds (Frawley *et al.*, 1952a).

Stimulation of the activity or production of plasma cholinesterase has been reported in volunteers receiving parathion orally at rates ranging from 0.003 to 0.025 mg/kg/day (Rider *et al.*, 1958). The largest dosage that produces no inhibition of this enzyme in humans is about 0.07 mg/kg/day. This phenomenon of tolerance and eventually rebound of cholinesterase levels also has been observed in workers exposed to methyl parathion, trichlorfon, and dimethoate during aerial spraying. The concentration of the compounds in air ($0.01–40$ mg/m^3) was not sufficient to cause symptoms. Blood cholinesterase increased during the first 2–5 days of exposure, then decreased sharply, but stabilized between days 7 and 10 in spite of continued exposure. After exposure stopped, there was a rebound of cholinesterase activity, sometimes reaching twice the normal level (Genina, 1974).

Myopathic Changes It has been known for some time that segmental, but sometimes very extensive, necrosis of voluntary muscle can be caused by certain venoms that are rich in acetylcholine. If the victim survives, regeneration and repair begin a week or two after the bite. Surviving nuclei multiply, and each muscle fiber is regenerated within its original sarcolemmal sheath. Repair is remarkably complete (Marsden and Reid, 1961). Later it was shown that similar lesions can be produced in the diaphragm of rats by intravenous injection of sublethal doses of DFP, paraoxon, and some other cholinesterase inhibitors. Swelling, eosinophilia, and loss of striations can be observed in the end-plate region of striated muscle 2 hr later. The change is fully developed in 12 hr. Recovery begins in 2 days and is almost complete 10 days after injection. The injury is caused by prolonged depolarization of the end-plate region. It can be promoted by stimulation via the nerve and can be prevented by denervation, oximes, or sufficiently great doses of tubocurarine or α-bungarotoxin (Ariëns *et al.*, 1968, 1969; Salpeter *et al.*, 1979). Using an electron microscope, the lesion may be detected as early as 30 min after a subcutaneous injection of paraoxon at the rate of 0.25 mg/kg (Laskowski *et al.*, 1976). Emphasizing the importance of acetylcholine, the myopathy can be produced by guanidine, which does not inhibit cholinesterase but does cause an increased release of acetylcholine by each nerve impulse. However, carbamylcholine, an analog of acetylcholine that depolarizes the end plate and causes contraction, does not induce myopathy, even when given in near-fatal doses. It seems possible that muscle necrosis is not simply the result of excessive depolarization and contraction but is related to a disturbance in the trophic effect mediated by acetylcholine (Fenichel *et al.*, 1974).

Lesions identical to those in the rat were demonstrated in the diaphragm of a man who died of cardiac arrest 9 days after drinking parathion. He had remained in coma and had required respiratory assistance during the entire period. No cholinesterase or nonspecific esterase activity could be demonstrated in the myoneural junctions of any skeletal muscle examined, but muscle necrosis was restricted to the diaphragm. Each focus involved one to four sarcomeres of both types of fibers and varied from acute swelling to vacuolar disintegration of the fibers. In some places there was an invasion by histiocytes, and regeneration of small basophilic muscle fibers was seen. The nerve endings in the segmental necrotic zones of the muscle fibers were degenerated. There was no loss of oxidative enzyme activity in nonnecrotic muscle fibers. An increase in 5-nucleotidase and of acid phosphatase activity was present in the zones of myolysis. An increase in alkaline phosphatase activity was observed in the capillary walls near degenerating sarcomeres (De Reuck and Willems, 1975).

It is unclear what the interpretation should be of certain electron microscopic changes that have been reported in rats following a very large but nonfatal dose. Specifically, it is not known how much hypoxia may have contributed to the changes or whether more extreme changes of the same kind contribute to death in fatal poisoning of animals or humans. It is assumed but not proved that the changes are typical of anticholinesterase organic phosphorus compounds and are not peculiar to the compound studied. Asanuma (1973) reported that electron microscopic examination of rats killed 5 days after a single oral dose of fenitrothion at the rate of 300 mg/kg revealed changes in the synaptic vesicles of the neurolemma and "denaturation" of muscle fibers. Even in rats killed 15 days after poisoning, flattening and thickening of the junctional fold at the motor end plate and vacuolations of Schwann cells were seen. Emphasis was placed on the external ocular muscles and their nerve end plates (Asanuma *et al.*, 1974).

Although electromyographic (EMG) changes would be expected in connection with the muscle necrosis under discussion, it is not clear what relation, if any, the necrosis has to the rapidly reversible EMG changes discussed in Section 7.4.1 (Hayes, 1975) that have been reported in a high proportion of some groups of healthy workers. In fact, there is a question as to whether any direct relationship exists. One of the proponents of the idea (Roberts, 1977) has reported that exposure insufficient to cause any symptoms can cause either an *increase* or *decrease* in EMG voltage. On the contrary, Jusic and Milic (1978) have reported that in two cases of severe poisoning, the electromyographic results did not differ significantly from those obtained in healthy adults.

Most investigations regarding the relations of acetylcholine to muscle injury involve voluntary muscle. Separate reports (Biernat and Giermaziak, 1976; Giermaziak and Andrze-jewski, 1976) concern degenerative and necrotic changes in cardiac muscle following toxic doses of thiomethon. That these changes are similar to those in skeletal muscle is indicated by the report that 2-PAM but not atropine was protective.

Myopathies have a number of causes, of which excessive acetylcholine is only one. The entire subject of experimental myopathy and its contribution to an understanding of spontaneous myopathies in humans has been reviewed by Laskowski and Dettbarn (1977). However, even this review contains little bearing directly on the chronic myopathy that has been observed rarely in cases of polyneuropathy associated with neurotoxic organic phosphorus compounds and some other conditions with no recognized relationship. The lesion is characterized by dramatic target, targetoid, and targetoid/core structures visible even with a light microscope in affected muscle fibers. With the electron microscope, greatly disorganized muscle striations and absence of mitochondria may be seen directly adjacent to essentially normal parts of the same fiber. A case of such myopathy associated with delayed polyneuropathy following ingestion of trichlorfon was described and beautifully illustrated by Fukuhara *et al.* (1977). It must be pointed out that such myopathy is related to a lack of acetylcholine, if it has any relation to acetylcholine whatever.

Relation of Cholinesterase Inhibition to Other Effects

Some anticholinesterase organic phosphorus compounds interfere with temperature control and make the body temperature of rats and mice abnormally dependent on the environmental temperature. Following intravenous, or in some instances subarachnoid, injection of just sublethal doses into rats, the body temperature fell 4°C or more in about 2–3 hr and then returned to normal in 12–20 hr. No such effect was observed in guinea pigs or rabbits. The effect in rats (Meeter and Wolthuis, 1968b) and in mice (Ahdaya *et al.*, 1976) was partially prevented by atropine, suggesting that it is related to cholinesterase inhibition. The hypothermal action is thought to be on the central nervous system (Meeter *et al.*, 1971). Rats develop thermoregulatory tolerance following the third injection of DFP, probably due to altered sensitivity of the anterior hypothalamus to acetylcholine (Overstreet *et al.*, 1973). Neither the rate of recovery from hypothermia after a single dose of DFP nor the rate at which tolerance to repeated doses appeared was influenced by an inhibitor of protein synthesis. It was concluded that these rates were not influenced by synthesis of new acetylcholinesterase (Overstreet *et al.*, 1977).

Hypothermia has been reported in humans (see Section 16.7.7.3).

The behavioral effects of anticholinesterases have been studied extensively in the hope of learning the action of acetylcholine in the brain and in the hope of developing more sensitive toxicological tests. Such studies have been reviewed in detail (Bignami and Gatti, 1967). Very briefly, behavioral studies with anticholinesterases have yielded theoretically important results, confirming other evidence of cholinergic mediation in inhibitory pathways in the central nervous system.

Behavioral methods are not obviously superior to other

available methods for routine toxicological investigations on organic phosphorus compounds. Behavioral changes are not observed except at dosage levels that produce easily measurable changes in cholinesterase, especially in the brain. Biochemical measurements are technically easier to make, are much more directly related to clinical effects, and may be detected at lower dosage levels (Pan'shina, 1963b).

Behavioral methods can be used with success when studying possible antagonists of the cholinesterases. This type of experimentation could prove particularly useful in studying the relative importance of central and peripheral changes in determining behavioral disturbances. The anticholinesterase-intoxicated, methylatropine-protected animal, showing no peripheral signs but a marked depression of conditioned behavior, could be used for systematic investigation of centrally acting antagonists.

Of course, some behavioral effects, although not fully understood may depend on physiological changes directly linked to enzyme inhibition. A possible example is the finding of Reiter *et al.* (1973a) that a sufficiently daily dosage of parathion disrupts visual discrimination performance in monkeys and that the maximal effect corresponds with peak inhibition of acetylcholinesterase.

Cause of Death The cause of death in poisoning by organic phosphorus compounds is usually respiratory failure and consequent anoxia but may be cardiovascular in origin. Four factors (excessive secretion of the respiratory tract, bronchoconstriction, weakness of the muscles of respiration, and failure of the respiratory center) may contribute to respiratory failure. The relative importance of these factors depends mainly on the compound, route of administration, and species. For example, direct inhibitors are capable of producing local as well as systemic effects. Some compounds are capable of passing the blood–brain barrier while others, such as schradan, pass it with great difficulty. Single fatal doses of schradan have no significant effect on brain cholinesterase of rats (DuBois *et al.*, 1950; Frawley *et al.*, 1952a), but the brain enzyme of these animals is reduced more than 50% by a dietary level of 100 ppm for 15 weeks (Frawley *et al.*, 1952a). Thus, central effects are not necessary for a lethal outcome but may contribute to it.

In a few instances, death has followed profound brain damage that occurred, usually early in the course of poisoning, as a result of severe anoxia (see Section 16.2.2.2).

16.2.1.4 Relation of Toxicity to Chemical Structure

Direct and Indirect Inhibitors Some organic phosphorus insecticides are able to inhibit cholinesterase effectively and are said to have a direct action; many other compounds have only slight activity until they have been altered either by chemical or enzymatic change and, therefore, are called indirect inhibitors. Direct inhibitors tend to have more prominent local

effects (see Section 16.2.2.1) and to produce systemic poisoning more rapidly.

Pure compounds containing the $=S$ are indirect inhibitors. The most common reaction leading to their activation is oxidation to the corresponding $=O$ compound. This reaction is promoted by ultraviolet light and by certain microsomal enzymes of the liver and other organs including the brain. Thus, residues of indirect inhibitors may be converted chemically to direct inhibitors. If absorbed, indirect inhibitors are always converted biochemically to direct inhibitors. The fate of the sulfur atom released in the biotransformation of $=S$ to $=O$ compounds has been studied in connection with parathion (see Section 16.7.1.2).

In some instances, isomerization of the form

$$(aklyl-O)_2P(S)X \rightarrow (aklyl-S)(alkyl-O)P(O)X$$

or

$$(aklyl-O)_2P(S)OX \rightarrow (aklyl-O)_2P(O)SX$$

leads to activation of an $=S$ compound. Isomerization may occur during storage. It is not known to occur in the body.

Complete purification of most organic phosphorus compounds is extremely difficult because their lability to heat interferes with their separation by distillation, and many are liquids that cannot be crystallized. Even preparations that are crystalline regularly contain oxidation products that are direct inhibitors and that are difficult to remove (Ackerman, 1969). Really accurate determination of the cholinesterase inhibitory activity of $=S$ compounds is defeated by a trace of the corresponding $=O$ compound. Thus, the difference between the two is likely to be greater than measured. Even so, the observed difference may be great. For example, the inhibitory action of paraoxon is approximately 9090 times greater than that of parathion (Fallscheer and Cook, 1956).

Not all $=O$ organic phosphorus compounds are strong inhibitors. Some [e.g., $(C_2H_5O)_3 P(O)$] are not inhibitors at all. Of far greater interest, however, is the fact that some $=O$ compounds, such as schradan (see Section 16.9.1) undergo change of one or more side chains to form more inhibitory compounds. The change may be *in vitro, in vivo,* or both.

Commercial formulations of indirect or weak inhibitors frequently contain a small percentage of related compounds, some of which are direct inhibitors. Thus, local effects (miosis, local sweating, respiratory symptoms, etc.) may be seen after exposure to a commercial product whose label indicates an indirect inhibitor only.

When a pure inactive inhibitor was administered to rats by mouth, the onset of symptoms was found by measurement to correspond precisely with the appearance of the oxon in the muscles, especially the abdominal muscles, and with inhibition of cholinesterase in this tissue but not plasma (Ackerman, 1970).

Rate of Reaction The organic phosphorus compounds under discussion are esters but may be regarded as acid anhydrides also. In a nucleophilic displacement reaction of the molecule shown in Section 16.1, the most acidic group (X) attached to the phosphorus atom is removed, while the more basic groups

(R_1 and R_2) remain attached. The rate may be predicted by the electronic theory for such reactions, and can be summarized as follows:

1. Molecules containing $=S$ are very much less reactive than corresponding molecules containing $=O$.
2. The rate of reaction corresponds to the acidity or, more accurately, the electron-withdrawing power of X. For example, $(C_2H_5-O)_2P(O)F$ reacts faster than $(C_2H_5-O)_2P(O)-O-C_6H_5NO_2$ because the fluorine atom has greater electron withdrawing power than the $-O-C_6H_5NO_2$ group. In most instances, the electron-withdrawing power of X can be judged by considering the strength of the acid formed. In connection with the example just given, hydrofluoric acid is a stronger acid than p-nitrophenol. However, this simple test may be completely misleading, as it is in connection with the metabolite formed by the action of carboxyesterase on malathion. Here the production of a $-COOH$ group on the side chain reduces the electron-withdrawing power of the side chain and renders the compound incapable of phosphorylating enzymes, even though the acid potentially formed by cleavage of the side chain from phosphorus is stronger than the one formed from unmetabolized malathion.
3. Where X remains constant, the rate of reaction increases in the following order corresponding to increasing instability of the R_1 and R_2 groups: amino $<$ isoproproxy $<$ propoxy $<$ ethoxy $<$ methoxy.

Prediction of the nucleophilic displacement reaction rate is rather accurate when the reaction involves the hydroxyl ion or water, that is, hydrolysis of the phosphorus compound. Prediction of the reaction rate is less satisfactory but still useful when the reaction involves esterases *in vitro*. The reaction of organic phosphorus compounds with these enzymes is complicated because it involves the formation of an enzyme-inhibitor complex, which then permits the nucleophilic displacement reaction to occur. The formation of the complex depends more on the steric fit of portions of the organic phosphorus compound to the enzyme surface or on electronic charges in a side chain than on electronic properties of the phosphorus atom and of the groups immediately surrounding it. For example, compounds that resemble acetylcholine, the natural substrate of acetylcholinesterase, by having a positive charge in the acid side chain, react with the enzyme faster than do otherwise identical compounds that lack the charge. Of a pair of diethoxy compounds identical except for the side chain, the one with a positive charge [$-S-CH_2-CH_2-S^+(C_2H_5)-CH_3$] is 1000 times more toxic intravenously than the one without a charge [$-S-CH_2-CH_2-SC_2H_5$] (Vandekar and Heath, 1957).

Thus, compounds that are difficult to hydrolyze are weak inhibitors of cholinesterase, but compounds that are easily hydrolyzed vary greatly as inhibitors, depending on the fit of their side chains to the enzyme surface.

In a discussion of the relationship between toxicity and inhibition of cholinesterase, it is convenient to measure the inhibitory power of each compound in terms of its pI 50. The I 50 of a compound is the molar concentration causing 50% inhibition of enzyme activity. Measurements are usually expressed and used in the form of the pI 50, which is negative logarithm of the I 50 in the same way that pH is the negative logarithm of hydrogen ion concentration. The pI 50 values of a series of compounds increase in the order of increasing activity of the compounds. The pI 50 is of greatest value when measured for acetylcholinesterase because that is the enzyme related to toxicity. The I 50 is not a bimolecular rate constant for the compound and the enzyme. Since the enzyme has not been purified, the I 50 reflects the net effect of an initial association reaction, the subsequent nucleophilic displacement reaction, and, in addition, side reactions such as decomposition of the inhibitor, reactivation of the enzyme, and others. According to Homstedt (1963), I 50 values seem to be a better basis for a rough prediction of toxicity than the reaction velocity with the enzyme, mainly because the experimental situation in an I 50 determination on an impure enzyme preparation has a closer resemblance to the situation *in vivo* than do kinetic experiments where side reactions are avoided as much as possible. Comparisons between I 50 values reported in the literature and the few measured in human brain tissue are in good agreement (Patocka and Bajgar, 1971).

Figure 16.2 shows the relationship between toxicity *in vivo* and ability to inhibit the acetylcholinesterase *in vitro* for all direct inhibitors for which the intraperitoneal LD 50 in mice and the pI 50 for acetylcholinesterase in any species were tabulated by Holmstedt (1963). The coefficient of correlation of the pI 50 values and the logarithms of the corresponding LD 50 values is -0.71. The relationship is sufficiently dependable that it may be used to detect indirect inhibitors. For example, the coordinates for schradan and dimefox (not used in calculating the regression line or the coefficient of correlation) fall completely off the line. It is known that although they are $=O$ compounds, they are converted in the body to much more toxic materials, thus explaining the fact they are far more toxic than their pI 50 values would suggest.

The exact practicality of using the pI 50 to predict the toxicity of pesticides is unknown because so few pesticides have been studied in this way. Nearly all the values in Fig. 16.2 are for compounds not suitable for pesticides.

The observed variability in the relationship between pI 50 and the logarithm of LD 50 of direct inhibitors is explained by differences of absorption, distribution, and rate of detoxication of the compounds. Greater variation than that shown in Fig. 16.2 would be expected if oral, or especially dermal, toxicity rather than intraperitoneal toxicity were compared because oral, or especially dermal, absorption is more variable than intraperitoneal absorption. There is also the state of the organism to be considered. For example, damage to the epidermal barrier may make the difference between fatal or trivial absorption of poison from a contaminated area of skin.

The relation of absorption, distribution, and storage to chemical structure is discussed in Section 3.2.1.

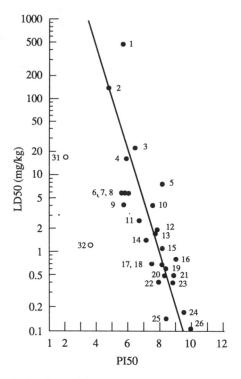

Figure 16.2 *In vivo* toxicity of some directly acting organic phosphorus insecticides as related to their ability to inhibit acetylcholinesterase *in vitro*. Values used for calculating the regression line were those for 1, dipterex; 2, *O,O*-diethyl-4-chlorophenylphosphate; 3, *O,O*-diethyl-bis-dimethyl pyrophosphordiamide (*sym*); 4, TIPP; 5, *O,O*-diethylphosphostigmine; 6, isodemeton sulfoxide; 7, isodemeton; 8, isodemeton sulfone; 9, DFP; 10, diethylamido-ethoxy-phosphoryl cyanide; 11, *O,O*-dimethyl-*O,O*-diisopropyl pyrophosphate (*asym*); 12, diethylamido-methoxy-phosphoryl cyanide; 13, tetramethyl pyrophosphate; 14, *O,O*-diethyl phosphorocyanidate; 15, *O,O*-dimethyl-*O,O*-diethyl pyrophosphate (*asym*); 16, soman; 17, TEPP; 18, *O*-isopropyl-ethylphosphono-fluoridate; 19, tabun; 20, amiton; 21, diethylamido-isopropoxy-phosphoryl cyanide; 22, *O,O*-diethyl-*S*-(2-diethylaminoethyl)phosphorothioate; 23, sarin; 24, *O,O*-diethyl-*S*-(2-triethylammoniumethyl)thiophosphate iodide; 25, echothiophate; 26, methylfluorophosphorylcholine iodide; 27, methylfluorophosphoryl-β-methylcholine iodide; 28, *O*-ethyl-methylphosphorylthiocholine iodide; 29, methylfluorophosphoryl-homo-choline iodide. The last three of these, which had LD 50 values in the range of 0.03–0.07 mg/kg, are not shown on the graph. Two additional compounds that are shown on the graph but whose values (for the reason explained in the text) were not used in calculating the regression line are 31, schradan, and 32, dimefox.

(Blaber and Creasey, 1960b). In connection with erythrocytes, new enzyme is formed only in connection with new cells, and the rate-limiting step depends on the formation of new red cells. In the sheep and rabbit this rate is 0.5–0.7%/day (Blaber and Creasey, 1960a).

Recovery of cholinesterase activity in different species may depend on different processes, even when the inhibiting compound is the same. Recovery of brain and plasma cholinesterase in the rat after inhibition by dichlorvos depended entirely on spontaneous reactivation of inhibited enzymes. On the contrary, recovery of red cell and plasma cholinesterase activity in humans after inhibition by the same compound depended on resynthesis (Reiner and Plestina, 1979).

Rate of Reversibility Phosphorylated enzymes, like acetylated acetylcholinesterase, are esters and may be hydrolyzed by nucleophilic agents, including water. The rate at which phosphorylated enzymes are reactivated by water is extremely low, compared to the rate for acetylcholinesterase combined with acetate. When inhibition is by isopropyl phosphate, the rate is essentially zero.

The rate of reactivation cannot be influenced by the acidic group of the original organic phosphorus compound, for that was split off by the reaction leading to inhibition of the enzyme. Aldridge and Davison (1952) demonstrated this point clearly by graphs showing that, under the same conditions, a particular enzyme is reactivated at the same rate following inhibition by a series of dimethoxy phosphates varying in their acidic groups from fluorine to *p*-nitrophenol.

The rate of reactivation does depend on the basic groups and on the enzyme involved. For rat brain acetylcholinesterase, the rate of reactivation decreases in the order dimethoxy > diethoxy > dipropoxy ≫ diisopropoxy = diisopropylamino. See Table 16.5 extracted from Davison (1955a). Rat plasma cholinesterase varies in the same way, except that the combination with dimethoxy phosphate is about as stable as the combination with the isopropyoxy phosphate. This exception may be related to the rapid aging of the dimethoxyphosphate to form hydrogen methoxyphosphate.

Even under the same conditions of temperature and pH, cholinesterases from different tissues or from the same tissue

Recovery of Cholinesterase Activity Once cholinesterase activity is inhibited *in vivo,* its recovery depends on reversal of inhibition, aging, and regeneration of new enzyme, as discussed in the next three sections. For most pesticides, the net effect of these factors is that there is an initial, rapid, partial recovery followed by a slower, linear return to normal activity. With some compounds such as DFP, the initial, rapid phase is lacking because there is no reversal of inhibition. When initial rapid recovery is present, it represents the algebraic sum of reversal of inhibition plus aging. The slow phase of recovery is exponential and depends on the regeneration of new enzyme. In the brain this regeneration occurs in preexisting cells, and the rate depends on the rate of formation of new enzyme

Table 16.5

Rates of Reactivation of Phosphorylated Rat Brain Acetylcholinesterase at 37°C in Bicarbonate Buffer at pH 7.8[a]

Moiety inhibiting enzyme	Time for 25% reactivation (hr)
dimethyl phosphate	1.3
diethoxy phosphate	20
di-*n*-propoxy phosphate	40
di-*i*-propoxy phosphate	>1000
di-*i*-propyl phosphoramid	>1000

[a] From data of Davison (1955a).

of different species usually are reactivated at different rates following inhibition by the same compound. The difference may be great. As an extreme example, acetylcholinesterase inhibited by schradan cannot be reactivated by water (Kewitz, 1957), but horse plasma cholinesterase inhibited by the same compound is half reactivated by water in 28 hr at 37°C (Davison, 1955b). The dimethylamino groups of schradan require partial oxidation before inhibition occurs, and the exact nature of the phosphorylated enzyme is not known (Heath, 1961). Under these conditions, there is some possibility that the phosphorylating moieties are different. However, rather large differences have been observed in connection with well-defined inhibitors. Twenty-five percent reactivation of diethoxyphosphorylated pseudocholinesterase from the hen requires only 0.9 hr while that from humans requires 310 hr (Davison, 1955a). Another example involves over 40% reactivation of rat diaphragm cholinesterase in 80 min following inactivation by paraoxon, contrasted with failure of reactivation of this enzyme from lobster leg during an even longer period (Welsch and Dettbarn, 1972).

Water is a weak nucleophilic reagent. The natural reactivation of acetylcholinesterase it accomplishes requires hours—often many hours. Dilute solutions of some hydroxylamine derivatives are capable of doing the same thing more completely in a few minutes, not only *in vitro* but also *in vivo*. The use of these compounds (oximes) in therapy is discussed in Section 16.2.2.7. It must be mentioned here, however, that all potent reactivators contain a positively charged atom capable of attaching to the anionic site of the enzyme and so positioned that dephosphorylation of the enzyme is facilitated.

Aging   Reactivation of phosphorylated acetylcholinesterase is almost complete if an appropriate oxime or other hydroxylamine derivative is used soon after inhibition. However, reactivation becomes progressively less efficient in proportion to the duration of inhibition and consequent delay in starting reactivation; a portion of the enzyme is reactivated at the original rate but an increasing portion is completely resistant to reactivation and is said to be aged (Hobbiger, 1955). The part capable of reactivation decreases exponentially with time (first-order reaction) at a given temperature. The rate of reaction is much higher at higher temperatures. Both of these facts indicate that a chemical reaction is involved. The reaction is now known to be the hydrolysis of one alkoxy group, leaving monoalkoxy phosphate attached to the enzyme and quite immune to oximes or other nucleophilic reagents. This relationship was demonstrated by finding that reactivation of cholinesterase previously inhibited by DFP released a diisopropylphosphoryl group and that initially almost all protein-bound ^{32}P was in the form of diisopropyl phosphate, but, as aging progressed, an increasing proportion of protein-bound ^{32}P was found as monoisopropyl phosphate, which could not be released from the enzyme even by an oxime. Aging of cholinesterase-inhibited [^{14}C]DFP released free [^{14}C]isopropanol into the reaction mixture (Berends *et al.*, 1959). Harris *et al.* (1966) made a similar demonstration *in vivo*.

The rate of aging depends on the enzyme involved and on the type of phosphorylation. Human plasma cholinesterase inhibited by a particular dialkoxy phosphate changes to the corresponding irreversible monoalkylphosphate about 5 or 10 times faster than human red cell cholinesterase inhibited by the same dialkoxy phosphate. Both enzymes age most rapidly if their inhibition involves isopropoxy phosphate. The rates of aging for mammalian acetylcholinesterase increase in the order diethyl < diisopropyl ≥ dimethyl < isopropyl-methyl (Hobbiger, 1955, 1956; Davies and Green, 1956; Witter and Gaines, 1963b).

It should not be supposed that either reversibility or aging operates independently. Easily reversible inhibitors that persist in the body either in their original form or as active metabolites produce almost irreversible inhibition because the continuing availability of inhibitor gradually exhausts the supply of uninhibited enzyme, and the inhibited enzyme gradually undergoes aging. By using prolonged intravenous infusion in order to maintain a steady level of a normally nonpersistent inhibitor in the blood, it is possible to produce the same clinical effects as those produced by a single dose of a persistent inhibitor (Vandekar and Heath, 1957).

Regeneration of Cholinesterase   Once a given molecule of cholinesterase has been inhibited irreversibly, the only means of replacing the activity is through synthesis of new enzyme. This synthesis does not occur in circulating red blood corpuscles, and the only way acetylcholinesterase activity is renewed in the blood is through synthesis of the enzyme in erythropoietic cells of the bone marrow and their subsequent entrance into the circulating blood. The plasma enzyme is synthesized in the liver. Following inhibition of brain cholinesterase in rats by DFP, acetylcholinesterase activity regenerated in the synaptosomes 24 hr after its regeneration in the microsomal fractions. From this it was concluded that this enzyme is synthesized primarily within the nerve cell body and then transported to the nerve ending by axonal flow (Austin and James, 1970).

Relation of Safety to Chemical Structure   Although the safety of chemicals is related as much to the way in which they are used as it is to their inherent toxicity, it is desirable to employ compounds of low toxicity where possible. Understanding of the relationship of toxicity to chemical structure requires consideration of all factors that contribute to toxicity. However, without evaluation, the collected data may be confusing. For example, as we have seen, dimethoxy compounds tend to be more toxic than diethoxy compounds because they react more rapidly but less toxic because acetylcholinesterase inhibited by a dimethoxy compound shows faster spontaneous reactivation than that inhibited by a diethoxy compound. Another difference is that alkyl-phosphorus hydrolysis is more prominent for dimethoxy than for diethoxy compounds (Plapp and Casida, 1958). The net effect of these and perhaps other variables is that dimethoxy compounds always are less toxic than their diethoxy analogs. As shown in Table 16.6, the degree of difference varies from little more than 1 to as much as

Table 16.6

Comparison of the Toxicity of Certain Methoxy and Ethoxy Organic Phosphorus Analogs of the Form $(alkoxy)_2 P (=S \text{ or } =O) X$

Double bond	X	Methoxy	Ethoxy
=O	$-O-P(alkoxy)_2$	tetramethylpyrophosphate 1.7, mice, ip[a]	tetraethyl pyrophosphate 0.7, mice, ip[a]
=O	$-S-CH_2-CH_2-S-C_2H_5$	isodemeton-methyl 60, rats, oral[a]	isodemeton 1.5, rats, oral[a]
=O	$-S-CH_2-CH_2-\overset{\overset{O}{\|\|}}{S}-C_2H_5$	isodemeton-methyl sulfoxide 30, rats, oral[a]	isodemeton sulfoxide 2.0, rats, oral[a]
=O	$-S-CH_2-CH_2-\overset{\overset{O}{\|\|}}{\underset{\underset{O}{\|\|}}{S}}-C_2H_5$	isodemeton-methyl sulfone 40, rats, oral[a]	isodemeton sulfone 2.0, rats, oral[a]
=S	$-O-CH_2-CH_2-S-C_2H_5$	demeton-methyl 250, rats, oral[a]	demeton 30, rats, oral[a]
=S	$-O-CH_2-CH_2-\overset{\overset{O}{\|\|}}{S}-C_2H_5$	demeton-methyl sulfoxide 600, rats, oral[a]	demeton sulfoxide 100, rats, oral[a]
=S	$-O-CH_2-CH_2-\overset{\overset{O}{\|\|}}{\underset{\underset{O}{\|\|}}{S}}-C_2H_5$	demeton-methyl sulfone 500, rats, oral[a]	demeton sulfone 90, rats, oral[a]
=O	—⟨benzene ring⟩—NO_2	paraoxon-methyl 1.4, mice, sc[a]	paraoxon 0.6–0.8, mice, sc[a]
=S	—⟨benzene ring⟩—NO_2	parathion-methyl 14, M rats, oral[b] 24, F rats, oral[b] 30, mice, sc[a]	parathion 13, M rats, oral[b] 3.6, F rats, oral[b] 10–12, mice, sc[a]
=S	$-S-CH_2-S-$⟨benzene ring⟩—Cl	carbophenothion-methyl 98, M rats, oral[b] 120, F rats, oral[b]	carbophenothion 30, M rats, oral[b] 10, F rats, oral[b]

[a] Toxicity values from Holmstedt (1963).
[b] Toxicity values from Gaines (1960).

40. In some instances, the dimethoxy compounds are almost as toxic as the others to insects and, therefore, present a real advantage.

A difference depending on the identity of the inhibiting compounds has been suspected in connection with cholinesterases inhibited by dimethoxy compounds. Evidence regarding this matter in humans is based on cases subject to so many different variables that interpretation is difficult. So far, the only objective evidence that not all compounds of the same group form identical reaction products with acetylcholinesterase is the finding in mice that oximes are effective in treating poisoning by either member of some pairs of analogs (parathion, methylparathion; demeton, methyldemeton) but effective for only the diethoxy member of some other pairs (Diazinon, methyldiazinon; phenkapton, methylphenkapton) (Stenger, 1960).

Table 16.7

Comparison of the Toxicity[a] of =S and =O Analogs of Organic Phosphorus Compounds of the Form (alkoxy)$_2$ P (=S or =O) X

Substituent groups		Name of compound and its LD 50 (mg/kg) in species and by route stated	
Alkoxy	X	=S	=O
methoxy	—O—⟨C$_6$H$_4$⟩—NO$_2$	parathion-methyl 30, mice, sc[a]	paraoxon-methyl 1.4, mice, sc[a]
ethoxy	—O—P(=S or =O)(C$_2$H$_5$)$_2$	sulfotepp 8, mice, sc[a]	TEPP 0.7, mice, ip[a]
ethoxy	—S—CH$_2$—CH$_2$—S—C$_2$H$_5$	disyston 5–6, mice, ip[a] 5, rats, oral[a]	isodemeton 5.6–5.9, mice, ip[a] 1.5, rats, oral[a]
ethoxy	—S—CH$_2$—CH$_2$—S(=O)—C$_2$H$_5$	disyston sulfoxide 6.5, rats, oral[a]	isodemeton sulfoxide 2.0, rats, oral[a]
ethoxy	—S—CH$_2$—CH$_2$—S(=O)$_2$—C$_2$H$_5$	disyston sulfone 7.5, rats, oral[a]	isodemeton sulfone 2.0, rats, oral[a]
ethoxy	—O—⟨C$_6$H$_4$⟩—NO$_2$	parathion 10–12, mice, sc[a]	paraoxon 0.6–0.8, mice, sc[a]
ethoxy	—O—⟨pyrazole ring CH—C—CH$_3$, C, N, H⟩	pyrazothion 12, mice, oral[a]	pyrazoxon 4, mice, oral[a]

[a] Toxicity values from Holmstedt (1963).

Presumably, different compounds of the same group could produce different esters if the inhibitors failed to cleave immediately when they phosphorylate the enzyme. Another possible explanation lies in complexity of the enzyme. It has been reported that plasma cholinesterase in the rat consists of 20 isoenzymes with different affinities for different organic phosphorus compounds (Yamanaka and Nishimura, 1979). If multiple isoenzymes were demonstrated in the acetylcholinesterase of mammalian nerve tissue, it would open a real possibility for explaining variable effectiveness of oximes in poisoning by different organic phosphorus compounds of the same group.

Although it probably has no bearing on the relative safety of diethoxy and dimethoxy compounds under practical conditions, a striking difference between parathion and parathion-methyl was demonstrated in mice pretreated with piperonyl butoxide. A dosage of 400 mg/kg increased the intraperitoneal toxicity of parathion twofold but decreased that of parathion-methyl 40-fold. Whereas piperonyl butoxide inhibited both oxidative toxication and detoxication of both insecticides, it was without effect on glutathione-dependent hydrolysis capable of detoxicating parathion-methyl but not parathion (Mirer et al., 1977). Whether all diethoxy and dimethoxy compounds demonstrate the same differences is unexplored, but azinphosethyl and azinphos-methyl do show some similarity to parathion and parathion-methyl in this regard (Levine and Murphy, 1977a,b).

Another constant difference is that indirect inhibitors are always less toxic than the corresponding direct inhibitors. This is true even though the less toxic =S compound is converted by the body to the =O compound. As shown in Table 16.7, the degree of difference varies from about 3 to as much as 21. The reason for the difference is at least twofold. First, a portion of absorbed =S compound may be destroyed by A-esterases or by oxidative enzymes, or it undergoes excretion or relatively harmless storage before it has time to be converted to the active form. Second, conversion requires time so that the action that finally results from an indirect inhibitor tends to be delayed and distributed over a longer period; this permits greater metabolism and excretion of the active derivative so that its peak of concentration in the blood and in critical tissues is not so high, although potentially more prolonged. The delay associated with an indirect inhibitor may permit greater adaptation to increased concentrations of acetylcholine, as well as greater elimination of the poison. Indirect inhibitors may be as injurious as corresponding direct inhibitors to insects, resulting in an improved "therapeutic index."

Over and above the general advantage of indirect inhibitors, it is desirable to employ those (*a*) that are detoxicated by mammals with ease and by insects with difficulty or (*b*) that react more readily with insect cholinesterase. No real rules exist for selecting such compounds, although some examples are known. Malathion appears to be a compound more easily detoxicated by mammals. Mammalian A-esterases, including a carboxylase, can remove not only the acidic group but also just part of it; in either case the resulting molecule is not toxic.

Isopropylparathion is another compound that is more readily detoxicated by mammals than by insects. Here, the difference arises largely from the ability of mammals to remove an isopropyl group from the molecule either before or after its conversion to isopropylparaoxon (Camp *et al.*, 1969).

Fenitrooxon appears to be more effectively detoxicated by mammals and more selective for insect cholinesterase than is its analog methylparaoxon. Fenitrothion is only 2.6 times less toxic than methylparathion to houseflies but is 54.5 times less toxic to mice. A smaller proportion of fenitrothion than of methylparathion is converted to P=O metabolites. Desmethylation is of greater importance in the metabolism of fenitrothion, and the difference increases at higher doses. Finally, fenitrooxon is 5.7 times less effective than methylparaoxon as an inhibitor of mouse brain cholinesterase but is more effective as an inhibitor of housefly cholinesterase (Hollingworth *et al.*, 1967a,b).

Differences in chemical structure account for differences in partition coefficients, and this difference, in turn, is an important factor in determining distribution and storage, the clinical implications of which are discussed in Section 16.2.2.1.

There is a broad tendency for the safest organic phosphorus insecticides to be of low toxicity to many insects as well as to humans. In other words, they tend to be selective insecticides with more than average variation in their toxicity to different species of insects. To be sure, malathion has a broad spectrum of effectiveness, but temephos and the various compounds used for systemic treatment of bots and other endoparasites are of little value in treating the wide range of pests that attack crops and forests.

Nonetheless, it is remarkable that any anticholinesterase can be used as a drug for treating not only parasites in the gastrointestinal tract but also parasites in the tissues (see Section 2.4.7.1). This kind of use is entirely different from the use of some organic phosphorus compounds for treatment of glaucoma, wherein a regulated anticholinesterase action is wanted, and excessive action is avoided only by vigorous regulation of dosage.

16.2.1.5 Treatment of Poisoning in Animals

Atropine, enzyme reactivators, and symptomatic care constitute the most important means of treating poisoning by organic phosphorus compounds in humans (see Section 16.2.2.7). Their value is so firmly established by pharmacological theory and clinical experience that there is no need to review studies in animals that first explored and later confirmed their value. It is desirable to review animal experiments exploring certain other compounds that may be useful for treating poisoning by organic phosphorus compounds.

Glucose   Glucose apparently gave some protection when 3 ml of a 20% aqueous solution was injected intraperitoneally in rats poisoned by parathion, parathion-methyl, and demeton (Deichmann and Rakoczy, 1953). Glycogen stores may be depleted during poisoning, but this is more likely to be significant in small animals.

Cysteine   It was reported that cysteine protected animals intoxicated by parathion (Botescu *et al.*, 1970), but the pharmacological basis is not clear and the finding apparently has not been reinvestigated.

Vitamin C   According to Karimov (1974), there is a significant reduction in the concentration of vitamin C in the blood and urine of people considered to have sequelae of acute poisoning or to be chronically poisoned. The same was true of rabbits receiving 3.8 mg/kg/day of dimethoate plus 3.1 mg/kg/day of lindane for 3 months. Vitamin C at the rate of 30 mg/kg/day restored the normal blood level of this vitamin, reduced the abnormally high blood alkaline phosphatase level, and was considered to improve the detoxifying power of the liver. It was recommended that vitamin C, unlike vitamin B$_1$, should be used in treating chronic poisoning by pesticides. In another study, large doses of vitamin C were found to counteract growth retardation produced in rats by repeated administration of parathion and malathion at selected levels (Chakraborty *et al.*, 1978).

Reduced Glutathione (GSH)   What was apparently the first paper reporting the use of GSH to treat poisoning by parathion-methyl (Matsueda *et al.*, 1972a) began with a discussion of glutathione transferase but reported only on the response of cholinesterase to a single intravenous dose of 600 mg. There was little or no effect on red blood cell cholinesterase, but a definite but limited increase of plasma cholinesterase. This positive response seemed too prompt to be explained by promotion of detoxification, but no other mechanism for the increase in plasma enzyme activity was advanced. In pigs, plasma cholinesterase activity that had been depressed by parathion-methyl was increased temporarily by GSH (Matsueda *et al.*, 1972b). Further study involved the relationship between plasma cholinesterase activity and GSH (Matsueda *et al.*, 1973a). The reported results do not yet justify use of multiple doses of GSH in human therapy, but further studies should focus on influences of GSH on the rate of metabolism of different organic phosphorus compounds and on the survival of poisoned animals.

Chlorella Extract   Although apparently untested in animals, chlorella extract was reported to restore red cell cholinesterase activity *in vitro* (Matsueda *et al.*, 1974).

16.2.2 CLINICAL CONSIDERATIONS

16.2.2.1 Absorption, Distribution, Metabolism, and Excretion

Routes of Absorption   Organic phosphorus insecticides are absorbed by the skin, as well as by the respiratory and gastrointestinal tracts. Absorption by the skin tends to be slow, but, because the insecticides are difficult to remove, such absorption is frequently prolonged. Skin absorption is somewhat greater at higher temperatures and may be much greater in the presence of dermatitis. Thus, dermatitis may lead to serious poisoning following exposure that would ordinarily cause no inconvenience.

Distribution and Storage   It has been recognized for a long time that there is much more involvement of the central nervous system in connection with poisoning by some compounds than in connection with equally severe poisoning by others. Clearly, compounds vary in the ease with which they cross the blood–brain barrier. There also may be variation in the ability of a given compound to inhibit brain cholinesterase activity. Using standard conditions (measurements of brain cholinesterase 150 sec after an intravenous dose), Reiff *et al.* (1971) showed that the median inhibitory dose (ID 50) of a wide range of compounds varied directly with the water–lipid partition characteristic (expressed as Rm) and inversely with *in vitro* brain enzyme inhibiting power (expressed as bimolecular rate constant).

The distribution of an organic phosphorus compound is not always closely related to the signs of illness it produces, but knowledge of the distribution is useful in understanding the complete clinical picture, including the duration of illness. The distribution of parathion containing ^{32}P was studied in mice by radioautography (Fredriksson and Bigelow, 1961). Following subcutaneous injection, the level of radioactivity in the major blood vessels and the chambers of the heart never became high. However, with $\frac{1}{2}$ hr the material had accumulated to the highest degree in the cervical brown fat and the salivary glands; to a marked degree in the liver, kidney, and ordinary adipose tissue; a fairly high degree in the gastric and intestinal walls, thyroid, spleen, and lungs; to an even lower degree in the central nervous system, musculature, and bone marrow; and to an undetectably low degree in the thymus, adrenals, skin, bile, and intestinal lumen. In the kidney there was an initial concentration of activity in the cortical region, and 1 hr after injection there was high activity (undoubtedly from water-soluble metabolites) in the renal pelvis and noticeable

activity in the bladder. Activity in the bladder and in the adipose tissue increased gradually through the period of observation (4 hr). Distribution in the central nervous system was low and equal from one structure to another.

The observed high concentration of parathion in the intestinal wall and the ability of that tissue to oxidize parathion to paraoxon (Kubistova, 1959) are consistent with the observation that increased peristalsis and abdominal cramps are very early signs of systemic poisoning by the compound. In a similar way, the affinity of parathion for the salivary glands is consistent with profuse salivation as an early sign of poisoning and with morphological changes in these organs in cases of accidental poisoning (Klein, 1956).

In early studies, some animals relapsed several hours after an initial success of treatment with 2-PAM, but responded favorably to a second treatment. This rather prompt relapse was attributed to continuing formation of a direct inhibitor from the indirect one administered (Svetličić and Vandekar 1960). When relapse occurs after several days instead of several hours, continuing absorption or release from storage, or both, must be involved, in addition to continuing bioactivation. In cases of human poisoning, it may not be possible to distinguish toxicant still being absorbed from the skin or intestine from that stored very early in the illness and later mobilized from fat. Certainly, organic phosphorus compounds have been demonstrated on the skin or in the intestine long after exposure stopped. The importance of early and thorough clearing of the intestine following ingestion has been emphasized (see Section 16.6.1.3). Some compounds have been measured in the fat of persons poisoned by them (see Section 16.7.11.3). In studies with [^{32}P]dicrotaphos, Menzer and Casida (1965) found no radioactivity in the fat. This was attributed to the fact that the compound is water soluble and is rapidly excreted. It may be that no significant storage of dicrotaphos or of its toxic metabolites is possible. However, the fact that a man very severely poisoned by this compound relapsed on day 10 but responded to greatly increased doses of 2-PAM chloride (see Section 16.6.12.3) is strong evidence that he was still mobilizing unmetabolized compound from some source at that late time.

There is no model for the severely poisoned person. The reason is that no one has time to keep an animal alive following a dosage that some human beings survive either for many days or indefinitely as a result of assisted respiration, carefully adjusted medication, and continuous nursing care. Thus storage and later mobilization of toxicants in severely poisoned people may be more important than it is practical to demonstrate in animals.

Metabolism   The biotransformation of organic phosphorus compounds is discussed in several subdivisions of Section 16.2.1.3. In contrast to the metabolism of some chlorinated hydrocarbon insecticides, the metabolism of organic phosphorus insecticides is rapid. Both groups of compounds are subject to storage. One gets the impression that it is storage and, therefore, unavailability for metabolism that sometimes delays the excretion of organic phosphorus compounds, whereas it is slow metabolism *per se* that is the limiting factor for those chlorinated hydrocarbon insecticides that are stored tenaciously.

Excretion Excretion of organic phosphorus insecticides is discussed in Section 16.2.2.3 under Other Measures of Absorption.

16.2.2.2 Signs and Symptoms of Poisoning in Humans

Typical Poisoning Signs and symptoms are, at least to a very great extent, secondary to cholinesterase inhibition. The usual symptoms include headache, giddiness, nervousness, blurred vision, weakness, nausea, cramps, diarrhea, and discomfort in the chest. Signs include sweating, miosis, tearing, salivation and other excessive respiratory tract secretion, vomiting, cyanosis, papilledema, uncontrollable muscle twitches followed by muscular weakness, convulsions, coma, loss of reflexes, and loss of sphincter control. The last four signs are seen only in severe cases but do not preclude a favorable outcome if treatment is prompt and energetic. Cardiac arrhythmias, various degrees of heart block, and cardiac arrest may occur (Singh *et al.*, 1969; Namba *et al.*, 1970; Chhabra *et al.*, 1970; Khandekar, 1971). On the other hand, tachycardia and ST-wave abnormalities may be induced by large doses of atropine required in treatment; these effects can be corrected by propranolol, thus eliminating any need to reduce the rate of atropine administration (Valero and Golan, 1967). Bradycardia is seen occasionally (Singh *et al.*, 1969; Cecconello, 1968) but not as often as animal experiments might lead one to expect.

Following a massive oral dose associated with murder or suicide, death has occurred in 5 min or less after ingestion. Following smaller doses swallowed accidentally, onset of illness was sometimes delayed an hour or more. In occupational cases, illness is frequently delayed several hours so that the worker may first become sick at home after supper. However, if symptoms begin more than 12 hr after the last known exposure to an insecticide, illness probably is not due to parathion. In rare instances, onset of poisoning by a very few compounds may be more delayed but for reasons that are far less clear. For example, a 62-year-old man showed minimal cholinergic signs for the first 29 hr after he ingested dichlofenthion (see Section 16.7.11.3). Two men in their sixties had no characteristic signs when admitted to hospital after drinking demeton-methyl, and one of them showed no change for the first 60 hr (see Section 16.6.3.3). In spite of markedly delayed onset, these were extremely severe cases. The first survived after more than a month of hospitalization; the last two died after prolonged treatment.

In ordinary occupational cases, relatively incapacitating symptoms of nausea, cramps, discomfort in the chest, muscular twitching, etc. often follow the initial giddiness, blurred vision, and headache only after a period of 2–8 hr, but the onset of serious symptoms may be more rapid. Undue emphasis has been given to miosis as a diagnostic sign. Miosis may appear late; in fact, the opposite condition, mydriasis, may be present initially (Dixon, 1957; Castedo and Bruno, 1966), perhaps as a nonspecific reaction to the discomfort and apprehension associated with poisoning. Treatment of significant illness following excessive exposure to these compounds should not be delayed merely because miosis is absent.

There have been several reported cases (Christensen, 1959;) and several unpublished cases in which artificial respiration was required but was inadequate, so that the patient survived temporarily but showed severe brain injury as a result of the anoxia. Some of the difficulties leading to inadequate artificial respiration were beyond medical prevention. The patients gradually recovered from the specific signs of poisoning but remained comatose and tended to continue to have inadequate spontaneous respiration. Two of them showed temporary hyperthermia after the acute episode, presumably as a result, rather than as a cause, of brain injury. Death occurred 6 days to 4 weeks after onset. Extensive necrosis of the brain was present in the cases that came to autopsy.

There have also been a few cases of prolonged illness in which significant brain injury from hypoxia appeared unlikely and could be ruled out entirely when recovery was complete. Prolonged illness and/or delayed exacerbations have been observed in cases of poisoning by dichlofenthion, dicrotophos, dimethoate, fenthion, and malathion. Protracted illness of this kind depends at least in part on persistence of unmetabolized insecticide in the body, especially in fat, as has been demonstrated in connection with dichlofenthion. Prolonged absorption may be another factor. Apparently, prolonged illness has not been produced by schradan or other compounds that cause truly irreversible inhibition of acetylcholinesterase, except in the presence of myasthenia gravis or other complications.

Regardless of the kind of compound, the major cause of prolonged illness in the absence of major brain damage undoubtedly has been improved therapy, permitting the survival of persons who otherwise would have died promptly. Therapy improved partly because oximes became available and partly because the nature and importance of proper treatment became more generally known.

No matter what the cause, prolonged illness often involves complications seen less frequently in patients who either recover or die rapidly. These complications can include liver dysfunction (Barckow *et al.*, 1969; Boelcke and Erdmann, 1969; Prinz, 1969; Boelcke and Gaaz, 1970; Boelcke and Kamphenkel, 1970), heart dysfunction (Singh *et al.*, 1969; Schorn, 1972), psychosis (Seybold and Braeutigam, 1968; Wender and Owsianowski, 1969), and delayed convulsions (Pukach and Shakov, 1971). There is considerable evidence that many of the complications of poisoning are the result of hypoxia and are not directly related to cholinesterase inhibition (Heering, 1970). Infusion of paraoxon into the left renal artery of anesthetized dogs showed that the toxic action of this compound on the kidney is entirely indirect; it occurs only as an extension of systemic poisoning (Williams and Pearson, 1970).

The same applies to liver damage, as indicated by infusion experiments (Ganz *et al.*, 1974).

It has been claimed that a substantial proportion of persons who have been poisoned acutely by an organic phosphorus insecticide continue for years to suffer ill effects. These may take the form of an asthenovegetative syndrome (Faerman, 1967) or of hypertension, gastrointestinal disturbances, and a variety of other complaints (Watanabe, 1972c). However, other investigators, some of whom considered larger series of cases, found no evidence for any sequelae (Tabershaw and Cooper, 1966).

Whereas the initial symptoms of anticholinesterase poisoning have some resemblance to asthma, Ganelin *et al.* (1964) found by epidemiological and laboratory study that environmental exposure to parathion had a negligible effect on the general population, including persons known to suffer from asthma.

Behavioral Effects As discussed in Section 7.4.1 (Hayes, 1975), it has been suspected that otherwise mild poisoning by organic phosphorus compounds has been associated with lapses of attention or judgment that led to accidents, especially in pilots. Durham *et al.* (1965) showed that brief lapses of attention may increase after exposure but only in persons who have absorbed enough of an anticholinesterase compound to produce other signs or symptoms. When volunteers were given parathion-methyl for a week at a rate of 2 or 4 mg/person/day or parathion at a rate of 1 or 2 mg/person/day, no effect was detected on plasma or red cell cholinesterase activity, and there was no worsening of the results of tests of memory, vigilance, information processing, language, proprioceptive feedback performance, anxiety level, or depression. In fact, the only trend following exposure was one of improvement, but the change was so small that the significance was unclear (Rodnitzky *et al.*, 1978).

Decrements in alertness and memory have been associated with chronic industrial and agricultural exposures to organic phosphorus pesticides. Increased irritability, memory deficits, lethargy, and lack of energy have also been associated with multiple or severe acute exposures. Electroencephalographic analysis found narcoleptic sleep patterns and unusually long stage I sleep in some of these cases. This provides support for the occasional observations of excessive drowsiness following organic phosphorus pesticide exposures (Metcalf and Holmes, 1969).

So far there is no evidence that anticholinesterases such as mevinphos and physostigmine that are capable of crossing the blood–brain barrier and affecting hippocampal inhibitory phenomena and visual integrative neurons in the thalamus of pigeons (Revzin, 1976a,b) would affect human behavior at dosages that do not produce mild illness. On the other hand, the fact that atropine produces the same changes in neuronal function and is at least additive with the effects of anticholinesterases justifies a warning against any prophylactic use of atropine.

Another kind of mental derangement occurs during only a few cases of poisoning, frequently in the course of recovery. It may be reported as delirium, combativeness, hallucinations, depression, or psychosis. Instances have been reported in connection with parathion (see Section 16.7.1.3), trichlorfon (see Section 16.6.3), dichlorvos (see Section 16.6.5.3), fenthion (see Section 16.6.16.3), and dimethoate (see Section 16.6.13.3). There is not enough information to exclude the possibility that some organic phosphorus compounds or impurities in some batches of them predispose to delirium or related conditions. However, in most cases in which these conditions occurred at all, they appeared late and were probably a result of earlier anoxia or, in a few instances, a side effect of atropine used in therapy. This complication, of whatever origin, apparently never has contributed to a fatal outcome and never has failed to resolve completely in patients who survived.

Visual Effects The typical anticholinesterase visual effects of organic phosphorus insecticides constitute a minor aspect of poisoning, but blurred vision may offer an early warning which, if heeded, can stop exposure and initiate therapeutic management. The pharmacologically expected changes may also have special importance for the safety of workers. The inability of the pupils of both eyes to expand in dim light (bilateral miosis) could be a cause of an accident as a worker enters a dimly lit area. (Miosis as such does not interfere with vision in bright light.) Of far more importance for safety is unilateral miosis, commonly caused by the local effect of getting an anticholinesterase dust or liquid into one eye as a result of wind or splashing. Unilateral miosis greatly interferes with judging distances and this, in turn, can interfere with driving vehicles, especially piloting aircraft. Of course, unilateral miosis leads to unequal illumination of the two eyes. That such unequal illumination leads to a misinterpretation of the path of a moving object has been known for a long while. The effect can be produced experimentally either by placing a neutral filter in front of one eye or a red filter in front of one and a green filter in front of the other. Under these circumstances, the path of a swinging pendulum appears to follow an elliptical path rather than to follow a simple arc in one plane. This phenomenon is called the Pulfrich stereo effect after Pulfrich (1922), who first explained it. A more quantitative explanation has been developed by subsequent investigators, as discussed in detail by Duke-Elder and Weale (1968). However, it was not until Upholt and his colleagues studied the effect of TEPP on the eyes of volunteers (see Section 16.7.5.3) that the relationship of the early ophthalmological findings to the experience of pilots who had sprayed or dusted anticholinesterase insecticides was recognized.

There is a separate set of literature dealing with organic phosphorus compounds used as drugs to treat glaucoma. Some of these compounds (echothiophate, DFP) are not insecticides, but one of them, paraoxon (called Mintacol as a drug), is the active metabolite of parathion.

Long-acting cholinesterase inhibitors can control many cases of glaucoma which cannot be controlled by maximal conventional therapy. Unfortunately, the long-acting inhibitors, which are more convenient for the patient, are cataractogenic. The effect is not confined to patients but has been demonstrated in guinea pigs and monkeys. Cataract is a serious side effect in many—possibly even the majority—of patients in whom ocular hypertension does not progress to a pronounced loss of visual field. Cataract is not a serious side effect in patients whose condition otherwise would progress to optic nerve damage and blindness. Surgery to correct glaucoma also has its complications. In spite of their drawback, long-acting cholinesterase inhibitors are indicated in cases where maximal conventional therapy fails to prevent the progression of nerve damage in glaucoma, and surgery is indicated only when these drugs, too, prove insufficient to prevent progression (Axelsson, 1969; Kaufman and Axelsson, 1975). On the contrary, long-acting cholinesterase inhibitors should only be used with caution in young people, even though the side effects tend to be reversible in them (Axelsson and Nyman, 1970).

The ophthalmological experience is a warning of a possibility of injury in heavily exposed workers. However, the dosage to the eyes of workers is far less than that of patients. Although cataracts resulting from occupational exposure to organic phosphorus insecticides has been reported (Pietsch *et al.*, 1972), it has not been confirmed.

Both the well-recognized visual effects of organic phosphorus compounds and atypical effects that have been reported were reviewed in detail by Pleština and Piukovič-Pleština (1978).

Other Local Effects Not only may some visual effects be local but also effects on the respiratory system, skin, and even muscles and gastrointestinal system may be local, provided the cholinesterase inhibitor involved is direct acting (see Section 16.2.1.4).

Besides visual effects, respiratory effects are the only local ones likely to be of clinical importance. The inhalation of anticholinesterase vapors or aerosols may lead rapidly to illness characterized at first almost exclusively by respiratory signs and symptoms and only later by a full range of effects of systemic absorption.

Local effects on sweat glands and muscles from dermal absorption in the area involved indicate the peripheral nature of signs frequently seen in systemic poisoning. Intradermal injection of paraoxon or surface application of maloxon or dichlorvos to human skin produced after a few minutes a long-lasting local sweating response (McLaughlin and Sonnenschein, 1960). Prolonged local sweating followed dermal application of technical parathion (Funckes *et al.*, 1963a).

Atypical Cases of Various Origins At least as early as 1970 Ishikawa and Oto described "Saku strange disease," which they first observed about 1965 among students of primary schools in the Saku district of Japan. The condition was said to be characterized by amblyopia, constriction of visual fields, and optic neuritis; astigmatism was common; pupils often were dilated and sometimes unequal; and intraocular pressures were slightly elevated in some patients. Plasma cholinesterase was low in about 30% of cases, and the condition was attributed to chronic poisoning by organic phosphorus and carbamate insecticides. Ishikawa (1970) reported the effectiveness of prolonged treatment of the condition with PAM, prifinium, and atropine. Even in these early papers, the eye trouble was more or less clearly linked to peripheral paresthesias of the extremities, extrapyramidal disorders, and liver dysfunction. However, later in the same year, Kito (1970) reported his inability to confirm the syndrome among 71 young patients referred by Dr. Oto as suffering from Saku disease. Kito did observe some abnormalities, including abnormal electroencephalogram (EEG) patterns in 16 of 70 children, but these patterns were quite different from those obtained during poisoning by organic phosphorus compounds. Dr. Kito proposed that the difficulties he did find might be the result of consanguineous marriages. There followed what has been termed a barren controversy. A great many papers were published reporting Saku disease in adults as well as in children. At least one other paper reported failure to find this disease or any other ophthalmologic disorder among patients referred by Dr. Oto. In fact, no severe ophthalmologic disorder was found among nearly 300 students in Nagano Prefecture (Kato, 1971). Because particular emphasis had been placed on visual field abnormalities in diagnosing Saku disease, visual field screening was incorporated into the school health program. Of 13,351 children examined, 32 had visual field abnormalities, and this was confirmed in 12 cases when the 32 children were reexamined under hospital conditions. One child had retinitis pigmentosa and one was suffering the aftereffects of meningitis; one had a history of carbon monoxide poisoning at 9 months of age, and another had suffered asphyxia neonatorum. Five cases were attributed to psychological difficulty, and these abnormalities disappeared after elimination of psychological disturbances. Three children declined follow-up (Futenma, 1973).

Because of the reports that organic phosphorus compounds cause serious eye injuries in people and that these injuries are of a kind that could be measured objectively in animals, a number of studies have been carried out in animals to explore the problem. Some of the animal studies were based on the assumption that the injury was real, and they attempted to explore the mechanism. For example, Imaizumi *et al.* (1973) reported changes in the fatty acids of the optic nerve, retina, iris, and lens of rabbits that had received oral doses of fenitrothion for 6 months at the rate of only 0.5 mg/kg/day, which they considered 0.00055 of an LD 50 per day. They reported similar changes in the ocular tissues of rabbits intoxicated by organochlorine and organic·mercury pesticides. Clearly, the possibility is remote that such different chemicals will have the same effect.

Other studies simply explored the action of organic phosphorus compounds on the eye. For example, the effects of fenitrothion and fenthion on the eye were tested by feeding each compound to dogs at the rate of 2 mg/kg/day for 1 year. Plasma and red cell cholinesterase activities were depressed, and there was some increase in ocular secretions, salivation, and diarrhea. However, no significant change in refraction, corneal curvature, ocular tension, or conditions of the eye grounds was revealed by repeated examinations during the year, and no gross or microscopic morphological change was seen at autopsy (Ogata, 1972; Maebashi *et al.*, 1972). In a later study, fenitrothion was administered to three beagles at the rate of 5 mg/kg/day for 10 months. The results were the same, except that the corneal radius of curvature was noticeably reduced in experimental animals and controls until the growth stopped and the values were identical. Results of muscle, liver, and kidney function were also normal (Kawamura *et al.*, 1974). Considering the same parameters, the findings were essentially similar in rabbits receiving fenitrothion at rates of 1, 3, or 10 mg/kg/day for 3 months or in monkeys receiving 0.1, 0.5, or 2.0 mg/kg/day for the same period. However, the motor end plate changed conspicuously, especially on the outer ocular muscles of rabbits given 10 mg/kg/day and in monkeys given 2 mg/kg/day (Matsushima *et al.*, 1972).

In rabbits sprayed with high concentrations of fenitrothion, a decrease in the radius of curvature of the cornea was the only change recognized (Kawai and Naito, 1974).

If there is such a thing as Saku disease, there is no reason to think that it is related to organophosphorus insecticides.

16.2.2.3 Laboratory Findings

Clinical Laboratory Findings Leukocytosis and moderate albuminuria, acetonuria, and glycosuria are frequent, and hemoconcentration may occur. Less common findings include microscopic hematuria.

Increased stability of human erythrocytes to hypotonic challenge has been noted in cases where serum or erythrocyte cholinesterase levels were inhibited by 40–60%. Reductions in serum or erythrocyte cholinesterase levels exceeding 60% were accompanied by increased hemolysis upon hypotonic challenge, as well as a significant increase in phosphatidylcholine levels. Although further investigation is required to explain these observations convincingly, it appears that altered fixed charge densities on the erythrocyte membranes could render them impermeable to hemoglobin and electrolytes, resulting in hemolysis (de Potas and de D'Angelo, 1987).

Bradycardia; A-V block and dissociation, exaggeration, and inversion of the T wave; and disappearance of the P wave have been observed in experimental animals poisoned by TEPP and are likely to be encountered with the other organic phosphorus insecticides under suitable conditions.

Hypertension has been found in animals and might be predicted on the basis of stimulation of the adrenals. Increased excretion of catecholamines in the urine of rats has been measured (Brzezinski, 1969). In human cases, mild hypertension has been remarked on only infrequently (Mutalik *et al.*, 1962). The possibility is not excluded that some compounds are more likely than other to produce this effect, but there is no decisive evidence.

In a similar way, moderate azotemia has been reported (Mutalik *et al.*, 1962) but apparently not at a level that significantly influenced the clinical course. Again, whether some com-

pounds are more likely than others to produce azotemia is unknown.

In poisoning by parathion and by a wide range of unrelated compounds, serum creatine, creatine phosphokinase, and serum glutamic-oxaloacetic transaminase (SGOT) frequently are elevated. The fact that lactate dehydrogenase (LDH) and serum glutamic-pyruvic transaminase (SGPT) do not undergo a parallel change and the fact that creatine occurs almost exclusively in the muscles suggest that the striated muscles undergo hypoxic damage during poisoning and exclude substantial liver involvement (Prellwitz *et al.*, 1970). However, temporary liver damage (increased serum bilirubin, increased urinary urobilogen, or delayed excretion of bromosulfophthalein) may occur (Lutterotti, 1961).

Animals poisoned by organic phosphorus compounds develop a variety of electroencephalographic abnormalities which, interestingly enough, tend to be corrected by atropine (Mitra, 1966; Vajda *et al.*, 1974). In animals, EEG changes are not specific for anticholinesterase compounds, as compared to chlorinated hydrocarbon insecticides (Santolucito and Morrison, 1971). EEG changes apparently have never been found valuable in the management of persons with occupational exposure to or clinical poisoning from any anticholinesterase compound. However, EEG results should be considered in the differential diagnosis of any patient who has had substantial exposure to an organic phosphorus insecticide but who is suspected of having an organic brain lesion.

In a similar way, X-ray examination generally does not contribute to the management of people poisoned by organic phosphorus insecticides. When X-ray pictures were made, it was found that the diffuse density in the lungs appeared to be confined to the peripheral areas. The fact that the heart was not enlarged served to distinguish pulmonary edema associated with poisoning from that associated with myocardial disease (Blesdoe and Seymour, 1972).

Methods of Measuring Cholinesterase Activity Anyone interested in measuring blood cholinesterase should consult the critical reviews by Witter (1963) and Holmstedt (1971). For practical purposes, the procedures may be divided into three classes: methods especially suitable for research, methods suitable for the adequate assay of large numbers of clinical samples, and field methods. The most accurate and sensitive methods are the recording titrimetric and Warburg manometric procedures, in which the amount of acid is measured stoichiochemically. Both of these methods are of great versatility and can be applied to the study of kinetics of inhibitors or activators and to the study of a variety of other experimental conditions, since rate curves are obtained. The Warburg procedure cannot be used for the study of the effect of pH beyond the range 7.2–7.7; the titrimetric method can be used to study the entire useful pH range. Because rate curves can be obtained within a period of 2 min, the titrimetric method is of particular value in studying the kinetics of the initial phase of the reaction between inhibitor (or activator), substrate, and cholinesterase. The titrimetric method not only offers special advantages for biochemical research but also is sufficiently simple that it is being employed increasingly for clinical applications. Directions for its use have been given by Nabb and Whitfield (1967).

The manometric technique originally used for the determination of cholinesterase activities of whole blood samples (Augustinsson, 1955) has been replaced by a more convenient and less laborious method, making it a viable option as a routine clinical laboratory procedure (Augustinsson et al., 1978).

The most used method of measuring cholinesterase probably still is that of Michel (1949). This method does not yield rate curves, and it is not sufficiently sensitive to measure the inherently low cholinesterase activity found in the blood of many experimental animals. However, its dependability and convenience for clinical determinations have made the Michel method essentially standard for this purpose. Consequently, much of what is known about normal variations in blood cholinesterase in humans and about the relation of enzyme activity to exposure and to clinical conditions was gathered by this method.

A variety of field methods have been proposed for measuring blood cholinesterase, and kits for this purpose are commercially available. They have a valid place in following the exposure of workers, such as the members of antimalaria spray teams, in areas remote from a laboratory. The most used field method is that employing a Tintometer, as described by Edson (1958). It permits the recognition of eight steps (12.5%) in human blood cholinesterase activity between normal and complete inhibition. Some of the other field methods are inherently even less precise. It is open to question whether there is any valid justification for using a field method to measure cholinesterase when a laboratory is available, permitting use of a better method.

The way in which blood is collected for measuring cholinesterase activity following exposure to dichlorvos has an important effect on the accuracy of the result. Although this detail apparently has been explored only in connection with this one compound and although the relationship may depend in part on the higher vapor pressure of dichlorvos, the possibility that precaution should be exercised with other direct inhibitors cannot be excluded. Briefly, Rasmussen et al. (1963), in studying the safety of dichlorvos vapor, found that measurements of plasma cholinesterase indicated consistently lower activity when carried out on blood collected by skin puncture as compared with blood collected by intravenous puncture from the same people at corresponding times. This was true even though the results for the two kinds of samples varied in a predictable and parallel way, corresponding to the duration and intensity of exposure. A number of possible explanations were explored. Eventually it was found that the usual methods for cleaning the skin prior to puncture were inadequate to remove dichlorvos, and no effective method was found. When an exposed person was taken to a room where dichlorvos had not been used and drops of blood from normal, unexposed people were placed on the person's "cleaned" skin, the cholinesterase activity of plasma later separated from the blood was rapidly and progressively inhibited, corresponding to the brief but increasing intervals during which the drops were left on the skin.

Units for Measurement of Cholinesterase Activity Unfortunately, cholinesterase activity is expressed in different units when measured by different methods. In a few instances the units are accurately convertible from one to another in the same sense that one can convert inches to centimeters. In other instances, the units are not strictly convertible because the kinetics of the methods are not identical; even in these instances, an empirical conversion may be possible under practical conditions. Theoretically, the results of any method can be expressed as percentages of normal and thus can be compared with values determined by any other method. However, because there is so much normal variation in cholinesterase levels, this method of comparison lacks precision.

Normal Blood Cholinesterase Activity The most extensive study of normal blood cholinesterase values is that of Rider et al. (1957), using the method of Michel (1949) and summarized in Table 8.4. The ranges shown are based on samples from 400 normal men and 400 normal women. The means are for persons 40 years old. Other studies, including unpublished ones, have shown that values exceeding the ranges reported by Rider et al. (1957) are encountered in normal people, but only rarely. Agreement is satisfactory regarding the mean values also (Vorhaus and Kark, 1953; Fremont-Smith et al., 1952; Wolfsie and Winter, 1952; Sealey, 1951; Sumerford et al., 1953; Ganelin, 1964; Michel, 1949; Grob et al., 1950; Kay et al., 1952; Fryer et al., 1955; Reinhold et al., 1953).

The cholinesterase activity of normal human blood as measured by the recording titrimeter method is shown in Table 8.5, based on a study by Nabb and Whitfield (1967). Although the number of samples analyzed by Nabb and Whitfield was small, the values reported by Cavagna et al. (1969), based on many samples, fell within the same range. A variant of the method (Spiers and Juul, 1964) gives essentially the same results for normal plasma enzyme but distinctly lower normal values (4.9–8.5 with a mean of 6.7 $\mu M/min/ml$ for red cell enzyme). The coefficient of variation of this method, based on repeated analysis of the same sample, is only 2.9% (Spiers and Juul, 1964).

Physiological Sources of Variation in Cholinesterase Activity Within the normal range, blood cholinesterase activity is subject to certain variation, regarding both individual and group levels. Since the work of Sawitsky et al. (1948), it is generally agreed that there is greater variation between samples from different individuals than between samples taken at intervals from the same person. Augustinsson (1955) found that the coefficient of variation for erythrocyte cholinesterase in both men and women varied from 13.3 to 15.6% for different groups of determinations by the manometric method. Corresponding values for plasma enzyme were 14.7–26.8%. In a review of many earlier studies using different methods, he found that the coefficient of variation for red cells enzyme ranged from 10.2 to 39.5% and that for plasma enzyme from 12.1 to 46%.

So far as groups are concerned, there is (in the normal range) no correlation between red cell and plasma values ($r = +0.09$ for men and $+0.02$ for women). The two enzymes vary independently in the absence of a specific inhibition (Rider *et al.*, 1957).

Wetstone and LaMotta (1965) studied 82 normal adults for 1–250 weeks and found very little variation in serum values for the same individual. Correlation (r) between the first and second tests was $+0.80$ for females and $+0.94$ for males. The average difference between two succeeding samples was only 0.6%. The coefficient of variation for 6–25 tests run on 19 adults during periods ranging from 18 to 247 weeks varied from 5.0 to 11.5%. There was no correlation between the degree of variation and the average values for different individuals. The same paper contains a valuable table of the range and mean of normal values for serum cholinesterase, as determined by different investigators employing manometric, titrimetric, colorimetric, and electrometric methods.

Lippi (1950) measured the serum cholinesterase activity of 14 men and 16 women at seven approximately equal intervals throughout one 24-hr day. The lowest average value, found at 7:30 in the morning, was 92% of the mean of all values at other sampling times. The next lowest value was 98.7% of the same mean. The author concluded that the small variation observed did not take the form of a regular curve but was entirely individual without correspondence to hour.

In an investigation that apparently was never published, Dr. Ernest M. Dixon found the opposite result, namely, that a diurnal rhythm existed. Samples were taken at 7:00 a.m., 11:45 a.m., 4:45 p.m., and 9:45 p.m. For both plasma and red blood cells and for both men and women, the values were highest just before noon (11:45 a.m.) and lowest in the evening (9:45 p.m.). The degree of difference was much greater for plasma than for red cell values. By calculation from the available data it was estimated that the peaks for plasma values of men and women occurred at or a little after noon, and the nadirs occurred at or a little after midnight.

Several investigators have systematically sampled one or more persons at intervals of a day or more for periods ranging from 4 weeks to 5 years and found that the average coefficient of variation of individuals around their own means is 7.6% (Callaway *et al.*, 1951), 10.3% (Gage, 1955), 11.3% (Kane, 1958), and 8.4% (Wetstone and LaMotta, 1965). Those who studied both enzymes found no difference in the coefficient of variation for plasma and red cell enzyme (Callaway *et al.*, 1951; Gage, 1955). The degree of variation does not depend on the initial activity (Wetstone and LaMotta, 1965). In spite of the statistical regularity in the cholinesterase values of any unexposed, normal individual, he or she may show striking and unpredictable variation from one sample to another. Maximal fluctuations of 13–25% in red cell values and 20–23% in plasma values have been reported (Klonglan *et al.*, 1956; Fryer *et al.*, 1955; Callaway *et al.*, 1951). Ganelin (1964) reported

that the plasma activity of one normal unexposed individual varied from 0.61 to 1.37 ΔpH/hr in the course of 8 months. Augustinsson (1955) followed one man for 2.25 years. The plasma values sometimes remained relatively constant but at other times varied sharply by at least 25%. The red cell levels were more stable.

In a normal, healthy person, there is no reason to think that the observed variation in cholinesterase levels is caused by a cycle of destruction and repair. The rhythmic fluctuations seen in series of values from some individuals (Gage, 1955) do not correspond to the period necessary for replacement of plasma cholinesterase (about 50 days) or to the average life of the red cell (about 120 days). Furthermore, in some persons many of the fluctuations are abrupt. Regardless of pattern, the fluctuations obtained by most analytical methods exceed the variation (about 4%) involved in multiple analysis of the same sample or analysis of multiple samples taken immediately one after the other from the same person (Gage, 1955; Witter, 1963). There is no objective reason why there should be greater variation in the sampling technique of an experienced technician from day to day than from moment to moment. Thus all present evidence suggests that day-to-day fluctuation in cholinesterase activity is physiological, but its basis is entirely unknown.

Some authors have failed to detect differences in enzyme activity related to age and sex, probably because their samples were too small to measure the minor differences that exist.

There is no change in red cell cholinesterase activity in adults associated with age (Rider *et al.*, 1957; Shanor *et al.*, 1961). It has been claimed variously that activity of this enzyme increases progressively during the first year of life (Barsegyan, 1967), that it is higher in children under 3 years of age than in older children (Kats and Gabuchiya, 1964), and that it is markedly higher in 5-year-old children than in 3-year-olds (Safiulina *et al.*, 1962).

There is disagreement also about the change of plasma enzyme activity of men; some find that it increases with age (Rider *et al.*, 1957; Spiers and Juul, 1964), others that it decreases (Shanor *et al.*, 1961; Augustinsson, 1955; Barrows *et al.*, 1958). Plasma enzyme activity does not vary with age in women (Shanor *et al.*, 1961).

Cholinesterase activity of plasma is significantly higher in men than in women (Rider *et al.*, 1957; Reinhold *et al.*, 1953; Augustinsson, 1955; Kaufman, 1954; Smith *et al.*, 1952; Butt *et al.*, 1942; Spiers and Juul, 1964; Wetstone and LaMotta, 1965), and this is true no matter which of several choline esters are used as substrate in measuring the enzyme activity (Shanor *et al.*, 1956). According to some (Shanor *et al.*, 1961), the difference is confined to young people.

There is no sex difference in the red cell enzyme activity (Augustinsson, 1955; Rider *et al.*, 1957; Shanor *et al.*, 1961).

Serum cholinesterase activity of blacks tends to be lower than that of whites of the same sex (Reinhold *et al.*, 1953). Whether the difference is of genetic or nutritional origin is unknown.

Most normal physiological processes have no influence on blood cholinesterase activity. The plasma enzyme activity of women fluctuates during the menstrual cycle (Augustinsson, 1955).

Kaufman (1954) reported that red cell, but not plasma, enzyme always is decreased after meals. The same author's claims that the plasma enzyme increases immediately postoperatively or may drop during periods of stress do not seem supported by his data. Wetstone *et al.* (1960) reported that the plasma enzyme increased after meals.

Callaway *et al.* (1951) reported that servicemen had significantly higher red cell activity than male civilians of comparable age. Whether the difference was due to greater exercise of the servicemen, their preselection, or some other factor is not clear. Some authors (Croft and Richter, 1943; Frugoni *et al.*, 1959; Lalli and Cascino, 1961) have found experimentally that exercise causes an increase in plasma cholinesterase activity, ranging from 3 to 27%. A transient rise has been reported also after electroshock therapy (Ravin and Altschule, 1952), but was attributed to hemoconcentration rather than "exercise." Other authors (Vahlquist, 1935; Hall and Lucas, 1937; Stoner and Wilson, 1943) have failed to note a change after exercise. Some and perhaps all of the failures were associated with different experimental conditions. In discussing the matter, Croft and Richter (1943) noted that the increase may appear within 3 min and may return to normal within 10–15 min. They suggested that failure to find a change might result from taking samples after the change had disappeared. They thought that the increased activity in the plasma resembled that of red cells rather than that of normal plasma and was released from the red cells through an unidentified mechanism. They considered that the mechanism associated with exercise was different from that associated with circulatory stasis caused by a ligature.

Even those who have found a consistent increase in plasma cholinesterase activity following exercise have reported a unidirectional change no larger than the change that may occur in either direction by chance. This fact may be the real basis for the continuing lack of agreement about the effect of exercise.

In the absence of specific inhibition, there is a simple, positive correlation between the activity of serum cholinesterase and the concentration of serum albumin, another material formed by the liver (Faber, 1943; Scudamore *et al.*, 1951). There is considerable evidence that the rate of synthesis of protein by the liver is determined in part by the level of circulating albumin. When this level is artificially raised above normal, the liver "rests" in a way analogous to that of an endocrine gland when the corresponding hormone is injected. The production of plasma cholinesterase corresponds to the production of serum albumin. Thus, the production of plasma cholinesterase can be reduced by overloading the serum with albumin. The enzyme activity of volunteers declined sharply and progressively in response to daily infusion of 50 gm of human serum for 18 days but gradually returned to normal as soon as the infusions were stopped. Conversely, in nephrosis, a condition in which serum albumin is depleted, production of both albumin and cholinesterase is increased, and the enzyme usually reaches high levels in the plasma because its larger molecule, unlike that of albumin, is not lost in the urine (Vorhaus and Kark, 1953). However, Wetstone *et al.* (1960) pointed out that concentrations of plasma cholinesterase and albumin are correlated only imperfectly in different pathological states.

Genetic Sources of Variation in Cholinesterase Activity

Succinylcholine (suxamethonium) and related drugs are widely used as muscle relaxants in surgery and in electroconvulsion therapy. It was observed that a few persons exhibit an abnormally prolonged period of muscular paralysis after such a drug has been administered at the usual rate. These persons proved to have serum cholinesterase activity much lower than that of most normal people (Bourne *et al.*, 1952; Evans *et al.*, 1952, 1953). Not only is there less enzyme activity per unit volume of plasma, but also the enzyme is less reactive with certain inhibitors (Kalow and Genest, 1957; Kalow and Davies, 1958) and has greater than normal Michaelis constants when tested with a variety of substrates (R. O. Davies *et al.*, 1960). These and other differences lead to the conclusion that the abnormal enzyme is qualitatively different from the normal. The usual test for it depends on its lesser inhibition by dibucaine.

Use of the dibucaine test shows that the usual phenotype has dibucaine numbers averaging about 79%, the intermediate phenotype has dibucaine numbers averaging about 62%, and the atypical phenotype has dibucaine numbers averaging about 16% (Kalow and Staron, 1957). (The percentage is the degree of inhibition under specified conditions.) A similar trimodal distribution is found if initial cholinesterase activity, rather than inhibition by dibucaine, is taken as the basis of classification (Kaufman *et al.*, 1960).

Kalow and Staron (1957) suggested that the three phenotypes are determined by two autosomal allelic genes without dominance, individuals with the usual phenotype being homozygous for the one and individuals with the atypical phenotype being homozygous for the other. The intermediate phenotype is thought to involve the heterozygous condition and the presence of a mixture of normal and atypical enzymes in the plasma. The exact frequency of the three phenotypes in the population is unknown. The frequency of the atypical gene has been estimated as being in the order of 1 in 2000 to 1 in 4000 (Harris and Whittaker, 1962). If the latter value (0.025%) is accepted, then (on the basis of a pair of allelic, autosomal genes) the frequency of the heterozygous phenotype may be calculated as 3.106% and that of the usual phenotype as 96.865%. The value of 3.106% corresponds, within the accuracy of measurement, with values of 2.8–4.3% (Kalow and Staron, 1957) and 3–4% (Harris and Whittaker, 1962) observed in different populations. Essentially the same is true if the ratio of 1 : 2,000 is accepted. This value (0.05%) is consistent with values of 4.36 and 95.40% for the intermediate and usual phenotypes, respectively.

Kalow and Staron (1957) concluded that some of their observations pointed to "additional factors which may be variants of the normal gene, or modifying genes which influence the expressivity of the normal gene." Harris and Whittaker

(1962), using two tests based on inhibition by dibucaine and fluoride, respectively, obtained evidence for two new phenotypes which was consistent with inheritance involving three allelic genes. However, the data were not adequate to exclude the possibility of a pair of alleles plus a pair of modifying genes. As indicated in a thorough review, more recent research indicates that there may be as many as five genes (Lehman and Liddell, 1969).

Apparently hypersusceptibility to organic phosphorus or carbamate anticholinesterases has never been associated with a genetic defect in cholinesterase, although some search for such a relationship was made by William F. Durham and perhaps others. The fact that only about one person among several thousand is homozygous for the genetic trait clearly limits the frequency with which a relationship might be expected. However, the trait would never have been discovered if some of these unusual people had not required treatment with succinylcholine—an experience perhaps no more common than heavy exposure to anticholinesterases. It seems likely that there are more than statistical reasons for the lack of an observed relationship between genetically abnormal plasma cholinesterase and poisoning by an anticholinesterase. First, persons with the abnormal trait have normal acetylcholinesterase, which is the enzyme critical in anticholinesterase poisoning. Second, the genetically defective plasma enzyme is less reactive than normal; its inefficiency in metabolizing succinylcholine as a substrate is a source of danger, but its relative failure to react with an inhibitor is a source of no danger and is likely to be attributed to failure of exposure.

In one small series, the plasma cholinesterase activity of unexposed persons who were homozygous for abnormal enzyme varied from 8 to 21% of the mean for normal people in the same study, and the abnormal and normal values did not overlap. In the same study, the plasma cholinesterase values of unexposed persons who were heterozygous for abnormal enzyme varied from 35 to 74% of the mean for normal people; some but not all of the values for the heterozygous ones overlapped the lower range of normal. Under some circumstances, it may be desirable to determine whether low plasma cholinesterase activity is genetic in origin or caused by inhibition. A convenient way of doing this has been described; it consists of using a recording titrimeter to measure sequentially the cholinesterase activity of the same sample before and after the addition of dibucaine hydrochloride (Bonderman and Bonderman, 1971).

Disease as a Source of Variation in Cholinesterase Activity Little information about the relationship between cholinesterase activity and disease has been added since the observations and review by Vorhaus and Kark (1953) or, in fact, since the work of Grob *et al.* (1947a,b,c), but their findings have been confirmed frequently. In general, low plasma cholinesterase values are found in patients ill with parenchymal liver disease, malnutrition, chronic debilitating diseases, acute infections, and some anemias. Of various sorts of malnutrition, those involving deficiencies of protein or thiamine are especially likely to reduce plasma cholinesterase activity (Casterline *et al.*, 1969). Contrary to some early reports, normal levels are observed in patients ill with uncomplicated obstructive jaundice, myasthenia gravis, hyperthyroidism, asthma, hypertension, epilepsy, diabetes mellitus, and many other diseases. Of course, persons with these conditions may reach such a state of debility that their plasma enzyme activity is depressed. High levels of plasma cholinesterase occur in the nephrotic syndrome.

Patients with liver disease not only have low plasma cholinesterase values but also may show a further reduction as a result of a level of exposure to an organic phosphorus insecticide that causes no change of enzyme activity in normal persons or in persons sick with other diseases (Cavagna *et al.*, 1969). After adminsitration of DFP to volunteers, the regeneration of serum cholinesterase in those with liver damage was significantly slower than in normal persons (Wescoe *et al.*, 1947). Measurement of the activity may help to determine whether a known carcinoma elsewhere has metastasized to the liver (Molander *et al.*, 1954; Moore *et al.*, 1957). Plasma enzyme activity is reduced sharply in acute myocardial infarction; it may gradually fall to even lower levels in those who die but recovers promptly in those destined to survive. In either case, the activity of the enzyme presumably reflects the degree of circulatory adequacy. The activity is below normal in dermatomyositis but not in other collagen diseases (Moore *et al.*, 1957).

Serum cholinesterase activity shows little or no relation to mental disease (Ravin and Altschule, 1952). Small increases may occur in conditions involving agitation (Isoshima, 1960), but this effect, if real, may be secondary to muscular activity rather than mental state.

Generally, the red cell enzyme is subject to less variation than the plasma enzyme. However, it is known that the enzymatic activity of reticulocytes is several times greater than that of mature cells (Allison and Burn, 1955). Thus, the cholinesterase activity of circulating red cells is increased by reticulocytosis, for example, that accompanying recovery from hemorrhage or the successful treatment of pernicious anemia or the megaloblastic anemia of pregnancy and the puerperium (Pritchard and Weisman, 1956). The enzyme level does not parallel the number of reticulocytes *per se* (Meyer *et al.*, 1948; Scudamore *et al.*, 1951) but does reflect the accumulation of young, relatively normal cells in the circulation. No other physiological change or disease is known to affect the red cell enzyme significantly.

Abnormal Cholinesterase Values and Their Interpretation For practical purposes, exposure to organic phosphorus or carbamate insecticides is the only cause of significant depression of cholinesterase activity among people who are fully active. Certain diseases cause a reduction of the enzyme in the plasma, but these diseases are rarely if ever consistent with active work. An abnormal decrease in cholinesterase activity in a worker is almost always a result of absorption of an anticholinesterase compound. It is sometimes an indication of poisoning. The distinction depends largely on the rate at which activity of the enzyme is depressed. Slow depression often has no clinical effect.

Because of the great variation in cholinesterase activity from one person to another, it is desirable to measure the normal level of each person before occupational exposure to one or more really toxic anticholinesterases begins. Even when this is done, interpretation of enzyme levels measured during exposure is complicated by (a) the recognized normal variability in the activity of this enzyme in each person and (b) the fact that the seriousness of a particular degree of chemical inhibition depends on the rate at which it was reached. The cholinesterase content of various tissues is not affected equally in the same poisoned animal, and the level in all tissues, including even the brain, can be lowered markedly from the prepoisoning level without seriously affecting normal function, especially if the reduction is gradual.

It is believed that cholinesterase values of 0.5 ΔpH/hr or less for either cells or plasma represent abnormal depressions for most individuals. However, workers who are exposed daily over a period of weeks but whose exposure at any one time is kept at a minimum may experience depression of both enzymes to 0.1 ΔpH/hr (a reduction from normal of about 90% for plasma enzyme and 87% for red cell enzyme) without clinical signs or symptoms (Grob *et al.*, 1947a; Sumerford *et al.*, 1953; Bruaux, 1957; Ganelin, 1964; Horiguchi *et al.*, 1978).

Some absorption of an organic phosphorus insecticide may occur in one or a few exposures without producing any measurable reduction of blood cholinesterase (Edson *et al.*, 1962; Erdmann and Clarmann, 1963; Arterberry *et al.*, 1961). Greater absorption does lead to inhibition of cholinesterase and, if inhibition is sufficiently great, illness will occur. In fact, mild poisoning can occur in the presence of blood cholinesterase values within the range of normal, although some depression of the enzyme values of the individual patient probably accompanies even the mildest illness (Kay *et al.*, 1952; Holmes and Gaon, 1956; Sumerford *et al.*, 1953; Hayes *et al.*, 1957). In such instances, the mild symptoms involved are suggestive, but not diagnostic, of poisoning in the individual case. Consistent illness can be identified as poisoning only on a statistical basis by comparison of exposed and unexposed groups, preferably by a study during preexposure, exposure, and postexposure periods. The same symptoms combined with a definite depression of cholinesterase activity are essentially diagnostic.

A further complication is that the degree of blood cholinesterase inhibition that can be tolerated without illness apparently varies according to compound, even though the effect of the exposure schedule is eliminated by considering only cases involving one or a few doses. Perhaps this is what one would expect. Some compounds preferentially inhibit plasma cholinesterase, while others inhibit red cell cholinesterase earlier and to a greater degree (see Table 16.8). For a particular compound (e.g., dichlorvos or parathion) the relationship may be different in different species. Inhibition of cholinesterase in the brain and nerves must be subject to similar variation, even for compounds with identical capacity to pass the blood–brain barrier.

The situation is more complex if repeated doses are involved. Compounds that preferentially inhibit plasma cholinesterase inhibit the red cell enzyme also if absorbed in sufficient dosage for a sufficient period. Irreversibly inhibited red cell enzyme is replaced more slowly than the plasma enzyme in the circulation. A characteristic sequence of cholinesterase change is (a) depletion of plasma enzyme, followed by (b) depletion of both plasma and red cell enzymes, followed by (c) depletion of red cell enzyme only, and it is often seen during the course of repeated occupational exposure and the subsequent recovery period. Condition *a* reflects recent, slight, or moderate exposure. Condition *b* reflects continued slight or moderate exposure, or a single substantial exposure. Condition *c* reflects the postexposure state with incomplete recovery of red cell cholinesterase or slight to moderate exposure to a compound that preferentially inhibits the red cell enzyme.

In nearly all of the cases of severe poisoning by whatever compound, the cholinesterase activity of both plasma and red cells is greatly reduced. If death occurs, the depression of enzyme activity may be demonstrated by testing blood collected at autopsy within a few days of death (Petty *et al.*, 1958). Marked depression of the enzyme activity of other tissues may also be demonstrated if fresh unfixed material is employed. Table 16.9 shows the range of cholinesterase activity of different parts of the brain in persons killed by parathion.

There has been a very small number of cases in which death followed exposure to an anticholinesterase, but the blood enzyme activity measured after death was within the normal range. In a high proportion of these cases the evidence is circumstantial or incomplete. This was true of a case that led Edson *et al.* (1962) to explore the matter in experimental animals. They gave special attention to the possibility that, under some conditions of storage, either in dead bodies or *in vitro*, blood cholinesterase activity might be regenerated in such a way that values obtained on autopsy samples would appear normal. However, no such conditions were found, and the cause of death was never explained in the case that led to the study.

However, in another case observed by William F. Durham, the cause of death seemed all too clear, for the victim left several suicide notes and a large amount of parathion was found in his stomach. The plasma and red cell cholinesterase activity of blood taken at autopsy and measured less than 12 hr after death was within the normal range. Thomas B. Gaines (unpublished studies) failed to duplicate the phenomenon in animals. The negative results of Edson and his colleagues were confirmed. In addition, (because contemplation of suicide might lead to stimulation of the sympathetic nervous system), Gaines explored the possibility that parathion administered just after a dose of epinephrine might cause death by an unknown mechanism not involving cholinesterase inhibition. These and other experiments failed to throw any light on the mechanism of death in the suicide. The matter remains a complete myste-

Table 16.8
Selected Organic Phosphorus Compounds Arranged According to Their Ability to Inhibit Either Plasma or Red Cell Cholinesterase

Compound	Kind of exposure	Reference
Plasma enzyme most inhibited		
bromophos	single and repeated doses in rats	Muacevic *et al.* (1970)
chlorpyrifos	sprayers	Eliason *et al.* (1969)
	2-yr feeding in dogs	McCollister *et al.* (1974)
demeton	30-day experiment in humans	Moeller and Rider (1965)
DFP	treatment of glaucoma in humans	Leopold and Comroe (1946)
diazinon	32–43-day experiment in humans	FAO/WHO (1967)
dichlorvos	2-week experimental intermittent exposure in humans	Rasmussen *et al.* (1963)
echothiophate iodide	short-term therapy for glaucoma in humans	Spiers and Juul (1964)
fenitrothion	spraying homes	Vandekar (1965)
malathion	living in sprayed homes	Elliott and Barnes (1963)
mipafox	exposure of production workers	Bidstrup *et al.* (1953)
parathion	experimental, dog	Frawley and Fuyat (1957)
trichlorfon	short-term therapy for *S. hematobium* and *S. mansoni* in children	Abdel-Aal *et al.* (1970)
Red cell enzyme most inhibited		
dichlorvos	continuous exposure for 1 wk in monkey	Durham *et al.* (1959)
dimefox	70-day experiment in humans	Edson (1964)
malathion	2-yr feeding in rats	Hazleton and Holland (1953)
mevinphos	30-day experiment in humans	Rider *et al.* (1972, 1975)
parathion	experimental—rat	Frawley *et al.* (1952a); Matsueda *et al.* (1973b)
	accidental dermal poisoning in humans	Hayes (1963; unpublished records)
parathion-methyl	4-wk experimental in humans	Rider *et al.* (1970)
schradan	experimental feeding in rats	Barnes and Denz (1954)
temephos	extended experimental feeding in rats	Gaines *et al.* (1967)
thiometon	12-mo study in rats, 6-mo study in dogs	FAO/WHO (1970)

ry. It must be emphasized that death caused by an organic phosphorus compound without significant inhibition of blood cholinesterase is a very rare phenomenon.

The greatest value of measuring cholinesterase activity is to aid in the evaluation of exposure and of techniques for handling organic phosphorus and carbamate insecticides (Barnes and Davies, 1951; Gage, 1967). However, because of the complexities discussed above, there is real difficulty in determining the degree of change that may be interpreted with confidence ($P < 0.05$) as due to inhibition rather than random variation. Statistically, such a threshold depends on the number of preexposure measurements available. If no preexposure measurement has been made for a particular person, the postexposure value must be evaluated by population norms. Only changes in plasma cholinesterase of about 30% or greater and differences in red cell enzyme of about 20% or greater can be recognized with assurance as not due to normal variation (see statistical threshold in Table 16.10).

The wide range of normal human erythrocyte and serum cholinesterase levels complicates the diagnosis of organic phosphorus pesticide poisoning in cases where decreased cholinesterase levels remain in the normal range. A unique approach to the problem involves the back extrapolation of erythrocyte cholinesterase values based on measurements taken at a number of intervals following the suspected exposure time (Midtling *et al.*, 1985; Hodgson and Parkinson, 1985). This procedure has been particularly useful in cases where a substantial time has lapsed following the exposure.

If preexposure measurements are available for a person, a

Table 16.9
Range of Cholinesterase Activity of Different Parts of the Brain in Persons Killed by Parathion and in Those Killed in Accidents Unrelated to Anticholinesterases[a,b]

Part of brain	Parathion	Normal
putamen	39–104	290–300
head of caudate nucleus	4–76	220–300
thalamus	0–12	12–21
pons	2–15	20–30
medulla oblongata	0–11	13–27
cerebellum	10–35	58–158
cerebrum	0–12	5–9

[a] Translated and condensed from Wirth (1956) by permission of Springer-Verlag.
[b] All values measured manometrically and expressed as mm³ CO_2/30 min/12.5 mg brain substance.

Table 16.10

Percentage Reductions from Mean Values for Plasma and Red Cell Cholinesterase That Permit Recognition of the Reduction or Indicate the Need for a Worker to Stop Exposure

| Kind of threshold | Percentage difference | | | Reference |
	Blood	Plasma	Cells	
Statistical		38	22	Callaway *et al.* (1951)
		33	20	Gage (1967)
Action				
examine hygiene		25	25	Hayes (1961)
		25[a]	25[a]	Gage (1967)
			30	Zavon (1965); Menz *et al.* (1974)
stop exposure	25[b]			Bouilliat and Duperray (1964)
		30[a]	30[a]	Gage (1967); Simpson and Penney (1974)
	40			
			60	Zavon (1965); Menz *et al.* (1974)
Danger		75	50	Gage (1967)
	65[c]			Simpson and Penney (1974)

[a] Based on individual normal.

[b] Actually a cutoff of 65 units, where the range of normal was 86–126 units.

[c] Hospitalize.

somewhat smaller percentage decrease in cholinesterase can be recognized with statistical assurance as being caused by exposure to an anticholinesterase, as illustrated in Table 16.11, taken from Callaway *et al.* (1951). The estimate of some other investigators (Wetstone and LaMotta, 1965; Gage, 1967) are similar to those in this table.

The statistical thresholds just discussed are based on hundreds of determinations of normal cholinesterase values in many laboratories. They reflect the facts of normal variation. Two other kinds of thresholds have been proposed that involve a greater measure of personal judgment, namely, thresholds of action and danger (see Table 16.10).

Some investigators have suggested, in effect, that the exposure of a worker should be stopped temporarily if the worker's depletion of cholinesterase activity exceeds the statistical range of normal variation. Some have been so cautious that they would exclude from work numerous persons with low normal cholinesterase values. For simplicity, the threshold may be set at the same percentage for both plasma and red cell enzymes. As Gage (1967) put the matter:

If the threshold inhibition of 30 percent is exceeded, and if this can be confirmed by another determination made on the following day, then the worker concerned should be removed from the risk of any further exposure until the activity of his blood has returned to normal. At the same time, the process should be carefully investigated to ascertain the origin of the excessive exposure. If the reduction in activity cannot be confirmed by a second test, or if the reduction is between 25 and 30 percent of normal, then there is a case for an investigation of the safety precautions, but an interruption of the process

or the removal of the man concerned from his occupation could hardly be justified.

It must be emphasized that the removal of a man from his employment when either his red cell or his plasma enzyme falls to 70 percent of its normal value is not required because the health of the individual is thereby affected, but rather to ensure that further absorption does not lead to a deterioration of the man's condition. There is evidence that at this level of inhibition, some increased sensitivity to further exposure may occur. A man removed from his occupation for this reason, or because he has been subjected to a more serious exposure leading to toxic effects, may return to his work when his blood enzyme activity has recovered to 80 percent of its normal value.

Other authors have suggested, in effect, that there is no need to cry alarm where no danger exists, and they have taken more account of the fact that a gradual depression of cholinesterase activity without any signs and symptoms does not place a worker in a precarious state in which he or she is more subject to poisoning than normal persons. This difference of approach explains the range of estimates of the threshold requiring that a worker be removed from exposure. The views quoted from Gage represent an ideal policy in terms of both conservatism and ease of application. The use of somewhat less conservative standards is just as satisfactory, provided the policy is administered by someone really familiar with the subject.

No matter what threshold is selected, the schedule of sampling should be adapted to the compound and the kind of occupational exposure. No surveillance is necessary with malathion, except under the most extraordinary circumstances. Routine surveillance of people with occupational exposure to parathion is highly desirable.

Before beginning to make or apply a compound that requires or may require surveillance, a worker should have at least two cholinesterase determinations. If the degree of hazard is unknown, either because the compound or the nature of its application is new, each worker should undergo frequent cholinesterase determinations after work is begun. Thus, tests should be daily if danger is considerable and weekly if danger is small or improbable. If no depression of cholinesterase is found, the interval between tests may be increased from daily

Table 16.11

Minimal Differences for Statistical Recognition of Abnormal Plasma and Red Cell Cholinesterase Values

| Number of preexposure estimations | Percentage differences | |
	Plasma	Cells
1	19.9	15.3
2	17.3	13.3
3	16.3	12.5
4	15.7	12.1
5	15.5	11.9
10	14.7	11.3
∞	14.1	10.9

to weekly to monthly, and if no significant decrease is found after several months, the tests may be discontinued. If a significant decrease is found for several workers, the need for improved hygiene should be examined. If a significant decrease is found for only an exceptional person, that person's work habits should be examined, and if no correction proves possible, it may be decided he or she is unsuited to the job.

Measurement of cholinesterase activity is of some value in clinical evaluation, as well as in occupational hygiene. However, it should be used only in association with thorough clinical and exposure histories and a careful physical examination. The final decision as to when a person who has been poisoned should return to work must be made by the individual's physician only after evaluating the severity of the illness, the length of exposure, the degree of cholinesterase inhibition and the rapidity of its return toward normal, and the intelligence and reliability of the patient and the employer in regard to safety precautions.

Other Measures of Absorption   At least in theory, surveillance of workers could be carried out through measurement of blood or urinary levels of the compound to which they are exposed, or through measurement of a metabolite.

It is possible to estimate absorption of some of the organic phosphorus insecticides by analysis for their metabolic products in urine (Gardocki and Hazleton 1951; Mattson and Sedlak, 1960; Waldman and Krouse, 1952). Urinary levels of *p*-nitrophenol have been used in this way to provide an estimate of parathion exposure (Elliott *et al.,* 1960; Arterberry *et al.,* 1961; Geldmacher-von Mallinckrodt and Deinzer, 1966). There is a broad correlation between the excretion of biotransformation products and the occurrence of illness. Figure 16.3 illustrates the relationship among excretion of paranitrophenol, red cell and plasma cholinesterase activity, and state of health. It may be seen that paranitrophenol may be excreted at a rate of about 0.09 mg/hr, corresponding to a rate of 0.18 mg/hr for parathion, with little or no change in cholinesterase activity. (This result is in good agreement with those in which parathion has been fed to volunteers; see Section 16.7.1.3). However, if absorption of parathion and consequent excretion of *p*-nitrophenol is increased much beyond this level, blood cholinesterase is progressively inhibited and poisoning becomes increasingly likely.

In connection with Fig. 16.3, it should be pointed out that meaningful measurement of the excretion of *p*-nitrophenol by workers is easy because the rate of excretion decreases only slowly after exposure stops. However, corresponding measurements in patients are difficult because the rate of excretion usually decreases rapidly so that a brief delay in collecting the sample results in a value that is not representative of maximal absorption and excretion.

Under circumstances that led to numerous cases of poisoning, urinary *p*-nitrophenol levels remained at 3 ppm in operator-farmers and at 2 ppm in their assistants for about 2 weeks after spraying stopped. In the same area, urinary *p*-nitrophenol values of about 0.6 ppm were found in boys attending school

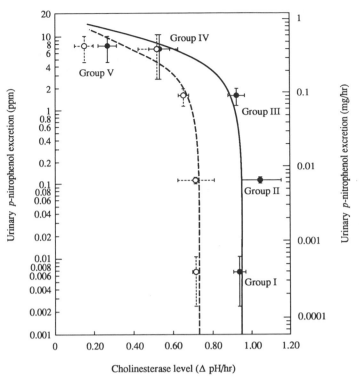

Figure 16.3   Relationship between urinary excretion of *p*-nitrophenol and inhibition of red blood cell (○) and plasma (●) cholinesterases among people with different degrees of exposure to parathion. Group I, planned survey, preexposure period (56 cases); group II, residents near orchard during exposure period (3 cases); group III, planned survey, exposure period (25 cases); group IV, poisoning cases, mild to moderate (7 cases); group V, poisoning cases, severe to fatal (3 cases). Each point represents the mean and associated standard error for a group of cases. Only cases for which both cholinesterase and *p*-nitrophenol values were known are included. The vertical portion of each curve is not related directly to the points shown but represents the average normal cholinesterase value found in the laboratory where the study was made. Modified from Arterberry *et al.* (1961) and reproduced by permission of the American Medical Association.

(Watanabe, 1972c). The latter finding appears to indicate a high level of contamination of much of the area.

Gas chromatographic measurement of metabolites of organic phosphorus compounds in serum or urine is so sensitive that some of them can be detected in people of the general population and at least six can be measured in workers. The most recent improvements in methods for measuring these metabolites are those of Shafik (1973).

Any measurement of compounds or metabolites in blood or urine will give a different kind of information from that derived from measurement of cholinesterase activity because excretion occurs rather rapidly while enzyme activity recovers more slowly. Thus analysis of compounds or metabolites gives information on recent exposure, whereas measurement of cholinesterase values, especially red cell values, gives a kind of summary of the physiological effect of exposure during the preceding month or more. Both kinds of information may be valuable. In view of recent analytical developments, measurement of unchanged compounds in plasma or of compounds or metabolites in urine is a much more sensitive indicator of exposure than is measurement of cholinesterase (Arterberry *et al.*, 1961; Roan *et al.*, 1969). Furthermore, with one exception involving a brain sample, the measurement of metabolites was a more sensitive indicator of exposure than was analysis for intact pesticides. The metabolites permitted a distinction between ethoxy and methoxy compounds. Of course, only successful analysis of the intact compound contributed to specific identification. These conclusions were based on studies of blood, tissue, urine, and/or stomach contents in one very serious and three fatal cases of poisoning (Lores *et al.*, 1978a).

Using a method that revealed no acetylcholine in the plasma of normal persons, concentrations as high as 0.036 ppm were found in the plasma and as high as 0.055 ppm in the cerebrospinal fluid of patients during the acute phase of severe poisoning. The patient with the highest plasma level still had the compound detectable on day 11 of illness and she died suddenly of cardiac complications on day 23 (Okonek and Kilbinger, 1974). Whereas the measurement of acetylcholine is of great theoretical interest, it so far is not helpful in the care of patients.

16.2.2.4 Effects of Other Variables

Diets deficient or excessive in protein, calcium, or magnesium cause a complex pattern of changes in cholinesterase and aliesterase in some but not all tissues of rats that receive no foreign compound; the degree of inhibition of these enzymes by anticholinesterase compounds also is modified by these diets, and the degree of change is different for different compounds (Casterline and Williams, 1969). The activities of some other but not all enzymes are decreased by protein deficiency, and this may influence the interaction of these enzymes with an anticholinesterase (Casterline and Williams, 1971). These findings emphasize the importance of standardizing experimental conditions, but it is questionable whether they have any practical bearing on human safety.

The learning ability of rats was reduced by protein deficiency and reduced even further in rats receiving parathion or carbanolate in a diet containing only 5% protein. The pesticides had no effect on learning when offered in an 18% protein diet (Casterline *et al.*, 1971).

Water deficiency had little effect on the susceptibility of rats and mice to parathion, although it increased their susceptibility to water-soluble drugs (Baetjer, 1973).

16.2.2.5 Pathology

Acute emphysema, pulmonary edema, pink froth in the trachea and bronchi, and considerable congestion of the organs are found at autopsy. Slight microscopic changes may occur in the liver and kidneys (Chadli *et al.*, 1970; Jonecko and Jonecko, 1973). Petechial hemorrhages in the organs may be present, especially if convulsions occurred during life. The findings are not diagnostic.

In a few cases in which death occurred unexpectedly after several days of survival, multiple pericapillary and periprecapillary hemorrhages were noted in the myocardium and medulla oblongata (Fazekas, 1971). Whereas these observations were made in connection with parathion-methyl, there is no reason to think they are peculiar to that compound. To what extent they were the result of prolonged hypoxia is unclear.

Diminished cholinesterase activity in the motor end-plate region in the intercostal muscles of a man whose death was attributed to demeton was demonstrated histochemically (Petty, 1958b). Although poisoning in this particular case undoubtedly was acute, there should be a study of cholinesterase activity of the motor end plates of animals and persons who are clinically well but whose blood cholinesterase activity has been gradually and severely depressed through repeated absorption of moderately heavy but tolerated doses of an anticholinesterase. Furthermore, unpublished records related to the case described by Petty indicated that it was more complex than reported. There is a real question whether demeton was involved, although the depression of cholinesterase and certain clinical aspects of the case leave little doubt that one or more organic phosphorus compounds were at least contributing causes. Evidence brought out the inquest indicated that the victim had been exposed to a mixture of dinitro compounds, and this was confirmed by yellow stains on his hands and one foot. That the dinitro compounds may have contributed to death is suggested by the fact that the patient, who had complained only of dizziness, collapsed and had a convulsion only a few minutes after taking two atropine tablets, that extensor-type rigidity of the muscles was observed during life, and that at death the degree of rigor mortis was extreme.

Whereas myopathic changes associated with excessive acetylcholine (see under Myopathic Changes in Section 16.2.1.3) can be produced dependably in animals and have been reported in human cases, they are not found in all cases, and their demonstration is not necessary for diagnosis.

Enteritis is another change that has been found in experimental studies but is not prominent and certainly is not necessary for diagnosis in humans. In dogs, enteritis was produced by both an organic phosphorus and a carbamate anticholinesterase compound, and the extent and severity of the lesion corresponded well with both the dosage and the degree of illness. The lesion may have been due to local ischemia, as measurement showed that mesenteric arterial blood flow was reduced in dogs with the lesion (Kirkland *et al.*, 1974).

Pancreatitis has been noted occasionally at autopsy, and it was the focus of one paper concerning poisoning by fonofos (see Section 16.11.5). In animals, injury of the pancreas has been noted in dogs and pigs poisoned by Diazinon (Earl *et al.*, 1971), and it has been the subject of continuing research to determine the mechanism of this injury produced by Diazinon (Dressel *et al.*, 1979a,b). Briefly, it was shown that inhibition of acetylcholinesterase increased the secretion of pancreatic juice and increased the intraductal pressure, just as is true of vagal stimulation. The increases of secretion and pressure could be blocked by atropine. It was possible to produce acute pancreatitis characterized by interstitial edema, acinar cell vacuolization, and increased serum amylase and lipase in dogs treated with Diazinon and infused with secretin.

16.2.2.6 Differential Diagnosis

In the absence of laboratory facilities for cholinesterase determinations, brain hemorrhage, heat stroke, heat exhaustion, hypoglycemia, gastroenteritis, and pneumonia or other severe respiratory infections have been confused at times with poisoning by these compounds. Mild poisoning must frequently be distinguished from asthma and from simple fright with various psychosomatic manifestations, particularly among the associates of known poisoning cases. In the past, a number of cases were provisionally diagnosed as poisoning by one of the less toxic organic phosphorus insecticides before a complete investigation of the exposure history and clinical course changed the diagnosis to poisoning by more toxic insecticides, mercury fungicides, or solvents, or even to disease unrelated to pesticides. See Section 8.1.

16.2.2.7 Treatment of Poisoning in Humans

Recommendations In very serious cases of poisoning by organic phosphorus insecticides, the order of treatment should be as follows: (a) artificial respiration, preferably by mechanical means and, of course, with a patent airway; (b) atropine sulfate (2–4 mg) intravenously and repeated at 5–10-min intervals until signs of atropinization appear; (c) pralidoxime chloride (1 gm) slowly, intravenously; (d) decontamination of the skin, stomach, and eyes as indicated; and (e) symptomatic treatment (e.g., inhalation of oxygen).

In the more usual cases, the procedure should be as follows: (a) atropine sulfate (1–2 mg) if symptoms appear, and repeated doses as required by excessive secretions; (b) decontamination of the skin, stomach, and eyes; (c) pralidoxime chloride (1 gm) slowly, intravenously if the patient fails to respond satisfactorily to atropine; and (d) symptomatic treatment.

The sublingual administration of oximes as first aid has been recommended (Luzhnikov and Pankov, 1969).

Pralidoxime chloride is recommended because of its excellence and availability. This oxime and others of real merit have been discussed by Briggs and Simons (1986) and also in Section 8.2.3.3. The following remarks are concerned with problems peculiar to treating poisoning by organic phosphorus compounds.

The recommended dosage of atropine sulfate is greater than that conventionally employed for other purposes but is within safe limits. Atropine sulfate relieves many of the distressing symptoms, reduces heart block, and dries secretions of the respiratory tract. A single dose of as much as 10 mg of atropine sulfate has been inadvertently administered to normal adults without endangering life, although it has, of course, produced very marked signs of overdosage. However, people poisoned by anticholinesterase organic phosphorus compounds have an increased tolerance for atropine sulfate (Freeman and Epstein, 1955). In the presence of severe anticholinesterase poisoning, 600 mg of atropine sulfate was given in a day to one patient

and 1600 mg to another without producing symptoms attributable to it (Hopmann and Wanke, 1974; Warriner et al., 1977). Total doses as high as 240 mg (Zavon, 1962), 453 mg (Milthers et al., 1963), 850 mg (Richards, 1964), 2620 mg (Jax et al., 1977), 3911 mg (Warriner et al., 1977), 11,442 mg (Hopmann and Wanke, 1974), and 30,730 mg (LeBlanc et al., 1986) have been given in severe cases in which the patients recovered from poisoning, although one died later from an unrelated cause. Worrell (1975) successfully treated a 2-year-old, 13.6-kg boy poisoned by Diazinon with a total of 707.2 mg of atropine administered during 19 days. The boy received 32.5 mg during the first 12 hr; the largest single dose was 15 mg. A 14-year-old girl had essentially recovered from parathion poisoning following treatment, including 1122 mg of atropine, but she died of massive hemorrhage from erosion of her innominate artery by her tracheotomy tube (Wyckoff et al., 1968).

The effects of intravenous atropine sulfate begin in 1–4 min and are maximal within 8 min. A mild degree of atropinization should be maintained in all cases for 24 hr and in severe cases for as long as necessary.

Miosis and headache may persist after recovery from poisoning by organic phosphorus insecticides is otherwise largely complete. In some cases, the systemic administration of atropine sulfate is followed by partial or temporary dilatation of the pupils (Chamberlin and Cooke, 1953; Smith et al., 1955; Quinby and Clappison, 1961). Miosis responds more dependably to oximes. If further systemic treatment is not necessary, the miosis and associated headache will respond to the instillation of 0.5–1% atropine sulfate solution or 0.5% atropine sulfate ointment into the eyes (Sachs et al., 1956).

The only practical question about the value of pralidoxime chloride that remains partially unresolved concerns its value in relation to different compounds and especially different groups of compounds. The predominant effect of the oximes is to promote breaking of the bond between acetylcholinesterase and the phosphorus moiety derived from an insecticide. As discussed in Section 16.2.1.3, phosphorylation of the enzyme is thought to be accompanied by cleavage of the insecticide with the most acidic portion as the leaving group. Because the active forms of most organic phosphorus insecticides are dimethoxy or diethoxy phosphates, it follows that enzymes inhibited by them will be mostly dimethoxy- and diethoxy-phosphate esters. A few inhibited enzymes (derived from EPN, leptiphos, dimefox, mipafox, and others) will be other esters.

There is essentially universal agreement that poisoning by diethoxy compounds is treated effectively by oximes (Karlog et al., 1958; Namba and Hiraki, 1958; Imo, 1959; Quinby, 1964). There is also general agreement that the effects of oximes are less spectacular in treating poisoning by dimethoxy compounds as a group (Quinby, 1964). However, there are many cases in which oxime treatment of patients poisoned by dimethoxy compounds was clearly beneficial (Quinby, 1964; Warriner et al., 1977). Thus pralidoxime in particular and oximes in general are recommended when poisoning by either a diethoxy or dimethoxy phosphorus compound is sufficiently severe.

Pralidoxime was given in a total dose of 92,000 mg over a period of 23 days to a patient who recovered without sequelae (Warriner *et al.*, 1977).

The value of oximes for treating poisoning by other groups of organic phosphorus compounds is less clear. The available information is considered in connection with individual compounds.

The action of succinylcholine is greatly potentiated by inhibition of esterases that ordinarily metabolize it. The danger was illustrated by at least two cases in which poisoned patients had to be maintained by artificial respiration for extended periods after receiving the drug (Quinby *et al.*, 1963; Seybold and Braeutigam, 1968). The onset of apnea is sudden. Use of succinylcholine may be indicated in a few patients poisoned by organic phosphorus insecticides, but obviously it should not be administered unless an anesthetist is present and all preparations for assisted respiration are complete.

Definite Contraindications Never give morphine, theophylline, and theophylline ethylenediamine (Johns *et al.*, 1951).

Large amounts of intravenous fluids generally are contraindicated because of the threat of pulmonary edema.

Management of the Patient If pulmonary secretions have accumulated before atropine sulfate has become effective, they should be removed by suction and a catheter. If the stomach is distended, empty it with a Levin tube.

If the patient has not yet shown symptoms or they have been allayed by treatment, he or she must be completely and quickly decontaminated. Smith *et al.* (1955) are apparently the only authors to report injury to attendants in a case involving TEPP. Remove the patient's clothing and, with due regard for his or her condition at the moment, bathe the patient thoroughly. Remove any visible insecticide gently with lots of water and soap or other detergent, if available. Avoid abrasion. When the skin appears clear, bathe or swab with ethyl or isopropyl alcohol. Parathion and many of the other organic phosphorus insecticides are very much more soluble in alcohol than in water, and significant amounts can be removed with alcohol from skin that already has been washed thoroughly with soap and water.

If there is any suspicion that the poison has been ingested or inhaled and if the patient is still responsive, induce vomiting; give some neutral material such as milk or water, and induce vomiting again. The reason for mentioning inhaled material is, of course, that a large portion of such material may be deposited in the upper respiratory tract and subsequently may be carried to the pharynx and swallowed. Nausea may be anticipated, of course, on the basis of the systematic action of organic phosphorus compounds, but if vomiting is not profuse, gastric lavage may be used. It is also important that the intestine be cleared thoroughly.

If there is any reason to think that the eyes may have been contaminated, irrigate them with physiological saline or water. The absorption of some of the organic phosphorus insecticides by the eye is remarkably rapid.

Atropine sulfate does not protect against muscular weakness. Because the usual mechanism of death is respiratory failure, the use of an oxygen tent or even the use of oxygen under slight positive pressure is advisable and should be started early. This may help to prevent injury of the liver and kidneys (see Typical Poisoning in Section 16.2.2.2). Watch the patient constantly, since the need for artificial respiration may appear suddenly. Equipment for oxygen therapy and for artificial respiration should be placed by the patient's bed in readiness while the patient is on the way to the hospital. Cyanosis should be prevented by the most suitable means, since continued hypoxia aggravates the depression of the respiratory center caused directly by the poison. Complete recovery may occur after many hours of artificial respiration have been necessary. Milthers *et al.* (1963) reported complete recovery of a patient who had to be maintained for 5 hr on artificial respiration. (Their fatal cases were given artificial respiration for 10–149 hr.) More recently, patients have recovered completely, although it was necessary to assist their respiration for days (Kramer, 1972; Guenther *et al.*, 1972; Warriner *et al.*, 1977).

The acute emergency may last 24 hr or more. The patient must be watched continuously for several hours after recovery appears essentially complete but for a minimum of 24 hr in any case. Favorable response to one or more doses of atropine sulfate, frequently given as a first-aid measure, does not guarantee against sudden and fatal relapse. Medication must be continued during the entire emergency.

Any person who is ill enough to receive a single dose of atropine sulfate should remain under medical observation for 24 hr because the atropine sulfate may produce only a temporary relief of symptoms in what may prove to be serious poisoning. Freeman and Epstein (1955) mention five patients poisoned with parathion who improved with atropine at first but relapsed and died, evidently because of inadequate maintenance of atropinization.

Following exposure heavy enough to produce symptoms, further organic phosphorus insecticide of any sort should be avoided. The patient may remain susceptible to relatively small exposures to the same or other organic phophorus compounds until regeneration of cholinesterase is nearly complete.

Therapeutic Procedures Requiring Evaluation and a Discussion of Some Old Warnings A dihydroderivative of 2-PAM called Pro-2-PAM was found far superior to 2-PAM in treating poisoning by DFP in mice, rats, and rabbits (Rump *et al.*, 1978). However, a later evaluation involving mice and guinea pigs poisoned by soman, sarin, and DFP concluded that Pro-PAM was not a significant improvement over PAM (Clement, 1979).

Some organic phosphorus compounds are sufficiently water soluble that it is practical to remove them from blood by dialysis. Probably more important, progress has been made in the dialysis of blood against activated charcoal, a process now spoken of as hemoperfusion.

Using concentrations of pesticides that are known to occur in the blood of severely poisoned patients, it was shown (by pumping blood from a tank, through a commercially available unit, and back into a tank) that demeton-S-methyl sulfoxide and dimethoate could be cleared by dialysis from blood at rates of 53 and 59 ml/min, respectively, at a flow rate of 100 ml/min. Dialysis was not effective for parathion. However, hemoperfusion through a column of coated activated charcoal was effective for all three compounds; clearance rates for them (in the order named) were 84, 88, and 59 ml/min. Hemoperfusion was carried out for 7 hr on a patient who had attempted suicide with parathion and who already had suffered irreversible brain damage as the result of hypoxia during cardiorespiratory arrests. Although there was no possibility of saving the man, measurements made on blood withdrawn at intervals from the inlet and outlet of the charcoal column served to show that clearance occurred at a rate of 73 ml/min at a flow rate of 161 ml/min. This indicated 31 liters "cleared" during the 7 hr this treatment was continued or, put another way, the elimination of about 0.4495 mg of parathion. The concentration of parathion in the blood averaged 0.0145 ppm, much less than in some patients who have survived. One hour after hemoperfusion, the concentration in the blood returned to its original level, as a result of either redistribution from the tissues or continuing absorption from the intestine, or both (Okonek, 1976a).

Whether the presently possible rate of removal of parathion from the blood would make a sufficient contribution to the survival of persons severely poisoned by it remains to be determined. However, it must be emphasized that the clinical value of hemoperfusion in the management of severe liver failure based on either infection or any of several drugs or other poisons (Gazzard et al., 1974) or in the management of poisoning by barbiturates, glutethimide, and methyl salicylate (Vale et al., 1975) already is well documented. In fact, marked success was claimed in the treatment of three men poisoned by parathion-methyl. The blood was separated, and the plasma line was carried through columns containing uncoated charcoal (Luzhnikov et al., 1977). Favorable results also have been reported in connection with hemodialysis against soybean oil (Jax et al., 1977).

Although the practical value of hemoperfusion in the treatment of poisoning by different organic phosphorus compounds remains to be determined, it appears to be safe. In one case, a slight reduction of red cells and platelets was the only side effect observed (Inoue et al., 1979).

Prompt clinical improvement has been reported following repeated injections of purified human cholinesterase (Klose and Gutensohn, 1976; Jax et al., 1977). However, the value of the method remains unproved.

Lopez (1970) gave a very glowing account of the benefit of various corticosteroid compounds in treating acute poisoning by both organic phosphorus and carbamate insecticides. He administered atropine and 2-PAM only to patients who failed to respond promptly to one or more corticosteroids. The method appears to deserve further evaluation without, of course, neglecting the proven benefits of atropine and 2-PAM.

The Soviet literature (e.g., Lapushkov, 1973) reports the value of camphor, potassium chloride, vitamin C, and a variety of other vitamins. Certainly, potassium chloride or other salts

should be administered to any patient whose blood chemistry demonstrates this particular need. However, the specificity of these remedies in treating poisoning by organic phosphorus insecticides remains to be proved.

Ganglionic blocking agents (discussed in Section 16.2.1.2) have been used in treating patients (Luzhnikov, 1966), but information is inadequate for evaluating them either separately or in combination with other kinds of drugs.

A protein-free calf serum extract of low molecular weight had no antidotal effect in rats poisoned by various organic phosphorus compounds when given alone, but it potentiated the effects of atropine and Toxogonin (Bruener et al., 1977).

It has been reported that the inhibition of cholinesterase activity in the liver and brain of rats was reversed when L-histidine was administered along with an inhibitor, phosphamidon (Vyas et al., 1977).

A paper by Wood (1950) is the origin of the usual warning: Do not give atropine to a severely cyanotic patient; give artificial respiration first and then give atropine sulfate. In dogs poisoned by intravenous injection of TEPP, delay in administration of atropine for longer than 4–5 min may result in rapid death from ventricular fibrillation following injection of atropine. If respiratory paralysis has occurred before atropine administration, ventricular fibrillation follows that therapy in every instance. In the dog with paralyzed respiration, administration of artificial ventilation before atropine therapy allows recovery (Wills et al., 1950). In treating human cases, a decision on whether to give atropine immediately or wait until respiration is restored must be based on medical judgment. It is hoped that few patients will be in such an advanced state of poisoning when first seen that atropine cannot be given at once. The fact that no reports of cases of sudden death following administration of atropine have been found indicates that there may be a marked species difference so that the danger of giving atropine in the presence of cyanosis in human cases is small or simply that few, if any, patients have the degree of cyanosis involved in the animal studies.

Another warning in the literature has been against the use of phenothiazine derivatives in cases of poisoning by organic phosphorus compounds. This warning grew out of the unusual and complicated case of a mentally deficient man who was poisoned by a mixture of insecticides; the illness was inexplicably prolonged, although it was so mild at first that the patient was treated at home. The major complication was the patient's agitation, to combat which promazine was first administered on the ninth day of illness. The appearance of other complications and persisting if not increased restlessness led to hospitalization on the evening of the eleventh day; the promazine was continued. Next morning the patient had a convulsion, became incontinent, went into shock, and died at 1:20 a.m. It was concluded that the death might have represented potentiation of the organic phosphorus poisoning by promazine (Arterberry et al., 1962). This hypothesis was tested in rats using both promazine and chlorpromazine. A small but statistically significant potentiation of the toxicity of parathion but not of mevinphos was found (Gaines, 1962; Orzel and Weiss,

1966). Potentiation of the effects of dichlorvos by chlor-promazine in rats has been reported (Michaelek and Stavinoha, 1977). However, it was concluded that this potentiation was not necessarily related to the cholinergic systems of the brain (Michaelek and Stavinoha, 1978). The interaction of chlor-promazine with parathion may involve permeability of the blood–brain barrier (Vukovich et al., 1971). Because the degree of potentiation in rats was small, one must consider the possibility that the death of the patient under discussion may have been entirely a side effect of the phenothiazine tranquilizer. Certainly, a severe hypotensive reaction has followed small doses of these drugs in persons never exposed to an organic phosphorus compound (Burnstein and Sampson, 1955). On the other hand, phenothiazines have been used in the treatment of patients poisoned by organic phosphorus compounds without observed injury and with the clinical impression that they were beneficial (Luzhnikov, 1966). It seems unlikely that decisive evidence will be forthcoming regarding possible potentiation by phenothiazine drugs of human poisoning by organic phosphorus compounds. The question is moot. In the meantime, it would seem best to administer diazepam to those few patients poisoned by organic phosphorus compounds who require tranquilization. Diazepam increased the therapeutic effect of atropine and an oxime in rats poisoned by phosphamidon (Gejewski, 1974).

16.2.3 PREVENTION OF POISONING

Essentially all of the measures discussed in Chapter 9 should be employed to prevent injury by the more toxic organic phosphorus insecticides.

Perhaps more than any other group of pesticides, these compounds have been subject to regulation of use. Some compounds of this group may be the only ones for which medical surveillance has been required as a condition of use, as is done in California. Similar surveillance of these materials has been carried out elsewhere without legal requirement. At its best, the system leads to education of the physician as well as the user, and it generally involves some kind of test to help regulate exposure (see Abnormal Cholinesterase Values and Their Interpretation and Other Measures of Absorption under Section 16.2.2.3).

16.3 POTENTIATION AND ANTAGONISM

16.3.1 POTENTIATION

A general discussion of potentiation and methods for measuring it is presented in Section 2.4.3.1. The following re-emphasizes a few points and offers further details regarding potentiation by certain pairs of organic phosphorus compounds.

Apparently, the first report of potentiation involving an organic phosphorus insecticide was that of Rider et al. (1951), who found that a combination of schradan and neostigmine led to "toxic side effects."

The discovery of potentiation of the toxicity of malathion by EPN (Frawley et al., 1957) led to a ruling by the Food and Drug Administration that no tolerance would be granted for an organic phosphorus insecticide until its ability to participate in potentiation had been tested in connection with every organic phosphorus compound for which a tolerance was in effect. This ruling, as well as the scientific interest of the subject, generated a large number of tests. The results of some that were published are summarized in Table 16.12, which is concerned almost entirely with pesticides. Extensive studies were made of the interaction of malathion with other organic phosphorus compounds, many of them not pesticides (Casida, 1961; Casida et al., 1963). Briefly, it was found that many combinations with malathion exhibit a moderate degree of potentiation but, whereas no combination of malathion with another insecticide gave as much potentiation as that with EPN, a combination of malathion with tri-o-cresyl phosphate (TOCP) produced an 88- to 134-fold potentiation (Murphy et al., 1959). [Incidentally, TOCP interacts in a very complex way with many other insecticides but the alterations of toxicity are not dramatic (Lynch and Coon, 1972).]

Most combinations of other compounds have only an additive reaction. When potentiation does occur, it is restricted to the effects of one or a few doses and generally is of small magnitude and doubtful clinical significance. The only potentiation of possible importance involved malathion and TOCP. The latter is not a pesticide, and the two are unlikely to be encountered together.

In general, potentiation depends on interference with the detoxication of a compound that ordinarily is not highly toxic but is rendered toxic by anything that prevents its usually rapid detoxication. Most of the compounds that are potentiated contain a carboxy ester group (e.g., malathion) or carboxamide group (e.g., dimethoate), and the potentiating compounds inhibit the enzymes normally responsible for detoxication (Seume and O'Brien, 1960b). Most attention has been given to malathion. Many papers (Murphy and DuBois, 1957; Cook et al., 1958; DuBois, 1958; Rosenberg and Coon, 1958; Casida, 1961; Casida et al., 1963; DuBois et al., 1968; Su et al., 1971; Cohen and Murphy, 1971a) have been devoted to its potentiation by compounds that inhibit carboxylesterase and to the measurement of this and related enzymes. In the case of malathion, the metabolite, whose rapid formation under ordinary conditions accounts for the low toxicity of malathion, is a monoacid formed by the removal of one alcohol group from the diethylsuccinate portion of the molecule (Cook and Yip, 1958).

Inhibition of a normally protective enzyme such as carboxylesterase depends, of course, on the dosage of the inhibitor. As an exception that proves the rule, it was shown that potentiation of the toxicity of malathion by parathion (a compound that does not potentiate under practical conditions) can be demonstrated in animals protected by atropine and oximes (Ramakrishna and Ramachandran, 1977).

Carboxyesterase inhibition alone is not adequate to predict the relative capacities of various compounds to potentiate the toxicity of malathion (Cohen and Murphy, 1971b). Dosages of

Table 16.12
Potentiation of Insecticides

Compounds	Degree of potentiation		Reference
	Positive	Negative	
azinphos-methyl			
+ demeton		<additive	DuBois (1958)
+ parathion		<additive	DuBois (1958)
+ trichlorfon	1.5×		DuBois (1958)
chlorothion + Phostex®	some		Rosenberg and Coon (1958)
demeton + methyl parathion		yes	Zatatzian *et al.* (1960)
demeton + methyl parathion		questionably	Williams *et al.* (1958c)
diazinon + DDT		yes	Kocher and Treboux (1957)
EPN			
+ acethion	80%[a]		Seume and O'Brien (1960a)
+ acethionamide	80%[a]		Seume and O'Brien (1960a)
+ azinphos-methyl		additive	DuBois (1958)
+ chlorothion	some		Rosenberg and Coon (1958)
+ *cis*-mevinphos		0[a]	Seume and O'Brien (1960a)
+ *cis*-thionomevinphos	15%[a]		Seume and O'Brien (1960a)
+ demeton		<additive	DuBois (1958)
+ demeton	some		Williams *et al.* (1958c)
+ diazinon		10[a]	Seume and O'Brien (1960a)
+ dimethoate	100%[a]		Seume and O'Brien (1960a)
+ EL-241	*in vitro*		Hoffman *et al.* (1968)
+ endoate-methyl	100%[a]		Seume and O'Brien (1960a)
+ fenitrothion	10×		Ramakrisna and Ramachandran (1978)
+ methyl methprothion	100%[a]		Seume and O'Brien (1960a)
+ Narlene®	100%[a]		Seume and O'Brien (1960a)
+ parathion		additive	DuBois (1958)
+ parathion		yes	Rosenberg and Coon (1958)
+ parathion	10×		Ramakrisna and Ramachandran (1978)
+ schradan		yes	Rosenberg and Coon (1958)
+ *trans*-mevinphos		0[a]	Seume and O'Brien (1960a)
+ *trans*-thionomevinphos	85%[a]		Seume and O'Brien (1960a)
+ trichlorfon		<additive	DuBois (1958)
+ trichlorfon		0[a]	Seume and O'Brien (1960a)
fraction commercial dimethoate			
+ pure dimethoate	3–4×		Casida and Sanderson (1961)
+ malathion	some		Casida and Sanderson (1961)
+ *O,O*-dimethyl *S*-carbamoylmethyl phosphorodithioate	some		Casida and Sanderson (1961)
malathion			
+ azinphos-methyl		<additive	DuBois (1958)
+ azinphos-methyl	*in vitro*		Cook *et al.* (1958)
+ azinphos-methyl	some		Williams *et al.* (1958c)
+ azinphos-methyl	some		Knaak and O'Brien (1960)
+ azinphos-methyl	*in vivo*		Seume and O'Brien (1960a)
+ bis(dimethylamido)fluorophosphate		yes	Rosenberg and Coon (1958)
+ chlorothion	*in vitro*		Cook *et al.* (1958)
+ chlorothion	some		Rosenberg and Coon (1958)
+ demeton	*in vitro*		Cook *et al.* (1958)
+ demeton		additive	DuBois (1958)
+ diazinon	*in vitro*		Cook *et al.* (1958)
+ dichlofenthion	*in vitro*		Cook *et al.* (1958)
+ dichlorvos	some		Tracy (1960)
+ EPN	"very toxic"		Anonymous (1956)
+ EPN	*in vitro*		Cook *et al.* (1958)
+ EPN	50× (dogs)		Frawley *et al.* (1957)
+ EPN	10× (rats)		Frawley *et al.* (1957)
+ EPN	100%[a]		Seume and O'Brien (1960a)
+ EPN	*in vitro*		Murphy and DuBois (1957)
+ EPN	1.8×		DuBois (1958)
+ EPN	some		Rosenberg and Coon (1958)

(*continued*)

Table 16.12 (*Continued*)

Compounds	Degree of potentiation		Reference
	Positive	Negative	
+ EPN	some		Awad and Karczmar (1960)
+ malathion	*in vitro*		Cook *et al.* (1958)
+ methyl cellosolve	severalfold		Casida and Sanderson (1961)
malathion			
+ mevinphos	*in vitro*		Cook *et al.* (1958)
+ paraoxon	*in vitro*		Cook *et al.* (1958)
+ paraoxon	*in vitro*		Cook *et al.* (1958)
+ paraoxon		<additive	DuBois (1958)
+ paraoxon		yes	Rosenberg and Coon (1958)
+ paraoxon		at least additive	Seume *et al.* (1960)
+ parathion-methyl	*in vitro*		Cook *et al.* (1958)
+ phorate	*in vitro*		Cook *et al.* (1958)
+ Phostex®	some		Rosenberg and Coon (1958)
+ physostigmine		yes	Rosenberg and Coon (1958)
+ ronnel	*in vitro*		Cook *et al.* (1958)
+ schradan		yes	Rosenberg and Coon (1958)
+ sulfotepp	*in vitro*		Cook *et al.* (1958)
+ TOCP	88–134×		Murphy *et al.* (1959)
+ TOCP	100%[a]		Seume and O'Brien (1960a)
+ TOCP	8×		Casida (1961)
+ trichlorfon	*in vitro*		Cook *et al.* (1958)
+ trichlorfon	2.2×		DuBois (1958)
methyl cellosolve			
+ Dow ET 15	some		Casida and Sanderson (1961)
+ ronnel	some		Casida and Sanderson (1961)
parathion + parathion-methyl	minimal		Williams *et al.* (1958c)
Phostex® + EPN	some		Rosenberg and Coon (1958)
schradan			
+ neostigmine	"toxic side effects"		Rider *et al.* (1951)
+ parathion		yes	Rosenberg and Coon (1958)
TOCP			
+ acethion	100%[a]		Seume and O'Brien (1960a)
+ acethion amide	60%[a]		Seume and O'Brien (1960a)
+ diazinon	30%[a]		Seume and O'Brien (1960a)
+ dimethoate	100%[a]		Seume and O'Brien (1960a)
+ endoate-methyl	30%[a]		Seume and O'Brien (1960a)
+ methyl methprothion	100%[a]		Seume and O'Brien (1960a)
+ Narlene®	100%[a]		Seume and O'Brien (1960a)
+ trichlorfon	20%[a]		Seume and O'Brien (1960a)
TPT			
+ acethoin	90%[a]		Seume and O'Brien (1960a)
+ acethion amide	100%[a]		Seume and O'Brien (1960a)
+ diazinon		10%[a]	Seume and O'Brien (1960a)
+ dimethoate	100%[a]		Seume and O'Brien (1960a)
+ endoate-methyl	60%[a]		Seume and O'Brien (1960a)
+ malathion	100%[a]		Seume and O'Brien (1960a)
+ methyl methprothion	100%[a]		Seume and O'Brien (1960a)
+ Narlene®	80%[a]		Seume and O'Brien (1960a)
+ trichlorfon		10%[a]	Seume and O'Brien (1960a)
trichlorfon			
+ demeton		<additive	DuBois (1958)
+ parathion		additive	DuBois (1958)

[a] Seume and O'Brien injected half an LD 10 of each compound simultaneously. The result is expressed as percentage mortality observed in a group.

TOCP greater than that necessary to produce maximal inhibition of carboxylase produce a dosage-related inhibition of maloxon binding in the liver, thus freeing the active agent for inhibition of cholinesterase (Cohen *et al.*, 1972).

The action of an inhibitor is likely to extend beyond any one class of enzymes (Casida *et al.*, 1963). For example, EPN, which inhibits cholinesterase and various aliesterases, also inhibits isocarboxazid amidase. Isocarboxazid is a monoamine oxidase inhibitor. Its hydrolysis by its amidase was consistently inhibited by EPN at dosages of 0.5–2.5 mg/kg for 3 days, although this caused no inhibition of cholinesterase. The amidase was almost completely inhibited after a single dose of EPN in the range of 5 to 15 mg/kg, and this inhibition occurred sooner and persisted longer than cholinesterase inhibition (Satoh and Moroi, 1973).

It appears that some compounds must be metabolized in order to potentiate (Cook *et al.*, 1958) or in order to potentiate more fully (Casida, 1961), but this relationship has not been explored fully.

Because different classes of enzymes may be inhibited, the effects may be complex and potentially at least could extend to interactions with drugs as well as interactions with other insecticides. Potentiation also may involve solvents or other components of formulated pesticides. Thus, of four compounds (tetrachlorvinphos, chlorpyrifos, leptophos, and phosfolan) chosen for study, all were more toxic as formulations than as technical materials (El-Sebae *et al.*, 1978). Another example is that associated with demeton (see Section 16.7.3.2).

Potentiation may be demonstrated not only in intact adult mammals but also in the chick embryo (Marliac and Mutchler, 1963). However, potentiation must ultimately be judged by direct evidence concerning the species in question. If evidence regarding humans is not available, evidence from experimental animals must be considered with the usual caution. Evidence based on enzyme inhibition *in vitro* may be of great value in identifying modes of action. However, *in vitro* studies never can be depended on for a quantitative evaluation of potentiation between a pair of compounds. Cohen and Murphy (1971b) established this point by comparing the ability of EPN, parathion, and temephos to inhibit the metabolism of diethyl succinate, triacetin, methyl butyrate, and malathion *in vitro* and the ability of the same compounds to potentiate malathion *in vivo*. Even the use of malathion as an *in vitro* substrate was not a satisfactory substitute for *in vivo* testing.

Finally, caution must be exercised in interpreting *in vitro* studies of enzyme inhibition as mechanisms of *in vivo* potentiation. For example, Knaak and O'Brien (1960) confirmed that EPN potentiated the toxicity of malathion *in vivo* in both dogs and rats but found that, contrary to expectations, the concentration of malaoxon was not increased and in the dog the overall rate of urinary excretion was increased rather than decreased. The authors reached the not entirely satisfying conclusion that potentiation of malathion by EPN must be caused by increased persistence of malaoxon at the target site, rather than by its increased concentration there.

Separate reasons for questioning the idea that potentiation of malathion toxicity by EPN depends simply on protection of

malathion from decarboxylation were supplied by Karzcmar *et al.* (1962). They found some potentiation when EPN was administered intravenously 45 min after an otherwise subeffective, intravenous dose of malathion and reasoned that much of the malathion already had been metabolized during this interval. They found that the toxicity of EPN alone depends on a high degree of inhibition of central, especially medullary, cholinesterase, but malathion action is mainly peripheral. This raises the possibility that potentiation by the two compounds depends on combining central and peripheral action.

The interval between administration of another compound and administration of malathion that leads to maximal potentiation varies from less than 1 hr to more than 24 hr, depending on the compound. However, by 72 hr after a single dose, the degree of potentiation is greatly reduced (Casida *et al.*, 1963).

Actual potentiation requires not only that the interacting compounds be present simultaneously or almost simultaneously but also that both be present at toxic or near-toxic levels. It was pointed out by DuBois (1961) that there is no danger from residues of potentiating compounds in food, provided the individual tolerance levels are not exceeded. Apparently, the only instance in which potentiation was the cause of poisoning under occupational conditions involved malathion formulations that had deteriorated during tropical storage (see Use Experience in Section 16.6.1).

16.3.2 ANTAGONISM

Antagonism sufficient to combat poisoning by organic phosphorus compounds has been discussed in Section 2.4.3.1 in connection with drugs useful for that purpose. In addition, it has been known for many years that chlorinated hydrocarbon insecticides show a small but measurable antagonism to the action of organic phosphorus insecticides. Undoubtedly the main basis for this interaction is the induction of mixed-function microsomal enzymes by the chlorinated hydrocarbon insecticides. However, in addition, Mayer and Himel (1972) have shown that chlorinated hydrocarbon insecticides compete with certain fluorescent probes for a hydrophilic site adjacent to the anionic site on horse serum cholinesterase. This binding of a large chlorinated molecule, although it does not inhibit cholinesterase, may reduce access of organic phosphorus molecules to the esteratic site.

16.4 NONANTICHOLINESTERASE EFFECTS OF ORGANIC PHOSPHORUS COMPOUNDS

16.4.1 POLYNEUROPATHY

16.4.1.1 Background

A thorough review of the neurotoxic effects of various organic phosphorus compounds is beyond the scope of this book. Tens of thousands of people have been severely crippled by tri-*o*-cresyl phosphate, a compound without any known pesticidal action. Likewise, most compounds studied in the laboratory to determine whether they are capable of producing neurotoxicity either are not pesticidal or are too toxic in other ways to consider for this application. By contrast, not more than about 100 cases (including those of doubtful diagnosis) have resulted from compounds used as pesticides or considered for that use. The following paragraphs emphasize information on the neurotoxicity of organic phosphorus pesticides and offer only as much background information as seems essential to provide perspective. Those interested in the broader aspects of the matter should consult reviews by Cavanagh (1964, 1973), Aldridge and Barnes (1966a,c), Johnson, (1975b,c), and Freemon (1975).

A Perspective on Neuropathy Neuropathy is an abnormal, noninflammatory condition of peripheral nerves and/or tracts within the central nervous system. The cell bodies may or may not be severely involved. Mononeuropathy is confined to a single nerve and may have an origin as obvious as trauma, neoplasm, or vascular damage. Multiple local injuries, such as multiple emboli, may cause a condition called mononeuropathy multiplex. Whereas this can occur on both sides of the body, it is inherently asymmetrical.

Polyneuropathy is a symmetrical neuropathy of systemic origin. Before the noninflammatory character of the lesions was emphasized, it often was referred to as multiple neuritis. Polyneuropathy in humans usually begins with burning and tingling, especially in the feet. Motor weakness, which is the cardinal symptom, begins a few days later in the feet. Both sensory and motor difficulty may extend to the legs and to the hands. Objective signs of sensory loss, in a stocking and glove distribution, usually are present. The gait is high stepping and involves some ataxia. Patients suffer little spasticity if they recover completely or almost completely within a few months. However, patients who are more severely and permanently affected usually develop spasticity as well as ataxia.

Some old causes of polyneuropathy undoubtedly antedate history, and they have been recognized medically for a long while. The underlying causes include nutritional deficiency (e.g., beriberi and, at least to some extent, alcoholic polyneuropathy), hereditary defect (e.g., Freidreich's ataxia and the polyneuropathy of acute intermittent porphyria), infection (e.g., poliomyelitis), the toxic effects of infection (e.g., diphtheria), and various toxicants (e.g., mercury, lead, thallium, and arsenic). Palsies of workers exposed to mercury and lead were mentioned by Ramazzini (1713), who cited Roman authors to the same effect. An early medical discussion of polyneuropathy associated with alcohol is that of Jackson (1822).

Where people are well fed on the average, most polyneuropathy now is associated with diabetes and alcoholism (Freemon, 1975). Nearly all other cases are of idiopathic origin. There is no indication that the proportion of idiopathic cases is increasing. However, the fact that a growing number of compounds, mainly drugs, clearly have been associated with human polyneuropathy increases the ever-present temptation to assign a cause to each idiopathic case. The result is that a large number of compounds have been alleged to be the cause of occasional cases, often in persons who had little or no exposure, rather than in those with heavy exposure.

More constructively, increasing awareness of the dosage-related danger of polyneuropathy of toxic origin has contributed to greater care in the testing and use of drugs and other chemicals. At least as important in the long run, each effective toxicant constitutes a tool for exploring the nature of the underlying biochemical lesions associated with different classes of etiological agents and perhaps eventually gaining better understanding and control of those forms of polyneuropathy that affect substantial numbers of people.

A review of peripheral neuropathy (Cavanagh, 1973) reveals not only the diversity of etiological agents mentioned above and displayed in Table 16.13, but also a variety of morphological lesions. The nerve cell as a whole may be attacked (poliomyelitis infection and mercury poisoning). The Schwann cell (lead) or the oligodendrocyte, its counterpart in the brain, may be attacked, leading to secondary segmental disintegration of the axon. Finally, the axon may be subject to Wallerian degeneration that begins in the part most distant from the cell body and may extend a variable distance toward the cell body, a process simply described by Cavanagh as "dying back" and more recently, but no more informatively, called "distal axonopathy" (Spencer and Schaumburg, 1976). This kind of degeneration may be associated secondarily with degeneration of myelin, and it was this aspect of the whole change that was seen and correctly described in connection with the first great outbreaks of poisoning by tri-o-cresyl phosphates (Smith and Lillie, 1931).

However, Goodale and Humphreys (1931) early recognized that the axon as well as the myelin sheaths are fragmented in people poisoned by TOCP. Later, it was shown that in hens poisoned by TOCP (Cavanagh, 1954), or by DFP (Fenton, 1955), the earliest functional disturbances coincided with the appearance of structural change in the most distal, nonmyelinated portion of the nerves. Although demyelination occurs a little later in association with degeneration of more proximal portions of nerves, it is largely Wallerian in pattern, and not segmental, as is seen in primary demyelinating conditions such as diphtheria and lead neuropathy (Cavanagh, 1954, 1973). The same kind of selective involvement is seen in axons within the spinal cord.

By use of an electron microscope it is possible to visualize changes in the axons of small myelinated motor nerve terminals in the foot muscles and in small myelinated fibers in the spinal gray matter of cats treated with TOCP a week or more before the onset of neurological signs and several weeks before changes can be seen with the light microscope. Similar changes, confined essentially to large-diameter fibers, appear later.

The ultrastructural changes occurring in TOCP neuropathy do not indicate whether the mechanism leading to distal degeneration of axons in this neuropathy is due to a direct attack by the chemical on the axon or is secondary to a metabolic failure at the level of the nerve cell body (Prineas, 1969). Experiments

Table 16.13
Some Causes of Polyneuropathy in Humans[a]

Principal injuries and conditions or compounds causing them	Onset	Duration	Animal model	Remarks
Cell death				
poliomyelitis		permanent	monkey	
organic mercury	7–30 days		rat, cat	
Schwann cell injury				
diphtheria toxin	7–12 days	weeks	hen, rabbit	injury mainly paranodal
lead	variable	weeks	guinea pig	
Dying back of axon				
Freidreich's ataxia	adolescence	progressive	none	
beriberi	insidious	prolonged		vitamin B_1 involved
alcohol	insidious	prolonged		
nitrofurans	10–14 days			vitamin B_1 involved
arsenic		prolonged	none	pyruvate metabolism involved
isoniazid[b]			rat	vitamin B_6 preventive
carbon disulfide		prolonged	cat, monkey	vitamin B_6 involved
porphyria[c]				
tri-o-cresyl phosphate	7–14 days	very prolonged	hen[d]	see text for mechanism
p-bromophenylacetyl urea			rat[e]	
tetraethylthiuram disulfide		prolonged		
diethydithiocarbamate			hen, rabbit	
thalidomide	90+ days	very prolonged	none	
thallium			dog	
acrylamide				
vinca alkaloids	3 days		rodents	
plasmocid			rat, monkey	
trichlorethylene		prolonged		
n-hexane				
chlorobiphenyl				
methyl-n-butyl ketone			rat, cat	
chlorinated hydroxyquinolines (e.g., cliquinol)				

[a] This table summarizes information, most of which was reviewed by Cavanagh (1973), where references may be found.

[b] Other B_6 antagonists that cause polyneuropathy are hydralazine, L-penicillamine, and the hydroxylamine group.

[c] See pyrroloporphyria in Table 2.12.

[d] Does not work well in partridge, rat, or guinea pig.

[e] Does not work in chicken.

with cats (Pleasure *et al.*, 1969) and chickens (James and Austin, 1970) rule out the possibility that the injury involves interference with slow axonal transport of protein. The studies do not exclude the possibility of interference with axonal transport of some other necessary substance. In the cat, transport of protein was at an average rate of 1.3–1.6 mm/day. Apparently, fast axonal transport (approximately 410 mm/day in sensory nerves and 930 mm/day in motor nerves) demonstrated in the cat (Ochs *et al.*, 1969) has not been explored in animals suffering from neurotoxicity.

Of course, the dying back may be so extreme that the entire neuron dies. However, more commonly the dying of the axonal tips is accompanied by a reparative process in the cell body and in the living part of the axon relatively near the cell body. The reaction within the cell body is called chromatolysis. The nucleus increases in size, and dry mass, and the synthesis of nuclear RNA increases. The orderly blocks of nucleoprotein (Nissl bodies) in the cytoplasm are broken up, so that the rough endoplasmic reticulum and ribosomal arrays are dispersed. The cell increases in size and in water content at such a rate that its concentration of RNA remains constant in spite of increased production. All of this is considered an indication of heightened metabolic activity directed to restitution of the damaged axon. Chromatolysis is considered a response of an essentially healthy cell (Cavanagh, 1973).

Eosinophilic swellings may be seen in long fiber pathways. Such swellings seem to be due to accumulations of smooth membranes and other intraaxonal organelles within greatly dilated axons and terminals. They tend to be located just proximal to nodes of Ranvier. Cavanagh (1973) has suggested that these swellings represent frustrated attempts at axonal repair. Some others have emphasized the contribution the swellings may make to necrosis of that part of the axon distal to them.

Later studies demonstrated that, at least in the cat, the initial lesion was focal and subterminal but later spread to involve the entire distal part of the axon. Degeneration was preceded by nerve fiber varicosities and paranodal demyelination (Bouldin and Cavanagh, 1979a,b).

There have been great improvements in methods for studying the light and electron microscopic changes associated with different kinds of neuropathy. Cavanagh (1973) has furnished a list of useful procedures and references to the major techniques involved. However, while acknowledging the very real advances in methods of observing dying back, it must be emphasized that its effects have been recognized for a long while. Sharkey (1896) stated it this way: "It is a somewhat remarkable thing that in multiple neuritis the terminal portions of the nerves are nearly always first affected."

A study using intraarterial injection of DFP and the most modern morphological techniques showed that no change was detectable in the terminal of motor nerves until extensive changes had occurred in the postjunctional apparatus (first seen at 7 days) and then begun to resolve (14 days). Only in conjunction with extensive axonal degeneration was secondary postjunctional atrophy noted. Reinnervation of the neuromuscular junctions occurred 28–56 days after DFP was injected. It was accomplished by sprouting from the undamaged portions of the original axon to that end plate (Glazer, 1976).

As pointed out by Cavanagh (1973), the functional effect at a particular nerve ending is identical, whether the extent of the break is 10 μm or 1 m. However, the time required for recovery depends greatly on the extent of the lesion. First, regrowth occurs at a rate of approximately 1 mm/day, so that a 1-mm lesion may recover in 1 day, whereas a 1-m lesion will require at least 2.74 years. Second, in order to be effective, the axon must grow back to its original point of synapse. To do this, it follows the supporting structures of the peripheral nerve or central tract of which it is a part. In practice, functionally effective regrowth becomes disproportionately more difficult the greater its extent, and it is far less efficient in the central nervous system than in the peripheral nerves. Thus a 1-m lesion that theoretically might be repaired in 2.74 years may last a lifetime.

That dying back can be the end result of completely different biochemical lesions is suggested by the fact that different animal models are effective for studying different compounds, all of which cause polyneuropathy in humans (see Table 16.13). For example, rodents are sensitive to several of the compounds but are quite useless for studying the polyneuropathy caused by certain organic phosphorus compounds. That dying back can have fundamentally different causes is suggested also by the fact that different toxicants produce different distributions of lesions, both as regards sensory and motor and as regards the central and peripheral nervous systems. There is direct evidence also. Beriberi is caused by a deficiency of vitamin B_1 and can be corrected by small dosages of it, even the amounts present in nutritious food. Several compounds that interfere with pyruvate metabolism, which depends on thiamine, cause polyneuropathy. It is thought that the polyneuropathy caused by some other compounds is the result of interference with vitamin B_6 (pyridoxime), and patients show a deficiency of this vitamin, as evidenced by positive tryptophan-load tests. The administration of pyridoxal or pyridoxamine has a clear-cut protective effect in both humans and animals against the polyneuropathy caused by isoniazid (Cavanagh, 1973).

No significant disturbance in pyruvate metabolism has been found in birds poisoned by TOCP or its metabolites (Earl *et al.*, 1953; Baron and Casida, 1962), or by any other neurotoxic organic phosphorus compound. Polyneuropathy caused by these compounds has not been prevented or alleviated by large dosages of vitamin (Johnson, 1975b). On the contrary, these compounds inhibit an enzyme that is linked to polyneuropathy but is not known to be influenced by other classes of compounds or by diseases associated with polyneuropathy.

Early History of Polyneuropathy Associated with Organic Phosphorus Compounds The history of paralysis due to organic phosphorus compounds dates back to the last years of the nineteenth century, when phosphocreasote was used to treat pulmonary tuberculosis (Lorot, 1899). At that time the exact chemical nature of the material producing paralysis was unknown. However, as early as 1930, Smith and his colleagues (1930a,b) established that TOCP, which had been used to fortify certain lots of extract of Jamaica ginger, was the etiological agent of a large number of cases of paralysis occurring in the United States. In the following year, Smith and Lillie (1931) showed that this "ginger paralysis" or "jake leg" was accompanied by a demyelination of the nerve sheaths. It was estimated by the U.S. Bureau of Prohibition that some 20,000 persons became paralyzed during 1930 as a result of drinking contaminated Jamaica ginger (Kidd and Langworthy, 1933). Whereas some of the victims recovered fairly promptly, some remained affected for life. Eleven such men were the subject of medical reexamination 47 years after they consumed TOCP. All of them had suffered some degree of paresis of both lower and upper extremities, usually involving footdrop plus wristdrop combined with clawed hands. All had experienced complete or nearly complete recovery of hand and arm function. However, only one of the 11 was able to walk without crutches or a cane. Only one suffered any type of impotence for a time after onset. At the time of reexamination, the men showed mild dementia that may have been explained by advanced age and cerebrovascular atherosclerosis but that may have been influenced by TOCP directly (Morgan and Penvich, 1978).

An outbreak involving approximately 10,000 persons occurred in Morocco in 1959 after a mixture of olive oil and aircraft lubricating oil was sold as food (Smith and Spalding, 1959; Geoffroy *et al.*, 1960). Some other outbreaks have involved entirely accidental contamination of food during shipping or storage (Sorokin, 1969) or the substitution of TOCP for cooking oil (Jordi, 1952).

The 1930 outbreak of poisoning led to a very thorough study. It was soon learned that different species show extreme variation in their susceptibility to the paralytic affects of TOCP (Smith *et al.*, 1930a,b, 1932; Koelle and Gilman, 1946). The hen was found to be most susceptible and has remained the preferred laboratory animal for studying this kind of injury. According to a personal communication from Dr. John Barnes, chickens do not become fully susceptible to paralytic effects until they are 55–70 days old. The essential difference between the chick and adult hen in their responses to neurotoxic organophosphorus compounds is not understood. It does not, as one might expect, involve the degree of activity of what is now called neuropathy target esterase (NTE) (see Section 16.4.1.3), which is not greatly different in the brains of chicks and hens (Johnson and Barnes, 1970). The rates of excretion in chickens of different ages may have some bearing on the matter. The half-lives of leptophos were 1.5 and 4.9 days in 6- and 21-day-old hens, respectively (Konno et al., 1977; Konno and Kinebuchi, 1978a).

Some difference between species can be explained on the basis of absorption. If this is taken into account, a fairly typical paralysis can be produced in dogs, monkeys, and especially cats. Rabbits and guinea pigs given enough TOCP to produce any effect do not show the characteristic delay and go on to die in 5–14 days. Rats are virtually immune to poisoning by TOCP, but histological study shows that they may develop distal, axonal degeneration, even though ataxia and paralysis are not evident. Leptophos was found neurotoxic in lambs and mice, and EPN was positive in mice (El-Sebae et al., 1977), but there are few reports of neurotoxicity in mice.

It has become customary to speak of both the polyneuropathy caused by certain organic phosphorus compounds and also of the entire process leading to this polyneuropathy as "neurotoxicity." Compounds are said to be neurotoxic if they produce polyneuropathy in one or more species. Contrary to the root meaning, the terms neurotoxicity and neurotoxic are avoided in connection with other forms of injury to the nervous system, for example, convulsions. In a completely different context, a few authors have used the word neurotoxicity to mean behavioral changes induced by a toxicant. This aspect of toxicity is reviewed briefly in Section 16.2.2.2.

16.4.1.2 Structure–Activity Relationships in the Neurotoxicity of Organic Phosphorus Compounds

It is an observed fact that a few organic phosphorus compounds produce neurotoxicity, but the majority do not. It is possible that some compounds that failed to produce this affect when tested would be able to do so if administered at a higher dosage level. However, it is customary to make the test in animals protected by atropine, oximes, or a combination of the two in order to minimize anticholinergic effects. Thus, there is no direct way to test substantially higher doses *in vivo* than those already investigated. Furthermore, some of the compounds that have not produced neurotoxicity are of low toxicity in other ways also and have been given in massive dosages, whereas some compounds that do produce neurotoxicity do so at very low dosage levels, some at less than 1 mg/kg (see Table 16.14).

Triphenyl Compounds of Category IV   The discovery that TOCP produces paralysis in humans and animals led to several studies of its analogs. Most of the analogs that produce neurotoxicity contain one or more 2-methylphenyloxy groups. In fact, O-2-methylphenyl-O,O-4-methylphenyl phosphate, and

O,O-2-methylphenyl-O-4-methylphenyl phosphate are both somewhat more active than O,O,O-2-methylphenyl phosphate. However, not all 2-methylphenyl compounds are active. For example, O-2-methylphenyl-O,O-diethyl phosphate, O-2-methylphenyl-O,O-2-ethylhexyl phosphate, O,O-2-methylphenyl chlorophosphate, and O,O-2-methylphenyl hydrogen phosphate are all inactive at dosage levels of 1000 mg/kg or higher (Hine et al., 1956).

Although O,O,O-2-ethylphenyl phosphate (Hine et al., 1956) and O,O,O-2-propylphenyl phosphate (Bondy et al., 1960) are inactive, several compounds with one or two 2-ethylphenyl or 2-isopropylphenyl moieties and with no 2-methylphenyl moiety are active (Bondy et al., 1960).

Activity is not limited to compounds with one or more phenyl groups substituted at the 2-position. O,O,O-4-Ethylphenyl phosphate is neurotoxic (Bondy et al., 1960; Silver, 1960; Aldridge and Barnes, 1961). However, with this exception, no triphenyl compound is known to be neurotoxic without an alkyl substitution at the 2-position of at least one of the phenyl rings and no other substitution on that ring (Smith et al., 1932; Hine et al., 1956; Bondy et al., 1960). Phosphites (e.g., O,O,O-2-methylphenyl phosphite) and phosphine oxides (e.g., 2-methylbenzyl phosphine oxide) are inactive (Hine et al., 1956).

Neurotoxicity is not entirely confined to phosphorus compounds; it is produced by O,O,O-2-methylphenyl borate (Hine et al., 1956).

Aldridge (1954) showed that the neurotoxicity of TOCP could be greatly enhanced by incubation with a liver homogenate, and enhancement by intact rats was established by Myers et al., (1955). Later, it was shown (Casida et al., 1961; Eto et al., 1962) that the active metabolite is a cyclic compound called o-cresyl saligenin phosphate (see Table 16.14). The lowest effective dosage of this compound is 4–8 mg/kg, compared to 200 for the parent compound. The exactly comparable cyclic compound derived from O,O-2-methylphenyl-O-4-methylphenyl phosphate is even more active, its lowest effective dosage being 0.25 mg/kg (Casida et al., 1963). Several other cyclic compounds are active also (Casida et al., 1963; Aldridge and Barnes, 1966a).

It may be that the marked difference in the ability of different triphenyl phosphates to produce neurotoxicity is the result of the ability of some and the inability of others to form ring compounds similar to the two just mentioned. However, this is speculative. So far, no one has proposed a way by which one dependably could predict the neurotoxicity of a triphenyl phosphate from examination of its structural formula.

The situation was revealed as immeasurably more complicated by the discovery of other classes of organic phosphorus compounds that are neurotoxic.

Fluorine Compounds of Category II   It was shown by Koelle and Gilman (1946) and later confirmed by others that diisopropyl phosphofluoridate (DFP) is neurotoxic. The occurrence of neurotoxicity in humans following exposure to another fluorine compound, mipafox (Bidstrup and Hunter, 1952;

Table 16.14
Neurotoxicity to Hens or Lack of It in Pesticides and a Few Other Selected Compounds[a]

Compound	Route	Lowest lethal dosage (mg/kg)[c]	Highest dosage not neurotoxic (mg/kg)[c]	Compounds found neurotoxic[b]			Reference
				Lowest neurotoxic dosage (mg/kg)[c]	Delay in onset (days)	Duration of ataxia (days)[d]	
Fluorine-containing organic phosphorus compounds of category II (Table 16.15)[e]							
DFP[f]	sc			1	yes	per.	Barnes and Denz (1953)
	sc			1	yes	per.	Davison (1953)
	—			1	yes	per.	Fenton (1955)
	im			0.3	yes	per.	D. R. Davies et al. (1960)
	—			0.4	yes	per.	Lancaster (1960)
mipafox	po			20	yes	per.	Barnes and Denz (1953)
	sc			20	yes	per.	Davison (1953)
	sc			60[g]	yes	per.	Durham et al. (1956)
Dimethoxy compounds of category IV (Table 16.16)[e]							
azinphos-methyl	sc	150	20	40	<1	3–5	Gaines (1969)
carbophenothion-methyl	sc	800	160	320	<1	7–26	Gaines (1969)
chlorothion	sc	1,200	1,600	—	—	—	Durham et al. (1956)
crotoxyphos	sc	200	50	100	<1	ca. 1	Gaines (1969)
dicapthon	sc	300	100	200	<1	3–30	Gaines (1969)
dichlorvos	sc	20[g]	160	—	—	—	Durham et al. (1956)
	sc		30	—	—	—	Aldridge and Barnes (1966a)
				100 + 100[h]	yes	per.	Johnson (1975c)
dicrotophos	sc	15	15	—	—	—	Gaines (1969)
dimethoate	sc	175		—	—	—	Gaines (1969)
fenitrothion	sc			—	—	—	Gaines (1969)
	po		500		—	—	Kadota et al. (1975b)
	po				—	—	Freed et al. (1976)
fenthion	sc	40		25[g]	<1	3–10	Gaines (1969)
malathion	sc	1,400[g]	50	100	<1		Durham et al. (1956)
	sc	1,000		100	<1	4–14	Gaines (1969)
	po			10,000 ppm	yes	?	Frawley et al. (1956); Frawley (1976)
menazon	sc	600		400[g]	<1	4–11	Gaines (1969)
mevinphos	sc	3	3	—	—	—	Gaines (1969)
oxydemeton-methyl	sc			—	—	—	Gaines (1969)
parathion-methyl	sc			—	—	—	Barnes and Denz (1953)
	sc	200	32	64	<1	3–28	Gaines (1969)
phosphamidon	sc	20	20	—	—	—	Gaines (1969)
ronnel	sc	1,600	800	1,600	<1	4–24	Witter and Gaines (1963a); Gaines (1969)
SD-7438	sc	300	100	200	<1	3–20	Gaines (1969)
temephos	sc	1,000		125[g]	<1	6–31	Gaines (1969)
trichlorfon	sc	125	125	—	—	—	Witter and Gaines (1963a); Gaines (1969)
	sc		200	200 + 100[i]	yes	per.	Johnson (1970)
Diethoxy compounds of category IV (Table 16.35)[e]							
carbophenothion	sc			640	2–7	15–49	Witter and Gaines (1963a)
	sc	640	320	640	<1	35–>53	Gaines (1969)
chlorfenvinphos	sc	200	200	—	—	—	Gaines (1969)
chlorpyrifos	sc	200	100	200	3–18	10–20	Gaines (1969)
coumaphos	sc	100[g]		100	<1	16–24	Gaines (1969)
demeton	sc	20[g]	80	—	—	—	Durham et al. (1956)
	po		1,600 ppm	—	—	—	Frawley et al. (1956)
diazinon	sc	15[g]	80	—	—	—	Durham et al. (1956)
dioxathion	sc	320	160	320	<1	3–31	Gaines (1969)
disulfoton	sc	>50	16	32	<1	3–13	Gaines (1969)
ethion	sc	1,200	200	400	<1	7–71	Gaines (1969)
methosfolan		2.8	2.8	—	—	—	Abou-Donia et al. (1974)
parathion[j]	—			—	—	—	Barnes and Denz (1953)
	po		1,600 ppm	—	—	—	Frawley et al. (1956)

(continued)

Table 16.14 (*Continued*)

| Compound | Route | Lowest lethal dosage (mg/kg)[c] | Highest dosage not neurotoxic (mg/kg)[c] | Compounds found neurotoxic[b] | | | Reference |
				Lowest neurotoxic dosage (mg/kg)[c]	Delay in onset (days)	Duration of ataxia (days)[d]	
phorate	sc	48	16	32	<1	4–14	Gaines (1969)
phosfolan		5.2	5.2	—	—	—	Abou-Donia *et al.* (1974)
TEPP			100	—	—	—	D. R. Davies *et al.* (1960)
Other dialkoxy compounds of category IV (Table 16.49)[e]							
isopropyl paraoxon	sc			—	—	—	Barnes and Denz (1953)
isopropyl parathion	sc			—	—	—	Barnes and Denz (1953)
	sc		15	—	—	—	Davison (1953)
TIPP	sc		8	—	—	—	
	sc			—	—	—	
Diamino compounds of category IV (Table 16.49)[e]							
schradan	sc		320	—	—	—	Durham *et al.* (1956)
	sc		300	—	—	—	Davison (1953)
Chlorethoxy compounds of category IV[e]							
O,O-di(2-chloroethyl)-p-nitrophenyl phosphate[k]				100[g]	yes	per.	Aldridge and Barnes (1966a)
haloxon	po			200 × 3	yes	per.	Aldridge and Barnes (1966a)
	po			500[l]	—	—	Johnson (1975c)
	iv			13[l]	—	—	Johnson (1975c)
Trithiobutyl compounds of category IV (Table 16.49)[e]							
DEF	ip	100		50 × 5	14	per.	Baron and Johnson (1964)
	sc	200		200[f]	14–28	30	Gaines (1969)
	sc		200	1,100[m]	yes	per.	Johnson (1970)
merphos	ip			100 × 10[n]	yes	per.	Baron and Johnson (1964)
	sc	600	400	600	3–21	90	Gaines (1969)
Triphenyl compounds of category IV and their derivatives[e]							
TOCP[o]				50	yes	per.	Smith *et al.* (1930a,b)
	po			500	yes	per.	Barnes and Denz (1953)
	po			500	yes	per.	Cavanagh (1954)
	—			200	yes	per.	Hine *et al.* (1956)
	sc	200	100	200	yes	per.	Durham *et al.* (1956)
	po			2,500 ppm	yes	per.	Frawley *et al.* (1956)
	po			100 ppm	yes	per.	Frawley (1976)
o-cresyl saligenin phosphate	ip			4–8	9–11	yes	Baron and Casida (1962)
p-cresyl saligenin phosphate	ip			0.25–0.50	yes	per.	Casida *et al.* (1963)
Mixed constituent compounds of category IV (Table 16.49)[e]							
crufomate	sc	400		400	<	4–64	Gaines (1969)
cyanofenphos	po			10	yes	per.	Reichert and Abou-Donia (1979)
DMPA	—				yes	per.	Casida and Baron (1976)
EPBP	po		400	800	yes	per.	Abou-Donia *et al.* (1979)
EPN	po			600 ppm	yes	per.	Frawley *et al.* (1956)
	sc	80	20	40	1	6–330	Durham *et al.* (1956); Gaines (1969)
	po			50 ppm	yes	per.	Frawley (1976)
	po	10	10	25	20–22	per.	Abou-Donia and Graham (1979)
ethyl-O-ethyl-2,4,5-trichlorophenyl phosphonothionate[p]	ip			100	yes	per.	Aldridge and Barnes (1966a)
	po	140	160	180	8–14	per.	Abou-Donia *et al.* (1974) Abou-Donia and Preissig (1976a)
	po			500	yes	per.	Johnson (1975c)
	po			250	12	per.	Kinebuchi *et al.* (1976)
	po			200	7	per.	Yatomi *et al.* (1978)

(*continued*)

Table 16.14   (Continued)

Compound	Route	Lowest lethal dosage (mg/kg)[c]	Highest dosage not neurotoxic (mg/kg)[c]	Lowest neurotoxic dosage (mg/kg)[c]	Delay in onset (days)	Duration of ataxia (days)[d]	Reference
				Compounds found neurotoxic[b]			
desbromoleptophos	po			50	yes	per.	Abou-Donia (1979a)
methyl-O-ethyl-2,4-dichlorophenyl phosphonothionate	—			100	yes	per.	Aldridge and Barnes (1966a)
Carbamates (Table 19.3)[e]							
carbaryl	sc	800	800	1,600	<1	4–24	Gaines (1969)
propoxur	sc			—	—	—	Gaines (1969)
aminocarb	sc			—	—	—	Gaines (1969)
4-benzothienyl-N-methylcarbamate	sc	48	16	32	<1	4–14	Gaines (1969)
3,5-diisopropylphenyl-N-methylcarbamate	sc			—	—	—	Gaines (1969)
isolan	sc			—	—	—	Gaines (1969)
mexacarbate	sc			—	—	—	Gaines (1969)
2-(2-propynyloxy)phenyl-N-methylcarbamate	sc			—	—	—	Gaines (1969)
3,4,5 trimethylphenyl-N-methylcarbamate	sc	400	—	200	<1	1–3	Gaines (1969)

[a] Organic phosphorus compounds are arranged according to the classification in Section 16.1.

[b] A series of dashes (—) in the three columns headed "Compounds found neurotoxic" indicates that the compound was *not* neurotoxic at the highest dosage tested. An "x" in the column headed "Lowest neurotoxic dosage" indicates that the compound was found neurotoxic but the dosage was not reported. The word "yes" in the column headed "Delay in onset" indicates that a classic delay (about 10–15 days) was reported. The abbreviation "per." in the column headed "Duration of ataxia" indicates that the neurotoxicity was permanent within the limits of the experiment.

[c] Dosage expressed as mg/kg unless stated otherwise; ppm indicates a dietary level.

[d] Duration from onset, even in instances where onset is significantly delayed.

[e] Structural formulas are shown in the table indicated.

[f] Doses that caused severe ataxia caused greater than 90% inhibition of NTE. *In vitro* the I 50 was 0.7 μM (Johson, 1975c).

[g] Lowest dosage reported.

[h] Massive doses of dichlorvos caused high inhibition of NTE.

[i] This dosage caused 68% inhibition of NTE activity.

[j] A 15 mg/kg dosage given subcutaneously caused only trivial inhibition of NTE, and *in vitro* the I 50 was over 100 μM (Johson, 1975c).

[k] The lowest neurotoxic dosage caused marked inhibition of NTE; *in vitro* the I 50 was 10 μM (Johson, 1975c).

[l] Inhibited NTE by only 22 or 23%.

[m] Inhibited NTE activity by 77%.

[n] Baron and Johnson (1964) reported that hens tolerated repeated oral or intraperitoneal doses at the rate of 100 mg/kg with signs of weakness only.

[o] An oral dosage of 250 mg/kg inhibited NTE by 96% (Johson, 1975c).

[p] The compound apparently requires biotransformation for neurotoxicity. *In vitro* it showed no significant inhibition of NTE; *in vivo* it inhibited this enzyme only moderately (Johnson, 1975b,c).

Bidstrup *et al.*, 1953), led to a number of studies of this compound and, of course, the demonstration that it was neurotoxic to chickens. Later it was shown that a whole series of fluorophosphates containing either one or two alkyloxy side chains were neurotoxic to chickens, several of them at the level of 1 mg/kg or less (D. R. Davies *et al.*, 1960; Lancaster, 1960). Even dicyclohexylphosphorofluoridate is neurotoxic (D. R. Davies *et al.*, 1960). Nearly all of the compounds tested were of the =O sort, but diethylphosphorofluorodithioate is also neurotoxic (D. R. Davies *et al.*, 1960; Lancaster, 1960). On the contrary, a series of phosphenic fluorides, that is, compounds with two alkyl groups rather than at least one alkoxy group, were found not to be neurotoxic (D. R. Davies *et al.*, 1960).

The members of category III (see Section 16.1) are not

fluorine compounds and, according to D. R. Davies *et al.*, (1960), they are not neurotoxic, even though some of them, like category II compounds, are highly toxic and have other properties characteristic of chemical warfare agents.

Chlorinated Dialkoxy Compounds of Category IV   Of the compounds reported, most but not all of the small number containing one or two $ClCH_2CH_2O$ groups cause irreversible neurotoxicity (Aldridge and Barnes, 1966a). Why this group is neurotoxic in combination with certain moieties with no neurotoxic action of their own but not with others is not understood. The relationships are as inexplicable at present as those among the triphenyl compounds. It is clear, of course, that great caution is indicated in the use of chlorethoxy compounds as pesticides.

Chloro-*n*-propoxy compounds have not proved neurotoxic (Aldridge and Barnes, 1966a).

Trithioalkyl Compounds of Category IV All trithiobutyl compounds tested are neurotoxic in hens (Table 16.14), and merphos and DEF have produced polyneuropathy in workers (see Sections 16.10.1.3 and 16.10.2.3).

Mixed Substituent Compounds of Category IV Frawley *et al.* (1956) and Durham *et al.* (1956) apparently were the first to show that a compound of category IV with nonidentical basic constituents (EPN) produced permanent paralysis in hens. The most thorough single study of the group is that of Aldridge and Barnes (1966a). Studies of EPN and other compounds of the group are outlined in Table 16.14. Compounds that have been studied in regard to neurotoxicity or other effects in humans are discussed in Section 16.11.

Why compounds of category IV with nonidentical basic groups tend to be neurotoxic is entirely unknown. It is true that such compounds contain a phosphorus–carbon bond, and the same is true of trichlorfon (see Section 16.6.6), which (perhaps because of contaminants) is neurotoxic under certain circumstances. As reviewed by Menn and McBain (1974), the P—C bond of methyl-, ethyl-, and phenyl phosphates resists metabolism by mammals. However, it seems unlikely that the P—C bond is directly related to neurotoxicity, inasmuch as many fluoride, chlorinated dialkoxy, trithioalkyl, and substituted triphenyl compounds lack the P—C bond but are neurotoxic.

Discussion It is true that, in homologous series of alkyl phosphorus esters that contain a neurotoxic member, the activity increases rapidly as the size and/or the hydrophobic nature of the alkyl group is increased, until near maximal activity is reached at *n*-butyl (Johnson 1975a). It is interesting but not necessarily illuminating that antiacetylcholinesterase activity does not change greatly in the series from methyl to *n*-butyl, and, therefore, the ratio of neurotoxicity to lethality increases upward in a homologous series (Johnson, 1975c).

The ease with which some triaryl phosphates form saligenin compounds offers a neat explanation of their neurotoxicity. Knowledge of chemistry offers some possibility of explaining why other triaryl compounds have little tendency to form such compounds or are likely to form excretable compounds before a critical concentration of saligenin can be reached.

In spite of some progress, there is still much mystery about why some compounds of phosphorus or of boron are neurotoxic and others are not.

16.4.1.3 Characteristics of Polyneuropathy Caused by Organic Phosphorus Compounds

Kinds of Polyneuropathy The only kind of neurotoxicity associated with organic phosphorus compounds that unques-

tionably has occurred in humans is the classic form involving an initial delay in onset and a prolonged course. Many cases fit the stereotype of a 10–14-day delay in onset, followed by paralysis lasting the remainder of the victim's life. However, there are exceptions. Even with TOCP, some cases recover within a year (Bermejillo, 1971), but the proportion of severe cases with such rapid recovery is less than 2% (Geoffroy *et al.*, 1960). Furthermore, there seems to be no doubt that the syndrome varies in humans, depending on the toxic agent as well as on the dose. The variation in duration of human illness associated with different compounds is discussed further in Section 16.4.1.4.

Although not confirmed in human patients, an immediate neuropathy characterized by relatively rapid reversibility has been described in the hen by Durham *et al.* (1956). Further examples were reported by Frawley *et al.* (1956), Frawley (1976), Witter and Gaines (1963a), and Gaines (1969). In this condition, which they spoke of as "muscle weakness," paralysis typically appears within the first 24 hr and lasts for only a few days or weeks, the hen going on to complete recovery. Although the use of a separate name for this rapidly reversible condition is justified, the term "muscle weakness" was an unhappy selection because while hens are suffering from the condition, their clinical state is indistinguishable from that seen in classical neurotoxicity; the muscles do not appear involved in the primary action, although muscle wasting eventually takes place in the classical form of the disease.

It is interesting that, under laboratory conditions, the effects of DFP, which always are delayed and usually are permanent, can be made temporary. Close intraarterial injection of DFP in cats produced some changes detectable in as little as 2 weeks, and the cats showed weakness of the affected leg 3–4 weeks after injection. Deficiency of motor nerve terminal function was maximal in 3 weeks. Recovery was essentially complete in 8 weeks (Lowndes, 1973; Lowndes *et al.*, 1973). This suggests that the process of dying back depends primarily on a direct toxic action on the distal part of the axon but that simultaneous injury to the nerve cell body prolongs the process of repair.

Following intraarterial injection of DFP, a change in reaction to endrophonium can be detected in 24 hr (Lowndes *et al.*, 1975). Apparently, this test has not been run on systemically dosed cats or chickens.

In spite of the striking difference in chronicity, it is difficult to believe that immediate and delayed neurotoxicity are unrelated in their biochemical lesions. However, the nature of the lesion is incompletely known in one instance and unstudied in the other. It has been reported (Frawley *et al.*, 1956; Frawley, 1976) that demyelination does not occur in animals suffering from reversible neurotoxicity caused by malathion; this was confirmed by unpublished results in another laboratory. It would be interesting to see whether there is any disintegration of the unmyelinated nerve endings in immediate neurotoxicity, such as that in those described by Cavanagh (1964, 1973) in connection with delayed neurotoxicity.

Although most compounds that produce neurotoxicity of

any sort produce either the delayed irreversible or the immediate reversible form just described, there is really a spectrum of effects. As shown in Table 16.14, there is no delay in the onset of paralysis caused by carbophenothion and EPN, but the injury produced by these compounds appears irreversible, at least in most hens, and typical demyelination was found by Frawley *et al.* (1956) in hens fed EPN. In addition to these clear-cut instances, there are others in which a difference in syndrome has been claimed. For example, it was considered by Silver (1960) that O,O,O-4-ethylphenyl phosphate produced somewhat different effects from those of TOCP (O,O,O-2-methylphenyl phosphate). Other examples might be found.

Some investigators have failed to accept immediate, temporary neurotoxicity seen in hens as a real phenomenon, viewing it as merely the weakness that constitutes a part of acute anticholinesterase poisoning. Apparently, those who hold this view have never taken the trouble to examine affected chickens. The two conditions are quite distinct clinically, although words have sometimes been used in a way that could not have been more confusing. As already noted, Durham *et al.* (1956) referred to temporary neurotoxicity in hens as muscle weakness, although the muscles were strong and only their control was lacking. Conversely, Wadia *et al.* in 1974 used the term "type II paralysis" and in 1977 used the term "delayed paralysis" in referring to the profound weakness that characterizes some human cases of acute poisoning. The delay they specified varied from 2 to 96 hr, and one of the paralytic signs they specified was "inability to sit up with arms folded." Certainly, one cannot quarrel with this use of "delayed paralysis" as a clinical description, but the condition described must not be confused with polyneuropathy, and was not so confused.

A set of neurotoxic symptoms have been observed in humans prior to those of delayed neuropathy and clearly following those of acute toxicity. It occurs from 1 to 4 days after organophosphate poisoning and is characterized by muscle weakness primarily in the neck flexors and proximal limb muscles, cranial nerve palsies, perfuse diarrhea (where severe loss of potassium and fluids appears to complicate the poisoning), and respiratory depression which, if not treated immediately, could lead to death. Respiratory difficulty appeared in patients who were conscious and not suffering from miosis or fasciculation. Thus, with the inclusion of this "intermediate syndrome," the sequelae of human organophosphate intoxication may now be considered to be triphasic. The respiratory systems signaled the onset of the syndrome in the 10 cases observed, all of which had a well-defined acute cholinergic phase. Knee and ankle reflexes were substantially impaired or absent in the majority of cases, with transient dystonic movements of the limbs noted in some patients suffering from fenthion poisoning. Electromyographic analysis of muscle function, however, showed a tetanic fade as opposed to the characteristic denervation associated with polyneuropathy. Recovery time from onset of the syndrome ranged between 4 and 18 days. Treatment included atropine at doses up to 40 mg in 24 hr and pralidoxime at the rate of 1 gm every 12 hr for 24–48 hr. In some cases, immediate endotracheal intubation and mechanical ventilation were required for varying periods up to 28 days. Administration of intravenous fluids and electrolyte therapy were usually required to maintain circulatory function inhibited by the effect of persistent diarrhea. Initial atropine therapy for acute cholinergic symptoms did not alter the development of the syndrome (Senanayake and Karalliedde, 1987; Karalliedde and Senanayake, 1988).

Pesticides primarily responsible for this syndrome include fenthion, monocrotophos, dimethoate, and methamidophos. Dicrotophos has been reported to cause respiratory paralysis 6 days following intoxication (Perron and Johnson, 1969). Malathion and Diazinon have also been associated with symptoms resembling those of intermediate syndrome (Gadoth and Fisher, 1978; Wadia *et al.*, 1974). While central nervous system components may contribute to this syndrome, postsynaptic dysfunction at the neuromuscular junction seems to be the predominant factor at this time (Senanayake and Karalliedde, 1987).

Neurotoxicity, whether delayed or immediate, prolonged, or reversible, is characterized by incoordination; muscle weakness, if any, is secondary. The hind legs mainly are affected. The forelimbs show less or even no effect. The muscles of respiration are almost always spared. The person or animal is alert until starvation intervenes.

By contrast, acute poisoning involves true muscle weakness, which is far more generalized than the incoordination just discussed. The muscles of respiration often are involved in severe cases, and this may be the immediate cause of death.

Mode of Action   It was not until the antiesterase activity of TOCP and related compounds was noted by Bloch (1941) and emphasized by Koelle and Gilman (1946) that a long series of studies was begun to explore the possibility that inhibition of plasma cholinesterase or some other esterase might be responsible for neurotoxicity. Briefly, it was found that some compounds that produce moderate, brief inhibition of cholinesterase are neurotoxic, whereas others that produce profound, prolonged inhibition are not neurotoxic. When neurotoxicity occurs, its course does not parallel the degree of cholinesterase inhibition (Cavanagh, 1964, 1973). The ataxia is not prevented or modified by atropine, eserine, or cholinesterase reactivators administered before or after the neurotoxic agent. Finally, it was found that O,O,O-2-methylphenyl phosphate is neurotoxic, even though it does not inhibit either true or pseudocholinesterase (Aldridge and Barnes, 1961).

Some compounds that potentiate the anticholinesterase action of malathion are neurotoxic to hens, but there are many exceptions (Casida, 1961).

The idea that inhibition of cholinesterase is related to neurotoxicity has been dropped (Aldridge and Barnes, 1966b), but it is difficult to abandon the idea that some antiesterase activity is of importance. This is especially true because a few carbamate anticholinesterases, which appear to have little in common with organic phosphorus compounds except their ability to inhibit enzymes, are capable of producing reversible neurotoxicity (see Section 16.4.1.4), whereas others discussed below are capable of blocking the action of compounds that otherwise produce permanent neurotoxicity.

Until recently, no chemical reaction, whether *in vitro* or *in vivo*, was known by which a neurotoxic compound could be distinguished from one lacking that property. The first progress to this end was reported in a preliminary way by Aldridge *et al.* (1969) and in greater detail by Johnson (1969a). Incubation of radioactive DFP with nervous tissue and subsequent washing to remove unreacted reagent was used as a test in searching for a tissue component that reacts with neurotoxic compounds but not with otherwise similar organic phosphorus compounds. Since it was recognized that neurotoxic compounds react with a wide range of esterases, an effort was made to block non-specific reaction sites by means of nonneurotoxic compounds. It was shown that when each of several neurotoxic compounds of different types was administered to living hens, it was bound to a constituent of nervous tissue not affected in a parallel experiment by a close but nonneurotoxic analog. Paired samples of a soluble fraction from the brains of hens previously dosed with a neurotoxic compound combined with essentially the same amount of radioactive DFP, no matter whether they were preincubated with TEPP or TEPP plus mipafox, the difference being only 2–10 pmol/gm. On the contrary, soluble fractions from the brains of hens previously dosed with a non-neurotoxic analog and then incubated with TEPP plus mipafox bound significantly less DFP than fractions incubated with TEPP alone, the difference being 14–43 pmol/gm. It was clear from the chemical procedure that the specific binding site was on a large molecule, most likely a protein, although proof of its exact chemical nature as an esterase was not established until a little later (Johnson, 1969b). Evidence was given that the specific binding site is present in brain in a concentration of about 68 pmol/gm, as compared to 136–156 pmol/gm for cholinesterases in the same tissue. The specific site constitutes 4–5.5% of all phosphorylation sites (about 700 pmol/gm) in the brain and spinal cord of hens and in ox brain but is completely undetectable in plasma, the only nonnervous tissue tested. About 70% of the esterase in question was recovered in a microsomal fraction of adult hen brain, and there was some evidence that this fraction contained many small synaptosomes. Nuclear and mitochondrial fractions were low in esterase. It was concluded that early events of organic phosphorus neuropathy involve the axonal and perhaps the synaptic surface (Richardson *et al.*, 1979). Indicative of a causal relationship is the fact that the degree of inhibition of the specific esterase corresponded to the severity of the pharmacological response (Olajos *et al.*, 1978). The fact that progress has been made toward identification of an enzyme or other reactive site specifically associated with neurotoxicity offers hope that the physiological function of this entity may be found and the mechanism of neurotoxicity can be explained.

The esterase phosphorylated by neurotoxic organic phosphorus compounds has been renamed neuropathy target esterase (NTE) (Johnson, 1987) because the original name "neurotoxic esterase" could be misconstrued as a natural toxin (Johnson, 1969b). Since the original name was frequently used in the literature, it must be understood that inhibition of the enzyme, not its normal function, is associated with polyneuropathy. NTE activity has been found in the hen spinal cord, sciatic nerve (Olajos *et al.*, 1978; Olajos and Rosenblum, 1978), lymphocytes (Dudek *et al.*, 1979), and other tissues of the adult bird (Dudek and Richardson, 1982). However, human NTE activity appears to have a comparatively wider tissue distribution (Moretto *et al.*, 1983).

While the minimum dose of organic phosphorus compounds required to induce anticholinesterase effects is a function of the alkoxy and aryl groups attached to the central phosphorus atom, the production of delayed neuropathy seems to be associated with a number of phosphonate compounds containing a variety of leaving groups (see Sections 16.4.1.2 and 16.4.1.4).

Some compounds are direct inhibitors of NTE; others are indirect inhibitors, requiring metabolic change in order to become active. The nature of the metabolism is understood in some instances, as illustrated in the case of TOCP (see Triphenyl Compounds in Section 16.4.1.2). However, why the precursor is inactive and the metabolite is active is not clear, as is true in the case of inactive =S— and active =O— inhibitors of cholinesterase. Furthermore, the time necessary for metabolism of neurotoxic compounds contributes only about a day to the delay of about 2 weeks that is characteristic of classical neurotoxicity.

The present understanding of the initiation of organophosphate-induced delayed neuropathy is based on the inhibition and modification of NTE in an "aging" process outlined in Fig. 16.4 (Johnson, 1987). Although the exact mechanism of the NTE aging process is presently unknown and is probably much more complex than a simple hydrolysis reaction, the reaction is rapid for simple dialkyl phosphates ($t_{1/2} = 1$–4 min) (Johnson, 1987).

Further evidence that permanent inhibition of an enzyme is involved in irreversible ataxia is the finding that some carbamates that react with the "neurotoxic" site *in vitro* are protective when given to living hens prior to administration of a neurotoxic compound. It may be assumed that such a carbamate temporarily occupies the critical site while the neurotoxic compound is available for reaction but later releases the enzyme, leaving it free to perform its normal function. Phenyl benzylcarbamate and phenyl phenylcarbamate were found especially effective (Johnson and Lauwerys, 1969).

Certain sulfonates and phosphinates also have a protective action, presumably for the same reason. However, the fact that phosphinates behave in this way indicates that mere phosphorylation of the active site of neurotoxic enzyme cannot be the cause of irreversible neurotoxicity. A hypothesis has been proposed that phosphates, phosphoramidates, and phosphonates bound to the enzyme undergo aging, whereas phosphinates do not. Aging would yield an ionized acidic group on the phosphorus and, according to the hypothesis, it is this combination of an ionized group on the phosphorus bound to the enzyme that leads to ataxia (Johnson, 1974). Further study confirmed that aging occurs. Reactivation of neurotoxic esterase was possible only immediately after a brief inhibition,

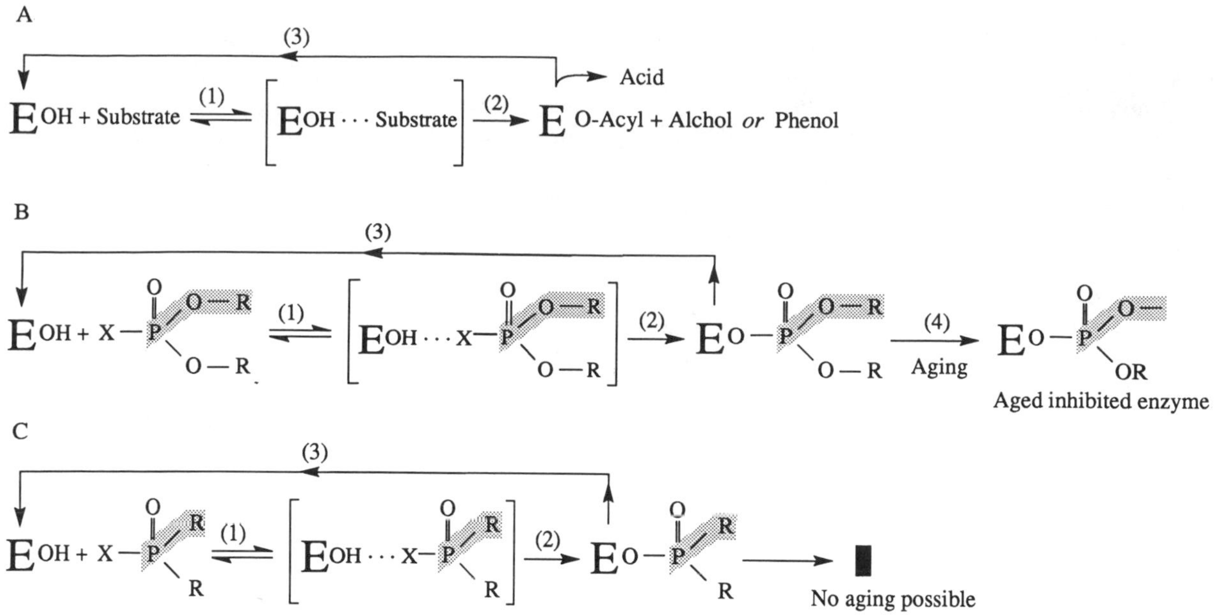

Figure 16.4   Reaction steps for a typical β-esterase (organophosphate-sensitive serine hydrolase). A. Reaction with substrate. (1) is the reversible formation of a Michaelis complex. (2) is the formation of the acyl enzyme and one product. (3) is the liberation of the other product and free enzyme to repeat the cycle. Good substrates [acetylcholine for acetylcholinesterase and phenyl valerate (a nonphysiological ester) for NTE] complete the cycle more than 10,000 times per minute. B. Reaction with an organophosphate. Reactions (1)–(3) are analogous to those in A except that, for most organophosphates, (3) proceeds at a negligible rate unless aided by nucleophilic reactivators. Reaction (4) is a chemical change which can be monitored enzymically as "aging" (time-dependent loss of responsiveness to reactivators). Aging rates of organophosphate-inhibited esterases depend on both the organophosphate and the enzyme but, for most esterases, the R group is liberated into the medium. For NTE, however, aging involves intramolecular transfer of R to a secondary site (commonly called site Z) on the NTE molecule. The presence in the inhibited NTE of a residual hydrolyzable bond (such as P-O-C from phosphates or phosphonates or P-NH-C from phosphorami-dates) is obviously necessary for aging to occur and has been found to be an absolute requirement for neuropathic organophosphate esters. The intimate molecular mechanism of aging of inhibited NTE is not known and may be more complex than simple hydrolysis; the rate depends on steric factors but is very high ($t_{1/2}$ = 1–4 min) for simple dialkyl phosphates. C. Reaction with a protective organophosphinate. Reactions (1)–(3) take place but aging [reaction (4)] cannot occur because the residual R—P bonds in the inhibited esterase are not hydrolyzable.

and the half-life was about 2–4 min. When the enzyme reacted with [^{3}H,^{32}P]DFP, no radioactivity was released to the medium during aging, but hydrolysis revealed a decreasing concentration of diisopropyl phosphate and an increasing concentration of monoisopropyl phosphate plus a volatile tritiated compound (possibly propan-2-ol). It was concluded from this and other evidence that aging NTE involves molecular rearrangement rather than the formation of a charged monosubstituted phosphoric acid residue, as in the case of cholinesterase (Clothier and Johnson, 1979).

Apparent exceptions prove the rule. For example, a subcutaneous dose of dichlorvos at a rate of 100 mg/kg caused 90% inhibition of NTE but failed to cause paralysis in chickens. When hens were given a second dose 2 days after the first, delayed neurotoxicity occurred (Johnson, 1975a).

All neurotoxic compounds examined by the test cause 75% or more inhibition of NTE, usually within 24 hr (Johnson, 1975a, 1981). A second apparent exception involves 2,4,5-trichlorophenyl ethyl phenylphosphonothioate, which is metabolized to an active inhibitor so slowly that the brains of chickens to which it has been administered must be sampled after 48 hr rather than after 24 hr in order to demonstrate extensive inhibition of the enzymes (Johnson, 1975c).

Certain dimethyl phosphates have been shown to produce

anomalous results in the *in vivo* inhibition of NTE; under certain conditions, the brain but not the spinal cord enzyme may be strongly inhibited without the production of ataxia. This unusual situation is the only one found so far in which the reaction of brain NTE is not a perfect biochemical monitor (Johnson, 1978).

At this time, the adult hen is the most reliable predictor of delayed neuropathy in humans. Biochemical comparisons of brain and lymphocyte NTE in hens and humans have demonstrated that the enzyme is the same in both species. Presence of NTE in human erythrocytes has also been confirmed. The ratio of NTE inhibition in brain and lymphocytes is not necessarily 1 : 1 and may vary depending on the compound tested. Inhibition of human lymphocytic NTE as a precursor to delayed neuropathy has been demonstrated by Lotti (1986). Although the threshold of NTE inhibition required for delayed neuropathy remains undetermined, its discovery in these tissues will allow more accurate establishment of no-effect levels for long-term exposures to subtoxic doses (Lotti, 1987).

The improved NTE test procedure developed by Johnson (1977) marked the first of a series of advances that have made the test more selective, sensitive, and easier to perform. A good correlation between the *in vivo* reactivity of brain NTE derived from hens and humans (Lotti and Johnson, 1978) and a correlation coefficient of $+0.88$ for inhibition of NTE in brain and lymphocytes introduced the possibility of using the test in humans (Dudek *et al.*, 1979). Although human lymphocyte NTE levels appear to be a reliable indicator of NTE inhibition in the nervous system (Lotti *et al.*, 1983; Bertoncin *et al.*, 1985), the procedure has some problems. First, separation of lymphocytes requires a considerable amount of time. Second, NTE activity levels determined by this procedure are often erroneously high due to presence of platelets (which also possess NTE activity) not removed from the lymphocyte sample. Because of this finding, the measurement of NTE activity in human platelet samples is now being considered. This alternative is especially attractive since the purity of platelet separation is much higher than that of lymphocytes, and a strong correlation has been shown between NTE levels in the brain, lymphocytes, and platelets. However, further confirmation of these findings is needed in both humans and animals before this method is accepted as the alternative of choice in the determination of human NTE activity (Maroni and Bleecker, 1986).

So far, the NTE test has two limitations that may be eliminated by further study. First, the test does not explain the delay inherent in classical neurotoxicity. In some cases, the enzyme becomes inhibited within 1 hr of dosing (Johnson, 1987). So far, no chain of events has been found to explain sufficiently the 2 weeks or so from dosing to paralysis. In fact, following a neurotoxic dose, the enzyme activity of the tissue returns nearly to normal before the onset of clinical effect (Johnson, 1969a). That such a problem could be solved is illustrated by the dicoumarols that act by inhibiting the formation of prothrombin; it is not the inhibition *per se* but the depletion of existing prothrombin that leads to hemorrhage, and it takes time to exhaust the supply.

Second, the test is carried out on tissues that are not directly linked to the changes in polyneuropathy. NTE inhibition apparently has not been demonstrated specifically in the axonal tips, where injury is maximal. As already noted, intraarterial injection of DFP shows that recovery of the axonal lesion is faster when the nerve cell body is relatively spared. This permits the speculation that inhibition of NTE interferes with some normal process of continuous maintenance or repair, both in the cell body and in the axon, rather than producing primary damage to axonal tissue.

Obvious advantages of the NTE test are speed and quantitation. Whereas the dosage–response relationship of neurotoxic compounds represents quantitation, this quantitation can be extended by the NTE test in two ways. First, doses too small to produce a neurotoxic effect *in vivo* may cause a measurable inhibition of NTE. Second, doses may now be tested that hens could never survive long enough to complete the previously used *in vivo* test. This could also facilitate the determination of possible clinical effects of nonfatal exposures in humans by back-extrapolation of NTE and acetylcholinesterase levels from cases of fatal organic phosphorus pesticide exposures (Lotti, 1986).

An entirely different but little-explored approach to explaining neurotoxicity involves the critical role of Na^+,K^+-stimulated Mg^{2+}-dependent ATPase in maintaining energy metabolism in neurons. This enzyme is inhibited by a much lower concentration of TOCP than of mevinphos, a highly toxic but not neurotoxic organic phosphorus compound (Brown and Sharma, 1975).

Another entirely separate approach was the demonstration that, following repeated subcutaneous injections of three compounds that inhibited brain cholinesterase, only the two (mipafox and leptophos) that are neurotoxic lowered the level of dopamine in the corpus striatum (Freed *et al.*, 1976). Apparently, this test has not been extended to a wide range of neurotoxic compounds and to a range of similar compounds that lack this property.

A third alternative approach to neurotoxicity involved inhibition of fast axioplasmic transport. Leptophos, disbromoleptophos, EPN, and two other neurotoxic insecticides, as well as TOCP, caused marked inhibition of transport, but parathion did not (Reichert and Abou-Donia, 1979). It may be that the observed change in transport is secondary to inhibition of one or more enzymes. A feature of any transport is that it requires time so that its inhibition would tend to explain delay in final effect.

Dosage Response   As documented in Section 2.3.2 and by Olajos *et al.* (1978), neurotoxic organic phosphorus compounds show definite dosage–response relationships for single or repeated doses above a threshold level. Dosage levels that are a substantial fraction of the minimal effective single dosage are approximately additive in their effects, and (at least for DFP) the interval between doses leading to neurotoxicity may be as long as 16 days (Davies and Holland, 1972). Kinebuchi *et al.* (1977) found that, for a carefully chosen total dosage, a higher proportion of hens were paralyzed when leptophos was administered in divided doses on four or five succeeding days than when administered as a single dose or as half doses on two succeeding days. However, when the total dosage remained the same but five divided doses were administered to groups of hens on succeeding days and at increasing intervals, the neurotoxicity was lessened if the interval of administration was greater than 3 days (Kinebuchi and Konno, 1977, 1978).

One of the few long-term studies of neurotoxic compounds that would simulate repeated, prolonged, heavy exposure of workers at daily levels that do not constitute a substantial fraction of the minimal effective acute dosage but are far greater than those encountered by the general population was that of Frawley (1976). In feeding tests with TOCP and EPN, the onset of neurotoxicity was delayed as much as 5 months in some hens, but never more. In a 7-month study, neurotoxicity of some degree was seen in one of four hens fed TOCP at a dietary level of 100 ppm and in three of four fed EPN at 50 ppm (about 2.9 mg/kg/day). A smaller dosage of EPN was not investigated. In another study, delayed neurotoxicity developed in hens receiving technical EPN at an oral dosage of only 0.1 mg/kg/day by capsule for only 3 months. In these birds, ataxia appeared in 17–21 days (total dose 1.7–2.1 mg/kg).

One hen went on to paralysis and died on day 117; the other five showed some degree of clinical recovery when dosing was stopped after 90 days. A dosage of 0.01 mg/kg for the same 3-month period (total of 0.9 mg/kg) did not produce ataxia. Dosages ranging from 0.1 to 10 mg/kg/day produced, on the average, progressively more severe illness, ranging from only ataxia to paralysis and death (Abou-Donia and Graham, 1978a). Results with leptophos were similar, except that higher dosages were required to produce neurotoxicity and the latent periods were longer. The severity of illness and pathology was proportional to dosage. At 1.0 mg/kg/day, ataxia appeared in 62–68 days, that is, after 62–68 mg/kg. At 20 mg/kg/day, ataxia appeared in 22–29 days (total dosages 240–580 mg/kg). A dosage of 0.5 mg/kg/day for 78 days (total dosage of 39 mg/kg) did not produce ataxia (Abou-Donia and Preissig, 1976b). Ataxia was produced by smaller dermal than oral dosages of leptophos, suggesting more effective absorption when leptophos was applied to the combs of hens than when they ingested it. At 0.5 mg/kg/day, ataxia appeared in 50–94 days (total dosage 25–47 mg/kg); at 20 mg/kg/day, ataxia appeared in 17–28 days (total dosage 340–560 mg/kg). A dosage of 0.1 mg/kg/day for 183 days (total dosage 18.3 mg/kg) was without effect on gait or behavior. Unlike oral administration, dermal application did not produce weight loss or decreased egg production (Abou-Donia and Graham, 1978b).

In a study of the pharmacokinetics of leptophos given at a single nonneurotoxic dose, the half-life for elimination was 11.55 days, but even though the proportion of the dose stored in brain, spinal cord, and nerve was small, it remained unchanged for 20 days (Abou-Donia, 1976a). This lack of clearance from nervous tissue probably has a bearing on the cumulative neurotoxic action.

16.4.1.4 Polyneuropathy Associated with Pesticides

Table 16.14 lists most insecticides that have been tested for neurotoxicity and representative compounds mentioned in Section 16.4.1.2 and elsewhere that are not insecticides but are neurotoxic. It may be seen from the table that most of the pesticides and also the drug haloxon that produce ataxia in the hen do so only at dosage levels approaching the lethal. This is true even though the lethal dosages were determined in hens protected by atropine to minimize anticholinergic affects. In comparison, with some flurophosphates or the cyclic metabolite of O,O-2-methylphenyl-O-4-methylphenyl phosphate, no highly neurotoxic compound has been found among the insecticides in general use. On the other hand, several of the compounds produce neurotoxicity in hens at a dosage not much greater than the neurotoxic dosage of mipafox and lower than those of TOCP, leptophos, merphos, and trichlorfon, compounds that have produced paralysis in humans. It must be emphasized that the compounds that have produced human illness produce delayed, prolonged polyneuropathy in hens, but so do some other pesticides, notably DEF and EPN.

Caution seems indicated in the use of any pesticide that is neurotoxic in the hen, but caution in interpreting the test is indicated also. Certainly, the high dosage of some pesticides necessary to produce neurotoxicity may be one reason why they have produced no cases in humans. The chance is small that such a large dosage of a little-used compound would be absorbed in a brief period. However, it is also possible that humans are inherently less susceptible than the hen to some of the compounds. This seems most likely in connection with DFP and EPN. The first has been used as a drug in single intramuscular dosages of 0.05 mg/kg and in dosages of 0.02 mg/kg/day for 25 or more days (Grob et al., 1947b). Not only has EPN been used extensively as an insecticide (leading no doubt to substantial exposure of many formulators and applicators), but its ingestion has produced severe cholinergic poisoning. Humans may also be inherently less susceptible to paralysis by caresin, edifenphos, and fonophos, which have caused cases of cholinergic poisoning (as discussed in Sections 16.11.3.3, 16.11.4.3, and 16.11.5.5, respectively) but without indication of paralysis. However, in spite of their chemical similarity to neurotoxic compounds, their ability to paralyze chickens apparently remains untested.

Temephos is one of the compounds that produce temporary paralysis in hens. It has been given orally to volunteers at a rate of about 4.0 mg/kg/day for 5 days and a rate of about 1.0 mg/kg/day for 28 days (Laws et al., 1967), but even these heavy rates were not as great as that required to produce ataxia in the hen.

The only pesticides or candidate pesticides that clearly have caused classical neurotoxicity in people are merphos (see Section 16.10.1), mipafox (see Section 16.5.1), trichlorfon (see Section 16.6.6), and perhaps leptophos (see Section 16.11.2) and chlorpyrifos (see Section 16.7.9). Insufficient information is available to compare the effective dosages of these compounds in people and in the hen. On the other hand, it is clear that all of the affected persons had occupational or accidental exposure. Apparently, all cases caused by trichlorfon involved ingestion but exposure in the one merphos case was entirely dermal.

One other case that presumably represented classical neurotoxicity occurred in an organic chemist whose work involved development of new organic phosphorus insecticides. The illness was characterized by gradual onset of weakness and muscle atrophy (Namba et al. 1971). Some of the compounds involved were known to be neurotoxic.

The small number of persons poisoned by mipafox have remained crippled. Almost complete, albeit slow, recovery has been the rule with persons who developed polyneuropathy from trichlorfon or from an unrecognized impurity in some batches of it (see Section 16.6.6.3). One of the many cases attributed to trichlorfon was unusual in that there was a definite deterioration of the patient's neurological condition 5 months after onset, which had been about 2 weeks after ingestion and was followed by some improvement; the deterioration, too, was followed by partial recovery (Eljasz and Krzyston-Przkop, 1975). It is too early to reach any conclusion about the duration of human polyneuropathy associated with leptophos.

The other organic phosphorus compounds alleged to cause polyneuropathy in humans pose different and incompletely resolved problems. Because sufficient dosages of malathion cause polyneuropathy of rapid onset and rapid resolution in hens (see Table 16.14), there is no reason to exclude the possibility that it might cause a similar condition in people, and cases have been reported. However, the human cases were dissimilar from one another, and all were reported in people with trivial exposure, never in people with heavy exposure (see Section 16.6.1.3). There is, therefore, reason to question whether malathion contributed to these conditions ascribed to it.

The relation between polyneuropathy and parathion or demeton (see Sections 16.7.1.3 and 16.7.3.3) is also obscure. These compounds do not cause neurotoxicity in hens. Paraoxon, apparently the only clearly related compound yet tested, does not effectively inhibit NTE (see Mode of Action). These compounds do not cause polyneuropathy in the vast majority of persons who suffer anticholinesterase poisoning as a result of absorbing large dosages. Thus the small number of cases of polyneuropathy that have been reported in persons exposed to parathion and demeton probably should be viewed as idiopathic. As pointed out by Namba *et al.* (1971), a causal relationship never has been established in cases that involved them.

16.4.2 NARCOTIC EFFECTS

Some organic phosphorus compounds produce an immediate narcotic effect, ranging from incoordination to deep anesthesia following intravenous injection. At the same time respiration may be affected. A large dosage is required for all compounds for which the effect has been demonstrated and, by necessity, all of them are of low toxicity. Although some of these compounds, such as malathion, demeton-*S*-methyl, demeton-*O*-methyl, and dimethoate inhibit cholinesterase, others such as trimethyl phosphate, triethyl phosphate, tributyl phosphate, and triethyl phosphorothionate do not inhibit it (Vandekar, 1957; Brown and Murphy, 1971). The mechanism of the narcotic actions is not known. However, the effects are marked only after injection into the blood has resulted in concentrations estimated to be about 10^{-3} M, which is high enough to block nerve conduction and motor end plates and thus to produce anesthesia and paralysis. The action probably depends on a block in sodium ion transport across membranes (Heath, 1961).

Apparently, the narcotic action has not been observed in clinical cases and probably is not to be expected.

16.4.3 TERATOGENIC EFFECTS

Although some anticholinergic compounds are teratogenic, most are not. It has been reported that electrophoresis can be used to separate from the chicken egg yolk sac membrane enzymes that are inhibited *in vivo* by teratogenic treatment schedules but not by nonteratogenic schedules. This postulated mode of action is analogous to that of the esterase involved in delayed neurotoxicity (Flockart and Casida, 1972), but its bearing in teratogenesis caused by an excess or deficiency of other compounds or caused by physical or living agents remains unexplored.

16.4.4 ALKYLATING EFFECTS

That organic phosphorus compounds are chemical alkylating agents has been recognized at least since the work of Schrader (1963a,b). Therefore, it is not self evident, in the absence of any indication that these compounds are significant alkylating agents in mammals, why a warning about akylation and consequent mutagenesis caused by dichlorvos (Löfroth *et al.*, 1969) was indicated. As might have been expected, alkylation by organic phosphorus compounds *in vitro* and mutation in unprotected cells were demonstrated. For example, when calf thymus DNA was allowed to react with dichlorvos *in vitro* for 66 hr at room temperature, the yield of N-7-methylguanine was about 1% of the available guanine (Löfroth, 1970). The ratio of dichlorvos to nucleotide units was $50:1$, compared to a ratio of about $1:1,000$ that might be expected *in vivo*.

Dichlorvos can methylate guanine in bacterial or other cells in culture (Fahrig, 1973; Lawley *et al.*, 1974; Wennerberg and Löfroth, 1974).

When dichlorvos tagged with radioactive carbon or hydrogen was administered to mice intraperitoneally, 62–70% of the radioactivity was recovered in the urine during the first 24 hr, and an additional 2.1–4.2% was recovered during the second 24 hr. A small fraction of this radioactivity was extracted from the urine along with 7-methylguanine, and it was concluded on the basis of chromatography that the purine was methylated (Wennerberg and Löfroth, 1974). While assuming without strict proof that they were dealing with a single compound rather than two compounds that were chromatographically inseparable, the authors did point out that it was unclear whether methylation had occurred at the polymeric (DNA and RNA) level. The proportion of the dose of dichlorvos recovered in association with 7-methylguanine was 3 to 6×10^{-5}, compared to 2×10^{-3} for similar studies with methyl methanesulfonate or dimethyl sulfate. Results were obtained following respiratory exposure to dichlorvos of the same order of magnitude as were obtained by the intraperitoneal route, but calculation of recovery factors was not justified because the retained inhaled dose was not known.

Even strong alkylating agents differ in what purine is methylated to an important degree. For the nitrosamines and nitrosamides, which are a real threat to health, the critical reaction involves 6-O-alkylation of deoxyguanosine (Loveless, 1969). The biological significance of 7-*N*-alkylation of guanine is less clear.

By far the most thorough studies of the problem are those of Bedford and Robinson (1972) and Wooder *et al.* (1977). They showed that a laboratory test designed to emphasize alkylation and suppress phosphorylation did reveal that dichlorvos, paraoxon-methyl, tetrachlorfenvinphos, mevinphos, crotoxyphos, parathion-methyl, dicrotophos, malathion, monocrotophos, and trichlorfon were chemical alkylating agents. Their relative rates of reaction ranged (in decreasing order) from 34 to about 0.5, compared to 2400 for dimethyl sulfate, a recognized biological alkylating agent. No alkylating reaction was observed for chlorfenvinphos or for the metabolites of dichlorvos. The authors provided convincing evidence that anticholinesterase organic phosphorus insecticides are unlikely to be important biological alkylating agents and convincing biochemical evidence that these compounds in general (and dichlorvos in particular) are unlikely to persist long enough *in vivo* to exert any alkylating ability they may possess. Using dichlorvos at concentrations encountered in practical use situations and methods sensitive to one methyl group per 6.0×10^{11} units of DNA and 2×10^9 units of RNA, no methylation of the N-7 atom of guanine moieties was detected. Under these conditions, only 0.000001% of the dose of dichlorvos would have had to react with DNA in order to produce detectable methylation.

Studies regarding the mutagenic or carcinogenic action of different organic phosphorus insecticides are discussed in connection with the individual compounds. It may be noted that alkylation may not be the only mechanism capable of producing mutagenesis or carcinogenesis.

16.4.5 OTHER PHARMACOLOGICAL ACTIONS

Santolucito and Whitcomb (1971) found that 0.002 *M* paraoxon abolished the oxygen uptake of red blood cells *in vitro* but that this inhibition required 2 hr and was reversed by 0.002 *M* glutathione (GSH) within 15 min. Oral dosing with parathion also resulted in inhibition of oxygen consumption (measured *in vitro*) when blood samples were taken at the appearance of severe poisoning; again, *in vitro* GSH restored oxygen uptake but had no influence on acetylcholinesterase activity, which was undetectable. Apparently, the possibility that GSH may have therapeutic value has not been explored.

Oxygen uptake is inhibited not only in red blood cells but also in the brain. In rats dosed *in vivo,* the reduction of oxygen uptake (measured *in vitro*) was accompanied by inhibition of several enzymes (Jovic *et al.,* 1971). Apparently, the relationship of this phenomenon to glutathione has not been explored.

Whereas the injury of striated muscle associated with prolonged depolarization of the end-plate region can be prevented by oximes (see Section 16.2.1.3), injury to the heart produced by supralethal dosages is not blocked by these compounds (Wolthuis and Meeter, 1968). This may mean that the two injuries are inherently different, or it may be merely a dosage effect. The effects on the heart may determine an upper limit of successful therapy with oximes and atropine, as the authors suggest. On the other hand, no single recognizable cause of therapeutic failure in cases where treatment was the best

known has been recognized, and it is not certain that the harmful effects of imperfect oxygenation of the tissues had been excluded in the animal studies.

According to Nikolayev (1973) and Poloz and Nikolayev (1973), trichlorfon and dimethoate inhibit Na^+, K^+-ATPase and acetylcholinesterase to approximately the same degree, both *in vitro* and *in vivo*.

A number of clinical and immunotoxic anomalies in laboratory animals have been associated with *O,S,S*-trimethyl phosphorodithioate and *O,O,S*-trimethyl phosphorothioate, which are contaminants of technical malathion, parathion, fenitrothion, and acephate.

Delayed toxicity including a distinct cytotoxic effect on the lungs of treated rats has been associated with *O,S,S*-trimethyl phosphorodithioate (Konno *et al.,* 1984). In mice observed for 90 days following a single oral dose, the LD 50 for this compound has been estimated as approximately 118 mg/kg, although an acute oral dosage of only 10 mg/kg caused temporary immunosuppression (Rodgers *et al.,* 1987). Acute dosages of 20 and 40 mg/kg caused significant decreases in thymic weight and thymic nucleated cell number, an increased primary cytotoxic T-lymphocyte response to an alloantigen, and elevated primary and secondary humoral immune responses. Acute dosages of 60 and 80 mg/kg caused lethargy and decreases in body weight, plasma cholinesterase levels, thymic nucleated cell numbers, and primary and secondary humoral immune responses. However, the observed immunosuppressive responses were not as great as those associated with *O,O,S*-trimethyl phosphorothioate (Rodgers *et al.,* 1987).

The LD 50 for acute oral doses of *O,O,S*-trimethyl phosphorothioate has been estimated as 35 mg/kg. Dosages near or above the LD 50 caused some hemoconcentration (probably due to dehydration), decreased serum potassium levels, bronchopneumonia, and morphological alterations in the heart, adrenal tissue, small intestine, liver, and kidney (Hammond *et al.,* 1982). Acute exposures below the LD 50 resulted in reversible suppression of mitogenic, humoral, and cell-mediated immune responses, enhanced production of interleukin 2, weight loss, and an increase in delayed mortality (Umetsu *et al.,* 1981). Weight loss and malaise have been noted in the absence of serum cholinesterase depression (Rodgers *et al.,* 1986a; Devens *et al.,* 1985). Oral dosage at or above 20 mg/kg caused a transient decrease in splenic white pulp and lymphocyte numbers, thymic lymphocyte numbers, and repairable thymic necrosis (Devens *et al.,* 1985). Acute dosages as low as 1 mg/kg decreased the cytotoxic T-lymphocyte response and the ability of splenocytes to produce antibody-secreting cells, with macrophages being the most affected cell type (Rodgers *et al.,* 1986b).

Although these contaminants may account for some of the initial observations in severe human poisonings, their relatively transient nature and large required doses relative to those present in technical grade products do not provide substantial support for any long-term effects, such as increased disease susceptibility and tumor development, which may be associated with prolonged occupational exposures.

16.5 FLUOROPHOSPHATES OF CATEGORY II

Very few fluorophosphates have been considered or used as pesticides. One of them, mipafox, caused neurotoxicity in three persons when it reached the pilot-plant step. Therefore, it is important to discuss mipafox and the other two fluorophosphates that have been given to people in measured doses. The identity and chemical structure of these compounds are shown in Table 16.15.

16.5.1 MIPAFOX

16.5.1.1 Identity, Properties, and Uses

Chemical Name Mipafox is N,N'-bis(1-methylethyl)-phosphordiamidic fluoride.

Structure See Table 16.15.

Synonyms Trade names for mipafox (B51, 150) have included Isopestox®, Pestox 15®, and Pestox XV®. The CAS registry number is 371-86-8.

Physical and Chemical Properties Mipafox has the empirical formula $C_6H_{16}FN_2OP$ and a molecular weight of 182.20. The pure material forms crystals.

16.5.1.2 Toxicity to Laboratory Animals

Basic Findings The acute toxicity of mipafox is not greatly different from that of parathion. The intraperitoneal LD 50 is 105.7 mg/kg in rats, 13.5 mg/kg in mice, and 35.4 mg/kg in chickens (Chattopadhyay *et al.*, 1986).

Phenylmethylsulfonyl fluoride administered to rats at 250 mg/kg subcutaneously 4 hr before an intraperitoneal dose of 15 mg/kg mipafox protected the animals from neurological damage normally associated with mipafox exposure. However, mortality among animals at this dose sequence was abnormally high (50%) (Veronesi and Padilla, 1985).

A daily dosing regimen to rats involving subcutaneous administration of 0.05 mg/kg mipafox followed by 0.5 mg/kg DFP 30 min later significantly potentiated cholinergic activity in the muscle, brain, and liver, while inhibiting liver aliesterse activity. This combined treatment degraded DFP tolerance to such an extent that no animal survived more than 5 days (Gupta *et al.*, 1985).

It is of interest that pretreatment with phenobarbital gives marked protection against single doses (O'Brien, 1967).

16.5.1.3 Toxicity to Humans

Accidents and Use Experience Three persons involved in the pilot-scale production of mipafox all developed typical acute intoxication accompanied by marked inhibition of cholinesterase (Bidstrup *et al.*, 1953). Although no spillage or

Table 16.15
Structure of Fluorophosphates (Category II) of the Form $R_2P(O)F$

Name	R
mipafox	$(CH_3)_2CH—NH—$
dimefox	$(CH_3)_2N—$
DFP	$(CH_3)_2CH—O—$

other accident was mentioned, onset of the two most serious cases was within a period of something less than 24 hr, suggesting a period of overexposure. The plasma enzyme was slightly more depressed than the red cell enzyme in the two patients in whom both were measured. The degree of acute illness corresponded to the degree of enzyme inhibition. One man recovered uneventfully, and no delayed effects developed. The other two persons required hospitalization and received large doses of atropine for 4 and 6 days, respectively. Their signs and symptoms during the acute phase were not remarkable, with the possible exception that the 28-year-old woman complained of cramps in the muscles of her legs. Both she and the 39-year-old man experienced muscle weakness, but it was not unusual in degree, and both of them maintained respiration without difficulty.

After what appeared to be a full recovery from acute illness, the woman and man experienced a gradual, delayed onset of weakness. The degree of chronic illness corresponded to the degree of both acute illness and cholinesterase inhibition and presumably reflected a difference of initial dosage.

On day 16 after her illness began, the woman first noticed weakness and unsteadiness of her legs. Three or four days later, this weakness increased, and she first noticed weakness of her hands and arms. These symptoms gradually became worse, and she was readmitted to hospital. One month after initial onset there was complete flaccid paralysis of the legs. The knee and ankle jerks were absent, and the plantar reflexes could not be elicited. Tone and power of the arms and hands were greatly reduced. The trunk muscles also were weaker than normal. Cranial nerves were normal; there were no signs of involvement of the central nervous system, and no disturbances of cutaneous sensation could be demonstrated. All muscles, particularly those of the calf, were tender to palpation, and twitches were observed in the deltoids and the muscles of the face and legs. Power gradually returned to the thighs and arms. About 2 months after initial onset, the knee jerks not only had returned but were exaggerated, and clonus of the patella could be elicited easily. The ankle jerks were still absent, and there was wasting of the small muscles of the feet. Fasciculations were still present in some muscles. Alternating vasodilation and vasoconstriction resulted in subjective burning and coldness and visible flushing and pallor or cyanosis. During the next several months, the recovery already mentioned continued, but wasting of the small muscles of the hands became increasingly obvious. However, these muscles too began to improve about 7.5 months after initial onset.

Within another month there was some improvement of the muscles of the feet, the ankle jerks returned, and slight movement of the toes became possible.

The man noticed weakness of his legs and cramplike pains of his calves and feet 21 days after initial onset and immediately after riding a bicycle. He was readmitted to hospital 5 days later. By this time dorsiflexion of both feet was impossible, and plantar flexion was absent on the right and weak on the left. The ankle jerks were diminished, and plantar reflexes could not be elicited. The patient's condition improved gradually, but wasting of the small muscles of the feet increased for a time. He was discharged in less than a month and returned to work within 10 months after initial onset. After a year he could walk 2 miles before noticing difficulty, but prolonged standing led to low back pain. Even with sedentary work, he complained of a dull aching pain in the right foot and calf severe enough to wake him from sleep.

Treatment of Poisoning Treatment of acute poisoning by mipafox is the same as that of poisoning by other organic phosphorus compounds (see Section 16.2.2.7). Unfortunately, only symptomatic care can be given for the neurotoxic effects of the compound.

16.5.2 DIMEFOX

16.5.2.1 Identity, Properties, and Uses

Chemical Name Dimefox is tetramethylphosphorodiamidic fluoride.

Structure See Table 16.15.

Synonyms The common name dimefox (BSI, ISO) is in general use. Other nonproprietary names have included BFPO, DIFO, and DMF. Trade names include Hanane®, Pestox IV®, and S-14®. Code designations include CR-409 and ENT-19,109. The CAS registry number is 115-26-4.

Physical and Chemical Properties Dimefox has the empirical formula $C_4H_{12}FN_2OP$ and a molecular weight of 154.13. The pure material is a colorless liquid with a boiling point of 67°C at 4 mm Hg. The vapor pressure is 0.36 mm Hg at 25°C. The density is 1.115 at 20°C. Dimefox is miscible with water and most organic solvents. It has a chloroform/water partition coefficient of 15:1 in favor of chloroform. Dimefox is resistant to hydrolysis by alkali. It is hydrolyzed by acids, slowly oxidized by vigorous oxidizing agents, and rapidly oxidized by chlorine. Like other amidophosphates, dimefox is stable in aqueous solution (DuBois and Coon, 1952). This undoubtedly contributes to persistence on surfaces, but whether it has any direct bearing on its duration of effect in animals is obscure.

History, Formulations, and Uses Dimefox was first introduced by Pest Control, Ltd., in 1949 as a Pestox IV®. It is a systemic insecticide and acaricide used for soil treatment to control aphids and red spider mites on hops.

16.5.2.2 Toxicity to Laboratory Animals

The oral LD 50 in rats is approximately 7.5 mg/kg (Okinaka *et al.*, 1954) or, in another strain, 1.8 mg/kg (Sanderson and Edson, 1959). The intraperitoneal LD 50 is 5 mg/kg in rats, 1.4 mg/kg in mice, 2.5 mg/kg in guinea pigs, and between 5 and 10 mg/kg in dogs (DuBois and Coon, 1952; Okinaka *et al.*, 1954).

Repeated intraperitoneal administration of dimefox to rats at a rate of 0.5 mg/kg/day killed half of them within 10 doses; 0.1 mg/kg/day produced marked inhibition of cholinesterase but no deaths following 30 injections.

The no-effect dosages of dimefox based on the most sensitive criterion, red cell cholinesterase, are 0.003, 0.006, and 0.002 mg/kg/day in rat, pig, and human, respectively (Edson, 1964).

Unmetabolized dimefox is a moderately strong inhibitor of cholinesterase *in vitro;* the molar concentration required to cause 50% inhibition is 4×10^{-5}. It undoubtedly is converted to an active metabolite (as well as being detoxified) *in vivo*, for the fall in cholinesterase is gradual, requiring in rats 2 hr following administration of one-half an LD 50. Its action is mainly peripheral, that on the brain being slower in onset and less marked than the action of DFP (Okinaka *et al.*, 1954).

Oximes were found ineffective for treating rats poisoned by dimefox (Sanderson and Edson, 1959).

16.5.2.3 Toxicity to Humans

Apparently, the only direct information about the effect of dimefox in humans comes from studies of volunteers. In a study lasting 70 days, whole-blood cholinesterase was not inhibited in a total of four men and women who ingested the compound at a dosage of 0.002 mg/kg/day, but it was reduced about 25% by a dosage of 0.0034 mg/kg/day. In another study, a dosage of 0.004 mg/kg/day gradually caused a 40% reduction in whole-blood cholinesterase by day 49 of exposure when inhibition stabilized until dosing ended on day 95. This effect was entirely due to lowering of red cell cholinesterase, since the plasma enzyme remained unchanged. Whole-blood activity recovered to 90% of normal within 56 days after dosing stopped (Edson, 1964).

In spite of its high toxicity, dimefox has not been an important cause of poisoning. Even more interesting, there has been no indication of neurotoxicity among people working with it.

Treatment of Poisoning See Section 16.2.2.7.

16.5.3 DFP

16.5.3.1 Identity, Properties, and Uses

Chemical Name DFP is the acronym for diisopropyl fluorophosphate.

Structure   See Table 16.15.

Synonyms   In addition to variants on the chemical name, DFP has been called fluostigmine and isofluorphage. Trade names include Diflupyl®, Dyflos®, Dyphlos®, Floropryl®, and Fluropryl®. The CAS registry number is 55-91-4.

Chemical and Physical Properties   DFP has the empirical formula $C_6H_{14}FO_3P$ and a molecular weight of 184.15. DFP is a liquid at temperatures above −82°C. The vapor pressure at 20°C is 0.579 mm Hg. The compound is soluble in vegetable oils and soluble to the extent of 1.54% in water at 25°C.

16.5.3.2 Toxicity to Laboratory Animals

Basic Findings   The intraperitoneal LD 50 for DFP in mice is 4 mg/kg (Holmstedt, 1959).

Studies of animals receiving repeated doses were made in preparation for a proposed clinical trial of DFP for treatment of myasthenia gravis and glaucoma. Intramuscular dosages as low as 0.05 mg/kg twice per week in dogs, 0.03 mg/kg twice per week in monkeys, and 0.50 mg/kg twice per week in rats led to muscular fasciculations soon after individual doses but to no other typical signs of poisoning. Three of four monkeys developed bronchopneumonia, which investigators (rightly or wrongly) associated with excessive secretions. Cardiospasm often associated with dilation of the esophagus was seen in three dogs receiving dosages of 0.1, 0.3, and 0.5 mg/kg twice per week, and this led to malnutrition at the higher dosages. Partial urinary incontinence was observed in the dogs on the two higher dosage levels. Both cardiospasm and urinary incontinence were considered related to inhibition of cholinesterase. Finally, hind leg paralysis developed during or before the tenth week of dosing in dogs receiving 0.3 and 0.5 mg/kg twice per week; some functional improvement occurred after dosing was stopped, but recovery was incomplete (Koelle and Gilman, 1946). This would seem to be the first observation of neurotoxicity produced by DFP.

Newborn rats are much more sensitive than adults to DFP; resistance increases until the animals are about 120 days old (Freedman and Himwich, 1948).

Acute doses of DFP decreased the magnitudes and durations of slow-wave and REM sleep while increasing wakefulness in a dosage-dependent manner (Gnadt et al., 1986). This contrasts with findings of an earlier repeated dose study in which a single initial injection of 1.0 mg/kg DFP followed by injections of 0.5 mg/kg every third day for a total of five injections over 13 days was found to increase the number of REM sleep episodes, although the total length of REM sleep was unaffected (Gnadt et al., 1985).

Rats given daily injections of 1 mg/kg DFP for 14 days had a 71–77% decrease in acetylcholinesterase activity in the cortex, hippocampus, and striatum, along with a significant decrease in body weight and decreased muscarinic receptor density and spatial memory impairment (as determined by their ability to perform the spontaneous alteration task in a T-maze). (McDonald et al., 1988).

Rats receiving three to five subcutaneous doses of DFP at 0.5 mg/kg/day experienced signs of cholinergic toxicity similar in severity to those observed in another experimental group 15 min following a single dose of 1.5 mg/kg. Repeated daily doses of 0.5 mg/kg/day DFP inhibited cholinesterase to the greatest extent in the diaphragm, followed by the soleus, and least in the extensor digitorum longus. The same dose regimen caused the greatest inhibition of brain cholinesterase in the brain stem, followed by the striatum, cortex, and hippocampus. When these daily doses were continued for 17 days, some recovery of cholinesterase activity was noted in the muscle tissue but not in the brain. This is probably the result of *de novo* esterase synthesis in these areas. A recovery of aliesterase activity was also noted by the end of the 17-day dosing period (Gupta et al., 1985).

A daily subcutaneous dose of 0.05 mg/kg mipafox or 3 mg/kg iso-OMPA followed by 0.5 mg/kg DFP 30 min later significantly potentiated cholinergic activity in muscle, brain, and liver, while inhibiting liver aliesterase activity. No animal survived more than 5 days on the combined treatments (Gupta et al., 1985).

Absorption, Distribution, Metabolism, and Excretion   Following intravenous injection of hydrogen-labeled DFP, the concentration in arterial serum declined in two exponential phases with half-lives of about 7 and 200 min, respectively, reflecting (a) fast accumulation of the compound and its metabolites in the tissues and (b) elimination. DFP is rapidly metabolized to diisopropylphosphate and is excreted, mainly in the urine. Less than 1% is eliminated by bile and lung within the first 2 hr (Hansen et al., 1968).

Effects on Reproduction   DFP is toxic to the fetus but is not teratogenic (Fish, 1966).

Pathology   The pituitaries of most rats treated with DFP for more than 12 months were macroscopically abnormal, and all contained hyperplastic chromophobes (Glow, 1969). Whereas the author viewed this effect as a result of prolonged inhibition of brain cholinesterase, it may be peculiar to DFP, for it apparently has not been noted in connection with other compounds. The dilation of the esophagus in dogs that has been observed at autopsy as well as clinically appears peculiar to DFP.

16.5.3.3 Toxicity to Humans

Experimental Exposure   [^{32}P]DFP was used at single dosages of 0.69–2.2 mg/person/day to study the survival of platelets in normal volunteers and in patients with hypersplenic thrombocytopenia or polycythemia vera. It was concluded that the compound became bound covalently to protein in platelets of all ages in the peripheral circulation without interfering with their normal function. It was further concluded that average platelet life span is 11.5 days with a linear decay curve based on age of the platelets (Cooney and Fawley, 1968).

Therapeutic Use DFP has had only limited use as a pesticide and, therefore, will be discussed briefly. Its great interest in connection with the safety of pesticides lies in the fact that dosages of it as great as about one-tenth of the minimal dosage that produces neurotoxicity in hens (see Table 16.14) have been administered to people as a drug or experimentally. The patients often experience symptoms associated with inhibition of cholinesterase, but neurotoxicity did not occur. This may be simply because they did not receive a sufficient dosage.

When DFP was used for glaucoma and other ophthalmological conditions, solutions of it were placed directly into the eye (Marr, 1947; Leopold and McDonald, 1948; Stone, 1950) so that, even though the local concentration was relatively high, the systemic dose was low, specifically about 0.123 or 0.246 mg for the treatment of one eye with 0.1 or 0.2% solution. Ordinarily, only a slight decrease in plasma cholinesterase was found after instillation of DFP, indicating that only minimal systemic absorption had occurred (Leopold and Comroe, 1946). However, even ophthalmological use may have led, on rare occasions, to systemic poisoning. In one instance, a 12-month-old boy, who had received one drop of 0.1% DFP in each eye daily for 2 months, experienced two brief apneic spells, with probable seizure activity for 1 or 2 min each time. When examined in the hospital, he was alert and seemed normal, except for miotic, unreactive pupils, profuse nasal discharge, and possible motor weakness. Eight hours after admission, he had a typical grand mal convulsion lasting 2–3 min. For 3 days after admission, he had a temperature of 39.5°C, and cultures of the nose and throat yielded *Pneumococcus*. During this period and for two more days, he continued to be miotic, and he developed more marked motor weakness. The cholinesterase activity of serum collected 60 hr after the last eye drops was below the range of normal and 44% of the average normal (Verhulst and Crotty, 1965). Clearly, the miosis, rhinorrhea, and slight cholinesterase inhibition were the result of DFP; whether the seizures in this infant were caused by the drug or by infection is not clear.

Intramuscular administration of DFP to people with schizophrenia, to people with manic–depressive psychosis, and to normal controls at a dose of 1 mg/person/day produced marked inhibition of both red cell and plasma cholinesterase; a rate of 2 mg/person/day (about 0.028 mg/kg/day) for 7 days produced anorexia, vomiting, and diarrhea, somewhat more severe in normal than in psychotic people (Rowntree *et al.*, 1950).

Other studies showed that even a single intramuscular dose of 0.6 mg produced approximately 50% inhibition of plasma cholinesterase but no sign of toxicity (Munker *et al.*, 1961).

There is some indication that persons suffering from myasthenia gravis are more tolerant than normal persons to DFP; certainly the drug produced clinical improvement in some cases. The difference between the reaction of the myasthenic and the normal person was best illustrated by the injection of 1.5 mg into the brachial artery so that most of the effects were confined to one arm and systemic effects were minimal or absent. Under these conditions, normal persons experienced marked sweating, numerous spontaneous fasciculations, and pronounced motor weakness in the arm. By contrast, patients with myasthenia gravis experienced no fasciculations, and there was a striking increase in muscle strength that was still detectable 8–10 days later (McGehee *et al.*, 1946; Harvey *et al.*, 1947). Even so, daily intramuscular doses at the rate of 0.5–2 mg/person/day for as much as 3 months produced tightness in the chest in patients with the disease, and this side effect was not counteracted by atropine (Gaddum and Wilson, 1947). Other side effects have included nausea and vomiting (Comroe *et al.*, 1946a). DFP was less effective and produced more side effects than neostigmine (Comroe *et al.*, 1946b; Harvey *et al.*, 1947).

For abdominal distension without organic obstruction, DFP has been used at a single intramuscular dose of 2 mg, sometimes followed by two or three doses of 1 mg at 12-hr intervals. Neostigmine or pitressin was added after DFP as required (Grob *et al.*, 1947c).

Accidental and Intentional Poisoning Autopsy findings in a case of poisoning by DFP were reported by Mozes (1977). The lung findings were nonspecific.

Treatment of Poisoning See Section 16.2.2.7.

16.6 DIMETHOXY COMPOUNDS OF CATEGORY IV

About half of all organic phosphorus insecticides are dimethoxy compounds. The identity and chemical structure of those known to have affected people or to have been studied in volunteers are listen in Table 16.16. The only injury that any of these compounds have produced in humans is typical cholinergic poisoning. The compounds range from highly toxic ones to temephos, the acute toxicity of which is less than that of table salt.

16.6.1 MALATHION

16.6.1.1 Identity, Properties, and Uses

Chemical Name Malathion is O,O-dimethyl-S-(1,2-dicarbethoxyethyl)phosphorodithioate.

Structure See Table 16.16.

Synonyms The common name malathion (BSI, CSA, ESA, ISO) is in general use. Other nonproprietary names include carbophos (USSR), maldison (Australia and New Zealand), and mercaptothion (Republic of South Africa). Trade names include Chemathion®, Cython®, Emmaton®, Karbophos®,

Table 16.16
Structure of Dimethoxy Organic Phosphorus Compounds of the Form $(CH_3-O)_2P(R)X$

Compound	=R	X	Compound	=R	X
azinphos-methyl	=S	$-S-CH_2-N$ (benzotriazinone ring with C=O, N=N)	endothion	=O	$-S-CH_2-$ (pyranone ring with $O-CH_3$)
bromophos	=S	$-O-$ (phenyl, Cl, Br, Cl substituents)	famphur	=S	$-O-$ (phenyl)$-S(=O)_2-N(CH_3)_2$
carbophenothion-methyl	=S	$-S-CH_2-S-$ (phenyl)$-Cl$	fenitrothion	=S	$-O-$ (phenyl)$-NO_2$, CH_3
chlorothion	=S	$-O-$ (phenyl)$-NO_2$, Cl	fenthion	=S	$-O-$ (phenyl)$-S-CH_3$, CH_3
chlorpyrifos-methyl	=S	$-O-$ (pyridine ring, Cl, Cl, Cl)	formothion	=S	$-S-CH_2-C(=O)-N(CH_3)(CH=O)$
crotoxyphos	=O	$-O-C(CH_3)=CH-C(=O)-O-CH(CH_3)-$(phenyl)	jodfenfos	=S	$-O-$ (phenyl, Cl, I, Cl)
demeton-O-methyl	=S	$-O-CH_2-CH_2-S-C_2H_5$	malathion	=S	$-S-CH(C(=O)-O-C_2H_5)-CH_2-C(=O)-O-C_2H_5$
dementon-S-mehtyl	=O	$-S-CH_2-CH_2-S-C_2H_5$			
dicapthon	=S	$-O-$ (phenyl)$-NO_2$, Cl	menazon	=S	$-SCH_2-$ (triazine ring with NH_2, NH_2)
dichlorvos	=O	$-O-CH=CCl_2$	methidathion	=S	$-S-CH_2-N$ (thiadiazolone ring, $C=O$, S, $O-CH_3$)
dicrotophos (E isomer)	=O	$-O-C(CH_3)=CH(H)-C(=O)-N(CH_3)_2$			
dimethoate	=S	$-S-CH_2-C(=O)-NH-CH_3$	mevinphos E isomer	=O	$-O-C(CH_3)=CH(H)-C(=O)-O-CH_3$

(continued)

Table 16.16 *(Continued)*

Compound	=R	X	Compound	=R	X
Z isomer	=O	$-O-C(CH_3)=C(H)-C(=O)-O-CH_3$	pirimifos-methyl	=S	$-O-$ pyrimidine (4-CH$_3$, 2-N(C$_2$H$_5$)$_2$)
monocrotophos (E isomer)	=O	$-O-C(CH_3)=C(H)-C(=O)-N(H)-CH_3$	ronnel	=S	$-O-$ 2,4,5-trichlorophenyl
naled	=O	$-O-CHBr-CBrCl_2$	SD-7438	=O	$-S-C(H)(C_6H_5)-S-P(=O)(O-CH_3)_2$
oxydemeton-methyl	=O	$-S-CH_2-CH_2-S(=O)-C_2H_5$			
parathion-methyl	=S	$-O-C_6H_4-NO_2$	temephos	=S	$-O-C_6H_4-S-C_6H_4-O-P(=S)(O-CH_3)_2$
phenthoate	=S	$-S-CH(C_6H_5)-C(=O)-O-CH_2CH_3$			
phosphamidon	=O	$-O-C(CH_3)=C(Cl)-C(=O)-N(C_2H_5)_2$	thiomethon	=S	$-S-CH_2-CH_2-S-CH_2-CH_3$
			trichlorfon	=O	$-CH(OH)-CCl_3$

Malaspray®, Malathiozol®, Malathiozoo®, and Malathon®. Code designations include EI-4049, ENT-17034, and OMS-1. The CAS registry number is 121-75-5.

Physical and Chemical Properties Malathion has the empirical formula $C_{10}H_{19}O_6PS_2$ and a molecular weight of 330. The pure material forms a clear amber liquid with a boiling point of 156–157°C at 0.7 mm Hg. The density is 1.23 at 25°C. The vapor pressure is 4×10^{-5} mm Hg at 30°C. The melting point of malathion is 2.85°C. The solubility of malathion in water at room temperature is 145 ppm. It is miscible with many organic solvents, although its solubility in petroleum oils is limited. Malathion is rapidly hydrolyzed at pH above 7.0 or below 5.0 but is stable in aqueous solution buffered at pH 5.26. It is incompatible with alkaline pesticides.

History, Formulations, Uses, and Production Malathion was introduced in 1950 by the American Cyanamid Company. The technical product is 95% pure. It is a nonsystemic insecticide and acaricide. Malathion is used in control of mosquitoes, flies, household insects, animal ectoparasites, and human head and body lice. Malathion is formulated as 25–86% emulsifiable concentrates, as 25–50% wettable powders, as dusts (usually at 4% concentration), and as ultralow-volume concentrates of 96%.

Problems of Formulation and Storage Eleven impurities of malathion were separated by column and thin-layer chromatography, and their structures were determined by nuclear magnetic resonance, by infrared and mass spectroscopy, and by gas and thin-layer chromatography. Several of the impurities potentiated malathion; the highest activity was observed with *O,S,S*-trimethyl phosphorodithioate and *S*-methyl malathion. When the concentration of various impurities varied from 0.05 to 5%, the factor of potentiation for the rat varied from 1.4 to 10. Potentiating effects were significantly smaller in the mouse than in the rat. Storage of technical malathion for 3–6 months at 40°C resulted in materials that were noticeably more toxic to mice (Umetsu *et al.*, 1977).

There is no evidence that any commercial preparation of malathion is totally free of impurities, but it seems possible that their initial concentrations are higher in the products of some factories than in those of others. Certainly, all preparations, but especially water-wettable powders, are subject to chemical change during storage. The change is fastest under tropical conditions. Whether it can be retarded by techniques of formulation does not seem to have been the subject of a published report. What has been reported is an epidemic of occupational poisoning, in which the frequency and intensity of illness correlated with the concentration of an impurity and with the place of manufacture (see Section 16.6.1.3).

16.6.1.2 Toxicity to Laboratory Animals

Basic Findings The anticholinergic effects of malathion are entirely similar to those of other organic phosphorus compounds (DuBois *et al.*, 1953). By an entirely different mechanism, malathion produces reversible ataxia in hens (Durham *et al.*, 1956) (see Section 16.4.1). However, the dosage necessary to achieve this effect is large (100 mg/kg subcutaneously), and the compound is practical for the control of ectoparasites of chickens, the most susceptible test species.

Very early samples of malathion were only 65–70% pure, and they were more toxic than commercial samples made since about 1952. The toxicity of any particular sample is increased by solution, especially solution in vegetable oil (Hazleton and Holland, 1953). Malathion of recent manufacture is not faultless. Umetsu *et al.* (1977) identified 11 impurities in a technical product and noted that storage of the mixture for 3–6 months at 40°C resulted in materials that were noticeably more toxic to mice. Several of the impurities potentiated the toxicity of pure malathion to rats. Most active were *O,S,S,*-trimethyl phosphordithioate and the *S*-methyl isomer. There was less potentiation in mice. In spite of these variables, malathion that has been made properly and stored under favorable conditions has a low acute toxicity when administered by any natural route (see Table 16.17 and Use Experience in Section 16.6.1.3). Technical malathion of good quality has an oral LD 50 value in the rat of not less than 1000 mg/kg. Corresponding values for highly purified samples lie between 8000 and 12,500 (Pellegrini and Santi, 1972).

An increase in mitogenic and humoral immune responses in female mice 5 days following an oral dose of 715 mg/kg has been reported by Rodgers *et al.* (1986a). Doses of 143 mg/kg/day for 14 days decreased thymic cell numbers. These

Table 16.17
Single-Dose LD 50 Values for Malathion

Species	Route	LD 50 (mg/kg)	Reference
Rat, M	oral	5,843	Hazelton and Holland (1953)
Rat	oral	1,400	DuBois *et al.* (1953)
Rat, M	oral	1,375	Gaines (1960)
Rat, F	oral	1,000	Gaines (1960)
Rat, M	oral	2,830	Shaffer and West (1960)
Rat	oral	1,401	Boyd *et al.* (1970)
Rat	oral	8,000	Pellegrini and Santi (1972)
Rat	oral	12,500	Umetsu *et al.* (1977)
Rat	oral	10,700	Aldridge *et al.* (1979)
Rat, M	dermal	4,444	Gaines (1960)
Rat, F	dermal	4,444	Gaines (1960)
Rat	intraperitoneal	750	DuBois *et al.* (1953)
Mouse	oral	4,059	Hazelton and Holland (1953)
Mouse	oral	400–500	Kagan (1957b)
Mouse	intraperitoneal	985	Menzer and Best (1968)
Puppy	intraperitoneal	1,857	Guiti and Sadeghi (1969)
Chicken	oral	525	Gupta and Paul (1971)

and other immunotoxic effects have been associated with the malathion contaminants *O,O,S*-trimethyl phosphorothioate and, to a lesser extent, *O,S,S*-trimethyl phosphorodithioate (see Section 16.4.5)

In 2-year feeding studies, even a dietary concentration of 5000 ppm did not increase mortality of rats, although food intake was reduced (so that the dosage was somewhat less than the predicted 250 mg/kg) and weight gain was subnormal. The rats remained asymptomatic, even though plasma cholinesterase activity was reduced to about 5–40% of normal, red cell enzyme activity was reduced to approximately 0, and brain acetylcholinesterase was reduced to about 5–40% of normal (Hazleton and Holland, 1953).

A dietary concentration of 1000 ppm (50 mg/kg) for 2 years was accepted by rats. It produced no inhibition of growth but did reduce plasma cholinesterase activity to about 64%, red cell enzyme activity to 5–40%, and brain enzyme activity to about 63% of normal (Hazleton and Holland, 1953).

A dietary level of 100 ppm for 2 years (about 5 mg/kg/day) produced little or no inhibition of cholinesterase and no other detectable effect in rats (Hazleton and Holland, 1953). Results in short-term feeding studies were consistent. In fact, rats tolerated dietary levels of highly purified malathion as high as 500 ppm without inhibition of blood cholinesterase.

Absorption, Distribution, Metabolism, and Excretion The most striking difference between the metabolism of malathion and that of the majority of organic phosphorus compounds used as insecticides depends on the presence of two carboxy groups in malathion. The compound is subject to the various kinds of metabolism that other organic phosphorus insecticides undergo. In addition, the splitting of either carboxy ester linkage renders the compound nontoxic. Details of the metabolism have been reported by O'Brien (1960) and by Heath (1961).

Malathion B-esterase responsible for hydrolyzing the carboxyethyl ester groups arises from a different part of the cell and is biochemically distinct from malathion A-esterase, which degrades malathion at the P—S linkage to form O,O-dimethyl phosphorothioate (Bhagwaat and Ramachandran, 1975).

The excretion of absorbed malathion is prompt. When 25 mg of ^{14}C-labeled malathion was administered to each of six male rats, activity appeared in the urine within 2 hr, and 91.72% was eliminated within 24 hr while an additional 7.75% remained in the gastrointestinal contents. Excretion was mainly via the urine (83.44%) and partly by the feces (5.51%), but 2.77% was exhaled as carbon dioxide. No unmetabolized malathion could be detected 8 hr or longer after dosing (Bourke *et al.*, 1968).

In *in vitro* studies of human and rat liver, no important difference was found in ability to degrade malathion (Matsumura and Ward, 1966).

Biochemical Effects Malathion and other organic phosphorus insecticides are inhibitors of liver microsomal enzymes *in vitro*, probably acting as alternative substrates. Depending on circumstances, malathion may or may not affect hexobarbital sleeping time or zoxazolamine paralysis *in vivo* (Gundu Rao and Anders, 1973; Stevens, 1972; Stevens *et al.*, 1973). In fact, as shown by Murphy (1967), a metabolite of malathion and certain impurities in technical malathion inhibit the hydrolysis of malathion in rats. This may mean that hydrolysis is relatively less important as a detoxicating mechanism following large doses than following small ones. The dosage of malathion necessary to inhibit carboxylesterase activity is less than that necessary to inhibit red cell and brain cholinesterase (Murphy and Cheever, 1968). The impurities just mentioned may be the same as those that Pellegrini and Santi (1972) found increased the toxicity of malathion and of some other compounds to mammals and that could be neutralized without reducing the toxicities of the main ingredients to insects.

The critical importance of the carboxylesterase titer in serum and especially liver in determining susceptibility to malathion was demonstrated by measuring the activity of this enzyme and malathion LD 50 values in rats, in three strains of mice, and in five groups of one of these strains pretreated with different dosages of O,S,S-trimethyl phosphorodithioate to inhibit the enzyme to different degrees. The equation for the best regression line for all the data ($r = 0.995$) was LD 50 = $42.4(S + 2L) - 429$, where 422.4 was the slope of the regression line, $S + 2L$ was the sum of carboxylesterase activity in serum plus twice that in liver (in milligrams of malathion hydrolyzed per minute per kilogram of body weight), and 429 was the y intercept in milligrams per kilogram of body weight. Use of this equation and measurements of carboxylesterase activity in samples of human liver (the serum being devoid of activity) permitted the calculations of human LD 50 values ranging from 2282 to 5239 mg/kg and averaging 3655 mg/kg.

The fact that these estimates indicate far lower toxicity of malathion to humans than is indicated by the clinical record of dosage response may be related to the presence of carboxylesterase-inactivating impurities in those formulations that caused poisoning (Talcott *et al.*, 1979c).

The difference in susceptibility of male and female rats to malathion is associated with differences in their aliesterase activity (Brodeur and DuBois, 1964). Newborn rats are much more sensitive than preweanling or adult rats to malathion (Lu *et al.*, 1965) and this, too, probably involves aliesterase activity.

In rats, toxicity is greater in those maintained on diets deficient in protein, but even at protein levels that do not permit survival, much less growth, the difference is less than threefold (Boyd and Tanikella, 1969; Boyd *et al.*, 1970; Webb *et al.*, 1973).

Husain and Matin (1986b) have reported hyperglycemia in female rats following intraperitoneal administration of 500 mg/kg malathion. Although the mechanism remains unknown, the observed decrease in cerebral glycogen and increase in blood glucose levels are apparently in response to the need for additional energy (based on increased glycogen use) in tissues following malathion exposure (see Section 16.2.2.3).

Potentiation of the toxic action of malathion is discussed in Section 16.3.1. Although malathion more than any other pesticide is subject to this kind of interaction, the outbreak in Pakistan described in Section 16.6.1.3 under Use Experience seems to have been the only documented example of its occurrence in people.

Effects on Organs and Tissues An *in vitro* concentration of 23 or 50 ppm inhibited the growth of human hematopoietic cells but did not increase chromosome aberrations; normal growth was renewed when the medium was replaced to reduce the malathion concentration (Huang, 1973). An opposite result, that is, an increase in the frequency of sister chromatid exchange, was found in cultured human fetal fibroblasts exposed twice to concentrations of 5 ppm or higher (Nicholas *et al.*, 1979). Concentrations as high as 40 ppm were not cytotoxic under the conditions of the test.

Effects on Reproduction A dietary level of 4000 ppm (about 53 mg/kg/day), although tolerated by both male and female rats, reduced the size of their litters and the number of those born that survived the first week of nursing (Kalow and Marton, 1961). Malathion at a dosage of 0.1 mg/kg was found not to cause changes in reproductive function or in the viability of offspring in rats (Leybovich, 1973).

Using conventional teratological techniques and dosages ranging from 105 to 356 mg/kg/day, Dobbins (1967) produced in rats mild changes of the kidney and ureter characteristic of retarded development and, in one group, a few mild examples of hydrocephalus. The insecticide was used as a commercial solution involving an unknown solvent. The estimated LD 50 in the pregnant female was 370 mg/kg, indicating toxicity far greater than that of pure malathion.

Whereas there is no evidence that malathion is teratogenic in mammals, it does cause a characteristic syndrome of deformity in chickens that apparently depends on tryptophan metabolism and may be peculiar to the egg, which is a closed system. When 1.17–29.20 mg of malathion was injected directly into the yolk of each egg, it often killed the embryo and deformed many of those that survived. When injections were on days 8–12, half of the survivors lacked feathers or had only a few feathers on the abdominal region. When injections were on day 6 or 7, 95% of the survivors were smaller than normal. When injections were on day 4 or 5, the legs were half the proper size and the phalanges were permanently flexed in 95% of the survivors, and the maxilla was curved downward over the shortened mandible in 50% of cases. All of the hatched chicks had abnormal feathers, and some lacked feathers completely or in some areas. Most of the hatched chicks were about two-thirds normal size, and 6% were only one-fourth normal size (Greenberg and LaHam, 1969). What was truly unexpected was the report that tryptophan prevented the hindlimb, beak, and feather defects and overall growth retardation in malathion-dosed embryos (Greenberg and LaHam, 1970).

Essentially similar results were reported by Walker (1971), who found nicotinamide protective. These results were confirmed and extended by Wenger and Wenger (1973), who showed that application of 3 μl of malathion directly to the *area vasculosa* of chick embryos on day 4 and again on day 5 of incubation produced the characteristic parrot beak syndrome in 100% of survivors without increasing mortality above that of controls. Application of 0.1 ml of 0.2 *M* nicotinamide or 0.1 ml of 0.1 *M* tryptophan simultaneously with malathion prevented development of the syndrome in all survivors, although the nicotinamide increased mortality. Tryptophan was also effective when injected into the yolk, and it was not toxic. It was speculated that malathion interferes with mobilization of tryptophan from yolk proteins, consequently decreasing synthesis of nicotinamide, which is essential for pyridine nucleotide-dependent reactions involved in differentiation of legs, beak, feathers, and other organs.

Deformities of chicks can also be produced by feeding malathion to laying hens for 3 weeks at dietary concentrations up to 600 ppm (Ghadiri *et al.*, 1967). However, the most likely problem for poultry is not teratogenicity but simple toxicity. The hatchability of eggs was reduced when the hens were fed dietary levels of 1.0 ppm or higher but not 0.1 ppm (about 0.0058 mg/kg/day) (Sauter and Steele, 1972).

Treatment of Poisoning in Animals Atropine, 2-PAM, and other oximes are effective in treating malathion poisonings. In rats, Agarwal and Matin (1981) have demonstrated the effectiveness of immediate atropine and oxime treatment in the prevention of malathion-induced hyperglycemia (associated with acetylcholine accumulation) over delayed treatment (30

min following poisoning) or the prophylactic administration of reserpine (Matin and Husain, 1984).

16.6.1.3 Toxicity to Humans

All experimental studies have been carried out with malathion that was properly manufactured and stored under favorable conditions. Not only did the experimental studies indicate low toxicity, but this has been confirmed by most occupational experience. However, there has been at least one important exception traced to impurities in formulations available under field conditions and described under Use Experience below. Of course, accidents and suicides have occurred with formulations that did not contain more than the usual traces of impurities and, no doubt, with some that did.

Experimental Oral Exposure A single dose of 58 mg (0.84 mg/kg) produced no clinical effect, and 23% of it was recovered from the urine in the form of organic phosphorus (Mattson and Sedlak, 1960).

Dosages up to 16 mg/person/day for 47 days produced no significant effect on either plasma or red cell cholinesterase activity. Plasma cholinesterase was reduced to as low as 75% about 3 weeks after malathion had been given at a rate of 24 mg/person/day for 56 days but not during the dosing period. The volunteers remained asymptomatic throughout (Moeller and Rider, 1962a). The change in cholinesterase was statistically significant, but its causal relation to malathion is uncertain because of the timing.

No inhibition of plasma or red cell cholinesterase activity occurred when malathion and EPN were given simultaneously at rates up to 16 and 3 mg/person/day, respectively, for 32 or more days. The enzymes were also unaffected by a dosage combination of 8 and 6 mg/person/day, respectively. However, a malathion–EPN dosage combination of 16 and 6 mg/person/day, respectively, for 42 days produced a slight depression of both plasma and red cell cholinesterase activity, even though EPN alone is tolerated at a rate of 6 mg/person/day for 88 days (Rider *et al.*, 1959). The lowest combination of malathion and EPN known to produce a slight inhibition of cholinesterase activity is 16 and 5 mg/person/day, respectively (Moeller and Rider, 1962a).

Experimental Dermal Exposure In order to test the safety of single applications of 1% malathion dust for controlling human body lice, concentrations of 0, 1, 5, and 10% were applied to volunteers and their clothing five times a week for 8 or more weeks, using 90 gm of powder per person per day. The powder was left on for more than 23 hr/day but was removed on weekends. Complaints about odor and skin irritation were minor but approximately proportional to dosage; a few men exposed to plain talc also complained. Concentrations of 1 and 5% malathion produced no change in red cell cholinesterase, while 10% caused a depletion which approached, but did not reach, statistical significance. No dosage-related change in plasma cholinesterase occurred. The excretion of malathion-derived material in the urine was variable but proportional to dosage. On the average, a little more than 2% of the dose actually available for absorption (28 gm of powder) was recovered in the urine, but on one occasion a man reached a value of 18%, corresponding to a rate of 9.57 mg of malathion equivalent per hour. The average recovery of malathion equivalent from the urine of men receiving 10% powder was 2.15 mg/hr or 51 mg/person/day, or (taking the limited recovery of malathion from urine into account) 224 mg/person/day. No changes other than statistically insignificant inhibition of cholinesterase attributable to malathion were found (Hayes *et al.*, 1960). Malathion powder (1%) was found both safe and effective for louse control when tested among hundreds of people under village conditions (Shawarby *et al.*, 1963). Malathion powder (1%) eventually became standard for louse control (Steinberg *et al.*, 1972). Although originally studied for louse control, malathion is fairly effective for treatment of scabies. An 83% cure rate was obtained in one study in which a 0.5% liquid formulation was used (Hanna *et al.*, 1978).

When [^{14}C]malathion was applied to the ventral forearm of 12 volunteers, radioactivity equivalent to a "corrected" average of 8.2% of the total dose was recovered from urine produced during the first 5 days (Feldmann and Maibach, 1970). This percentage is an essentially accurate indication of absorption during the period because almost all (90.2%) of the radioactivity was recovered in the urine following intravenous injection of malathion.

Milby and Epstein (1964) found that nearly half of 87 volunteers developed contact sensitization following a single exposure to 10% malathion and that many of them responded to dilutions as little as 1 ppm. Similar results were reported by Kligman (1966). However, it was found as part of the first study that only about 3% of people with occupational exposure to the compound reacted to a patch test with 1% formulation, and no worker was sufficiently affected to require a change of work.

Experimental Respiratory Exposure In rooms with no ventilation, groups of four men received 84 exposures to aerosols on 42 consecutive days. The men in each group remained in the closed room for 1 hr following each application of aerosol. The control formulation contained pyrethrins, piperonyl butoxide, solvent, propellant, and perfume. The experimental formulations were identical, except that a portion of the propellant was replaced by 5 and 20%, respectively, malathion. The four groups of volunteers were exposed to aerosols applied as follows: group 1, 3 gm of control formulation per 1000 ft^3; group 2, 3 gm of 5% malathion per 1000 ft^3; group 3, 3 gm of 20% malathion per 1000 ft^3; and group 4, 12 gm of 20% malathion per 1000 ft^3. Careful observation failed to reveal any adverse effect of this extremely high exposure; red cell and plasma cholinesterase showed no dosage-related change, and they were as stable for men receiving the highest dosage as they were for the controls (Golz, 1959).

According to Danilow (1968), one volunteer was able to detect the odor of carbophos at a concentration of 0.052 mg/m^3, and all detected it at 0.096 mg/m^3. Furthermore, a concentration of 0.044 mg/m^3 (not detectable by smell) affected sensitivity to light as measured by a special device. Finally, EEG changes were found by a special technique at malathion concentrations of 0.025–0.032 mg/m^3 in inspired air. As a result, the maximum permissible concentration of carbophos was set at 0.014 mg/m^3.

A worker exposed to an average concentration of 0.014 mg/m^3 would inhale about 0.14 mg of compound during an 8-hr workday. This may be compared to a discrete oral dosage of 16 mg/person/day and a dermal dosage of approximately 224 mg/person/day, absorbed gradually throughout the day; both of these dosages failed to influence cholinesterase to a statistically significant degree or to produce any clinical effect. Under the circumstances, the significance of the highly specialized tests or the purity of the carbophos formulation or both are open to question.

Accidental and Intentional Poisoning Whereas most serious poisoning by malathion in the United States has been accidental and has involved young children, poisoning by this compound in some developing countries has been largely suicidal and has involved mainly adults (Mootoo, 1965; Nalin, 1973; Amarasingahm and Ti, 1976).

Almost all confirmed cases, whether fatal or not, have involved proved or possible ingestion as determined by history or the finding in stomach washings, or both. Rare cases of dermal poisoning prove the rule; for example, a number of children suffered typical poisoning when their hair was washed with a 50% solution of malathion in xylene to eliminate lice (Galzon and Levin, 1968; Ramu *et al.*, 1973). Whether the danger of this practice, in contrast to the tested safety of malathion powder for combating lice, depended on the higher concentration and presence of an irritant solvent or on the presence of impurities in the formulation or on all of these is unknown. In any event, if one excludes the cases in which a concentrated solution was applied to people intentionally, most of the small number of cases of systemic illness ascribed to dermal and/or respiratory exposure to malathion (Parker and Chattin, 1955; McLaughlin and Snyder, 1956; Petty, 1958a; Healy, 1959; Sare, 1972) showed little resemblance to confirmed cases or to one another, and, as Namba *et al.* (1970) suggested, the reported exposures did not appear sufficient to cause illness.

In valid cases following ingestion, illness sometimes has begun within a few minutes (Tuthill, 1958) and apparently never has begun more than 3 hr after exposure (Walters, 1957). On the other hand, in one of the few instances of poisoning by dermal absorption, illness began some 12–14 hr after the hair was washed to combat lice (Ramu *et al.*, 1973).

Broadly speaking, poisoning by malathion is similar to poisoning by parathion and other organic phosphorus compounds. However, it appears that some conditions are relatively more common in connection with malathion: (*a*) unconsciousness and marked flaccidity of the limbs, often accompanied by cyanosis but in the absence of life-threatening respiratory or cardiac involvement (Walters, 1957; Goldman and Teitel, 1958; Hayes, 1963; Richards, 1964; Amos and Hall, 1965); (b) convulsions (Gitelson et al., 1966; Wenzl and Burke, 1962; Hayes, 1982); and (c) prolonged, sometimes gradually worsening illness in the absence of initial, anoxic brain damage (Mathewson and Hardy, 1970). Instances of relapse with final recovery have been reported (Ekin, 1971; Amos and Hall, 1965; Goulding, 1968; Urban and Sando, 1965; Gadoth and Fisher, 1978). The relative disassociation of coma and flaccidity from life-threatening respiratory and cardiac involvement suggests that malathion poisoning may involve "side effects" not seen in connection with more toxic organic phosphorus compounds.

A number of cases of severe malathion poisoning have involved a prolonged course, even though recovery was eventually complete. In some instances, an intermediate syndrome developed 1–4 days following poisoning in spite of an early, encouraging response to treatment. The symptoms of this syndrome are pharmacologically distinct from those of acute neurotoxicity and delayed neuropathy (Wadia et al., 1974; Gadoth and Fisher, 1978; Senanayake and Karalliedde, 1987) and include weakness of proximal limb muscles, cranial nerve palsies, and respiratory depression, which could be fatal if not treated immediately with pralidoxime, atropine, and assisted respiration (see Section 16.4.1.3).

Dagli and Shaikh (1983) reported 63% of all patients admitted to a hospital in Bombay with malathion poisoning to have elevated amylase levels. This may be the result of hormones released in response to cholinergic stimulation or of direct cholinergic stimulation of pancreatic acinar and ductal cells. This effect was relatively mild and transient (lasting 3–4 days) and required no special treatment.

Because detoxification and excretion of malathion is rapid in volunteers, the recurrence of coma and the occurrence of prolonged illness without initial anoxia suggest recurrent or continuing absorption of the compound. Quinby (1964) has emphasized the importance of emptying the intestine as rapidly as possible following ingestion of malathion.

Use Experience   An outbreak of poisoning by malathion was associated with impurities in the formulation being used to control malaria. The result stands in sharp contrast to the generally excellent record of occupational safety of malathion, and it calls attention to the necessity of considering formulation problems in connection with prevention of any future difficulty.

In 1976 an epidemic of poisoning due to water-wettable powder occurred among 5350 sprayers, 1070 mixers, and 1070 supervisors in the malaria control program in Pakistan. Some cases began within a few days after spraying commenced in June in one sector and in August in another. In July, the peak month, there were approximately 2800 cases. During the entire epidemic there were five deaths, but they occurred before special study began and details about them are scant. The systemic symptoms in the nonfatal illnesses were entirely typical, and many of the workers were sick enough to resign and seek other employment. Treatment at first was inadequate. One of the

deaths involved a man who was treated with atropine in a local dispensary and sent home; he died shortly after being returned to the same dispensary for further treatment.

A careful study begun in late August revealed that the three brands of malathion that had been in use in Pakistan differed substantially in (a) toxicity to rats, (b) content of isomalathion, and (c) degree of inhibition of cholinesterase produced in sprayers who applied them. The relationships are summarized in Table 16.18. Evidence that malathion formulations were responsible for the epidemic and, more specifically, that the contamination of some brands was responsible included findings that signs and symptoms were typical of anticholinesterase poisoning; the degree of cholinesterase inhibition corresponded to the degree of exposure to insecticide; cholinesterase levels of workers with each of several symptoms were significantly lower than those of workers who lacked the symptoms; and cholinesterase levels decreased during the work week, especially in workers exposed to preparations containing 2 or 3% isomalathion. The investigators attributed the epidemic to the combination of inappropriate techniques of handling the insecticide and the toxicity of two of the three brands. Elimination of use of the two more toxic preparations and special instructions on proper safety measures halted the epidemic in September 1976 (Baker et al., 1978).

It was assumed, no doubt correctly, that concentrations of 2–3% isomalathion contributed to the toxicity of the preparations in which they occurred, not so much through their inherent toxicity as through their demonstrated potentiation of the toxicity of malathion (Aldridge et al., 1979). The relatively great importance of isomalathion under field conditions is consistent with the finding that a soluble, stable, partially purified preparation of human liver malathion carboxylesterase was susceptible to inhibition by isomalathion but not by three other impurities isolated from technical malathion (Talcott et al., 1979a,b).

It was shown that formation of isomalathion occurred at high temperatures (either in the laboratory or in the tropics) but only to a significant degree in formulations with improper "inert" ingredients (Miles et al., 1979).

There may still be some question as to why formulations with oral LD 50 values in the rat of 500–600 mg/kg should

Table 16.18

Mean Oral LD 50 Values, Isomalathion Levels, and Postspray Cholinesterase Activities by Malathion Brand[a]

Brand	Rat oral LD 50[b] (mg/kg)	Isomalathion content (% of weight)	Postspray cholinesterase activities[c] (ΔpH/hr)
1	1940	0.3	0.58
2	626	2.1	0.38
3	651	3.1	0.24

[a] From data of Baker et al. (1978).
[b] For 50% malathion powder.
[c] Mean level in sprayers using each brand during workday.

cause illness and especially death in occupationally exposed people. Studies in volunteers and the majority of use experience indicate a relatively low level of toxicity to humans. However, the ultimate dosages involved in fatal and near-fatal cases suggest that humans are inherently more susceptible than the rat to malathion. A further answer may lie in species differences in potentiation, a parameter that has been little explored in connection with malathion or other compounds.

In the very small number of other instances of occupational poisoning by malathion (e.g., Japanese cases cited without detail by Namba *et al.*, 1970), it is not known whether a relatively high concentration of impurities or some other unusual circumstance was responsible.

Grech (1965) concluded that agricultural workers exposed to malathion for 6 months were mildly poisoned, even though their plasma cholinesterase and a number of clinical laboratory measurements did not differ statistically from those of controls. On the contrary, when malathion was used for spraying the entire inside of every home and other building in Nigerian villages for control of malaria, the inhabitants showed a moderate decrease of blood cholinesterase activity. However, there was no detectable illness, and cholinesterase activity returned to normal within 6 weeks (Elliott and Barnes, 1963). Safety of good formulations was confirmed by later malaria control tests involving a population of about 26,000 in Uganda (Najera *et al.*, 1967).

Properly manufactured malathion is safe for application to cities for the control of vector-borne disease, as exemplified by the experience in Africa. No symptoms or inhibition of cholinesterase was found among men exposed to a malathion aerosol dispensed by ground equipment for control of mosquitoes that transmit western equine and St. Louis encephalitis (Culvert *et al.*, 1956). In another instance, a group of 119 citizens were studied before and after aerial application of 95% malathion concentrate to a city and its suburbs using the low-volume technique in a successful effort to curb an outbreak of St. Louis encephalitis. Some of the people were not in the sprayed area, some were outdoors and under the spray planes during several passes, and the majority had intermediate exposure. The plasma cholinesterase values showed no decrease related to the degree of exposure. Six persons reported minor symptoms, but they were nonspecific, and there were no pathognomonic signs (Gardner and Iverson, 1968).

Atypical Cases of Various Origins The most interesting cases attributed to malathion are those involving paresis without earlier or simultaneous occurrence of signs and symptoms typical of anticholinesterase poisoning. Such cases were reported during the 1950s (Parker and Chattin, 1955; Petty, 1958a; Healy, 1959) but apparently have not been reported since. If humans were as susceptible as the chicken to the ataxia produced by malathion, one would expect to see cases among people with heavy occupational exposure and especially among those who have survived accidental or suicidal poisoning. However, nothing resembling the ataxia of chickens has been observed among people who received very large doses.

The alleged cases followed trivial, often dermal exposure. Several involved fever, and no two cases were really alike clinically or in their time relationship to malathion exposure.

Great interest was excited many years ago by a report (Gershon and Shaw, 1961) of 16 cases of mental illness (schizophrenia, depression, and impairment of concentration) among people exposed to organophosphorus insecticides, especially malathion, in the course of their work in fruit orchards and greenhouses. Several letters to the editor of the journal that published the report drew attention to deficiencies in both its epidemiological and clinical aspects. Extensive experience in many countries and a reinvestigation in the country of origin (Stoller *et al.*, 1965) failed to substantiate any of the fears that the report aroused.

Aizenshtad *et al.* (1971) reported impaired nervous function, gastrointestinal illness, altered blood proteins, and many subjective complaints among workers who showed only moderate inhibition of cholinesterase.

Severe fatty degeneration of the liver, necrosis in the gastrointestinal tract, and microscopic lesions of the nervous system were reported in a fatal case attributed to "Foszfothion," of which malathion was said to be the active ingredient (Varnai, 1971). If identification of the active ingredient was accurate, it would seem that some other ingredient must have been responsible for destruction of tissue.

Rivett and Potgieter (1987) reported a case of diaphragmatic weakness requiring continuous positive pressure ventilation for 3 months following the ingestion of malathion, brodifacoum (a vitamin K antagonist), and alcohol in a suicide attempt. Recovery from the weakness was complete 6 months after the patient was weaned from the respirator, as the absence of diaphragmatic weakness was confirmed by fluoroscopic screening.

A clinical study of 57 persons associated with the manufacture of carbophos revealed only two cases of occupational dermatitis and no systemic illness; however, numerous depressions of cholinesterase were found (Trefilov *et al.*, 1968). The presence of inhibition raises the question of whether the material being made was identical in composition to technical malathion as manufactured in the United States. A similar question is raised by a report (Bychkovskiy and Pisarchik, 1972) of mild to severe illness of children attributed to their having eaten malathion residues on cherries.

Dosage Response Dosages ranging from 350 to 1000 mg/kg were ingested in five cases of suicide that proved fatal in all cases in spite of treatment in three of them (Farago, 1967; Namba *et al.*, 1970). An estimated 3855 mg (about 56 mg/kg) led to the death of a 75-year-old man about 1.5 hr after he ingested malathion that he mistook for cough medicine (Paul, 1960).

On the contrary, a younger man, who also had mistaken malathion for a medication, survived a dosage of 615 mg/kg (Crowley and Johns, 1966). A 34-month-old boy survived a dosage of about 190 mg/kg (Goldman and Teitel, 1958), and a boy only 40 days old lived in spite of a dose of approximately 1750 mg (about 407 mg/kg) (Freundlich and Steinlauf, 1964).

Other survivals involved dosages ranging from about 100 to 1000 mg/kg (Walters, 1957; Goldin *et al.,* 1964; Richards, 1964; Gitelson *et al.,* 1966; Valero and Golan, 1967; Goulding, 1968; Mathewson and Hardy, 1970). Vomiting and gastric lavage may have reduced the retained dose in many of these instances and certainly did in an attempted suicide in which the amount of malathion missing from a bottle and presumably ingested was 44,360 mg. However, in this near-fatal case, 1106 mg of malathion was recovered from the urine over a period of 123 hr. Judging from the proportion of an oral dose recovered from the urine of a volunteer, the amount recovered in the attempted suicide indicated absorption of 4800 mg; that is, an absorbed dosage of about 68 mg/kg (Hayes, 1963). It must be emphasized that the high dosages that were survived would have been fatal in the absence of aggressive treatment.

The dosage that would lead to mild illness has not been defined. As discussed in connection with experimental exposure, people tolerate a single oral dosage of 0.84 mg/kg, repeated oral dosage of 0.34 mg/kg/day, or a repeated dermal, absorbed dosage of 3.2 mg/kg/day, all with no statistically significant degree of cholinesterase inhibition. These dosages are of the same order of magnitude as 1.4 mg/kg/day, the occupational intake considered safe on the basis of the threshold limit of 10 mg/m³.

Laboratory Findings The urinary metabolite present in greatest concentration after ingestion of about 100,000 mg of malathion was malathion monocarboxylic acid; a sample collected during the second 24 hr after ingestion contained 223 ppm. Other metabolites measured in the same sample were dicarboxylic acid, 12 ppm; dimethylthiophosphate, 96 ppm; dimethyldithiophosphate, 20 ppm; dimethylphosphate, 50 ppm; and monomethylphosphate, 8 ppm (Bradway and Shafik, 1977).

Treatment of Poisoning Treatment is the same as for other organic phosphorus compounds (see Section 16.2.2.7). The benefit of oximes is striking in some cases (Amos and Hall, 1965), and one of these drugs should be used in every case of serious poisoning by malathion.

16.6.2 PARATHION-METHYL

16.6.2.1 Identity, Properties, and Uses

Chemical Name Parathion-methyl is *O,O*-dimethyl *O*-(4-nitrophenyl)phosphorothioate.

Structure See Table 16.16.

Synonyms The common name parathion-methyl (BSI, ISO) is in general use, except that methyl parathion and metaphos are used in the United States and USSR, respectively. Trade names have included: Bladan M®, Dalf®, Folidol-M®, Metacide®, Metron®, and Nitrox®. Code designations include

BAY-E-601, E-601, ENT-17292, and OMS-213. The CAS registry number is 298-00-0.

Chemical and Physical Properties Parathion-methyl has the empirical formula $C_8H_{10}NO_5PS$ and a molecular weight of 263.23. The pure material forms a white crystalline powder melting at 37–38°C. The technical product is light to dark tan, crystallizes at about 29°C, and is about 80% pure. The density of parathion-methyl at 20°C is reported variously from 1.20 to 1.36. The vapor pressure is 0.97×10^{-5} mm Hg at 20°C. Parathion-methyl is soluble in water at 25°C to the extent of 55–60 ppm. It is slightly soluble in light petroleum and mineral oils and soluble in most other organic solvents. Parathion-methyl is hydrolyzed by alkali at a higher rate than parathion and readily isomerizes on heating.

History, Formulations, Uses, and Production Parathion-methyl first was described by Schrader in 1952. It was introduced under several trade names by Bayer Leverkusen. Formulations include emulsifiable concentrates, wettable powders, and dusts of various concentrations. Parathion-methyl is a nonsystemic contact and stomach insecticide with some fumigant action. Its range of usefulness is similar to that of parathion, but its mammalian toxicity is lower.

16.6.2.2 Toxicity to Laboratory Animals

Basic Findings Although parathion-methyl is considerably less toxic than parathion, it is still a dangerous compound from the standpoint of acute toxicity (see Table 16.19). A method that permitted actual measurement of LD 1 values and extrapolation of LD 0.1 values showed that the oral LD 50, LD 1, and LD 0.1 values were 14.5, 8.46, and 7.07 mg/kg, respectively, in male mice and 19.5, 9.58, and 7.63 mg/kg, respectively, in female mice (Haley *et al.,* 1975a).

When methylnitrophos was fed to rabbits at a level of 10 mg/kg/day for 3 months, they lost weight and showed considerable pathology; a dosage of 5 mg/kg/day produced only slight effect (Abbasov, 1971).

When parathion-methyl was fed to dogs for 12 weeks, a dietary level of 50 ppm soon caused a significant depression of red cell and plasma cholinesterase, 20 ppm inhibited red

Table 16.19
Single-Dose LD 50 for Parathion-Methyl

Species	Route	LD 50 (mg/kg)	Reference
Rat, M	oral	20	Shaffer and West (1960)
Rat, M	oral	14	Gaines (1960)
Rat, F	oral	24	Gaines (1960)
Rat, M	dermal	67	Gaines (1960)
Rat, F	dermal	67	Gaines (1960)
Rat, M	intraperitoneal	5.8	Benke and Murphy (1975)
Rat, F	intraperitoneal	8	Benke and Murphy (1975)
Mouse, M	oral	14.5	Haley *et al.* (1975a)
Mouse, F	oral	19.5	Haley *et al.* (1975a)

cell but not plasma cholinesterase, and 5 ppm (about 0.1 mg/kg/day) was a no-effect level [Food and Agriculture Organization/World Health Organization (FAO/WHO), 1969].

Absorption, Distribution, Metabolism, and Excretion
^{32}P-labeled parathion-methyl was rapidly absorbed following oral administration; the maximal tissue level was attained in 1–2 hr (Gar *et al.*, 1958).

The intraperitoneal LD 50 for parathion-methyl is slightly less than 1 mg/kg. During the first 35–40 days after birth, there is a marked decrease in susceptibility in both sexes. Benke and Murphy (1975) found that the age difference did not depend on the susceptibility of cholinesterase to inhibition by paraoxon-methyl *in vitro*. Increases in LD 50 values with age correlated better with increased detoxification of paraoxon-methyl than with any direct metabolism of the parent compound.

Effects on Organs and Tissues Parathion-methyl at concentrations of 23 and 50 ppm inhibited the growth of three human hematopoietic cell lines, but normal growth usually resumed after substitution of a medium lacking the compound. The occurrence of chromosome aberrations was not increased. Dosages of 5–100 mg/kg in mice did not increase the incidence of bone marrow cells with chromosome aberrations (Huang, 1973). Feeding the compound for 7 weeks failed to produce dominant lethals in male mice (Jorgenson *et al.*, 1976).

Effects on Reproduction A three-generation study in rats fed dietary levels of 30, 10, and 0 ppm parathion-methyl revealed at the higher dosage (about 1.5 mg/kg/day in nonlactating, adult rats but higher in young or lactating rats): lower weanling survival rate in the F_{1a}, F_{1b}, and F_{2a} generations; increased stillbirth rate in F_{1b} and F_{3a} generations; reduced mean weanling rate in the F_{2a} generation; and reduced reproductive performance in the F_{1a}, F_{1b}, F_{2a}, and F_{3b} generations. Defects of reproduction were entirely sporadic at 10 ppm. There was no increase in anomalies at either rate of intake (FAO/WHO, 1969).

A single intraperitoneal injection of parathion-methyl into rats on day 12 and into mice on day 10 at LD 50 rates (15 and 60 mg/kg in rats and mice, respectively) caused suppression of fetal growth and of ossification in the young of rats that survived. It caused reduced ossification, high fetal mortality, and a 14.9% incidence of cleft palate in the young of mice that lived. Lower dosages (5 and 10 mg/kg in rats and 20 mg/kg in mice) also caused severe systemic symptoms and transient decrease in intake of food and water, but few deaths. These dosages did not cause statistically significant changes in the young (Tanimura *et al.*, 1967).

The young of rats that received parathion-methyl orally at a rate of 4 or 6 mg/kg on day 9 or 15 showed no anomalies or other indication of fetal toxicity (Fish, 1966). In another study, no injury was produced by repeated dosages less than 3 mg/kg; 3 mg/kg was fetatoxic but not teratogenic (Fuchs *et al.*, 1976).

Whether the latter preparation was more toxic by reason of contaminants is unclear.

16.6.2.3 Toxicity to Humans

Experimental Exposure Parathion-methyl was administered by mouth to groups of five volunteers for about 4 weeks. At 22 mg/person/day, it produced no effect. At 24 mg/person/day, two subjects showed a depression of 24 and 23%, respectively, in plasma cholinesterase and 27 and 55% in red cell enzyme; the maximal mean decreases were 17% for plasma and 22% for red cell enzyme. At 26 mg/person/day, plasma cholinesterase was not significantly changed; the red cell enzyme was decreased to 25 and 37% in two subjects only. The maximal mean decrease was 18% (Rider *et al.*, 1970). At 28 mg/person/day, parathion-methyl produced a significant decrease in red cell cholinesterase in three subjects only, and the maximal mean decrease was only 19%. At 30 mg/person/day, the maximal mean depression was 37%. Thus, the level of minimal incipient toxicity for parathion-methyl is 30 mg/person/day or about 0.43 mg/kg/day (Rider *et al.*, 1971). These investigations followed a long series of others in which groups of volunteers received dosages ranging from 1 to 22 mg/person/day, all with negative results (Moeller and Rider, 1961, 1962b, 1963, 1965; Rider and Moeller, 1964; Rider and Puletti, 1969; Rider *et al.*, 1966, 1968, 1969). The most complete single description of the early work is that of Rider *et al.* (1969).

Studies in four volunteers showed that dosages of 2 and 4 mg/person/day resulted in distinctly different average rates of excretion. It is possible to measure excretion following intakes that do not lead to cholinesterase inhibition and, of course, after larger doses. Excretion of *p*-nitrophenol was 60% complete in 4 hr, 86% complete in 8 hr, and essentially complete in 24 hr. Excretion of dimethylphosphate was more protracted (Morgan *et al.*, 1977).

Accidental and Intentional Poisoning Whereas parathion-methyl is clearly safer than parathion, it is not harmless. Several papers reported multiple cases of poisoning (Grigorowa, 1960; Lanyi and Horvath, 1966; Gal *et al.*, 1970). Kawashiro (1959) reported 113 successful suicides and four occupational deaths associated with parathion-methyl. Fazekas (1971) reported on 30 fatal cases, of which 26 were suicides involving ingestion and 4 were accidents involving skin and respiratory contact. Only if such poisoning were common in one area could one author collect such a long series of cases. Survival in this series reported by Fazekas varied from 2 hr to 9 days.

Exposure that was almost exclusively dermal has led to poisoning (Petty, 1957). A combination of dermal, respiratory, and perhaps oral exposure led to the poisoning of 7 of 13 members of a rural family. Nine days after symptoms appeared, one 26-year-old man died and a 17-year-old woman was hospitalized and successfully treated with atropine. The clinical illness suggested poisoning by an organic phosphorus compound, and investigation revealed depressed cholinesterase levels in members of the family and the presence of an abnormal amount of organophosphate in the liver of the deceased. The father said that he had obtained parathion-methyl from a discarded drum and applied it inside his home with a hand nebulizer to kill cockroaches. Application started a few days before illness appeared and was stopped at that time. Other formulations sold for the control of household insects were found in the house. These had been sprayed into the air periodically during the day and night to reduce the number of mosquitos and flies. Whether the parathion-methyl formulation also had been sprayed into the air was unknown. Following cleaning of the house, no further illness occurred (Blakey *et al.*, 1977).

Use Experience   Use experience has been good. In most if not all instances, occupational poisoning has been associated with excessive, definitely accidental exposure.

In a survey carried out in the 1957 crop-dusting season among a total of 245 tractor drivers, pilots, crop insect checkers, insecticide mixers, farmers, and others mainly in that part of Louisiana where the cultivation of cotton is most intense, none of 511 blood samples was found to have cholinesterase activity depressed significantly below normal. During the survey four cases of occupational poisoning occurred in the state, three of them involving factory workers exposed to parathion-methyl (Petty *et al.*, 1959). The findings were entirely similar in another survey carried out during the same summer in the delta area of Mississippi. Contributing to the safety of cotton checkers was the fact that the half-life of parathion-methyl on cotton leaves is less than 1 hr. One case of nonfatal poisoning and three cases of asymptomatic cholinesterase depression associated with parathion-methyl were encountered (Quinby *et al.*, 1958).

Two entomologists checking cotton plants treated with parathion-methyl experienced a marked depression of cholinesterase but no symptoms when they worked in fields beginning only 2 hr after application of an ultralow-volume spray (Nemec *et al.*, 1968).

Dosage Response   One person consumed about 50 ml of a solution of unstated concentration but survived following treatment (Flesch, 1958).

The daily dosage that causes distinct inhibition of cholinesterase but no discomfort is 0.43 mg/kg/day. This value is over 10 times greater than 0.029 mg/kg/day, the dosage considered safe for occupational intake on the basis of the threshold limit value of 0.2 mg/m^3.

Treatment of Poisoning   See Section 16.2.2.7.

16.6.3 DEMETON-METHYL

16.6.3.1 Identity, Properties, and Uses

Chemical Name   At least in the past, commercial formulations have contained two related compounds: *O,O*-dimethyl-*O*-ethylthioethyl phosphorothioate (demeton-*O*-methyl) and *O,O*-dimethyl-*S*-ethyl-thioethyl phosphorothioate (demeton-*S*-methyl).

Structure   See Table 16.16.

Synonyms   Demeton-*O*-methyl (ISO) has been called mercaptophos (USSR), P=S isomer, S=P isomer, and SPOG compound. The CAS registry number is 867-27-6.

Demeton-*S*-methyl (BSI, ISO) has been called methyl mercaptophos teolovy (USSR), O=P isomer, P=O isomer, and SPSC compound. It is sold under the proprietary names of Metaisosystox®, Meta-Systox I®, and Azotox®. Code designations have included Bayer-18436 and Bayer-25/154. The CAS registry number is 916-86-8.

A mixture of O and S isomers, at first in a ratio of about 70:30, has been called methyl demeton and methyl Systox and sold under the proprietary name Meta-Systox®. The CAS registry number of the mixture is 8022-00-2. Later the mixture was replaced by demeton-*S*-methyl, which is more toxic to insects. Another derivative, demeton-*S*-methyl sulfone, was introduced as an insecticide in 1965, but information regarding its toxicity to humans apparently is lacking.

Physical and Chemical Properties   Both isomers have the empirical formula $C_6H_{15}O_3PS_2$ and a molecular weight of 230.30. Both isomers are yellowish oils with an unpleasant odor. The O isomer is more volatile but less soluble in water (333 ppm) than the S isomer (3.6×10^{-4} mm Hg at 20°C and 3333 ppm). The O isomer boils at 74°C at 0.15 mm Hg; its density at 20°C is 1.190. The S isomer boils at 89°C at 0.15 mm Hg; its density at 20°C is 1.207. Both isomers are soluble in organic solvents. They are hydrolyzed by alkali.

The technical mixture undergoes a series of complicated changes that are gradual during storage and more rapid in water. Briefly, about 30% of the O isomer goes to the S isomer, and the rest is hydrolyzed to harmless products. The S isomer is oxidized to the sulfoxide and eventually the sulfone before it finally decomposes. At the same time, both isomers form several sulfonium compounds, which vary in stability but are powerful cholinesterase inhibitors (Heath and Vandekar, 1957). Conversion of the S isomer to sulfoxide and sulfone also occurs in plants (Fukuto *et al.*, 1955, 1956, 1957). Formulations of the technical products may vary in toxicity, depending on the duration and conditions of storage. By the same token, it is virtually impossible to know the exact composition of formulations associated with accidental human poisoning.

History, Formulations, and Uses   Demeton-methyl was first introduced in 1954 as a mixture of both isomers. The S isomer was introduced in 1957. For a time, both products were sold. Both are systemic and contact insecticides and acaricides. The material is available as an emulsifiable concentrate of different concentrations.

16.6.3.2 Toxicity to Laboratory Animals

Basic Findings Demeton-O-methyl is considerably less toxic than demeton-S-methyl. The latter is remarkable in that the oral and intravenous LD 50 values are essentially the same, although the intraperitoneal toxicity is somewhat greater (see Table 16.20).

Effects on Organs and Tissues Rats receiving 15 daily dermal applications of demeton-methyl at 5 mg/kg/day did not show any overt signs of toxicity. However, partially reversible degeneration and necrosis of the liver, as well as reversible cholinesterase inhibition in the brain and serum, were noted (Dikshith *et al.*, 1980).

16.6.3.3 Toxicity to Humans

Use Experience Among a series of 33 cases described by Tarashchyuk (1966a,b), the signs and symptoms were similar to those caused by other organic phosphorus insecticides.

According to Hegazy (1965), there were 673 occupational cases, including three deaths, about 1 week after demeton-S-methyl began to be used for spraying cotton in one region of Egypt. As a result he examined the serum cholinesterase activity of 121 men with occupational exposure and also of three children and two young adults whose exposure was incidental to the spraying but not strictly occupational. Most of the spraying was done with knapsack sprayers, but a few men used power sprayers. Personal hygiene was imperfect. In general, the symptoms were characteristic and had the usual relationship to cholinesterase inhibition. There were, however, some workers who had intention tremor, ataxia, Parkinsonism, and/or hiccough. It was thought that these conditions were caused by the insecticide but might not be the result of cholinesterase inhibition *per se*. Two of the children were unconscious for a few minutes, although their cholinesterase activities were normal. It was concluded by Hegazy that atropine was beneficial in all instances, and all the patients recovered without sequelae. Whether all the cases were valid instances of poisoning is impossible to judge from the evidence available.

Table 16.20
Single-Dose LD 50 for Demeton-Methyl

Compound and species	Route	LD 50 (mg/kg)	Reference
Demeton-O-methyl			
Rat, F	oral	676	Heath and Vandekar (1957)
Fat, F	intravenous	216	Heath and Vandekar (1957)
Demeton-S-methyl			
Rat, F	oral	62.5	Heath and Vandekar (1957)
Rat, F	oral	80	DuBois and Plzak (1962)
Rat, F	intraperitoneal	7.5	DuBois and Plzak (1962)
Rat, M	intraperitoneal	7.5	DuBois and Plzak (1962)
Rat, F	intravenous	64.6	Heath and Vandekar (1957)
Guinea pig	oral	110	DuBois and Plzak (1962)
Guinea pig	intraperitoneal	12.5	DuBois and Plzak (1962)

A man who had been an agricultural applicator for 5 years began working with demeton-S-methyl, mainly as a flagman in aerial spraying but also in preparing the spray and in cleaning containers after spraying. Symptoms gradually increased in severity during the week and subsided during the weekend. Later, he developed anorexia and loss of ability to concentrate. At the end of 6 weeks his symptoms became worse while he was driving a tractor applying disulfoton. After 2 hr, he became dissatisfied with his control of the machine and sought medical aid. Clinical findings were normal, but cholinesterase activity was low. The patient responded promptly to treatment with atropine. Inquiry showed that he always had adhered strictly to safety regulations (Readhead, 1968).

It has been claimed that most teenagers living near cotton fields showed a small to moderate but definite inhibition of blood cholinesterase activity when cotton fields near their houses were treated with demeton-methyl. This was attributed to air contamination (Khasanov and Li, 1970).

Atypical Cases of Various Origins In a suicide attempt, a 60-year-old man drank two liqueur glasses of demeton-methyl and two bottles of beer. He was hospitalized within 2 hr and given conventional treatment, including gastric lavage and a cathartic, even though he showed no toxic signs at the time of admission and there was no change in his condition during the first 60 hr. The man was known to suffer from brucellosis, emphysema, bronchitis, rheumatoid arthritis, diabetes mellitus, and chronic alcoholism. For his underlying illness he received insulin, tolbutamide, and digitoxin. After 60 hr, the patient developed numbness, followed in 12 hr by diarrhea and then sudden cardiocirculatory collapse 81 hr after entering hospital. Autopsy revealed extensive chronic as well as acute pathology (Tilsner, 1966). Because of the great delay in onset and the absence of typical signs of poisoning by an organic phosphorus compound, the possibility must be considered that the identity of the poison was misrepresented by the patient.

A totally different kind of case is intriguing because it, too, involved unusual delay in onset. A 65-year-old man with a history of mental depression, who drank an estimated 15 ml of a mixture of demeton-methyl (25%) and benzene methyl chloride, had no characteristic signs and, in fact, no serious illness of any kind when admitted to hospital. However, 32 hr after he ingested the insecticide, his condition suddenly deteriorated. All signs and symptoms were consistent with anticholinesterase poisoning and some, especially copious bronchial secretions and profuse sweating, were characteristic. Following a stormy course, the patient seemed to be well on his way to recovery, but 9 days following ingestion he died suddenly as the result of a massive pulmonary embolus (Barr, 1964). The cause of the sudden deterioration of the patient's condition 32 hr after ingestion is unknown, regardless of whether it represented poisoning by demeton-methyl or not. Also unknown is whether the benzyl chloride (the purpose of which in the formulation is obscure) contributed to the clinical course. It seems strange that no irritation was mentioned because benzyl chloride is intensely irritating. The author mentioned the possibility of some synergism between the insecticide and antidepressive drugs given to the patient, but again no proof is possible.

Dosage Response   A farmer drank about 90 ml of one of the older formulations in which about 70% of the active ingredient was demeton-*O*-methyl. He was hospitalized within 30 min. He was restless, salivating, and coughing up mucus, and there was some muscle twitching. He recovered following conventional treatment, including gastric lavage. No assistance of respiration was required (Great Britain Ministry of Agriculture, Fisheries and Food, 1969). This is a poor indication of dosage but enough to show a sharp contrast to demeton, which is more toxic.

A 26-year-old man injected his upper arm at a rate of 44.6 mg/kg. Surgical drainage released some of the fluid, so that the retained dosage was unknown. The patient survived following a protracted illness (Klose and Gutensohn, 1976).

Laboratory Findings   Klimmer and Pfaff (1958) found an average increase of 40.0% in reticulocytes in the blood of four volunteers who applied demeton-methyl for several days in large, heated greenhouses under physically exhausting conditions. Their hemoglobin levels and red and white blood cell counts were unchanged, as were their cholinesterase levels. The authors suggested that the reticulocyte count might be more sensitive than cholinesterase measurement as an indicator of exposure. It is not clear whether the failure of others to find an increase in reticulocytes reflects a lack of change or a lack of search.

Treatment of Poisoning   Treatment should be the same as that for poisoning by other organic phosphorus insecticides (see Section 16.2.2.7). Whereas no benefit from an oxime has been observed in some cases (Milthers *et al.*, 1963; Barr, 1964, 1966), distinct improvement has been noted in others (Molphy and Rathus, 1964).

16.6.4 OXYDEMETON-METHYL

16.6.4.1 Identity, Properties, and Uses

Chemical Name   Oxydemeton-methyl is *O,O*-dimethyl-*S*-2-(ethylsulfinyl)ethyl phosphorothioate.

Structure   See Table 16.16.

Synonyms   Oxydemeton-methyl (BSI, ISO) is only one of several common names in use. Although this name has ISO approval, the compound can be accurately described as demeton-*S*-methyl sulfoxide by reference to the ISO-approved name of the parent compound, and this term is sometimes used as a name. The "S" in this instance, refers to sulfur in the acidic group. However, in Germany, a different convention has been used by which reference is made to ═O, and thus one sees the term demeton-*O*-methyl sulfoxide applied to the compound under discussion. However, the term demeton-*S*-methylsulfoxyd also is used in

Germany. Ossidemeton-metile is the term used in Italy, and metilmekaptophrosoksid is used in the USSR. Other common names include isomethylsystox-sulfide and metaisosystox sulfoxide. A trade name for oxydemeton-methyl is Meta-Systox R®. Code designations for oxydemeton-methyl have included Bayer-21097, ENT-24964, and R-2107. The CAS registry number is 301-12-2.

Physical and Chemical Properties   Oxydemeton-methyl has the empirical formula $C_6H_{15}O_4PS_2$ and a molecular weight of 246.29. The pure material forms a clear, amber-colored liquid with a boiling point of 106°C at 0.01 mm Hg and a melting point of −10°C. The density at 20°C is 1.289. Oxydemeton-methyl is soluble in water and most organic solvents, except light petroleum. It is hydrolyzed in alkaline media.

History, Formulations, and Uses   Oxydemeton-methyl was introduced as a separate compound by the Bayer Leverkusen Company in 1960. It is a systemic pesticide for control of sucking insects and mites. Oxydemeton-methyl is available as a 50% solution concentrate and a 25% emulsifiable concentrate.

16.6.4.2 Toxicity to Laboratory Animals

Oxydemeton-methyl is a compound of moderate acute toxicity, as shown in Table 16.21.

Rats given dietary levels of 200 and 100 ppm (about 10 and 5 mg/kg/day) showed not only marked inhibition of cholinesterase activity but also signs of intoxication during the first 3 weeks (Vandekar, 1958). In another study, no illness or pathology was produced by 5 mg/kg for 3 months (Wirth, 1958). A dietary level of 50 ppm also inhibited cholinesterase but produced no signs of illness and did not interfere with growth (Vandekar, 1958).

Table 16.21
Single-Dose LD 50 for Oxydemeton-Methyl

Species	Route	LD 50 (mg/kg)	Reference
Rat, M	oral	65	Heath and Vandekar (1957)
Rat, M	oral	65	DuBois and Plzak (1962)
Rat, F	oral	75	DuBois and Plzak (1962)
Rat, M	oral	30–75	Schrader (1963a)
Rat, M	oral	47	Gaines (1969)
Rat, F	oral	52	Gaines (1969)
Rat	dermal	250	DuBois and Plzak (1962)
Rat, M	dermal	173	Gaines (1969)
Rat, F	dermal	158	Gaines (1969)
Rat	intraperitoneal	20	DuBois and Plzak (1962)
Rat	intraperitoneal	47	Heath and Vandekar (1957)
Mouse	oral	30	DuBois and Plzak (1962)
Mouse, M	intraperitoneal	12	DuBois and Plzak (1962)
Mouse, F	intraperitoneal	8	DuBois and Plzak (1962)
Guinea pig	oral	120	DuBois and Plzak (1962)
Guinea pig	intraperitoneal	30	DuBois and Plzak (1962)
Rabbit	oral	104	Khaitov *et al.* (1971)

No paralysis was observed in hens given the maximal dosage of oxydemeton-methyl that they could survive (Gaines, 1969).

A significant increase in the number of micronucleated cells among polychromatic erythrocytes in mice was observed when oxydemeton-methyl was administered in two intraperitoneal doses of 1 mg/kg 24 hr apart. The number of micronucleated cells increased with dose. Although the clastogenic mechanism of oxydemeton-methyl remains unknown, the possibility of DNA alkylation cannot be ruled out (Vaidya and Patankar, 1980).

Effects on Organs and Tissues   Oxydemeton-methyl has been shown to cause chromatid and isochromatid breaks among human leukocytes *in vitro* at concentrations as low as 10^{-9} *M*. The amount and types of chromosome damage increased with concentration. The mechanism for this clastogenic action remains to be determined (Vaidya and Patankar, 1980).

16.6.4.3 Toxicity to Humans

Accidental and Intentional Poisoning   Some cases of poisoning by oxydemeton-methyl involved relapse in the course of a long illness. In one instance, a 17-year-old girl was found unconscious with an empty bottle beside her. She was hospitalized 12–15 hr after the estimated time of ingestion. On admission, she was in a coma and had nearly all the signs of anticholinesterase poisoning, except pulmonary edema. She received immediate treatment, including gastric lavage, assisted respiration, atropine, and 2-PAM. After a brief amelioration, her condition began to deteriorate on the second day so that artificial respiration had to be reinstituted. There was no further change in spite of vigorous treatment until days 7 and 9, when pulmonary edema developed. A blood transfusion of 350 ml was performed on day 10, and between days 10 and 12 a partial blood exchange was carried out. The patient was released after 41 days with all clinical and laboratory findings normal (Goebel *et al.*, 1969).

Another poisoning involving relapse was the result of injection of a mixture of 20% oxydemeton-methyl and 17.5% parathion with suicidal intent. Approximately ½ hr after injection, the 29-year-old man complained of feeling unwell, excessive salivation, perspiration, and vomiting. On admission to the hospital, he was pale, weak, and dyspneic and his lips were cyanotic. The site of injection at the elbow was tender and surrounded by a swollen reddish area 5.5 cm in diameter. Appropriate treatment with atropine and obidoxime relieved the cyanosis. He was intubated, and later a tracheotomy was performed. Artificial respiration was continued until day 10 and symptomatic treatment until day 15. The patient was discharged on day 25, and he remained normal when followed up 1 year later (Knolle, 1970).

A third example involved a suicide attempt by a 40-year-old woman. She received gastric lavage 2 hr after ingestion and was hospitalized 4.5 hr after ingestion. Appropriate treatment

with drugs had led to a regression of miosis; however, the patient suffered cardiac arrest at 48 hr and again at 72 hr after admission. Heart action was restored each time by external cardiac massage. Clinical recovery was essentially complete by day 8. Plasma cholinesterase had returned to normal by day 13 and red cell cholinesterase by day 50 (Gaultier *et al.*, 1975).

Dosage Response   In the two unsuccessful suicides by ingestion described above, the dosage was thought to be 357 mg/kg for the 17-year-old girl and 71 mg/kg for the 40-year-old woman. Gastric lavage was performed in both instances, but it was necessarily 12–15 hr late in the case of the girl. In addition, the woman had vomiting and diarrhea. The dosage retained could not be known. Retention was complete in the unsuccessful suicide by injection. The dosage was 5.7 and 5.0 mg/kg for oxydemeton-methyl and parathion, respectively. It appears obvious that all three patients would have died except for treatment.

Treatment of Poisoning   See Section 16.2.2.7.

16.6.5 DICHLORVOS

16.6.5.1 Identity, Properties, and Uses

Chemical Name   Dichlorvos is *O,O*-dimethyl-*O*-2,2-dichlorovinyl phosphate.

Structure   See Table 16.16.

Synonyms   The common name dichlorvos (BSI, ISO) generally is accepted, except in the USSR, where DDVF was used and dichlorfos is used now. The acronym DDVP was used extensively until supplanted by dichlorvos except in Japan. Trade names include Canogard®, Crossman's Fly-Cake®, Dedevap®, De-Pester Insect Strip®, Estrosol®, Hercol®, Herkol®, Kill-Fly Resin Strip®, Lethalaire®, Mafu®, Misect®, Nogos®, No-Pest Strip®, Nuvan®, Oko®, Phoracide®, Phosvit®, Vapona®, Vaponicide®, and Vaporette Bar®. The compound in the form of a resin granule formulation is sold as an anthelmintic under the names Atgard®, Dichloroman®, Equigard®, and Task®. Code designations include BAY-19149, ENT-20738, OMS-14, and SD-1750. The CAS registry number is 62-73-7.

Physical and Chemical Properties   Dichlorvos has the empirical formula $C_4H_7Cl_2O_4P$ and a molecular weight of 220.98. The pure material forms a colorless to amber liquid with a mild chemical odor. The density of dichlorvos at 25°C is 1.415. The boiling point is 35°C at 0.05 mm Hg. The vapor pressure of dichlorvos is 1.2×10^{-2} mm Hg at 20°C. Dichlorvos is miscible with alcohol and in aromatic and chlorinated hydrocarbon solvents. Its solubility is about 1% in water and 3% in kerosene and mineral oils. Dilute dichlorvos hydrolyzes rapidly in the presence of moisture. A saturated aqueous solution (1%) hydrolyzes at a rate of about 3% per day. Concentrates are readily decomposed by strong acids and bases.

History, Formulations, and Uses Dichlorvos was first described in 1952 (Perkow *et al.*, 1952) and a further report appeared in 1954 (Perkow, 1954). It was not until 1955 (Mattson *et al.*, 1955) that its potential application as an insecticide was brought to light. The initial discovery of its value grew out of the striking insecticidal action of vapor from crystalline trichlorfon. This vapor was shown to consist of dichlorvos, a breakdown product of trichlorfon. The fact that the vapor pressure of dichlorvos is higher than that of any other organophosphorus compound commonly used as an insecticide (see Table 16.22) makes it practical to produce insecticidal concentrations of it in closed spaces. Further studies (Tenhet *et al.*, 1957) revealed the remarkable ability of dichlorvos vapor to penetrate in several hours the interstices of a large space, even though the liquid insecticide was applied initially to a small area within the space.

A series of studies performed in 1961 (Maddock and Sedlak, 1961; Maddock *et al.*, 1961) revealed the concentration–time relationships necessary to kill insect vectors of disease. Briefly, it is now concluded that exposure to a concentration of 0.015 mg/m³ for several hours kills both flies and mosquitoes, but concentrations at or above 0.15 mg/m³ are required to produce 100% mortality of houseflies and mosquitoes if the exposure is limited to half an hour.

A device capable of producing the necessary concentration without exceeding 0.25 mg/m³ was developed in 1964 (Jensen *et al.*, 1965) for use in aircraft with the ventilation system in operation. A unique way of using dichlorvos is to impregnate it in polyvinyl chloride resin from which vaporizers and animal collars are cast. When worn by dogs and cats, the collars control fleas. A similar formulation prepared in granular form has been investigated as an anthelmintic in humans and is used extensively for this purpose in domestic animals. Finally the granular formulation has been given to sows to increase the weight of their litters at the time of marketing.

Dichlorvos is used mainly for the control of insects in tobacco and other warehouses, mushroom houses, greenhouses, animal shelters, homes, restaurants, and other food-handling establishments. It was recommended by the Twenty-First World Health Assembly for the control of flies, mosquitoes, and other disease vectors in aircraft. It has been tested for the control of malaria mosquitoes in houses, but with little success, at least in part because the open construction of the houses prevented achievement of an adequate concentration. Dichlorvos has limited use on outdoor crops, but it is used for postharvest treatment of grain.

Technical dichlorvos contains not less than 93% of the pure material, and the remainder is related, insecticidally active materials.

The insecticide is available in oil solutions (50 and 90%), emulsifiable oil concentrates, aerosol formulations, and baits.

16.6.5.2 Toxicity to Laboratory Animals

Basic Findings Illness caused by dichlorvos is generally similar to that caused by other organic phosphorus insecticides but is remarkable for the rapidity of onset and especially recovery (see Absorption, Distribution, Metabolism, and Excretion below).

Dichlorvos is not neurotoxic and, when administered by natural routes, is not teratogenic. It is not irritating or sensitizing to laboratory animals. However, Muller (1970) has reported dichlorvos to cause dermal irritation in domesticated dogs and cats when impregnated flea-collars were held in close contact with their necks. Although the majority of these dermatitis cases were restricted to the site of contact, cases of sensitization involving widespread reactions have also been reported (Muller, 1970).

The acute toxicity of dichlorvos is summarized in Table 16.23. By using large groups of mice at lower dosage levels, Haley *et al.* (1975c) were able to measure oral LD 1 values of 84 and 95 mg/kg in males and females, respectively. The corresponding LD 0.1 values were 70 and 82. The compound is of moderate toxicity—far less dangerous than TEPP or parathion but more toxic than malathion, for example.

Table 16.22
Molecular Weight and Vapor Pressure of Selected Compounds

Compound	Molecular weight	Vapor pressure (mm Hg)	Temperature (°C)
Sarin	140	1.57	20
Dichlorvos	221	0.025	25
		0.032	32:2
Parathion	291	0.0000378	20
Malathion	330	0.00004	30
Phosphine (PH_3)	34	29,200	25
Cyanide (HCN)	27	760	26
Carbon tetrachloride	154	100	25
Tetrachlorethylene	166	18	25

Table 16.23
Single-Dose LD 50 for Dichlorvos

Species	Route	LD 50 (mg/kg)	Reference
Rat, M	oral	46.5 ± 6.09	Vrbovský *et al.* (1959)
Rat, M	oral	80	Gaines (1969)
Rat, F	oral	56	Gaines (1969)
Rat, M	dermal	107	Gaines (1969)
Rat, F	dermal	75	Gaines (1969)
Rat, M	intraperitoneal	18.5 ± 1.31	Vrbovský *et al.* (1959)
Mouse, M	oral	90 ± 5.81	Vrbovský *et al.* (1959)
Mouse	oral	124	Yamashita (1962)
Mouse	oral	75–175	Vashkov *et al.* (1966)
Mouse, M	oral	145	Wagner and Johnson (1970)
Mouse, M	oral	135	Wagner and Johnson (1970)
Mouse, M	oral	145	Haley *et al.* (1975c)
Mouse, F	oral	148	Haley *et al.* (1975c)
Mouse, F	subcutaneous	24	Yamashita (1962)
Mouse	subcutaneous	22	Jaques (1964)
Mouse	intraperitoneal	28	Casida *et al.* (1962)
Mouse, M	intraperitoneal	28.5 ± 2.39	Vrbovský *et al.* (1959)
Chick, F	oral	14.8	Sherman and Ross (1961)

A single dermal dose at the rate of 100 mg/kg produced onset of poisoning within 10 min but was not fatal to a monkey. A dose at the rate of 50 mg/kg produced illness after a delay of 20 min, and when this smaller dosage was repeated for 8 days it killed the monkey (Durham et al., 1957).

Dogs that received dichlorvos by capsule at rates of 0.13–0.37 mg/kg/day showed no detectable effect, but those receiving 0.65 and 1.30 mg/kg/day had brain cholinesterase activity 88 and 33%, respectively, of normal and were considered more active than usual (FAO/WHO, 1967).

Respiratory exposure to a concentration of 30 mg/m³ for more than 4 hr was necessary to kill rats (Durham et al., 1957). Miosis and a rapid drop in blood cholinesterase but no illness occurred in monkeys exposed for 2 hr/day for 4 days to concentrations greater than 7 mg/m³ (Witter et al., 1961). Continuous exposure for a week to concentrations initially in the range of 1.4–2.0 mg/m³ produced marked depression of blood cholinesterase in monkeys but little depression in rats. Only slightly lower initial concentrations (0.8–1.8 mg/m³ for 22 days) produced no cholinesterase inhibition in either monkeys or rats but both species showed recognizable depression of red cell cholinesterase when exposure was continued for 50 days. Continuous exposure for 4 days to concentrations that did not exceed 0.27 mg/m³ produced no effect on cholinesterase levels of either monkeys or rats (Durham et al., 1959).

Feeding studies indicated that a dosage very much larger than that sufficient to inhibit plasma cholinesterase was required to produce illness. In fact, rats were shown to tolerate a dietary level of 1000 ppm for at least 90 days without any clinical sign of injury, although a dietary level of 5 ppm produced a detectable reduction of blood cholinesterase in only 4 days, and this change was persistent in rats maintained at a dietary level of 50 ppm (Durham et al., 1957).

Animals tolerate somewhat higher dosages of active ingredient administered in slow-release formulations rather than in the uncombined form. The dosage of slow-release formulation necessary to treat internal parasites generally produces some inhibition of red cell cholinesterase, occasional softening of feces, but no sign of illness in domestic animals (Ward and Glicksberg, 1971; Brglez and Skubic, 1971; Snow, 1971, 1974; Drudge and Lyons, 1972; Bello et al., 1974; Bossen et al., 1973; Hass, 1973). Monkeys treated with a slow-release formulation as dosages up to 80 mg/kg/day showed complete inhibition of cholinesterase and some anorexia, diarrhea, salivation, and emesis, but remained vigorous and agile. Even this high dosage was ineffective in treating schistosomiasis (Hass et al., 1972). On the other hand, oral doses of dichlorvos were effective in treating demodectic mange in dogs (Hughes and Lang, 1973) even though dosing was oral and the parasites infest the skin. Thus direct contact with the formulation is not necessary for all kinds of parasites.

Dichlorvos is one of the organic phosphorus insecticides sufficiently selective in its action that it can be used effectively for the treatment of certain internal parasites of animals and humans. The susceptible organisms include bots and some but not all nematodes infesting cattle (Bris et al., 1968), camels (Wallach and Frueh, 1968), chimpanzees and monkeys (Wallach and Frueh, 1968), and humans (Cervoni et al., 1968). When used for these purposes, the dichlorvos may be mixed in the feed directly, or it may be administered in the form of plastic containing about 20% dichlorvos to provide slow release of the compound in the gastrointestinal tract. The use of one or a few large doses has produced side effects (diarrhea and debility). Repeated small doses are without side effect.

Dichlorvos fed to cattle in their feed was successful in greatly reducing or eliminating the development of flies in their feces. The insecticide was given as polyvinyl chloride resin formulations. Dosages of these formulations up to 4 mg/kg produced no clinical toxicity, but dosages of 2 mg/kg or higher of a rapid-release formulation and dosages of 1 mg/kg or higher of a slow-release formulation did reduce blood cholinesterase (Pitts and Hopkins, 1964). No insecticidal residue appears in the milk (Lloyd and Matthysse, 1971).

Cattle tolerated dichlorvos at a dietary level of 110 ppm (about 3.2 mg/kg/day) for 84 days without clinical injury. Half that dosage was found equally effective as an anthelmintic in the animals (Bris et al., 1968). Chimpanzees and a monkey tolerated two doses totaling 7.5 and 8.0 mg/kg. Some camels suffered severe diarrhea but survived following two doses totaling 10 mg/kg. Other camels were unaffected by the same dosage (Wallach and Frueh, 1968).

Absorption, Distribution, Metabolism, and Excretion Absorption from the gastrointestinal tract is by way of the portal blood rather than the lymph (Laws, 1966). In the intact animal, the compound is rapidly detoxified by the liver (Gaines et al., 1966). Following a subcutaneous dose at the rate of 1.52 mg/kg, cholinesterase inhibition in a goat was almost maximal at 0.25 hr, slightly greater at 0.5 hr, slightly less at 1 hr, and well on the way to recovery at 2 hr after injection (Casida et al., 1962). If poisoning occurs by the oral route, the onset is rapid and recovery is prompt (Durham et al., 1957; Yamashita, 1962; Modak et al., 1975). Rats administered an oral or dermal dose at the LD 50 level survive less than an hour or recover completely (Gaines, 1960). Dichlorvos is not stored in the body and has not been detected in the milk of cows or rats, even when given in doses that produce severe poisoning (Tracy et al., 1960).

No dichlorvos could be detected in the blood of rats, mice, or people after exposure to atmospheric concentrations of it up to 17 times that normally attained for insect control in homes. Exposure of rats to 10 mg/m³ (250 times normal exposure) for 4 hr was required before dichlorvos was detectable, and then only in the kidneys. At 90 mg/m³ (2000 times normal exposure) dichlorvos could be detected in most tissues of the rat. Following exposure at 50 mg/m³, the half-life in the rat kidney was 13.5 min. Distribution of dichlorvos in mice was qualitatively similar to that in rats but, under similar conditions, the concentrations in mice were only about one-tenth as great. The reason for the rapid disappearance of dichlorvos is the presence of degrading enzymes not only in the tissues but also in the plasma (Blair et al., 1975).

Continuous exposure of experimental animals to dichlorvos vapor inevitably entails not only respiratory exposure but also dermal exposure to vapor and oral exposure to the compound adsorbed by feed. Actual measurement indicated that only half of the absorption by rats continuously exposed to vapor was by the respiratory route (Stevenson and Blair, 1977).

Only during the first 2 hr after intravenous or oral administration of [^{32}P]dichlorvos was there a trace of organosoluble phosphorus in the milk. Later (chiefly between 4 and 48 hr) substantial amounts of ^{32}P-labeled metabolites that could not be extracted with organic solvents were found in the milk (Casida et al., 1962).

The goat excretes about 15% of the metabolized compound in the feces following subcutaneous administration, and the cow excretes more than 50% of it by this route after oral administration. However, in the rat, the proportion of dichlorvos excreted in the feces is the same (about 3%) whether the insecticide is administered orally or intraperitoneally (Casida et al., 1962). Thus, the principal difference in route of excretion involves species rather than route of administration.

The major in vitro pathways for the metabolism of dichlor-

vos were defined first by Hodgson and Casida (1962). Their results, together with some more recent additions, are shown in Figure 16.5.

The initial metabolites of dichlorvos in vivo are O,O-dimethyl phosphate and O-methyl-O-2,2-dichlorovinyl phosphate (desmethyldichlorvos). They are rapidly excreted or further degraded. The intraperitoneal toxicity of identified metabolites in mice varies from 250 to more than 3000 mg/kg, as compared to 28 mg/kg for the parent compound. The 1-carbon of the 2,2-dichlorovinyl group is excreted in urine predominantly as a conjugate of dichloroethanol, probably the glucuronide, in the feces as unknown derivatives, and in the expired air as carbon dioxide (Casida et al., 1962), and it enters various normal metabolic pools (Loeffler et al., 1976).

Although all of the chlorinated organic compounds shown in Fig. 16.5 have been found in the intestinal lumen of intact animals and one of them (dichloroethanol) has been found in the blood, none of them has been found in the tissues. Not even dichlorvos itself has been found in the tissues; the only evidence for its presence is the inhibition of cholinesterase. This reemphasizes the remarkably rapid metabolism and excretion

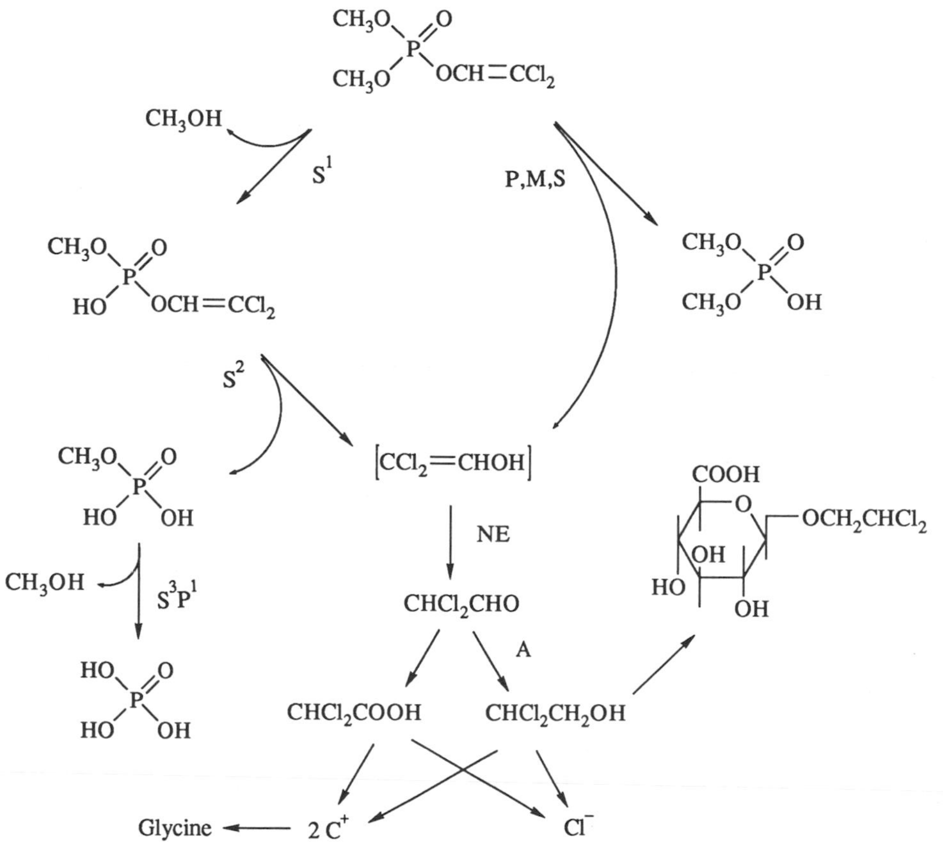

Figure 16.5 Metabolic pathways of dichlorvos in the rat based on in vitro and in vivo studies. From Hodgson and Casida (1962) by permission of the American Chemical Society. Symbols: P, plasma enzyme hydrolyzing dichlorvos to dimethyl phosphate; P^1, plasma enzyme hydrolyzing monomethyl phosphate to inorganic phosphate; S, soluble liver enzyme hydrolyzing dichlorvos to dimethyl phosphate, activated by Mn^{2+}; S^1, soluble liver enzyme hydrolyzing dichlorvos to desmethyl dichlorvos; S^1, soluble liver enzyme hydrolyzing desmethyl dichlorvos to monomethyl phosphate, activated by $1 \times 10^{-4} M$ Co^{2+}; S^3, soluble liver enzyme hydrolyzing monomethyl phosphate to inorganic phosphate, no known activators, inhibited by —SH inhibitors, pH optimum 6.8–7.2; M, liver mitochondrial enzyme hydrolyzing dichlorvos to dimethyl phosphate, activated by Ca^{2+}; A, reduction of dichloroacetaldehyde to dichloroethanol by alcohol dehydrogenase, requiring DPNH; NE, nonenzymatic.

of dichlorvos. Of course, once the various portions of the molecule have been converted to normal metabolites (two-carbon fragments; phosphorus ion, chlorine ion) their turnover rate is the same as that for identical materials of other origins. Thus, small fractions of the carbon, phosphorus, and chlorine derived from dichlorvos are retained in the body for several days (Hutson *et al.*, 1971; Loeffler *et al.*, 1971; Hutson and Hoadley, 1972a,b; Page *et al.*, 1972; Potter *et al.*, 1973a,b). Use of ^{14}C-labeled dichlorvos has shown that the most important normal carbon metabolites are glycine and serine (Loeffler *et al.*, 1976).

Biochemical Effects Dichlorvos is a direct inhibitor of cholinesterase. Its pI 50 is 5.66 (Durham *et al.*, 1957) compared to 7.2 for paraoxon (Holmstedt, 1959). The kinetic constants for its inhibition of acetylcholinesterase have been measured (Braid and Nix, 1969). Its mode of action does not differ from that of other direct inhibitors, but its relatively high vapor pressure makes it unique among organic phosphorus insecticides. A direct result of this is that it inhibits cholinesterase of bronchial tissues at a lower air concentration than that necessary to inhibit blood cholinesterase. For example, in rats, acetylcholinesterase activity of bronchial homogenate was reduced to 63 and 51%, respectively, by air concentrations of 0.8 and 1.8 mg/m^3, whereas acetylcholine activity of blood was unaffected. Histochemical preparations showed that acetylcholinesterase of the bronchial glands was lost even at a concentration of 0.2 mg/m^3 (Schmidt *et al.*, 1975). It is interesting that this inhibition occurs even though the destruction of dichlorvos is so rapid that, at levels of exposure encountered in use, only the metabolites have been recovered from lung tissue (Loeffler *et al.*, 1971). It is not clear what significance the inhibition of bronchial cholinesterase has.

Rats given a single dose of dichlorvos at half the LD 50 rate developed hyperglycemia and abnormal glucose tolerance tests that could be prevented by insulin. The effect of dichlorvos seemed to be due to simultaneous stimulation of glycogen phosphorylase and inhibition of glycogen synthesis. Whether the changes depend ultimately on increased release of catecholamines or on blocking of the glucose receptor of the β cells of the pancreas remains to be learned (Teichert-Kuliszewska and Szymczyk, 1979).

In humans, dichlorvos inhibits plasma cholinesterase more readily than red cell cholinesterase (Rasmussen *et al.*, 1963; Cavagna *et al.*, 1969). The two enzymes are about equally susceptible in the guinea pig (Guyot, 1958). In the monkey (Durham *et al.*, 1957) and in the horse (Tracy *et al.*, 1960), the red cell enzyme is more easily inhibited by this compound.

Dichlorvos potentiates the toxicity of malathion but only by a small factor (Tracy *et al.*, 1960).

The reason why susceptibility to dichlorvos is far greater in insects than in mammals was studied in detail by Van Asperen and Dekhuijzen (1958). Briefly, the I 50 of mouse brain cholinesterase is 10^{-7} M, whereas that of fly head cholinesterase is 10^{-9} M. Inhibition of mouse cholinesterase by this compound is slowly reversible, but inhibition of the fly enzyme is irreversible. Dichlorvos has a much greater affinity for the insect cholinesterase. An unidentified compound in mouse brain homogenates competes significantly with cholinesterase for binding of the compound.

Effects on Organs and Tissues The possibility that dichlorvos is mutagenic has been examined extensively because of emphasis (see Section 16.4.4) on the fact that it is a chemical alkylating agent. The compound caused a dosage-related increase in the back-mutation rate of two strains of *Serratia marcescens* and *Escherichia coli* WP2 (Dean and Thorpe, 1972a). *In vitro* results with *Saccharomyces cerevisiae* were positive at a concentration of 4000 ppm but negative at 2000 ppm (Dean *et al.*, 1972). The positive results have been confirmed with the same or different test organisms (Ashwood-Smith *et al.*, 1972; Voogd *et al.*, 1972; Buselmaier *et al.*, 1973; Dyer and Hanna, 1973).

Host-mediated tests with *S. cerevisiae* were negative in mice that had received dichlorvos orally at 50 or 100 mg/kg or had breathed a vapor concentration of 60 or 99 mg/m^3 (Dean *et al.*, 1972). This negative result of a host-mediated test was confirmed (Voogd *et al.*, 1972; Buselmaier *et al.*, 1973).

At 5–40 ppm but not at 1 ppm, dichlorvos was cytotoxic for human lymphocytes in culture, but it did not cause cytogenic changes (Dean, 1972b). Respiratory exposure of mice and oral exposure of hamsters failed to cause chromosomal aberration (Leonard, 1976). The compound also failed to increase chromosome abnormalities in the bone marrow and spermatocytes of mice and Chinese hamsters that had been exposed for 16 hr to air containing dichlorvos at concentrations from 64 to 72 mg/m^3 or for 21 days to a concentration of 5 mg/m^3 (Dean and Thorpe, 1972a).

Dichlorvos was not mutagenic in *Drosophila* (Sobels and Todd, 1979).

Dominant lethal mutation tests were negative in mice exposed to air containing dichlorvos at concentrations of 30 and 55 mg/m^3 for 16 hr or to concentrations of 2.1 and 5.0 mg/m^3 for 4 weeks (Dean and Thorpe, 1972b). This result in mice has been extended and confirmed (Dean and Blair, 1976). That dichlorvos is not mutagenic in the intact organism may be due to its extremely rapid and complete metabolism.

The question of whether dichlorvos is a biological alkylating agent in mammals is discussed in Section 16.4.4.

No tumors attributable to dichlorvos were found at the end of 2-year feeding tests in rats that had received 0.005, 0.05, 0.5, 5, and 25 mg/kg/day or in dogs that had received 0.002, 0.02, 0.2, 2, and 10 mg/kg/day (Witherup *et al.*, 1971). The carcinogenicity of dichlorvos later was tested by feeding two dietary levels for 80 weeks to rats and mice. The rats were killed and examined at the end of 110–111 weeks, and the mice were killed after 92–94 weeks. The initial dietary levels were 150 and 1000 ppm for rats and 1000 and 2000 ppm for mice. Levels of 1000 ppm or more produced severe illness; the animals receiving 1000 ppm were changed to 300 ppm, and the mice receiving 2000 ppm were changed to 600 ppm. The "time-weighted average" levels for the whole study were 150 and 326 ppm for rats and 318 and 635 ppm for mice. These levels are equivalent to about 7 and 16 mg/kg/day for rats and 41 and 81 mg/kg/day for mice. After the high dietary levels were reduced, no toxic signs directly attributable to the compound were observed except that average weights of high-dosage animals were slightly depressed. Survival was not dosage related. No statistically significant increase in the incidence of tumors was found in male or female rats and mice exposed to dichlorvos [National Cancer Institute (NCI), 1977].

In order to test the carcinogenicity of dichlorvos using the route by which people receive their greatest and usually only dosage, 50 rats of each sex were exposed for about 23 hr/day for 2 years to air containing 5, 0.5, 0.05, or 0.0 mg/m^3. Clinical poisoning did not occur. The growth rate of all treated rats, especially males, was depressed, but there were no consistent differences in food intakes, organ weights, or hematological or blood chemistry measurements, except cholinesterase activity, and a higher proportion of the treated rats than controls survived the treatment period. No compound-related differences in acetylcholine or choline concentrations were found in the brains of a small number of female rats examined in this regard. There were no gross or microscopic compound-related changes in the tissues. Electron microscopic examination of respiratory tissues of rats from the control and the 5 mg/m^3 groups showed no changes attributable to dichlorvos. There was no dosage-related increase in tumor risk for rats of either sex (Blair et al., 1976).

Dichlorvos is not neurotoxic in hens protected by atropine (Durham et al., 1956; Aldridge and Barnes, 1966a). Johnson (1975c) reported positive results in hens that received two doses, each at the rate of 100 mg/kg, and he attributed the difference to dosage. However, a study of dichlorvos analogs showed that compounds with both methyl groups replaced by longer carbon chains (C$_3$ to C$_{10}$) or by —CH$_2$—CH$_2$Cl were neurotoxic in unprotected hens at less than lethal dosage levels. Highly purified analogs that were mixed isomers (e.g., methyl, octyl) were not neurotoxic, but impure mixed isomers containing only 0.6–4% of the corresponding bis- compound (e.g., octyl, octyl) were neurotoxic when administered to atropine-protected hens in sufficiently high dosages (Albert and Stearns, 1974). The result with pure and impure mixed isomers raises the possibility that the positive results reported for massive doses of some samples of dichlorvos were the result of traces of impurities. An "ataxia–depression" syndrome in cats exposed to dichlorvos vapor has been reported (Padgett et al., 1975) but not studied in sufficient detail to determine its relationship to neurotoxicity.

Intraperitoneal dosages of dichlorvos that caused mortality of 7 and 81% in mice led to increases of 21 and 43%, respectively, in the weights of the adrenals in survivors, as measured 10 days after injection. The epinephrine and norepinephrine content was depleted. The increase in adrenal weight was considered secondary to stimulation by the pituitary gland (Ramade and Roffi, 1976).

Effects on Reproduction   Isolated reports on the effects of dichlorvos cover the spectrum from implied sterility to statistically confirmed improvement in performance. All tests of actual reproduction indicate that dichlorvos does not interfere, except at dosage levels that threaten the life of the mother. The question of possible benefit has been explored in one species only and can be discussed in that context only.

Extensive injury to the seminal epithelium of mice following a single oral dose at the rate of 40 mg/kg has been reported; similar, although less extensive, changes were found in animals given 10 mg/kg/day for 18 days (Krause and Homola, 1972, 1974). This report is inconsistent with the reproductive success of several species heavily exposed to dichlorvos.

Compared to controls, estrus was delayed 10 days in female rats apparently delivered and kept in a common cage with a small dichlorvos vaporizer on top of it (Timmons et al., 1975). Although no effort was made to measure the concentration of the compound in the air in the cage, the concentration must have been exceedingly high, for the compound was reported to have been measured in all but one sample of blood and in many samples of tissues.

Dichlorvos has proved nonteratogenic where administered by a natural route. Dosages of 34 mg/kg or more in the form of a slow-release formulation during the critical days of organogenesis were poorly tolerated by rabbit dams. Maternal toxicity was associated with cholinesterase inhibition. At dosages of 12 mg/kg, dichlorvos was not teratogenic in rabbits and did not interfere with reproduction in any way (Vogin et al., 1971).

Rabbits and rats were exposed throughout pregnancy to concentrations of 0.25, 1.25, and 6.25 mg of dichlorvos per cubic meter of air. In another experiment rabbits were exposed to 2 and 4 mg/m^3. There was no indication from either experiment that the compound was teratogenic even at concentrations that killed some rabbits and caused depression of cholinesterase activity of the plasma, erythrocytes, and brain of both species (Thorpe et al., 1972).

In a separate study, dichlorvos was not teratogenic when administered orally to rats (Baksi, 1978). However, when the compound was given intraperitoneally to rats on the eleventh day of pregnancy at a rate of 15 mg/kg, umbilical hernias were found in 3 of 41 fetuses. A dosage of 20 mg/kg by the same route was fatal to pregnant rats, although 40 mg/kg was the lowest dosage that killed nonpregnant ones (Kimbrough and Gaines, 1968). Without further study, it seems impossible to exclude direct transamniotic absorption as the reason for teratogenesis following intraperitoneal injection.

In conventional reproduction studies, male and female rats were given a diet containing 100 ppm dichlorvos just prior to and during mating, and for the females this diet was continued throughout gestation and lactation. There were no harmful effects on reproduction or on the survival or growth of the young, even though the diet produced almost complete inhibition of plasma and red cell cholinesterase in the mothers and marked inhibition of these enzymes in the young at the time of weaning [World Health Organization (WHO), 1967]. An even larger oral dosage (30 mg/kg) that produces severe acute poisoning but permits survival of female rats does not injure their litters (Tracy *et al.*, 1960). The same negative result was reported in a three-generation test in rats with dietary levels of 0, 0.1, 1.0, 10.0, 100, and 500 ppm (Witherup *et al.*, 1971).

Dichlorvos at dietary levels up to 500 ppm does not interfere with the reproduction of pigs. Females, whose parents had been fed the compound and who themselves had received it continuously from conception onward, were themselves bred. There was no reduction in the number, viability, or growth of the young and there was no evidence of teratogenesis (Collins *et al.*, 1971). Dosages of the slow-release formulation several times the one recommended for therapeutic use were safe for sows and piglets (Stanton *et al.*, 1979).

Although it is not conventional to report any beneficial effects of toxic materials, considerable evidence has accumulated that the administration of dichlorvos as a slow-release formulation to sows during the latter part of gestation results in an increase in the weight of their litters at birth, weaning, and market. The dosage of active material involved usually has been in the range of 700–1000 mg/sow/day for 20–50 days. The observation is not new. An extensive search for a biochemical basis appeared early (Tumbleson and Wescott, 1969), but understanding of the phenomenon is still incomplete. It has been found conclusively that the effect is not dependent on the anthelmintic action of dichlorvos (Keasling *et al.*, 1974; Young *et al.*, 1979a).

Even though the cause remains obscure and the existence of the effect has been denied on the basis of limited studies (England, 1974; Stanton *et al.*, 1979), the reality of the effect is difficult to refute. One statistical analysis involving 1543 control litters and 1613 treated litters revealed an average increase of 11.7% in the litter weight at weaning (Fogg *et al.*, 1974). The improvement was due, at least in part, to better survival. Although the treatment did not change the number of piglets born, it increased the number born alive and the number surviving to market age (DeKay *et al.*, 1974; Siers *et al.*, 1974). The lipid content of the colostrum from treated sows was higher than that of controls, and the response of many physiological parameters to temperature stress was changed (Siers *et al.*, 1976).

Pathology   The only tissue change (other than the pulmonary edema, congestion, and petechial hemorrhages often associated with the agonal state) is an increase in liver size. This increase has been reported in pigs maintained for a long period on concentrations as high as 500 ppm (Collins *et al.*, 1971).

"Disorder in the content and distributions of RNA and DNA" and other histochemical changes were described in the viscera of chickens that died with typical signs and within 5–30 min after dosing with dichlorvos (Mukhamedshin, 1969). The same author (1970b) found an even greater variety of pathology after repeated doses. These reports remain unconfirmed.

Treatment of Poisoning in Animals   Studies in mice have shown that both atropine and oximes are effective in the treatment of poisoning by dichlorvos and that the actions of the two types of antidote are additive (Jaques, 1964; Natoff and Reiff, 1970).

16.6.5.3 Toxicity to Humans

Experimental Oral Exposure   The plasma cholinesterase of five men who received dichlorvos orally at a rate of 2.0 mg/man/day for 28 days was depressed to 71% of the control value. There was no change in the red cell enzyme (Rider *et al.*, 1967). A slightly smaller dosage (1.5 mg/man/day) inhibited plasma cholinesterase when continued for 60 days. In both studies, involving a total of 30 men plus controls, the red cell enzymes remained normal and there were no clinical effects. The plasma enzyme activity returned to control levels when dichlorvos feeding was discontinued (Rider *et al.*, 1968).

Experimental Respiratory Exposure   In studies designed to test the safety of using dichlorvos for the disinsection of aircraft, a group of 15 volunteers underwent intermittent exposure totaling 5 hr/night, 4 nights/week, for 2 weeks, at a concentration of 0.5 mg/m^3 of air; this produced a gradual, moderate reduction of plasma cholinesterase but no illness, no impairment of visual performance, no increase in airway resistance or complex reaction time, and no change in physical condition or neurological function. There was no inhibition of red cell cholinesterase activity, and the lowest single plasma value observed was 34% of normal. Exposure to half that concentration for ten $\frac{1}{2}$-hr periods each night for 10 weeks was tolerated without any effect, even on plasma cholinesterase (Rasmussen *et al.*, 1963).

During this series of tests, the following functions of factors were investigated at frequent intervals: complex reaction time (including not only measurement of reaction time in units of 0.2 sec but also separate counting of errors of omission and commission), airway resistance, near and distant visual acuity, visual accommodation, stereoscopic vision, phorias, prism vergence, flicker fusion, pupil size following adaptation to the dark, peripheral and central vision, color vision, physical condition, and neurological function. None of these was affected at any time. Thus, these studies confirmed the conclusion established in literature on organophosphorus compounds, namely that there is no test more sensitive than the inhibition of cholinesterase for detecting changes in physiological functions.

In these tests, which involved higher concentrations and more frequent applications than would ever be encountered in practice, the dichlorvos was applied with the same equipment that would be used in aircraft, and the concentration was regulated much more carefully than was possible in earlier studies in humans or animals.

Studies of volunteers carried out at operational cabin altitudes (2438 m) reached the same results regarding safety (Smith *et al.*, 1972) as had been reached in the earlier study carried out at ground level.

The earliest in-flight tests of the disinsection system were made in DC-6B and DC-7B aircraft in 1961 (Schoof *et al.*,

1961, 1965; Jensen *et al.,* 1965). Since the collection of air samples would inconvenience passengers, such samples were collected only on flights without passengers. Measurement of dichlorvos concentrations in the air and biological tests on houseflies were followed by modifications of the vapor distribution system in such a way that 100% mortality of flies was obtained throughout the aircraft without exceeding a concentration of 0.25 mg/m³; the need for a double system to produce concentrations as high as 0.35 mg/m³ was thus eliminated. Blood cholinesterase activity determinations on the men who carried out the complete series of 24 tests showed no changes (Schoof *et al.,* 1961).

Studies of hospital patients, including normal mothers and babies as well as patients suffering from a wide range of diseases, showed that use of dichlorvos dispensers at recommended rates constituted no danger to health and caused detectable reduction in cholinesterase only in persons already suffering from serious liver disease (Cavagna *et al.,* 1969, 1970).

As discussed in Section 7.4.1 in Hayes (1975) and again (under Myopathic Changes) in Section 16.2.1.3, the relationship of EMG changes to organic phosphorus insecticides remains obscure. Regardless of what conclusion eventually may be reached on the general relationship, it was demonstrated that exposure of normal volunteers was insufficient to cause a biologically or statistically significant change from preexposure values in their EMG results following 1.5 and 3 months of exposure to dichlorvos vapor from properly installed resin strips (Ottevanger, 1975).

Field Tests Involving Respiratory Exposure   Initial tests of the safety of dichlorvos in flight were made with only the crew and professional personnel aboard. Later tests were made on a limited number of regular commercial flights on a DC-6B aircraft between Miami and Nassau. Passengers and crew experienced no discomfort and, in fact, the former were unaware of the disinsection process (Schoof *et al.,* 1961; Jensen *et al.,* 1965).

In June 1964, the automatic disinsection system was installed in a Boeing 720 jet aircraft assigned to passenger service between the United States, Mexico, and Central and South America. During the next 12 months, personnel of the U.S. Public Health Service and of the airline made five inspection trips on the aircraft to observe the operation of the system, to evaluate its effectiveness, and to observe passenger reactions. In no instance did any of the passengers manifest a reaction to the disinsection, and they appeared completely unaware that such an operation was in progress. The only evidence of the procedure was that flies that had entered the aircraft during servicing and loading fell to the floor and died. Crew personnel expressed their satisfaction with the operation of the system and used it routinely to meet quarantine requirements until, as part of the investigation, the equipment was removed for examination at the end of 1 year of use. Regular use of the equipment for a full year confirmed its efficiency and safety. During this period, no adverse reactions were observed in pilots or other crew members (WHO, 1967).

A different kind of use experience involves malaria control. There have been at least four studies of the value of dichlorvos for this purpose. In three of them, the concentration of the insecticide in the air of treated dwellings was measured. In Upper Volta, the concentration ranged from 0.007 to 0.840 mg/m³ (Funckes *et al.,* 1963b) and exposure continued for 3 years. In Western Nigeria, the variation was only 0.004–0.56 mg/m³ and exposure continued for 18 months (Gratz *et al.,* 1963). In Haiti, concentrations measured in the presence of fresh dispensers were 0.09–0.17 mg/m³ (Stein *et al.,* 1966) and the exposure period lasted 2 years. The differences in the range of concentrations in the four studies were partly the result of differences in construction and ventilation of the houses and partly the result of intentional differences in dosage of dichlorvos. The earliest studies involved small villages, but the work in Haiti (Stein *et al.,* 1966) and Northern Nigeria (Foll and Pant, 1964) involved large villages in which 10,000 and 25,200 people, respectively, were living. People of all ages and conditions were represented in all the studies. In no instance was there a complaint or observed illness among the residents of treated houses referable to dichlorvos. In two of the studies it was possible to measure cholinesterase activity, but no abnormality was found among residents, even in the plasma enzyme (Funckes *et al.,* 1963b; Gratz *et al.,* 1963).

The situation was somewhat different among men who prepared the dispensers or installed them in the houses to be treated in Haiti. Daily dermal exposure plus exposures to air concentrations of dichlorvos ranging from 0.29 to 2.13 mg/m³ during working hours produced no effect on the red cell cholinesterase of workers and no illness among them. These concentrations did gradually reduce the men's plasma enzyme levels to about 32% of normal in 16 days, after which there was no further decrease in spite of continued exposure for 5 additional days (Stein *et al.,* 1966).

No depression of plasma or red cell cholinesterase and no physical abnormality was found among 12 men who spent 16 hr per week for 2–4 months applying 4% dichlorvos as a fog to tobacco warehouses (Witter, 1960). Thirteen male and female workers employed in the production and processing of dichlorvos showed an average reduction of plasma activity to 40% of normal but no symptoms or signs attributable to the compound. The average exposure over a period of 8 months was 0.7 mg/m³. One month after exposure stopped, cholinesterase levels had returned to normal (Menz *et al.,* 1974). Workers involved in the fumigation of greenhouses in Japan were reported to show a marked decrease of cholinesterase activity (Hanyu and Tsuji, 1974). In studies of workers, apparently no study has been made of the relative importance of dermal and respiratory exposure.

Dichlorvos vaporizers have been used extensively in homes for several years without adverse effect. Measurement of cholinesterase and other observations failed to reveal any alteration resulting from handling the vaporizers much more than would be required for their installation or from their use in ordinary homes, even those homes with air conditioning and, therefore, little ventilation with outside air (Zavon and Kindel, 1966). In test homes where, contrary to the usual practice, vaporizers were used in all rooms and were replaced frequently, the maximal concentrations of dichlorvos were 0.13 mg/m³ in air and 0.12 ppm in food; the only physical or laboratory change was a very slight inhibition of plasma cholinesterase (Leary *et al.*, 1971, 1974).

Therapeutic Use   Dichlorvos is an effective broad-spectrum anthelmintic. In a carefully controlled investigation, a granular-resin, slow-release formulation was administered in hard gelatin capsules to men and women so that the dosage of active ingredient was either 6 or 12 mg/kg. One hundred and eight patients, who varied in age from 16 to 75 years, were selected because they were heavily infested with hookworm, ascaris, and whipworm. The drug did cause a reduction in plasma cholinesterase levels but, with the exception of brief mild headache in a few patients, no clinical side effects were noted. The cure rate for a single dose at the rate of 12 mg/kg ranged from 77.8 to 87.8% for the three main species of worms. Egg counts were reduced by 83.7% or more in cases where cure was not achieved (Peña Chavarría *et al.*, 1969). Essentially similar results were obtained in a separate study of 705 patients, some of whom received other drugs or a placebo. In this study dichlorvos produced no side effects. A dosage less than 6 mg/kg was inadequate (Cervoni *et al.*, 1969).

As might be expected, the dosage relationships for a slow-release, polyvinyl chloride formulation of dichlorvos were entirely different from those for the uncombined compound. Single doses of slow-release formulation providing active ingredient in excess of 4 mg/kg decreased red cell cholinesterase activity with a maximum of 46% reduction at 32 mg/kg, the highest dosage tested. Plasma cholinesterase was more sensitive, its reduction being 50 and 74% at dosages of 1 and 32 mg/kg, respectively. Side effects of the drug and of a placebo were principally related to the gastrointestinal tract but were not dosage related. Similar side effects accompanied repeated dosing, but this also caused intermittent giddiness, increased salivation, and shortness of breath. However, all subjects were able to do their normal work throughout the testing period. Following repeated doses at the rate of 16 mg/kg/day, depression of both red cell and plasma cholinesterase reached 90%. All other laboratory tests were normal. The largest total dose was 8318 mg (117.6 mg/kg) (Hine and Slomka, 1970). The possibility that the gastrointestinal side effects may be related to granulated polyvinyl chloride needs to be considered.

Accidental and Intentional Poisoning   Dichlorvos causes typical symptoms of poisoning by organophosphorus insecticides (Hayes, 1963; Dinman, 1964). Although the compound is rapidly metabolized and excreted, the danger may last more than a few hours in very serious poisoning; a young woman who drank dichlorvos died the next morning in spite of prompt and aggressive treatment (Shinoda *et al.*, 1972).

Onset was delayed at least 3 hr and respiratory arrest was delayed an additional 3 hr in the case of a 19-month-old girl who ate part of a cakelike bait labeled as containing dichlorvos. The ingested material was not available for analysis, but

each of two identically labeled baits contained approximately equal quantities of dichlorvos and malathion. This raises the possibility that the clinical course was atypical for dichlorvos because of an interaction with malathion. The patient never regained the power of spontaneous respiration and died in 4 days. Both the clinical course during the last 3.5 days and marked cerebral edema found at autopsy suggested that brain damage, rather than intoxication, was the primary cause of death. This possibility receives some indirect support from another case in which a child ate an identically labeled bait but never became sick. Gastric lavage was carried out early in both cases. Since the cases were widely separated in time and place, the possibility seems remote that the bait that produced no injury also contained malathion not declared on the label.

Two workers in Costa Rica died after splashing a concentrated formulation on their bare arms and failing to wash it off promptly. In a serious, nonfatal case following dermal exposure, the victim developed slurred speech and drowsiness slightly more than 1.5 hr after the accident. He collapsed suddenly after reaching a hospital. Prompt use of oxygen, a total of 15 mg of atropine sulfate (mostly intravenously), artificial respiration, and other supportive treatment saved him (Hayes, 1963). The time of onset was more poorly defined in another case in which the history was inconsistent, the compound involved was not positively identified, and suicide may have been a factor (Dinman, 1964).

In one case, the patient developed periodic hallucinations and violent combativeness during the fourth and fifth days after his accident (Hayes, 1963). Because he had stopped breathing for a poorly defined period during the acute illness and because of a history of drinking, there was no way to judge whether his delayed agitation was a response to dichlorvos or to anoxia or alcohol. Recovery was complete in any event.

Four cases of primary irritant contact dermatitis resembling mild poison ivy dermatitis have been reported among persons in contact with dogs wearing "flea collars." The patients and some other persons gave positive patch tests to fragments of collar and to a 0.25% solution of dichlorvos (Cronce and Alden, 1968). General experience with the collars indicates that few people are susceptible to this kind of irritation and raises a question of the possibility of a nonspecific reaction in the tests reported.

Atypical Cases of Various Origins   A case of contact dermatitis was clearly associated with leakage of a 1% solution of dichlorvos over the left shoulder of a pest control operator. After some delay, the man changed his overalls but did not bathe and did not change his undershirt. Instead, he placed a plastic sheet between the sprayer and his back to intercept any further leakage, and he completed his day's work. During the day he noticed increasing local irritation and later tiredness, weakness, dizziness, and difficulty in breathing. By the end of the day large bullae had formed. He was never seriously sick and did not miss a regular day of work. On the fourth day he consulted the Division of Occupational Health. The distribution or erythema and bullae still showed the pattern of the undershirt he had worn. Signs of systemic illness were not present, although whole-blood cholinesterase was 36% of normal. No treatment was given but complete rest and total avoidance of exposure were advised (Bisby and Simpson, 1975). What is remarkable about the case is that significant systemic illness did not occur; the possibility that the skin burn was associated with the solvent confined under the plastic sheet apparently was not considered.

A case described as peripheral neuropathy was reported in a 32-year-old woman who had worked with dichlorvos, benomyl, and aldicarb for 1 year and still was working with them when she developed weakness of her arms and legs accompanied by intense physical asthenia. No sensory changes were mentioned. She improved after her employer changed her assignment. Her cholinesterase, which was only slightly depressed, returned to normal within 3 months, and her motor difficulty regressed almost completely within 2 years (Fournier *et al.*, 1976). Whether the condition was true polyneuropathy and whether it was causally related to dichlorvos or to any pesticide are unclear.

Jablecki *et al.* (1983) report a case in which a 16-year-old male was exposed to dichlorvos and chlorpyrifos vapors when he entered his house for 5 min to eat lunch shortly after an extermination. Weakness and incoordination of the upper extremities, along with abdominal cramps and diarrhea, occurred for 1–2 days following the incident. Approximately 1 week following exposure, the patient experienced cramping in both calves. Over the next 2 weeks, atrophy of both upper extremities and loss of 20 pounds occurred. Neurological symptoms stabilized during the fourth week following exposure. At this time, the patient experienced bilateral weakness of the long finger flexors, all intrinsic hand muscles, and hip flexors and extensors. Distal muscles of the lower extremities and all cranial nerves were normal, however. Serum cholinesterase was normal, and red cell cholinesterase activity was within the lower limits of the normal range. This case is atypical in that the symptoms associated with delayed neuropathy developed much sooner and were restricted primarily to the upper body. Furthermore, the circumstances surrounding the time of exposure suggest the observed toxicity might be the result of a combination of oral and inhalation exposures. On the other hand, the authors failed to consider the possibility that the illness was really a Guillain–Barré syndrome only circumstantially related to dichlorvos and/or chlorpyrifos.

Blakey *et al.* (1977) attributed the illnesses of 10 of the 36 employees of a restaurant to insecticides, mainly dichlorvos, applied for the control of cockroaches while the restaurant was closed and only professional pest control operators were present. All food preparation and service utensils were removed from the spaces to be treated, and there were no exposed food items. The food service manager was advised that all food contact surfaces would require washing prior to reopening the restaurant. Pyrethrum and chlorpyrifos were applied as spot treatments to cracks, crevices, and voids; propoxur was applied as a bait in voids; and dichlorvos was applied as a mist. After the misting, the ventilation fans were turned on. The area was

first reentered and cleaning started at 5:30 a.m., about 12 hr after application had been completed, and illnesses consisting of nausea, light headiness, dizziness, headache, and burning sensations of eyes, nose, and throat started between 9:30 a.m. and 12:30 p.m. No symptoms were reported among customers or among the pest control operators. Close surveillance for 14 days revealed no further illnesses among the employees. The published account was erroneous in several particulars; specifically, approximately 1 gallon of <0.5% dichlorvos was applied as a mist instead of 3 gallons of 5% dichlorvos applied as a fog. All of the formulations were approved for use in food-handling establishments, and all were applied according to label directions. Whereas nausea is typical of poisoning by an organic phosphorus compound, burning of the eyes, nose, and throat is not typical of poisoning by any of the pesticides used in the restaurant. Poisoning by these compounds under the conditions recommended for treatment of food-handling areas would not be expected. No attention seems to have been given to the possibility that the entire syndrome of the cleaners, including burning of the eyes, nose, and throat, was caused by the cleaning agents. Chlorine gas or chlorinated ammonias (e.g., NH_2Cl, NCl_3) may be formed, depending on what improper combination of cleaners is made.

Dosage Response   A suicide that succeeded in spite of proper treatment involved a dosage of about 400 mg/kg (Shinoda *et al.*, 1972). The maximal dosage ingested by the child who ate a cake bait and died was about 20 mg/kg for both dichlorvos and malathion, but the probable ingested dosage was less and the retained dosage was much less.

A woman who ingested dichlorvos at an estimated rate of about 100 mg/kg survived following intensive care for 14 days. It was concluded that if the dosage was estimated correctly, the toxicity of the compound for humans appears less than that for the rat (Watanabe *et al.*, 1974).

Spillage of only about 4 ounces of a 3% oil solution of DDVP on a man's lap (about 72 mg/kg) resulted in poisoning which apparently would have been fatal had it not been for unusually vigorous treatment. There was no previous exposure, and no effort was made to remove the poison until the man noticed a burning of the skin about $\frac{1}{2}$ hour after the accident. Even then, washing was very superficial, and a bath was delayed another hour. In still another case, a man spilled a smaller amount of the same 3% formulation on his arm. He removed his shirt at once and washed with soap and water as soon as possible, about 15 min later. He developed dizziness and nausea as the only symptoms (Hayes, 1963).

The results of experimental and carefully observed occupational respiratory exposure are shown in Table 16.24. The results of different observers are remarkably consistent, even though the range of concentration available to some investigators was so wide that it was difficult to draw a conclusion from them. In spite of this limitation, it appears that the threshold for inhibition of plasma cholinesterase without inhibition of red cell cholinesterase is approximately 0.10 mg/m³ for 24 hr/day, 0.15 mg/m³ for 16 hr/day, 0.4 mg/m³ for 5 hr/day,

Table 16.24
Factors Influencing the Inhibition of Plasma Cholinesterase in Persons Exposed to Dichlorvos Vapor

Concentration (mg/m³)	Schedule (hr/day)	Duration (weeks)	Persons, number, health, and age	Plasma cholinesterase (%)	Reference
0.008–0.09	16	1–2	2 adults with liver disease	35–57	Cavagna et al. (1969)
0.02–0.10	24	0.5–2	4 sick adults	100	Cavagna et al. (1969)
0.04–0.10	24	1–4	5 sick babies	100	Cavagna et al. (1969)
0.15–0.25	5[a]	10	15 normal men	100	Rasmussen et al. (1963)
0.10–0.21	16	1–4	6 sick babies	100	Cavagna et al. (1969)
0.10–0.28	16	0.5–2	17 sick adults	100	Cavagna et al. (1969)
0.17–0.84	unknown	2	23 normal adults and children	100	Funckes et al. (1963a)[b]
0.095–0.25	18–24	1	29 normal women[b]	100	Cavagna et al. (1969)
0.10–0.28	24	0.5–2	5 sick adults	54	Cavagna et al. (1969)
0.10–0.21	24	1–4	11 sick babies	25	Cavagna et al. (1969)
0.1–0.5	8	0.57	9 normal men	100	Durham et al. (1959)
0.40–0.55	5[a]	2	15 normal men	65	Rasmussen et al. (1963)
0.26–0.88	1	0.57	7 normal men	100	Witter et al. (1961)
0.7–1.0	8	0.14[c]	4 normal men	78–92	Durham et al. (1959)
0.29–2.13	8	3	4 normal men	32	Stein et al. (1966)
0.9–3.5	2	0.57	3 normal men	70–88	Witter et al. (1961)
6.9	1	0.14[c]	3 normal men	100	Durham et al. (1959)

[a] Ten 0.5-hr periods.
[b] During labor and puerperium.
[c] Single exposure.

and 1.0 mg/m³ for 1 hr/day, but a concentration of 6.9 mg/m³ is tolerated for a single hour. This generalization applies to babies and adults, including women at the time of delivery. It applies to adults and babies with a wide range of diseases but not those with severe liver disease. Thus, response to respiratory exposure to dichlorvos appears to correspond reasonably well to a straight line when the log of concentration in air is plotted against the log of hours of daily exposure.

Rasmussen et al. (1963) found that a total of 5 hr of respiratory exposure per 24-hr day to an average concentration of 0.25 mg/m³ produced no inhibition of cholinesterase, but equal duration of exposure to an average concentration of 0.51 mg/m³ did produce slight inhibition of plasma enzyme. From these values it may be calculated that a dosage of 0.013 mg/kg/day produces no inhibition but a dosage of 0.026 mg/kg/day produces slight inhibition. The calculation takes into account that the men did light work during two releases of dichlorvos each night and rested during the remaining eight releases.

Based on similar calculations, Cavagna et al. (1969) estimated from their respiratory studies that the dosage necessary to inhibit plasma but not red cell cholinesterase is 0.028 mg/kg/day in adults and 0.030 mg/kg/day in children. Lower dosages did not cause plasma cholinesterase inhibition, except in persons with severe liver disease, in whom a dosage of 0.006 mg/kg/day was effective. These respiratory dosages may be compared with an oral dosage of about 0.02 mg/kg/day found by Rider et al. (1968) to produce a decrease in plasma but not red cell cholinesterase.

The slow and partial release of dichlorvos from polyvinyl chloride formulations permits toleration of considerably larger oral doses. One such formulation produced marked inhibition of plasma cholinesterase but no inhibition of red cell enzyme at a dosage of 2–4 mg/kg. Dosages averaging 5.6 mg/kg/day over a period of 21 days produced moderate to marked inhibition of red cell cholinesterase but no side effects distinguishable from those of volunteers who received placebos (Hine and Slomka, 1968).

Laboratory Findings The first sample of blood for cholinesterase determination in the serious, nonfatal case mentioned above was taken the day after the accident. The enzyme activity, though reduced, was surprisingly high in view of the near-fatal outcome. Animals show a rapid recovery of cholinesterase activity, especially of the plasma, following poisoning with dichlorvos. The same may occur in humans.

Dichlorethynol, a known metabolite of dichlorvos, was detected in β-glucuronidase-treated urine following exposure of a person to air containing dichlorvos at a concentration of 38 mg/m³ (Hutson and Hoadley, 1972a).

Pathology A perforation extending from the cardiac portion to the greater curvature of the stomach was found in a 1-year-old girl who had been murdered by dichlorvos at a dosage of about 1300 mg/kg. It was concluded that the poison had affected the mucosa, leading to a rupture after death (Hara et al., 1977). This finding was most unusual, but so was the dosage. Autopsy findings usually are meager and nonspecific.

Treatment of Poisoning   See Section 16.2.2.7.

16.6.6 TRICHLORFON

16.6.6.1 Identity, Properties, and Uses

Chemical Name   Trichlorfon is *O,O*-dimethyl(2,2,2-trichloro-1-hydroxyethyl)-phosphonate.

Structure   See Table 16.16.

Synonyms   The common name trichlorfon is approved by ISO, but many countries use other nonproprietary names. Chlorophos is used in the USSR, dipterex in Turkey, and trichlorphon (BSI) in Great Britain. When the compound is used as a drug, it is called metrifonate or metriphonate. Trade names include Anthon®, Dipterex®, Dylox®, Dyrex®, Foschlor®, Neguvon®, Masoten®, Proxol®, and Tugon®. Neguvon® usually applies to preparations for veterinary use. Code designations include Bayer-15,922 and Bayer-L13/59. The CAS registry number is 52-68-6.

Physical and Chemical Properties   Trichlorfon has the empirical formula $C_4H_8Cl_3O_4P$ and a molecular weight of 257.45. The pure material forms a white crystalline powder with a melting point of 83–84°C. The density is 1.73 at 20°C. The solubility of trichlorfon in water at 25°C is 15.4 gm/100 ml. Trichlorfon is soluble in benzene, ethanol, and most chlorinated hydrocarbons. It is insoluble in petroleum oils and poorly soluble in diethyl ether and carbon tetrachloride. Trichlorfon is stable at room temperature but is decomposed at higher temperatures and at a pH less than 5.5 to form dichlorvos.

History, Formulations, and Uses   Trichlorfon was introduced in 1952 by Bayer Leverkusen. It is used to control flies and roaches; it is also an anthelmintic. Trichlorfon is available as a 50% wettable powder; as 50, 80, and 95% soluble powders; as a 50% soluble concentrate; as 5% dust; and as 5% and 25% granules. Trichlorfon is also available in ultralow-volume concentrates with 250, 500, and 750 gm of active ingredients per liter, respectively.

16.6.6.2 Toxicity to Laboratory Animals

Basic Findings   Signs of poisoning in animals are entirely typical of organic phosphorus compounds in general. Trichlorfon is not allergenic (Viyevskiy, 1974).

Trichlorfon is a compound of moderate to low toxicity in several species of mammals (see Table 16.25). The dosage–response curve is rather steep. Haley *et al.* (1975b) measured not only the oral LD 50 in mice (800 mg/kg in both sexes) but also the LD 1 (430.23 and 458.28 in males and females, respectively). Their data were of sufficient quality that extrapolation of the LD 0.1 was justified; it was 362.18 and 371.85 mg/kg in males and females, respectively.

Table 16.25
Single-Dose LD 50 for Trichlorfon

Species	Route	LD 50 (mg/kg)	Reference
Rat	oral	450	DuBois and Cotter (1955)
Rat, M	oral	432 ± 26.87	Vrbovský *et al.* (1959)
Rat, M	oral	649	Edson and Noakes (1960)
Rat, M	oral	630	Gaines (1969)
Rat, F	oral	560	Gaines (1969)
Rat	oral	438	Crawford and Dull (1970)
Rat	oral	630	Stuneyeva (1974)
Rat, M	dermal	>2800	Edson and Noakes (1960)
Rat	dermal	>2000	Gaines (1969)
Rat	intraperitoneal	225	DuBois and Cotter (1955)
Rat, M	intraperitoneal	351 ± 24.88	Vrbovský *et al.* (1959)
Rat[a]	intraperitoneal	190	Brodeur and DuBois (1963)
Rat[b]	intraperitoneal	250	Brodeur and DuBois (1963)
Mouse, M	oral	660 ± 25.71	Vrbovský *et al.* (1959)
Mouse	oral	579	Kirichek and Kharchenko (1968)
Mouse	oral	650	Belyayev (1969)
Mouse	oral	1370	Crawford and Dull (1970)
Mouse, M	oral	727	Haley *et al.* (1975b)
Mouse, F	oral	866	Haley *et al.* (1975b)
Mouse	intraperitoneal	500	DuBois and Cotter (1955)
Mouse, M	intraperitoneal	650 ± 25.99	Vrbovský *et al.* (1959)
Mouse, F	intraperitoneal	575 ± 20.13	Vrbovský *et al.* (1959)
Guinea pig	intraperitoneal	300	DuBois and Cotter (1955)
Calf	oral	600	Belyayev (1969)
Chicken	oral	125	Belyayev (1969)

[a] Weanling.
[b] Adult.

Pure trichlorfon is less toxic than technical material (Petrova and Arestov, 1968).

Puppies are slightly more susceptible than grown dogs to poisoning by trichlorfon (Zhivoglyadova, 1968).

Repeated doses of trichlorfon at a rate of 100 mg/kg/day reduced the cholinesterase activity of rats to less than half of normal, and 50 mg/kg/day reduced the activity to 50–75% of normal during a 60-day period (DuBois and Cotter, 1955). In the same species a dietary level of 125 ppm (about 5.6 mg/kg/day) for 16 weeks had no effect on red cell cholinesterase, food consumption, growth, or appearance of the organs at autopsy (Edson and Noakes, 1960).

In the dog, 45 mg/kg/day for 3 months reduced serum cholinesterase to 60% of normal (Deichmann and Lampe, 1955). A dietary level of 500 ppm (about 10.5 mg/kg/day) for 12 weeks had about the same effect, and 200 ppm produced a borderline depression of both plasma and red cell cholinesterase, but 50 ppm (about 1 mg/kg/day) was without effect (Williams *et al.*, 1959).

Hens receiving acute subcutaneous doses of 100 or 300 mg/kg trichlorfon showed little if any visible sign of acute neurotoxicity. Although brain, spinal cord, and plasma cholinesterase activities were significantly inhibited, no significant reductions of NTE activity in these tissues were observed. Subcutaneous doses of 100 mg/kg trichlorfon every 3 days for a total of six doses resulted in little or no sign of overt neurotoxicity. No inhibition of spinal cord or brain NTE occurred (Slott and Ecobichon, 1984).

The limited toxicity of trichlorfon for mammals and its greater toxicity for some external and internal parasites have made it possible to employ the compound as a drug for treating both people and domestic animals. Trichlorfon is one of the compounds used for treating bots and other internal parasites in domestic animals. Although usually administered orally or dermally (Anderson and Machin, 1969), it has been used as an aerosol in a closed room in which animals were confined for 1 hr after spraying. This procedure was 94.1% effective, even though cholinesterase activity of the animals was not inhibited (Nepoklonov and Bukshtynov, 1969).

Absorption, Distribution, Metabolism, and Excretion When [^{32}P]trichlorfon was injected subcutaneously into pigs, the maximal concentration in blood (10–11 ppm) was reached in 15–60 min and the maximal concentration in gut contents (4–5 ppm) was reached in 20–150 min. After 5–7 hr, both blood and gut contents still contained radioactivity equivalent to about 1 ppm trichlorfon. During the first 3 hr, dichlorvos could be identified in the blood by paper chromatography (Schwarz, 1965). Dichlorvos also could be identified in the blood of sheep following the dermal application of ^{32}P-labeled trichlorfon (Dedek and Schwarz, 1970b) or following exposure to an aerosol (Nepoklonov and Bukshtynov, 1971). Dichlorvos occurs in the tissues and is excreted in the milk of cows following "pour-on" application of trichlorfon (Nepoklonov and Metelitsa, 1971a,b).

Biochemical Effects Reiner et al. (1975) presented biochemical evidence that trichlorfon is not an inhibitor of cholinesterase but that its entire anticholinesterase action is the result of its decomposition to form dichlorvos. Thus trichlorfon may be viewed as a mechanism for the slow release of dichlorvos. However, this kind of slow release potentially has different effects from mechanisms that depend on wax or polyvinyl chloride because trichlorfon might reach a tissue and release the active agent there at a concentration that might not be possible for dichlorvos absorbed from either the respiratory or gastrointestinal tract. A different kind of experiment (Nordgren et al., 1978) led to the same conclusion. Dichlorvos formed in vivo was found to have its maximal concentration a few minutes after the maximum for metrifonate.

Rats that received chlorophos by stomach tube at rates of 1, 2.5, 5, 10, and 15 mg/kg/day for 6 months showed changes of serotonin in the blood and enterochromaffin cells earlier and more clearly than they showed changes of blood cholinesterase activity (Kolosovskaya, 1971).

Effects on Organs and Tissues When trichlorfon was administered subcutaneously or orally to rats, papillomas developed in the forestomach. Animals surviving 6 months showed varying degrees of liver damage, including steatosis, cell necrosis, and cirrhosis. Subcutaneous application failed to induce

local tumors. In rats and mice dosed by various routes, with or without croton oil, two hepatic carcinomas and one soft tissue sarcoma were found (Lohs and Gibel, 1971; Gibel et al., 1971), but it was not clear whether the findings were statistically significant. Presumably because of the very large dosages given to the animals, the authors considered that a hazard to people from trichlorfon residues on food was unlikely. No indication of carcinogenicity was found when trichlorfon was administered orally or intraperitoneally to rats for 90 weeks and the experiment was terminated at 118 weeks (Teichmann et al., 1978) or when the compound was administered orally, intraperitoneally, or dermally to mice (Teichmann and Hauschild, 1978). A similar negative result was found in hamsters injected intraperitoneally with trichlorfon for 90 weeks at a rate that reduced body weight and survival in the males (Teichmann and Schmidt, 1978). In a later study (Gibel et al., 1973; Stieglitz et al., 1974) in which the stomach tube or intermuscular dosage was 15 mg/kg twice per week (that is, one-third the rate used earlier), the findings were essentially the same, except that marked hyperplasia of the hematopoietic parenchyma of the bone marrow plus myeloid hyperplasia of the liver and spleen were reported in one-third of the animals. Hyperplasia involved all cell types, although granulocytopoiesis predominated. The absence of a dosage–response relationship compared to the earlier study was noteworthy.

When injected subcutaneously at high dosage once per week, trichlorfon produced local sarcomas in only 2 of 24 rats and the latent period was almost 800 days (Preussman, 1968).

Trichlorfon has no influence on the growth of implanted tumors (Hoffman et al., 1973).

Using the highest tolerable single dose or smaller repeated doses, Schiemann (1975) found that trichlorfon produced dominant lethal mutations in mice. Dedek et al. (1975) found that demethyl trichlorfon (at intraperitoneal dosages of 405 mg/kg once and 54 mg/kg/day for 3 weeks) was at least as mutagenic as the parent compound. They concluded, quite rightly, that the injury caused by trichlorfon is not likely due to alkylation. See Section 16.4.4.

Effects on Reproduction In a three-generation study of reproduction in rats, a dietary level of 3000 ppm (about 150 mg/kg/day) caused a marked decrease in the pregnancy rate; pups that were born were small, and none survived to weaning. A dietary level of 1000 ppm reduced the number of pups per litter and the weight of individual pups. A dietary level of 300 ppm (about 15 mg/kg/day) had no detectable effect on reproduction. There was no indication of teratogenesis, even at dosages that were highly toxic (FAO/WHO, 1972). The results of two other three-generation studies in which trichlorfon was administered in drinking water had the same result; poisoning occurred at the higher dosages but teratogenesis was not observed (Ryback, 1973; Wojcik, 1975). Metabolic studies also indicate the toxicity, but not teratogenicity, of large dosages (50 and 75 mg/kg/day) in rabbits (Andrashko et al., 1975).

When dosages approaching the LD 50 level were administered during the critical period of gestation, fetal anomalies were produced. This was achieved, and the dams were permitted to survive by using three daily doses at a total rate of 480 mg/kg/day in rats and 400 mg/kg/day in hamsters and mice. The apparent no-effect level was 200 mg/kg/day (Staples and Goulding, 1979).

An entirely opposite result was reported by Gofmekler and Tabakova (1970), who exposed pregnant rats to chlorphos concentrations of 9, 0.2, 0.02, and 0.005 mg/m³ of air. All concentrations were associated with external and internal anomalies, changes in the weight of the pups and in the relative weights of their organs, histopathological changes in the placentas, and various biochemical changes. The occurrence of similar results in spite of an 1800-fold range of dosage suggests that the observed injuries may have been the result of an unrecognized variable. Severe gonadotoxic effects in rats from a dosage of only 1.5 mg/kg/day for 2 months were reported by Martson and Badayeva (1975). Clearly, such findings are not consistent with normal reproduction for three generations at a much higher dosage.

Although Leybovich (1973) did not report teratogenic effects, he did report toxicity not only to young rats but also to their mothers at a maternal dosage of 0.1 mg/kg/day, suggesting that the compound tested was very different from trichlorfon investigated elsewhere.

A marked species difference was revealed when congenital ataxia and tremor occurred in piglets in some herds in which the sows had been treated with Nequvon during pregnancy (Dobson, 1976; Kronevi, 1977; Knox et al., 1978). Usually, all of the piglets were affected and many died in litters that were involved at all; autopsy revealed marked cerebellar and spinal hypoplasia. Retrospective study showed that fetuses approximately 45–63 days old were susceptible. Approximately 92 litters treated within this period were all abnormal; litters treated either earlier or later were all normal. The therapeutic dose for each sow had been about 10 gm. When trichlorfon was administered to sows experimentally on day 55 of pregnancy, all four litters suffered ataxia and tremor. One of two litters was affected when treatment was on day 56. Neither of two litters was affected when treatment was on day 66. The smallest dosage used (teratogenic in one litter) was 59 mg/kg (Knox et al., 1978).

When injected into the yolk sac of 7-day-old chicken embryos, trichlorfon at a rate of 0.0008 of the rat LD 50 only decreased viability somewhat (Dinerman et al., 1970) and, in view of the small number of eggs used, the difference was uncertain.

16.6.6.3 Toxicity to Humans

Experimental Exposure and Therapeutic Use   In connection with its possible use as an anthelmintic, a highly purified sample of trichlorfon was studied in volunteers. Two doses at the rate of 7.5 mg/kg given on succeeding days produced nausea, colic, and sweating in one and no significant ill effects in the others. The affected person recovered after a single dose

of atropine sulfate. The plasma cholinesterase activity fell to below 10% of normal and the red cell enzyme activity fell to about 50% in all subjects (Lebrun and Cerf, 1960).

In another study, nine persons who received two daily doses of 1320 mg each (about 18.8 mg/kg/day) experienced abdominal pain, and four of them vomited. Seven persons given 1000 mg/day (about 14.2 mg/kg/day) for 2 days had abdominal discomfort. No symptom or laboratory finding not fully explained by cholinesterase inhibition was found. Seven adults had no symptoms following a dose of 500 mg (about 7 mg/kg/day) on each of 2 days (Beheyt et al., 1961). Later, two daily dosages ranging from 7.5 to 20 mg/kg/day were administered to over 2000 patients suffering from a variety of helminthic infections. Side effects were infrequent and mild (Cerf et al. 1962).

Side effects occurred in some patients when trichlorfon was used to treat people infested with Onchocerca volvolus at dosages of 7.5–15 mg/kg/day with 4–16 doses at 2-week intervals. However, even under these conditions, 7 of 19 patients, including two who received 15 mg/kg/day, had no symptoms. The inflammation caused by dying worms was tolerable. The treatment reduced the size of 25–65 nodules and caused a 7-fold average decrease in the number of microfilaria in the skin. However, some new nodules appeared during treatment, so success was incomplete (Salazar Mallen et al., 1971).

When trichlorfon was given daily at the rate of only 5 mg/kg for 12 days, plasma cholinesterase was sharply reduced; side effects became more pronounced each day through the third day and then became no worse, even though the drug was continued. All of ten 16- to 28-year-old male patients developed one or more side effects, mainly in the morning after treatment. All of the men suffered from Schistosoma haematobium, and several of them were infested with other worms. In the dosage used, the drug did not have a lasting curative effect (Hanna et al., 1966).

Two to six single doses at monthly intervals at the rate of 10 mg/kg caused no side effects in 13- to 16-year-old children treated for urinary schistosomiasis (Forsyth and Rashid, 1967). Another regimen was studied in greater detail. Thirty 4- to 12-year-old children infected with Schistosoma haematobium, S. mansoni, or both were treated with trichlorfon at rates of 5 or 10 mg/kg/day for 10 days. The serum cholinesterase activity, already depressed by the disease, was reduced even further by the drug; the red cell enzyme activity was also reduced to 66% of normal. Both enzyme activities returned to true normal within 4 weeks after treatment. Both regimens were curative. As a result, liver function improved, the erythrocyte count increased, the normoblast and myeloid series counts remained about the same, and the eosinophil count decreased significantly. There was no significant effect on kidney functions (Abdel-Aal et al., 1970). Somewhat greater inhibitions of plasma and red cell cholinesterase but no side effects were seen in another clinical trial that confirmed the efficacy of trichlorfon against S. haematobium and its partial efficacy against hookworm. Oral dosages of 7.5, 10.0, and 12.5 mg/kg were administered up to three times at intervals of 14 days (Plestina et *al., 1972).* The World Health Organization has estimated that at least 1 million people have been treated by this regimen. Cure rates of schistosomiasis increase with dose from 28% after the first dose to 84% following the third dose (WHO, 1985).

In summary, the formulations of trichlorfon that have been used for treating people infested by worms frequently have produced mild, rapidly reversible side effects that were no worse, on average, than those caused by other, chemically diverse anthelmintics. The effectiveness of trichlorfon in combating different species of *Schistosoma* apparently has varied greatly under different circumstances. A review of the treatment of *S. mansoni* is that of Kutz (1977). There is considerable evidence that a substantial therapeutic effect is obtained only in infections by *S. haematobium.*

A review (Holmstedt *et al.,* 1978) provides far more detail not only on the therapeutic use of trichlorfon but also on its toxicology than can be covered in this book.

Accidental and Intentional Poisoning There is an important question as to whether poisoning by trichlorfon should be described as a single spectrum of disease subject to the usual variation imposed by differences in dosage and susceptibility or whether it should be described as two distinct conditions, one of which is uncomplicated trichlorfon poisoning and one of which is trichlorfon poisoning complicated by some as yet unrecognized contaminant or additive.

Briefly, all reports agree that poisoning by this compound is initially similar to that caused by other dimethoxy compounds. Onset is rapid, and early signs and symptoms are typical. Following large dosages, unconsciousness is disproportionately common and prolonged or, conversely, cardiorespiratory function is disproportionately good compared to that in poisoning by parathion. Papers dealing with this simple or primary form of poisoning with little or no mention of complications include those by Bordiug (1968), Martynov (1970), Titova and Badiugin (1970), Barkov and Glukhovets (1971), and Luzhnikov and Kosarev (1971).

The first indication that poisoning by trichlorfon is different from that caused by most, if not all, organic phosphorus compounds was the frequency with which mental disturbance was mentioned. Among 379 accidents and attempted suicides, a minimum of 12 cases involved such disturbance. Some clinical variability undoubtedly existed in these cases, but the true variation may have been less than the different descriptions might suggest. In any event, one author stated that the disturbances, which usually lasted only a few days, were otherwise similar to those encountered in endogenous psychoses. Loss of memory and problem-solving ability correspond to the toxic origin. Terms used in connection with the condition have included delirium, depression and anxiety, psychomotor stimulation, hallucinations, and paranoid delusions. Whereas similar difficulties have been noted in connection with poisoning by a wide range of compounds, such reports have been less frequent.

The main indication that poisoning by trichlorfon or by some batches of it is different from poisoning caused by other organic phosphorus compounds is the occurrence of severe polyneuropathy. Among a total of 379 cases of all degrees of severity mentioned in different papers, there were at least 82 cases of polyneuropathy, that is, at least 21%. Although an occasional case of polyneuropathy has been attributed to other organic phosphorus compounds that were not promptly established as neurotoxic, the reported frequency has never been so high nor the relationship to poisoning so clear in connection with any other compound. However, the literature on trichlorfon is not internally consistent. Even if one excludes works (Kosik, 1968; Shutov and Varavkina, 1969; Belenkii and Landesman, 1970; Vatulin *et al.,* 1971; Vernik, 1971; Voiculescu *et al.,* 1971; Zhabin and Litvishchenko, 1971; Demochowsha-Mroczek *et al.,* 1972; Kazakevich *et al.,* 1972; Petrova *et al.,* 1972; Ikuta, 1973; Marchenko, 1973; Pollinger *et al.,* 1973; Ishihara *et al.,* 1974; Irányi, 1975; Takahashi *et al.,* 1975; Eljasz and Krzyszton-Przkop, 1975; Mori *et al.,* 1976; Fukuhara *et al.,* 1977; Kazakevich and Shamrai, 1977; Hierons and Johnson, 1978; Vasilescu *et al.,* 1984) concerned entirely with cases of polyneuropathy, it seems significant that Lobzin and Tsinovoi (1969) found eight instances of polyneuropathy among 41 cases of poisoning (19.5%). Barabach (1971) reported polyneuropathy among a series of 82 cases. Akimov *et al.* (1975) found 38 instances among a total of 160 cases (23.7%) and, perhaps more important, all of the polyneuropathy was among 67 cases of serious poisoning. In a later work presumably based on additional patients, Akimov *et al.* (1977) reported on 136 cases, of which 73 were severe and 25 (18.4%) developed polyneuropathy. By contrast, Gembitskii *et al.* (1970) reported 100 cases of poisoning without any mention of polyneuropathy. This contrast in frequency in large series raises the possibility that fundamentally different materials were involved. However, reports of polyneuropathy have not been confined to one place and time. Most of the cases have been reported from the Soviet Union, where positive results span at least the period 1968–1977 (Kosik, 1968; Kazakevich and Shamrai, 1977). However, positive reports have involved Poland (Dmochowska-Mroczek *et al.,* 1972; Cichecki, 1971), Romania (Voiculescu *et al.,* 1971; Pollinger *et al.,* 1973), Hungary (Irányi, 1975; Eljasz and Krzyszton-Przkop, 1975), Japan (Ikuta, 1973; Takahashi *et al.,* 1975; Mori *et al.,* 1976; Fukuhara *et al.,* 1977), and Iran (Hierons and Johnson, 1978). The Iranian patient came to London for further examination 4 months after onset. He brought with him a sample of granular trichlorfon said to have been taken from the same large container in a wholesale store as the one from which the ingested material had been taken several weeks earlier with suicidal intent. Extensive study of the available sample revealed no difference between it and a high grade of trichlorfon in their clinical effects on chickens or in their *in vitro* effect on neuropathy target esterase. The report emphasized the impossibility of establishing whether or not the sample supplied for study was identical to the one that had been ingested. No information was given on what manufacturer(s) had supplied trichlorfon to the wholesale store.

There is no better way to introduce the clinical picture of polyneuropathy associated with trichlorfon than by a case history. A 26-year-old woman drank 200 ml of a trichlorfon formulation. This resulted in coma for 11 hr followed by headache, vomiting, stomach pain, frequent liquid stools, and general weakness. She improved in a clinic and was discharged in 10 days. However, she noted general fatigue and especially tiredness of the muscles of the legs. Seven to 10 days after discharge, the patient began to notice burning and stabbing pains in her feet. The paresthesia gradually increased and extended to include the legs, hands, and arms. There was an increased tendency to sweat, and discoloration of the hands and feet appeared. Two months after initial poisoning, the patient could not walk or hold a spoon. A slight improvement began after an additional month, but 4 months after original poisoning she still walked with difficulty (Shutov and Varavkina, 1969).

The onset of polyneuropathy has been as early as 3 days after ingestion (Belenkii and Landesman, 1970) and as late as 26 days (Zhabin and Litvishchenko, 1971). In a series of six cases, the average time from ingestion until the first symptom of polyneuropathy (pain in the feet and calves) was 12.8 days; weakness began 1 to 3 days after the start of pain. Involvement of the legs was more severe than that in the arms in all instances, but paralysis of the hands occurred in half of the cases. Reflexes were absent in the legs for 2–6 months but usually persisted in the arms. There was marked atrophy of the lower legs in five of the six cases. Furthermore, in half of the cases there was evidence of involvement of the cranial nerves indicated by limitation of movement of the eyeballs, reduction in visual acuity, and dysarthria. One patient displayed weakness of the respiratory muscles with subjective respiratory insufficiency, which lasted about a week. Recovery began in 1–4 months, with an average of 2.5 months. However, 1.5 years after poisoning, recovery was incomplete in all six instances and special orthopedic shoes were required (Vernik, 1971). At least one instance of horizontal nystagmus has been seen (Petrova *et al.*, 1972).

One would expect early onset of polyneuropathy to be associated with a severe and protracted course. In general, this seems to have been true. However, a patient, who noticed pronounced weakness of her hands and feet on day 3, began to improve by day 13, could stand alone by day 18, and was discharged on day 38 (Belenkii and Landesman, 1970).

Voiculescu *et al.* (1971), who reported a single case of polyneuropathy following accidental exposure to trichlorfon, considered this sequela unusual and attributed it to alcohol, which the patient had ingested on the day of exposure. This relationship may have been significant, for it has been noted specifically in other cases (Kosik, 1968; Babchina, 1972; Petrova *et al.*, 1972; Marchenko, 1973; Irányi, 1975; Takahashi *et al.*, 1975; Fukuhara *et al.*, 1977), and alcohol may have been consumed in yet other cases without any record having been made. The relationship was discounted by Irányi (1975).

Muscle changes were described in one case (Fukuhra *et al.*, 1977) that presumably was typical of polyneuropathy, although

there was little or no recovery about $1\frac{1}{2}$ years after ingestion. Whereas cases of slower recovery are on record, one cannot be certain that some permanent (and, therefore, atypical) changes were not involved. In any event, the onset was typical. A 52-year-old farmer accidentally drank 7 ml of 50% solution of trichlorfon and became unconscious. He was cyanotic, sweating profusely, and wheezing with excessive salivation and bronchial secretion. He was hospitalized and diagnosed promptly, and he was treated appropriately. Following recovery and 16 days after ingestion, he noticed paresthesia pain and slight weakness of his legs. The weakness progressed so that he had difficulty in walking and his hands were affected. When he was first hospitalized for this condition 36 days after ingestion, he had a burning sensation and hyperesthesia in the feet, footdrop, weakness, and atrophy of the muscles of the extremities, especially the legs and feet, and he was unable to sit up or to walk. Biopsies of the left and right gastrocnemius muscles were taken 70 and 220 days, respectively, after ingestion. The tissue was studied by both light and electron microscopy. The observed changes were described in such tremendous detail that even a summary of them cannot be attempted here. The fact that extensive histochemical studies were made in the case under discussion but in few of the other studies makes any comparison difficult.

Most cases of poisoning by trichlorfon, whether complicated by polyneuropathy or not, have been associated with ingestion. In many instances, the ingestion was suicidal in intent. Several instances of poisoning through skin contact have been reported (Svetličić and Wilhelm, 1968; Fukel'man and Afonin, 1971), and at least two associated with application of the compound in an effort to cure scabies were fatal (Titova and Badiugin, 1970).

Use Experience Relatively few instances of occupational poisoning by trichlorfon have been reported. However, in some cases the degree of illness was greater than would have been predicted on the basis of dosage–response relationships observed in accidental and intentional poisoning. For example, agricultural workers who were in an area that was being machine-sprayed with chlorophos and others who weeded crops the day after the crops were sprayed promptly suffered cholinergic illness that was mild in most cases but moderate to severe in a few persons. An interval of recovery was followed by polyneuropathy (Simkin and Mironov, 1971).

In another situation, only very slight cholinesterase inhibition was found in sprayers applying trichlorfon (Lebrun and Cerf, 1960).

Veterinarians treating grub infestations in cattle with pour-on applications of trichlorfon and other organic phosphorus pesticides in poorly ventilated areas experienced nausea, headaches, and irritations of the throat and facial skin. However, blood cholinesterase activity was not reduced in any of these cases, and alkyl phosphate metabolites were only occasionally found in the urine (Beat and Morgan, 1977).

Dosage Response Gembitskii *et al.* (1970) considered 30,000–90,000 mg a fatal dose. Based on their own experience and on a review of the Soviet literature, Titova and Badiugin (1970) concluded that severe poisoning had followed dosages of 80–700 mg/kg and higher, and light to moderate poisoning had occurred at an average dosage of 40 mg/kg. This is consistent with the report of a man who survived a dosage of about 540 mg/kg taken with suicidal intent but combated with vigorous treatment (Ikuta, 1973) and is also consistent with the results of the use of trichlorfon as an anthelmintic. When used as a drug, a total dosage as high as 37.7 mg/kg produced very mild poisoning and a dosage of 10 mg/kg/day had no untoward effects. Depending on unidentified factors, trichlorfon produced mild poisoning among other persons receiving daily doses as low as 5 mg/kg/day for 12 days. A single dose at the rate of 10 mg/kg was tolerated. In no instance have the side effects of trichlorfon been severe enough to interfere with its therapeutic use.

On the other hand, a dosage of only about 50 mg/kg swallowed accidentally produced immediate unconsciousness and other signs of severe acute poisoning, followed in 16 days by severe polyneuropathy (Fukuhra *et al.*, 1977). This case seems to indicate that the preparation involved was not only neurotoxic but also quantitatively more toxic than trichlorfon available in Western Europe and especially the preparations used for treatment of people and animals.

The occurrence of only moderate symptoms in a woman thought to have ingested 20,000 mg with suicidal intent (Okuyama *et al.*, 1975) is unexplained.

Discussion Poisoning by trichlorfon in areas from which polyneuropathy has not been reported has been described by Molphy and Rathus (1964). Whether the small number of cases from these areas is the result of less extensive use of trichlorfon or is the result of using purer preparations is unknown. Certainly, in many parts of the world its agricultural use causes little or no poisoning, and its use as an anthelmintic in humans and animals has been associated with only minor side effects. These circumstances make it very tempting to speculate that the compound that frequently has caused poisoning and especially polyneuropathy is not identical to trichlorfon. It may be recalled that, contrary to the findings of others, one report from the Soviet Union found chlorphos teratogenic, one found it toxic to the young at an extremely low dosage, and another report found that this material has a more clear-cut effect on serotonin than on cholinesterase. Finally, a few cases of polyneuropathy have been associated with dosages that one would expect to be harmless (Fukuhara *et al.*, 1977) or with unexpected effects such as hepatitis and nephritis (Kazakevich and Shamrai, 1977); these cases suggest that a contaminant was responsible for the untoward results. However, simple toxicity studies in animals offer no support for this speculation. Most Soviet LD 50 values for rats and mice are in good agreement with those reported elsewhere (see Table 7.25). Of course, the difficulty could arise from something included in certain formulations. This modified speculation would be consistent with the fact that, when polyneuropathy has occurred at all, it has

shown a reasonably satisfactory dosage–response relationship, but the problem remains unsolved.

Another unsolved problem involves the exact nature of the polyneuropathy. According to Vasilescu (1972), nerve conduction velocities and EMG values in a patient suggested that the lesion was perikaryal in nature. An opposite conclusion was reached by Kazakevich *et al.* (1972), who considered that the injury was predominantly an affection of the myelin membrane and of the axial cylinders.

There is a general discussion of polyneuropathy in Section 16.4.1. As shown in Table 16.14, several investigators failed to produce neurotoxicity in hens with large doses of trichlorfon. Johnson (1970) succeeded by using repeated massive doses. However, this throws no light on whether trichlorfon is a very weak neurotoxic agent or whether the sample Johnson used contained a trace of some strong agent.

Treatment of Poisoning The basic treatment for poisoning by trichlorfon is the same as that for other organic phosphorus compounds. A discussion of this treatment offers reason for caution in the use of chlorpromazine and related drugs. These general cautions must be balanced by the physician against the view (Nazardinov and Spicin, 1974) that chlorpromazine eliminates not only muscular fasciculations but also the acute psychosis that they considered common in poisoning by trichlorfon, although they tended to attribute it to atropine used in treatment.

16.6.7 MEVINPHOS

16.6.7.1 Identity, Properties, and Uses

Chemical Name Mevinphos is *O,O*-dimethyl 1-carbomethoxy-1-propen-2-yl phosphate.

Structure Mevinphos exists in two isomeric forms (Fukuto *et al.*, 1961), shown in Table 16.16. The *cis* isomer also has been designated α and E; the *trans* isomer has been called β and Z. The two differ greatly in NMR spectra, in melting point, in stability, in toxicity to insects and mammals, and probably in other properties too.

Synonyms The common name mevinphos (BSI, ISO) is in general use, except in the USSR, where no common name has been adopted. The trade name Phosdrin® also is used quite generally. Code designations include OS-2,046. The CAS registry number is 7786-34-7.

Physical and Chemical Properties Mevinphos has the empirical formula $C_7H_{13}O_6P$ and a molecular weight of 224.16. The pure material forms a pale yellow to orange liquid that has a very mild odor or is odorless. The boiling point of mevinphos is 99–103°C at 0.003 mm Hg. The melting point of the *cis* isomer is 21°C, and that of the *trans* isomer is 6.9°C. The density of mevinphos is 1.25, with a density of 1.2345 and

1.245 for the *cis* and *trans* isomers, respectively. Technical mevinphos is miscible with water, alcohols, ketones, chlorinated hydrocarbons, and aromatic hydrocarbons but is only slightly soluble in aliphatic hydrocarbons. Mevinphos is stable at ordinary temperatures. It is hydrolyzed in aqueous solution with a half-life of 1.4 hr at pH 11, 3 days at pH 9, 35 days at pH 7, and 120 days at pH 6. Decomposition of mevinphos by lime sulfur is rapid.

History, Formulations, and Uses Phosdrin is 100% insecticidally active with at least 60% of the product being the *cis* isomer. Most commercial products contain about 30% of the *trans* isomer. Although soluble in water, mevinphos is available as emulsifiable concentrates of 10, 18, 24, 48, and 50% of the technical product.

16.6.7.2 Toxicity to Laboratory Animals

Basic Findings Mevinphos is a compound of high toxicity not only orally but dermally (see Table 16.26). It is a direct inhibitor of cholinesterase.

In one study, all rats were killed within 3 weeks on a dietary level of 100 ppm and, at 50 ppm for 60 days, rats showed reduced growth, slight tremor, and brain cholinesterase only 20% of normal. Even at 6.3 ppm, the rats showed slight tremor, and brain cholinesterase was only 90% of normal (Kodama *et al.*, 1954). Because of unknown factors, some rats survived 13 weeks in another study at a dietary level of 400 ppm, but they showed signs of poisoning, nonspecific degeneration of the liver and kidneys, and degeneration of the epithelial cells lining ducts and acini of salivary, lacrimal, and other exocrine

Table 16.26
Single-Dose LD 50 for Mevinphos

Species	Route	LD 50 (mg/kg)	Reference
Rat, M	oral	6.1	Gaines (1960)
Rat, F	oral	3.7	Gaines (1960)
Rat, M	oral	6.0–6.8	Kodama *et al.* (1954)
Rat, M	oral	7	Shaffer and West (1960)
Rat, M	dermal	4.7	Gaines (1960)
Rat, F	dermal	4.2	Gaines (1960)
Rat, F	intraperitoneal	1.5	Kodama *et al.* (1954)
Rat	intraperitoneal	0.35[a]	Casida (1955)
Rat	intraperitoneal	35[b]	Casida (1955)
Mouse	oral	4.3–6.8	Kodama *et al.* (1954)
Mouse	oral	10.8[c]	Sato (1959)
Mouse	oral	12.9[d]	Sato (1959)
Mouse	dermal	40[c]	Sato (1959)
Mouse	dermal	50.2[d]	Sato (1959)
Gerbil, M	intraperitoneal	0.45	Steen *et al.* (1976)
Gerbil, F	intraperitoneal	0.54	Steen *et al.* (1976)

[a] *Cis* isomer.
[b] *Trans* isomer.
[c] Technical phosdrin.
[d] Phosdrin emulsion.

glands. A level of 200 ppm produced similar but lesser injury. A level of 25 ppm for 13 weeks produced minimal signs of toxicity. No significant clinical effect or effect on brain cholinesterase was produced by 2 ppm (about 0.1 mg/kg/day), but erythrocyte cholinesterase was reduced to 75% of normal (Cleveland and Treon, 1961).

When dogs were fed mevinphos at a dietary level of 5 ppm (about 0.1 mg/kg/day) for 14 weeks, erythrocyte and plasma cholinesterase were reduced to 70 and 90% of controls, respectively; brain enzyme remained normal. A level of 0.03 ppm was without effect on cholinesterase (Cleveland and Treon, 1961).

16.6.7.3 Toxicity to Humans

Experimental Exposure Mevinphos at a dosage of 2.5 mg/person/day (about 0.036 mg/kg/day) produced a maximal decrease of 25% in red cell cholinesterase by day 27 but did not affect plasma cholinesterase activity or cause any symptom. Dosages of 1.5 and 2.0 mg/person/day also reduced red cell cholinesterase. A dosage of 1 mg/person/day for 30 days produced no detectable effect. After dosing was stopped, the return of red cell cholinesterase to normal was determined entirely by the rate of replacement of red cells in the circulation, indicating that inhibition had been irreversible (Rider *et al.*, 1972, 1975). In a separate study of eight treated and eight control volunteers, dosage at the rate of 0.025 mg/kg/day (approximately 1.75 mg/person/day) for 28 days caused average decreases of 19% in red cell cholinesterase and of 13% in plasma cholinesterase. The corresponding decreases for individuals were 15–25% and 4–19%. There was no tendency of the red cell values to approach a steady state within the 28-day period; the plasma values did approach and possibly reach a steady state. None of the subjects demonstrated signs or symptoms that could be ascribed to mevinphos. There was no change in SGOT, SGPT, or alkaline phosphatase activity (Verberk, 1977). At the end of the exposure period, a 7% decrease in slow motor fiber nerve conduction velocity and an increase of 38% or less in Achilles tendon reflex force were reported (Verberk and Salle, 1977). However, examination of the graphs raises a serious question as to whether the differences between experimental and control values were real.

Accidental and Intentional Poisoning The use of mevinphos for suicide sometimes has been followed by rapid death (Lewin and Love, 1974) and sometimes by complete recovery (Bennett and Best, 1962).

The most interesting accident, although not the most severe illness, was that involving the poisoning of six children who wore pants that were contaminated by mevinphos during shipment and were later sold as damaged goods (Warren *et al.*, 1963).

Use Experience In many instances, onset of poisoning has been less than 2 hr after exposure (Stoeckel and Meinecke,

1966; Holmes *et al.*, 1974; Hayes, 1963, 1982). In one instance, onset was within 15 min after a bag broke, releasing 25% mevinphos on the clothing of a workman operating a bagging machine. In this case and at least one other, impairment of judgment was an early and important feature of poisoning. In spite of the accident, the man continued to work; after he had vomited twice and stopped work, his foreman noticed that he had removed bags from the machine before they were full. In another case, a pilot ran into power lines and crashed only 45 min after he started applying 2% mevinphos dust. He survived and reported later that, after the second of four loads, he noticed that his depth perception was becoming impaired and he had trouble seeing where the field was. After his third load, he looked in a mirror and learned that his pupils were contracted to pinpoint size. After the fourth load, he thought the aircraft was losing power; he knew that he was going to hit wires but just did not care. He said that normally he would have landed but his reasoning ability was lost. Observers on the ground reported that there was no indication of power loss but that the pilot's flying during his fourth load was very erratic.

The observed impairment of judgment is not explained by studies in animals which indicate that penetration of mevinphos into the brain is slow and limited and that brain cholinesterase is less susceptible to the compound than the enzymes derived from plasma and red cells (Sharma *et al.*, 1973).

From four cases of poisoning among formulators, it was concluded that symptoms may occur up to 48 hr after last contact (Roche *et al.*, 1961). However, in another case in which onset was delayed 2 days after initial exposure, poisoning was attributed to continuing exposure to unwashed clothing and to the contaminated tractor on which the 17-year-old youth worked. There was little or no improvement for 3 days, but the patient improved steadily after his hair was cut and he was given a thorough shower (Brachfeld and Zavon, 1965).

In addition to signs and symptoms observed by others, Gonzalez Laprat *et al.* (1966) reported high fever and cramping of the lower extremities in three heavily exposed agricultural spraymen who recovered following unusually large doses of atropine.

Atypical Cases of Various Origins A leak led to sudden, gross overexposure of a mevinphos formulator; the typical poisoning that followed began in one-half hour and required intensive treatment for 2 days. Following discharge from hospital, the man continued to have a cough productive of white, frothy sputum. He improved somewhat during the next winter but had an attack of pneumonia when activity in the plant began next season. He claimed that following his initial attack, even the slightest contact with chemicals in the plant caused coughing and wheezing (Weiner, 1961).

In another case in which typical acute signs and symptoms lasted 2 days after occupational exposure, anxiety, depression, vertigo, and spontaneous vertical nystagmus without tinnitus

or hearing loss persisted for 4 months (Huelse and Federspil, 1975).

Dosage Response The dose in a successful suicide was unknown (Lewin and Love, 1974). The dose in an attempted suicide in which the patient was saved by heroic treatment was thought to have been at least 3 ounces of an unstated concentration (Bennett and Best, 1962).

An orchardist, who had had no exposure to pesticides for 2 months, suffered mild but typical poisoning 10 hr after a patch test with mevinphos applied at a rate later estimated as 14 mg/kg. The illness lasted 5 days (Bell *et al.*, 1968). Actually, some of the material applied was taken up by the gauze pad placed on the skin. Contrary to what the authors supposed, the use of an adhesive over the pad would reduce rather than increase absorption (see Section 4.3.5.3).

In two cases of moderate poisoning following combined respiratory and dermal exposure, the absorbed doses of mevinphos (based on recovery of a metabolite from the urine) were 7.7 and 9.2 mg (Holmes *et al.*, 1974), only 3.0–3.7 times more than an oral dose volunteers tolerated daily without symptoms. It may be that recovery of the metabolites was incomplete.

A dosage of 0.036 mg/kg/day produced no clinical effect in volunteers but did reduce red cell cholinesterase activity; 0.014 mg/kg/day was without effect, as is consistent with the threshold limit value of 0.1 mg/m^3.

Laboratory Findings The concentrations of mevinphos found in samples taken at autopsy from a man who had died within 45 min after drinking the compound were: stomach wall, 3400 ppm; blood, 360 ppm; liver, 240 ppm; brain, 3 ppm; skeletal muscle, 86 ppm; kidney, 20 ppm; and urine 8 ppm. Inhibition of blood cholinesterase was essentially complete (Lewin and Love, 1974).

In cases of moderate poisoning associated with occupational exposure to mevinphos, the concentration of dimethyl phosphate (DMP) in urine samples collected during the first 12 hr after onset was 0.4 ppm. The concentration declined rapidly until about 36 hr after onset, and excretion was essentially complete within about the first 50 hr (Holmes *et al.*, 1974). The dimethylphosphate concentration was 2.0 ppm in the urine of a farmer exposed to both parathion and mevinphos who was mildly poisoned 2 hr after a hose broke and filled his boots with mevinphos emulsion (Haley *et al.*, 1978; E. R. Reichert *et al.*, 1978).

Treatment of Poisoning Treatment is the same as that for poisoning by other organic phosphorus compounds (see Section 16.2.2.7). The beneficial effects of oximes in people poisoned by mevinphos have been noted in several cases (Bennett and Best, 1962; Quinby, 1964; Bell *et al.*, 1968), but not in all (Stoeckel and Meinecke, 1966; Holmes *et al.*, 1974). The importance of thorough bathing is emphasized by a case in which continuing illness suggested continuing dermal absorption (Brachfeld and Zavon, 1965).

16.6.8 AZINPHOS-METHYL

16.6.8.1 Identity, Properties, and Uses

Chemical Name   Azinphos-methyl is *O,O*-dimethyl-*S*-[4-oxo-1,2,3-benzotriazin-3(4*H*-yl) methyl] phosphorothioate.

Structure   See Table 16.16.

Synonyms   The common name azinphos-methyl (BSI, ISO) is in general use. Trade names include Cotnion-methyl®, Gusathion®, Guthion®, and Methyl Guthion®. Code designations include BAY-90278, Bayer-17147, ENT-23233, OMS-186, and R-1582. The CAS registry number is 86-50-0.

Physical and Chemical Properties   Azinphos-methyl has the empirical formula $C_{10}H_{12}N_3O_3PS_2$ and a molecular weight of 317.3. The pure material forms a white crystalline solid with a melting point of 73–74°C. The density of azinphos-methyl at 20°C is 1.44. The vapor pressure is below 3.8×10^{-4} mm Hg at 20°C. The technical material forms a brown waxy solid with a melting point of 65–68°C. The solubility of azinphos-methyl in water at 25°C is 33 ppm. Azinphos-methyl is also soluble in most organic solvents. Azinphos-methyl decomposes at temperatures above 200°C. It rapidly is hydrolyzed by cold alkali to form anthranilic acid, and it is subject to hydrolysis by acids.

History, Formulations, and Uses   Azinphos-methyl was introduced in 1953 by Bayer Leverkusen as a nonsystemic insecticide and acaricide of long persistence. Azinphos-methyl is available as 20% emulsifiable concentrates; 20, 25, 40, and 50% wettable powders; and 5% dusts.

16.6.8.2 Toxicity to Laboratory Animals

Basic Findings   Illness produced by azinphos-methyl is similar to that produced by other dimethoxy organic phosphorus insecticides. The pure material is an indirect inhibitor of cholinesterase, easily absorbed by the skin as well as by other natural routes. Its acute toxicity by several routes is shown in Table 16.27.

Rats fed azinphos-methyl for 2 years at rates of 50 ppm and later 100 ppm (about 5–10 mg/kg/day) ate and grew normally, and their renal and erithropoietic functions were indistinguishable from those of controls. However, some females had convulsive episodes; and plasma, red cell, and brain cholinesterase activity were depressed in all of them. Dietary levels of 5 ppm (about 0.5 mg/kg/day) or less were without effect. There was no tumorigenic effect at any dosage level (Worden *et al.,* 1973).

Dogs receiving 300 ppm in their feed (about 9 mg/kg/day)

Table 16.27
Single-Dose LD 50 for Azinphos-Methyl

Species	Route	LD 50 (mg/kg)	Reference
Rat, F	oral	16.4	DuBois *et al.* (1957)
Rat	oral	15	Shaffer ad West (1960)
Rat, M	oral	13	Gaines (1960)
Rat, F	oral	11	Gaines (1960)
Rat	oral	12	Crawford and Dull (1970)
Rat, M	oral	26	Pasquet *et al.* (1976)
Rat, F	oral	24	Pasquet *et al.* (1976)
Rat, F	intraperitoneal	5.1	DuBois *et al.* (1957)
Rat, M	intraperitoneal	11.6	DuBois *et al.* (1957)
Rat, M	dermal	220	Gaines (1960)
Rat, F	dermal	220	Gaines (1960)
Rat, F	dermal	90	Pasquet *et al.* (1976)
Mouse	oral	8	Sato (1959)
Mouse	oral	3.4	O'Brien (1967)
Mouse	oral	20	Crawford and Dull (1970)
Mouse, M	oral	7.15	Haley *et al.* (1975a)
Mouse, F	oral	6.35	Haley *et al.* (1975a)
Mouse, M	intraperitoneal	5.4	DuBois *et al.* (1957)
Mouse, F	intraperitoneal	3.4	DuBois *et al.* (1957)
Mouse	intraperitoneal	8–10	Murphy (1966)
Guinea pig, M	oral	80.0	DuBois *et al.* (1957)
Guinea pig, M	intraperitoneal	40.0	DuBois *et al.* (1957)

showed tremors, weakness, abnormal quietness, and some weight loss; one of eight died of cholangitis apparently unrelated to azinphos-methyl. Half that concentration (about 4.7 mg/kg/day) was without clinical effect, and 5 ppm for 2 years (0.25–0.15 mg/kg/day as the dogs grew older) was without effect on plasma or red cell cholinesterase (Worden *et al.,* 1973).

Rats that inhaled azinphos-methyl at a concentration of 4.72 mg/m³, 6 hr/day, 5 days/week for 12 weeks showed a significant depression of red cell and plasma cholinesterases, and the males had a low gain of body weight. Concentrations of 0.195 and 1.24 mg/m³ were without effect (Kimmerle, 1976).

Effects on Organs and Tissues   An increased incidence of chromosomal abnormalities was found in cultured Chinese hamster cells exposed to azinphos-methyl at concentrations of 60 ppm or more (Alam and Kasitiya, 1974; Alam *et al.,* 1974). Of course, it is unlikely that concentrations of this order of magnitude will be reached in the tissues of poisoned animals, much less in the tissues of those that remain well. Exactly the same may be said of the chromosomal aberrations reported (Alam and Kasitiya, 1975) in human cells in culture. The compound did not produce dominant lethal changes in mice (Jorgenson *et al.,* 1976).

In a study of possible carcinogenicity, azinphos-methyl was given to male rats at time-weighted average dietary levels of 78 and 156 ppm, to female rats at average levels of 62.5 and 125 ppm, and to mice at 3.13 and 62.5 ppm for males and 62.5 and 125 ppm for females. It was concluded that carcinogenicity was not demonstrated in rats or mice, although a possible relationship of the compound and tumors of the pancreas and of the follicular cells of the thyroid was suggested (NCI, 1978a; Milman *et al.*, 1978).

16.6.8.3 Toxicity to Humans

Experimental Exposure Dosages given to volunteers for approximately 30 days each have included 4, 4.5, 6, 7, 8, 9, 10, 12, 14, 16, 18, and 20 mg/person/day, which did not produce clinical effects or a significant change in cholinesterase levels (Rider and Puletti, 1969; Rider *et al.*, 1970, 1971, 1972). Apparently, a level high enough to inhibit cholinesterase remains to be studied.

Use Experience In a study of groups of persons selected because of occupational exposure to azinphos-methyl or parathion-methyl, Quinby *et al.* (1958) found no clinical evidence of poisoning and no significant depletion of cholinesterase activity. However, they did report a case that illustrates how even a compound of moderate toxicity such as azinphos-methyl can cause serious injury unless used with all recommended precautions. (Some details from the original record are added herewith.) Actually, we know of this case only because a serious effect was barely missed. Briefly, a pilot, who already had several days exposure to parathion-methyl, became ill while applying azinphos-methyl. Work on the day of near disaster began at 9:30 a.m. There was a small leak so that the pilot could feel liquid hit his face while he flew, and it smeared his goggles; he spilled concentrate on his hand while loading but washed it off in 2 min. While flying, he began to experience headache, tightness in the chest, nausea, and excess salivation. He tried to avoid vomiting while airborne but retched anyway. However, it was difficulty in seeing, which he described as "stovepipe vision," that gave most trouble, and he made at least two passes at the landing strip before he saw well enough to land. He reported that he almost fainted in the process. His chief complaint when admitted to hospital about 48 km from the landing strip was that he "couldn't see to fly." His recovery was uneventful.

Its threshold limit value of 0.2 mg/m³ indicates that azinphos-methyl is considered safe for occupational intake at a rate of about 0.03 mg/kg/day.

Laboratory Findings When radioactive azinphos-methyl was administered intravenously to volunteers, radioactivity equivalent to about 1.5% of the administered dose per hour was recovered in the urine during the first 12 hr. Recovery decreased gradually but was still slightly over 0.1% 96 to 120 hr after injection. The total recovery during 120 hr was 69.5% of the dose following intravenous administration and 15.9% (corrected) following dermal application (Feldmann and Maibach, 1974). Because the correction factor differed little from 1.0, it is clear that the compound is easily absorbed by the human skin.

Treatment of Poisoning See Section 16.2.2.7.

16.6.9 BROMOPHOS

16.6.9.1 Identity, Properties, and Uses

Chemical Name Bromophos is *O,O*-dimethyl-*O*-(2,5-dichloro-4-bromophenyl)-phosphorothioate.

Structure See Table 16.16.

Synonyms The common name bromophos (ISO, BSI) is in general use. The homonym bromofos sometimes is used. Trade names include Brofene®, Brophene®, and Nexion®. Code designations have included CELA-1942, ENT-27162, OMS-658, S-1942, and SHG-1942. The CAS registry number is 2104-96-3.

Physical and Chemical Properties Bromophos has the empirical formula $C_8H_8BrCl_2O_3PS$ and a molecular weight of 366.00. The pure material forms yellowish crystals with a faint, characteristic odor. The melting point of bromophos is 53°C. Its boiling point is 140–142°C at 10^{-2} mm Hg. The vapor pressure is 1.3×10^{-4} mm Hg at 20°C. The technical material is at least 90% pure and has a melting point of at least 51°C. Bromophos is soluble in most organic solvents such as toluene, carbon tetrachloride, and diethyl ether. It is slightly soluble in low-molecular-weight alcohols. The water solubility of bromophos is 40 ppm at 27°C. Bromophos is stable in aqueous suspension. It hydrolyzes in a distinctly alkaline medium.

History, Formulations, and Uses Bromophos was introduced in 1964 by C. H. Boehringer Sohn. It is available as 25 and 40% emulsifiable concentrates, 25% wettable powders, 2–5% dusts, 5–10% granules, 20% dips, 40% atomizing concentrates, and 3% coarse powders.

16.6.9.2 Toxicity to Laboratory Animals

Basic Findings The signs of poisoning by bromophos are similar to those caused by other organic phosphorus compounds. The onset tends to be delayed and some deaths occur late (Kinkel *et al.*, 1966). However, these delays, although great compared to those seen with dichlorvos and TEPP, are little or no greater than those seen with several other compounds, notably diazinon, dursban, manazon, and mevinphos. In fact, some deaths caused by malathion and mevinphos were considerably later (Gaines, 1960, 1969). Delayed effects of organic phosphorus compounds tend to be associated with low toxicity and a consequent increase in the relative importance of storage in fat. Bromophos is a compound of low acute toxicity; see Table 16.28.

Rats survived dietary levels of 10,000 ppm (about 500 mg/kg/day) for 100 days, but they grew poorly and showed

Table 16.28
Single-Dose LD 50 for Bromophos

Species	Route	LD 50 (mg/kg)	Reference
Rat	oral	3750–6180	Kinkel *et al.* (1966)
Rat, M	oral	1600	Gaines (1969)
Rat, F	oral	1730	Gaines (1969)
Rat, M	dermal	>5000	Gaines (1969)
Rat, F	dermal	>5000	Gaines (1969)
Rat	intraperitoneal	1625–3125	Kinkel *et al.* (1966)
Mouse	oral	2829–5850	Kinkel *et al.* (1966)
Mouse	intraperitoneal	1040	Kinkel *et al.* (1966)
Guinea pig	oral	1500	Kinkel *et al.* (1966)
Rabbit	oral	720	Kinkel *et al.* (1966)

some degenerative changes of the liver and kidneys. Failure of growth and liver injury were less, kidney damage was absent at 6000 ppm, and no injury was detected at 1500 ppm (about 75 mg/kg/day) (Kinkel *et al.*, 1966). Other investigators have reported relative enlargement of the liver at dietary levels as low as 500 ppm but not 100 ppm (Desi *et al.*, 1971a).

A reduction in cholinesterase activity was observed in rats that received dietary levels of 500 or 100 ppm for 6 weeks but not in those receiving 30 or 10 ppm (Desi *et al.*, 1971b). The authors considered EEG and behavioral tests more sensitive than cholinesterase tests in detecting the effects of small dosages. However, at 10 ppm (about 0.5 mg/kg/day), learning was more rapid than in the controls, so the interpretation is obscure.

Bromophos may be unusual in the range of dosage between that necessary to inhibit cholinesterase and that necessary to produce illness. In rats, a single oral dosage of only 6 mg/kg caused slight but measurable inhibition. However, activity was inhibited only 70–78% in red cells, plasma, and brain following a dosage of 4000 mg/kg. A dosage of 1.25 mg/kg/day for 100 days caused no inhibition of plasma or red cell cholinesterase activity of rats, and 2.5 mg/kg/day produced no effect on red cell enzyme in males. Within 2 weeks the inhibited plasma enzyme activity returned to normal. Similar results were obtained in a 2-year study of rats. A dosage of 3 mg/kg/day for 100 days produced no statistically significant inhibition of red cell, plasma, brain, or liver cholinesterase activity in dogs. One dog was mildly poisoned after receiving bromophos for a year at a rate of 175 mg/kg/day; 4 months later cholinesterase activity had returned to normal. Dosages of 11, 44, and 88 mg/kg/day for 2 years produced no detectable illness but did cause marked and approximately proportional inhibition of cholinesterase activity in dogs (Muacevic *et al.*, 1970).

Dogs given bromophos at dietary levels of 38.4 mg/kg/day experienced decreases in food consumption; body weight; cholinesterase levels of the plasma, erythrocyte, and brain; and frequency of estrus. Dogs receiving 9.6 mg/kg/day for 1 year showed decreased erythrocyte and plasma cholinesterase levels, whereas those receiving 2.4 mg/kg/day experienced only a decrease in plasma cholinesterase levels. No adverse effects were noted among dogs receiving 0.6 mg/kg/day [World Health Organization/Food and Agriculture Organization (WHO/FAO), 1984a,b].

Single dermal applications of bromophos to rats resulted in the following ID 50 values for cholinesterase inhibition: plasma, 10 mg/kg; brain, 567.1 mg/kg; and erythrocyte, 1938 mg/kg (Shivanandappa *et al.*, 1988).

Absorption, Distribution, Metabolism, and Excretion Bromophos is absorbed by the skin as well as by the respiratory and gastrointestinal tracts.

On days 1, 8, and 22, respectively, following the last of nine weekly dippings of lambs in 0.5% bromophos, the concentration of the compound in their omental fat was 9.75, 2.5, and 0.33 ppm (Clark *et al.*, 1966).

The detoxification of bromophos takes place at both the methyl and the phenyl phosphate bonds (Stiasni *et al.*, 1967; Palut *et al.*, 1969). Following dermal application to cows, bromophos could be detected in the blood at a concentration of about 0.01 ppm, but bromoxon was not detectable. The main metabolite in this species was desmethylbromophos, which was detected in concentrations of 0.4–0.7 ppm in both milk and blood (Dedek and Schwarz, 1969). Following ingestion of bromophos, guinea pigs excrete a substantial proportion of insecticidal material in their feces (Ising, 1971), either as the parent compound or as some unidentified, insecticidal metabolite.

Effects on Organs and Tissues In mice, acute intraperitoneal bromophos doses of 1000 mg/kg did not cause any cytogenic effects in spermatogonia or bone marrow cells. No adverse genetic effects were observed in the dominant lethal mutation assay at this dose (Degraeve *et al.*, 1984).

Statistically significant increases in chromosomal breaks, gaps, and actinic fragments were observed 24 and 48 hr following intraperitoneal administration of 183.0 mg/kg bromophos to mice. An intraperitoneal dose of 73.2 mg/kg caused a significant increase in the number of cells with aberrations at both time intervals (Nehéz *et al.*, 1986).

Effects on Reproduction Although an increase in postimplantation losses in mice has been associated with oral administration of four doses of 73.2 mg/kg bromophos on days 6, 8, 10, and 12 of gestation (total dose 292.8 mg/kg), no significant increase in total implantation loss was associated with a total intraperitoneal dose of 219.6 mg/kg (73.2 mg/kg on days 6 and 8 of gestation, 36.6 mg/kg on days 10 and 12) (Nehéz *et al.*, 1986).

16.6.9.3 Toxicity to Humans

Use Experience Because of experimental indication of safety for laboratory animals and of value for malaria control, the safety of bromophos was tested in an African village. Eight sprayers and two supervisors applied the compound to the inside surfaces of the houses during a period of 4 hr on one day and 2.5 hr on the next day. Sprayers wore overalls, sou'westers, and rubber boots and all wore masks while weighing or spraying the compound. No clinical effects that could be related to spraying were observed in either sprayers or villagers. Plasma cholinesterase activity of the sprayers the day after spraying averaged 94.9% of preexposure levels. A statistically significant depression of plasma cholinesterase activity to 92% of normal was measured in the villagers 1 week after the spraying, and a statistically significant depression to 94.4% was found 4 weeks later (Vandekar and Svetličić, 1966).

Treatment of Poisoning   See Section 16.2.2.7.

16.6.10 DICAPTHON

16.6.10.1 Identity, Properties, and Uses

Chemical Name   Dicapthon is *O,O*-dimethyl *O*-(2-chloro-4-nitrophenyl) phosphorothioate.

Structure   See Table 16.16.

Synonyms   The common name dicapthon (ANSI, ESA, ISO) is in general use. Trade names have included Dicaptan®, Isomeric Clorthio®, and Isomer of Clorthioh®. Code designation have included AC-4,124, ENT-17,035, Exp. Insecticide-4,-124, and OMS-214. The CAS registry number is 2463-84-5.

Physical and Chemical Properties   Dicapthon has the empirical formula $C_8H_9ClNO_5PS$ and a molecular weight of 297.68. The pure material forms white crystals with a melting point of 53°C. Dicapthon is soluble in acetone, cyclohexane, ethyl acetate, toluene, xylene, ethylene glycol, propylene glycol, and some oils. It is pratically insoluble in water.

History, Formulations, and Uses   Dicapthon was introduced in 1954 as an aphicide and insecticide.

16.6.10.2 Toxicity to Laboratory Animals

Oral LD 50 values of 400 and 460 mg/kg were measured in male rats (Gaines, 1960; Shaffer and West, 1960). The oral value for females was 330 mg/kg and the dermal values were 790 and 1250 mg/kg for males and females, respectively (Gaines, 1960).

A relatively high proportion of the total metabolism in the rat involves alkyl-phosphate hydrolysis, as is true of other dialkyl compounds, in contrast to diethyl compounds (Plapp and Casida, 1958).

16.6.10.3 Toxicity to Humans

In an African village, dicapthon was tested for safety and for its ability to control malaria mosquitoes. The 50% water-wettable powder was applied as a 5% suspension of active ingre-

dient at a rate of 2 gm/m² to the inside of 219 homes and 262 other structures. The buildings had mud walls and thatch roofs. The workers wore waterproof hats, rubber gloves, shoes, and overalls that were washed daily. Workers who weighed out individual pump charges into bags wore respirators in addition to the other protective equipment. No complaints attributable to dicapthon were received from either the workers or the inhabitants of sprayed houses. Whole-blood cholinesterase activity was slightly depressed in the workers but not in the inhabitants (WHO, 1968).

Treatment of Poisoning   See Section 16.2.2.7.

16.6.11 MONOCROTOPHOS

16.6.11.1 Identity, Properties, and Uses

Chemical Name   Monocrotophos is the *E* isomer of *O,O*-dimethyl-*O*-(1-methyl-3-oxo-1-propenyl) phosphate. It also has been called the cis isomer (see Section 16.1.2).

Structure   See Table 16.16.

Synonyms   The common name monocrotophos (BSI, ISO) is in general use. Trade names have included Azodrin® and Nuvacron®. Code designations have included C-1,414, ENT-27,129, and SD-9,129. The CAS registry numbers are as follows: *E* isomer, 6923-22-4; *Z* isomer, 919-44-8; and mixed isomers, 2157-98-4.

Physical and Chemical Properties   The empirical formula of both isomers is $C_7H_{14}NO_5P$, and they have a molecular weight of 223.16. The pure material forms crystals with a melting point of 54–55°C. The vapor pressure is 7×10^{-5} mm Hg at 20°C. Monocrotophos is soluble in water, acetone, and alcohol but only slightly soluble in mineral oils. The technical material forms a reddish brown solid with a melting point of 25–30°C. Monocrotophos is unstable in low-molecular-weight alcohols and glycols. It is stable in ketones and higher-molecular-weight alcohols and glycols. It is stable when stored in glass and polyethylene containers. The half-life of monocrotophos in a 2 ppm solution at pH 7 and 38°C is 23 days; at pH 4.6 and 100°C, the half-life is 80 min.

History, Formulations, and Uses   Monocrotophos was introduced in 1965. It is a fast-acting systemic and contact insecticide of short persistence.

16.6.11.2 Toxicity to Laboratory Animals

Basic Findings   The signs of poisoning by monocrotophos are similar to those caused by other dimethoxy organic phosphorus insecticides. Its toxicity is moderately high. In male and female rats Gaines (1969) found oral LD 50 values of 18 and 20 mg/kg, respectively, and corresponding dermal values of 126 and 112 mg/kg. Intraperitoneal LD 50 values of

5 mg/kg were found in the male rat (Bull and Lindquist, 1966) and values of 3.8 and 8.0 in mice (Menzer and Casida, 1965; Menzer and Best, 1968).

In view of the fact that the oral LD 50 in rats is about 20 mg/kg, it is interesting that these animals survived a 2-year test at a dietary dosage level of 100 ppm, resulting in a dosage approaching 5 mg/kg/day. Understandably, their food consumption was reduced, their growth rate was depressed, and their plasma, red cell, and brain cholinesterase activity was markedly inhibited. Growth depression was recorded at dietary levels as low as 45 ppm, and cholinesterase inhibition was significant at various lower levels, including 1 ppm (about 0.05 mg/kg/day) (FAO/WHO, 1973).

Dogs survived dietary levels of monocrotophos starting at 135 ppm for 8 weeks and increasing by steps to 1080 ppm during week 13 of feeding. Decreased body weight and marked cholinesterase inhibition were present at the end of 10 weeks when the dogs were receiving 270 ppm (about 5.67 mg/kg/day). Even a dietary level of 100 ppm for 1 year caused tremors, increased salivation, and cholinesterase inhibition. A dietary level of 16 ppm (about 0.03 mg/kg/day) for 2 years caused only marginal inhibition of brain cholinesterase (FAO/WHO, 1973).

Absorption, Distribution, Metabolism, and Excretion The only metabolite of monocrotophos that is likely to have a significant anticholinesterase action is the unsubstituted amide. However, only traces of it are produced (Menzer and Casida, 1965; Bull and Lindquist, 1966).

Excretion of radioactive phosphorus by rats injected intraperitoneally with [^{32}P]monocrotophos was rapid. In 6 hr 45% was excreted, and in 24 hr 58.4 and 5.1% had been recovered from urine and feces, respectively. Dimethyl phosphate exceeded O-desmethyl monocrotophos in the excreta by a ratio of approximately 4 : 1 (Bull and Lindquist, 1966).

Treatment of Poisoning in Animals Injection of 2-PAM produced marked reactivation of inhibited whole-blood cholinesterase if done within 30 min after a short, intravenous infusion of monocrotophos but had only slight effect if done 2–3 hr after infusion (Gough and Shellenberger, 1971).

16.6.11.3 Toxicity to Humans

Experimental Exposure When radioactive monocrotophos was applied to human skin, the rate of excretion was maximal during the first 24–48-hr period, and it decreased only slightly during the third and fourth days. A total of 14.7% of the radioactivity was recovered in the urine within 120 hr and only a small correction factor was involved (Feldmann and Maibach, 1974).

Volunteers who worked for 5 hr in cotton fields treated with monocrotophos either 48 or 72 hr earlier experienced no symptoms and not more than 14% inhibition of blood cholinesterase activity (Ware *et al.*, 1975).

When monocrotophos was administered orally to six volunteers for 30 days at rates of 0.0036 and 0.0057 mg/kg/day,

plasma cholinesterase was lowered by 15 and 24%, respectively. There was no effect on red cell cholinesterase. Plasma cholinesterase reached a steady state within 10–15 days at the lower dosage but continued to decline slightly at the higher dosage. No subject demonstrated any sign or symptom that could be ascribed to the compound (Verberk, 1977).

Accidents and Use Experience A case that involved gross accidental dermal contamination with monocrotophos apparently was unmatched in the long delay between exposure and the onset of serious illness. Factors may have included slow dermal absorption combined with an unusually large dose and poor decontamination. Briefly, a 19-year-old man, while pumping a liquid emulsion concentrate from a 25-gallon-drum into a 2-gallon bucket, splashed about 570 ml on his bare chest and arms. He immediately attempted to wash off the material with water from a drum but did not remove his pants in the process, much less take a proper shower. (The report gives no indication of any later attempt at decontamination before or after hospitalization.) The man then put on a shirt and went about his work on the night shift. He detected no effect that night but felt vaguely unwell next morning, and he vomited during the afternoon. While driving into town 28 hr after exposure, he became aware of difficulty in controlling his truck because of muscular weakness and blurred vision. He also had some chest pain. Somewhat later he started having "blackouts" with intervening brief, relatively lucid intervals. It was only on the second morning, 38 hr after exposure, that the man was hospitalized. At that time he could not stand unaided, and he was troubled by dry retching. He was pale, perspiring profusely, confused, and unable to give any detailed history. His pupils were constricted. Treatment with atropine and pralidoxime led to marked recovery in 48 hr, and the patient was essentially symptom-free on the third day. However, as a precaution, pralidoxime was continued through the eighth day. The patient continued to complain of headaches and some numbness of the hands and arms, even after discharge on the tenth hospital day. Headache had not been an important part of his early symptoms. Red cell cholinesterase activity actually fell slightly during the first 2.5 days in the hospital and then increased very slowly, requiring 8 weeks to reach the normal range (Simson *et al.*, 1969).

Accidental ingestion of monocrotophos produced unconsciousness lasting 4 days; the case was complicated by bronchopneumonia and thrombophlebitis, but recovery was complete on day 33 (Przedziak and Wisniewska, 1975).

Peiris *et al.* (1988) report a case of a 32-year-old male admitted to a hospital approximately 45 min after receiving a 2-inch laceration above his left eyebrow caused by the shattering of a 100-ml bottle of 60% monocrotophos thrown at him. The spilled liquid was wiped off with his shirt, although the skin was not washed. Three to 4 hours after the wound was closed and oral penicillin was administered, the patient ate without washing his hands. Several hours later, an intravenous administration of furosemide was started after the patient experienced abdominal pain, nausea, vomiting, muscle fasciculations, excessive sweating, and small pupils. A diagnosis of organic phosphorus poisoning was made and atropine and pralidoxime therapy commenced 22 hr after exposure, although his blood pressure was normal and pulse rate was 92/min. The initial intravenous administration of furosemide was discontinued following a total dose of 120 mg.

During the second day, the patient developed diarrhea. Bradycardia, cyanosis, and respiratory distress started on the fourth day, warranting the use of endotracheal intubation and assisted ventilation. Grade 4 weakness of the limbs was noted.

Although acute cholinergic signs and symptoms subsided by day 6, respiratory difficulty and generalized muscle weakness persisted. Examination of the patient on day 10 found a continuation of grade 4 weakness of the limbs, symmetrically decreased deep tendon reflexes, and a spontaneous vital capacity of 200 cm^3. The serum sodium level was 130 mmol/liter, and serum potassium was 3.0 mmol/liter. Capillary blood gas analysis found a bicarbonate value of 28.2 mmol/liter, pH of 7.41, Po_2 of 120 mm Hg, and Pco_2 of 45.9 mm Hg. Prominent U waves were also found in all leads of the electrocardiogram, which became less prominent several hours following intravenous administration of Hartmann's solution and large amounts of king coconut water (containing high concentrations of potassium) via nasogastric tube.

Intermittent positive-pressure ventilation was discontinued on day 15, and the patient was able to move about with near-normal muscle power by day 16. However, blood cholinesterase activity remained between 37.5 and 50% of normal on day 21.

The case mentioned above characterizes the recently defined *intermediate syndrome,* a clinically and pharmacologically distinct entity of acute organic phosphorus pesticide poisoning separable from acute toxicity and delayed polyneuropathy. Intermediate syndrome has been associated with monocrotophos and other organic phosphorus pesticides in studies of a variety of acute poisoning cases; it is characterized by a number of symptoms which appear 1–4 days following poisoning and include diarrhea, proximal limb muscle weakness, motor cranial nerve palsies, and sudden respiratory distress, which could lead to death if not treated immediately with atropine (Gadoth and Fisher, 1978; Karalliedde and Senanayake, 1988; Senanayake and Karalliedde, 1987; Wadia *et al.,* 1974). Additional discussion of the intermediate syndrome is found in Section 16.4.1.3.

Dosage Response Death of a woman followed her ingestion of exactly 1200 mg of monocrotophos and smaller amounts of two other much less toxic compounds.

The threshold limit value of 0.25 mg/m^3 indicates that occupational intake of about 0.007 mg/kg/day is considered safe.

Laboratory Findings Following ingestion of 1200 mg of monocrotophos, the concentrations of it found in tissues were: 12 ppm in blood, 13 ppm in lungs, 13 ppm in brain, 11 ppm in kidney, and 1.8 ppm in liver (Gelbke and Schlicht, 1978).

Treatment of Poisoning See Section 16.2.2.7.

16.6.12 DICROTOPHOS

16.6.12.1 Identity, Properties, and Uses

Chemical Name Dicrotophos is the *E* isomer of *O,O-*dimethyl - *O* - (3-dimethylamino-1-methyl-3-oxo-1-propenyl) phosphate. It also has been called the *cis* isomer (see Section 16.1.2).

Structure See Table 16.16.

Synonyms The common name dicrotophos (BSI, ISO) is in general use. Trade names include Bidrin®, Carbicron®, and Ektafos®. Code designations include ENT-24,482 and SD-3,562. The CAS registry number for the mixed isomers is 3725-78-2, for the *E* isomer is 141-66-2, and for the *Z* isomer is 18250-63-0.

Physical and Chemical Properties Dicrotophos has the empirical formula $C_8H_{16}NO_5P$ and a molecular weight of 237.21. The pure material forms a brown liquid. The technical material consists of 85% *E* isomer. It has a boiling point of 400°C and a vapor pressure of 1×10^{-4} mm Hg at 20°C. Dicrotophos is miscible with water, acetone, diacetone, alcohol, 2-propanol ethanol, and other organic solvents. Dicrotophos is stable when stored in glass or polythene containers up to 40°C but is decomposed after 31 days at 75°C or 7 days at 90°C. The half-life of an aqueous solution at 38°C and pH 9.1 is 50 days, and at pH 1.1 it is 100 days.

History, Formulations, and Uses Dicrotophos was introduced in 1956 as a systemic pesticide with a wide range of applications. The *E* isomer is more insecticidally active than the *Z* isomer. Dicrotophos is available as 24 and 85% concentrates and as 50 and 40% emulsifiable concentrates.

16.6.12.2 Toxicity to Laboratory Animals

Basic Findings Dicrotophos is a compound of rather high oral and dermal toxicity. In the rat, oral LD 50 values of 21 and 16 mg/kg were found in males and females, respectively; corresponding dermal values were 43 and 42 mg/kg (Gaines, 1969). In the mouse, the intraperitoneal LD 50 was 11.2 mg/kg (Menzer and Best, 1968).

Absorption, Distribution, Metabolism, and Excretion Dicrotophos is metabolized in part to monocrotophos. In fact, the concentration of monocrotophos in tissues may be higher than that of the parent compound in a few hours after administration, as reflected by analysis of rat urine and goat milk. Residues of both compounds are dissipated almost entirely within 24 hr, as indicated by a rapid decrease in unhydrolyzed metabolites in urine or milk. Hydrolysis of the vinyl-phosphate bond of dicrotophos or its oxidative metabolites to produce dimethyl phosphate is the predominant detoxicating reaction. The proportion of dimethyl phosphate in the urine of rats increases rapidly after dosing, reaching 50% of all metabolites present in less than 4-hr and over 80% in 20 hr. During this interval, there is a corresponding rapid decrease in the excretion of the parent compound and its oxidation products. Desmethyl dicrotophos and inorganic phosphate also are found in minor concentrations in the urine of treated rats (Bull and Lindquist, 1964). The major paths of biotransformation are now well known (Bull and Lindquist, 1964; Menzer and Casida, 1965).

Dicrotophos is excreted rapidly in rats. After 6 hr, 65% of the injected dose was excreted, and after 24 hr, 83% was out in the urine alone (Bull and Lindquist, 1964). Similar results have been obtained in other studies of rats and other species. In fact, elimination of the compound and of its metabolites capable of inhibiting cholinesterase may be more complete than studies with ^{32}P and ^{14}C tend to show, for some inorganic ^{32}P-labeled phosphate becomes incorporated into bone, and some of the carbon is exhaled as $^{14}CO_2$ (Menzer and Casida, 1965).

Effects on Reproduction   Intraperitoneal injection of dicrotophos into pregnant mice at dosages of 1, 2, 4, and 7.5 mg/kg on day 11, day 13, or days 10–12 of gestation caused no morphological anomaly. A dosage of 5 mg/kg/day on days 8–16 of gestation caused no change in the developmental patterns of brain acetylcholinesterase or choline acetyltransferase, even though this dosage on day 11 reduced embryonic or fetal acetylcholinesterase to 1.8% of control levels. The fetal brain enzyme level returned to normal by day 19 following dosing of the mother on days 8–16 of gestation (Bus and Gibson, 1974).

Whereas avian teratogenesis is a poor predictor of the same effect in mammals, it is interesting that nicotinic acid, nicotinamide, and some of their precursors largely alleviate the teratogenic effect of dicrotophos in dosages of 0.1 mg/egg or even higher (Roger, 1964; Roger *et al.*, 1969). In spite of extensive study, the antidotal mechanism remains unknown. Dicrotophos is not neurotoxic (Gaines, 1969).

16.6.12.3 Toxicity to Humans

Accidental and Intentional Poisoning   It may or may not be a coincidence that the only two reported cases of poisoning by dicrotophos involved relapse 7 or more days after onset. In the first case, a 41-year-old tractor driver, who had applied dicrotophos to crops and who for the last 2 or 3 weeks had sprayed inside his house every day with the same compound to control mosquitoes, had abdominal cramps, nausea, vomiting, and diarrhea on one day and entered hospital the next day with complaints of increased sweating, salivation, dyspnea, coarse tremor of both legs, and generalized weakness. Physical examination confirmed poisoning but showed that the man was alert and in no immediate danger, although his plasma and red cell cholinesterase activities were both 0.00 mol/min/ml. The patient responded to atropine and pralidoxime. Atropine dosage was reduced gradually as he began to improve. However, on the sixth hospital day, he relapsed, and respiratory paralysis

occurred. He required artificial respiratory support for 5 days. He was discharged on day 22. He returned to work and was fit when seen 1 year after the episode (Perron and Johnson, 1969).

In the second case, a man without detectable respiration or pulse was brought by public ambulance to the emergency room of a hospital. He had been given artificial respiration in the ambulance after having been picked up in an unconscious condition in front of a house. His name and the circumstances leading to his illness were learned only gradually—some only after he recovered.

Briefly, this 52-year-old man had been drinking heavily and ran out of whiskey. At that point he thought of a gallon jug he had put away several months earlier but failed to recall effectively that the jug contained turpentine to which he had added an insecticide so that he would have something to kill "bugs." He had acquired the insecticide from an almost empty drum that he had cleaned at a drum salvaging company where he worked. Although the drum undoubtedly was fully labeled, it required gas chromatography and mass spectrometry to identify the active ingredient in the jug, which the ambulance drivers had picked up and brought along with the patient. Although the patient required assisted respiration for over a week, he showed definite improvement after treatment with atropine sulfate and pralidoxime chloride. In fact, medication was being reduced gradually when the patient began on day 10 to show renewed evidence of anticholinesterase poisoning. Dosage of atropine was increased moderately and dosage with pralidoxime was returned to its highest previous level. The patient responded, and the dosage of both drugs was reduced gradually again. The last medication was on hospital day 23. The total dose of atropine sulfate was 3911.5 mg, and that of pralidoxime chloride was 92,000 mg. He also had received an antibiotic for pneumonia that followed aspiration; transfusion, folate, and iron for anemia; and other medication, as well as continuous nursing care. The patient was discharged on hospital day 33 as good as new. Arrangements had been made for his continued employment by the salvage company from which he had been fired for drunkenness (Warriner *et al.*, 1977).

Treatment of Poisoning   See Section 16.2.2.7.

16.6.13 DIMETHOATE

16.6.13.1 Identity, Properties, and Uses

Chemical Name   Dimethoate is *O,O*-dimethyl *S*-2-(methylamino)-2-oxoethyl phosphorodithioate.

Structure   See Table 16.16.

Synonyms   The common name dimethoate (BSI, ESA, ISO) is in general use except in the USSR, where the name fosfamid is used. Another common name is phosphamide. Trade names include Cygon®, De-Fend®, Dimetate®, Ferkethion®, Fostion MM®, Perfekthion®, Rogor®, and Roxion®. Code designations include AC-12,880, E.I.-12,880, ENT-24,650,

L-395, OMS-94, and OMS-111. The CAS registry number is 60-51-5.

Physical and Chemical Properties   Dimethoate has the empirical formula $C_5H_{12}NO_3PS_2$ and a molecular weight of 229.28. The pure material forms colorless crystals with a camphor-like odor. The melting point is 51–52°C. The density is 1.281 at 50°C. Dimethoate has a vapor pressure of 8.5×10^{-6} mm Hg at 25°C. The solubility of dimethoate in water at 21°C is 2.5 gm/100 ml. The compound is soluble in most organic solvents, except saturated hydrocarbons such as hexane. Dimethoate is stable in aqueous solution, but it readily is hydrolyzed by aqueous alkali and is unstable in alkali media. Heating converts dimethoate to the —SCH₃ isomer.

History, Formulations, and Uses   Dimethoate was introduced as an experimental pesticide in 1956 by both the American Cyanamid Company and Montecatini S.p.A. The early technical product was formulated with a monohydroxylic solvent, methyl Cellosolve. In field use it was found that dimethoate was sometimes more toxic than laboratory testing would have indicated. In 1961, Casida and Sanderson reported results of LD 50 testing of dimethoate after storage under various conditions. From an original LD 50 or 150–250 mg/kg, the technical product increased in toxicity to an LD 50 of 30–40 mg/kg after 7 months of storage under English conditions. After 9 months of storage under tropical conditions the LD 50 was lowered to 15 mg/kg, and after storage at 100°C under laboratory conditions the LD 50 was lowered even further to 8 mg/kg. All of these changes took place without changing the insecticidal properties of the compound. The stored compounds had undergone actual chemical change during storage and contained compounds much more toxic in combination than any one of the compounds by itself. Of several monohydroxylic solvents tested, only methyl and ethyl Cellosolve resulted in formulations highly toxic to mammals on short-term storage at 70°C. Formulations containing the Cellosolve solvents were discontinued, and a newer formulation with more stability was distributed.

Dimethoate is a contact and systemic insecticide and acaricide. It is available in emulsifiable concentrates of 20, 40, and 50% technical dimethoate, 30% technical product for ultralow-volume applicators, 20% wettable powders, and 5% granules.

16.6.13.2 Toxicity to Laboratory Animals

Basic Findings   Dimethoate is sufficiently nontoxic to mammals that it has been administered to livestock with considerable success for the control of bots (Marquardt and Lovelace, 1961; Meleney and Peterson, 1964).

Early batches of dimethoate tended to become more toxic than later batches that were either more stable or more free of toxic contaminants, or both. The difference is illustrated by the fact that one 1959 sample was over seven times more toxic, both orally and dermally, than a 1962 sample examined in the

same laboratory under identical conditions (see Table 16.29). At least in some instances, the increase in the toxicity of dimethoate to mammals was the result of its storage in certain hydrolytic solvents, particularly 2-alkoxyethanols. This aspect of the problem was thoroughly studied by Casida and Sanderson (1961, 1963). The changes just mentioned involved laboratory or commercial grade compounds and were in addition to a change that occurred in highly purified dimethoate when stored under ordinary conditions. The oral LD 50 of highly purified dimethoate in rats was 600–700 mg/kg, and this very low toxicity was retained if the compound was stored in ampules that had been flushed with nitrogen, evacuated, sealed, and stored at 3°C (Sanderson and Edson, 1964). Change in the

Table 16.29
Single-Dose LD 50 for Dimethoate

Species	Route	LD 50 (mg/kg)	Reference
Rat, M	oral	215	Shaffer and West (1960)
Rat, M	oral	247	Edson and Noakes (1960)
Rat, M	oral	185	West *et al.* (1961)
Rat, F	oral	245	West *et al.* (1961)
Rat	oral	230	Pan'shina (1963a)
Rat, M	oral	500–600[a]	Sanderson and Edson (1964)
Rat, M	oral	280–350[b]	Sanderson and Edson (1964)
Rat, M	oral	180–325[c]	Sanderson and Edson (1964)
Rat, F	oral	570–680[a]	Sanderson and Edson (1964)
Rat, F	oral	300–356[b]	Sanderson and Edson (1964)
Rat, F	oral	240–336[c]	Sanderson and Edson (1964)
Rat, M	oral	28[d]	Gaines (1969)
Rat, F	oral	30[d]	Gaines (1969)
Rat, M	oral	215[e]	Gaines (1969)
Rat, F	oral	245[e]	Gaines (1969)
Rat, M	oral	360[a]	Schubert (1970)
Rat, F	oral	355	Schubert (1970)
Rat, M	dermal	443	Edson and Noakes (1960)
Rat	dermal	100	Pan'shina (1963a)
Rat, M	dermal	61[d]	Gaines (1969)
Rat, F	dermal	55[d]	Gaines (1969)
Rat, M	dermal	610[e]	Gaines (1969)
Rat, M	intraperitoneal	175–325[c]	Sanderson and Edson (1964)
Rat, F	intraperitoneal	350[c]	Sanderson and Edson (1964)
Rat, M	intravenous	450[c]	Sanderson and Edson (1964)
Mouse	oral	135	Pan'shina (1963a)
Mouse, F	oral	60[a]	Sanderson and Edson (1964)
Mouse, F	oral	60[c]	Sanderson and Edson (1964)
Mouse, M	oral	165	O'Brien (1967)
Mouse	intraperitoneal	198	Menzer and Best (1968)
Guinea pig	oral	550[a]	Sanderson and Edson (1964)
Guinea pig	oral	600[b]	Sanderson and Edson (1964)
Guinea pig	oral	350–400[c]	Sanderson and Edson (1964)
Rabbit	oral	500[a]	Sanderson and Edson (1964)
Rabbit	oral	450[b]	Sanderson and Edson (1964)
Rabbit	oral	approx. 300[c]	Sanderson and Edson (1964)
Rabbit	dermal	1500	Pan'shina (1963a)
Cat	oral	100	Pan'shina (1963a)

[a] Pure compound.
[b] Laboratory grade.
[c] Technical product.
[d] 1959 product.
[e] 1962 product.

toxicity of dimethoate formulations during storage sometimes was of practical importance. In extensive trials of dimethoate for control of larvae of *Oestrus ovis*, some 4675 sheep were given intramuscular doses at different times between September 1958 and November 1961. In one test, involving over 800 sheep, there was no intoxication; the dosage ranged from 15 to 21 mg/kg. However, in some other tests the rate of intoxication was as high as 50 or even 66% and there were a few deaths, even though the dosage was no higher than 25 mg/kg and in most instances was less. It was eventually realized that the formulation manufactured for injections was safe when it was not over 2 months old but toxic when it had been stored for 2 years (Meleny and Peterson, 1964).

The compound is not irritating to the skin or eyes. Erythrocyte cholinesterase is more susceptible than plasma cholinesterase to inhibition by dimethoate (West *et al.*, 1961; Sanderson and Edson, 1964).

A dietary level of 800 ppm (about 20 mg/kg/day) leads to toxic effects in rats in a few days (Sanderson and Edson, 1964). Minor toxic effects are produced by a dietary level of 125 ppm.

Reports of the no-effect dietary level in rats have varied from 32 ppm (West *et al.*, 1961) to 5–10 ppm (Sanderson and Edson, 1964) to 1 ppm (about 0.05 mg/kg/day) (Edson and Noakes, 1960). The difference probably depended on the same factors that have produced marked differences in acute toxicity.

In dogs, the no-effect dietary level for erythrocyte and plasma cholinesterase is 10 and 50 ppm (0.2 and 1.0 mg/kg/day), respectively (West *et al.*, 1961).

When rats were given 24 intraperitoneal injections in 34 days, the highest rate producing no toxic effects was 3 mg/kg/day, and the rate producing no significant inhibition of plasma, erythrocyte, or brain cholinesterase was 0.7 mg/kg/day. In similar but subcutaneous testing, guinea pigs showed no toxic effects at 16 mg/kg/day and no cholinesterase inhibition at 4 mg/kg/day.

No morphological change or cholinesterase inhibition was found in calves fed dietary levels of 6.3 and 3.5 ppm, respectively (Yašnova *et al.*, 1971).

Absorption, Distribution, Metabolism, and Excretion
Following application of ^{32}P-labeled dimethoate to the backs of cattle at the rate of 30 mg/kg, the concentration of active ingredient reached a maximum level of 0.02 ppm in blood and milk in about 3 hr and then dropped to 0.01 ppm by 9 hr (Dedek and Schwarz, 1970a).

Dimethoate was degraded rapidly by rat liver but very little by other rat tissues. The ability of the livers of different species decreased in the order rabbit > dog = sheep > rat > cow > hen > mouse = guinea pig > pig At least for the rat, sheep, mouse, cow, and hen, there was a reasonably good straight-line relationship between the LD 50 values and the products of the rate of metabolism multiplied by the proportion of the body constituted by the liver (Uchida *et al.*, 1964).

Dimethoate is rapidly metabolized. In one very thorough study in rats, about 60% of the administered dose was excreted in 24 hr in the urine and expired air. It was concluded that

dimethoxon is 75–100 times more potent than dimethoate as an inhibitor of rat brain acetylcholinesterase and that toxicity of the insecticide is due mainly to its conversion to dimethoxon (Hassan *et al.*, 1969). Another study (Lucier and Menzer, 1970) concluded that, compared to P=S derivatives, P=O derivatives of dimethoate and certain of its analogs were at least 1000 times more potent inhibitors of fly head and human plasma cholinesterases. Both papers contain extensive details on the biotransformation of dimethoate.

Cleavage of dimethoate by rats and cows occurs initially at the methyl-phosphate, phosphate-sulfur, sulfur-carbon, and particularly carbonyl-nitrogen bonds. In 24 hr, 81% of an oral dose of dimethoate was excreted by male rats, compared with 19% of a dose of the separately administered P=O derivative. Dimethoate is more readily attacked at the C—N bond than is true of the P=O derivative, and this is a major route of degradation. Within 48 hr after dosing, almost 90% of [^{32}P]dimethoate was recovered in the urine of male rats, and most of the rest was recovered in the feces. Only a little over a total of 50% was excreted by female rats in 48 hr, but later excretion was approximately as slow in females as in males. At 168 hr after treatment, the total ^{32}P remaining in the tissue was two to five times greater in female than in male rats. After 24 hr, the highest concentration of dimethoate equivalent was in the liver, but at 72 and 168 hr the highest concentrations were in the skin and bones, reflecting the conversion of ^{32}P to inorganic phosphate (Dauterman *et al.*, 1959).

Another evidence of the rapid excretion of dimethoate was given by Sanderson and Edson (1964). Following oral administration of [^{32}P]dimethoate, rats excreted 50% of the activity in the urine and 25% in the feces in 24 hr. Nine days after dosing, only 0.9–1.1% of the ^{32}P remained in the animals.

Biochemical Effects   It has been observed by several authors (O'Brien, 1967; Menzer and Best, 1968) that pretreatment of mice with phenobarbital increases their susceptibility to dimethoate, whereas it has little effect or even decreases their susceptibility to various other organic phosphorus compounds. The reason for the difference remains obscure. At least in houseflies, the des-*N*-methyl analog of dimethoxon is the most toxic of all known metabolites of dimethoate (Lucier and Menzer, 1970). However, whether it is an increase in the rate of formation of this metabolite, of dimethoxon, or of some unidentified metabolite is unknown.

Dimethoate is an indirect inhibitor of cholinesterase but, as in many other instances, the commercial product contains direct inhibitors (see Section 16.2.1.4).

When weanling rats were maintained on diets containing 3.5 and 26% protein as casein and were later poisoned with dimethoate, there was no difference in their susceptibility (LD 50, 147 and 152 mg/kg, respectively). However, other groups maintained on a normal proportion (24%) of protein derived from various plant and animal sources were distinctly less susceptible to the compound (LD 50, 358 mg/kg). Dimethoate was the only insecticide studied by Boyd that was not at least somewhat more toxic when administered in association with a diet severely deficient in protein. It was Boyd's view that, for a range of compounds, the difference between casein and mixed protein changed the toxicity by a factor of no more than 0.5–2.0 (Boyd and Muis, 1970).

No potentiation of toxicity was found when dimethoate was administered orally to rats with any one of several other organic phosphorus insecticides, including EPN (West *et al.*, 1961; Sanderson and Edson, 1964). However, potentiation between the effects of dimethoate and EPN was found in mice and guinea pigs injected intraperitoneally, and this was attributed to a blockade of metabolism of dimethoate (Seume and O'Brien, 1960a; Uchida *et al.*, 1966).

It may be that dimethoate induces its own metabolism. Unlike the situation with other compounds studied, the concentration of recoverable metabolites, especially dimethyl dithiophosphate, decreased from day 1 to day 3 in rats that received the compound by gavage on these days (Bradway *et al.*, 1977).

Effects on Organs and Tissues   Gibel *et al.* (1973) reported an increase in malignant tumors but no increase in benign tumors in rats receiving dimethoate at rates of 5, 15, and 30 mg/kg orally and 15 mg/kg intramuscularly for 511–627 days. The increase did not correspond to dosage. Changes in the liver and blood were also reported. In what seems to have been the same experiment, Stieglitz *et al.* (1974) described severe hyperplasia of the hematopoietic parenchyma of the bone marrow and myeloid metaplasia, especially in the liver and spleen. All types of blood cells were involved, but the greatest effect in most animals was on granulocytopoiesis. The material studied was a commercial product, presumably of eastern European origin.

Dimethoate had no influence on the growth of implanted tumors (Hoffman *et al.*, 1973).

Dominant lethal tests were more positive in male mice that received a single sublethal dose of dimethoate than in those that received one-twelfth of that dose daily for 30 days. It was concluded that the compound is a potential mutagen (Gerstengarbe, 1975).

Effects on Reproduction   The addition of dimethoate to the drinking water of mice at a concentration of 60 ppm (9.5–10.5 mg/kg/day) interfered with reproduction, survival of pups, and growth rate of those that did survive. It had no teratogenic effect. This dosage caused a 66% reduction of plasma cholinesterase activity of the adults and a reduction in their rate of weight gain during the first 2 weeks of exposure, but it did not increase mortality among them. In a three-generation study, the slightly lower concentration of 50 ppm did not decrease reproductive performance or increase mortality of the pups (Budreau and Singh, 1973b).

A dosage of 12 mg/kg/day during the critical period of pregnancy increased the incidence of polydactyly in cats and wavy ribs, extra ribs, fused sternebrae, hydroureter, dilated bladder, and runted fetuses in rats; dosages of 3 and 6 mg/kg/day were without teratogenic effect in either species (Khera, 1979; Khera *et al.*, 1979b).

16.6.13.3 Toxicity to Humans

Experimental Oral Exposure   For 21 days one adult ingested dimethoate at the rate of 18 mg/day (about 0.26 mg/kg/day) and another ingested 9 mg/day; neither showed any cholinesterase inhibition. For 4 weeks 20 adults ingested 2.5 mg/day (about 0.04 mg/kg/day), again with no toxic effect and no inhibition of cholinesterase (Sanderson and Edson, 1964). In later studies, actual does of 7, 21, 42, 63, and 84 mg were administered 5 days per week so that the average intakes were 5, 15, 30, 45, and 60 mg/day, respectively, for the men and women in different groups. Twelve persons who received 5 mg/day for 28 days and 9 persons who received 10 mg/day for 39 days showed no significant change in plasma or erythrocyte cholinesterase activity. Eight persons who received 30 mg/day began to show a decrease in cholinesterase activity by day 20, and the depression lasted until the end of the test on day 57. Depression of cholinesterase occurred earlier and to a somewhat greater degree in groups of six persons, each of whom received 45 and 60 mg/day, respectively. None of the volunteers experienced any clinical effect from the dimethoate (Edson *et al.*, 1967).

When [^{32}P]dimethoate was given to volunteers orally, it was absorbed and excreted rapidly, 76–100% of the radioactivity appearing in the urine in 24 hr (Sanderson and Edson, 1964).

Accidental and Intentional Poisoning   A suicide accomplished by drinking a large amount of dimethoate illustrated the possibility of relapse. The 51-year-old man who drank the compound was taken promptly to a hospital, where his stomach was washed out at 2:00 p.m. Vomiting, apparently his greatest difficulty during the afternoon, stopped at 7:00 p.m. Next morning his general condition appeared quite good. He retained food but had several loose bowel movements. He suddenly collapsed at 12:15 p.m. while having lunch. When a physician arrived, the patient was unconscious, his pupils were pinpoint, and coarse rhonchi and rales were present in his chest. Emergency treatment was started, but he died at 12:30 p.m. (Molphy and Rathus, 1964).

LeBlanc *et al.* (1986) reported a case in which a 68-year-old male ingested approximately three ounces of Cygon 2-E® (23.4% dimethoate). Upon reaching the local emergency room approximately 20 min after the incident, the patient was coherent and lucid with a regular pulse of 120 and a temperature of 35.9°C. There was no evidence of heart failure, lungs were clear, pupils were symmetrical, round, and responsive to light stimulus, and neurologic examination found no abnormalities. Following dermal decontamination, the patient was given 30 ml syrup of ipecac, 60 gm activated charcoal, 4 ml/kg magnesium citrate, and several 1-mg atropine boluses. However, the patient became unconscious over the next 30 min as his blood pressure dropped to 46/0 and pulse remained at 116/min. One gram of pralidoxime was administered, and an endotracheal intubation was done. The patient regained normal sensorium and was extubated as his condition stabilized over the next 24 hr. However, the patient relapsed during the next 8 hr, necessitating reintubation and parenteral atropinization. Atropine and pralidoxime treatment was continued over the following 24 hr. The patient was then started on an atropine infusion for the next 24 hr, requiring at least 50 mg/hr to maintain systolic pressure above 100 and a pulse rate between 130 and 140/min. A third respiratory and cardiac event on day 16 of the atropine drip warranted another increase in atropine administration. Complete weaning from the atropine drip could not be accomplished until day 35 of the therapy, at which time gastrointestinal, cardiac, renal, and pulmonary functions were normal and there were no further relapses. Electroencephalographic analysis 1 week following discontinuation of atropine therapy showed an abnormality characteristic of diffuse encephalopathy of metabolic or toxic origin. The patient was discharged 42 days following admission with some spastic rigidity, a sensorineural hearing deficit, and a slight, nonspecific personality change. This case is remarkable in that the patient received a total of 30,730 mg atropine in daily doses that ranged as high as 3600 mg.

Intermediate syndrome, exemplified by symptoms clinically and pharmacologically distinct from acute toxicity and delayed polyneuropathy, has been associated with dimethoate and other organic phosphorus pesticide poisonings. It is characterized by diarrhea, proximal limb muscle weakness, motor cranial nerve palsies, and respiratory distress of sudden onset 1–4 days after poisoning (Gadoth and Fisher, 1978; Karalliedde and Senanayake, 1988; Senanayake and Karalliedde, 1987; Wadia *et al.*, 1974). Additional information on this syndrome may be found in Section 16.4.1.3.

Use Experience   Dimethoate itself has not been an important cause of irritation. However, severe irritation of the eyes occurred in workers who manufactured the compound. During neutralization of the acid intermediate $[(CH_3\text{—}O)_2P(S)SH]$ some of the molecules combined to form bis(dimethoxythiophosphoryl) disulfide. Tests in animals showed that both the acid and the disulfide were irritating (Wenzel and Dedek, 1971).

Atypical Cases of Various Origins   After he had worked for 2 weeks picking hops previously treated with dimethoate, a 16-year-old boy developed weakness, nausea, headache, and severe depression. The depression was characterized by psychomotor retardation, inability to concentrate, suicidal thoughts, guilt, loss of interest, and anxiety. Laboratory study revealed (in addition to moderate inhibition of cholinesterase activity consistent with the patient's history of exposure): indirect bilirubin, 3.08 mg %; SGOT, 85 units; SGPT, 60 units; and cadmium, 2+. Recovery was said to coincide with the normalization of cholinesterase activity in 2.5 months (Masiak and Olajossy, 1973). Apparently, no treatment for poisoning by an organic phosphorus compound was needed or administered, no effort was made to account for the reportedly increased cadmium level, and no diagnostic study was directed toward the common causes of hepatitis in young people.

Two boys, 14 and 17 years old, played with dead pigeons one day and awoke next morning with nausea, vomiting, abdominal cramps, diarrhea, and considerable dehydration. Examination revealed mucocutaneous purpura and nystagmus. Miosis was absent, and muscular fasciculations were not observed. Treatment was nonspecific, but recovery was prompt. A diagnosis of dimethoate poisoning was made on the strength of a report of finding this compound in the gastrointestinal tract of one of the pigeons (Rampelberg, 1975). There were no clinical or laboratory findings diagnostic of poisoning in these cases. The possibility that food poisoning may have caused these gastrointestinal upsets seems to have been ignored.

A 24-year-old male experienced abdominal pain, nausea, vomiting, increased salivation, generalized muscle weakness, excessive lacrimation, and muscle fasciculations 4 hr after cleaning spray equipment used to apply a mixture of dimethoate and triphenyltin hydroxide without wearing gloves or a mask. Physical examination upon arrival at a local emergency room 12–16 hr following exposure revealed a blood pressure of 137/70, a pulse of 112, and diffuse abdominal tenderness in the epigastric area. A diagnosis of anticholinesterase toxicity and acute pancreatitis secondary to organic phosphorus compound exposure was made after serum amylase and lipase levels were found to be elevated. Following a period of clinical improvement several days after conservative management of the condition, the nausea, vomiting, and abdominal pain worsened, warranting the use of parenteral hyperalimentation. Although blood cholinesterase activities returned to normal levels 8 weeks following exposure, attempts at dietary intake continued to result in hyperamylasemia and exacerbation of abdominal pain. The patient was able to tolerate an elemental dietary formula at 10 weeks and was totally asymptomatic 3 months following exposure, at which time he was placed on a low-fat diet. Although a normal diet was started at 4 months, anorexia, mild hyperamylasemia, abdominal pain, and nausea recurred in the fifth month following exposure. However, these symptoms resolved 1 week following conservative treatment including a return to the low-fat diet. The patient was asymptomatic with normal serum amylase values at 7 months, and no further complications occurred (Marsh *et al.*, 1988). There was apparently no consideration of excessive consumption of alcohol, a common cause of acute pancreatitis.

Dosage Response   A 35-year-old man died after drinking approximately 200 ml of a solution of unstated concentration (Gaultier *et al.*, 1975). After a very stormy course and as a result of intensive care, a 62-year-old woman recovered completely after drinking an entire 250-ml bottle of a 20% formulation (about 714 mg/kg) (Chiantera *et al.*, 1968), but how much may have been lost by vomiting was unknown.

Based on a demonstrated relationship between LD 50 values for several species and the rate at which dimethoate is hydrolyzed by the livers of the same species, Uchida and O'Brien (1967) estimated from the measurements of the hydrolysis produced by frozen samples of human liver that the oral LD 50 for humans is 15–30 mg/kg. Unfortunately, there is no body of data that permits an evaluation of this kind of estimate in humans. Obviously, considerably higher dosage levels can be counteracted by appropriate treatment.

Studies in volunteers showed that a dosage of 0.4 mg/kg/day or above will cause a slow decrease in blood cholinesterase activity, but that 0.2 mg/kg/day is a no-effect level (Edson *et al.*, 1967).

Treatment of Poisoning   See Section 16.2.2.7.

16.6.14 ENDOTHION

16.6.14.1 Identity, Properties, and Uses

Chemical Name   Endothion is O,O-dimethyl-S-[(5-methoxy-4-oxo-4H-pyran-2-yl)methyl]phosphorothioate.

Structure   See Table 16.16.

Synonyms   The common name endothion (BSI, ISO) generally is used except in Portugal. A trade name is Endocide®. Code designations have included AC-18737, ENT-24653, FMC-5767, NIAgara-5767, and 7175-R.P. The CAS registry number is 2778-04-3.

Physical and Chemical Properties   Endothion has the empirical formula $C_9H_{13}O_6PS$ and a molecular weight of 280.24. The pure material forms a white crystalline solid with a melting point of 96°C. Endothion is soluble in water, acetone, benzene, and chloroform but insoluble in ether, cyclohexane, or carbon tetrachloride.

History, Formulations, and Uses   Endothion was introduced by Rhone-Poulene, S. A., in 1958. It also was introduced by the American Cyanamid Company and FMC Corporation. It is a systemic aphicide and acaricide effective for the control of sap-feeding insects and mites of orchard, field, and market garden crops. Endothion is available as a 25% soluble powder and a 50% water soluble powder. It is not sold in the United States or Canada.

16.6.14.2 Toxicity to Laboratory Animals

Endothion is a compound of moderate toxicity. The oral LD 50 values are 30 and 36 mg/kg in male and female rats, respectively, and 17 mg/kg in mice. The compound is reported not to increase in toxicity on storage (Schuppon, 1961).

16.6.14.3 Toxicity to Humans

Apparently the only poisoning by endothion involved a 27-year-old chemist and his 25-year-old assistant and was the result of an explosion in their laboratory. A hot, vaporized solution of endothion in acetone reached the face and clothed trunk of one and the head of the other. Each of them washed, received an injection of 1 mg of atropine sulfate, and then entered hospital so rapidly that cholinesterase activity of one of them was still normal. It became somewhat decreased later.

During the next few hours the men developed moderate poisoning characterized in one or both of them by sweating, weakness, myosis, headache, diarrhea, and intermittent fasciculations. They recovered in 3 and 4 days, respectively (Célice *et al.*, 1961).

Treatment of Poisoning   See Section 16.2.2.7.

16.6.15 FENITROTHION

16.6.15.1 Identity, Properties, and Uses

Chemical Name · Fenitrothion is O,O-dimethyl-O-(3-methyl-4-nitrophenyl)-phosphorothioate.

Structure   See Table 16.16.

Synonyms   The common name fenitrothion (BSI, ISO) is used, except in eastern Europe, where methylnitrophos is employed. A less common term is SMT. Trade names include Accothion®, Agrothion®, Cyfen®, Cytel®, Danathion®, Debucol®, Docofen®, Fenstan®, Folithion®, Metathion®, Sumithion®, and Verthion®. Code designations have included AC-47300, Bayer-41841, ENT-25715, OMS-43, S-1102A, and S-5600. The CAS registry number is 122-14-5.

Physical and Chemical Properties   Fenitrothion has the empirical formula $C_9H_{12}NO_5PS$ and a molecular weight of 277.25. The pure material forms a yellowish brown liquid with an unpleasant odor. Fenitrothion has a density of 1.3084 at 20°C and a vapor pressure of 6×10^{-6} mm Hg at the same temperature. The boiling point of fenitrothion is 140–145°C at 0.1 mm Hg. Fenitrothion is soluble in alcohols, ethers, ketones, and aromatic hydrocarbons. It is insoluble in water and has low solubility in aliphatic hydrocarbons. Fenitrothion is completely stable for 2 years if stored at temperatures between 20 and 25°C. Storage temperature should not exceed 40°C. Fenitrothion is unstable in alkaline media.

History, Formulations, and Uses   Fenitrothion was introduced in 1959 by both Sumitomo Chemical Company and Bayer Leverkusen and later by American Cyanamid Company. It is a contact insecticide effective against rice stem borers and a wide range of other pests (Hattori *et al.*, 1976). Fenitrothion is available as a 95% concentrate, 50% emulsifiable concentrate, 40 and 50% wettable powders, and 2, 2.5, 3 and 5% dusts.

16.6.15.2 Toxicity to Laboratory Animals

Basic Findings   Fenitrothion, at sufficient dosage, produces typical cholinergic poisoning. It produces little or no irritation, and it is not neurotoxic. Its acute toxicity is low (see Table 16.30). In one study, enough mice were used to measure the oral LD 1 (674 and 693 mg/kg in males and females, respectively) and to estimate corresponding LD 0.1 values (578 and 607 mg/kg) (Haley *et al.*, 1975a).

Table 16.30
Single-Dose LD 50 for Fenitrothion and Fenitrooxon

Compound and species	Route	LD 50 (mg/kg)	Reference
Fenitrothion			
rat, M	oral	740	Gaines (1969)
rat, F	oral	570	Gaines (1969)
rat, M	oral	607.9	Camargo *et al.* (1970a)
rat	oral	571.3	Camargo *et al.* (1970b)
rat	oral	200	Suzuki (1970)
rat, M	dermal	1001.5	Camargo *et al.* (1970a)
rat, F	dermal	1001.5	Larini *et al.* (1970)
rat	intravenous	33	Miyamoto *et al.* (1963)
mouse	oral	870	Suzuki (1970)
mouse, M	oral	1045	Haley *et al.* (1975a)
mouse, F	oral	1220	Haley *et al.* (1975a)
mouse	intravenous	220	Miyamoto *et al.* (1963)
guinea pig	oral	1850	Miyamoto *et al.* (1963)
guinea pig	intravenous	112	Miyamoto *et al.* (1963)
Fenitrooxon			
rat	oral	24	Miyamoto (1969)
rat	intravenous	3.3	Miyamoto (1969)
mouse	oral	120	Hollingworth *et al.* (1967b)
mouse	oral	90	Miyamoto (1969)
guinea pig	oral	221	Miyamoto (1969)
guinea pig	intravenous	32	Miyamoto (1969)

Except for one rat that may have died of other causes, rats tolerated fenitrothion at a dietary level of 500 ppm for 90 days, and they grew normally; cholinesterase in plasma, red cells, and tissues was decreased (Misu *et al.,* 1966; Suzuki, 1970). A dietary level of 30 ppm for 6 months decreased the red cell and brain cholinesterase of female but not male rats; neither sex showed any sign of toxicity. A dietary level of 5 ppm (about 0.25 mg/kg/day) for 92 weeks was a no-effect level (Kadota *et al.,* 1975a).

Mice that received fenitrothion at a dietary level of 1000 ppm (about 12.8 mg/kg/day) developed symptoms within a week and at the end of a 20-day feeding period had cholinesterase activity in brain, red cells, and plasma reduced to 45, 26, and 5% of normal, respectively; body weight and liver weight were not affected. Dietary levels of 100 and 10 ppm also inhibited cholinesterase activity to a lesser degree, corresponding to intake. A dietary level of 1 ppm (about 0.128 mg/kg/day) caused no inhibition but rather a significant increase above normal for brain and plasma enzyme. The results for aliesterase in the same groups were similar; a dosage response was present. A dietary level of 1 ppm was a no-injurious-effect level and may have caused a slight increase in enzyme levels above normal (Tsumuki *et al.,* 1970).

Monkeys are more susceptible than dogs. A dosage of 2 mg/kg produced no effect on serum or erythrocyte cholinesterase in dogs but after 2 months of administration did cause a reduction of erythrocyte enzyme activity in monkeys, and the effect was greater at 4 mg/kg (Matsushima *et al.,* 1976, 1978).

A dietary concentration of 5 ppm was found to be a no-effect level in calves (Yasnova *et al.,* 1971).

Rats survived exposure for 1 hr to a concentration of 3.030–4.890 mg/m^3, but cholinesterase was inhibited (Sakama *et al.,* 1975).

Caged rats exposed to fenitrothion spray at ground level during an aircraft application of the pesticide experienced signs of toxicity, and on autopsy scattered areas of alveolar involvement were noted. However, this was not evident in a recovery group 2 months after exposure. No cholinergic crisis or alterations in pseudocholinesterase activity were observed in any of the animals (Coulombe *et al.,* 1986).

Technical fenitrothion contains variable concentrations of *S*-methyl fenitrooxon, depending on the conditions of manufacture. However, it is less toxic and much less stable than fenitrooxon and is unlikely to pose an environmental problem (Ecobichon *et al.,* 1975). Apparently, it has not been determined whether some formulations of fentrothion tend to form the *S*-methyl isomer on tropical storage, as is true with malathion. Some formulations do contain the isomer. In any event, *S*-methyl-fenitrothion is two to three times stronger than fenitrothion as an inhibitor of cholinesterase *in vitro,* and its acute toxicity to rats is higher; however, its metabolism is more rapid (Rosival *et al.,* 1976; Hladka, 1977).

Absorption, Distribution, Metabolism, and Excretion
Following application of [^{32}P]fenitrothion to the skin of rats, it disappeared most rapidly during the first hour, suggesting an absorption rate of slightly over 1%. Some radioactivity was found in the urogenital tract and other tissues but, 31 hr after application, the highest concentration, except on the skin, was in the cartilaginous parts of the bones (Hendrichova *et al.,* 1972). This result suggests that the phosphorus had been metabolized to an inorganic state, but the finding has not been explored further.

In another study, the concentration of fenitrothion in the blood of rats reached a maximum 8 hr after a single dermal application of the compound (Kohli *et al.,* 1974). Fenitrothion is far less toxic than parathion-methyl, but the difference apparently cannot be explained by a difference in metabolism. In general, the metabolism of the two compounds is similar in both rats and guinea pigs. In fact, following equal intravenous dosages, more fenitrothion than parathion-methyl was converted to the ═O analog (Miyamoto, 1964a). The difference in toxicity is correlated with a lesser ability of fenitrothion than of paraoxon-methyl to penetrate the blood–brain barrier, even though penetration of the barrier by the insecticides themselves is not significantly different (Miyamoto, 1964b).

The proportion of different metabolites formed from a single dose of [^{32}P]fenitrothion was the same in previously undosed mice and in those that had received the nonradioactive compound for 45 days (Tsumuki *et al.,* 1970).

One day after a near-fatal dose of 300 mg/kg to rats, the concentration of fenitrothion was 0.363 ppm in blood and ranged from 1.392 in the brain to 13.23 ppm in the kidney. Greatest excretion occurred during the first 3 days. By the fifth day, the highest concentration detected in any tissue was 0.086 ppm, found in the kidney. By the tenth day none could be detected (Asanuma, 1973; Asanuma *et al.*, 1974). By contrast, three-quarters of the radioactivity was excreted within a hour after an oral dosage of 15 mg/kg, and within 24 hr hardly any could be detected. Metabolism and conjugation were extensive (Miyamoto *et al.*, 1975). Excretion was slower in monkeys even after an oral dosage of only 2 mg/kg (Asanuma *et al.*, 1976; Wakasuki, 1976).

Rats receiving intraperitoneal doses of 500 and 50 mg/kg fenitrothion experienced significantly decreased hepatic glutathione concentrations. However, the expected potentiation of hepatotoxicity following oral administration of 600 mg/kg acetaminophen did not occur, as fenitrothion was also found to inhibit significantly hepatic mixed-function oxidase activity (Ginsberg *et al.*, 1982).

Biochemical Effects   The half-life of fenitrothion was noticeably longer after 10 doses at the rate of 30 mg/kg/day than after a single dose at the rate of 300 mg/kg. It was concluded that this effect was caused by suppression of metabolism of the compound during its repeated administration and was associated with inhibition of demethylation and hydrolysis by microsomal enzymes (Uchiyama *et al.*, 1973). Unlike the parent insecticide, fenitrooxon did not inhibit microsomal enzymes (Uchiyama *et al.*, 1974). Furthermore, the degree of inhibition of microsomal enzymes by fenitrothion or its derivatives was small (Hosokawa and Miyamoto, 1975).

Effects on Organs and Tissues   Damage to the nuclear membrane, decreases in staining capacity of cells, and an increase in anomalous mitoses were reported in monolayer cultures of fibroblasts taken from fetuses of rats that had received 0.1 or 0.2 of the LD 50 level of fenitrothion daily during the first 15 days of pregnancy. However, these results were not related to dosage, and no change in the rate of proliferation of the cells and no change in mitotic phase distribution compared with that of controls were observed (Rashev, 1972). The fact that proliferation and mitotic phase remained normal raises a question of the statistical significance of the reported injuries.

Fenitrothion is known to contain a number of contaminants produced in the manufacture of the compound. The most active of these compounds include *O,O,S*-trimethyl phosphorothioate, which has been found to alter transiently humoral and cell-mediated immune responses in rats at doses that do not produce an overt toxic response (Devens *et al.*, 1985). These compounds have not been found to alter the toxicity of fenitrothion in rats (Miles *et al.*, 1979). However, *O,S,S*-trimethyl phosphorodithioate has a distinct cytotoxic effect on the lungs of rats and is known to modulate immune responses in mice (Rodgers *et al.*, 1987). Further information on these contaminants can be found in Section 16.4.5.

Fenitrothion had no mutagenic effect in *Drosophila melanogaster* or mice (Sram, 1974) or in rats (Benes *et al.*, 1975).

Treatment of Poisoning in Animals   A combination of 2-PAM chloride and atropine raised the LD 50 of fenitrothion in rats from 197 to 809 mg/kg (Saxena *et al.*, 1974). This is an important finding, even though the preparation used was more toxic than high-grade fenitrothion.

16.6.15.3 Toxicity to Humans

Experimental Exposure   When volunteers were given single oral dosages ranging from 2.5 to 20 mg/person, the maximal concentration of *p*-nitro-*m*-cresol in the urine was reached within 12 hr, and nearly the entire amount discharged was eliminated during the first 24 hr. Although the amount recovered was directly dosage-related, the proportion recovered was inversely dosage-related; that is, at doses of 2.5, 5, 10, 15, and 20 mg, the proportions recovered were 70.4, 58.7, 51.9, 49.5, and 48.1%, respectively. With one exception, cholinesterase activity remained normal following these doses. When fenitrothion was given at rates of 2.5 and 5 mg/person/day for 5 days, nearly all the insecticide was excreted within 12 hr, and there was no indication of cumulation (Nosal and Hladka, 1968).

Use Experience   Because of its probable value for the control of malaria, the safety of fenitrothion has been studied in village trials. Eight sprayers and two supervisors applied fenitrothion indoors for 6 hr on each of two succeeding days. The men wore overalls, waterproof hats, and rubber boots; when actually weighing out insecticide and spraying, they wore masks. No clinical effects were observed in either the sprayers or the villagers, although the villagers did complain about the odor of the insecticide. A very slight but statistically significant depression of plasma cholinesterase activity was found in the sprayers the day after they finished work. Among villagers, depression of plasma cholinesterase activity was very slight and statistically significant only in the 7- to 14-year-old age group (Vandekar, 1965). In another study, three sprayers and one supervisor spent part of 2 days under identical conditions. The results were similar, except that no mention was made of odor and the cholinesterase activity of the villagers increased slightly rather than decreasing slightly (Vandekar and Svetličić, 1966). In neither of these trials was there any medically important change in cholinesterase activity.

Safety experience with the agricultural uses of fenitrothion has been good. This stands in contrast to experience with parathion, which it largely replaced in Japan. It also stands in contrast to a report of moderate poisoning of 25 workers in Czechoslovakia. The episode was attributed to a formulation containing 50% of the compound, which was applied by aircraft during a strong wind that blew the insecticide 500 yards from the field. Onset was 2.5–6 hr after inhalation; symptoms were typical; blood cholinesterase was decreased by 48%, and recovery required 3 days in spite of treatment with atropine (Kalas, 1978). Evidence apparently is lacking on whether *S*-methyl-fenitrothion contributed to this episode. The presence of this contaminant in Czech formulations has been recognized, but safety experience with fenitrothion has been good in Czechoslovakia (Hladka *et al.*, 1977).

Atypical Cases of Various Origins Three young men who had worked as pest control operators for 3 months and who had recently applied fenitrothion for periods varying from 2 to 8 hr complained of general malaise, fatigue, headache, loss of memory and of ability to concentrate, anorexia, nausea, thirst, and loss of weight. With the exception of proteinuria in one case, all laboratory tests, including serum cholinesterase and EEG, were normal (Matushima, 1972).

Within 2 days after using absorbent tissue in wiping up some approximately 7.5% formulation of fenitrothion that had leaked onto the floor of her automobile, a 33-year-old female technician asked that her blood cholinesterase activity be measured because she was experiencing nausea, cramps, muscular weakness, mental confusion, and tremors. Based on earlier tests, the red cell cholinesterase was thought to be 86% of normal and the plasma enzyme activity 56% of normal. She was hospitalized and treated with pralidoxime chloride but no atropine. She was discharged after 16 days but readmitted within 24 hr and treated with diazepam, acetaminophen, amitriptyline hydrochloride, and calcium. She was discharged from hospital 35 days after exposure, but she continued to complain for several months of episodes of fatigue and muscular weakness (Ecobichon *et al.*, 1977).

Laboratory Findings The blood of a man who killed himself by drinking an unknown amount of fenitrothion (after drinking alcohol) contained 1.09 ppm of the compound, and his urine contained 0.50 ppm of the metabolite *p*-nitro-*m*-cresol (Furuno *et al.*, 1975). In a similar case, the concentrations of fenitrothion equivalent in blood and urine were 1.1 and 0.9 ppm, respectively (Sugahara and Oki, 1976). Fenitrothion also can be detected at 0.001–0.043 ppm in the plasma of persons poisoned by it less severely (Watanabe, 1972a,b).

In two workers who applied fenitrothion and another organic phosphorus insecticide that does not form the metabolite, averages of 0.362 and 0.575 mg of *p*-nitro-*m*-cresol were found in 24-hr urine samples. The concentration of fenitrothion in the serum was 0.0065–0.0200 ppm immediately after application, and it was a trace or undetectable after 36 hr (Nishiyama *et al.*, 1974). However, low values must be viewed with skepticism because a peak with the same *R* value has been found in the gas chromatographs of persons who were never exposed to the compound (Nishimura *et al.*, 1974).

Treatment of Poisoning See Section 16.2.2.7.

16.6.16 FENTHION

16.6.16.1 Identity, Properties, and Uses

Chemical Name Fenthion is *O,O*-dimethyl-*O*-(4-methyl-mercapto-3-methylphenyl)thiophosphate.

Structure See Table 16.16.

Synonyms The common name fenthion (BSI, ISO) is in general use, having replaced the acronym DMTP. Trade names include Baycid®, Baytex®, Entex®, Lebaycid®, Mercaptophos®, Queletox®, Spotton®, and Tiguvon®. Code designations include BAY-29493 and S-1752. The CAS registry number is 55-38-9.

Physical and Chemical Properties Fenthion has the empirical formula $C_{10}H_{15}O_3PS_2$ and a molecular weight of 278.34. The pure material is a colorless liquid with a boiling point of 87°C at 0.01 mm Hg. The density of fenthion is 1.250 at 20°C. The vapor pressure at the same temperature is 3×10^{-5} mm Hg. The technical material is a brown oily liquid of 95–98% purity with a weak garlic odor. Fenthion is practically insoluble in water but readily soluble in most organic solvents and glyceride oils.

History, Formulations, and Uses Fenthion was introduced in 1957 by Bayer Leverkusen. It is a contact and stomach insecticide effective against fruit flies, leafhoppers, and cereal bugs. Fenthion is available as 25 and 40% wettable powders, 60% fogging concentrates, 50% emulsifiable concentrates, 100% ultralow-volume spray, 3% dust, and 2% granules.

16.6.16.2 Toxicity to Laboratory Animals

Fenthion is of sufficiently low toxicity (see Table 16.31) that it has been administered to dogs (Fowler *et al.*, 1970; Garlick, 1971) and cows (Galdney *et al.*, 1972) to study its possible value for the treatment or prevention of parasites.

Table 16.31
Single-Dose LD 50 for Fenthion

Species	Route	LD 50 (mg/kg)	Reference
Rat, M	oral	250	Francis and Barnes (1963)
Rat, F	oral	615	Francis and Barnes (1963)
Rat, M	oral	190	DuBois and Kinoshita (1964b)
Rat, F	oral	310	DuBois and Kinoshita (1964b)
Rat	oral	250	Shimamoto and Hattori (1968)
Rat, M	oral	215	Gaines (1969)
Rat, F	oral	245	Gaines (1969)
Rat	dermal	500	Francis and Barnes (1963)
Rat, M	dermal	330	Gaines (1969)
Rat, F	dermal	330	Gaines (1969)
Rat, M	intraperitoneal	260	DuBois and Kinoshita (1964b)
Rat, F	intraperitoneal	325	DuBois and Kinoshita (1964b)
Mouse, M	oral	150	Francis and Barnes (1963)
Mouse, F	oral	190	Francis and Barnes (1963)
Mouse, M	intraperitoneal	125	DuBois and Kinoshita (1964b)
Mouse, F	intraperitoneal	150	DuBois and Kinoshita (1964b)
Guinea pig, M	oral	>1000	Francis and Barnes (1963)
Rabbit	oral	150–175	Francis and Barnes (1963)
Hen	oral	30–40	Francis and Barnes (1963)

Fenthion differs from a number of other well-known phosphorothionates of the same general type in that the signs of poisoning develop rather slowly in rats but persist several days. This is true even if the material is injected intravenously. For these and other reasons, it is thought that a substantial proportion is converted to the sulfoxide and sulfone before P=S is oxidized to P=O. The complexity of the metabolism is consistent with the observed wide species difference in susceptibility and makes it difficult to predict how susceptible humans would be. The prolonged action of a single dose of fenthion suggests that much of it is stored and later released for metabolism, and this is consistent with the continuing effectiveness of repeated doses of oximes (Francis and Barnes, 1963).

A dietary level of 250 ppm (about 12.5 mg/kg/day) in rats caused weight loss without change in food intake and an inhibition of brain cholinesterase activity to about 15% of normal in 4 weeks. The effect of 20 ppm was similar but less marked, the brain cholinesterase being inhibited to 60–70% of normal. There was even a slight inhibition at 5 ppm (about 2.5 mg/kg/day) (Francis and Barnes, 1963).

Rats were killed by intraperitoneal injection of fenthion at the rate of 40 mg/kg/day for 5–10 days, and most were killed by 20 mg/kg/day for a slightly longer period; all survived 10 mg/kg/day for 60 days (DuBois and Kinoshita, 1964b).

The toxicities of the sulfoxide and sulfone of fenthion are similar to those of the parent compound. The toxicity of the *S*-methyl isomer is about 6 times greater and that of the oxygen analog 13 times greater, but the *S*-methyl isomer may not be formed. The toxicity of the sulfoxide of the oxygen analog is about the same as that of the oxygen analog, but the sulfone is more toxic, being about 36 times more toxic than fenthion itself (DuBois and Kinoshita, 1964b).

Absorption, Distribution, Metabolism, and Excretion
The metabolic pathway of fenthion is generally similar to that of other phosphorothioates and phosphorodithioates having a thioether group, but no evidence of *S*-methyl isomerization was found. Cleavage of the *O*-methyl ester appeared to be a minor degradative mechanism (Brady and Arthur, 1961). It is interesting that in cows, about the same percentage of various metabolic fractions derived from [^{32}P]fenthion appeared in the feces following dermal application as appeared after intramuscular injection, indicating that the dermally applied material had been truly absorbed, whether from the skin or from the gastrointestinal tract, after being licked from the skin (Knowles and Arthur, 1966). Following dermal application of [^{32}P]fenthion at the rate of 9 mg/kg, 45–55% of the radioactivity (primarily in the form of water-soluble hydrolysis products) was recovered in the urine, 2.0–2.5% in the feces, and 1.5–2.0% in the milk (Avrahami and White, 1975). The parent compound, fenthion sulfoxide, fenoxon, and fenthion sulfone were stored in the fat of steers slaughtered 3 days after dermal application, and the first three were found in the fat of those slaughtered 10 days after application (Wright and Riner, 1979).

Biochemical Effects   The ability of fenthion and of its P=O metabolite, sulfoxide, and sulfone to inhibit cholinesterase var-

ies according to the tissues from which the enzymes are taken. However, none of the compounds interfered with neuromuscular transmission, ventilatory activity, or the duration of the PR interval or QRS complex when administered in intravenous doses up to 10 mg/kg (Groblewski *et al.*, 1975).

Single, large doses of fenthion in combination with 13 other anticholinesterase insecticides produced additive or less than additive effects. However, slight potentiation was observed in combination with malathion (1.8 times), dioxathion (1.7 times), and cumaphos (2.8 times) (DuBois and Kinoshita, 1964b).

Effects on Organs and Tissues   Rats that received 1 mg of fenthion (about 4 mg/kg) presented a supernormal electroretinogram (ERG) characterized by shortened time intervals and increased amplitudes. Time intervals were prolonged, and the wave pattern was progressively disorganized at progressively higher doses. These changes are the result of cholinesterase inhibition, and they correspond to the overstimulation and later depression observed in other functions (Imai *et al.*, 1973). There was a dosage-related decrease of acetylcholinesterase activity in the retina and cerebellum in rats receiving more than 0.5 mg/kg fenthion. When inhibition was <50%, the ERG was stimulated, but when inhibition was >50%, the ERG was depressed. It was considered that changes in the ERG could be recognized at dosages as low as 0.005 mg/kg (Miyata *et al.*, 1973, 1974; Imai, 1974a,b).

Fenthion at a dosage of 25 mg/kg produced neurotoxicity lasting 3–10 days in atropinized hens (Gaines, 1969). A similar paralysis occurred among young laying hens that ingested fenthion that had been applied in their living area for fly control (DiModugno *et al.*, 1973).

Effects on Reproduction   A single intraperitoneal injection of fenthion at rates of 40 or 80 mg/kg on one day, especially days 10–12, of gestation was embryotoxic in mice. There was a statistically significant increase in fetal anomalies in the young of dams that received 40 mg/kg on day 8 or 10, but both the percent of resorptions and the percent malformed were less at 80 mg/kg. Dosages of 120–160 mg/kg on day 8, 9, or 10 of gestation had no effect on litter size at birth or on survival rate of the young. Fetuses were injured mainly by dosages that produced toxicity in the dam (Budreau and Singh, 1973a).

The use by five generations of mice of drinking water containing 60 ppm fenthion had little or no effect on mating success, slightly increased the time from pairing to delivery of young, and caused a slight but statistically significant increase in mortality in some but not all litters. It was not teratogenic and did not result in any histological change in the liver or kidney. It is of interest that greater inhibition of plasma cholinesterase was caused by fenthion than by dimethoate, but dimethoate was more harmful to reproduction (Budreau and Singh, 1973b).

16.6.16.3 Toxicity to Humans

Accidental and Intentional Poisoning   Borowitz (1988) has reported a case of a 26-month-old male exposed to an unknown amount of Spotton, a flea killer whose active ingredient is fenthion, via the dermal and possibly the ingestion routes. His mother removed the pesticide from the skin by washing with soap and water, but his clothes were not changed. Eight hours later, he experienced abdominal pain and vomiting and was taken to the local emergency room, where he was released with the diagnosis of a viral infection. Eighteen hours later, when he became increasingly lethargic and the intermittent pain and vomiting persisted, he was admitted to the local hospital with the diagnosis of organic phosphorus poisoning. Although he was carefully bathed and given atropine intravenously at 0.05 mg/kg every 2–4 hr, he went into respiratory arrest 24 hr later, requiring the use of an endotracheal tube and transfer to a more advanced facility.

Upon arrival at the intensive care unit of the new hospital, the child had pinpoint pupils, hyperactive bowel sounds, diffuse crackles in both lungs, mild pulmonary edema, diminished muscle tone and reflexes, no spontaneous respirations, a rectal temperature of 37.8°C, a pulse rate of 116 beats/min, and a blood pressure of 13/82 mm Hg. Erythrocyte and plasma cholinesterase activities were 0.06 and 0.04 ΔpH/hr, respectively. He was given a continuous atropine infusion at the rate of 0.025 mg/kg/hr. 2-PAM at a rate of 50 mg/kg was given intravenously 12 hr later and every 12 hr thereafter. The first dose caused irregular spontaneous respirations, and involuntary movement was great enough to warrant the use of diazepam for sedation. On day 4, the child's alertness improved to the point where he could recognize his mother. Mechanical ventilation was removed 17 days after admission, although atropine was still required at 0.05 mg/kg every 4–8 hr due to bradycardia and excessive oral and pulmonary secretions. Atropine and 2-PAM were discontinued on day 22 of hospitalization, and the patient was discharged on day 30 with plasma and erythrocyte cholinesterase activities in the lower reaches of the normal range. Follow-up examination findings were normal.

An attempted suicide with an unknown quantity of fenthion was treated successfully by atropine, oximes, and artificial respiration for 9 days. The case was interesting because of delay in the onset of really serious illness and also a relative sparing of the function of nonrespiratory, voluntary muscles. Although the patient was unable to breath without assistance, he retained considerable strength in his trunk and limbs and, because of marked agitation, required heavy sedation (Dean *et al.*, 1967). Another attempted suicide that was treated successfully was interesting because of temporary myocardial damage indicated by ECG and by an increase in serum creatine phosphatase. The myocardial damage was attributed to hypokalemia (von Clarmann and Geldmacher-von Mallinckrodt, 1966).

Five employees at a veterinary hospital were complaining of various degrees of neurologic symptoms ranging from occasional tingling and numbness of the hands and feet at night to multiple shooting pains, back pain, numbness, and generalized muscle weakness. However, plasma and red blood cell cholinesterase activities were normal for all patients. An investigation of the hospital found the workers routinely using topical applications of a 20% fenthion solution on dogs for flea infestation control, with no special precautions being taken by the employees to avoid dermal contact. The conditions of the patients improved following discontinuation of fenthion exposure (Metcalf *et al.*, 1985).

Use Experience   Four out of six sprayers, who applied fenthion 6 hr/day for 5 days at rates of 1.5 and 2 gm/m² in Nigerian villages, showed no fall in whole-blood cholinesterase activity on the final day. The other two showed falls of 37.5 and 12.5%, the latter being that of the foreman, who did not wear rubber gloves, waterproof hat, and overalls as the others did. There was slight inhibition of whole-blood cholinesterase activity among inhabitants of sprayed villages. This was somewhat greater in a community with houses with nonabsorbent surfaces sprayed at the rate of 1.5 gm/m² than in another village with mud-walled houses sprayed at 2 gm/m². No correlation appeared to exist between age or sex and the degree of enzyme inhibition. In no instance was there any illness attributable to fenthion (Elliott and Barnes, 1963). The authors stressed that, until more was known about the significance of cholinesterase reduction, fenthion should be used with caution for malaria control. In a separate study of a village sprayed at a rate of 1.5 gm/m², it was found that inhibition of cholinesterase activity did not occur in erythrocytes but only in plasma. No illness attributable to fenthion was found. Changes in hemoglobin and hematocrit were similar in the sprayed and the control village. Changes in the peak expiratory flow rate were erratic but may indicate a need for further study (Taylor, 1963).

In the United States, eight of nine workers using fenthion for mosquito control showed a progressive decline in plasma but not erythrocyte cholinesterase activity during the season of exposure. No illness occurred. Extensive measurement indicated that contact was much greater when granules were used than when the insecticide was applied as a spray using either power or hand equipment (Wolfe *et al.*, 1974).

Nausea, headaches, and irritations of the throat and facial skin were occasionally reported by veterinarians treating grub infestations in cattle with pour-on applications of fenthion and other organic phosphorus pesticides in poorly ventilated areas. Blood cholinesterase values were not reduced in these cases, and alkyl phosphate metabolites were only occasionally found in the urine (Beat and Morgan, 1977).

Atypical Cases of Various Origins   Two cases of mental disturbance lasting over 2 months and attributed to fenthion have been described (Kim *et al.*, 1967).

During somewhat more than 2 years, a 57-year-old farmer was hospitalized repeatedly for hemolytic crises thought to coincide with the application of pesticides to his fields. His last admission followed exposure to fenthion, DDT, lindane, and 2,4-D but, after some improvement, he had further crises without additional exposure, and he died. The authors acknowledged that an inborn defect of the erythrocytes may have existed (Kotlarek-Haus *et al.*, 1971). No effort apparently was made to distinguish the effects of the very different compounds mentioned, and there was no objective test to associate any of them with the illness.

Dosage Response A 71-year-old farmer who swallowed a little fenthion by mistake while drunk was thought to have received about 83 mg/kg. Although he suffered nausea, there was no record of vomiting, and he was not hospitalized until 13 hr after ingestion. On the third day the patient recovered consciousness and was able to eat, but his condition began to deteriorate next morning, and he died on the afternoon of the fourth day (Endo *et al.*, 1974).

A 40-year-old man who attempted suicide by drinking fenthion at a rate of about 25 mg/kg received gastric lavage, atropine, and 2-PAM promptly. Although he did not become fully conscious for 4 days, he did not require artificial respiration, and he survived without sequelae (Kondo *et al.*, 1973). It is not clear how much of the difference between these cases should be attributed to the age of the patients, to promptness of treatment, or to unrecognized factors. In another attempted suicide, a 44-year-old man was thought to have ingested 310 mg/kg. He showed only a few mild signs of poisoning when hospitalized 3 hr after ingestion. However, he experienced two relapses in spite of adequate drug therapy and required tracheotomy during his long stormy course to recovery (Haavik and Ihlen, 1974). In yet another attempted suicide, a 33-year-old woman was thought to have swallowed only about 0.5 gm of a 2% dust. The patient received appropriate treatment beginning 8.3 hr after ingestion and lasting for 10 days (Kanda and Matsushima, 1974). The illness never reached a critical stage. Even so, the true dosage may have been greater than the approximate 0.17 mg/kg as estimated.

Treatment of Poisoning See Section 16.2.2.7.

16.6.17 FORMOTHION

16.6.17.1 Identity, Properties, and Uses

Chemical Name Formothion is *O,O*-dimethyl-*S*-(*N*-formyl-*N*-methylcarbamoylmethyl)phosphorodithioate.

Structure See Table 16.16.

Synonyms The common name formothion (BSI, ISO) is in general use, except in Germany. Trade names include Aflix® and Anthio®. Code designations include J-38 and OMS-968. The CAS registry number is 2540-82-1.

Physical and Chemical Properties Formothion has the empirical formula $C_6H_{12}NO_4PS_2$ and a molecular weight of 257.29. It has a density of 1.361 at 20°C. The pure compound melts at 25–26°C and has a vapor pressure of 8×10^{-7} mm Hg at 20°C. Formothion is soluble in alcohols, ether, chloroform, ketones, and aromatic solvents; it is insoluble in paraffin solvents and water. It is stable in apolar solvents but is unstable in alkali and incompatible with alkaline pesticides.

History, Formulations, and Uses Formothion was introduced in 1959 by Sandoz Limited. It is a contact and systemic insecticide. Available formulations include 25 and 33% emulsifiable concentrates.

16.6.17.2 Toxicity to Laboratory Animals

As shown in Table 16.32, formothion is a compound of low to moderate toxicity. Rats fed the compound did not develop cholinesterase inhibition at dosages less than 9 mg/kg/day. Dogs tolerated 100 mg/kg/day for 46 days without acute illness, but some died after only a few more weeks of dosing; a survivor made rapid recovery of weight and cholinesterase after withdrawal of formothion. Dogs given 32 mg/kg/day showed slight weight loss after the 11th week, but other findings were normal. The no-clinical-effect level was 16 mg/kg/day. No neurotoxicity appeared in atropine-protected hens given large intramuscular doses of formothion (Klotzsche, 1966).

Rats were fed dietary levels of 160, 40, 10, and 0 ppm for 4 weeks, after which they were fed 320, 80, 20, and 0 ppm for the remainder of 2 years with the result that their intakes of approximately 16, 4, 1, and 0 mg/kg/day were essentially constant throughout their lives. At the highest dosage level, slight tremor and muscle fasciculations were observed intermittently in individual rats between months 3 and 12 but not during the remainder of the study. In males but not females there was a significant impairment of growth during this same period with a tendency to recovery during the second year. Mortality was not increased in any group. At the highest dosage level, red cell, plasma, and brain cholinesterase activities were decreased. At 4 mg/kg/day, red cell cholinesterase activity was decreased in both males and females, but plasma and brain cholinesterase activities were unaffected. A dosage of 1 mg/kg/day was a no-effect level for all parameters exam-

Table 16.32
Single-Dose LD 50 for Formothion

Species	Route	LD 50 (mg/kg)	Reference
Rat, M	oral	330[a]	Klotzsche (1961)
Rat, M	oral	375[b]	Klotzsche (1961)
Rat, F	oral	350[b]	Klotzsche (1961)
Rat, M	oral	370–400	Klotzsche (1966)
Rat, F	oral	500–540	Klotzsche (1966)
Rat	oral	218	Vorob'yeva and Lapchenko (1973)
Rat	oral	332	Kur (1974)
Rat, M	dermal	1650	Klotzsche (1961)
Rat, M	dermal	700–1500	Klotzsche (1966)
Rat, M	intravenous	35.5	Klotzsche (1966)
Mouse, M	oral	190	Klotzsche (1966)
Mouse, F	oral	195	Klotzsche (1966)
Mouse	oral	83.3	Vorob'yeva and Lapchenko (1973)
Cat	oral	310	Vorob'yeva and Lapchenko (1973)
Sheep	oral	180	Khaitov *et al.* (1976)

[a] Active substance.
[b] 25% preparation.

ined. None of the dosages studied caused an increase in the incidence of spontaneous tumors or any other form of gross or microscopic pathology. A few abnormalities of clinical chemistry were observed, but they were not dosage-dependent (FAO/WHO, 1974).

In a 2-year study, male and female dogs were fed dietary levels of 640, 160, 40, and 0 ppm, resulting in dosages of about 13.44, 3.36, 0.84, and 0 mg/kg/day. All dogs appeared normal, and the weight gains, hematological findings, urinalyses, and gross and histological morphologies of the different groups were similar throughout the study. The only abnormality of clinical chemistry involved cholinesterase; activity of that enzyme in red cells and liver but not brain was reduced at the highest dosage level. Red cell cholinesterase activity was inhibited at a dosage of 3.36 but not 0.84 mg/kg/day (FAO/WHO, 1974).

Some Soviet preparations may not be identical to those available elsewhere. In rats and mice, the acute toxicity of one Soviet product was relatively high (see Table 16.32). Rats that received daily oral dosages greater than 0.38 mg/kg/day showed significant inhibition of cholinesterase of plasma, red blood cells, liver, and brain; disturbances of carbohydrate and protein metabolism; fatty degeneration of the liver; and dystrophy of fibers of the myocardium (Vorob'yeba and Lapchenko, 1973). The Soviet product also was reported to produce immunological changes when administered either in a single dose (Aripdzhanov, 1973b) or in repeated doses (Aripdzhanov, 1973a). Whereas a dosage of 1/5000 of an LD 50 (about 0.044 mg/kg/day) for 8 months did not affect cholinesterase levels of rats and rabbits at ordinary temperatures, it did reduce activity of this enzyme in animals exposed to 36–40°C for 2 hr daily. Animals exposed to 1/50 of an LD 50 (about 4.36 mg/kg/day) and also to the intermittent high temperature showed 1.5–2.0 times greater abnormality of cholinesterase activity and electrolyte disturbance than animals exposed either to the insecticide or to high temperature alone (Demidenko and Mirgiyazova, 1974). Animals that received acute toxic doses or repeated daily doses at rates of 5 or 10% of the LD 50 level were reported to show disturbances of carbohydrate metabolism, reduction of detoxification in the liver, and dystrophy and karyolysis of liver cells (Vorob'yeva and Lapchenko, 1970).

Absorption, Distribution, Metabolism, and Excretion According to an unpublished report cited by FAO/WHO (1970), autoradiographic studies showed that formothion was rapidly absorbed from the stomach of rats. Within 30 min after a dose at the rate of 10 mg/kg, greatest activity still was in the stomach, but activity already was high in the liver and kidney. Six hours after administration, activity was low in the stomach, highest in the kidneys, and noticeable in liver, intestine, pancrease, and thymus. After 24 hr, distinct radioactivity was found in the thymus only.

A major metabolite rapidly excreted in the urine is an acid tentatively identified as O,O-dimethyl-S-carboxymethyl phosphorodithioate or its oxygen analog. Although there is some question whether dimethoate is formed from formothion in animals, it certainly occurs as a residue in plants treated with formothion (FAO/WHO, 1970; Konyukhov et al., 1974).

In studies with radioactive formothion, 98–99% was recovered in the urine and only 1–2% in the feces. A total of 51% of the radioactivity was excreted in the urine within 4 hr and 96% in 24 hr. There was considerable radioactivity in the bile, indicating the excretion of the compound or its metabolites by that route, but most of this activity was reabsorbed and not excreted in the feces (FAO/WHO, 1970).

Effects on Reproduction No evidence of teratogenic or embryotoxic effects was seen when rabbits were given formothion by stomach tube from day 6 to day 18 of pregnancy at rates of 6 and 30 mg/kg/day (Klotzsche, 1970).

16.6.17.3 Toxicity to Humans

Accidental and Intentional Poisoning A 36-year-old tractor driver was exposed directly to a 0.00025% solution of formothion while repairing a sprayer. Headache, dizziness, weakness, and palpitation, which appeared after 3–4 hr, were followed by an itching rash on his face, trunk, and hands. A test with the same formulation produced erythema, edema, and isolated papules. Recovery required 20 days in spite of treatment (Karimov, 1979).

Use Experience In the Soviet Union, depression of cholinesterase and disturbance of plasma electrolytes have been reported in workers exposed to low concentrations of formothion at high ambient temperatures (Demidenko and Migiyazova, 1974).

Atypical Cases of Various Origins Collective farm workers became sick within 6 hr after starting to weed cotton in a field that had been sprayed 4 days earlier with formothion at a rate of 2 kg/ha. Symptoms included extreme weakness, vertigo, nausea, and stomach pains; signs included vomiting, pallor, and tachycardia. Cholinesterase activity initially was depressed 30–70%. Treatment involved atropine and other measures of questionable relevance. In spite of atropine and symptomatic care, hospitalization lasted 9–12 days (Rozin, 1969). Although the initial episode would appear to be a typical instance of reentry poisoning, its severity and unusual duration suggest that some other compound or a highly toxic contaminant was involved.

Treatment of Poisoning See Section 16.2.2.7.

16.6.18 JODFENFOS

16.6.18.1 Identity, Properties, and Uses

Chemical Name Jodfenfos is O,O-dimethyl O-(2,5-dichloro-4-iodophenyl)-phosphorothioate.

Structure   See Table 16.16.

Synonyms   The common name jodfenfos (ISO) is in use, except in Canada, New Zealand, the United Kingdom, and the United States, where the name iodofenphos (BSI) is used. Trade names have included Alfacron®, Nivano 1-N®, and Nuvanol N®. Code designations include C-9491 and OMS-1211. The CAS registry number is 18181-70-9.

Physical and Chemical Properties   Jodfenfos has the empirical formula $C_8H_8Cl_2IO_3PS$ and a molecular weight of 412.97. The pure material forms colorless crystals with a mild odor. The melting point is 76°C. The vapor pressure is 8×10^{-7} mm Hg at 20°C. At 20°C the solubility of jodfenfos in water is less than 2 ppm. Its solubility in acetone is 48%; in benzene, 68%; in hexane, 3.3%; in 2-propanol, 2.3%; and in dichloromethane, 86%. Jodfenfos is relatively stable in neutral or weakly acidic or alkaline media but unstable to concentrated acids and alkalies.

History, Formulations, and Uses   Jodfenfos was introduced in 1966 as a broad-spectrum, nonsystemic contact and stomach insecticide and acaricide. It is toxic to bees. Jodfenfos is available as 50% wettable powders, 20% dip concentrates, 20% emulsifiable concentrates, and 5% powders.

16.6.18.2 Toxicity to Laboratory Animals

Basic Findings   The oral LD 50 is about 2000 mg/kg (Melnikov, 1971).

Absorption, Distribution, Metabolism, and Excretion   Ninety-two percent of [^{32}P]jodfenfos was eliminated by rats within 24 hr after an oral dose. A trace of jodfenoxon was found in the urine, but over 98% of the total radioactivity in the urine was in the form of metabolites (Johannsen and Knowles, 1970).

Although irradiated solutions of jodfenfos in many solvents are relatively stable, the compound reacted almost completely to form a compound that chromatographed with jodfenoxon when dissolved in carbon tetrachloride or chloroform and exposed to sunlight for 4 hr (Shrivastava and Knowles, 1972). If the oxon was formed under these conditions, it might also be formed from residues on crops. However, it seems unlikely that the derivative was really the oxon because free iodine was released in the solution.

16.6.18.3 Toxicity to Humans

Use Experience   While wearing protective clothing, five sprayers and one mixer applied 50% water-wettable jodfenfos powder as a 5% suspension of active ingredient at an intended rate of 2 gm/m². They treated a village of 874 homes and 412 other structures. Most of the walls were of mud and the roofs of thatch. The work required 5 to 6 hr/day for 8 days. No complaints attributable to the insecticide were elicited from the 6 workers or the 1819 inhabitants of the village. There was no significant depression of whole-blood cholinesterase among the workers or among over 30 inhabitants who were tested 1 and 10 days after spraying (WHO, 1969).

Treatment of Poisoning   See Section 16.2.2.7.

16.6.19 METHIDATHION

16.6.19.1 Identity, Properties, and Uses

Chemical Name   Methidathion is O,O-dimethyl S-(2,3-dihydro-5-methoxy-2-oxo-1,3,4-thiadiazol-3-ylmethyl) phosphorodithioate.

Structure   See Table 16.16.

Synonyms   The common name methidathion (ANSI, BSI, ISO) is in general use except in Japan, where DMTP (JMAF) is employed. Trade names include Supracide®, Ultracide®, and Ustracide®. Code designations include GS-13,005. The CAS registry number is 950-73-8.

Physical and Chemical Properties   Methidathion has the empirical formula $C_6H_{11}N_2O_4PS_2$ and a molecular weight of 302.31. The pure material forms colorless crystals with a melting point of 39–40°C. The density is 1.495 gm/cm³ at 20°C. The vapor pressure at the same temperature is 1×10^{-6} mm Hg. Methidathion is soluble in water at 25°C to 240 ppm. It is readily soluble in acetone, benzene, and methanol. Methidathion is stable in neural or weakly acid media but much less stable in alkali. It is compatible with captan, thiram, zineb, and acaricides.

History, Formulations, and Uses   Methidathion was introduced in 1966 by J. R. Geigy S.A. It is used in the control of scale insects, leaf eaters, and some mites. Methidathion is available in 20 and 40% emulsifiable concentrates and wettable powders.

16.6.19.2 Toxicity to Laboratory Animals

Basic Findings   Methidathion is a compound of moderate to high acute toxicity (see Table 16.33). All rats were killed within 2 weeks by a dosage of 33.2 mg/kg/day administered by stomach tube. In similar tests lasting 4 weeks, 90, 40, and 0% were killed by dosages of 20, 10, and 8.3 mg/kg/day; inhibition of cholinesterase activity and reduction in growth were detectable at dosages as low as 2.5 mg/kg/day. The same 2.5 mg/kg/day dosage administered in the diet (50 ppm) caused only inhibition of erythrocyte cholinesterase, but a dosage of 0.5 mg/kg/day did the same to a slightly lesser degree. A dosage of 0.25 mg/kg/day by stomach tube was a no-effect level in rats (FAO/WHO, 1973).

Dogs survived a 2-year test at a dietary level of 64 ppm (about 1.35 mg/kg) with inhibition of erythrocyte but not brain cholinesterase activity; however, there was evidence of liver

Table 16.33
Single-Dose LD 50 for Methidathion

Species	Route	LD 50 (mg/kg)	Reference
Rat, M	oral	31	Gaines and Linder (1986)
Rat, F	oral	32	Gaines and Linder (1986)
Rat[a]	oral	21	Gaines and Linder (1986)
Rat, M	dermal	94	Gaines and Linder (1986)
Rat, F	dermal	85	Gaines and Linder (1986)
Mouse, F	oral	18	FAO/WHO (1973)
Guinea pig, F	oral	25	FAO/WHO (1973)
Rabbit, M	oral	80	FAO/WHO (1973)
Dog	oral	200	FAO/WHO (1973)

[a] Male weanling.

injury, including an increase in SGPT, serum alkaline phosphatase, sulfobromophthalein retention, and liver pigmentation. Similar but slightly lesser effects were present at a dietary level of 16 ppm, but 4 ppm (about 0.08 mg/kg/day) caused only a slight increase in SGPT in males and was considered a no-effect level (FAO/WHO, 1973).

Absorption, Distribution, Metabolism, and Excretion
Details of the metabolism of the acidic group of methidathion have been explored using insecticide in which every carbon atom in this group was marked with ^{14}C. Up to 36% of the dose applied to rats was recovered as carbon dioxide (Esser *et al.*, 1968). In another study in rats, it was shown that averages of 22.4, 25.8, and 17.7% of the applied dose were recovered as carbon dioxide when the 2-methoxy, carbonyl, and methylene carbons, respectively, of the acidic groups were labeled with ^{14}C. Dimethyl phosphate (33.6%) and dimethyl phosphorothioate (24.2%) were the main urinary metabolites of methidathion, but 11.1% was recovered during the first 48 hr as desmethyl methidathion. Almost 80% of intraperitoneal doses of [^{32}P]methidathion was excreted in 48 hr, including 7.1% in the feces (Bull, 1968).

Methidathion with a [^{14}C]carbonyl group was rapidly metabolized and eliminated by lactating cows. Not only did ^{14}C appear in the urine, but a substantial proportion was exhaled as carbon dioxide. Milk from the cows contained 1–2% of the radioactivity; of this, a small proportion was sulfoxide and sulfone, but no parent compound was detected. Most of the radioactivity was nonextractable, indicating complete metabolism and incorporation into natural, nonfat solids (Polan and Chandler, 1971). Failure of the compound to be excreted in milk has been confirmed (St. John and Lisk, 1974).

Biochemical Effects *In vitro*, methidathion, but not methidaoxon, inhibits acetylcholine synthesis by choline acetyltransferase and also inhibits the uptake of choline by synaptosomes. It has been speculated that the parent compound may affect neuromuscular transmission *in vivo* through inhibition of choline acetyltransferase (Hemsworth and Cholakis, 1972).

Effects on Organs and Tissues In the cat, intravenous injection of methidathion causes an immediate, nonmuscarinic, temporary depressor effect and a slowly developing and fairly rapidly disappearing block of neuromuscular transmission. Oximes differ in their ability to counteract this effect. Indirect evidence was obtained that decreased release of acetylcholine at nerve endings is not a component contributing to the paralysis (Wills and Chalakis, 1968).

Effects on Reproduction In a preliminary study, male and female rats were fed for 12 weeks prior to mating on diets containing 0–50 ppm methidathion. Compared to controls, those receiving the insecticide showed no difference in gestation period, fertility, number of young, survival at weaning, or average weight at 25 days of age. In a second study, rats received dietary levels of 0, 2, or 16 ppm for 3 weeks and thereafter 0, 4, or 32 ppm. This was a conventional three-generation study, except that the F_{1b} and F_{2b} litters did not receive the test diets until 26 and 22 days, respectively, after weaning. The P, F_{1b}, and F_{2b} animals did receive the test diets for 27–28 weeks, during which each produced two litters. The number of young surviving at weaning was reduced in all generations from dams receiving 32 ppm, and the mean liver weight of F_{3b} weanlings was slightly increased. The body weight, reproductive capacity, and mortality of the parents and the number of litters, size of litters, mean birth weight, and mean weight at weaning were comparable to those in controls. Stillbirths and congenital abnormalities were not increased. No histological damage was found in the F_{3b} animals. The no-effect level was 4 ppm (about 0.2 mg/kg/day) (FAO/WHO, 1973).

16.6.19.3 Toxicity to Humans

One man took a dosage of 0.04 mg/kg/day for 17 days and 0.08 mg/kg/day for 8 days without any adverse effect on red cell or plasma cholinesterase activity or on clinical condition. In a separate study, groups of four, eight, and eight men received methidathion in capsules at the rate of 0, 0.04, and 0.11 mg/kg/day, respectively, for 6 weeks. All dosages were without effect on clinical condition, EEG patterns, plasma or erythrocyte cholinesterase levels, SGPT, SGOT, or other clinical laboratory findings (Wills *et al.*, 1971; FAO/WHO, 1973).

A 25-year-old farmer was found unconscious in a field. Eventually, it was learned that he had swallowed methidathion about 2 hr earlier. It was not until 5 hr after he was found that he received gastric lavage. He was treated for many days with substantial doses of atropine and abidoxime; artificial respiration was required until day 15. The early, critical part of the illness was characterized not only by deep coma but also by high fever, an unusual and unexplained finding. Jaundice, another unusual finding, appeared on the fourth day and regressed 4 days later. Prothrombin time increased, but other liver functions remained within normal limits. No cause for the jaundice was assigned. Treatment with obidoxime "was stopped after day 3 due to its known hepatotoxicty," but it was reinstituted on days 7 and 8, during which time bilirubin in the serum increased. Follow-up examinations 2, 5, and 10 months after hospitalization showed no delayed neuropathy or other abnormality (Teitelman *et al.,* 1975).

Treatment of Poisoning   See Section 16.2.2.7.

16.6.20 NALED

16.6.20.1 Identity, Properties, and Uses

Chemical Name   Naled is *O,O*-dimethyl-*O*-1,2-dibromo-2,-2-dichloroethyl phosphate.

Structure   See Table 16.16.

Synonyms   The common name naled (ANSI, BSI, ESA, ISO) is in general use. However, it is called bromchlophos in the Republic of South Africa and dibram in Denmark. Trade names include Bromex® and Dibrom®. Code designations include ENT-24,988, JSR-381, OMS-75, and RE-4,355. The CAS registry number is 300-76-5.

Physical and Chemical Properties   Naled has the empirical formula $C_4H_7Br_2Cl_2O_4P$ and a molecular weight of 380.79. The melting point of the pure material is 26°C. The technical material forms a yellow liquid with a slightly pungent odor. Its boiling point is 110°C at 0.5 mm Hg. The vapor pressure of the technical material is 2×10^{-3} mm Hg at 20°C. Nales is practically insoluble in water, slightly soluble in aliphatic solvents, and readily soluble in aromatic solvents. Naled is stable under anhydrous conditions but is rapidly hydrolyzed in the presence of water (90–100% in 48 hr at room temperature) and by alkali. Naled is degraded by sunlight and should be stored in lightproof containers. It is stable in brown glass containers but in the presence of metals and reducing agents rapidly loses bromine and reverts to dichlorvos.

History, Formulations, and Uses   Naled was introduced in 1956 by Chevron Chemical Company as a fast-acting, nonsystemic contact and stomach insecticide and acaricide. It is used against adult mosquitoes and flies and on many field crops, as well as on plants under glass and in mushroom houses. Naled is available as a 4% dust and a 96% emulsifiable concentrate.

16.6.20.2 Toxicity to Laboratory Animals

The acute toxicity of naled is low. Oral LD 50 values of 250 mg/kg have been reported in male rats (Gaines, 1969), 281 mg/kg in female rats (Brzezicka-Bak and Bojanowska, 1968), and 59 mg/kg in the chicken (Mukhamedshin, 1970a). The dermal LD 50 in male rats was 800 mg/kg (Gaines, 1969). By using large numbers of mice at the lower dosages, it was possible not only to measure the oral LD 50 and LD 1 but also to estimate the LD 0.1. The values were 375, 205, and 168

mg/kg, respectively, for males and 360, 195, and 159 mg/kg for females (Haley *et al.,* 1975c).

Berteau and Deen (1978) reported respiratory LD 50 values of 7.7 and 156 mg/kg for female rats and mice, respectively. Unfortunately, the values may lack precision, for they were calculated using tabular values for respiratory volume and the proportion of aerosol retained. The oral LD 50 values for naled reported in the same paper are lower than those measured by other investigators. Furthermore, rats tolerated a dosage of 28 mg/kg/day for 9 weeks without clinical effect and with only moderate inhibition of blood and brain cholinesterase (Brzezicka-Bak and Bojanowaka, 1969). The compound has been used as an anthelmintic in dogs; it is effective against several nematodes but entirely ineffective against tapeworms. The recommended dosage is 16.7 mg/kg, but administering twice as much was slightly more effective and produced soft feces and diarrhea, as the only side effects (Kobayashi *et al.,* 1964).

16.6.20.3 Toxicity to Humans

Use Experience   At least two papers have attributed dermatitis to naled. In some cases there was strong evidence for sensitization. In other cases, the dermatitis was attributed to irritation, but sensitization was not ruled out.

Within a few hours after they had worked with chrysanthemum plants, 9 of 12 women complained of burning arms, face, neck, and abdomen. It was eventually found that, 2 hr before the women worked among the plants, the field had been sprayed with a mixture of naled (10.8%), captan (6%), and dicofol (2.4%). Four of the women were examined 4 days after onset, and they had eruptions diagnosed as contact sensitization dermatitis. These patients were patch-tested 2 weeks later when there was no evidence of dermatitis; the results in three of the four patients gave strong evidence that naled had been the cause of the trouble (Edmundson and Davies, 1967).

Four cases interpreted as direct irritation were reported by Mick *et al.* (1970). In the most severe case, naled entered through an unnoticed hole in the elbow-length gloves worn by a pilot during loading and cleaning operations. When discovered, the formulation was wiped off, not washed. The exposed area became red and had a burning sensation. Later, the area became edematous and blistered. When the blisters became dry, the skin itched. The man continued to work but reduced his exposure; recovery required 3 weeks.

Laboratory Findings   When a 1376-ha area was sprayed by aircraft with naled and temephos for mosquito control, there was no increase in the concentration of urinary metabolites of the compounds in persons who were indoors during spraying. However, for people who were outdoors in the area at the time, the concentration of dimethyl phosphate increased from a maximum of 0.06 ppm before spraying to a maximum of 0.50 ppm within 3 hr after spraying; the corresponding values for dimethyl thiophosphate was 0.30 and 1.60 ppm (Kutz and Strassman, 1977).

Treatment of Poisoning   See Section 16.2.2.7.

16.6.21 PHENTHOATE

16.6.21.1 Identity, Properties, and Uses

Chemical Name   Phenthoate is *O,O*-dimethyl *S*-α-ethoxy-carbonylbenzyl phosphorodithioate.

Structure   See Table 16.16.

Synonyms   The common name phenthoate (BSI, ISO) is in general use. Occasionally, the names dimephenthioate, dimephenthoate, dimethenthoate, and fenthoate was used. Trade names have included Cidemul®, Cidial®, Elsan®, Erucin®, Erusan®, PAP®, Papthion®, Phendal®, Rogdial®, Tanone®, and Tsidial®. Code designations have included Bay-33051, Bayer-18510, ENT-23438, ENT-27386, L-561, OMS-1075, S-2940, and TH-346-1. The CAS registry number is 2597-03-7.

Physical and Chemical Properties   Phenthoate has the empirical formula $C_{12}H_{17}O_4PS_2$ and a molecular weight of 320.37. The pure material forms a colorless crystalline solid with an aromatic odor. Its melting point is 17.0–18.0°C. Its density is 1.226 at 20°C. The technical material forms a reddish-yellow oily liquid with an aromatic odor. In water at 24°C, phenthoate is soluble to 11 ppm. Phenthoate is stable in acid and in neutral media in a buffer solution. At a pH of 9, about 25% of the phenthoate were hydrolyzed after 20 days.

History, Formulations, and Uses   Phenthoate was introduced in 1961. It is a nonsystemic pesticide with contact and stomach action. Phenthoate is used to protect from lepidopterans, leafhoppers, aphids, and soft scales. It also is effective against mosquito larvae and adults. Phenthoate is available in concentrations ranging from 2 to 100%.

16.6.21.2 Toxicity to Laboratory Animals

The acute toxicity of phenthoate is shown in Table 16.34. Commercial products vary in purity. Those containing the least active ingredients and the most impurities are most toxic to mammals. A preparation that was 98.5% pure had an extremely low toxicity to rats and a slightly increased toxicity to houseflies. Unfortunately, such a product is not available commercially.

Phenthoate, like malathion but unlike most other organic phosphorus insecticides, contains a carboxylic ester in the acidic side chain. This means that the compound can be detoxified by mammals by splitting this ester, as well as by other means effective for other compounds. It also means that the toxicity of the compound may be potentiated by any compound that is relatively effective in inhibiting carboxylesterase. The potentiating compound may be an impurity normally present in the technical product. The impurities of phenthoate may be

Table 16.34
Single-Dose LD 50 for Phenthoate

Species	Route	LD 50 (mg/kg)	Reference
Rat	oral	77.7[a]	Pellegrini and Santi (1972)
Rat	oral	118[a]	Pellegrini and Santi (1972)
Rat	oral	242.5[a]	Pellegrini and Santi (1972)
Rat	oral	4728[b]	Pellegrini and Santi (1972)
Rat	oral	246	Gupta (1976)
Rat	dermal	4498	Gupta (1976)
Mouse	oral	350–400	WHO/FAO (1982a)
Guinea pig	oral	377	WHO/FAO (1982a)
Rabbit	oral	210	WHO/FAO (1982a)
Hare	oral	72	WHO/FAO (1982a)
Dog	oral	500	WHO/FAO (1982a)

[a] Commercial products varying in purity from 61.2 to 90.5%, respectively.
[b] Purified product containing 98.5% active ingredient.

destroyed by reaction with acetyl bromide so that the technical product is less toxic to rats and other warm-blooded animals, including mice, guinea pigs, rabbits, hares, pheasants, quail, and chickens, but is essentially unchanged in toxicity to insects (Pellegrini and Santi, 1972). The difference depends, of course, on the relative lack of carboxylesterase activity in insects.

In the mouse, ^{14}C- and ^{32}P-labeled phenthoate is metabolized to a wide variety of less toxic compounds and to an insignificant amount of phenthoate oxon. Most of the radioactivity appears in the urine within 2–4 hr (Takade *et al.*, 1976).

16.6.21.3 Toxicity to Humans

Use Experience   A 40% water-wettable powder of phenthoate was applied to the inside surfaces of houses at a rate of 2 gm/m². Five sprayers and one mixer applied the material during 5–6 hr/day for three consecutive days. The Nigerian village treated contained 213 homes and 172 other buildings. No complaints related to phenthoate were elicited from the operators, and they showed no significant decrease in whole-blood cholinesterase activity. There were no complaints from the 384 inhabitants of the village and, in a group of over 30 who were tested on day 1 and again on day 10, there was no enzyme inhibition (WHO, 1969).

No adverse effects were observed when an undisclosed number of young adult male military recruits wore clothing with sleeves treated with a 1% phenthoate solution for a total of 6 weeks at 34–48 hr/week (WHO/FAO, 1982a,b).

Treatment of Poisoning   See Section 16.2.2.7.

16.6.22 PHOSPHAMIDON

16.6.22.1 Identity, Properties, and Uses

Chemical Name   Phosphamidon is the *Z* isomer of *O,O*-dimethyl-*O*-(2-chloro-2-diethycarbamoyl-1-methylvinyl) phosphate.

Structure See Table 16.16.

Synonyms The common name phosphamidon (ANSI, BSI, ISO) is used, except in Italy and Turkey. In some languages, the word is spelled phosphamidone. The trade name is Dimecron®. Code designations have included C-570, CIBA-570, ENT-25,515, ML-97, and OR-1,911. The CAS registry number for the *trans* isomer is 297-99-4 and for the *cis* isomer is 23783-98-4. The number for the mixture is 13171-21-6.

Physical and Chemical Properties Both isomers of phosphamidon have the empirical formula $C_{10}H_{19}ClNO_5P$ and a molecular weight of 299.70. It is the Z isomer that has been defined by ISO as phosphamidon. The Z isomer (also known as the *cis* or β isomer) can be separated from the E isomer (also called *trans* or α isomer) by gas–liquid chromatography or countercurrent distribution. The Z isomer has greater insecticidal activity. The material usually available is a mixture of about 70% Z isomer and 30% E isomer. The mixture is a pale yellow oil with a faint odor. The boiling point is 162°C at 1.5 mm Hg. Its density is 1.2132 at 25°C. At 20°C the vapor pressure is 2.5×10^{-5} mm Hg. Phosphamidon is miscible with water. It is readily soluble in most organic solvents except paraffins. Its solubility in hexane is 3.2% at 25°C. Phosphamidon is stable in neutral and acid media but is hydrolyzed by alkali with a half-life at 23°C of 13.8 days at pH 7 and 2.2 days at pH 10. Phosphamidon is compatible with all except highly alkaline pesticides although, for an unknown reason, its biological activity is decreased by copper oxychloride. The technical product is 90% pure with a density of 1.22 at 20°C.

History, Formulations, and Uses Phosphamidon was introduced in 1956 by CIBA AG as a systemic and contact insecticide and acaricide with a broad spectrum of activity. Phosphamidon is effective against sap-feeding insects, sugarcane and rice stemborers, and rice leaf beetles.

Phosphamidon is available in concentrations of 20, 40, 50, 75, and 100 kg/100 liters in 2-propanol, the water content being rigidly controlled to delay hydrolysis.

16.6.22.2 Toxicity to Laboratory Animals

Basic Findings Phosphamidon is a compound of moderate acute toxicity as shown in Table 16.35. Phosphamidon is a direct inhibitor of cholinesterase and produces typical anticholinesterase effects. The onset of poisoning is rapid. Experimental animals that survive single oral or intraperitoneal doses recover in a day or two, but recovery requires about 10 days following the dermal route, doubtless because of continuing absorption. Phosphamidon is slightly irritating to the skin and moderately irritating to the eyes (Sachsse and Voss, 1971).

In one short-term study, all rats that received phosphamidon by stomach tube at a rate of 10 mg/kg/day were killed within 33 days (Klotzsche, 1958a). In another test, rats survived this same dosage for 90 days or more when the material was administered in the food; the only untoward effects were reduced

Table 16.35
Single-Dose LD 50 for Phosphamidon

Species	Route	LD 50 (mg/kg)	Reference
Rat, M	oral	24	Gaines (1969)
Rat, F	oral	24	Gaines (1969)
Rat, M	dermal	143	Gaines (1969)
Rat, F	dermal	107	Gaines (1969)
Mouse	oral	13	Jaques and Bein (1960)
Mouse	oral	6.5[a]	Sachsse and Voss (1971)
Mouse	oral	220[b]	Sachsse and Voss (1971)
Mouse	subcutaneous	26	Jaques and Bein (1960)
Mouse	intraperitoneal	5.8	Menzer and Best (1968)
Mouse	intravenous	6	Jaques and Bein (1960)

[a] Z isomer.
[b] E isomer.

food intake and reduced rate of growth, and these occurred also at 5 mg/kg/day (Sachsse and Voss, 1971). It is not clear whether the difference in results was the result of differences in dosing schedule, formulation, or some other factor. In any event, rats on a dosage of 5 mg/kg/day survived as well as controls in a 2-year test, but they ate less and grew less, as was true in the short-term study. The next lowest dosage, 1.25 mg/kg/day, caused no abnormality in survival, growth, behavioral patterns, hematology, urology, organ weights and ratios, gross and microscopic pathology, or tumor incidence (Sachsse and Voss, 1971). The same investigators found that a dietary level of 7.5 ppm (about 0.367 mg/kg/day) caused a statistically significant inhibition of plasma, erythrocyte, and brain cholinesterase activity in rats but a dietary level of 2 ppm (about 0.098 mg/kg/day) was a no-effect level (Sachsse and Voss, 1971). Others found that 0.3 mg/kg/day was a no-effect level (Jaques and Bein, 1960).

Dogs that received phosphamidon by capsule survived 5 mg/kg/day for 90 days. Plasma and erythrocyte cholinesterase activities were depressed initially by a dosage of 1 mg/kg/day, but returned to normal before the end of the test. The no-effect level was 0.5 mg/kg/day. In a 2-year test, all dogs receiving 5 mg/kg/day eventually developed typical signs of poisoning and died between days 100 and 600 of the experiment. Dogs receiving 2.5 mg/kg/day showed signs of moderate poisoning but no change in hematology, clinical blood chemistry, urine, or organ function and no gross or histological pathology. A dosage of 0.1 mg/kg/day was a no-effect level (Sachsse and Voss, 1971). Apparently, dogs have not been tested for 2 years at 0.5 mg/kg/day.

Absorption, Distribution, Metabolism, and Excretion Phosphamidon was administered to rats and a female goat. Analysis revealed nine organoextractable metabolites in goat urine, eight in rat urine, and six in goat milk; however, over 90% of radioactivity in urine was in the form of unextractable polar metabolites assumed to be essentially nontoxic. Only trace amounts of phosphamidon were found. Among the extractable compounds, the following were identified: desethyl phosphamidon in urine only, phosphamidon amide in urine and milk, and deschloro phosphamidon amide, also in urine and milk. These three metabolites, formed oxidatively, are at least as toxic as phosphamidon itself. In addition, the hydrolytic product N,N'-diethylacetoacetamide was detected in urine and milk (Clemons and Menzer, 1968). Details of the oxidative metabolism have been studied *in vitro* (Lucier and Menzer, 1971).

Biochemical Effects   The respiration of slices of normal rat brain is stimulated by potassium ions. The oxygen uptake of brain slices taken from rats 45 min after subcutaneous injection of phosphamidon at the rate of 15 mg/kg was 20–35% below normal, but it was stimulated more than that of the controls by potassium. This effect was not seen with equitoxic doses of parathion or TEPP. The mechanism is not clear (Andjelkovic and Milosevic, 1969).

There was no significant potentiation when phosphamidon was administered to rats in combination with 20 other organic phosphorus compounds, including malathion (Sachsse and Voss, 1971).

Technical phosphamidon contains 1–2% of an impurity, γ-chlorophosphamidon, which differs from phosphamidon by having a chlorine atom on the first as well as on the second carbon of the acidic group. Although γ-chlorophosphamidon is from 10 to 20 times more active than phosphamidon in inhibiting different mammalian cholinesterases, technical phosphamidon is not significantly more toxic than the highly purified compound. The apparent paradox is explained by the faster degradation of the impurity (Rose and Voss, 1971).

Effects on Organs and Tissues   Phosphamidon is not neurotoxic to hens (Gaines, 1969; Sachsse and Voss, 1971).

It has been reported that intraperitoneal dosages of phosphamidon as low as 0.07 mg/kg cause chromosome aberrations in bone marrow cells of rats and mice and that the effect shows a dosage–response relationship (Georgian, 1975).

Effects on Reproduction   A three-generation test of reproduction was carried out using a mixture of phosphamidon (75%) and two of its metabolites considered to be of special significance (desethylphosphamidon, 22%, and N,N-diethyl-α-chloroacetoacetamide, 3%). Feeding levels were 0, 1, 7.5, and 15 ppm of the mixture. (The highest dietary level is equivalent to about 0.735 mg/kg/day for an adult rat, but it is about twice as great for young rats and about three times as great for dams during the latter part of lactation.) In the parental animals of all generations, behavior, mortality, body weight, and rate of gain were unaffected, and there were no pathological changes in the tissues. Reproductive performance (mating, fertility, incidence of pregnancy, and duration of gestation) was normal. There were no significant differences in the number of young born, the number of stillborns, or in body weight at weaning. Survival of young between days 4 and 21 of lactation was slightly less in the F_{1b}, F_{3a}, and F_{3b} litters of dams receiv-

ing 15 ppm (Sachsse and Voss, 1971). Whether a maternal dosage of about 2.2 mg/kg/day during lactation really affected the survival of half the groups of nursing litters but not the others is unclear. The lactation index of the controls was sometimes as low as 70%, indicating poor experimental conditions.

16.6.22.3 Toxicity to Humans

Experimental Exposure   In a test of the effect of direct exposure during agricultural spraying, 32 volunteers varying in age from 10 to 70 years stayed in paddy fields while phosphamidon was applied by aircraft and for 1 hr afterward. Cattle, goats, and chickens were tethered along the paths between the rice fields. The ultralow-volume application was at a rate of 550 gm/ha, that is, at almost twice the recommended rate. The volunteers wore their usual light clothing and no other protection. Most of the 32 people experienced irritation of their conjunctivae immediately after the application; that was the only clinical effect. The animals were unaffected. Plasma cholinesterase of the people showed a depression of 0–25% in 19 subjects, 26–50% in 19 subjects, and over 50% in 2 subjects. Maximal depression occurred from 1 to 3 days after exposure; recovery was complete by day 9. There was no significant effect on red cell cholinesterase (Kashyap and Gupta, 1976; Sachsse and Hess, 1973).

Accidental and Intentional Poisoning   It seems possible that, under other circumstances, an 18-year-old girl could have been saved from suicidal poisoning by phosphamidon because she lived 6 days; however, she was apneic and deeply cyanotic when she reached hospital, and her clinical course and the condition of her brain at autopsy made it clear that she had suffered irreparable brain damage before treatment could begin. Death was actually caused by severe bilateral bronchopneumonia with early abscess formation that developed on the fifth hospital day in spite of massive antibiotic treatment that had been given from the day of admission. Chief interest in the case lies in the evidence of liver damage revealed by tests on the fourth day, specifically, prothrombin, 37%; bilirubin, 2.5 mg %; cholesterol, 93 mg %; alkaline phosphatase, 4.2 B.L. units; albumin, 2.7 gm %; and globulin, 3 gm %. At autopsy, the liver was yellow and showed marked diffuse fatty change on histological examination (Gitelson *et al.*, 1965). The authors cited reports of liver injury attributed to poisoning by organic phosphorus compounds but also cited another report of similar injury caused by prolonged anoxia. They concluded that anoxia may have been a factor in causing or aggravating the liver damage they had observed.

Two operators were completely drenched with 50% phosphamidon, and six others had their feet soaked with the insecticide and their hands, arms, and clothes splashed with it when a pipe burst. They immediately washed themselves thoroughly with soap and water. Gastric pains, headache, and a burning sensation in the eyes were the only symptoms reported, and the operators were able to return to work without antidotal therapy (CIBA, 1967).

Another accident is discussed under Dosage Response.

Use Experience One case of poisoning has been reported in which the only recognized exposure was the uprooting and cutting of shrubs that 2 weeks previously had been sprayed with phosphamidon. The 50-year-old man had worked without gloves but for 1 day only. In the afternoon he suffered dizziness and repeated severe vomiting, and he collapsed. When brought to hospital he was sweating and showed excessive lacrimation; he was confused and very restless. Poisoning was diagnosed, even though serum cholinesterase activity 12 hr after admission was 80% of "normal." In spite of little treatment, the patient regained full consciousness in a few hours, regained full strength after 2 days, and recovered completely (Gitelson et al., 1965). The rate of application of phosphamidon to the shrubs was not stated, nor was it recorded why any treatment had been applied if the shrubs were to be eliminated in only 2 weeks.

Dosage Response A 10-year-old boy ingested 20% phosphamidon at a dosage thought to be within the range of 60 to 120 mg/kg. He was given an emetic immediately so that the retained dosage was even less certain. He required little treatment and was discharged from hospital next day (CIBA, 1967).

Treatment of Poisoning See Section 16.2.2.7.

16.6.23 PIRIMIPHOS-METHYL

16.6.23.1 Identity, Properties, and Uses

Chemical Name Pirimiphos-methyl is *O,O*-dimethyl *O*-(2-diethylamino-6-methylpyrimidin-4-yl) phosphorothioate.

Structure See Table 16.16.

Synonyms The common name pirimiphos-methyl (BSI, ISO) is in general use. The French spelling is pyrimiphos-méthyl. Trade names include Actellic®, Actellifog®, Blex®, Silosan®, and Silo-San®. Code designations have included OMS-1424 and PP-511 (discontinued name). The CAS registry number is 29232-93-7.

Physical and Chemical Properties Pirimiphos-methyl has the empirical formula $C_{11}H_{20}N_3O_3PS$ and a molecular weight of 305.3. The pure material is a straw-colored liquid with no characteristic odor and decomposes at temperatures above 100°C. Pirimiphos-methyl has a melting point of 15–18°C and a density of 1.157 at 30°C. Its vapor pressure is 1.1×10^{-4} mm Hg at 30°C. The solubility of pirimiphos-methyl in water at 30°C is 5 ppm. It is miscible or very soluble in most organic solvents. Pirimiphos-methyl is hydrolyzed by strong acids and alkalies.

History, Formulations, and Uses Pirimiphos-methyl was introduced in 1970 by ICI, Ltd. as a fast-acting insecticide and acaricide with both contact and fumigant action. Pyrimiphos is

able to penetrate leaf tissue to give translaminar action. It is suitable for stored products. Pirimiphos-methyl is available as 8, 25, and 50% emulsifiable concentrates, 10 and 50% ultra-low-volume sprays, 20% encapsulated forms, 2% dust, 90% solvent-free formulation, and a smoke generator formulation. Domestic sprays are available containing pirimiphos-methyl and synergized pyrethrins.

16.6.23.2 Toxicity to Laboratory Animals

With the few exceptions noted below, it appears that essentially everything known about the toxicity of pirimiphos-methyl to animals is the subject of unpublished reports that were summarized by FAO/WHO (1975) and WHO/FAO (1982b).

Basic Findings Pirimiphos-methyl applied to the skin was neither an irritant nor a sensitizing agent for rats and guinea pigs. It was not irritating to the eyes of rabbits and, what is much more unusual, it did not cause miosis when an undiluted drop was placed in the conjunctival sac. Most ═S─ organophosphorus compounds contain enough ═O─ isomers as impurities to cause miosis by local action.

Signs of poisoning are typical of cholinesterase inhibition. In rats that received large doses, signs were mild to moderate 12 hr after dosing but marked at 24 hr. Signs persisted as much as 12 days in rats that survived a single large dose.

The oral LD 50 is 1840–2260 mg/kg in female rats, 1450 mg/kg in male rats, 1030–1360 mg/kg in the male mouse, 1000–2000 mg/kg in the female guinea pig, 1154–2300 mg/kg in the female rabbit, 1500 mg/kg in the male dog, 575–1150 mg/kg in the female cat, and 30–60 mg/kg in the hen. The intraperitoneal LD 50 is only slightly less, being approximately 800 mg/kg in the male rat. The dermal LD 50 is approximately 2000 mg/kg in the female rat.

Ninety percent of male rats and 30% of females were killed by a dosage of 400 mg/kg/day for 2 weeks; poisoning was evident after only two doses. Half that dosage for 2 weeks was not fatal to rats but did produce mild poisoning after 7 days, reduced weight gain, and reduced hemoglobin while producing reticulocytosis and moderate hematopoiesis of the spleen. In a 90-day study, dietary levels of 360 ppm resulted in a rapid and severe onset of organophosphate toxicity, with reduced weight gain and inhibition of cholinesterase in the plasma and brain. Levels of 80 ppm caused the same symptoms, but they were milder, and onset was more gradual. With the exception of brain cholinesterase levels, all adverse effects were reversed following cessation of treatment. The group receiving 8 ppm experienced no adverse effects. In a 2-year study, no effect on the blood or blood-forming organs was reported at a dietary level of 300 ppm (about 15 mg/kg/day), although marked inhibition of plasma and red cell cholinesterase did occur and weight gain was reduced. At 50 ppm, only female rats showed a consistent depression of plasma cholinesterase. At 10 ppm, this inhibition was transient, and the dosage of approximately 0.5 mg/kg/day was considered a no-adverse-effect level.

In an 80-week study on mice of both sexes, plasma and

erythrocyte cholinesterase activities were inhibited by dietary concentrations of 500 and 250 ppm. No increase in mortality was observed at these dosages. No effects were reported at concentrations of 5 ppm, and 0.5 mg/kg was designated as the no-adverse-effect level for mice.

In a 90-day study of male and female dogs, daily dosages of 50 mg/kg in the diet did not result in any observed adverse effects. However, a dosage of 25 mg/kg/day caused some mild, reversible cases of bile duct proliferation and liver damage. This confirmed findings of an earlier study carried out under the same conditions. Brain cholinesterase activity was not inhibited at 25 mg/kg/day. Only females given 10 mg/kg/day suffered reduced weight gains, but no additional adverse effects were noted at this dosage or at 2 mg/kg/day.

Dogs given pirimiphos-methyl in gelatin capsules at the rate of 10 mg/kg/day for 2 years suffered 25% mortality among females but no mortality among males. The survivors had loss of appetite, reduced weight gain, increased liver weight, and marked reduction of plasma, red cell, and brain cholinesterase. Somewhat less cholinesterase inhibition and less clinical effect was seen in dogs receiving 2 mg/kg/day. A dosage of 0.5 mg/kg/day produced no clinical effect, no gross or microscopic pathology, and no laboratory changes, except for occasional reduction of red cell cholinesterase and a 20–25% depression of plasma cholinesterase activity.

Absorption, Distribution, Metabolism, and Excretion Whereas it was not practical to measure a dermal LD 50, pirimiphos-methyl is absorbed from the skin. Dermal application to rabbits at the rate of 1000 mg/kg/day for 14 days caused fibrillations, loss of body weight, and death of one of six animals.

When ^{14}C-ring-labeled pirimiphos-methyl was administered to rats orally or intraperitoneally at a rate of 0.6 mg/kg, 73–81% of the dose was excreted in the urine during the first 24 hr, indicating rapid absorption, metabolism, and excretion. At 120 hr after a single oral dose, the entire dosage could be accounted for in the urine (86%) and feces (15.2%). Excretion was similar, except slower, after intraperitoneal injection. Dogs given a much larger dosage (17–18 mg/kg) also excreted most of the material during the first 24–48 hr. In cows, 99% of a single dose was recovered from the urine and feces within 7 days; during the first 3 days 0.35% of the label was excreted in milk. The milk contained 0.04 ppm of pirimiphos-methyl equivalents, of which less than 2% was unchanged compound and phosphorus metabolites.

Twelve metabolites of pirimiphos-methyl were separated by thin-layer chromatography from the urine of rats and a dog. No unchanged compound was detected and no metabolite had anticholinesterase activity. Briefly, the P—O bond is cleaved extensively and N-dealkylation and/or conjugation is a further step in the metabolism of the pyrimidine leaving group.

Biochemical Effects Systemically, pirimiphos-methyl inhibits cholinesterase, and this is the only known mechanism of its toxic action. In spite of its rapid absorption, rats given a dosage of 1.450 mg/kg did not show clear signs of poisoning until 24 hr later, when their brain cholinesterase was inhibited by 46%. Recovery of cholinesterase activity began to be apparent in 72 hr; it was complete for plasma enzyme by 96 hr but was slower for the red cell enzyme.

The mechanism by which large repeated doses of pirimiphos-methyl reduce the hemoglobin of rats is unknown. It may be caused by 2-diethylamino-4-hydroxy-6-methylpyrimidine, a metabolite formed by both mammals and plants. Although this metabolite has an acute toxicity of the same order of magnitude as the parent compound, it was (unlike the parent compound) tolerated by rats at a dosage of 400 mg/kg for 2 weeks; even so, its action on the blood was indicated by an increase in reticulocytes and a decrease in lymphocytes.

A three-generation mutagenicity study on rats did not show pirimiphos-methyl to possess any mutagenic activity. A micronucleus test in female mice also showed a lack of mutagenic activity.

No gross or histopathological observations of carcinogenic activity in excess of background levels were made in the previously mentioned dietary study on mice.

No primary irritation or sensitization was observed on the dorsal skin of rats in a 24-hr patch test using undiluted pirimiphos-methyl. The same observations were made in an identical patch test on the dorsal skin of guinea pigs using a 50% pirimiphos-methyl solution in olive oil.

Effects on Reproduction In a three-generation test, rats received dietary levels of 200, 20, and 0 ppm, none of which produced illness among parent animals. Pregnancy rates were reduced in some but not all generations. Total litter loss, litter size, litter weight, average weight of pups, pup mortality, and the incidence of abnormalities showed no dosage-related change.

When rats were fed pirimiphos-methyl throughout pregnancy, mean fetal weight was reduced, but this may have been because there were more pups per litter. No increased incidence of skeletal abnormalities was observed. The only significant soft tissue abnormality was hydronephrosis, with an incidence as high as 17%; this was said to be within the normal limits for the strain and, in any event, is a sign of immaturity rather than teratogenesis.

Rabbits showed no teratogenic effects when given 1 or 16 mg/kg/day throughout pregnancy, even though these dosages caused considerable inhibition of cholinesterase activity.

Dosing of chicken eggs with 0.3 mg pirimiphos-methyl on day 4 of incubation resulted in abnormal feathering and the induction of micromelia.

16.6.23.3 Toxicity to Humans

Experimental Exposure Pirimiphos-methyl is known to be absorbed through intact skin, from the gastrointestinal tract, and by inhalation.

Five healthy male volunteers ingested 97.8% pure pirimiphos-methyl at the rate of 0.25 mg/kg/day for 28 days.

Increases and decreases of plasma cholinesterase activity were within 12% of the predosing values, except for one depression of 21.5% on day 28. Red cell cholinesterase activity did not change significantly during exposure (FAO/WHO, 1975). The dosage at which detectable cholinesterase inhibition occurs has not been determined.

Use Experience   Pirimiphos-methyl was applied to the inside of all buildings in a village at a rate of 2 gm/m². Monitoring of the cholinesterase activity of the six sprayers and six baggers, mixers, and helpers showed no significant change following the first round of spraying in March and a slight decrease in plasma (but not whole-blood) cholinesterase activity following the second round in June. There were no complaints of illness attributable to the spray from either the operators or the approximately 3000 inhabitants. Domestic animals were not injured (Rishikish *et al.*, 1977b).

No adverse effects were observed among sprayers or village inhabitants when a pirimiphos-methyl solution was applied at the rate of 1 gm/m² to control the malaria vector *Anopheles aconitus* in central Java, Indonesia (Suplain *et al.*, 1979).

Treatment of Poisoning   See Section 16.2.2.7.

16.6.24 TEMEPHOS

16.6.24.1 Identity, Properties, and Uses

Chemical Name   Temephos is *O,O,O′,O′*-tetramethyl-*O,O′*-thiodi-*p*-phenylene diphosphorothioate.

Structure   See Table 16.16.

Synonyms   The common name temephos (BSI, ISO) is in general use. Trade names have included Abat®, Abate®, Abathion®, Biothion®, Bithion®, Nimitex®, and Swebate®. Code designations have included AC-52160 and OMS-786. The CAS registry number is 3383-96-8.

Physical and Chemical Properties   Temephos has the empirical formula $C_{16}H_{20}O_6P_2S_3$ and a molecular weight of 466.46. The pure material forms a white crystalline solid with a melting point of 30–30.5°C. The technical material forms a brown viscous liquid which is 90–95% pure. Temephos is soluble in acetonitrile, chloroform, carbon tetrachloride, diethyl ether, ethylene dichloride, toluene, and lower alkyl ketones. It is essentially insoluble in water, hexane, and methylcyclohexane. Temephos undergoes hydrolysis at either high or low pH.

History, Formulations, and Uses   Temephos was introduced first by the American Cyanamid Company in 1965. It is a nonsystemic larvicide with long residual action. It is used in the control of larvae of mosquitoes, chironomid midges, blackflies (Simuliidae), biting midges (Ceratopogonidae), moths, and sand flies (Psychodidae). On crops, it is used for the control of cutworms, thrips on citrus, and lygus bugs. It is also effective in control of human body lice. Temephos is available as 10, 43, and 50% emulsifiable concentrates; 50% wettable powder; and 1, 2, and 5% granules.

16.6.24.2 Toxicity to Laboratory Animals

Basic Findings   Male and female rats showed typical signs of cholinesterase inhibition when given single oral doses of temephos at rates as low as 750 and 500 mg/kg, respectively, but death was observed only at 6000 mg/kg or higher. The oral LD 50 in males and females was 8600 and 13,000 mg/kg, respectively. In male mice it was 4700 mg/kg. The dermal toxicity was not measured so precisely because it is not possible to apply accurately to rats a dermal dosage higher than 4000 mg/day; clearly, the dermal LD 50 was higher than that (Gaines *et al.*, 1967).

In their original studies, Gaines and his colleagues found that batches of temephos differed somewhat in acute toxicity. The cause of the trouble was found and eliminated by the manufacturer. It is not known whether the higher toxicity (oral LD 50 of 1226 mg/kg in rats) reported by Ito *et al.* (1972) was associated with a difference of manufacture or with some unidentified factor. Even less easy to explain is the report (Levinskas and Shaffer, 1970) that both the oral and dermal LD 50 values in both rats and rabbits were about 2000 mg/kg. The same may be said of the report (Goncharenko, 1975) of oral LD 50 values of 1650 and 460 mg/kg in rats and mice, respectively, a dermal LD 50 value of 1200 mg/kg in rats, and air concentrations of 40 and 12.9 mg/m³ for single and repeated exposures leading to pronounced inhibition of cholinesterase. Actually, the toxicity observed in all laboratories has been low.

All rats fed temephos at a dietary level of 2000 ppm (about 100 mg/kg/day) developed 100% inhibition of red cell cholinesterase and signs of poisoning. Eight of them died between days 5 and 10, but two survived 99 days of dosing although red cell cholinesterase remained inhibited completely and the plasma enzyme was inhibited to a lesser degree. Rats, rabbits, guinea pigs, and chickens tolerated 10 mg/kg/day for extended periods without clinical effects, and dogs tolerated 3–4 mg/kg/day, the highest levels fed. These dosages produced some inhibition of cholinesterase. However, rats and rabbits tolerated an oral dosage of 1 mg/kg/day for 35 or more days without cholinesterase inhibition (Gaines *et al.*, 1967). Levinskas and Shaffer (1970) reported similar results in rats, namely cholinesterase inhibition, but no clinical signs in rats receiving about 17.5 mg/kg/day and no inhibition in those receiving about 0.29 mg/kg/day. Dogs on a dietary level of 700 ppm (about 14 mg/kg/day) showed severe signs that were greatly reduced when the dietary level was lowered to 500 ppm.

Temephos and malathion showed an approximately fourfold potentiation in rats when they were given together at levels approaching their LD 50 values (Gaines *et al.*, 1967). However, under other conditions no potentiation was observed between temephos and 23 other organic phosphorus compounds (Levinskas and Shaffer, 1970).

The potentiation of malathion toxicity by temephos is explained, at least in part, by the fact that temephos inhibits carboxylesterase, but 1 ppm in drinking water for 8 weeks produces only a slight inhibition of the enzyme in rats (Murphy and Cheever, 1972).

Temephos in a dosage of 500 mg/kg produced a rapid onset of leg weakness in chickens, from which survivors recovered within 36 days or less. An intake of 125 mg/kg produced very mild leg weakness, followed by prompt recovery. This sign was produced in 30 days at a dosage of 15.3 mg/kg/day but not in 108 days at a level of 7.4 mg/kg/day (Gaines *et al.,* 1967). Thus the effect of temephos in chickens is similar to that of malathion, and the lack of myelin loss in hens fed the compound at a dietary level of 920 ppm (about 53 mg/kg/day) for 30 days, as reported by Levinskas and Shaffer (1970), would be expected.

Effects on Reproduction Male and female rats maintained on a dietary level of 500 ppm (about 25 mg/kg/day), sufficient to produce marked inhibition of cholinesterase and some signs of poisoning, reproduced normally with no decrease in number of litters, litter size, or viability of the young and with no increase in congenital defects (Gaines *et al.,* 1967). In another laboratory, it was found that rats maintained on a dietary level of 125 ppm from weaning through reproductive age for three successive generations suffered no adverse effect (Levinskas and Shaffer, 1970).

Temephos at oral dosage levels as high as 2.5 mg/kg/day for 422 days or at 5 mg/kg/day for 186 days caused no ill effects in sheep or their lambs (McCarthy *et al.,* 1968).

Absorption, Distribution, Metabolism, and Excretion When [³H]temephos was administered to rats by mouth, radioactivity reached a peak in the blood between 5 and 8 hr and then dissipated with a half-time of about 10 hr. Appreciable radioactivity was found only in the gastrointestinal tract and fat. Both in the feces and in the fat, most of the activity came from unchanged insecticide, but small amounts of the sulfoxide were present also. Traces of temephos were found in the urine, but the principal urinary metabolites were sulfate ester conjugates of 4,4′-thiodiphenol, 4,4′-sulfinyldiphenol, and 4,4′-sulfonyldiphenol. At least 10 other components could be extracted but were not identified. In the guinea pig, absorption apparently was less than in the rat, and biliary excretion of metabolites was demonstrated (Blinn, 1969).

Over a 90-day period, rats tolerated a diet containing 9 ppm of the sulfoxide with no apparent effect except inhibition of red cell cholinesterase activity; no inhibition occurred at 3 ppm (Levinskas and Shaffer, 1970).

Pathology Mild pathological changes occurred in the liver of some rabbits receiving 10 mg/kg/day for 30 days but not in those receiving 1 mg/kg/day for 35 days nor in any other species studied, regardless of dosage (Gaines *et al.,* 1967).

16.6.24.3 Toxicity to Humans

Experimental Exposure Temephos is highly effective for the control of mosquitoes that transmit certain hemorrhagic fevers and other serious diseases. To determine whether it would be safe to prevent these diseases by controlling the breeding of mosquitoes in cisterns and other household stores of drinking water in the tropics, the compound was administered to volunteers. An effort was made to determine the dosage that produces definite but harmless inhibition of cholinesterase. However, this effort failed because when the dosage was increased to 256 mg/person/day, the 10 volunteers refused to take the material for more than 5 days because of the obnoxious taste (the concentration of the compound in the formulation was 6400 ppm). Therefore, a formulation of one-fourth the concentration was prepared so that the dosage was reduced to 64 mg/person/day (average of 0.91 mg/kg/day). Nine previously unexposed volunteers tolerated this for 4 weeks without clinical effect and without effect on plasma or red blood cell cholinesterase. The concentration of temephos in the men's urine was proportional to dosage, and the material could still be detected at a greatly reduced concentration 3 weeks after dosing stopped (Laws *et al.,* 1967).

As another step in learning the safety of adding temephos to drinking water, a 19-month study was made of a community of about 2000 people. All cisterns and other containers of potable water in the village were treated once a month with a formulation of 1% temephos adsorbed on sand. Each individual application was adjusted to the approximate volume of water to produce a nominal concentration of 1 ppm. However, because of the adsorption and other factors, only one water sample during the entire 19-month period had a concentration greater than 0.5 ppm. In addition to the treatment of all drinking water with temephos, all premises and all containers of nonpotable water were sprayed every 2 months with 2.5% malathion emulsion, and the entire area was sprayed with malathion from the air at the rate of 0.21 kg/ha. No significant change was measured in either plasma or red blood cell cholinesterase of the villagers at any time during the study. A steady state of urinary excretion of temephos was reached after about 4.6 months. No illness attributable to the insecticides occurred and, of eight babies born to the volunteer group, all were normal (Laws *et al.,* 1968).

Temephos has been successfully used in an eradication of mosquitos (*Aedes aegypti*) from Cayman Brac and Little Cayman in the West Indies between January 1970 and March 1972. Indoor walls of the houses were treated with a 1.5% emulsion, while a 1.5% wettable suspension was used on outdoor walls, unpainted surfaces, and areas around outdoor water containers. One percent granules were also used to produce a nominal concentration of 1 ppm in potable water sources of wells and roof catchments. No adverse effects have been reported among either residents or those who applied the temephos (Nathan and Giglioli, 1982).

A 2% formulation of temephos in pyrax powder was found both safe and effective for combating human lice. The material was applied to test subjects and their bedding from a shaker or to clothed subjects from a power duster using 56.7 and 33.9 gm per person, respectively (Steinberg *et al.,* 1972).

The threshold limit value of 10 mg/m³ indicates that occupational intake at a rate of 1.4 mg/kg/day is considered safe.

Treatment of Poisoning If treatment were required, it would need to be according to principles discussed in Section 16.2.2.7.

16.6.25 THIOMETON

16.6.25.1 Identity, Properties, and Uses

Chemical Name Thiometon is *O,O*-dimethyl *S*-ethylmercaptoethyl dithiophosphate.

Structure See Table 16.16.

Synonyms Although the common name thiometon (BSI, ISO) has wide popularity, it is not used in the USSR (M-81), France (dithiometon), West Germany, Portugal, or Turkey. Intrathion has been used as a common name in Eastern Europe. Trade names have included Ekatin® and Thiomethon®. The CAS registry number is 640-15-3.

Physical and Chemical Properties Thiometon has the empirical formula $C_6H_{15}O_2PS_3$ and a molecular weight of 246.35. The pure material forms a colorless oil with a characteristic odor. The boiling point is 110°C at 0.1 mm Hg. The density is 1.209 at 20°C. The vapor pressure at the same temperature is 3×10^{-4} mm Hg. The refractive index is 1.5515. Thiometon is hardly soluble in light in petroleum but is soluble in most organic solvents. Its solubility in water is 25°C is 200 ppm. In its pure state thiometon is of low stability, but it is stable in apolar solvents, especially xylene or chlorobenzene. Thiometon is unstable under alkaline conditions. Formulations are said to be stable for at least 2 years when stored below 40°C.

History, Formulations, and Uses Thiometon was introduced in 1953 by Bayer-Leverkusen and Sandoz AG. It is a systemic insecticide and acaricide suitable for controlling sucking insects—mainly aphids and mites. Thiometon is available as 20 and 25% emulsifiable concentrates and 2% dust.

16.6.25.2 Toxicity to Laboratory Animals

Basic Findings The acute toxicity of pure thiometon is only moderate, but formulations may be significantly more toxic than the pure material. Klotzsche (1958b) found oral LD 50 values of 225 mg/kg for the chemically pure material, 190 mg/kg for a commercial sample, and 120 mg/kg for the active ingredient in a formulation. Wilhelm *et al.* (1974) reported a comparable value of 75 mg/kg for a formulation.

The reported results of repeated dosing of rats are inconsistent without a reason being apparent. In one study in which groups of male rats were given 0, 5, 10, 15, and 20 mg/kg/day, respectively, all the animals showed mild to severe illness interpreted as poisoning; all died, except four receiving 5 mg/kg/day and a single rat receiving 10 mg/kg/day. The survivors recovered after 10 weeks while still receiving thiometon; when they were killed after 13 weeks, histological study failed to reveal specific pathology.

In another study lasting much longer (12 months), rats survived the daily administration of thiometon by stomach tube at rates as high as 18 mg/kg/day; the only untoward effect was a marked reduction in weight gain in males on 18 mg/kg/day and a slight reduction in those on 6 mg/kg/day. Dosages of 2, 6, and 18 mg/kg/day caused definite inhibition of plasma and red cell cholinesterase activity; a dosage of 1 mg/kg/day caused questionable inhibition of plasma enzyme but definite inhibition of red cell enzyme. Organ weights and histological findings were normal on autopsy (FAO/WHO, 1970).

Small groups of dogs received 0, 1, 2, 10, and 50 mg/kg/day for 6 months. All dogs in the 50 mg/kg/day group died within 1 week, and one died in the 10 mg/kg/day group, whereupon the dosage of the survivors was reduced to 5 mg/kg/day. All findings (including plasma cholinesterase) in dogs receiving 1, 2, or 5 mg/kg/day were normal, except that red cell cholinesterase was inhibited even at 1 mg/kg/day. Brain cholinesterase showed no depletion at the lowest dosage but definite and marked inhibition at 2 and 5 mg/kg/day, respectively (FAO/WHO, 1970).

A dosage of 0.008 mg/kg/day via drinking water was reported to slow down positive conditioned reflexes of rats (Cabejszek *et al.,* 1967). The relationship of this finding to cholinesterase inhibition under the same conditions is unknown.

Absorption, Distribution, Metabolism, and Excretion It has been reported that cats fed milk from cows acutely poisoned by thiometon developed typical anticholinesterase effects but recovered quickly (Balogh *et al.,* 1972). Apparently, no other study has been made of the transfer of the compound or its possibly toxic metabolites to milk.

Effects on Organs and Tissues Rabbits injected intraperitoneally with a Polish sample of thiometon at a rate of 100 mg/kg developed toxic lesions and proliferation of fibroblasts in the myocardium and endocardium within 24 hr. In addition to hyperemia, the myocardium showed foci of inflammatory, fatty, degenerative, and necrotic changes. In rabbits that received atropine and PAM at rates of 0.5 and 7 mg/kg, respectively, the lesions were more pronounced (Giermaziak, 1973; Biernat and Giermaziak, 1974). These results are unconfirmed.

Beagle dogs treated with thiometon at rates ranging from about 0.5 to 1.5 mg/kg/day for 2 years developed histological changes in the optic nerve, and a calf showed changes in a peripheral sensory nerve. Changes in motor nerves were very slight (Kono *et al.,* 1975), and functional change apparently was absent.

Effects on Reproduction   Thiometon, in the form of a commercial formulation, was administered to rabbits by stomach tube at rates of 1 or 5 mg/kg/day (active ingredient) during days 6–18 of pregnancy. There was no evidence of a teratogenic or embryotoxic effect (Klotzsche, 1970).

16.6.25.3 Toxicity to Humans

Use Experience   Lowered cholinesterase activity was found in the blood of several workers in a trimethon plant; some of them had transient subjective complaints, but there were no signs of illness (Katja *et al.,* 1973; Wilhelm *et al.,* 1974).

A case of contact dermatitis attributed to thiometon has been reported (Maric, 1970).

The compound has been mentioned as one capable of changing intraocular pressure and therefore to be avoided by agricultural workers with glaucoma, with only one eye, or with a wide range of other ophthalmological difficulties, including conjunctivitis and color blindness (Dugel'nyy, 1971). Apparently, there is no evidence that thiometon has any more effect on intraocular pressure than any other equally anticholinergic compound or that change in intraocular pressure has been a practical problem under conditions of agricultural use.

Atypical Effects of Various Origins   Twelve female agricultural workers exposed to thiometon were followed for at least 6 months. Changes were reported in catalase, cytochrome oxidase, and ceruloplasmin, and the changes persisted in some of the workers for the entire period (Jordanova *et al.,* 1974). Because these parameters are not commonly examined in persons poisoned by this or other organic phosphorus compounds, interpretation of the findings is difficult.

Treatment of Poisoning   See Section 16.2.2.7.

16.6.26 CHLORPYRIFOS-METHYL

16.6.26.1 Identity, Properties, and Uses

Chemical Name   Chlorpyrifos-methyl is *O,O*-dimethyl *O*--(3,5,6-trichloro-2-pyridyl) phosphorothionate.

Structure   See Table 16.16.

Synonyms   Chlorpyrifos-methyl (ANSI, BSI, ESA, ISO) is also known by the trade names Dowco® 214 and Reldan®. Code designations include ENT 27520. The CAS registry number is 5598-13-0.

Physical and Chemical Properties   Chlorpyrifos-methyl has the empirical formula $C_7H_7Cl_3NO_3PS$ and a molecular weight of 322.51. The pure material is a crystalline solid with a melting point of 45.5–46.5°C. Its solubility in water is 5 ppm at

25°C. The vapor pressure is 4.22×10^{-5} mm Hg at 25°C. Chlorpyrifos-methyl decomposes 110 times more rapidly than chlorpyrifos at pH 5 (Kenga, 1971). It also has a greater tendency to undergo hydrolysis than chlorpyrifos.

Uses   Chlorpyrifos-methyl is an insecticide and acaricide.

16.6.26.2 Toxicity to Laboratory Animals

Basic Findings   Chlorpyrifos-methyl has been found to be much less toxic to mammals than chlorpyrifos, with an oral LD 50 in rats of 1500 mg/kg (Eto, 1979).

16.6.26.3 Toxicity to Humans

Experimental Oral Exposure   Administration of chlorpyrifos-methyl tablets at rates of 0.03 or 0.10 mg/kg for 4 weeks did not cause any clinical toxicity or diminished cholinesterase activities in the erythrocytes or plasma (Griffin *et al.,* 1976).

16.6.27 FAMPHUR

16.6.27.1 Identity, Properties, and Uses

Chemical Name   Famphur is *O,O*-dimethyl-*O,p*-(dimethylsulfamoyl)phenyl phosphorothionate.

Structure   See Table 16.16.

Synonyms   The common name famphur (ESA) is generally accepted. It is also known by the trade names Bo Ana®, Famophos®, and Warbex®. Code designations include AC-38023 and ENT-26544. The CAS registry number is 52-85-7.

Physical and Chemical Properties   Famphur has the empirical fomrula $C_{10}H_{16}NO_5PS_2$ and a molecular weight of 325.36. The pure compound is in the form of crystals with a melting point of 52.5–53.5°C. Famphur is highly soluble in chlorinated hydrocarbons, slightly soluble in polar solvents, and insoluble in aliphatic hydrocarbons.

History and Uses   First introduced by the American Cyanamid Company in 1961, famphur is a systemic insecticide which may be applied by feeding, by pour-on, or intramuscularly to cattle to eliminate grubs.

16.6.27.2 Toxicity to Laboratory Animals

Basic Findings   Gaines and Linder (1986) reported the oral LD 50 values for rats to be 28 mg/kg in adult males, 51 mg/kg in adult females, and 73 mg/kg in weanling males. The acute dermal LD 50 values for rats are 400 mg/kg for adult males and 533 mg/kg for adult females (Gaines and Linder, 1986). The oral LD 50 for sheep is 400 mg/kg (Eto, 1979).

16.6.27.3 Toxicity to Humans

Use Experience   Veterinarians treating grub infestations in cattle with pour-on applications of famphur and other organic phosphorus pesticides in poorly ventilated areas occasionally reported nausea, headaches, and irritations of the throat and facial skin. Blood cholinesterase activities were not reduced in these cases, and alkyl phosphate metabolites were only occasionally found in the urine (Beat and Morgan, 1977).

16.6.28 RONNEL

16.6.28.1 Identity, Properties, and Uses

Chemical Name   Ronnel is O,O-dimethyl O-(2,4,5-trichlorophenyl)phosphorothioate.

Structure   See Table 16.16.

Synonyms   The common name ronnel (ANSI, ESA) is generally accepted. It is also known as fenchlorophos (BSI, ISO), as dimethyl trichlorophenyl thiophosphate, and by the trade names Ectoral®, Etrolene®, Korlan®, Nankor®, Trolene®, and Viozene®. The CAS registry number is 299-84-3.

Physical and Chemical Properties   Ronnel has the empirical formula $C_8H_8Cl_3O_3PS$ and a molecular weight of 321.57. It is a white powder with a melting point of 41°C and a boiling point of 97°C at 0.01 mm Hg. Vapor pressure is 8×10^{-4} mm Hg at 25°C. Ronnel is very soluble in acetone, carbon tetrachloride, ether, methylene chloride, toluene, and kerosene, although only slightly soluble (40 ppm at 25°C) in water. Demethylation occurs in slightly alkaline solutions, and hydrolysis occurs in strong alkali.

History and Uses   The Dow Chemical Company first introduced Ronnel in 1954. It was the first animal systemic insecticide and continues to be effectively used in livestock in oral and contact applications. Ronnel has also been successfully used in humans as a systemic antiparasitic (see Section 16.6.28.3). It is known to be effective on contact against cockroaches and flies.

16.6.28.2 Toxicity to Laboratory Animals

Basic Findings   Ronnel has low mammalian toxicity, with an acute oral LD 50 of 1250 mg/kg for male rats and 2630 mg/kg for female rats (Gaines, 1969).

16.6.28.3 Toxicity to Humans

Therapeutic Use   A group of 21 patients with creeping eruption (larva migrans) were given ronnel orally in doses of 10 mg/kg/day. After 5 days on the treatment, 80% of the patients were cured. This figure increased to 90% after 10 days. Although five of the patients reported side effects, which included nausea, weakness, blurred vision, and serpiginous

ulcers, none were of a serious or prolonged nature (Balthrop, 1966).

Use Experience   Nausea, headaches, and irritations of the throat and facial skin were occasionally reported by veterinarians treating grub infestations in cattle with pour-on applications of ronnel and other organic phosphorus pesticides in poorly ventilated areas. Blood cholinesterase activities were not reduced in these cases, however, and alkyl phosphate metabolites were only occasionally found in the urine (Beat and Morgan, 1977).

16.7 DIETHOXY COMPOUNDS OF CATEGORY IV

The diethoxy compounds constitute the next to largest group of organic phosphorus insecticides. The identity and chemical structure of those known to have affected people or to have been studied in volunteers are shown in Table 16.36. The only illness they have produced is acute, cholinergic poisoning.

16.7.1 PARATHION

16.7.1.1 Identity, Properties, and Uses

Chemical Name   Parathion is O,O-diethyl-O-(4-nitrophenyl)phosphorothioate.

Structure   See Table 16.36.

Synonyms   Parathion (BSI, ISO) also has been called AAT, DNTP, ethyl parathion, nitrostigine, and SNP. In the USSR, thiophos is the official name. Proprietary names are Alkron®, Alleron®, Aphamite®, Bladan®, Etilon®, Folidol®, Fosferno®, Niram®, Paraphos®, and Rhodiatox®. Code designations have included ACC-3,422 E-605, and OMS-19. The CAS registry number is 56-38-2.

Physical and Chemical Properties   Parathion has the empirical formula $C_{10}H_{14}NO_5PS$ and a molecular weight of 291.27. The pure material is a yellowish liquid at temperatures above 6°C. Parathion is freely soluble in alcohols, esters, ethers, ketones, and aromatic hydrocarbons, but is practically insoluble in water (20 ppm) or in petroleum ether, kerosene, or spray oil. Parathion is stable at a pH below 7.5.

History, Formulations, and Uses   Parathion currently is used as dilute sprays, which are prepared by the operator from 15 or 25% wettable powders or from emulsifiable concentrates of 50% or less. Dusts are used also. They may be purchased ready mixed in concentrations of 5% or less. Technical parathion, which is a deep brown to yellow liquid and is approximately 98% pure, may be encountered under industrial conditions and in formulating establishments. Aerosol formulations containing up to 10% parathion may be used in greenhouses.

Table 16.36
Structure of Diethoxy Organic Phosphorus Compounds of the Form $(C_2H_5-O)_2P(R)X$

Compound	=R	X	Compound	=R	X
azinphos-ethyl	=S	$-S-CH_2-N$ (3,4-dihydro-4-oxo-1,2,3-benzotriazin-3-yl)	dioxathion	=S	$-S-$ (1,4-dioxane ring) $-S-P(=S)(O-C_2H_5)_2$
carbophenothion	=S	$-S-CH_2-S-$ (phenyl) $-Cl$	disulfoton	=S	$-S-CH_2-CH_2-S-C_2H_5$
chlorfenvinphos	=O	$-O-C(=CHCl)-$ (2,4-dichlorophenyl)	ethion	=S	$-S-CH_2-S-\overset{\displaystyle S}{\overset{\|}{P}}-(O-C_2H_5)_2$
chlorphoxim	=S	$-O-N=C-$ (2-chlorophenyl), with $N\equiv C$	fensulfothion	=S	$-O-$ (phenyl) $-\overset{\displaystyle O}{\underset{\displaystyle O}{\overset{\|}{\underset{\|}{S}}}}-CH_3$
chlorpyrifos	=S	$-O-$ (3,5,6-trichloro-2-pyridyl)	mephosfolan	=O	$-N=C\big\langle\begin{smallmatrix}S-CH-CH_3\\S-CH_2\end{smallmatrix}$ (dithiolane ring)
coumaphos	=S	$-O-$ (3-chloro-4-methylcoumarin-7-yl)	parathion	=S	$-O-$ (phenyl) $-NO_2$
demeton-O	=S	$-O-CH_2-CH_2-S-C_2H_5$	phorate	=S	$-S-CH_2-S-C_2H_5$
demeton-S	=O	$-S-CH_2-CH_2-S-C_2H_5$	phosalone	=S	$-S-CH_2-N$ (6-chloro-2-oxo-benzoxazolin-3-yl)
dialifos	=S	$-S-\underset{ClH_2C}{\overset{}{CH}}-N$ (phthalimide ring)	phosfolan	=O	$-N=C\big\langle\begin{smallmatrix}S-CH_2\\S-CH_2\end{smallmatrix}$ (dithiolane ring)
diazinon	=S	$-O-$ (2-isopropyl-6-methylpyrimidin-4-yl)	phoxim	=S	$-O-N=C-$ (phenyl), with $C\equiv N$
dichlofenthion	=S	$-O-$ (2,4-dichlorophenyl)	TEPP	=O	$-O-\overset{\displaystyle }{\underset{\displaystyle O}{\overset{}{\underset{\|}{P}}}}-(O-C_2H_5)_2$

Cords impregnated with parathion for fly control contain about 100 mg/linear foot. Parathion finds almost its entire use in agriculture including nurseries and greenhouses.

16.7.1.2 Toxicity to Laboratory Animals

Basic Findings Signs of poisoning are typical of organic phosphorus anticholinesterases generally (see Section 16.2.2.2). Irritation and sensitization are not significant.

As shown in Table 16.37, the acute oral toxicity of parathion varies from about 2 to 30 mg/kg, depending on species and vehicle. Rats show a striking sex difference in susceptibility but other species do not. Estrogens increase the susceptibility of male rats, and androgens decrease the susceptibility of females to parathion (DuBois *et al.*, 1949).

Strains of rats apparently vary in their susceptibility. Some investigators have reported toxic symptoms, growth retardation, and death at dietary levels of 50 ppm (about 2.5 mg/kg/day) or above (Barnes and Denz, 1951). Others found no clinical effect in 2-year tests at 50 ppm and only slight toxic signs and retardation of growth but no decrease in food consumption or increase of mortality at 100 ppm

Table 16.37
Single-Dose LD 50 for Parathion

Species	Route	LD 50 (mg/kg)	Reference
Rat, M	oral	15	DuBois *et al.* (1949)
Rat, F	oral	3	DuBois *et al.* (1949)
Rat, M	oral	30	Frawley *et al.* (1952a)
Rat, F	oral	3	Frawley *et al.* (1952a)
Rat, M	oral	15	Shaffer and West (1960)
Rat, M	oral	13	Gaines (1960)
Rat, F	oral	3.6	Gaines (1960)
Rat, M	oral	16	Pasquet *et al.* (1976)
Rat, F	oral	6	Pasquet *et al.* (1976)
Rat, M	dermal	21	Gaines (1960)
Rat, F	dermal	6.8	Gaines (1960)
Rat, F	dermal	8	Pasquet *et al.* (1976)
Rat, M	intraperitoneal	7	DuBois *et al.* (1949)
Rat, F	intraperitoneal	4	DuBois *et al.* (1949)
Rat	intraperitoneal	5.5	DuBois and Coon (1952)
Mouse	oral	25	Frawley *et al.* (1952a)
Mouse, F	oral	12.8	Natoff (1967)
Mouse, F	subcutaneous	0.06	Natoff (1967)
Mouse, M	intraperitoneal	5[a]	DuBois *et al.* (1949)
Mouse, M	intraperitoneal	10[b]	DuBois *et al.* (1949)
Mouse, F	intraperitoneal	9–10[b]	DuBois *et al.* (1949)
Mouse, F	intraperitoneal	10.4–11.4[c]	Engbaek and Jensen (1951)
Mouse, F	intraperitoneal	2.29	Natoff (1967)
Mouse, F	intravenous	0.59	Natoff (1967)
Guinea pig	oral	32	Frawley *et al.* (1952a)
Guinea pig	intraperitoneal	12	Klimmer and Pfaff (1955)
Dog	oral	3.0–5.0[d]	Hazelton and Holland (1950)
Dog	intraperitoneal	12–20	DuBois *et al.* (1949)
Cat	intraperitoneal	3–5	DuBois *et al.* (1949)

[a] Tests performed in March.
[b] Tests performed in June.
[c] Different commercial preparations.
[d] Lethal dose.

(Hazleton and Holland, 1950; Lehman, 1951, 1952). There is no doubt that repeated ingestion of parathion at a dietary level of 125 ppm (about 6.25 mg/kg) causes severe illness, growth suppression, and death in rats (Edson and Noakes, 1960).

The 90-dose LD 50 was found in two studies to be 3.5 and 3.1 mg/kg/day, with corresponding chronicity factors of 1.03 and 1.16 (Hayes, 1967).

A dietary level of 5 ppm produces inhibition of red cell cholinesterase in rats (Frawley and Fuyat, 1957). This dietary level corresponds to about 0.25 mg/kg/day in the rat but to only 0.117 mg/kg/day in the dog. The red cell enzyme is more sensitive in the dog, which reacts slightly but significantly to 0.021 mg/kg/day (Frawley and Fuyat, 1957). Others have found rat acetylcholinesterase more sensitive only *in vitro* (Engbaek and Jensen, 1951).

A dietary level of 1 ppm (about 0.05 mg/kg/day) produces no change in cholinesterase or other indices in the rat (Edson and Noakes, 1960).

Protein-deficient rats are more susceptible than normal rats to acute poisoning by parathion (Boyd *et al.*, 1969).

Absorption, Distribution, and Excretion Absorption takes place readily through any portal. Fatal human poisoning has followed ingestion, skin exposure, and also inhalation with varying degrees of skin exposure. The vapor pressure of parathion is so low that respiratory exposure to vapor alone is not a likely cause of poisoning. Respiratory exposure to fine dust or aerosol preparations may be extremely hazardous.

On the basis of radioautographic studies in humans and animals, it appears that skin absorption is transepidermal (Fredriksson, 1961). The rate of dermal absorption of parathion in the rabbit is 0.059 μg/min/cm^2, while that of paraoxon is much higher (0.32 μg/min/cm^2). The animals exhibit about a 10-fold individual variation in permeability of the skin (Nabb *et al.*, 1966).

Respiratory absorption presumably is rapid and essentially complete. However, if aerosols are excluded, dosage is limited by the vapor pressure of parathion. A dosage of 0.88 mg/kg/day for young rats may be calculated from the tabular values for the vapor pressure at 25°C and their respiratory volume. (A similar calculation indicates a dosage of 0.14 mg/kg/day for a human adult at rest.) Rats tolerated for more than 2 days without any sign of discomfort air that had been carried through a saturation chain at room temperatures varying from 20 to 31°C. Actual exposure was for 23 hr/day, 1 hr being required for cleaning the exposure chamber. Some flies placed in the chamber with rats were knocked down in 95 min, and all were motionless in 230 min. This exposure caused a rapid depression of plasma and red cell cholinesterase in the rats, but there was little or no additional depression after day 6. In one replication, all rats died on day 13, and in the second test all died on day 16 (Hayes, 1982).

Other results illustrate how the marked differences in the rate of absorption by different routes require different dosage levels in order to achieve similar absorption, excretion, and outcome. Dosages that proved fatal to dogs had the following very different averages: 955, dermal; 20, oral; 4.0, respiratory;

and 4.6 mg/kg, intravenous; but they led to the following similar average rates of excretion of *p*-nitrophenol: 0.676, dermal; 1.468, oral; 1.003, respiratory; and 0.571 mg/hr, intravenous (Hayes, 1982).

The distribution of parathion in the tissues is discussed in Section 16.2.2.1.

The metabolism of parathion is shown in Fig. 16.6, modified from Plapp and Casida (1958). The conversion of parathion to paraoxon (reaction 1) was demonstrated early (Diggle and Gage, 1950; Gage, 1953). It is the only change known to occur *in vivo* that increases the toxicity of parathion. Reaction 1 is promoted by microsomal enzymes, requires NADPH and oxygen, and is inducible. The same enzyme system with the same requirement for NADPH and oxygen also produces diethyl hydrogen phosphorothionate (reaction 2) (Neal, 1967b). However, the two reactions (1 and 2) respond differently to various stimulators and inhibitors, suggesting either that two oxidative enzymes are involved or that there are two different binding sites for parathion which share a common electron transport pathway (Neal, 1967b). Both reactions occur in the rat lung and brain, as well as in the liver. In general, the enzymes from different tissues are induced and inhibited in similar ways, but those in the lung differ in not being induced by phenobarbital or 3-methylcholanthrene (Norman and Neal, 1976).

Later it was shown that diethylphosphoric acid may be formed by liver microsomes, and it was then concluded that all three metabolites are formed nonenzymatically via different breakdown pathways from a common enzymatically formed intermediate, namely a sulfine derivative of parathion (Kamataki *et al.*, 1976).

In vitro studies of intact rat liver microsomes and of a reconstituted mixed-function oxidase system from rat liver showed that the sulfur atom released in the metabolism of parathion to paraoxon becomes covalently bound predominantly, if not exclusively, to cytochrome P-450. At least 95% of this bound sulfur is free of the remainder of the parathion molecule. About 50% of the binding is to the side chain of the cysteine in the cytochrome P-450 apoenzyme to form a hydrodisulfide. The binding apparently leads to cross-linking of protein to form high molecular weight complexes (Kamataki and

Neal, 1976). Binding of sulfur results in progressive inhibition of parathion metabolism (Yoshihara and Neal, 1977). There is agreement that *in vitro* metabolism of parathion is characterized by progressive reduction of the rate of this metabolism (Yoshihara and Neal, 1977; Morelli and Nakatsugawa, 1978). However, there is some doubt regarding the mechanism. Evidence indicates that the reduction in rate is a direct result of the binding of sulfur to cytochrome P-450 (Yoshihara and Neal, 1977; Dalvi and Howell, 1978), but the explanation may be more complex (Morelli and Nakatsugawa, 1978).

Furthermore, only low levels of sulfur binding in liver were observed after parathion was administered to rats *in vivo*. This was explained by *in vitro* experiments indicating that some sulfur from parathion fails to bind to protein but forms water-soluble compounds and that some sulfur that is covalently bound initially is gradually removed by glutathione and other thiols, thus partially restoring activity of the enzymes (Morelli and Nakatsugawa, 1978).

Besides the metabolites already mentioned, parathion is metabolized to *O*-ethylphosphoric acid, phosphoric acid, and inorganic sulfate, as shown by using ^{35}S and ^{32}P as labels (Nakatsugawa *et al.*, 1969b).

The excretion of parathion metabolites has been demonstrated in the urine only (Fredriksson and Bigelow, 1961). In the monkey, *p*-nitrophenol is excreted faster than moieties containing the ethyl group. Under one set of experimental conditions, excretion of ^{14}C-ring-labeled compound was 75 and 90% complete in 6 and 24 hr, respectively, compared to 35 and 54% for ^{14}C-ethyl-labeled parathion at the same intervals (Copeland *et al.*, 1971). Although the matter has received little study, there is some indication that unchanged parathion is excreted on the skin surface, presumably in the sebum. Such excretion would represent a special case of the well-recognized distribution of the compound to neutral fat.

Effects on Reproduction   Radioactive parathion passes the placental barrier (Villenueve *et al.*, 1972). One-sixth or more of an LD 50 dose of parathion administered orally or intraperitoneally to pregnant rats caused prenatal and postnatal death of the young and reduced weight gain of the surviving young, but it caused no developmental abnormalities (Fish,

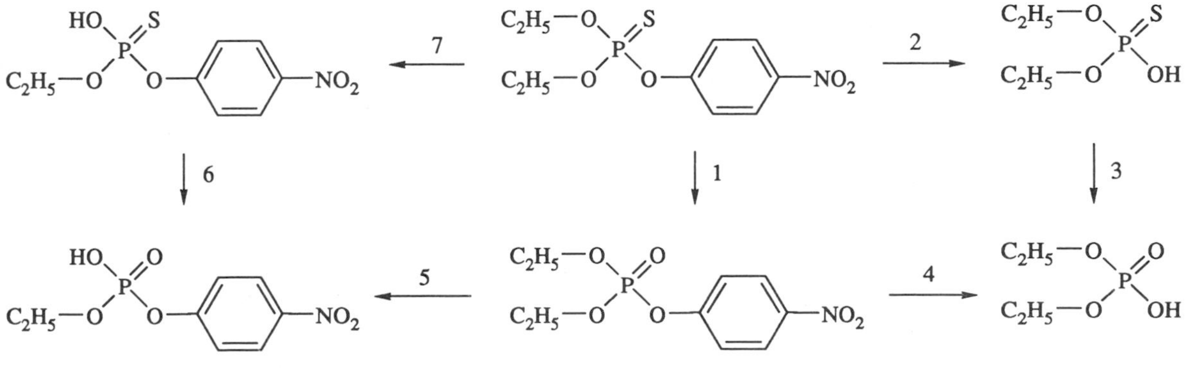

Figure 16.6   Metabolism of parathion.

1966). Other studies involving the same or other routes show that parathion is toxic to the fetus but not teratogenic (Kimbrough and Gaines, 1968; Noda *et al.*, 1972; Talens and Woolley, 1973). The greater susceptibility of the fetus is in spite of the fact that inhibition of cholinesterase activity in fetal blood is less than that in maternal blood following dosing of the mother (Villeneuve *et al.*, 1972).

At a dietary level of 10 ppm, reproduction is either normal (Hazleton and Holland, 1950) or borderline (Barnes and Denz, 1951). At higher dietary levels approaching those dangerous to adults, litters are produced but the young may die. Independent studies confirm that fetal or infant rats are more susceptible than adults to parathion, but pretreatment with phenobarbital antagonizes the toxicity of this compound (Harbison, 1975a,b). The greater susceptibility of weanlings is due to their poorly developed microsomal enzymes and also greater inherent susceptibility of the young brain (Gagne and Brodeur, 1972; Benke and Murphy, 1975).

Effects on Organs and Tissues Parathion in their diet failed to induce dominant lethal effects in mice (Jorgenson *et al.*, 1976).

Oral administration of 16 mg/kg parathion to mice resulted in 20% mortality, signs of cholinergic toxicity, and a significant but transiently reduced primary immune response to sheep red blood cells. A dose of 4 mg/kg did not cause the toxic response or immunosuppression. The mechanisms responsible for this action remain uncertain (Casale *et al.*, 1984).

16.7.1.3 Toxicity to Humans

Experimental Exposure Separate studies of repeated oral administration of parathion reached excellent agreement regarding the minimal dosage necessary to inhibit plasma cholinesterase (see Dosage Response below). No study was carried to the point of clinical effect or even inhibition of red cell cholinesterase.

Studies of four volunteers showed that oral dosages of 1 and 2 mg/person/day did not inhibit the cholinesterase but resulted in easily measurable, distinctly different rates of excretion. Excretion of paranitrophenol was 60% complete in 4 hr and 86% complete in 8 hr. Excretion of diethyl phosphate was more protracted (Morgan *et al.*, 1977).

Five grams of 2% parathion dust were applied to the right hand and forearm of each of several volunteers at different ambient temperatures. The dust was held within a narrow plastic bag, securely taped at the elbow and left in place for 2 hr. Following exposure, the arms were carefully washed. Maximal excretion of the metabolite, *p*-nitrophenol, occurred 5–6 hr after the dust was applied, regardless of temperature, and decreased to very low levels within 40 hr. The excretion was proportional to temperature, as shown by the average total recovery of *p*-nitrophenol: 0.196 mg/person at 14.4°C, 0.246 mg/person at 21.1°C, 0.287 mg/man at 27.8°C, and 0.804 mg/person at 40.6°C. The highest rate of excretion of *p*-

nitrophenol during a 2-hr interval was 0.155 mg/hr, and the highest rate at any one void was 0.174 mg/hr, both at the highest temperature (Funckes *et al.*, 1963a).

In addition to this very clear demonstration of the dependence of the rate of absorption of parathion on ambient temperature, Dr. Funckes and his colleagues carried out other studies on the effects of dermal and respiratory exposure, part of which were published (G. R. Hayes *et al.*, 1964; Hartwell *et al.*, 1964). Unfortunately, the exposures were carried out for different durations and under such a variety of conditions that they were difficult to summarize or interpret. Part of the difficulty arose from the fact that the concentrations of parathion in atmospheres breathed by volunteers were not measured, and the rates of excretion of *p*-nitrophenol were expressed in different time units, often as 24-hr averages. The situation was helped greatly by original records and other information supplied by Dr. Melvin H. Goodwin, Jr., who was director of the laboratory where the work was done but who was not personally involved in the toxicological investigations. This permitted the preparation of Table 16.38, in which the maximal rate of excretion of *p*-nitrophenol expressed as milligrams per hour makes it possible to compare diverse experiments and draw conclusions entirely consistent with what others have found regarding the toxicology of parathion in humans. Specifically, everything in Table 16.38 is consistent with the results summarized in Figure 16.3 and with the findings of Davies *et al.* (1967) discussed under Laboratory Findings.

Special interest attaches to the test designated No. 14 in Table 16.38, in which a volunteer became sick and vomited following only 10 min of respiratory exposure. That the maximal measured rate of excretion (0.264 mg/hr) was so low in association with clinical illness is easy to understand when one considers that exposure was so brief and the urine sample from which the rate was determined was collected over a 5-hr period. The time necessary for the metabolism of parathion to *p*-nitrophenol and excretion of the latter in the urine is several hours, and this leads to some relative reduction of the excretion peak following very brief absorption. Furthermore, the true peak must have been averaged out in a 5-hr sample. What was remarkable about the measured rate was not that it was so low but that it was so high. Because of its potentially cumulative effect and, especially, its final intensity, it is difficult to evaluate the respiratory exposure that led to illness in this test in terms of any conceivable occupational exposure. Hartwell *et al.* (1964) commented on the progressive increase in the excretion of *p*-nitrophenol during the first four of a series of five daily exposures to parathion vapor and concluded that it might have been associated with "unrecognized residues that accumulated as condensate in the generator after previous exposures." Be that as it may, the rate of generation of parathion vapor was increased in the fifth exposure, thus reinforcing whatever cumulative effect already was present. Although the concentration of the vapor was unmeasured, it seems likely that immediate evacuation of workers would be ordered if such vapor was released in an occupational situation. It was de-

Table 16.38
Summary of Certain Studies of Parathion in Volunteers

Test no.	Route[a]	Area	Duration of exposure (hr)	Temperature (°C)	Maximal excretion[b] (mg/hr)	Cholinesterase depression		Published designation[c]
						Red cell (%)	Plasma (%)	
1	d	forearm	2	14.4	0.015	0	0	I
2	d	forearm	2	21.1	0.025	0	0	I
3	d	forearm	2	27.8	0.024	0	0	I
4	d	forearm	2	40.6	0.155	0	0	I
5	d	forearm	2/day × 5	40.6	0.084	0	0	II, Ser. 1, A
6	d	forearm	1.7	27.2	0.068	0	0	II, Ser. 1, B + C
7	d	forearm	2.	20.6	0.021	0	0	II, Ser. 1, B + C
8	d	forearm	1.5	39.4	0.175	0	0	II, Ser. 1, D
9	d	body	7	15.6	0.508	10	59	II, Ser. 2, A
10	d	body	3	?	0.555	0	18	II, Ser. 2, B
11	d	back	3	11.1	0.094	0	0[d]	II, Ser. 3
12	d	back	3	26.7	0.411	0	0[d]	II,
13	d	back	3	40.0	0.537	0	50	II, Ser. 3
14	r		0.16		0.264[e,f]	98	83	III, Ser. 2
15	r		2.5		0.121	24	0	III, Ser. 3
16	d	back + chest	2.3	37.8	0.334			
17	r		2.3		0.121			
18	r + d	back + chest	2.3	37.8	3.044[g,h]			

[a] d, Dermal; r, respiratory.

[b] Excretion of p-nitrophenol.

[c] References: I, Funckes et al. (1963a); II, G. R. Hayes et al. (1964); III, Hartwell et al. (1964).

[d] Level was above normal, perhaps indicating overcompensation.

[e] Based on a 5-hr sample.

[f] Volunteer became ill.

[g] Based on a 0.75-hr sample.

[h] Volunteer severely poisoned.

scribed as follows: "When the face mask was removed from the volunteer, a heavy acrid fog was being emitted from the breathing tube and air-intake port of the chamber."

The illness resulting from the test designated No. 18 was more serious. It appeared unlikely that the man would have survived without the prompt and intensive treatment he received. It must be noted that maximal excretion of p-nitrophenol by the volunteer who received both dermal and respiratory exposure was many times greater than the sum of the maximal rates associated with dermal (test No. 16) and respiratory (test No. 17) exposure separately. No explanation was available. No skin injury was noted in the man who absorbed parathion at a high rate. However, as discussed in Section 3.2.2.5, injury to the superficial barrier of the skin may exist without being noticeable, and it may account for as much as a 40-fold increase in absorption rate.

Maximal urinary excretion of radioactive material came 8–12 hr after the application of a very small quantity of radioactive parathion to the ventral forearm, where it remained without washing for 24 hr. Some excretion was still detectable 96–120 hr after application of the material, which had been removed as well as possible by washing (Feldmann and Maibach, 1974). Other reports are in general agreement, and any small real differences that may exist are associated with unrec-

ognized differences of experimental conditions. Thus the following other intervals from first dermal exposure to maximal excretion have been reported: 5–6 hr (Funckes et al., 1963a) and 4–10 hr (Hayes et al., 1964).

Men who applied parathion to orchards and who volunteered for study absorbed from 0.1 to 2.8% (mean 0.9%) of the compound deposited on their exposed skin (Durham and Wolfe, 1963). The measured dermal exposure of such spraymen varied from 2.4 to 78 mg/person/hr.

Volunteers who worked in cotton fields 12, 24, and 72 hr after application of parathion experienced no signs or symptoms of poisoning and had only slight depression of blood cholinesterase activity. There was good correspondence between the magnitude of residues on the cotton, estimates of exposure of the men, and absorption, as evidenced by analysis of blood and urine (Ware et al., 1975).

Accidental and Intentional Poisoning   Hundreds of deaths associated with parathion have been reported. It is impractical even to list them, but outbreaks involving contaminated food or clothing are shown in Table 7.14. The problem continues. An outbreak leading to 79 cases and 17 deaths was reported by Diggory et al. (1977).

Our knowledge of the clinical picture of poisoning by

organic phosphorus compounds (see Section 16.2.2.2) in humans is drawn largely from poisoning by parathion. Any difference in the illness produced by adequate doses of other anticholinesterase organophosphates is, among other things, a difference from the syndrome produced by parathion. An exception to this statement is the tendency of dermal exposure to parathion to produce serious poisoning, the onset of which may be delayed for several hours. Few other organic phosphorus compounds exhibit a significant delay of onset in cases that prove severe. In occupational cases of poisoning by parathion, the delay seldom, if ever, exceeds 12 hr, and the same is true generally of cases associated with shampooing children's heads for the control of lice. However, a startling exception was the interval of 6 days between the last of several applications to a child's scalp and her sudden onset of illness leading to death (Introna, 1959). Because no similar case has been reported, the possibility of an unrecognized exposure not long before onset must be considered.

Once poisoning has begun, coma follows promptly; in fact, if coma does not occur, recovery usually is well advanced within 24 hr. However, in a few unexplained instances, coma was delayed until the day after onset of illness (Delons et al., 1964).

The use of parathion for control of lice or scabies has provided the most dramatic—and tragic—evidence for the dermal absorption of the compound in humans (Koeffler, 1958; Introna, 1959; El-Achrafi, 1963; Hristic and Milenkovic, 1961; Nameche and Bartman, 1964).

Nearly all of the victims have been children, partly because they are more likely to have head lice and, therefore, are more likely to be treated. However, epidemiological evidence indicates that parathion is more toxic to children than to adults (Klugman, 1959; Kanagaratnam et al., 1960).

Children 7 and 9 years old were killed by bathing in a tub in a house that had been sprayed several days earlier with 10% parathion intended for ornamental plants in a greenhouse (Anonymous, 1959).

A group of city children found a coarse cloth sack in a trash pile, stuffed it with rags, suspended it from a tree by a rope, and used it as a swing. Their bare arms, legs, and faces rubbed against the rough fabric as they clung to it and swung back and forth. The swing was used briefly on the day it was made and almost constantly from 1000 to 1730 hr the next day. Between 2000 and 2100 hr of the first full day of swinging, the children became sick and were taken to different hospitals. Three of them, a 10- and a 13-year-old boy and a 10-year-old girl, survived, but two, a 5-year-old boy and a 9-year-old girl, died. Parathion was identified in the bag and in the clothing of the dead. p-Nitrophenol was identified in the only sample of urine available. Red cell cholinesterase activity was greatly reduced. The bag was traced back to a farm, but how it became contaminated by parathion could not be determined (Hayes, 1963, 1982).

Another small epidemic of poisoning among children followed the use of flannelette sheets that had been contaminated by parathion during shipment. The symptoms were charac-

teristic but fortunately mild (Anderson et al., 1965). Other cases involving contact with contaminated bedclothing have been reported (Pilat et al., 1961; Meneses de Almeida and Pendroso S de Lima, 1964).

Finally, dermal contamination of adults through intentional application or direct splashing or spillage of parathion or its liquid formulations has led to poisoning (Hamlin and Marchand, 1951; Rosen, 1960; Prinz, 1969).

Some other instances of the purely dermal absorption of parathion might easily have been misdiagnosed because application of the compound was unintentional or unrecognized. The fact that so many recorded instances of dermal poisoning have involved small epidemics suggests that some single cases may have been missed.

Unlike most pesticides, except for the arsenicals, parathion frequently has been employed for suicide or murder. For example, of 361 deaths caused by parathion in Denmark between 1951 and 1963, 344 were suicides, 5 were murders, and one was a suspected murder (Friis, 1966). A significant proportion of deaths from parathion in some other countries have involved suicide (Posada and Valencia, 1966; Vercruysse and Deslypere, 1967; Kawashiro, 1959; Ohela et al., 1958; Ozgen, 1959; Vesileva and Abrasheva, 1960; Vethanayagam, 1962; Villares, 1968; Kashlan and Wagih, 1969; Kim et al., 1970; Kaye, 1970; Juhl, 1971; Ghachem and Hassen, 1973; Oarda, 1971).

Parathion has even been administered in multiple small doses (Luederitz et al., 1974), as has long been a common practice with arsenic intended for murder.

Use Experience In spite of the very real and continuing danger of parathion, its safety record has improved greatly. Soon after parathion was introduced, there were a number of occupational accidents (Hamlin and Marchand, 1951). Improved equipment and work practices soon reduced the number of serious accidents in manufacturing and formulating plants to a low level. The safety of parathion applicators was improved more slowly and may still be poor in countries with limited experience in the use of chemicals.

In the United States, parathion has been the main, if not exclusive, cause of crop-worker poisoning (Quinby and Lemmon, 1958). Apparently parathion has been the leading cause of this kind of poisoning in Bulgaria also (Kaloyanova-Simenova, 1970). Workers may be affected promptly when they first work in a field for only a few hours, beginning days or even weeks after the insecticide was applied. This delay is characteristic of crop-worker poisoning and serves to distinguish it from ordinary reentry poisoning, such as has occurred with carbofuran. It has become more clearly established that the toxicity of residues of parathion on tall crops in a very few isolated fields depends on an unusual degree of conversion of parathion to paraoxon or on an unusual retention of paraoxon residue, or on both. In a study of 32 California orange groves chosen at random, it was found that parathion residues disappeared with a half-life of 2.9 days but that paraoxon disappeared more slowly (half-life 5.55 days). The median ratio of paraoxon to parathion increased from 0.168 2 days after application of parathion to 0.825 on day 16. However, by day 16, the ratio was >1.0 in 30% of the groves; the largest ratio observed exceeded 4.0 (Spear *et al.*, 1975). In a similar way, the highest observed ratio (paraoxon to parathion on foliage) was 4.2, in connection with a study of volunteers who picked oranges in groves previously treated with parathion. The volunteers remained well, but they did show red cell cholinesterase inhibition proportional to their dermal exposure to paraoxon. Respiratory exposure to paraoxon and both dermal and respiratory exposure to parathion had essentially no influence on the cholinesterase levels under the conditions of the study (Spear *et al.*, 1977a). On the contrary, ratios as high as 30 : 1 were measured in groves where typical crop-workers' poisoning had occurred, and most of the ratios exceeded 10 : 1. The total residue present on the foliage was little, if any, more than that expected for the rate of application and waiting period involved. However, the paraoxon residue was far above expectation and entirely adequate to explain the injury of the workers (Spear *et al.*, 1977b). The investigators speculated that photochemical oxidants may have been involved in causing the abnormal production and persistence of paraoxon. They were careful to point out, however, that, regardless of their nature, the critical conditions occur rarely and unpredictably. This finding based on chemistry confirms what long has been evident from epidemiology.

Atypical Cases of Various Origins   Pericarditis occurred during treatment of one case that involved a large dose of parathion and otherwise typical signs and symptoms (Bianchi, 1966). Because this apparently is the only report of pericarditis associated with parathion, it may not have been causally related to poisoning.

A 29-year-old gardener dispersed a 0.01% formulation of parathion in closed greenhouses 10 or 12 times in the course of 4 weeks at temperatures of 40–50°C. Nausea, vomiting, and loss of appetite occurred several hours after each application but disappeared by the next day. Illness not obviously related to exposure occurred and led to hospitalization about 1.5 months after exposure stopped. It was not until about 1.3 months later (11 weeks after last exposure) that the patient noticed prickling, numbness, and weakness of his legs, and after another 3 weeks he could no longer walk. Almost 2 more years later, he still complained of weakness of his legs and other neurological difficulties (Petry, 1951). The condition was attributed to parathion after other causes of polyneuropathy were considered. However, the long delay from last exposure to onset made the diagnosis in his particular case highly questionable, and the rarity of suspected cases, even among people heavily exposed to parathion, makes it doubtful that the relation of parathion to polyneuropathy is more than circumstantial in any instance.

Following attempted suicide with parathion, one patient developed polyneuritis involving the distal limb muscles, and this was unimproved 4 months later. The unusual occurrence of this condition in association with parathion was attributed to alcohol consumed on the same day (Voiculescu *et al.*, 1971). For a general discussion of polyneuropathy associated with pesticides, see Section 16.4.1.4.

Two cases of persisting weakness and other complaints following exposure insufficient to cause acute poisoning have been reported (Petty, 1958a).

Parkinsonism developed in a 53-year-old man who said he had been poisoned several times by parathion and other organic phosphorus compounds when formerly employed as a crop duster (Davis *et al.*, 1978). No specific evidence for a cause-and-effect relationship was noted, and the circumstantial relationship apparently was peculiar to this case.

A case characterized mainly by narcolepsy and kleptomania lasting for 12 years after attempted suicide by parathion has been reported (Taneda and Hara, 1975). The possibility that the observed condition was a part of the total illness leading to suicide apparently was not considered.

Dosage Response   In a number of cases, the oral dose of parathion was known to be exactly 900 mg, and it was uniformly fatal. In one carefully studied case, the ingestion of 120 mg led rapidly to the death of a man (Goldblatt, 1950; Reinl, 1949). In spite of some improvement in methods of treatment, these facts make it difficult to explain how three patients survived doses of parathion estimated to be 20,000–40,000 mg (Okonek and Kilbinger, 1974) and bring the accuracy of the estimates into question. Treatment that involves oximes can save some patients who have ingested as much as 50,000 mg of parathion (Barckow *et al.*, 1969). Children 5–6 years old were killed by eating 2 mg of parathion, a dosage of about 0.1 mg/kg (Kanagaratnam *et al.*, 1960). On the contrary, a 14-year-old girl who was treated virogously had essentially recovered from poisoning by an estimated 67.5 mg (about 1.29 mg/kg) when she died of massive hermorrhage (Wycoff *et al.*, 1968). A 60-year-old man barely survived what was estimated to be 150 mg of parathion (Smerling, 1976).

In instances in which parathion-contaminated food was eaten by people of different ages, death occurred mainly or exclusively among children (Kanagaratnam *et al.*, 1960; Diggory *et al.*, 1977). In one outbreak, the death rate was higher among men than among women (Diggory *et al.*, 1977), but whether their average dosages were the same was not established.

In one instance, the purposeful application of 2000 mg to the skin produced illness within half an hour; unconsciousness, and respiratory failure followed promptly, but the patient was saved by treatment (Prinz, 1969). A similar onset but slower recovery resulted from subcutaneous injection of approximately the same dosage of a mixture of parathion and demeton (Knolle, 1970). Obviously, some workers survive larger doses, but there is no evidence that the amount of variation in absorption and/or susceptibility exceeds that found with many poisons.

There was no change in the erythrocyte count, white blood cell count, or differential count in one volunteer who at different times ingested 5 and 10 mg of parathion or in another who took 30 mg; however, the 30-mg dose did produce an unpleasant stomach cramp (Velbinger, 1949).

A daily oral dose of 7.2 mg produced no illness but a 33% fall in whole-blood cholinesterase of adult volunteers in 42 days. At the end of the period red cell and plasma cholinesterase activity were 84 and 63%, respectively, of normal. A dosage of 4.8 mg/person/day (about 0.07 mg/kg/day) for 63 days produced no effect, even on cholinesterase (Edson, 1964). In a separate experiment, a daily dosage of 3.5 mg/person/day for 21 days did not inhibit cholinesterase, and higher dosages were not tested (Rider *et al.*, 1958). In another study, ingestion of parathion at rates of 3.0–4.5 mg/person/day for 28 days did not produce a significant depression of red cell or plasma cholinesterase activity, but a dosage of 6.0 mg/person/day did produce a 10–15% depression of the activity of both enzymes (Moeller and Rider, 1961). Later, dosages of 3.0 and 4.5 mg/person/day for 35 days produced no effect of any kind; 6.0 mg/person/day slightly inhibited plasma cholinesterase of all subjects and reduced red cell cholinesterase to 63–86% of normal in three subjects but left it normal in two others (Rider *et al.*, 1969). These experimental results are consistent with tolerated dosages of workers that may be calculated from *p*-nitrophenol excretion rates. Men with occupational exposure leading to an average parathion intake of about 4.88 mg/person/day remained asymptomatic and had little or no depression of plasma cholinesterase activity. (The value for parathion was calculated from a measured average *p*-nitrophenol concentration of 1.56 ppm in the urine soon after each day's work and the excretion of 1.5 liters of urine in 24 hr.) Thus, a dosage of about 0.07 mg/kg/day is a no-effect level in adults.

The threshold limit value of 0.1 mg/m^3 indicates that occupational intake of 0.014 mg/kg/day is considered safe. A comparison with observed no-effect levels indicates that this standard is conservative.

Laboratory Findings Under certain circumstances, parathion may be isolated from exhumed bodies as well as fresh necropsy specimens (Hamada, 1955, 1956; Tajima and Todoriki, 1955; Vaesileva and Abrasheva, 1960; Dequeker, 1964; Elaikis *et al.*, 1966; Barquet, *et al.*, 1968; Poehlmann and Schwerd, 1976). More recently, it has become possible to measure the compound in plasma. Approximately 7 hr after ingesting a mixture of parathion, diazinon, and chlordane in doses estimated to be 1400, 558 and 254 mg, respectively, an 8-year-old girl had serum levels as follows: parathion, 1.000 ppm; diazinon, 0.384; and chlordane, 0.360 ppm; she died a few hours later in spite of vigorous treatment. Her 5-year-old brother, who had consumed less of the same mixture (an estimated 500 mg of parathion, 187 mg of diazinon, and 254 mg of chlordane) survived without sequelae in spite of reaching the following serum levels: parathion, 0.357 ppm; diazinon, 0.041 ppm; and chlordane, 0.72 ppm (DePalma *et al.*, 1970). In another case, 0.409 ppm was found one day after ingestion of parathion in an unsuccessful attempt at suicide (Okonek and Kilbinger, 1974). At the time of diagnosis, concentrations of 0.001–0.662 ppm were found in the plasma of

persons severely or very severely poisoned. No other organic phosphorus compound was found in the sample with most parathion, but values of 0.001–0.002 ppm were associated with other compounds (mainly fenitrothion at concentrations of 0.015–0.017 ppm), indicating a mixed intoxication (Watanabe, 1972a). In another instance, parathion was found in the gastric juice and plasma as late as day 7 after ingestion (Boelcke *et al.*, 1970).

Even more recently it was possible to detect paraoxon as well as parathion in the blood of five patients who were comatose, paralyzed, and without spontaneous respiration at the time. No red cell or plasma cholinesterase activity was detectable. Three of the patients survived. The highest concentrations of paraoxon in plasma was 6.3 ppm. Measurement was by gas chromatography and confirmation was by mass spectrometry (Okonek, 1976b).

Measurement of *p*-nitrophenol in the urine is a valuable tool for studying parathion absorption, whether occupational or otherwise (Arterberry *et al.*, 1961; Wolfe *et al.*, 1970) (see Fig. 16.3). The finding of an average initial *p*-nitrophenol concentration of 40.3 ppm in fatal cases and an average of 10.8 ppm in nonfatal cases of parathion poisoning (Davies *et al.*, 1967) is consistent with the values in Figure 16.3. Assuming urinary output at the usual rate of 1500 mg/day, these values are equivalent to rates of 2.52 and 0.68 mg/hr for fatal and nonfatal cases, respectively, under practical conditions of treatment. This does not exclude the possibility, of course, that some persons with exceptional treatment might survive at the higher level, and it certainly does not exclude death at the lower level, especially if good treatment were not available promptly. A 2-year-old boy seriously poisoned by parathion excreted *p*-nitrophenol at an initial concentration of about 8 ppm (Quinby and Clappison, 1961). A *p*-nitrophenol concentration of only 3.8 ppm was found in the urine of another poisoned child who also went on to recovery (Comer *et al.*, 1976).

Abnormal cholinesterase values and their interpretations are discussed in Section 16.2.2.3. The discussion includes the relationship between plasma and red cell cholinesterase and the urinary excretion of *p*-nitrophenol (Fig. 16.3) and also the levels of acetylcholinesterase found in different parts of the brains of normal people and those killed by parathion (Table 16.9).

In orchard sprayers, excretion of *p*-nitrophenol reached peak levels about 8.7 hr after exposure began and, therefore, several hours after work ended. Excretion tended to increase with an increase in ambient temperature. Excretion showed a diurnal variation after last exposure, the peaks becoming progressively lower and falling to undetectable levels by days 5–8 (Wolfe *et al.*, 1970).

According to Davies (1975), diethyl phosphate was the most sensitive indicator of dangerous exposure to parathion. Concentrations of >0.4 ppm were observed in the first urines collected in seven cases of poisoning accompanied by serious enzyme inhibition, whereas this concentration was reached in only one of 71 samples from exposed but unpoisoned workers.

Of perhaps even greater interest was the fact that the ratio of diethyl phosphate to diethyl thiophosphate averaged 4.14 in 20 samples from poisoned persons but only 0.88 in samples from unpoisoned workers, indicating a difference in the pattern of biotransformation. Whereas a difference of this sort is most likely to be caused by a difference in dosage, the data do not exclude the possibility of individual differences. This latter speculation finds support in the observation of Flugel and Geldmacher-von Mallinckrodt (1978) of substantial differences among people in their paraoxonase activity.

When a 12-year-old boy was hospitalized about 12 hr after he ingested parathion, his serum cholinesterase activity was undetectable, and the low-density lipoprotein and cholesterol levels were markedly decreased. The boy recovered following appropriate treatment. Later, animal experiments indicated that cholinesterase has a function in the synthesis of low-density lipoproteins (Kutty *et al.*, 1975).

Among 52 patients hospitalized for poisoning by insecticides, rodenticides, and various drugs, those poisoned by parathion showed greatest disturbance of liver function as judged by BSP retention and elevated SGOT, SGPT, and bilirubin levels (Kin *et al.*, 1977). There was no indication, however, that liver changes were critical in the outcome of these cases.

16.7.2 DIAZINON

16.7.2.1 Identity, Properties, and Uses

Chemical Name   Diazinon is *O,O*-diethyl *O*-(2-isopropyl-6-methyl-4-pyrimidinyl) phosphorothioate.

Structure   See Table 16.36.

Synonyms   The common name diazinon (BSI, ESA, ISO) is in general use. Trade names include Basudin®, Diazitol®, Dipofene®, Neocidol®, Nucidol®, and Spectracide®. Code designations include G-24480 and OMS-469. The CAS registry number is 333-41-5.

Physical and Chemical Properties   Diazinon has the empirical formula $C_{12}H_{21}N_2O_3PS$ and a molecular weight of 304.36. The pure material forms a colorless liquid with a faint esterlike odor. The boiling point is 83–84°C. The density at 20°C is 1.116–1.118. The vapor pressure is 1.4×10^{-4} mm Hg at 20°C and 1.1×10^{-3} mm Hg at 40°C. The refractive index (D^{20}) is 1.4978–1.4981. Diazinon is stable in alkaline formulations but is hydrolyzed slowly by water and by dilute acids. Diazinon decomposes above 120°C and is susceptible to oxidation. The solubility of diazinon in water at 20°C is 40 ppm. It is miscible with alcohol, ether, petroleum ether, cyclohexane, benzene, and similar hydrocarbons.

History, Formulations, Uses, and Production   Diazinon was first introduced in 1952, and its insecticidal properties were described by Gasser (1953). Formulations include wetta-

ble powder (25%), emulsifiable concentrates (25%), and dust (4%). Diazinon is used for the control of household and agricultural insects, including foliage and soil insects. The synthesis of technical diazinon, its purification, the by-products formed, and their respective properties have been described (Gysin and Margot, 1958).

16.7.2.2 Toxicity to Laboratory Animals

Basic Findings   There is nothing distinctive about the symptomatology of diazinon, except that reticulocytopenia and a high myloid-to-erythroid ratio were found in some animals killed in less than a month by large, repeated, oral doses. The ratio was greater than 100 : 1 in dogs receiving 20 mg/kg/day and greater than 3.4 : 1 in miniature swine receiving 10 mg/kg/day. It was not indicated that these changes were related to the cause of death, but nonfatal doses did not produce them (Earl *et al.*, 1968). See Pathology below.

Diazinon has not been found either irritating or sensitizing. The acute toxicity of diazinon is notable for its variability, both regarding different formulations and regarding species (see Table 16.39). Some formulations can be converted to much more toxic compounds, especially on contact with air (see Nonmetabolic Chemical Change in this section).

In calves, a dosage of 1 mg/kg produces signs of toxicity, and 10 mg/kg is lethal. In steers, 10 mg/kg is harmless; a dosage of 25 mg/kg is toxic but not lethal. Sheep are slightly less susceptible than steers (Radeleff, 1958).

Some birds have an inordinate susceptibility to diazinon (see Table 16.39).

Table 16.39
Single-Dose LD 50 for Diazinon

Species	Route	LD 50 (mg/kg)	Reference
Rat, M	oral	235	Gasser (1953)
Rat, M	oral	435	Shaffer and West (1960)
Rat, M	oral	108[a]	Gaines (1960)
Rat, F	oral	76[a]	Gaines (1960)
Rat, M	oral	250[b]	Gaines (1969)
Rat, F	oral	285[b]	Gaines (1969)
Rat, M	dermal	200[c]	Gaines (1960)
Rat, M	dermal	34[d]	Gaines (1960)
Rat, M	dermal	900[a]	Gaines (1960)
Rat, F	dermal	455[a]	Gaines (1960)
Mouse, M	oral	82	Bruce *et al.* (1955)
Mouse	oral	96	Gasser (1953)
Mouse	intraperitoneal	65	Klotzche (1955)
Guinea pig	oral	320	Gasser (1953)
Rabbit	oral	130	Gasser (1953)
Turkey	oral	6.81	FAO/WHO (1965)
Chicken	oral	40.8	FAO/WHO (1965)
Goose	oral	14.7	FAO/WHO (1965)
Gosling	oral	2.75	Egyed *et al.* (1974)

[a] 1959 technical product.
[b] 1965 technical product.
[c] 1953 technical product.
[d] Crystalline derivative of 1953 technical product.

Rats tolerated dietary levels as high as 1000 ppm (about 50 mg/kg/day) for 72 weeks without sign of toxicity. After only 4 weeks of feeding, a dietary level of 100 ppm produced marked inhibition of red cell cholinesterase, slight inhibition of plasma cholinesterase, and essentially no effect on brain cholinesterase. The enzymes responded in a different order to a dietary level of 1000 ppm for the same period—complete inhibition of red cell activity, marked inhibition of brain cholinesterase, and only moderate inhibition of plasma cholinesterase (Bruce *et al.*, 1955).

Dogs tolerated a dosage of 6.5 mg/kg/day for 43 weeks with no gross sign of toxicity, but even a dosage of 4.6 mg/kg/day produced marked inhibition of both plasma and red cell cholinesterase activity. Levels of 9.3 mg/kg/day and higher promptly resulted in excitement, tremor, and loss of appetite and weight (Bruce *et al.*, 1955).

Repeated dosages of diazinon failed to give a sharp dosage response in dogs and swine, at least partly because the results were confounded by malnutrition. Food consumption of animals receiving large doses dropped drastically soon after dosing began. However, pair-fed controls failed to develop lesions like those of the experimental animals discussed under Pathology below.

In other studies, a dosage of about 0.015 mg/kg/day (Williams *et al.*, 1959) or 0.02 (FAO/WHO, 1965) proved to be the no-effect level for cholinesterase inhibition in the dog. Even at a dosage of 0.015 there was a small inhibition of plasma cholinesterase, but the enzyme returned to normal activity despite continued intake. Only a moderate degree of inhibition was seen at 0.04 mg/kg/day. At a dosage of about 0.15 mg/kg/day, red cell as well as plasma cholinesterase was inhibited.

Rhesus monkeys tolerated daily stomach tube feeding with diazinon for 2 years without cholinesterase inhibition when the dosage was 0.05 mg/kg/day. Inhibition of both plasma and red cell cholinesterase was moderate or erratic at 0.5 mg/kg/day and marked at 5 mg/kg/day. Signs of poisoning were consistent with cholinesterase inhibition, but even the highest dosage produced no neurological, hematological, clinical chemical, or pathological effect (Woodard *et al.*, 1968).

Nonmetabolic Chemical Change Gaines (1960, 1969) reported great variation in the toxicity of different batches of diazinon and also that a formulation crystallized and became much more toxic when exposed to air. The fact that the sample gained weight suggests that oxidation rather than evaporation was responsible for the change (see Table 16.39). Radeleff (1964) also commented on the tendency of some emulsifiable concentrates (but not wettable powders) to become more toxic on standing. Many animals studies have been carried out with water-wettable powders and may, for this reason, fail to reflect the full spectrum of toxicity. According to Schrader (1963a), diazinon can form not only diazoxon but also tetraethyl monothiopyrophosphate. Margot and Gysin (1957) derived these compounds and also tetraethyl pyrophosphate from technical diazinon, but the methods used were artificial. Both of the

pyrophosphates are somewhat more active than diazoxon in inhibiting cholinesterase, and diazoxon itself is a strong inhibitor. Ultraviolet irradiation of diazinon for only 2 hr changed the isopropyl substitution on the ring to an acetyl group; the new compound was an indirect cholinesterase inhibitor apparently stronger than the parent compound (Machin *et al.*, 1971). This compound might help explain increased toxicity but cannot explain the increase of sample weight that occurred over a longer period of time but without special irradiation.

Modern formulations of diazinon in the United States are stabilized. Whether they are stable worldwide and under all conditions remains to be proved.

A different problem involves sulfotepp, which Meier *et al.* (1979) found to constitute 0.20–0.7% of the diazinon present in all formulations of diazinon that they examined. Sulfotepp is considerably more toxic than pure diazinon, and formulations containing a relatively high percentage of sulfotepp would be more toxic than those with low percentages. However, the investigators showed that sulfotepp could be formed during the synthesis of diazinon, and they did not consider that the concentration of this impurity in any given formulation increased with age.

Absorption, Distribution, Metabolism, and Excretion Diethyl thiophosphate and diethyl phosphate are recognized metabolites of diazinon in the cow (Robbins *et al.*, 1957), and in the rat (Plapp and Casida, 1958). A small percentage of the monoalkyl monoaryl derivatives is also formed (Plapp and Casida, 1958).

The acidic moiety of diazinon differs from those of many organic phosphorus insecticides in that it is subject to biotransformation that does not lead to detoxication but produces metabolites capable of inhibiting cholinesterase. Such metabolites have been demonstrated in mice and sheep (James *et al.*, 1973, and others cited by them). The compounds include two monohydroxy diazinons and a dehydration product of one of them (James *et al.*, 1973).

The metabolism of diazinon by microsomal enzymes leads to both toxication and detoxication, as is true of parathion (Nakatsugawa *et al.*, 1969a). The balance of the two in intact animals is unknown. However, excretion is rapid in the rat, requiring about 12 hr for 50% completion. Of either ^{14}C-ring-labeled or ^{14}C-ethyl-labeled compound, 69–80% was excreted in the urine and 18–25% in the feces. No cleavage of the ring and no production of CO_2 were detected (Muecke *et al.*, 1970). Furthermore, radiolabeled diazinon was excreted rapidly in the urine of the guinea pig (Kaplanis *et al.*, 1962), cow (Robbins *et al.*, 1957), dog (Iverson *et al.*, 1975), and goat (FAO/WHO, 1965).

Following weekly spraying with a 0.1% formulation for 16 weeks, cattle stored diazinon in their fat at concentrations up to 2.3 ppm one day after the last spraying, 0.7 ppm 7 days after spraying, but none after 14 days (Claborn *et al.*, 1963). Because of the instability of diazinon, it is unlikely that cattle will receive much of the compound in their food following ordinary use. Diazinon, sprayed on grass at rates of 10 and 100 ppm, disappeared rapidly in the silage during fermentation, with only 3% remaining after 22 days of storage. Residues of diazinon are not detectable in butterfat from cows fed daily at dietary levels as high as 500 ppm based on dry weight (Derbyshire and Murphy, 1962). Only a trace of diazinon is secreted in cows' milk for 24 hr after dermal application (Bourne and Arthur, 1967).

Gunner and Zuckerman (1968) reviewed earlier work indicating that certain species of *Arthrobacter* and *Streptomyces* can degrade the ^{14}C-tagged ethyl moiety of diazinon to carbon dioxide. They confirmed this finding for *Arthrobacter* and went on to show that neither of the organisms separately could convert the carbon of ring-labeled diazinon to carbon dioxide. However, when the two organisms were cultured together, complete biodegradation occurred, indicating a synergistic action.

Biochemical Effects Different authors agree that in rats, red cell cholinesterase is changed by repeated doses of diazinon too small to affect the plasma enzyme (Bruce *et al.*, 1955; Edson and Noakes, 1960). Brain cholinesterase is intermediate in response.

Different authors are not in good agreement about the dosage of the compound necessary to inhibit the enzymes. This probably reflects the variation in toxicity of different formulations already mentioned. For example, FAO/WHO (1965) reported that a dietary level of 4 ppm inhibited plasma cholinesterase of rats, whereas Edson and Noakes (1960) found a dietary level of 25 ppm inadequate to produce this effect, which with their material required 125 ppm.

There is no potentiation when diazinon and any of several other organic phosphorus compounds are administered to dogs (Lehman, 1965).

Although diazinon formulations may increase in toxicity on standing, there is no indication that they change in their mode of action. Thus, death is caused by diazinon in the same way that it is caused by other organic phosphorus anticholinesterase compounds.

Following a single intraperitoneal injection of diazinon at a rate of 75 mg/kg, the concentration of 3-glucuronidase in the serum of rats increased. This was accounted for by a decrease of the enzyme in the microsomal fraction of the liver, which reached its lowest level in 10 days and then required more than 30 days to return to normal. Both the increase in serum enzyme and the decrease in microsome enzyme were linear when plotted against the logarithms of dosage within the range of 1.5–50 mg/kg (Suzuki *et al.*, 1975).

Husain and Matin (1986a) have reported the depletion of cerebral glycogen and increased blood lactic acid levels in rats following intraperitoneal administration of 40 mg/kg diazinon. These alterations are apparently in response to the need for additional energy in cerebral and other tissues as a result of acute diazinon toxicity (see Section 16.2.2.3).

Of 11 biochemical determinations (excluding cholinesterase) made at monthly intervals on dogs fed 2.5–20 mg/kg/day

and on miniature swine fed 1.25–10 mg/kg/day, only amylase showed a dosage-related elevation (Earl *et al.*, 1968, 1971).

Diazinon is only about seven times more toxic to rats that have been maintained for 28 days on 0% protein than to those fed an approximately optimal proportion (26%); the difference is smaller at less than optimal levels that people are likely to encounter (Boyd *et al.*, 1969).

Effects on Organs and Tissues Cell division of cultured human lymphocytes was inhibited by concentrations of diazinon said to represent 1/40 to 1/800 of the LD 50 in rats. Some separate chromatids of chromosomes were broken (Tzoneva-Maneva *et al.*, 1971). Although the results were interpreted as an indication of mutagenic potential, all results may have reflected only cytotoxicity.

The pups of mice that received diazinon orally at a rate of 9.0 mg/kg/day during pregnancy had significantly small adrenals (Cranmer *et al.*, 1978).

Effects on Reproduction Diazinon is teratogenic to chick embryos when injected into the yolk sac before incubation or after 4 days of incubation at the rate of 1 mg/egg. The affected vertebral column is characteristically tortuous, shortened, and composed of abnormal vertebral bodies. In the neck region, these bodies have fused neural arches and lack most of the intervertebral joints (Khera and Bedok, 1967).

Diazinon was not teratogenic in rabbits receiving oral doses during organogenesis at rates of 7 or 30 mg/kg or in the hamster at a rate of 0.125–0.25 mg/kg. In the rabbit, 30 mg/kg produced cholinergic signs, as was true of both dosage levels in the hamster (Robens, 1969). In rats, dosages (e.g., 95.2 mg/kg on day 9) that increased maternal mortality reduced fetal development as indicated by reduced weight of litters and mild "hydronephrosis" but caused no real teratogenic effect (Dobbins, 1967). A similar result was reported for intraperitoneal dosages of 100 and 150 mg/kg on day 11 (Kimbrough and Gaines, 1968). Repeated administration (40, 50, or 60 mg/kg/day) on days 7–19 of gestation reduced the growth of the dams but had no effect on the number of resorptions or corpora lutea, on litter size, or on fetal weight. Of course, esterase activity of the fetal brain was reduced. A dosage of 75 mg/kg/day was fatal to dams in 4–5 days (Hoberman *et al.*, 1979).

Behavioral Effects When mice received diazinon orally at rates of 9.0, 0.18, and 0 mg/kg/day throughout gestation, all of the young were viable and overtly normal. However, pups from dams on the high dosage grew more slowly, showed several behavioral defects, and, when killed at 101 days of age, showed pathology of the forebrain. Pups from dams receiving 0.18 mg/kg/day grew normally and lacked brain pathology but did show small but measurable defects in behavior and slight delay in reaching maturity (Spyker and Avery, 1977).

Pathology Some dogs and swine receiving high daily dosages of diazinon (10 mg/kg or greater) showed marked edematous thickening (6 mm) of the small intestine on autopsy (Earl *et al.,* 1971). Similar findings were encountered earlier in connection with parathion. Rupture of the duodenum occurred in one dog and rupture of the pyloric part of the stomach in another. Duodenal ulcer occurred in some swine on 10 mg/kg/day. At a dosage level of 10 mg/kg/day, the liver was yellow and fatty in appearance and microscopic examination revealed cirrhosis. Some other organs showed some degree of atrophy confirmed by histopathology. Bone marrow smears revealed an increased myeloid/erythroid ratio in three of five dogs. However, no anemia was reported. Findings for swine were similar (Earl *et al.,* 1971).

When rats received a single intraperitoneal injection of diazinon at a rate of 21.6 mg/kg, there was no illness, but some degenerative changes were found in the liver and necrosis, edema, and reduction of tubular size were found in the testes (Dikshith *et al.,* 1975).

Treatment of Poisoning in Animals 2-PAM or other oximes are effective in treating poisoning by diazinon and/or restoring the activity of cholinesterase inhibited by it (Sanderson and Edson, 1959; Stenger, 1960; Harris *et al.,* 1968). The half-life for aging is 42.5 ± 5.5 hr (Harris *et al.,* 1968).

16.7.2.3 Toxicity to Humans

Experimental Exposure In an initial test, two men developed "marked" inhibition of plasma cholinesterase as a result of five doses at the rate of about 0.025 mg/kg/day. However, a dosage of 0.05 mg/kg/day for a total of 28 days reduced plasma cholinesterase of three men by only 35–40%. In three other tests, each involving three or four men and lasting 32–43 days, dosages ranging from 0.02 to 0.03 mg/kg/day led to reductions of plasma cholinesterase activity of 0, 15–20, and 14%, respectively—values indistinguishable from normal variation. In no instance was there any effect on red cell cholinesterase activity. Body weight; blood hemoglobin, hematocrit, cell count, prothrombin time, clotting time, and urea content; serum alkaline phosphatase and glutamic-pyruvic transaminase activities; and urinary constituents also remained normal (FAO/WHO, 1967). Thus, 0.02 mg/kg/day is a no-effect level in humans. Corresponding values for other species are: dog, 0.02; monkey, 0.05; and rat, 0.10 mg/kg/day.

Accidents and Use Experience Although the response of different persons to the same formulation of diazinon has been consistent, response to different formulations has varied enormously. There is a strong suggestion that some accidents involved unaltered diazinon whereas others involved formulations that had undergone change.

Three-week-old twins were hospitalized at 0700 hr one morning because of respiratory distress that had progressed since 2300 hr the previous night. One was cyanotic on admission, but both had rapid shallow breathing, profuse nasal and bronchial secretions, and pinpoint pupils; no muscle fasciculations were detectable. At 48 hr only the sicker twin had slightly reduced pseudocholinesterase. Treatment was appropriate and recovery uneventful. Investigation revealed that the babies lived in one side of a two-story house that had been divided into two apartments by partitions. About 1030 hr on the previous day the other apartment had been sprayed with 1% diazinon for cockroach control, using approved spot applications directed mainly at cracks. The weather had been hot and the windows of both apartments were kept open. Except for the twins, the members of both families (including one 2-year-old child) remained well, but apparently the twins were the only ones who had remained indoors (English *et al.,* 1970). This would appear to be a rare example of illness caused exclusively by respiratory exposure to a nonfumigant pesticide. The observed degree of respiratory distress in the presence of little or no inhibition of cholinesterase was consistent with exclusively respiratory exposure.

Accidents have involved dermal absorption of diazinon ointment and solution used for treatment of lice or of creeping eruption and also an oil formulation applied to a floor where children played and the bed where they slept (Muratore *et al.,* 1960; Hayes, 1963, 1982).

One accident involved eight elderly men who drank a solution of diazinon they mistook for wine. Three of them, with an average of 73 years, died (Hayes, 1963). In another instance, nine men survived the consumption of a beverage they prepared with diazinon emulsion concentrate as one ingredient (Kessler and Mracek, 1973). These examples and others (Mirza *et al.,* 1972), in which some people have survived the drinking of formulations with only moderate illness and sometimes with little or no treatment, suggest that diazinon is only moderately toxic. An opposite conclusion must be drawn from some other cases in which illness was severe in spite of limited exposure. A striking example involves the cases treated with diazinon for creeping eruption (see Dosage Response). The inconsistency of response in relation to dosage has been noted repeatedly (Sonejee *et al.,* 1969; Balani *et al.,* 1968; Karnick *et al.,* 1970).

Several other reports of ingestions of diazinon include suicides as well as accidents; a high proportion of the reports are from India (Gassmann, 1957; Bockel, 1957; Shankar, 1966, 1967; Mutalik *et al.,* 1962; Kabrawala *et al.,* 1965; Kamath *et al.,* 1964; Monseur, 1963; Gupta and Patel, 1968; Limaye, 1966; Sonejee *et al.,* 1969; Balani *et al.,* 1968; Karnik *et al.,* 1970; Mehta *et al.,* 1971; Reichert *et al.,* 1977; Klemmer *et al.,* 1978).

The symptoms in most reported cases of poisoning were similar to those caused by parathion. The onset of illness was less than an hour after dermal application of a 1% solution to two patients; both responded promptly to atropine. The deaths of three men who drank a diazinon solution they mistook for wine occurred in 1–2 days after ingestion and in spite of treatment with some atropine. One case with death 10 days after ingestion has been described (Monseur, 1963).

Pericarditis began on the second day and persisted for 2 days in a patient who eventually recovered in spite of a massive dose of diazinon (Banerjee, 1967). The same patient also developed pneumonia of the left lower lobe, perhaps due to aspiration of some solvent. Pericarditis and pneumonia are so unusual in connection with poisoning by any organic phosphorus compound that there is no reason to think they are peculiar to poisoning by diazinon. In fact, the possibility must be considered that the pericarditis and pneumonia had a common cause but were only circumstantially related to poisoning.

Slight, asymptomatic depletion of cholinesterase occurs in sprayers who have extensive occupational exposure to diazinon (Bruaux, 1957; Loddo, 1958; Hayes, 1982).

Atypical Cases of Various Origins   A formerly completely healthy 43-year-old farm worker was brought to hospital by his wife and his employer because of insomnia the night before and sudden loss of memory during the morning. He was found to have flushing of the abdominal wall; a firm, regular, nontender liver enlarged 2–3 cm below the costal margin; and a cholinesterase level only 33% of normal. By next morning he appeared completely recovered. His only known recent exposure to pesticides involved handling diazinon containers a day or two before admission, but there had been no recognized accident and no episode of typical cholinergic illness (Conyers and Goldsmith, 1971).

Dosage Response   Ingestion of the compound at a rate of about 90–444 mg/kg proved fatal, in some cases in spite of treatment (Kabrawala *et al.*, 1965). Dosages as high as 250 mg/kg (Bockel, 1957) or even 888 mg/kg or more (Banerjee, 1967; Bwibo, 1971) have been survived. Since vomiting often occurred and since many of the reported cases received gastric lavage (as well as other treatment), it is difficult to estimate the amounts retained. Certainly, many persons have been made severely sick by ingestion of the compound at rates as low as about 11 mg/kg (Kabrawala *et al.*, 1965) and, even in these cases, the dosage retained is unknown.

Although 0.02 mg/kg/day was accepted by an FAO/WHO Joint Meeting (WHO, 1967) as a no-effect level in humans, some episodes of poisoning cast doubt on this conclusion, either in connection with some formulations or in connection with the susceptibility of children, or both.

For example, two samples of oatmeal that had poisoned children were found to contain 244 and 2.5 ppm, respectively (Hirschy *et al.*, 1970). Assuming that a serving is cooked from 30 gm of dry oatmeal, the two samples would have determined doses of 7.32 and 0.075 mg, respectively, or, for half-grown children, dosages of 0.2 and 0.002 mg/kg. The contamination had occurred in a way that would offer maximal opportunity for oxidation. The illness produced by the lower dosage was characteristic of poisoning, even though distinctly milder than that produced by the higher dosage.

A man survived subcutaneous injection of diazinon at a rate of about 14 mg/kg (Rao, 1965). However, diazinon caused sweating, abdominal pain, nausea, and, in one instance, coma when 80 mg of active ingredient (in the form of a 1% solution) was applied to the skin of each of two men for control of creeping eruption (Hayes, 1963). This strong reaction to a

dosage of about 1.1 mg/kg is inconsistent with the other reports, especially those involving nonfatal illness following ingestion or subcutaneous injection. Thus, the diazinon used for therapy may have undergone change to a more toxic material. This was certainly the case in connection with a formulation responsible for intoxication of three applicators and a herd of cattle. The material was found to be 30 times more toxic than a recently formulated emulsion concentrate of equivalent concentration (Mello *et al.*, 1972).

A dosage of 0.02 mg/kg was a no-effect level in adult volunteers. The threshold limit value of 0.1 mg/m^3 indicates that occupational intake of about 0.014 mg/kg is considered safe, and it probably is sufficiently low to compensate for variation in the toxicity of different formulations.

Laboratory Findings   A woman drank diazinon and cut her wrists. Although the relative importance of poisoning and blood loss as causes of death is unclear, it is of interest that the following concentrations of unmetabolized diazinon were reported in the tissues: brain, 0.3 ppm; liver, 0.08 ppm; kidney, 0.04 ppm; and lung, 0.015 ppm (Heyndricks *et al.*, 1974). For the analytical results in a fatal and a nonfatal case involving ingestion of a mixture of diazinon, parathion, and chlordane, see Section 16.7.1.3

Even the relatively small dosage involved in the use of diazinon for cockroach control in an animal laboratory led to cholinesterase depression among the people working there as well as among the experimental animals (Koopman *et al.*, 1977).

Treatment of Poisoning   Treatment is similar to that for other organic phosphorus compounds (see Section 16.2.2.7). The value of 2-PAM in treating poisoning by diazinon in humans is clearly established (Shankar, 1966; Wadia *et al.*, 1971). In one series of cases, patients who could not be treated for 8 hr or more after they had ingested an estimated 15 ml of a diazinon formulation of unstated concentration died, whereas others survived who ingested the same volume of formulation but were treated not more than 3 hr later (Gupta and Patel, 1968).

16.7.3 DEMETON

16.7.3.1 Identity, Properties, and Uses

Chemical Name   Commercial formulations contain two related compounds: *O,O*-diethyl-*S*-2-ethylthioethyl phosphorothioate (demeton-S) and *O,O*-diethyl-*O*-2-ethylthioethyl phosphorothioate (demeton-O).

Structure   See Table 16.36.

Synonyms   Demeton (BSI, ISO) is the common name for a mixture of demeton-O (ISO) and demeton-S (ISO), except in the USSR, where there appears to be no common name for the mixture. In the USSR, demeton-O is called merkaptophos, and demeton-S is called merkaptophos teolovy. A trade name for the demeton mixture is Systox®. Demeton-S has been sold under the trade name Isosystox. Code designations for the mixture have included B-8,173, Bayer 10,756, and E-1,059. The CAS registry number for the mixture is 8065-48-3. The number for demeton-S is 126-75-0, and that for demeton-O is 298-03-3.

Physical and Chemical Properties Both isomers have the empirical formula $C_8H_{19}O_3PS_2$ and a molecular weight of 258.34. Both isomers are colorless oils. The boiling point of the mixture is 123°C at 1 mm Hg. The boiling points of the isomers at the same pressure are 128 and 118°C for the S-isomer and O-isomer, respectively. The vapor pressure of the mixture is 2.48×10^{-4} at 20°C. The vapor pressures of the isomers at the same temperature are 2.6×10^{-4} mm Hg and 2.48×10^{-4} mm Hg. Demeton is soluble in ethanol, propylene glycol, toluene, and similar hydrocarbons. It is hydrolyzed by boiling water and strong alkali, but it is compatible with most nonalkaline pesticides, except water-soluble mercury compounds. Demeton-S and demeton-O are soluble in water at room temperature to 2000 and 60 ppm, respectively.

History, Formulations, and Uses Demeton was introduced in 1951 by Farbenfabriken Bayer AG. It is a systemic insecticide and acaricide effective against sap-feeding insects and mites. It is available as emulsifiable concentrates of varying active ingredient contents.

16.7.3.2 Toxicity to Laboratory Animals

Basic Findings Demeton is highly toxic not only by the oral but also by the dermal route. Gaines (1960) reported oral LD 50 values of 6.2 and 2.5 mg/kg in male and female rats, respectively. His corresponding dermal values were 14 and 8.2 mg/kg. Shaffer and West (1960) found a similar oral toxicity (8 mg/kg in male rats). DuBois and Coon (1952) found an intraperitoneal LD 50 of 3 mg/kg in mice. The sulfoxide and sulfone derivatives of P=O demeton resemble the parent compound in their intraperitoneal and oral toxicity to rats, mice, and guinea pigs and in their anticholinesterase activities (DuBois *et al.*, 1956).

Formulation has a great influence on the dermal toxicity of demeton. An equal volume of an emulsifier changed the LD 50 from less than 24 to 620 mg/kg, whereas dilution of the mixture to the strength used for spraying greatly increased the toxicity. The lethal dosage was about 5 mg/kg (Deichmann *et al.*, 1952).

Female rats receiving demeton at a dietary level of 50 ppm became severely poisoned but after 3–4 weeks gradually recovered despite continued feeding. Feed intake was low at the beginning of the study but became greater than that of control rats for the latter part of the 16-week experiment. Blood and brain cholinesterase activities were severely inhibited, averaging only 8.2 and 7.1% of normal, respectively. Rats on 20 ppm appeared normal, although the cholinesterase activity of their

blood and brain was only about 15% of normal. Cholinesterase inhibition was progressively less at lower dietary levels but was only about 90% of normal in whole blood and brain at the lowest dietary level tested, namely 1 ppm (about 0.05 mg/kg/day) (Barnes and Denz, 1954). The observations of other investigators have been essentially similar (Deichmann and Rakoczy, 1955; Schrader, 1975).

Inhibition of erythrocyte cholinesterase of dogs was slight at a demeton dietary level of 5 ppm (0.149 mg/kg/day); inhibition of plasma cholinesterase activity was marked at 5 ppm and slight at 2 ppm. A dietary level of 1 ppm (0.025 mg/kg/day) was a no-effect level for both enzymes. When demeton and parathion were in the same diet at levels necessary for cholinesterase inhibition, the effects were additive (Frawley and Fuyat, 1957).

Rats that had been maintained for 28 days since weaning on a diet containing 3.5% protein as casein were about five times more susceptible than controls maintained on ordinary rat feed to a single dose of demeton. However, the protein deficiency was so severe that 17% of the rats on the low-protein diet died before receiving the insecticide (Boyd and Krupa, 1969).

Absorption, Distribution, Metabolism, and Excretion Radioactive phosphorus injected intraperitoneally into pregnant mice in the form of demeton resulted in heavy labeling of placental tissue, fetal muscle, and osteogenic mesenchyme within 20 min. Fetal tissue showed only a trace of activity after 3 hr, suggesting rapid metabolism and elimination (Budreau and Singh, 1973c).

Biochemical Effects A curious finding was that rats given fluoride by stomach tube at the rates of 16.8 and 33.6 mg/kg/day for 30 days had greatly increased susceptibility to demeton but only slightly increased susceptibility to parathion (Rice and Lu, 1963). It is tempting to speculate that fluoride inhibits an enzyme that is more important in detoxifying demeton than parathion, but such an enzyme has not been demonstrated.

Demeton does not potentiate the toxicity of other organic phosphorus compounds, including malathion (DuBois, 1958; Zaratzian *et al.*, 1960).

Effects on Organs and Tissues Ducklings hatched from eggs innoculated with demeton on day 13 of incubation at the rate of 0.01 mg/egg had partial to complete loss of voluntary control of one or both hind legs. Some were excitable and ataxic. The difficulties gradually disappeared about 1 week after hatching, but growth of treated ducklings remained retarded. The injury was more severe in ducklings inoculated at a high temperature. Histological examination of the skeletal muscles revealed areas of degenerative change and other areas of marked regenerative activity (Khera *et al.*, 1965a,b). Similar effects were produced by EPN, a compound that is neurotoxic in hens. Whether the condition seen in ducklings is etiologically similar to that seen in hens is unknown.

Effects on Reproduction Administration of demeton to mice as a single intraperitoneal dose at the rate of 7 or 10 mg/kg or as three consecutive doses of 5 mg/kg each between days 7 and 12 of gestation was embryotoxic, as evidenced by decreased fetal weight and slightly higher mortality of the young. Fetuses with intestinal hernias were found at 16 but not at 18 days. The circumstance and other evidence suggested that the hernias were the result of embryotoxicity and not teratogenicity (Budreau and Singh, 1973a).

16.7.3.3 Toxicity to Humans

Experimental Exposure Five men who received demeton orally at the rate of 7.125 mg/person/day (about 0.1 mg/kg/day) for 25 days showed maximal average depressions of 39.8 and 15.9% in plasma and erythrocyte cholinesterase activity, respectively (Moeller and Rider, 1965; Rider *et al.*, 1969). Earlier tests on other groups of men had been carried out at rates of 0.75–6.375 mg/person/day (Rider and Moeller, 1960, 1964; Moeller and Rider, 1959, 1962b, 1963). None of these rates produced any illness. One subject had marked plasma and red cell cholinesterase depression at 4.125 mg/day. Maximal average plasma cholinesterase depression at 6.375 mg/person/day (about 0.09 mg/kg/day) was 20% of the controls, whereas red cell values were not significantly changed (Rider and Moeller, 1964). The dosage producing no effect on cholinesterase was 0.05 mg/person/day (Rider *et al.*, 1969). It is not astonishing that Upholt *et al.* (1954) found no clinical or biochemical effect from heavy consumption of demeton-treated apples and peaches because, under those conditions, the maximal dosage was only 0.016 mg/kg/day.

Accidental and Intentional Poisoning Poisoning by demeton has been the cause of several deaths (Kaiser, 1953; Kleinman, 1960; Braito, 1959; Michelsen, 1958; Maresch, 1957).

Use Experience A number of cases of serious poisoning and a few deaths doubtless caused by demeton have been associated with occupational exposure without any recognized accident (Lyubetskii and Vengerskaya, 1961; Faerman *et al.*, 1961; Efendiev, 1961; Golubeva and Guglin, 1964; Salibaev, 1966, 1969; Bakhodirov, 1970; Rasuleva, 1970).

During aerial spraying of wheat and cotton, the concentration of demeton in the air breathed by agricultural workers approached 1 mg/m³. Twelve of 14 of the workers had lowered cholinesterase levels but no clinical evidence of poisoning. The authors considered that concentrations should not exceed 0.02 mg/m³ (Kagan, 1956).

Levels between 4.3 and 6 mg/m³ were reported later in the breathing zone of workers applying demeton to trees. Serum cholinesterase activity of the operators was reduced, but no symptoms were reported in spite of the much higher concentrations in the air (Kagan *et al.*, 1958).

Atypical Cases of Various Origins A 16-year-old boy suffered acute illness while spraying hops with demeton. He was

unconscious for 6 hr. He was treated mainly with atropine but did not recover promptly. Five weeks later, he still complained of difficulty in breathing, general weakness, and lack of coordination in walking. After 3 months he still had disturbances of the autonomic nervous system. The clinical course of a 17-year-old boy was similar (Klimková-Deutschová, 1959).

Seven of 25 workers examined in January and February had hemoconcentration, as did 8 of 30 examined in August and September. Four of those with hemoconcentration had 9–11% reticulocytosis. Leukopenia was found in two of the first group and five of the second (Yushkevich, 1958).

Dosage Response Recorded cases offer little information on the dosage of demeton required to produce poisoning in humans but are consistent with data from animal experiments indicating that the toxicities of demeton and parathion are similar.

At about 0730 hr a man spilled approximately 60 ml of concentrated liquid demeton on his left leg at the thigh. He rinsed it with water but continued wearing the pants. At 1500 hr, when he reported for a prearranged, routine blood sample, he felt fine. At 1630 hr, nausea, vomiting, and weakness began suddenly, and he was taken to hospital. He developed other typical signs of poisoning, but he responded rapidly to small doses of atropine and recovered uneventfully. The plasma and red cell cholinesterase activity 1½hr before onset was already severely depressed; in fact, all samples taken in hospital showed a gradual increase in both values (Hayes, 1982).

The highest dosage producing no effect on plasma and red cell cholinesterase of volunteers was 0.05 mg/kg/day. The threshold limit value of 0.1 mg/m³ indicates that an occupational intake of 0.014 mg/kg/day is considered safe.

Laboratory Findings In the near-fatal poisoning of a 3-year-old boy, metabolites equivalent to only 4.15 mg of demeton were recovered from his urine collected during the first 24 hr of hospitalization. Metabolites were detectable in greatly reduced amounts during the third hospital day, after which sampling was discontinued because recovery was essentially complete (Felsenstein *et al.*, 1976).

Treatment of Poisoning See Section 16.2.2.7.

16.7.4 PHORATE

16.7.4.1 Identity, Properties, and Uses

Chemical Name Phorate is *O,O*-diethyl-*S*-(ethylthiomethyl) phosphorodithioate.

Structure See Table 16.36.

Synonyms The common name phorate (ANSI, BSI, ISO) is in general use, except in the Soviet Union, where the name timet is used. Another common name found in the Eastern

European literature is cidial. Trade names include Granatox® and Thimet®. Code designations include American Cyanamid-3,911, E.I.-3,911, ENT-24,042, and L-11/6. The CAS registry number is 298-02-2.

Physical and Chemical Properties Phorate has the empirical formula $C_7H_{17}O_2PS_3$ and a molecular weight of 260.40. The pure material forms a clear mobile liquid with a boiling point of 118–120°C at 0.8 mm Hg. The melting point is −43.7°C. The vapor pressure is 8.4×10^{-4} mm Hg at 20°C. The technical material is over 90% pure and has a density of 1.167 at 25°C. The solubility of phorate in water at room temperature is 50 ppm. Phorate is miscible in carbon tetrachloride, dioxan, vegetable oils, xylene, alcohols, ethers, and esters. Phorate is stable at room temperature but is hydrolyzed in the presence of moisture and by alkalies; therefore, it is incompatible with alkaline pesticides.

History, Formulations, and Uses Phorate was introduced in 1954 by the American Cyanamid Company as a systemic and contact insecticide and acaricide. It is used primarily to protect crops, especially root and feed crops, cotton, brassicas, and coffee from sucking and biting insects, mites, and certain nematodes. Phorate also is used as a soil insecticide on corn and sugar beets. Phorate is available as a 20–25% emulsifiable concentrate and as 5, 10, and 15% granules.

16.7.4.2 Toxicity to Laboratory Animals

Basic Findings As shown in Table 16.40, phorate is highly toxic not only by the oral but also by the dermal route. It is so rapidly absorbed that some animals die within an hour or two following even dermal exposure (Gaines, 1960). The oral LD 50 of the most toxic metabolite, the sulfone of the oxygen analog, is in the range of 0.5–0.8 mg/kg (Wirth, 1958).

Absorption, Distribution, Metabolism, and Excretion Phorate is readily absorbed by the skin, as well as by the gastrointestinal tract.

The compound is metabolized by plants to very potent anticholinesterase agents, of which both the sulfoxide and the

Table 16.40
Single-Dose LD 50 for Phorate

Species	Route	LD 50 (mg/kg)	Reference
Rat	oral	2.1	Wirth (1958)
Rat, M	oral	2.2	Vrbovský et al. (1959)
Rat, M	oral	2	Shaffer and West (1960)
Rat, M	oral	2.3	Gaines (1960)
Rat, F	oral	1.1	Gaines (1960)
Rat, M	dermal	6.2	Gaines (1960)
Rat, F	dermal	2.5	Gaines (1960)
Rat, M	intraperitoneal	1.98	Vrbovský et al. (1959)
Mouse, M	oral	2.25	Vrbovský et al. (1959)
Mouse, M	intraperitoneal	2.1	Vrbovský et al. (1959)

sulfone of both phorate and its oxygen analog have been identified. The anticholinesterase activity of the compounds expressed as pI 50 values are as follows: phorate (P), 3.17; P-sulfoxide, 3.35; P-sulfone, 5.00; oxygen analog (PO) 5.87; PO-sulfoxide, 6.76; PO-sulfone, 7.02. Because of this oxidation by plants and in spite of some inevitable loss of total residue, residues on plants to which phorate had been applied increase in anticholinesterase activity for several days and only then gradually lose activity. Although phorate metabolites could be detected in foliage of 7.4-week-old cotton plants grown from treated seed, no metabolites (<0.03 ppm) could be found in the seeds gathered when the plants were 16 weeks old (Bowman and Casida, 1957; Metcalf et al., 1957).

Rats and cows not only form the same metabolites as plants but also cleave the P—S bond to form O,O-diethylphosphorothiolic and later O,O-diethylphosphoric acid, which are excreted in the urine. Rats given [^{32}P]phorate orally at the rate of 2.0 mg/kg excreted only 35% of the radioactivity in the urine and 3.5% in the feces in 6 days, while those treated at the rate of 1 mg/kg/day for 6 days excreted only 12% in the urine and 6% in the feces within 7 days. A cow that received a dosage of 3.04 mg/kg excreted 59% in the urine within 72 hr and only 0.8% in the feces. In both species most of the radioactivity remaining in the body when the animals were killed was bound to the tissues, especially liver and kidney, in an unidentified form (perhaps diethyl phosphorylated protein) that could not be extracted with either chloroform or acetones (Bowman and Casida, 1958).

Effects on Organs and Tissues Phorate was not mutagenic in bacterial systems (Simmon et al., 1976), and it did not produce dominant lethals in mice (Jorgenson et al., 1976).

16.7.4.3 Toxicity to Humans

Use Experience Several cases of poisoning were associated with the application of phorate to cotton seed or with the planting of the dressed seed. Special equipment was used to cover the seed with carbon dust impregnated with phorate to the extent of 44%. Cotton plants germinated from protected seed were toxic to aphids and mites for about 5 weeks after emergence. Those who treated the seeds usually wore respirators, rubber gloves, and long coveralls, and they escaped injury. Poisoning occurred among laborers who planted seeds, cleaned planting machines, or carried out related tasks while neglecting recommended protection. Considering the small number of reports available for study, it is remarkable that a large proportion of the patients were young (16–18 years old); their age may have influenced their susceptibility.

One of these cases referred to earlier (Hayes, 1963) lived through the most critical part of his illness in a physician's office. The 16-year-old youth, who had been working for several days with phorate-treated cotton seed, had gone to the physician one afternoon with typical but moderate symptoms and received an injection of atropine and some tablets of it to take orally. At home, the youth became worse and lapsed into coma; at 2000 hr about 3 hr after his first visit, he was taken back to the same physician, who administered oxygen for 3.5 hr and artificial respiration for 0.25 hr. During this period, the blood pressure became undectable for a time. By 2300 hr the patient's condition had stabilized, and he was transferred to a hospital. On arrival, the patient had pinpoint pupils; blood-tinged, frothy sputum; and occasional convulsions. With appropriate treatment, the excessive secretions diminished during the night, and the patient regained consciousness at 1115 hr the next morning. On the same day, red cell and plasma cholinesterase activities were 21 and 49%, respectively, of normal. Thirty-six hours after onset, the patient was much improved but tense, and restraints were required to control him during the following night. Intermittent periods of restlessness and drowsiness followed. Although physically essentially well, the patient became severely confused during days 7–10 of hospitalization, and at times he was noisy and uncooperative. A psychiatrist called as a consultant speculated whether the condition was the result of hypoxia suffered early in the illness or a direct result of poisoning, but he recorded no conclusion. By hospital day 12, the patient was mentally clear, and he was discharged on day 15. By this time, plasma cholinesterase activity had recovered completely but red cell enzyme activity was still depressed (24% of normal). In this case, treatment with atropine was continued through at least hospital day 7. Atropine, as well as hypoxia and phorate, may have contributed to the patient's psychotic reaction. The case illustrates the difficulty of evaluating the cause.

Two cases occurred at different times in the same formulating plant. No specific accident was recognized, but air samples collected at the plant after the first illness showed phorate concentrations ranging from 0.07 to 14.60 mg/m³, compared to the threshold limit value of 0.05 mg/m³. Treatment was appropriate, and recovery was prompt and uncomplicated in each case (Young *et al.*, 1979b).

Atypical Cases of Various Origins Phorate was blamed for chills, fever, and hypotension that a farmer experienced following self-administered hemodialysis. The trouble did not recur in hospital but did recur when hemodialysis was re-instituted at home. This time the symptoms included cardiac arrhythmia, alternating chills and fever, nausea, vomiting, and convulsions within minutes after the dialysis. A contamination of the home water supply was suspected. Gas chromatography revealed a compound interpreted as phorate in well water and also in blood. The concentrations in two samples of water were 0.016 and 0.001 ppm. The concentration interpreted as phorate was 0.111 ppm in the patient's blood and 2.3 ppm in the blood of one of his daughters, who was healthy. A new deeper well was drilled, and periodic checks of the water failed to reveal the contaminant. The patient recovered enough to resume farming. No source of phorate was found (Benson *et al.*, 1970). There is no reason to doubt that a contaminant in his well water caused the farmer's trouble. There is considerable question as to whether the contaminant was phorate because the man's symptoms were not diagnostic, the concentration in

the daughter's blood would have been fatal if the compound had been phorate, and no critical chemical test of the identity of the compound was reported. A woman was thought to have symptoms of poisoning 10 hr after she had traveled for 2 hr in a truck cab containing a sample of phorate-contaminated soil in a polyethylene bread wrapper. Her recovery over a period of 12 hr was attributed to atropine (Pugh, 1975). Exposure, if any, was respiratory. Her husband, who accompanied her in the cab, remained well, although he had collected the sample and had other potential exposure, which she lacked. Other possible diagnoses were not considered.

Treatment of Poisoning See Section 16.2.2.7.

16.7.5 TEPP

16.7.5.1 Identity, Properties, and Uses

Chemical Name TEPP is tetraethyl pyrophosphate.

Structure See Table 16.36.

Synonyms The common name TEPP (BSI, ISO) is in general use. Trade names have included Bladan®, Fosnex®, Gy-Tet 40®, HETP®, Hexaethyltetraphosphate®, Killex®, Kilmite®, Lethalaire®, Licophosphate®, Nifos T®, Pyfos®, Pyro-Phos®, Teep®, Tetradusto 100®, Tetron®, Tetraspa®, and Vapotone®. The British Pharmacopoeia Commission approved the name ethyl pyrophosphate for TEPP when used as a drug. The CAS registry no. is 107-49-3.

Physical and Chemical Properties TEPP has the empirical formula $C_8H_{20}O_7P_2$ and a molecular weight of 290.20. The pure material forms a colorless, odorless, hygroscopic liquid with a boiling point of 124°C at 1 mm Hg. TEPP has a density of 1.185 at 20°C and a vapor pressure of 1.5×10^{-4} mm Hg at the same temperature. TEPP is miscible with water and most organic solvents, but it is of low solubility in petroleum oils. TEPP is hydrolyzed rapidly by water with a half-life of 6.8 hr at pH 7 and 25°C. It is decomposed at 170°C with the evolution of ethylene.

History, Formulations, and Uses TEPP was patented in 1943 as a nonsystemic aphicide and acaricide. It is used in control of aphids, spiders, mites, mealybugs, leafhoppers, and thrips. For agricultural purposes, TEPP refers to a mixture of polyphosphates containing at least 40% tetraethyl pyrophosphate. As an aerosol, a solution in methyl chloride is used. TEPP is available as 0.66–1.2% dusts and 10–40% emulsifiable concentrates.

16.7.5.2 Toxicity to Laboratory Animals

TEPP is a compound of high acute toxicity. It is absorbed almost as effectively by the skin as by the gastrointestinal tract. Frawley *et al.* (1952a) reported that the oral LD 50 values in male and female rats were 2.0 and 1.2 mg/kg, respectively. In male rats, Gaines (1969) found an oral LD 50 of 1.1 mg/kg and a dermal LD 50 of 2.4 mg/kg. The intraperitoneal LD 50 in mice is 0.85 (DuBois and Coon, 1952).

16.7.5.3 Toxicity to Humans

Experimental Exposure   TEPP has been placed in the eyes of normal volunteers as a basis for exploring its possible use in the treatment of chronic glaucoma and also in an effort to investigate the visual difficulties that had occurred in crop-duster pilots. The reports do not agree regarding the concentrations of TEPP necessary to produce minimal and maximal miosis. This probably was because the earlier studies involved larger "drops," namely drops produced by a "standard eye dropper" (Marr and Grob, 1950) whereas a later study employed drops of about 0.01 ml each (Upholt *et al.*, 1956). A minim, commonly equated with a "drop," is 0.0616 ml. Either a 0.01- or a 0.06-ml drop might accidentally enter the eye of a worker, and the degree of contamination would be much greater in connection with a splash.

Grant (1948) found that TEPP is absorbed by the human eye from normal saline and peanut oil solution with about equal ease. A 0.01% solution produced definite miosis in 30 min, and it usually lasted 24 hr. A 0.1% solution produced more marked miosis in only 7 min, and it lasted to some degree more than 3 weeks. The higher concentration also produced twitching of the eyelids, moderate spasm of accommodation for near vision, and aching of the eye and supraorbital area. There was no change in intraocular pressure.

According to Marr and Grob (1950), one drop of 0.0125% TEPP in peanut oil produced a definite constriction of the pupil within 30 min, but no other changes. A 0.05% solution produced maximal miosis in 20–40 min, and some pupillary constriction remained for 2 days. In addition to the miosis, ciliary spasm developed and lasted 12–18 hr, but there was no significant change in ocular tension. Some subjects developed mild conjunctival injection lasting a few hours. One drop of 0.1 or 0.2% TEPP produced maximal miosis in 15–20 min, and some miosis remained for 2 weeks; twitching of the lids sometimes was noticed, and many of the subjects developed supraorbital pain that lasted 1–2 hr.

The physiological basis for the danger of unilateral miosis is discussed under Visual Effects in Section 16.2.2.2. TEPP was used to investigate this matter in volunteers because this compound more than others had been the cause of accidents and near accidents that pilots said were the result of their being unable to judge distance. Ability to judge distance correctly is probably more critical for crop-duster pilots than for any other group of workers because they must avoid trees and power lines while flying and often must land their planes on narrow, short runways.

In this study, it was found that two drops (about 0.02 ml) of 0.05% TEPP in peanut oil produced slight miosis and a slight increase in near accommodation, whereas a smaller dose had no effect. Maximal miosis in each eye, with the pupil fixed at 1 mm, was produced by placing in it drops of 0.1% TEPP at an interval of 30 min for a total of two drops (about 0.02 ml). This dosage was insufficient to cause any detectable change in blood cholinesterase, even when both eyes were treated. However, the maximal dosage in both eyes caused mild headache, a sensation of pressure in the eyeballs or over the frons, slight burning of the lids, running or stopped-up nose, and a sensation that things were getting darker. These symptoms passed their peak during the first or second hour. The experimentally induced miosis (as well as occupationally induced miosis in pilots) lasted 12–24 hr, after which the pupils began to react to light and accommodation. Subjective complaints lasted about the same length of time. Partial constriction of the pupil lasted 2 or 3 days. In addition to miosis, objective effects caused by two drops of 0.1% TEPP instilled into each eye of volunteers included an increase in near and far accommodation and a decrease in light perception, but there was no inability to judge distance. The same dosage in only one eye of seven volunteers produced unilateral miosis and all of the expected effects in the treated eye; in addition, four of them complained specifically of difficulty in judging distance, and six of them made sensorimotor errors that were clearly the result of this difficulty; all of them had difficulty by one measure or another (Upholt *et al.*, 1956).

Certain other results observed in normal volunteers were carried out in connection with therapeutic trials and are discussed in connection with Dosage Response.

Therapeutic Use   Treatment of myasthenia gravis requires systemic administration and effects of a drug, whereas treatment of glaucoma is entirely local.

Apparently, Burgen *et al.* (1948) were the first to report the treatment of myasthenia with TEPP. From a study of three patients, they concluded that TEPP was a completely satisfactory substitute for prostigmin but had the advantage of having a more even and persistent effect. The maintenance dosage of TEPP was 8–12 mg/day given in two or three doses by mouth. Side effects were controlled with atropine, as was true of the side effects of prostigmin.

In a very thorough paper, Grob and Harvey (1949) described the treatment of 11 patients with moderately severe and severe myasthenia gravis who had previously been treated with neostigmine. The main advantage of TEPP was that it required fewer doses per day but provided a more sustained increase of strength. The average dose of TEPP required to reach maximal or near-maximal strength was 41 mg administered orally over a period of 5 or more hours. The average daily amount for maintenance of strength was 16 mg orally in two or three divided doses. The difference distinguishing the dosage level of TEPP that produced a maximal increase in strength with a minimum of side effects, the dosage level that produced very little effect, and the dosage that produced prohibitive side effects (including increased weakness) was very narrow (2–4 mg above or below the optimum). Atropine sulfate (10 mg/day) was used concurrently with TEPP to minimize muscarinic side effects. Although the dosages used varied slightly, other reports confirmed the findings just discussed (Stone and Rider, 1949; Rider and Moeller, 1960).

Apparently, the first effort to treat glaucoma by means of

TEPP was that of Grant (1948), who reported 15 cases, most of which were refractive to other miotics. He noted several instances in which tension was more effectively lowered by 0.05–0.1% solutions of TEPP in peanut oil twice a day than by 4% pilocarpine nitrate several times a day. However, TEPP was not uniformly successful in lowering tension, and in two cases it actually increased the pressure.

Marr and Grob (1950) reported the treatment of 21 patients with chronic glaucoma that was uncontrolled by 2% pilocarpine, 0.25% eserine, or 10% furmethide. In most instances, the condition was wide-angle glaucoma. Most of the patients received TEPP for about 3 months; the longest period was 5 months. The concentrations used were 0.05, 0.1, and 0.2% in peanut oil; instillation of one drop varied from one to three times a day. Under these conditions there was no systemic effect. Among the 21 patients, only five glaucomatous eyes were treated successfully for 6 weeks or more by dosages ranging from one drop of 0.05% TEPP once a day to 0.1% three times a day. Treatment often was unsuccessful because (with or without local symptoms) the tension was not maintained within normal limits (20 eyes) or only because of local symptoms such as supraorbital pain or blurred vision (6 eyes).

Accidental and Intentional Poisoning   TEPP is a direct inhibitor of cholinesterase. This explains the main difference between poisoning by this compound and that produced by parathion, which depends on contaminants for any direct action it may show. Dermal and/or respiratory poisoning by TEPP often was well advanced within the hour, whereas occupational poisoning by parathion often was delayed until the worker was home and had had dinner (see Sections 16.2.2.2 and 16.7.1.3).

An occupational accident mentioned briefly by Hayes (1963) illustrates the speed of action. In the process of adding a gallon of TEPP concentrate directly to the spray tank of his plane, an apprentice pilot spilled some of the material on his right leg. He wiped it off but did not wash or change clothes. He did tuck his shirt under his shorts where the liquid had penetrated. By this time there was barely time to spray out the load before dark. He took off hurriedly and began spraying. After the third pass over the field, he ceased following the flagman and flew about the field erratically as though attempting to dump his load as quickly as possible. He actually made one pass at right angles to his flight pattern. His later recollection was that at about the eighth pass he became conscious of blurred vision, weakness, and lightheadedness, and he realized that the poison had affected him. He had trouble locating the landing strip but managed a rough landing in which the plane hit a ditch, and a spray boom was bent. The pilot climbed out of the plane but was unable to walk, and he fell down vomiting. He was taken to the nearest town but, because no physician could be located, he was carried an additional 14.5 km to the nearest hospital. On the way he became unconscious, and his condition deteriorated in other ways. On arrival at the hospital, less than an hour after spillage, he was cyanotic, his pulse was barely palpable, and foamy material filled his lungs and ran from his nose and mouth. Fortunately, the police had radioed ahead, and the emergency staff was ready to receive the patient. Vigorous treatment resulted in complete cure; he was released about 50 hr after admission. An interesting feature of the case was a first-degree burn of the skin that had been wet with TEPP.

Less fortunate was a 6-year-old boy also mentioned very briefly by Hayes (1963). While playing with his younger sister in a neighbor's orchard, he found and opened a 1-gallon bottle of TEPP concentrate that had been left in the orchard over winter and was now revealed because the cardboard carton that originally had contained four bottles was now almost disintegrated. In opening the bottle, the boy spilled enough of the contents to wet the front of his pants from the groin to the knees. Nothing got on his sister. About 10 min later the boy remarked that he noticed "two little girls walking down the road" when in reality there was only one such person. He then complained of abdominal cramps and an upset stomach. The children noticed a parked car and walked to it. The driver, seeing that the boy was sick, took both children to their home, arriving there an estimated 15 min after the exposure. The boy was clutching his abdomen and complaining of pain in his legs; he was ataxic, having difficulty in talking, frothing at the mouth, and gasping for breath, although his color was still good. While his father was removing the wet pants and putting on dry clothing, the boy lost consciousness and became limp. It required only about 10 additional minutes to reach a physician's office, but about 2 min before arrival the boy stopped breathing. The physician found the boy deeply cyanotic, unresponsive to painful stimuli, and without detectable respiration, heartbeat, or pulse. The physician considered the boy dead. However, manual artificial respiration, external pressure on the chest, and sucking out the upper respiratory tract brought a return of audible heart tones with a regular rhythm and an improvement in skin color. Artificial respiration was continued until spontaneous respiration returned in only about 2.5 hr. However, the harm had been done. Over a period of days, it became increasingly evident that poisoning was no longer the problem, but that the boy had suffered irreparable brain damage from anoxia. His fate had been sealed in less than 2 hr after exposure, although he survived 6 days.

A very different kind of accident involving people and animals exposed to static clouds of TEPP dust was described by Quinby and Doornink (1965). In the most serious outbreak, two planes dusted 18.6 ha of hops with 1% dust. They had applied 1043 kg at a rate of 56 kg/ha (that is, 0.56 kg of active ingredient per hectare) when they were stopped by the police. A thermal inversion existed during the application so that the dust settled among the 6-m-high hop vines, and some drifted at least 213 m over adjacent pastures, crops, and houses. It did not move from the hops or the nearby farmhouses for almost 2 hr. The temperature was 35.6°C. It was not unusual to apply insecticides during a thermal inversion, but it was unusual for an inversion to cause such still air for so long a period. The dust was so dense at one house that another house about 275 m away was not visible. No one involved could remember similar behavior of a dust cloud, although for many years they had seen dust applied in exactly the same way.

It seems likely that the entire episode would have escaped much attention if the cows at one farm in the cloud had not been seriously poisoned. Of particular interest was the different response of different species exposed to the same atmosphere. The condition of his cows caused the farmer and some others, including a veterinarian, to come to their assistance and some other members of the family to come outdoors to watch. Of a total of 11 people in the farmer's household, five, including a 7-month-old infant, coughed and became short of breath. These five had spent 30 min or more outside the house before shortness of breath occurred. None of those remaining inside had symptoms. All of the farmer's 15 cattle were affected. All of them coughed more than the people. Some stood with their legs far apart, drooling saliva and gasping for air. Some had their tongues out and showed different degrees of cyanosis. The cattle staggered when they moved, and several fell briefly to their knees. Small quantities of urine and feces were passed frequently. Two yearling heifers went down within 15 m of the house and soon began convulsing; they died within 2 hr after onset. It is possible that more of the cattle would have died if a veterinarian had not treated them with atropine. In contrast to the cattle, two geese and a cat in the area were not visibly affected, and chickens at an adjacent home were not harmed.

Subsequent investigation of neighbors raised to 14 the number known to have had shortness of breath plus an additional person who had a sensation of tightness in the chest but no shortness of breath.

It was after the dusting had been going on for half an hour that the farmer whose cattle were dying complained to the police. Apparently, no more dust was applied after the complaint. However, the immediate result of the complaint was not to remove affected people from the area but to bring in many more, including state and local police, firemen, civil defense workers, reporters, and those who were merely curious. The police ordered the area evacuated. However, all but three of the persons who had respiratory symptoms had recovered before they left the area or before they reached hospital. These three people were hospitalized overnight, even though they recovered promptly. As a precautionary measure the baby also was hospitalized until morning. Forty-one persons were examined in the emergency room, and five others were examined in the field. No treatment was required for anyone, but all were told to bathe and change clothes.

The authors reviewed a number of other episodes in which cattle had been poisoned by airborne TEPP dust; some of the cases were serious but none was fatal. People associated with the same episodes had either minor symptoms or none at all.

Even persons who made no complaint often noticed the sweetish smell of the TEPP, and many of them promptly experienced dryness of the throat and/or coughing, which—rightly or wrongly—was attributed to the talc that served as a vehicle for the TEPP. Those who developed tightness in the throat or chest or shortness of breath did so only after they had breathed the dust for about 30 min. These effects were almost certainly the result of local action of TEPP on the respiratory system. The degree of discomfort among the farm families was not greater than that frequently experienced by workers with occupational exposure to TEPP dust.

Local action undoubtedly played an important part in causing illness in the cattle, but it is difficult to evaluate the relative importance of hypoxia and the systemic action of TEPP in causing their nonrespiratory signs.

Use Experience   In spite of its high toxicity, the safety record of TEPP has been surprisingly good as far as truly occupational poisoning is concerned. Kawashiro (1959) reported that in Japan this compound had caused only eight cases of poisoning during spraying but 18 other accidents and 101 suicide attempts, of which 99 were successful. The number of cases and the ratios were completely different for parathion, which has a delayed and, therefore, more insidious action following occupational exposure.

Other occupational deaths, at least one of them the result of dermal exposure without any recognized "accident," have been reported (Smith *et al.*, 1968; Hearn, 1973).

If decontamination and treatment are started as soon as slight symptoms appear, serious illness often may be aborted (Reeder, 1961).

Dosage Response   What was estimated to be one mouthful of TEPP that had been stored in a wine bottle led to complete collapse in less than 5 min and death shortly thereafter (Davis, 1957).

Studies in normal people showed that a single dose of 5 mg, or 3.6 mg daily for 2 days or 2.4 mg daily for 3 days parenterally, or 7.2 mg every 3 hr orally for three to five doses produced symptoms that appeared suddenly about 30 min after the final dose (Grob and Harvey, 1949). These studies were preliminary to much more extensive ones in patients with myasthenia gravis who were slightly less susceptible to the drug, as discussed under Therapeutic Use.

The amounts of TEPP that produce miosis when instilled into the eye are discussed under Experimental Exposure.

The threshold limit of 0.05 mg/m³ indicates that occupational intake of TEPP at a rate of 0.007 mg/kg/day is considered safe.

Treatment of Poisoning   See Section 16.2.2.7.

16.7.6 CARBOPHENOTHION

16.7.6.1 Identity, Properties, and Uses

Chemical Name   Carbophenothion is O,O-diethyl-S-4-chlorophenyl-thiomethyl phosphorothionate.

Structure   See Table 16.36.

Synonyms   While carbophenothion (ANSI, BSI, ISO) is in general use, nephocarp also has been used as a common name. Trade names include Acarithion®, Garrathion®, and Trithion®.

Code designations include ENT-23708 and R-1303. The CAS registry number is 786-19-6.

Physical and Chemical Properties Carbophenothion has the empirical formula $C_{11}H_{16}ClO_2PS_3$ and a molecular weight of 342.85. The pure material forms an off-white to light amber liquid with a mild mercaptan-like odor. Its boiling point is 82°C at 0.01 mm Hg. The vapor pressure is 3×10^{-7} mm Hg at 20°C, and its refractive index is 1.590–1.597. Carbophenothion is slightly soluble in water (less than 4 ppm at 20°C). It is miscible with most organic solvents. Carbophenothion is stable to hydrolysis but is oxidized to the phosphorothiolate.

History, Formulations, and Uses Carbophenothion was introduced in 1955 by the Stauffer Chemical Company. It is a nonsystemic acaricide and insecticide with long residual action. It is used on deciduous fruits, in combination with petroleum oil, and as a dormant spray for the control of overwintering mites, aphids, and scale insects. Carbophenothion is available as 1, 2, 3, and 5% dusts; 25% wettable powders; and approximately 24, 48, 72, and 96% emulsifiable concentrates.

16.7.6.2 Toxicity to Laboratory Animals

Basic Findings Carbophenothion produces illness typical of cholinesterase inhibitors. It has a moderate acute toxicity as shown in Table 16.41. The dermal toxicity is only slightly less than the oral.

The compound was fed to hens at concentrations up to 100 ppm; although this dosage (about 5.8 mg/kg/day) affected egg production, it did not cause neurotoxicity (FAO/WHO, 1973).

In a 90-day study, tremors were seen in rats on dietary levels of 46 and 100 ppm but not at 22 ppm and lower. Cholinesterase inhibition occurred at 10 ppm but not at 5 ppm (Lehman, 1965).

A dietary level of 32.5 ppm (about 1.6 mg/kg/day) was the ED 50 for cholinesterase inhibition in the rat (Williams, 1961). A dietary level of 100 ppm for 90 days caused no mortality of rats but did produce cholinergic signs in both sexes and reduced growth in females; brain, red cell, and plasma cholinesterase activities were inhibited. The findings were similar

Table 16.41
Single-Dose LD 50 for Carbophenothion

Species	Route	LD 50 (mg/kg)	Reference
Rat, M	oral	55	Shaffer and West (1960)
Rat	oral	91	Hagan *et al.* (1961)
Rat	oral	28	Williams (1961)
Rat, M	oral	30	Gaines (1969)
Rat, F	oral	10	Gaines (1969)
Rat, M	dermal	54	Gaines (1969)
Rat, F	dermal	27	Gaines (1969)

in a 2-year study at a dietary level of 80 ppm; in addition, there was some reduction of hemoglobin and increased adrenal weights in females. Cholinergic signs and cholinesterase inhibition occurred at dietary levels as low as 20 ppm in the 2-year study, but there was no cholinesterase inhibition or other effect in either study at a dietary level of 5 ppm (about 0.24 mg/kg/day) (FAO/WHO, 1973).

In a 2-year test in dogs, brain, red cell, and plasma cholinesterase activity was depressed, and the females showed reduced growth and a relative increase in adrenal weight at a dietary level of 80 ppm (about 1.7 mg/kg/day). There was no effect on mortality, physical condition, neurological examination, food consumption, blood or other clinical laboratory measurements, or gross or histological examination of the tissues. Dogs were more irritable at dietary levels of 20 and 80 ppm but not at 5 ppm (about 0.1 mg/kg/day), even though plasma cholinesterase was depressed at this level (FAO/WHO, 1973). In a 90-day study, plasma cholinesterase was not affected at 0.8 ppm (about 0.017 mg/kg/day), although it was slightly inhibited at twice that intake (Lehman, 1965).

Absorption, Distribution, Metabolism, and Excretion Williams *et al.* (1962) showed by their measurement of whole-blood cholinesterase following dermal application that the time required for penetration of the skin of rats by carbophenothion is definitely less than 1 hr. Because they failed to measure inhibition associated with intravenous infusion (see Fig. 3.3) and because carbophenothion is an indirect inhibitor of cholinesterase, it cannot be concluded that penetration of rat skin by carbophenothion is slower than 12 min, the time found necessary for paraoxon to penetrate cat skin.

Excretion of carbophenothion is rapid. Following intraperitoneal injection, mice excreted over 75% of the dose within 24 hr (FAO/WHO, 1973). Carbophenothion is metabolized to the oxon, and both compounds are oxidized to the corresponding sulfoxide and sulfone. Each reaction renders the material more toxic, except that carbophenothion sulfone is less toxic than the parent compound. The pI 50 values for carbophenothion and carbophenooxon sulfone are 3.3 and 8.0, respectively (FAO/WHO, 1973). Reduction of the sulfoxide to carbophenothion also occurs, both *in vivo* and *in vitro* (DeBaun and Menn, 1975).

Biochemical Effects Following relatively large single doses, carbophenothion potentiates the toxicity of malathion about 3-fold. It does not potentiate other compounds tested (Lehman, 1965).

Effects on Reproduction Carbophenothion was fed to rats for three generations at a single dietary level of 20 ppm, which determines dosages of about 1 and 2 mg/kg/day in adults and weanlings, respectively. This procedure was toxic to the young but not teratogenic. Toxicity (reduced birth weight, increased stillbirths, decreased survival to weaning) was present in all generations but not in all litters (FAO/WHO, 1973).

16.7.6.3 Toxicity to Humans

Experimental Exposure Carbophenothion produced no clinical effect and no significant change in plasma or red cell cholinesterase values when administered orally to five volunteers at the rate of 0.8 mg/person/day (about 0.01 mg/kg/day) for 30 days (Rider *et al.*, 1972).

Accidental and Intentional Poisoning A 25-year-old workman was attacked by his colleagues during a lunch break and held down while carbophenothion dust was forced into his mouth. On the following morning he had symptoms of poisoning. Recovery was complete following repeated doses of atropine over 30 hr (Hearn, 1961). Even if symptoms started during the night (which was not reported), the delay in onset is remarkable, especially in view of the circumstances of exposure.

Seven members of a family became ill after eating tortillas made from flour which had been purchased from a salvage store and which apparently had been contaminated with carbophenothion during shipment. The onset of illness ranged from 4 to 6 hr after the meal. One woman experienced only nausea and vomiting and did not require hospitalization. Other members of the family developed more severe poisoning, including coma in four, and one remained critically ill for 4 days in spite of receiving 66 mg of atropine sulfate and 8 gm of pralidoxime chloride before he regained consciousness. All were fully recovered within 6 days. Animals to which leftover tortillas were distributed fared worse; eight chickens, one dog, and one cat died (Older and Hatcher, 1969).

Use Experience Nineteen cases of poisoning on one sugarcane plantation were reported (Hearn, 1961). With the exception of one case mentioned above, the cases presumably were caused entirely by occupational exposure.

Laboratory Findings In the episode described above, the serum cholinesterase of persons who ate three or four contaminated tortillas varied from 0.54 to 1.26 µmol/min/ml, while that of a person who ate only one was 2.16 µmol/min/ml, compared to a normal range of 3.3–7.7 µmol/min/ml. The serum samples were taken 48–72 hr after hospitalization.

Treatment of Poisoning See Section 16.2.2.7.

16.7.7 CHLORFENVINPHOS

16.7.7.1 Identity, Properties, and Uses

Chemical Name Chlorfenvinphos is the *trans* or β isomer of 2-chloro-1(2,4-dichlorophenyl) vinyl diethyl phosphate.

Structure See Table 16.36.

Synonyms The common name chlorfenvinphos (BSI, ISO) is in general use. The term CFVP was used earlier. Trade names include Birlane®, Dermaton®, Sapecron®, and Supona®. Code designations include C-0,949, Compound-4,072, GC-4,072, OMS-166 (also OMS-1,328), and SD-7,859. The CAS registry number for the *trans* isomer of chlorfenvinphos is 18708-86-6, and that for the *cis* isomer is 18708-87-7. The number for the mixture is 470-90-6.

Physical and Chemical Properties Chlorfenvinphos has the empirical formula $C_{12}H_{14}Cl_3O_4P$ and a molecular weight of 359.56. It is an amber-colored liquid with a mild odor. A typical example of the technical product contained 83.8% *trans* isomer, 9.7% *cis* isomer, and 6.5% of related compounds. The boiling point of chlorfenvinphos is 167–170°C; it has a vapor pressure of 4.0×10^{-6} mm Hg at 20°C. It melts at −19 to −23°C. It is soluble sparingly in water but is miscible with acetone, ethanol, kerosene, propylene glycol, and xylene. Chlorfenvinphos is stable when stored in glass- or polyethylene-lined containers but is hydrolyzed slowly by water. Its half-life at 38°C is more than 400 hr at pH 9.1 and more than 700 hr at pH 1.1.

History, Formulations, and Uses Chlorfenvinphos was introduced in 1963 by Shell Development Company. It is an insecticide for use on foliage and soil. When sold under the name Dermaton®, it is a miticide for veterinary use. Available formulations include a 24% emulsifiable concentrate, a 25% wettable powder, 5% dust, and 10% granules.

16.7.7.2 Toxicity to Laboratory Animals

Basic Findings Chlorfenvinphos shows an unusual degree of species variation in its acute toxicity. This applies to intravenous toxicity and even more to oral toxicity (see Table 16.42).

Table 16.42
Single-Dose LD 50 for Chlorfenvinphos

Species	Route	LD 50 (mg/kg)	Reference
Rat	oral	10–15	Hutson and Hathway (1967)
Rat, M	oral	15	Gaines (1969)
Rat, F	oral	13	Gaines (1969)
Rat	oral	9.66	Ambrose *et al.* (1970)
Rat, M	dermal	31	Gaines (1969)
Rat, F	dermal	30	Gaines (1969)
Rat	intraperitoneal	8.5	Hutson and Hathway (1967)
Rat	intravenous	6.6	Hutson and Hathway (1967)
Mouse	oral	150–200	Hutson and Hathway (1967)
Mouse	intraperitoneal	37	Hutson and Hathway (1967)
Guinea pig	oral	125–250	Hutson and Hathway (1967)
Rabbit	oral	500–1,000	Hutson and Hathway (1967)
Rabbit	oral	300[a]	Ambrose *et al.* (1970)
Rabbit	dermal	400	Ambrose *et al.* (1970)
Dog	oral	>5,000	Hutson and Hathway (1967)
Dog	oral	>12,000	Ambrose *et al.* (1970)
Dog	intravenous	50.4	Hutson and Hathway (1967)
Dog	intravenous	50.5	Ambrose *et al.* (1970)

[a] Approximate value.

Some hens survived 10 intraperitoneal injections of 100, 150, and 200 mg/kg/day, but none showed any neurotoxicity during observation lasting 20 days after the last injection, and their nerves were normal on histological examination.

Rats fed dietary levels ranging from 3 to 1000 ppm and dogs fed 1 to 1000 ppm for 12 weeks showed no clinical signs of intoxication. Growth was depressed in both sexes of rats fed 1000 ppm but not in dogs at the same dietary level.

Rats remained well when fed dietary levels of 10, 30, 100, and 300 ppm for 2 years. There was a clear dosage response in the degree of inhibition of both plasma and red cell cholinesterase activity. At the 10 ppm level, there was a tendency for the enzyme activity to return to normal during the course of the study (Ambrose et al., 1970). These results are entirely consistent with the findings that dosages of 10 mg/kg/day for 30 days or 30 mg/kg/day for 10 days had little or no effect on the intestinal absorption of a wide range of nutrients by rats (Barna and Simon, 1974).

The health of dogs was not influenced by dietary levels of 30, 200, and 1000 ppm for 2 years. Plasma cholinesterase was significantly depressed at all these levels; red cell cholinesterase was depressed only at the 1000 ppm level. Hematology, liver and kidney function tests, and histology remained normal (Ambrose et al., 1970).

Absorption, Distribution, Metabolism, and Excretion
Using ^{14}C-labeled vinyl chlorfenvinphos, it was shown that the main metabolites are desethyl chlorfenvinphos (32.3% in rats, 69.6% in dogs), [1-(2′,4′-dichlorophenyl)ethyl β-D-glucopyranosid] uronic acid (41.0% in rats, 3.6% in dogs), 2,4-dichlormandelic acid (7.0% in rats, 13.4% in dogs), 2,4-dichlorophenylethanediol glucuronide (2.6% in rats, 2.7% in dogs), and 2,4-dichlorohippuric acid (4.3% in rats). There was no sex difference in metabolites in rats or dogs.

Following a single oral dose of the ^{14}C-labeled vinyl chlorfenvinphos, rats excreted within 4 days 87.2% in the urine, 11.2% in the feces, and 1.4% in expired air. During the first day, excretion amounted to 67.5%. In dogs 94.0% was excreted in urine and feces within 4 days, with 86.0% in the urine and 4.1% in the feces during the first day (Hutson et al., 1967).

Biochemical Effects In spite of the considerable difference in acute intravenous toxicity and the astonishing difference in acute oral toxicity of chlorfenvinphos in dogs and rats, the difference following oral administration cannot be accounted for by any single factor. Instead, the relatively small differences observed in rates of absorption and metabolism, availability in the blood, rate of brain uptake, and sensitivity of brain acetylcholinesterase to the insecticide combine to explain the difference in toxicity (Hutson and Hathway, 1967).

Oral dosages as high as 1 mg/kg did not affect cholinesterase or the awake–sleep cycle of rats. At dosages over 2 mg/kg, the cholinesterase activities of both brain and red cells were significantly decreased, and the spontaneous EEG showed a prominent arousal pattern with suppression of curves characteristic of sleep. Maximal inhibition of brain cholinesterase

occurred 3 hr after dosing and lasted for more than 72 hr. Duration of the arousal pattern was proportional to dosage and was suppressed by atropine. This indicates that the arousal pattern depends on cholinergic activation (Osumi et al., 1975).

Effects on Reproduction In a three-generation study, rats were fed 300, 100, and 30 ppm. There was little or no reduction in the number of young born alive in either the first or second litter produced by the parent generation at the highest feeding level; however, few of these F_{1a} and F_{1b} pups survived. Production of living young was less successful in the next generation, and no young survived to weaning at the high dietary level. At a dietary level of 100 ppm, the same result tended to be delayed one generation; only a few young were weaned in the F_{3a} generation and none in the F_{3b}. The 30-ppm dietary level (2.9 mg/kg/day in adult, nonlactating rats) produced a small, statistically uncertain reduction in reproduction. No gross abnormalities were noted in the newborn in any generation. In rats that survived the 100- as well as the 3-ppm diets, the ovaries, Fallopian tubes, endometrium, and testes were histologically normal (Ambrose et al., 1970). There was strong evidence that the main or perhaps only difficulty lay in the inability of dams at the higher dietary levels to nourish their young after birth. Whether this depended on reduced production of milk, reduced suckling of the pups, or the presence of a toxicant in the milk was not explored.

16.7.7.3 Toxicity to Humans

Experimental Exposure Because of the unusually great difference in the toxicity of chlorfenvinphos in different species and because of the importance of dermal absorption associated with occupational exposure, the dermal toxicity of the compound was studied in nine volunteers (Hunter, 1969). Formulations were applied to the left forearm beneath a sealed aluminum-foil cover. After exposures of as much as 4 hr, the cover was removed, the exact area of contact was measured, and the remaining compound was removed with swabs and measured chemically. The absorbed dose was determined by difference and expressed in terms of unit area and time. Formulations used were 80 and 24% emulsifiable concentrates and 25% water-wettable powder. The report contains the raw data but presents the results in terms of dosages expressed as milligrams per square centimeter per hour, and it attempts to draw distinctions between the different formulations. A much improved relationship between absorbed dosage, inhibition of plasma cholinesterase, and blood levels of chlorfenvinphos may be obtained if the dosage is expressed as milligrams per hour. This is what one would expect, because absorption from each square centimeter of skin is additive. Dosage levels of 112 mg/hr/person reduced plasma cholinesterase by 67% or more and produced blood levels of 0.012 ppm or more measured 24 hr after exposure. The next highest dosage (70.8 mg/hr/person) caused a 53% inhibition of plasma cholinesterase and a blood level of 0.006 ppm 24 hr after exposure. These dosages involved the 24% emulsifiable concentrate, which contained trimethylbenzenes that may have promoted absorption. At lower dosage levels, the maximal decrease of plasma cholinesterase was 25%; red cell enzyme was inhibited in only one sample and then only by 9%. The men remained well. Tests of cardiovascular, nervous, and renal function remained unchanged from preexposure values, as did tests of blood and urinary glucose after a 10-gm load.

Accidental and Intentional Poisoning A 16-month-old died after drinking a chlorfenvinphos formulation (Felthous, 1978). This was the basis of a special plea for child-resistant packaging.

A 65-year-old man was accidentally poisoned by chlorfenvinphos. The patient had severe breathing disorders accompanied by acidosis. He was hyperglycemic when first seen but later became hypoglycemic. Treatment included trimedoxime, which made a distinct contribution to recovery (Jaros and Kratinova, 1973).

A 16-year-old boy said he had taken a full swallow of an antimange preparation prescribed by a veterinarian for his dog, mistaking it for cough medicine. He came to hospital about 90 min later because of abdominal cramps, nausea, vomiting, generalized weakness, muscle twitching, and apprehension. Physical signs were consistent with poisoning; the only unusual finding was a rectal temperature of 34.58°C. Gastric lavage was performed, and the boy was treated with atropine and pralidoxime chloride. He never became seriously ill, and he remained oriented. In spite of marked weakness of his grip, which improved soon after treatment was started, his respiratory muscles were never compromised. Red cell and plasma cholinesterase activities were about one-tenth of normal at first but almost up to the lower limits of normal 24 hr later. The hypothermia was almost alleviated 15 min after PAM was started; it had lasted at least 2 hr but was almost gone 4.5 hr after admission. Atropine was continued as a precaution. The day after admission, the patient began to give inappropriate answers to questions and later had hallucinations. Atropine was continued, and he was sedated with small doses of chlorpromazine. Next morning he was drowsy but oriented. At that time a full history revealed that some 24 or 48 hr before admission, the boy had taken capsules of tetrahydrocannabinol. It was thought that atropine contributed to the hallucinations, but a contribution from one or more other substances could not be excluded. His mental status cleared within 12–18 hr after atropine was stopped, and he was discharged without residuals 5 days after admission. The antimange formulation proved to be chlorfenvinphos sold under the trade name Dermaton®, and the compound was demonstrated in the boy's blood by gas chromatography (Cupp *et al.*, 1975). If one considers that marijuana has any bearing on the case, the possibility that it influenced ingestion of the miticide cannot be excluded.

The dosage of the miticide may be calculated as 85 mg/kg, of which much must have been lost through vomiting and lavage.

Laboratory Findings One metabolite of chlorfenvinphos in humans is desethyl chlorvinphos (DEC). Methylation of this compound permits measurement of the derivative by gas chromatography sensitive to 0.002 ppm of DEC. The method was tested in male volunteers who ingested the β isomer at the rate of 2.5 mg/person/day for 53 days. At this low level of intake, average daily excretion of the methylated derivative was 120 μg (approximately 0.08 ppm), which corresponded to 4.7% of the daily dose. Following a single oral dose of radioactive chlorfenvinphos at the rate of 12.5 mg/person, the proportion of the dose excreted as DEC was 23.8% (Hunter *et al.*, 1972). This difference in proportion of dose excreted as DEC indicates a difference in metabolism conditioned by adaptation to the compound or dosage, or both.

Treatment of Poisoning See Section 16.2.2.7.

16.7.8 CHLORPHOXIM

16.7.8.1 Identity, Properties, and Uses

Chemical Name Chlorphoxim is *O,O*-diethyl-*O*-2-chlorophenyl-glyoxylonitrile-oxime phosphorothioate.

Structure See Table 16.36.

Synonyms The common name chlorphoxim (BSI, ISO) is in general use. Code designations include B-78,182, ENT-27,449, and OMS-1,197. The CAS registry number is 14816-20-7.

Physical and Chemical Properties Chlorphoxim has the empirical formula $C_{12}H_{14}CIN_2O_3PS$ and a molecular weight of 332.73.

History, Formulations, and Uses Chlorphoxim was introduced in Europe in the late 1960s.

16.7.8.2 Toxicity to Laboratory Animals

According to the manufacturer, the oral LD 50 is greater than 2500 mg/kg in rats and more than 1000 mg/kg in both mice and guinea pigs. The dermal toxicity may be greater than the oral toxicity (WHO, 1977).

16.7.8.3 Toxicity to Humans

A village trial with chlorphoxim was carried out in Nigeria in 1972. Three baggers, four spraymen, and one mixer were engaged. Bagging was performed in a well-ventilated room and lasted for 4 hr. No hydrogen cyanide could be detected by the paper test method above freshly opened drums. Two out of three drums were used to prepare 169 bags. Spraying lasted for 5 consecutive days, during which 162 pump-charges were used to spray about 450 houses. No complaints were received, and no adverse effects could be detected among exposed baggers, spraymen, or inhabitants during this trial. Whole-blood cholinesterase in spraymen showed no depression when measured spectrophotometrically and tintometrically; neither could any inhibition be detected tintometrically among the exposed residents.

Since there were no complaints among exposed operators and villagers and no clinical or biochemical findings of adverse effects, the World Health Organization committee responsible for judging the matter concluded that chlorphoxim should be safe enough to warrant its use in larger trials, provided that simple protective clothing and good personal hygiene are employed. However, in view of the observation in a collaborating laboratory that the toxicity of chlorphoxim water-dispersable powder formulation increases when it is exposed to sunlight, the committee considered that the stability of the compound during storage and handling prior to spraying should be investigated before it can be recommended for really extensive testing (WHO, 1973).

A more extensive trial was carried out in 1975 when a group of Nigerian villages was sprayed three times at 3-month intervals. Twenty-one men were engaged in the operation, and they were observed and questioned frequently by a medical toxicologist. By the last day of spraying, plasma cholinesterase of the sprayers and mixers was reduced to about 75% of preexposure values, but whole-blood values were 90% of normal. No skin changes were detected. One man had a headache, but it was not considered to be related to the spraying. Inquiries failed to elicit any complaints from the villagers (Rishikesh *et al.*, 1977a).

Treatment of Poisoning   See Section 16.2.2.7.

16.7.9 CHLORPYRIFOS

16.7.9.1 Identity, Properties, and Uses

Chemical Name   Chlorpyrifos is *O,O*-diethyl-*O*-(3,5,6-trichloro-2-pyridyl) phosphorothioate.

Structure   See Table 16.36.

Synonyms   The common name chlorpyrifos (ANSI, BSI, ISO) is in general use. Another nonproprietary name, trichlorpyriphos, has been discontinued. Trade names include Dursban® and Lorsban®. Code designations include Dowco-179, ENT-27, 311, and OMS-971. The CAS registry number is 2921-88-2.

Physical and Chemical Properties   Chlorpyrifos has the empirical formula $C_9H_{11}Cl_3NO_3PS$ and a molecular weight of 350.57. The pure material forms white crystals with a mild mercaptan odor. The melting point is 42.5–43°C. The vapor pressure is 1.87×10^{-5} mm Hg at 25°C. At 35°C the solubility of chlorpyrifos in water is 2 ppm. In isooctane the solubility is 79%, and in methanol it is 43%. Chlorpyrifos is stable under normal storage conditions. The half-life in aqueous methanolic solution at pH 6 is 1930 days; at pH 9.96 it is 7.2 days.

History, Formulations, and Uses   Chlorpyrifos was introduced by Dow Chemical Company in 1965 as a broad-spectrum insecticide especially useful in controlling mosquitoes and household insects. Chlorpyrifos is used to control adult mosquitoes, flies, many foliage crop pests, household pests, and aquatic larvae. Chlorpyrifos is available as 25% wettable powders, 1–10% granules, and emulsifiable concentrates of 2 and 4 pounds per U.S. gallon.

16.7.9.2 Toxicity to Laboratory Animals

Basic Findings   When given in sufficient dosage, chlorpyrifos produces signs indistinguishable from those of other organic phosphorus compounds, and its speed of action is approximately the same as that of other =S diethoxy compounds. The acute toxicity is of moderate degree. The compound is only slightly less toxic when applied to the skin of rats than when administered to them by mouth (Gaines, 1969). There is considerable variation in the susceptibility of different species (see Table 16.43).

In hens protected from death by atropine, subcutaneous dosage of 200 mg/kg produced ataxia that lasted only 10–20 days but, unlike that caused by malathion, was delayed 3–18 days in onset. Recovery was complete. A subcutaneous dosage of 100 mg/kg did not cause neurotoxicity (Gaines, 1969). Oral dosages up to 150 mg/kg also failed to produce neurotoxicity (FAO/WHO, 1973; El-Sebae *et al.*, 1977).

In 2-year feeding studies in rats, dosages of 1 and 3 mg/kg/day produced moderate depression of plasma and red blood cell cholinesterase, and brain cholinesterase was depressed by 3 mg/kg/day. In 2-year feeding studies in dogs, the results were identical, except that there was some inhibition of plasma but not red cell cholinesterase by a dosage of 0.1 mg/kg/day. All cholinesterase levels recovered promptly when dosing was stopped. In both species, even the highest dosage studied (3 mg/kg/day) produced no clinically important effect, as judged

Table 16.43
Single-Dose LD 50 for Chlorpyrifos

Species	Route	LD 50 (mg/kg)	Reference
Rat, M[a]	oral	155	Gaines (1969)
Rat, F[a]	oral	82	Gaines (1969)
Rat, M[a]	oral	135	McCollister *et al.* (1974)
Rat, M[a]	oral	118	McCollister *et al.* (1974)
Rat, F[a]	oral	155	McCollister *et al.* (1974)
Rat, M[b]	oral	163	McCollister *et al.* (1974)
Rat, M[b]	oral	245	McCollister *et al.* (1974)
Rat, F[b]	oral	135	McCollister *et al.* (1974)
Rat, M[a]	dermal	202	Gaines (1969)
Mouse	oral	152	Berteau and Deen (1978)
Mouse	respiratory	94	Berteau and Deen (1978)
Guinea pig	oral	504	McCollister *et al.* (1974)
Rabbit	oral	>1000	McCollister *et al.* (1974)
Chicken, M	oral	34.8	Miyazaki and Hodgson (1972)
Chick	oral	32	McCollister *et al.* (1974)

[a] Sherman.
[b] Dow–Wistar.

by survival; growth; relative and absolute organ weights; blood, urine, and clinical chemical findings; and gross and microscopic pathology, including tumors. The no-effect levels are 0.10 and 0.03 mg/kg/day in rats and dogs, respectively (McCollister *et al.*, 1974).

When chlorpyrifos was administered to monkeys for 6 months, both plasma and red cell cholinesterases were inhibited at dosages of 2.0 and 0.4 mg/kg/day, but only the plasma enzyme was inhibited at a dosage of 0.08 mg/kg/day. Brain cholinesterase was not inhibited at any of these dosages, nor was there any clinical or morphological effect (Griffin *et al.*, 1976).

Cockerels tolerated repeated dosages at the rate of 1 mg/kg with only moderate inhibition of cholinesterase and with no illness or interference with growth. Very large repeated doses of a metabolite (the sodium salt of 3,5,6-trichloro-2-pyridinol) did cause an increase in liver size over a period of 25 weeks (Miyazaki and Hodgson, 1972). Five-week-old chickens tolerated a dietary level of 100 ppm (about 10 mg/kg/day) but with some loss in their efficiency of growth relative to feed intake (Schlinke, 1970). Not even interference with weight, feed efficiency, egg production, egg weight and quality, or shell thickness was observed in hens fed chlorpyrifos at a dietary level of 50 ppm (about 5.12 mg/kg), a level sufficient to provide control of the larvae of some but not all species of flies in the feces of the birds (Sherman and Herrick, 1973).

In a study of animals exposed to a thermal aerosol of chlorpyrifos used for adult mosquito control, it was concluded that use at recommended levels did not result in concentrations in the air sufficient to cause effects in rats, chicks, and various beneficial aquatic organisms tested (Oberheu *et al.*, 1970).

Absorption, Distribution, Metabolism, and Storage A single dose of [^{36}Cl]chlorpyrifos to rats led to rapid absorption and excretion in the urine (90%) and feces (10%). The products excreted were 3,5,6-trichloro-2-pyridyl phosphate (75–80%), 3,5,6-trichloro-2-pyridinol, and a trace of the unmetabolized material. In the initial distribution within the tissues, some of the [^{36}Cl]chlorpyrifos was trapped in the fat, and it was mobilized and excreted slowly with a half-life of about 62 hr (Smith *et al.*, 1967). Later study indicated that 3,5,6-trichloro-2-pyridinol constituted 96% of the urinary metabolites from chlorpyrifos in rats, but only 12% was free; the remainder was conjugated, 80% as the glucuronide and 4% as a glycoside (Bakke *et al.*, 1976).

Another metabolite was recovered from the liver of a person who had ingested chlorpyrifos. It was similar to the parent compound except for substitution of an —SCH$_3$ group for a chlorine on the pyridinol ring (Lores *et al.*, 1978b).

Slight storage of unmetabolized chlorpyrifos was found in the fat of cattle dipped repeatedly in 0.025% emulsion. No oxygen analog was detected in any tissue (Ivey *et al.*, 1972). In a similar way, the insecticide was excreted in the milk of cows that had been spray-dipped with a 0.15% emulsion. The maximal concentration in milk was 0.304 ppm, and detectable excretion continued through day 4. Pasteurization caused a 26–47% decrease in concentration (Leshev *et al.*, 1972).

Biochemical Effects Actual toxicity of chlorpyrifos is due almost exclusively to its oxygen analog. The I 50 values for the insecticide and the analog are approximately $2.5 \times 10^{-3} M$ and $2.5 \times 10^{-9} M$, respectively (Smith, 1966).

Effects on Reproduction Rats were fed chlorpyrifos at dosage levels up to 0.3 mg/kg/day for one generation and at rates up to 1.0 mg/kg/day for two generations. Neonatal mortality was somewhat higher at 1.0 mg/kg but reproduction and lactation indices were normal, and all parameters were normal at 0.3 mg/kg/day, even though cholinesterase inhibition was present. The compound was not teratogenic, even at the highest dosage (FAO/WHO, 1973).

16.7.9.3 Toxicity to Humans

Experimental Exposure Groups of four men each received chlorpyrifos tablets for 20 days or more at rates of 0.014 and 0.03 mg/kg/day and for 9 days at 0.1 mg/kg/day. No effects were noted on behavior, hematology, urinalysis, or blood biochemistry. Plasma cholinesterase was depressed at the highest level but returned to normal in 4 weeks. There was also possible depression at 0.03 mg/kg/day, but it did not reach statistical significance. Red cell cholinesterase was not effected at any dosage (FAO/WHO 1973; Griffin *et al.*, 1976). The no-significant-effect level is 0.03 mg/kg/day. This finding is consistent with the threshold limit (0.2 mg/m^3), which indicates that occupational intake at the rate of 0.028 mg/kg/day is considered safe.

No toxicity or erythrocyte cholinesterase inhibition was observed when six volunteers received chlorpyrifos in a single oral dose of 0.5 mg/kg followed in 2 weeks by a dermal dose of 0.5 or 5.0 mg/kg. Although a 15% reduction in plasma cholinesterase occurred following the oral dose, no significant changes were seen following the larger dermal dose. Chlorpyrifos concentrations in the blood never exceeded 30 ng/ml at any time during the study. Blood concentrations of the principal metabolite (3,5,6-trichloro-2-pyridinol) peaked at 0.93 μg/ml at 6 hr following the oral dose and 0.063 μg/ml at 24 hours following the 5.0 mg/kg dermal dose, and this metabolite was cleared from the blood and excreted in the urine with a half-life of 27 hr in both cases. Urinary excretion of approximately 70% of the oral dose but less than 3% of the dermal doses as 3,5,6-trichloro-2-pyridinol suggests minimal dermal absorption of chlorpyrifos. The rapid elimination of chlorpyrifos and its metabolite suggests minimal accumulation in those repeatedly exposed (Nolan *et al.*, 1984).

During 1966, 1967, and 1968, studies were made of sprayers applying 0.5% emulsion and 0.25 and 0.5% suspensions of water-wettable powder for control of pest mosquitoes. Much of the work was done with power sprayers equipped with hand guns operated at pressures as high as 250 lb/in.^{2} (17.6 kg/cm^2). Most of the workers showed more than 50% reduction of plasma cholinesterase values within 2 weeks after beginning the work, and one showed a reduction of more than 70%. No inhibition of red cell cholinesterase was observed at any time, and there was no sign or symptom or illness (Eliason *et al.,* 1969). In a later study using a nonthermal aerosol, no significant inhibition of cholinesterase was found, even in persons with maximal exposure (Lusk *et al.,* 1976).

Accidental and Intentional Poisoning An agitated 26-year-old male entered a hardware store and ingested 360 ml of Ortho Weed-B-Gone M (containing 10.8% dimethylamine salts of 2,4-D and 11.6% MCPP), 360 mL Dexol® (6.7% chlorpyrifos, 76.8% petroleum distillates), and some granules of D-Con® concentrate (0.025% warfarin). The patient gradually became unresponsive and had a blood pressure of 17/110, a pulse of 150 beats/min, and myoclonus. Analysis by electrocardiogram showed a prolonged QT interval, T-wave peaks, and sinus tachycardia. Paradoxically, he had miotic-reactive pupils, normal bowel sounds, and normal reflexes. Although no clinical improvement followed the primary treatment, which included activated charcoal lavage, atropine, dextrose, magnesium citrate cathartic, naloxone, and thiamine, no further cholinergic signs were observed. Supraventricular tachycardia with widened QRS occurred at 30 min and 4 hr following ingestion. Profuse diarrhea occurred from 2 to 6 hr. At 12 hr, a decrease in mean arterial pressure to 50 torr from the initial reading of 66 torr was noted. Fluids and bicarbonate were administered to counteract acidosis. A considerable amount (5.5 liters) of colloids was administered to treat fluid loss and hypotension. At 12 hr, lactate dehydrogenase was measured at 430 IU/liter and the level of serum potassium was 5.3 mEq/liter. Calcium level decreased from 2.5 mM on admission to 1.4 mM 21 hr later, while platelet counts were 109,000, 75,000, and 28,000/μl at 12, 26, and 28 hr following admission. Four episodes of asystole, bradycardia, and continued hypotension (38 torr) between 24 and 30 hr following ingestion warranted the use of additional pralidoxime and atropine, cardiac massage, and electrocardioversion. The patient expired during the fourth episode. No alcohol or drugs were found in analyses of urine and blood. On autopsy, diffuse mild necrosis of the liver, denuded duodenal mucosa with hemorrhage, and congested, edematous lungs were noted (Osterloh *et al.,* 1983).

Hodgson and Parkinson (1985) reported five cases of organic phosphorus pesticide poisoning among office workers in a cement bunker sprayed with chlorpyrifos and methylcarbamic acid. The workers experienced diarrhea and excessive salivation within 1 hr of the time the chemicals were used. However, the exterminator informed them that they probably had a virus. Following a series of referrals, erythrocyte cholinesterase activities were measured. Measurements at 17, 45, 80, and 112 days following exposure showed a significant upward trend. Conservative back-extrapolation indicated a 44% average decrease in cholinesterase activities immediately following exposure.

Atypical Cases of Various Origins A 23-year-old female with abnormal movements was initially discharged from a local emergency room with a diagnosis of hysteria after being found in a stupor near an empty chlorpyrifos container. She was later admitted when her condition deteriorated. At this time the patient was found to have a blood pressure of 120/100 mm Hg, a regular pulse of 100/min, pinpoint pupils, increased muscle tone, a sustained left ankle clonus, increased deep tendon reflexes, and significantly reduced serum cholinesterase and erythrocyte acetylcholinesterase activities. Unusually, the patient had episodic choreoathetosis in all limbs, accompanied by grimacing at approximately 3-min intervals. Atropine was administered at 2 mg/hr and reduced as cholinesterase activity increased and clinical improvement occurred. Abnormal movements resolved in 24 hr, although hyperreflexia, ankle clonus, and increased muscle tone continued for about 7 days. The patient was discharged on day 18 and was asymptomatic when examined 1 month later (Joubert and Joubert, 1984).

Jablecki *et al.* (1983) report a case of a 16-year-old male exposed to a combination of chlorpyrifos and dichlorvos when he entered his house to eat lunch shortly following an extermination of the premises. Abdominal cramps and diarrhea occurred for approximately 2 days following the incident. Weakness and incoordination of the upper extremities were noted. Cramping in both calves began about 7 days after exposure. Over the next 2 weeks, atrophy of both upper extremities and a weight loss of 20 pounds occurred. Neurological symptoms stabilized in the fourth week following exposure, although some weakness in the hip extensors and flexors was noted. Serum cholinesterase activity was normal, and erythrocyte cholinesterase activity was in the lower reaches of the normal range. This case was unusual in that symptoms associated with delayed polyneuropathy developed sooner and were restricted mainly to the upper body. Circumstances surrounding the time of exposure suggest that the observed toxicity might be the consequence of combined oral and inhalation exposures. However, the author failed to consider the possibility that the illness was a Guillain-Barré syndrome only circumstantially related to chlorpyrifos and/or dichlorvos exposure.

Laboratory Findings Unmetabolized chlorpyrifos at concentrations of 0.21, 0.47, and 0.08 ppm was found in the blood, brain, and liver, respectively, of a 61-year-old man who survived about 1 day after ingesting the compound accidentally. The parent compound was not detected in urine, but diethyl phosphate, diethyl thiophosphate, and the phenolic derivative were found at concentrations of 24.5, 23.6, and 13.8 ppm, respectively; traces of the first two were found in some tissues. As already mentioned, a new metabolite was isolated from the liver (Lores *et al.,* 1978a,b).

Treatment of Poisoning See Section 16.2.2.7.

16.7.10 DIALIFOS

16.7.10.1 Identity, Properties, and Uses

Chemical Name Dialifos is *O,O*-diethyl-*S*-(2-chloro-1-phthalimidoethyl) phosphorodithioate.

Structure See Table 16.36.

Synonyms The common name dialifos (BSI, ISO) is in general use, except in the United States and Japan, where dialifor (ANSI, JMAF) is used. A trade name is Torak®. A code designation is Hercules-14,503. The CAS registry number is 10311-84-9.

Physical and Chemical Properties Dialifos has the empirical formula $C_{14}H_{17}ClNO_4PS_2$ and a molecular weight of 393.84. The pure material is a colorless crystalline solid with a melting point of 67–69°C. Dialifos is insoluble in water; slightly soluble in aliphatic hydrocarbons and alcohols; and highly soluble in acetone, cyclohexane, isophorone, and xylene. The technical product and its formulations are stable for over 2 years under normal conditions but are hydrolyzed readily by strong alkali.

History, Formulations, and Uses Dialifos was introduced in 1965 by Hercules Incorporated. It is a nonsystemic insecticide and acaricide effective in controlling many insects and mites common to apples, citrus, grapes, nut trees, potatoes, and vegetables. Dialifos is available in formulations of 24–72% emulsifiable concentrate.

16.7.10.2 Toxicity to Laboratory Animals

Basic Findings Dialifos is a compound of high acute toxicity (see Table 16.44). The no-effect dietary level in rabbits is 3 ppm (Kenaga and Allison, 1969).

Effects on Reproduction Dialifos is a phthalimide derivative and hence an analog of thalidomide. It was in this context that the possible teratogenic effect of dialifos was studied in hamsters. However, the relevance of the study is obscure because most investigations, including the one under discussion, have found that thalidomide is not teratogenic in this species. Be that as it may, dialifos was administered by stomach tube on day 7 or 8 or repeatedly on days 6–8 or 6–10 at total dosages ranging from 100 to 500 mg/kg. The LD 50 for dams receiving single doses was 200 mg/kg. Mortality among the fetuses of surviving dams ranged from 20 to 100%, and the average weight of the fetuses ranged from 0.5 to 1.8 gm at different dosage levels, compared to 2.3 gm in the controls. In different

Table 16.44
Single-Dose LD 50 for Dialifos

Species	Route	LD 50 (mg/kg)	Reference
Rat, M	oral	24	Gaines and Linder (1986)
Rat, F	oral	6	Gaines and Linder (1986)
Rat[a]	oral	39	Gaines and Linder (1986)
Rat, M	dermal	45	Gaines and Linder (1986)
Rat, F	dermal	28	Gaines and Linder (1986)
Mouse	oral	39–65	Kenaga and Allison (1969)
Rabbit	dermal	145	Kenaga and Allison (1969)

[a] Male weanling.

groups, anomalies were found in 0–100% of the young, some of which were already dead when they were removed from the uteri; this effect corresponded poorly with dosage. There were seven instances of limb defects, five instances of short or curved tail, one umbilical hernia, and one ectopic heart (Robens, 1970).

16.7.10.3 Toxicity to Humans

Use Experience Among a crew of 120 grape pickers (110 men and 10 women), 15 became sick one day, 100 additional workers became sick the next day, and 3 more became sick the third day. Some were only dizzy or mildly weak. Others also had headaches, blurred vision, and tightness in the chest. Most plasma and red cell values were depressed more than 60%. Eighty-five of the workers received medical attention. Most were treated with atropine and some with 2-PAM. Three workers were hospitalized. Recovery was uneventful. The vineyard had been treated with dialifos and a less toxic compound, phosalone. On the basis of measurements made soon after the illnesses, it was concluded that the leaf residues of dialifos and of its oxon that caused poisoning were 100 and 2 ppm, respectively (Knaak et al., 1978b; Peoples and Maddy, 1978). Because of some evidence that the insecticide had been applied recently and in view of the relatively small proportion of oxon in the residues, this may have been an example of simple reentry poisoning.

In a separate episode, 32 men picked grapes for 3 days while exposed to dislodgeable residues of about 3 ppm ethion, 30 ppm phosmet, and 73 ppm phosalone and then for another day to foliage with residues of about 8 ppm dialifos. Some symptoms began to appear about midmorning on the last day. Twelve of the workers were so sick during the night that they did not work the next day, and six of the men were hospitalized for an average of 3 days. All or most of them complained of dizziness, nausea, vomiting, headache, numbness, and excessive salivation. None complained of dimness of vision. All available blood samples (29 men) showed significant depression of cholinesterase activity. The grapes had received the customary rates of pesticide applications more than 40 days prior to the men's entry, and the grapes met tolerance requirements for pesticide residues. In an effort to explain the illness, the possibility of interaction was raised (Maddy, 1976). This would seem to be a typical example of classical crop-worker poisoning, where present knowledge is inadequate to explain the cholinergic illness that occurs, and not an example of simple reentry poisoning, where observed exposure is adequate to explain observed illness. That crop-worker poisoning may be possible with dialifos was suggested by the finding of unexpectedly large amounts of the oxygen analog on foliage in a field where a worker recently became sick (Winterlin et al., 1978).

It should be understood that if interaction of chemicals is responsible for crop-worker poisoning, the interaction may not be confined to organic phosphorus compounds or to cholinesterase inhibitors of any kind.

Treatment of Poisoning   See Section 16.2.2.7.

16.7.11 DICHLOFENTHION

16.7.11.1 Identity, Properties, and Uses

Chemical Name   Dichlofenthion is *O,O*-diethyl-*O*-2,4-di-chlorophenyl phosphorothioate.

Structure   See Table 16.36.

Synonyms   The common name dichlofenthion (BSI, ISO) is in general use. Trade names include Bromex®, Hexa-nema®, Mobilawn®, Nemacide®, and V-C 13®. Code designations include ENT-17,470. The CAS registry number is 97-17-6.

Physical and Chemical Properties   Dichlofenthion has the empirical formula $C_{10}H_{13}Cl_2O_3PS$ and a molecular weight of 315.17. The pure material is a colorless liquid with a boiling point of 120–123°C at 0.2 mm Hg. Its density is 1.313 at 20°C. The technical material is 95–96% pure with a density of 1.30–1.32. The solubility of dichlofenthion in water at 25°C is 0.245 ppm, but it is miscible in most organic solvents, including kerosene. Dichlofenthion is stable to hydrolysis, except under strongly alkaline conditions.

History, Formulations, and Uses   Dichlofenthion was introduced in 1956 by the Virginia–Carolina Chemical Corporation as a nonsystemic nematicide and soil insecticide. Dichlofenthion is available as 25 and 75% emulsifiable concentrates and as 10% granules.

16.7.11.2 Toxicity to Laboratory Animals

Dichlofenthion is a compound of low to moderate toxicity (see Table 16.45). When it was fed to dogs at the rate of 0.75 mg/kg/day for 90 days, cholinesterase activity was not reduced significantly and no functional or morphological disturbances were found (Davies *et al.*, 1975).

The average time to onset from the application of a dermal, minimal toxic dose in the form of a spray or dip to cattle, goats, and sheep was 31–72 hr. The number of days from

Table 16.45
Single-Dose LD 50 for Dichlofenthion

Species	Route	LD 50 (mg/kg)	Reference
Rat, M	oral	185	Gaines and Linder (1986)
Rat, F	oral	172	Gaines and Linder (1986)
Rat, M	oral	270	Davies *et al.* (1975)
Rat, M	dermal	576	Gaines and Linder (1986)
Rat, F	dermal	355	Gaines and Linder (1986)
Rabbit	dermal	6000	Davies *et al.* (1975)
Chick	oral	148	Sherman *et al.* (1967)

application of a clinically harmless dose until depression of whole-blood cholinesterase activity became maximal varied from 2 to 11 days, depending partly on species (Younger *et al.*, 1962).

When laying hens were fed dichlofenthion at dietary levels of 50, 100, 200, and 800 ppm (range of about 2.9–46.4 mg/kg/day) for 55 weeks, there was no mortality attributable to the compound; feed consumption, weight gain, egg production, shell thickness, egg weight, and egg odor were unaffected, but the eggs from hens receiving 800 ppm had a less desirable flavor. Inhibition of cholinesterase activity corresponded to the concentration of the compound in the tissues. Enough anticholinesterase(s) appeared in the excreta of hens receiving 50 ppm to give excellent control of the housefly and the blowfly, but higher dietary levels were required to control the larvae of two other species of fly (Sherman *et al.*, 1972).

16.7.11.3 Toxicity to Humans

Accidental and Intentional Poisoning   Almost all we know about poisoning by dichlofenthion is recorded in a paper (Davies *et al.*, 1975) reporting five cases involving attempted suicide or the ingestion of the poison while drunk. Two men, aged 76 and 79 years, died; two other men, aged 25 and 62 years, and a 52-year-old woman survived. The interval from ingestion to hospitalization varied from 2 hr or less to 24 hr in four cases and was unclear in the fifth case. In four instances, typical cholinergic signs were present when the patient entered hospital. The 25-year-old man was cold and sweating and exhibited fecal and urinary incontinence; miosis was evident, and rhonchi were audible in both lungs. The other three were somewhat less severely affected when first seen. All were conscious, although the 76-year-old man, who had ingested chlordiazepoxide and diazepam as well as dichlofenthion, was disoriented and the 52-year-old woman, who had ingested a bottle of whiskey as well as dichlofenthion, was combative. The 62-year-old man showed no abnormal sign on admission, and he showed no clear anticholinesterase signs for 29 hr after ingestion. The cases were remarkably mild on admission when one considers that ingestion was involved in all instances. However, all of the patients showed one or more marked, delayed exacerbations. In four cases, the patient became distinctly worse 19–57 hr after ingestion. Two of them died during the third day of illness. The others had recurring crises, each of which responded to treatment. The fifth patient apparently became worse more gradually, but for many days she had a recurrence of cramps and difficulty in breathing secondary to profuse bronchial secretions whenever her atropine therapy was reduced; it finally was tapered off and discontinued 45 days after ingestion. The surviving patients received total doses of only 84, 659.6, and 33 mg of atropine sulfate and only 2, 1, and 5 gm of pralidoxime chloride. Administration of over 3000 mg of atropine sulfate and over 90 gm of 2-PAM chloride was followed by complete recovery in poisoning by another compound. The surviving patients apparently did not become comatose. Oxygen was administered but not artificial respiration. Thus, poisoning by dichlofenthion was characterized by relatively mild but prolonged illness in those who survived.

Among the five cases just discussed were two involving repeated bleeding from the gastrointestinal tract and three with hypokalemia. The relationship of these findings to intoxication was not investigated.

Dosage Response A patient who died had ingested dichlofenthion at a rate of about 1822 mg/kg, but another man who survived had ingested the same dosage while other survivors had received dosages of only 607 and 152 mg/kg. All of the patients vomited profusely or received gastric lavage, or both, so the retained dosage was unknown in all instances. The degree and duration of illness did not correspond to the dosage the patients reported; the first to recover had taken about 607 mg/kg (Davies *et al.*, 1975). The survivor who said he had ingested dichlofenthion at a rate of 1822 mg/kg excreted 2,4-dichlorophenol in his urine in a total amount that permits calculation of about 41 mg/kg of dichlofenthion-equivalent, which is a minimal estimation of retained dosage.

Laboratory Findings The concentrations of dichlofenthion in the tissues of a man who died on the third day after ingesting dichlofenthion were 19 and 0.83 ppm in serum and kidney, respectively. In a similar case the values were 174 ppm in fat, 37 ppm in bile, 4 ppm in liver, and 1.3 ppm in kidney. In a patient who survived, the concentrations of dichlofenthion in fat were 67, 58, and 0.63 ppm on days 4, 7, and 54 after ingestion. The concentration in the same person's whole blood was 0.660 ppm on day 1; it fell rapidly to about 0.018 on day 12 and then more gradually to 0.0017 on day 48. Another surviving patient, who was sampled less frequently, had higher values at comparable intervals after ingestion, as indicated by a dichlofenthion concentration of 36 ppm in fat on day 30 and serum levels of 0.1730 and 0.0022 ppm on days 14 and 75, respectively. Serum levels of this pesticide were approximately twice whole-blood levels. The survivor studied in greater detail excreted 2,4-dichlorophenol in his urine in concentrations of 274, 188, 77, 42, and 1.1 ppm on days 1, 2, 3, 9, and 34, respectively.

Inhibition of blood cholinesterase was prolonged in patients poisoned by dichlofenthion, as might be expected when the compound continued to circulate in the blood (Davies *et al.*, 1975).

Treatment of Poisoning See Section 16.2.2.7.

16.7.12 DIOXATHION

16.7.12.1 Identity, Properties, and Uses

Chemical Name Dioxathion is *O,O,O',O'*-tetraethyl-*S,S'*-1,4-dioxane-2,3-diyldi(phosphorodithioate).

Structure See Table 16.36.

Synonyms The nonproprietary name dioxathion (BSI, ISO) is used, except in Turkey and the USSR, where delnav is used as a common name. Trade names include Co-Nav®, Delnav®, Kavadel®, and Navadel®. Code designations have included ENT-22,897 and Hercules AC-528. The CAS registry number is 78-34-2.

Physical and Chemical Properties Dioxathion has the empirical formula $C_{12}H_{26}O_6P_2S_4$ and a molecular weight of 456.54. It is a brown liquid with a melting point of $-20°C$. Its density is 1.257 at 26°C. The technical material consists of about 48% *trans* isomer, 24% *cis* isomer, and 30% related compounds. Dioxathion is insoluble in water and less than 1% soluble in hexane and kerosene. It is soluble in most other organic solvents. Dioxathion is very stable, although it is hydrolyzed by alkali and decomposed by heating. It is unstable in contact with iron or tin surfaces.

History, Formulations, and Uses Dioxathion was introduced in 1954 by Hercules, Incorporated as a nonsystemic insecticide and acaricide for the treatment of livestock against external pests, including ticks. It also was recommended for use against citrus mites.

Dioxathion is available as a 25% wettable powder and a 48% emulsifiable concentrate. It is almost harmless to bees.

16.7.12.2 Toxicity to Laboratory Animals

Basic Findings Dioxathion is a compound of moderate toxicity, as shown by Table 16.46. Signs of poisoning are typical of those caused by organic phosphorus compounds. Dropped into the eye, it causes transient conjunctivitis but no corneal damage (Frawley *et al.*, 1963).

Dioxathion did not produce neurotoxicity in surviving hens that received single oral doses at the rate of 10–1000 mg/kg or subcutaneous doses at the rate of 25–200 mg/kg, even though

Table 16.46

Single-Dose LD 50 for Dioxathion

Species	Route	LD 50 (mg/kg)	Reference
Rat, M	oral	45–64[a]	Frawley *et al.* (1963)
Rat, M	oral	43	Gaines (1969)
Rat, F	oral	23	Gaines (1969)
Rat, M	dermal	235	Gaines (1969)
Rat, F	dermal	63	Gaines (1969)
Rat, F	intraperitoneal	30	Frawley *et al.* (1963)
Mouse, M	oral	176	Frawley *et al.* (1963)
Rabbit	dermal	106[b]	Frawley *et al.* (1963)
Rabbit	dermal	100[c]	Frawley *et al.* (1963)
Dog	oral	10–40	Frawley *et al.* (1963)
Chicken, F	oral	>316	Frawley *et al.* (1963)
Chicken, F	subcutaneous	>200	Frawley *et al.* (1963)

[a] Range for three strains.
[b] No solvent.
[c] Applied as xylene solution.

the higher rates killed some of the birds (Frawley *et al.*, 1963). However, a slightly larger subcutaneous dosage, namely, 320 mg/kg, in hens protected by atropine produced a temporary neurotoxic effect lasting 3–31 days (Gaines, 1969).

In rats, a dietary level of 500 ppm caused a marked food refusal and loss of body weight within the first week. Female rats on a dietary level of 100 ppm (7.5 mg/kg/day) showed hyperexcitability and slight tremor, but males remained well. Neither sex showed a change of food consumption or growth, an increase in mortality, or any pathology related to the compound. Both sexes showed marked inhibition of brain, plasma, and erythrocyte cholinesterase activity. A dietary level of 10 ppm (0.78 mg/kg/day) produced no inhibition of brain cholinesterase but significantly reduced plasma and erythrocyte cholinesterase activity. At dietary levels of 3 and 1 ppm (0.22 and 0.077 mg/kg/day) for 90 days, no statistically significant alteration of brain, plasma, or red cell enzyme activity was produced (Frawley *et al.*, 1963).

In dogs, a dosage of 8.0 mg/kg/day caused diarrhea, hypersalivation, tremor, ataxia, and depression, all of which subsided gradually until the animals were free of symptoms 10 days after the last dose. A dosage of 2.5 mg/kg/day caused no illness. Dosages of 0.25 mg/kg/day or greater decreased plasma cholinesterase activity, and dosages of 2.5 mg/kg/day or greater decreased red cell enzyme activity. A dosage of 0.075 caused a statistically insignificant decrease in plasma cholinesterase; dosages of 0.025 mg/kg/day or less were entirely without effect (Frawley *et al.*, 1963).

Absorption, Distribution, Metabolism, and Excretion   Dioxathion is effectively absorbed from the skin, as well as from the gastrointestinal tract. A high proportion (20.4%) was recovered from the urine, and traces were recovered from the feces of a steer within 7 days after dermal application of [^{32}P]dioxathion (Chamberlain *et al.*, 1960).

A small proportion of dioxathion, mainly unmetabolized, was found in the fat of a steer 7 days following dermal application (Chamberlain *et al.*, 1960).

Both the *trans* and *cis* isomers of dioxathion are rapidly and extensively metabolized by rat liver microsomes or by intact rats to the corresponding oxon and dioxon. The compound also undergoes oxidative *O*-deethylation and hydroxylation of the ring resulting in ring cleavage and loss of both phosphorus moieties. The more toxic *cis* isomer is metabolized more rapidly not only to form oxon and dioxon but also to form $^{14}CO_2$ from the labeled ethoxy group (Harned and Casida, 1976).

Biochemical Effects   Dioxathion showed additive or less than additive toxicity when administered in equitoxic ratios with 15 other anticholinesterase insecticides. However, when dioxathion was administered 4 hr before malathion, potentiation as great as 5.4-fold was observed (Frawley *et al.*, 1963). Dietary concentrations of dioxathion less than those necessary to inhibit red cell or brain cholinesterase activity did inhibit

liver and plasma carboxyesterases, and rats treated in this way were more susceptible than normal ones to inhibition of brain cholinesterase by a single 200 mg/kg dose of malathion (Murphy and Cheever, 1968).

Effects on Organs and Tissues   No indication of carcinogenicity was found when rats and mice were fed dioxathion at the maximal tolerated level for 78 weeks and then observed for an additional period (NCI, 1978b).

Effects on Reproduction   Administration of dioxathion to three generations of rats at dietary levels of 3–10 ppm (about 0.07–0.5 mg/kg/day) caused no measurable abnormality among either parents or their young (Kennedy *et al.*, 1973).

16.7.12.3 Toxicity to Humans

Experimental Exposure   Male and female volunteers showed slight inhibition of plasma cholinesterase activity as a result of 0.15 mg/kg/day for as much as 60 days. There was no effect on red cell enzyme activity and no clinical effect; a dosage of 0.075 mg/kg/day produced no effect on plasma cholinesterase. Plasma cholinesterase measurements showed slight but statistically uncertain decrease when dioxathion was administered daily for 60 days at a rate of 0.075 mg/kg/day and malathion was given at a rate of 0.15 mg/kg/day simultaneously for the last 30 of these days (Frawley *et al.*, 1963).

Accidental and Intentional Poisoning   Within 30 sec after he had received 0.75 teaspoonful of a dioxathion formulation mistaken for cough medicine, a 5-year-old boy vomited blue material that smelled like mothballs. The vomiting and profuse diarrhea continued after treatment with ipecac. Within 2 hr after ingestion, the child was mentally dull and unable to stand; he had shallow rapid respirations, muscle fasciculations, tearing, and miosis. Serum cholinesterase activity was less than 10% of normal. After 12 hr of appropriate treatment, most of the signs and symptoms cleared; a mild chemical pneumonitis resolved by the fifth day (Angle and Wermers, 1974a,b). It seems likely that the vomiting and diarrhea were largely the result of local action of the absorbed dioxathion. The formulation contained 60% of methylated naphthalenes, which may have been largely responsible for the pneumonitis.

Dosage Response   The dosage ingested by the 5-year-old boy was approximately 1100 mg of technical dioxathion or 57 mg/kg. The absorbed dosage was somewhat less; both the color and odor of the formulation were detected in the vomitus.

As already mentioned, people tolerate 0.075 mg/kg/day without inhibition of cholinesterase activity and 0.15 mg/kg/day without clinical effect. Thus the threshold limit value (0.2 mg/m^3) is conservative because it places the safe occupational intake at 0.028 mg/kg/day.

Treatment of Poisoning   See Section 16.2.2.7.

16.7.13 FENSULFOTHION

16.7.13.1 Identity, Properties, and Uses

Chemical Name Fensulfothion is *O,O*-diethyl *O*-[4-(methylsulphinyl)phenyl] phosphorothioate.

Structure See Table 16.36.

Synonyms The common name fensulfothion (BSI, ISO) is in general use. The acronym DMSP also has been used. Trade names include Dasanit® and Terracur P®. Code designations include Bayer-25,141, ENT-24,945, and S-767. The CAS registry number is 115-90-2.

Physical and Chemical Properties Fensulfothion has the empirical formula $C_{11}H_{17}O_4PS_2$ and a molecular weight of 308.35. The pure material forms an oily yellow liquid with a boiling point of 138–141°C at 0.01 mm Hg. Its density is 1.202 at 20°C. Fensulfothion is slightly soluble in water and soluble in most organic solvents. Fensulfothion is oxidized readily to the sulphone and apparently isomerizes readily to the *S*-ethyl isomer (Benjamini *et al.*, 1959).

History, Formulations, and Uses Fensulfothion was introduced in 1957 by Bayer Leverkusen as an insecticide and nematicide against free-living and root-knot nematodes. It is a systemic and contact insecticide with long residual action. Fensulfothion is available as 24 and 48% emulsifiable concentrates; 25% wettable powder; 10% dust; and 2.5, 3, 5, 10, and 15% granules.

16.7.13.2 Toxicity to Laboratory Animals

Basic Findings Fensulfothion produces signs typical of cholinesterase inhibition. Following suitable doses, the onset of poisoning is rapid, but death may be delayed (Gaines, 1969). As shown in Table 16.47, fensulfothion is highly toxic by the dermal as well as by the oral route. The acute toxicity of the sulfone is similar.

The compound did not produce neurotoxicity when given orally or intraperitoneally at rates up to 50 mg/kg to chickens protected by atropine and 2-PAM (FAO/WHO, 1973).

Repeated doses at the rate of 3, 2, and 1 mg/kg/day were fatal to yearling ewes in 2, 4, and 7 days, respectively; only a small proportion survived a dosage of 0.5 mg/kg/day for 20 days (Solly and Harrison, 1971).

According to unpublished reports (FAO/WHO, 1973), rats were killed within a week at an intraperitoneal dosage of 0.75 mg/kg/day. Most survived 0.5 mg/kg/day for 60 days, but their growth was reduced. In a 17-month study, the mortality of male rats was increased at dietary levels of 5 and 20 ppm, and the growth of both males and females was slightly impaired at 20 ppm. No effects were observed on gross or histological examination of the tissues. Cholinesterase of brain, red cells, and plasma was detectably inhibited at a dietary level of 1 ppm (about 0.053 mg/kg/day) in females. It is

Table 16.47
Single-Dose LD 50 for Fensulfothion

Species	Route	LD 50 (mg/kg)	Reference
Rat, M	oral	10.5	DuBois and Kinoshita (1964a)
Rat, F	oral	2.2	DuBois and Kinoshita (1964a)
Rat, M	oral	4.1	Gaines (1969)
Rat, F	oral	1.8	Gaines (1969)
Rat, M	oral	6–10	Solly and Harrison (1971)
Rat, F	oral	2–3	Solly and Harrison (1971)
Rat, M	dermal	30.0	DuBois and Kinoshita (1964a)
Rat, F	dermal	3.5	DuBois and Kinoshita (1964a)
Rat, M	dermal	19	Gaines (1969)
Rat, F	dermal	4.1	Gaines (1969)
Rat, M	intraperitoneal	5.5	DuBois and Kinoshita (1964a)
Rat, F	intraperitoneal	1.5	DuBois and Kinoshita (1964a)
Mouse, M	intraperitoneal	10.5	DuBois and Kinoshita (1964a)
Mouse, F	intraperitoneal	7.0	DuBois and Kinoshita (1964a)
Guinea pig, M	oral	9.0	DuBois and Kinoshita (1964a)
Guinea pig, M	intraperitoneal	5.4	DuBois and Kinoshita (1964a)
Sheep, F[a]	oral	3–4	Solly and Harrison (1971)

[a] Yearling.

interesting that male rats are reported to be less susceptible to single doses but more susceptible to repeated doses.

During the early weeks of a 2-year study, reduced food consumption, severe weight loss, and signs of cholinergic poisoning were evident in dogs receiving fensulfothion at a dietary level of 5 ppm, but after the second month food consumption increased and lost body weight was regained. Slight cholinergic signs were seen in dogs at 2 ppm (about 0.04 mg/kg/day), but they soon recovered. Slight reduction of cholinesterase occurred at 2 ppm but not at 1 ppm. None of the levels produced abnormality of the blood or other tissues (FAO/WHO, 1973).

Absorption, Distribution, Metabolism, and Excretion Sheep given [^{32}P]fensulfothion orally absorbed it rapidly, as indicated by peak blood levels 1–2 hr after dosing. However, poisoning was delayed about 12 hr in one that died and 30–35 hr in one that survived. Only 54% of the dose was excreted by the sheep that died, and significant residues were found in its organs. The surviving sheep excreted 65% of its dose in 24 hr and 96% within 7 days. Almost all the excretion was urinary, with little in the feces. Only negligible concentrations of fensulfothion and its oxidation and hydrolysis products were found in the organs of the sheep killed after 7 days (Avrahami and Gernert, 1973).

Biochemical Effects When given in half LD 50 doses, fensulfothion showed only additive effects with malathion and 16 other anticholinesterase pesticides (FAO/WHO, 1973).

Effects on Reproduction In a standard three-generation study, some female mice on a dietary level of 5 ppm died before mating but there was no effect on the reproduction, gestation, or lactation indices of the survivors, except a slight reduction in the lactation index of F_{3b} pups. A level of 1 ppm was without effect. Whereas there was a slight, nonsignificant increase of minor skeletal abnormalities in rabbits that received fensulfothion during pregnancy at 0.10 mg/kg/day, there was no effect whatever from 0.05 mg/kg/day (FAO/WHO, 1973).

Factors Influencing Toxicity   An ordinarily harmless dose (550 mg/kg) of tricaine caused loss of righting ability in all rats and 20% mortality when the anesthetic was given 1 hr after administration of 2.5 mg/kg fensulfothion (Cohen, 1984).

16.7.13.3 Toxicity to Humans

Accidental and Intentional Poisoning   In a case previously listed only as a statistic (Hayes, 1976), a 34-year-old black farmer, who had applied fensulfothion to potato plants one day, became ill with vomiting and diarrhea. Late that same evening he was taken to a hospital "where he was given a shot by a nurse on doctor's instructions." He returned home, where his body was found next morning at about 0630 hr. Autopsy revealed pulmonary edema; the cholinesterase activity of blood taken at autopsy was far below normal (Hayes, 1982).

The acute illness of a 7-year-old girl was linked circumstantially to fensulfothion by finding where the child had played with a weathered can that formerly had contained the compound but then contained rainwater. On the day she became ill, she had been making mud pies with water from this can, and she had sprayed some of the water from a plastic bottle onto her arms and into her mouth. During the evening, she began vomiting and grew weak so that walking was difficult. She was taken to an emergency room, where the trouble was diagnosed as gastroenteritis. An antispasmodic based on belladonna alkaloids was administered, and she was sent home, where she spent a restless night. By morning she had "lost sensation in her legs and experienced temporary blindness." By the time she was returned to the emergency room, she was in coma. For a time she alternated between coma and agitation. Findings included pinpoint pupils, moist rales in both lungs, fasciculations in the arms and legs, and undetectable serum cholinesterase. She improved dramatically after intravenous atropine sulfate and pralidoxime chloride (Gehlbach and Williams, 1975). According to a letter from Dr. Gehlbach, the loss of sensation and blindness were not confirmed medically and probably represented the child's way of expressing the obvious weakness of her legs and the blurring of her vision. It seems likely that the delay in onset and the relatively slow and limited progression were the result of the requirement for metabolism and the exposure's having been small and mainly dermal.

An entire family of five persons was poisoned following household application of a formulation made from an emulsifiable concentrate. It was estimated that about 12,000 mg of active ingredient was applied to 10 m² of surface in two rooms. After the family had slept in the home for only one night, the 38-year-old mother and her 5-year-old daughter suffered nausea, vomiting, and disorientation. However, the cause of the trouble apparently was not appreciated, and exposure was continued. After 3 days, the two females experienced diarrhea and abdominal pain, and the daughter died on the sixth day with a diagnosis of general debility and acute heart failure. Two sons aged 8 and 10 years were hospitalized with typical cholinergic symptoms, and their serum cholinesterase was depressed. They received appropriate treatment and recovered after 10 days in hospital. The 41-year-old father was less severely sick (Taya *et al.*, 1976).

Dosage Response   The accidents with fensulfothion suggest that it is significantly toxic, even by the dermal route. This is consistent with the threshold limit value of 0.1 mg/m³, indicating that occupational intake of only 0.014 mg/kg/day is considered safe.

Treatment of Poisoning   See Section 16.2.2.7.

16.7.14 PHOSALONE

16.7.14.1 Identity, Properties, and Uses

Chemical Name   Phosalone is *O,O*-diethyl-*S*-(6-chloro-2-oxobenzoxazolin-3-yl-methyl)-phosphorodithioate.

Structure   See Table 16.36.

Synonyms   The common name phosalone (ANSI, BSI, ISO, JMAF) is in general use, except in the Soviet Union, where the common name benzphos is used. Other common names have included bensophos and phosalon. Trade names include Rubitox® and Zolone®. Code designations include ENT-27, 163, NPH-1,091, and RP-11,974. The CAS registry number is 2310-17-0.

Physical and Chemical Properties   Phosalone has the empirical formula $C_{12}H_{15}ClNO_4PS_2$ and a molecular weight of 367.80. The pure material forms white crystals with a slight garlic odor. Phosalone has a melting point of 48°C. The vapor pressure of phosalone at room temperature is negligible. The technical product contains 93% active ingredient.

Phosalone is practically insoluble in water, cyclohexane, and light petroleum at room temperature. It is soluble in acetone, acetonitrile, benzene, chloroform, dioxan, ethanol, methanol, toluene, and xylene. Phosalone is stable under normal storage conditions. It is compatible with most other pesticides and is noncorrosive. It is incompatible with alkaline materials such as calcium arsenate and lime sulfur.

History, Formulations, and Uses   Phosalone was introduced in 1963 by Rhone-Poulenc Company as a nonsystemic insecticide and acaricide for use on deciduous fruit trees, market garden crops, cotton, potatoes, and rape. Phosalone is available in formulations of 30, 33, and 35% emulsifiable concentrate; 30% wettable powder; and 2.5 and 4% dusts.

16.7.14.2 Toxicity to Laboratory Animals

Basic Findings   Phosalone is a compound of moderate toxicity, as shown in Table 16.48. In rats, the oral and dermal LD 50 values for the oxygen analog, which may occur in residues or as a mammalian metabolite, are 35 and 400 mg/kg, respectively. Feeding of phosalone to rats at dietary levels of 25, 50, and 250 ppm and to dogs at 100, 200, and 1,000 ppm resulted in dosage-dependent inhibition of red cell and plasma cholinesterase but no signs of illness. In rats, 50 ppm or about 2.4 mg/kg/day was the highest level with no effect on cholinesterase (Gallo, 1976). In fact, rats and dogs tolerated oral dosages of 7.5 and 15 mg/kg/day for a month, and rats tolerated a dietary level of 250 ppm (about 12 mg/kg/day) for 1 year with no abnormality of growth, behavior, or hematology (Colinese and Terry, 1968).

Because of the low volatility of the compound, the danger of aerosols of it is almost restricted to the toxicity of particles small enough to be inhaled. Rats and cats tolerated repeated exposure to an atmospheric concentration of 9.34 mg/m^3 (Man'ko, 1970).

The compound is moderately irritating to the skin and eyes (Man'ko, 1970).

Absorption, Distribution, Metabolism, and Excretion   In general, the biotransformation of phosalone is similar to that of other organic phosphorus compounds. However, it is interesting that, when rats were given a single dose of ^{14}C-labeled phosalone (carbonyl carbon active) at the rate of 10 mg/kg, 65.4% of the labeled carbon was recovered within 4 days as carbon dioxide in the expired air, while only 32.4% of the activity was excreted in the urine and feces (Colinese and Terry, 1968). Of course, production of carbon dioxide from the carbonyl carbon indicates destruction of the heterocyclic ring.

Effects on Reproduction   Oral administration of a 30% phosalone formulation to rats at dosages up to 50 mg/kg/day on days 6–15 of gestation produced neither teratogenic effects nor maternal toxicity (Khera *et al.*, 1979a).

Table 16.48
Single-Dose LD 50 for Phosalone

Species	Route	LD 50 (mg/kg)	Reference
Rat	oral	135	Safonov (1968)
Rat	oral	108	Man'ko (1970)
Rat, M	oral	130	Pasquet *et al.* (1976)
Rat, F	oral	110	Pasquet *et al.* (1976)
Rat	oral	100	Gallo (1975)
Rat, F	dermal	1500	Pasquet *et al.* (1976)
Rat	dermal	1500	Gallo (1975)
Mouse	oral	180	Safonov (1968)
Mouse	oral	88	Man'ko (1970)
Cat	oral	112	Man'ko (1970)

16.7.14.3 Toxicity to Humans

Use Experience   Fourteen men worked in an orange grove beginning 14–17 and 21–23 days after application of phosalone at a rate of 13.5 kg/ha (twice the ordinary rate). No clinical effect was observed, and no phosalone or metabolite was found in the urine. Plasma cholinesterase remained normal. The red cell cholinesterase level was depressed by 15% compared to that of controls on day 15, but it returned to normal on day 17; although the dislodgeable residues on the trees on days 21–23 was equal to that on days 14–17, no change in red cell enzyme was detected during days 21–23 (Gallo *et al.*, 1976). The same or a related study had similar results, except that slight differences were found in plasma rather than red cell cholinesterase levels (Knaak *et al.*, 1978a). It seems doubtful whether any of the enzyme changes were biologically significant.

A study of peach pickers indicated that in spite of estimated dosage rates as high as 14 mg/person/hour the red cell cholinesterase was inhibited only about 4% if at all. It was estimated that 98–99% of the workers' exposure was dermal, mainly to the hands and upper extremities (Popendorf *et al.*, 1979). Four of six workers exposed to air concentrations of 5.32 mg/m^3 had their acetylcholinesterase depressed by only 16 to 29% (Man'ko, 1970).

Treatment of Poisoning   See Section 16.2.2.7.

16.7.15 PHOXIM

16.7.15.1 Identity, Properties, and Uses

Chemical Name   Phoxim is *O,O*-diethyl-phenylglyoxylonitrile oxime phosphorothioate.

Structure   See Table 16.36.

Synonyms   The common name phoxim (BSI, ISO) is in general use, although the French use phoxime. The trade name Baythion® has been used to indicate phoxim used against pests of humans and stored products, while Volaton® has been used to indicate phoxim for use in agriculture pest control. Other trade names include Valaxon® and Valexon®. Code designations have included BAY-5,621, BAY-77,488, and OMS-1, 170. The CAS registry number is 14816-18-3.

Physical and Chemical Properties   Phoxim has the empirical formula $C_{12}H_{15}N_2O_3PS$ and a molecular weight of 298.30. The pure material is a yellowish liquid with a melting point of 5–6°C. Its density is 1.176 at 20°C. The solubility of phoxim in water at 20°C is 7 ppm. It is soluble in alcohols, ketones, and aromatic hydrocarbons and less soluble in light petroleum.

History, Formulations, and Uses   Phoxim was introduced in 1969 by Bayer Leverkusen. It is a contact and stomach poison with a short residual life. It is nonsystemic. Phoxim is available as a 50% emulsifiable concentrate, 5 and 10% granules, and a concentrate for ultralow-volume spraying.

16.7.15.2 Toxicity to Laboratory Animals

Basic Findings In rats, the oral LD 50 of phoxim is 363 mg/kg for males and 300 mg/kg for females, while the dermal LD 50 is 1276 mg/kg for males and 1224 mg/kg for females (Gaines and Linder, 1986). The oral LD 50 of phoxim for mice is greater than 2000 mg/kg, and even the oxon has low toxicity, as indicated by an LD 50 of 1000 mg/kg (Vinopal and Fukuto, 1971).

No harmful effect was detected when phoxim was fed to rats and their young for as much as 5 months at dietary concentrations up to 10 ppm, a dosage of about 0.5 mg/kg/day (Lin, 1974).

Distribution, Metabolism, and Excretion Phoxim is metabolized rapidly in the mouse. Detoxication is accomplished in the usual way by formation of diethylphosphoric acid and desethyl phoxim and by unusually rapid metabolism of the oxon. In addition, the —C≡N group is metabolized, resulting in phoxim carboxylic acid. This essentially nontoxic compound apparently is not formed by flies and, of course, most organic phosphorus compounds are incapable of forming analogous compounds. The proportion of the original dose recovered in the urine as phoxim carboxylic acid increased from 2.8 to 23.6% when the dosage was increased from 114 to 955 mg/kg. Thus the formation of phoxim carboxylic acid contributes substantially to the safety of the insecticide for mammals (Vinopal and Fukuto, 1971).

Whereas metabolism of phoxim is rapid, excretion of the compound and its metabolites is unexpectedly slow. Forty-eight hours after a dosage of 114 mg/kg, when only about 43% of the dose had been recovered in the urine, 88.4% of the radioactivity in the carcass was in the urinary bladder and 8.77% was in the gut wall. In each instance, almost all of the material was in the form of water-soluble metabolites (Vinopal and Fukuto, 1971). The unexpected concentrations of metabolites in the bladder and gut may represent reabsorption, but it remains to be learned whether this is true, what specific compounds are involved, and what significance, if any, the concentration has.

16.7.15.3 Toxicity to Humans

Use Experience A village-scale trial of phoxim was carried out in Nigeria in 1971. The water-dispersible powder formulation smelled like cyanide when received. Test papers showed that hydrogen cyanide was present but at a low level. In order to assess this, an experimental hut was sprayed at 4 gm/m² (instead of the normally applied target rate of 2 gm/m²), and it was shown that no hydrogen cyanide was detectable by air sampling over a day and a night. It was only after this test that a decision to complete the trial was made.

The insecticide was bagged by three workers, none of whom was engaged as a spray operator. They wore overalls, plastic helmets, rubber gloves, and dust respirators. The bagging was carried out in a well-ventilated room, and the operators were placed upwind of the drum. Although test papers put above the insecticide in a freshly opened drum became cyanide-positive within 10 min, those placed at several points in the room used for bagging were negative. Two of the three men complained of weakness after completion of the work. No clinical signs or other symptoms were recorded, and the men had recovered fully by the next day without any treatment.

Four sprayers wearing overalls, sou'westers, and canvas shoes and one mixer who also wore rubber gloves sprayed a total of 93 pump charges over a period of 3 days. Two of them complained of pain in the face lasting for 1 hr after completion of daily work on days 1 and 3 of spraying. There were no visible changes in facial skin at that time. The first and third days of spraying were sunnier than the second. Except for these complaints, which appeared within 1 hr of spraying, no complaints or any clinical findings attributable to the insecticide were recorded among the spraymen and villagers exposed to phoxim. Very slight depression of whole-blood cholinesterase was detected spectrophotometrically in some of the exposed spraymen and tintometrically in some villagers.

The World Health Organization committee concerned with the matter discussed these findings and considered that, although there is apparently no hazard from the use of phoxim as far as its anticholinesterase activity is concerned, further investigation of this compound when used on a small scale is required to assess its pain-producing effect and the possible risk from liberation of hydrogen cyanide (WHO, 1973).

Treatment of Poisoning See Section 16.2.2.7.

16.7.16 AZINPHOS-ETHYL

16.7.16.1 Identify, Properties, and Uses

Chemical Name Azinphos-ethyl is S-(3,4-dihydro-4-oxobenzo(d)-(1,2,3-triazin-3-ylmethyl-O,O-diethyl) phosphorodithioate.

Structure See Table 16.36.

Synonyms Azinphos-ethyl (BSI, ISO) is also known as the benzotriazine derivative of ethyl dithiophosphate, ethylguthion, and guthion (ethyl). In the USSR, the name is triazothion. Trade names include Athyl-Gusathion®, Azinfos-ethyl®, Azinos®, Azinophos-aethyl®, Crysthion®, Ethylazinophos®, Ethyl-Gusathion®, Gusation®, Gusathion®, and Bay 16255, Bayer 16259, ENT 22,014, and R1513. The CAS registry number is 2642-71-9.

Physical and Chemical Properties Azinphos-ethyl has the empirical formula $C_{12}N_{16}N_3O_3PS_2$ and a molecular weight of

354.4. The pure material forms clear crystals having a melting point of 53°C and a boiling point of 111°C at 1×10^{-3} mm Hg. The density at 20°C is 1.284. The vapor pressure of azinphos-ethyl is 2.2×10^{-7} mm Hg at 20°C. Although azinphos-ethyl is not soluble in water, aliphatic hydrocarbons, or light petroleum, it is soluble in most other solvents. Azinphos-ethyl is thermally stable but is rapidly hydrolyzed by alkaline media.

History, Formulations, and Uses   Azinphos-ethyl was introduced in 1953 by Bayer AG as a nonsystemic insecticide and acaricide. Although it is no longer registered for use in many countries due to its extreme acute toxicity to humans, some countries still use azinphos-ethyl for fruits and vegetables, pastures, cotton, cereals, coffee, potatoes, grapes, citrus, tobacco, rice, hops, and other crops of the forest industry. Azinphos-ethyl is available in 20 and 40% emulsifiable concentrates, 25 and 40% wettable powders, and 50% dusts.

16.7.16.2 Toxicity to Laboratory Animals

Basic Findings   According to a series of unpublished reports cited by WHO/FAO (1984a,b), the oral LD 50 in rats is 7.2–15.2 mg/kg and the dermal LD 50 ranges from 72 to 280 mg/kg. The intraperitoneal LD 50 for female rats range from 7.5 to 9.2 mg/kg. In mice the intraperitoneal LD 50 is 3.8–4.0 mg/kg. The oral LD 50 for guinea pigs is 17.0 mg/kg.

Hens receiving single oral doses of 25 mg/kg azinphos-ethyl showed no overt signs of toxicity.

Male rats receiving 50 ppm (about 2.5 mg/kg/day) azinphos-ethyl in the diet for 16 weeks suffered a decrease in body weight. Rats of both sexes showed decreased cholinesterase activities at this dose. Daily dietary doses of 10 ppm resulted in decreased serum and erythrocyte cholinesterase activities. Only erythrocyte cholinesterase activity was depressed at dietary doses of 5 ppm (about 0.25 mg/kg/day).

Young dogs receiving 10 ppm azinphos-ethyl in the diet developed clinical signs of cholinesterase poisoning after 1 week, and those receiving 3 ppm developed the same symptoms after 6 weeks. Normal cholinesterase activity resumed 3–4 weeks following a return to a normal diet. Cholinesterase activities were reduced in these groups, as well as at doses of 2.1 and 0.5 ppm. Cholinesterase activities were not affected in the groups receiving 0.25 ppm (about 0.005 mg/kg/day).

In another study, rats of both sexes fed 8 ppm azinphos-ethyl in the diet exhibited steadily decreasing erythrocyte cholinesterase activity during the first 30 days of treatment. Plasma cholinesterase in this group also decreased but stabilized after the first week of treatment. A rate of 4 ppm caused a decrease in erythrocyte cholinesterase activity only. Clinical signs of toxicity were absent at all dosages.

Female rats receiving intraperitoneal doses of 2 or 3 mg/kg/day azinphos-ethyl for 60 days showed increased mortality and reduced weight gains. Groups receiving 0.5–1.0 mg/kg/day showed no weight changes or mortality compared with the control groups.

Male rats receiving an oral dosage of 1.0 mg/kg/day for 28 days showed no alterations in body weight gain and no overt signs of toxicity. However, erythrocyte cholinesterase activity was reduced 50% following 2 days, 82% following 3 days, and 90% at the conclusion of the treatment period. Cholinesterase activity returned to normal 35 days following the final dose.

Distribution, Metabolism, and Excretion   Azinphos-ethyl has not been shown to accumulate in body tissues. Male rats receiving acute oral and intravenous doses (0.1 and 2.0 mg/kg) of ^{14}C-ring-labeled azinphos-ethyl excreted 90% in 48 hr (60% in urine, 30% in feces). Of the radioactivity administered, 30% passed through the biliary route, while less than 0.1% was observed in respired air 24 hr following a 2.0 mg/kg dose. This suggests no significant degradation in the benzotriazine ring. Conversion to the anticholinesterase analog has been shown in hepatic tissue preparations *in vitro*. Although the metabolic pathway of azinphos-ethyl is assumed to be similar to that of azinphos-methyl, information on the exact pathway is not available.

Effects on Organs and Tissues   No azinphos-ethyl carcinogenic responses have been found, since no information on long-term exposure studies of mice or rats are presently available. A mouse dominant lethal test has not shown azinphos-ethyl to be an active clastogen.

Factors Influencing Toxicity   A twofold potentiation of toxicity was seen when azinphos-ethyl was used with ethion. Otherwise, no potentiation resulted when numerous other pesticides were used with azinphos-ethyl, including azinphos-methyl, chlorbenzilate, coumaphos, delnav, diazinon, di-syston, EPN, fenchlorofos, malathion, methyl-parathion, OMPA, parathion, phosdrin, Sevin, Systox, and trithion. Atropine and enzyme-reactivating compounds have been shown to counteract the effects of azinphos-methyl.

16.7.16.3 Toxicity to Humans

As of this printing, no reports have been found on occupational exposures, exposure in the general population, reported mishaps, voluntary experimental exposures, or dangerous doses. However, absorption of azinphos-ethyl is possible through intact skin, from the gastrointestinal tract, and by mist and dust inhalation.

Azinphos-ethyl at concentrations of 120–160 ppm has been shown to cause abnormally high rates of chromosome breakage and abnormalities in diploid and hyperploid human cell lines *in vitro* (Alam and Kasatiya, 1975), although no further investigation of this phenomenon has been done.

Treatment of Poisoning   Atropine and enzyme-reactivating agents counteract the effects of azinphos-ethyl.

16.7.17 COUMAPHOS

16.7.17.1 Identity, Properties, and Uses

Chemical Name Coumaphos is *O,O*-diethyl *O*-(3-chloro-4-methyl-7-coumarinyl) phosphorothioate.

Structure See Table 16.36.

Synonyms Coumaphos (BSI, ISO) is also known under the trade names Asuntol®, Baymix®, Co-Ral®, Meldane®, Muscatox®, and Resitox®. Code designations include Bayer-21/199.

Physical and Chemical Properties Coumaphos has the empirical formula $C_{14}H_{16}ClO_5PS$ and a molecular weight of 362.78. It is a colorless to brownish crystal with a melting point of 91°C. It is somewhat soluble in corn oil and chloroform; soluble in aromatic hydrocarbons, esters, and ketones; and stable over a relatively wide pH range in water.

History and Uses Initially synthesized in 1951 by Schrader, coumaphos is an insecticide with particular usefulness as an antiparasitic in livestock.

16.7.17.2 Toxicity to Laboratory Animals

Basic Findings Coumaphos is a compound of moderate to high toxicity. The oral LD 50 in male and female rats is 41 and 16 mg/kg, respectively (Gaines, 1969). The oral LD 50 in mice is 55 mg/kg.

16.7.17.3 Toxicity to Humans

Use Experience Veterinarians treating grub infestations in cattle with pour-on applications of Co-Ral® and other organic phosphorus pesticides in poorly ventilated areas experienced nausea, headaches, and irritations of the throat and skin. Blood cholinesterase activities were not found to be reduced in most cases, and alkyl phosphate metabolites were only occasionally found in the urine (Beat and Morgan, 1977).

16.7.18 PHOSFOLAN

16.7.18.1 Identity, Properties, and Uses

Chemical Name Phosfolan is 2-(diethoxyphosphinylimino)-1,3-dithiolane.

Structure See Table 16.36.

Synonyms The common name phosfolan (BSI, ISO) is generally accepted. It is also known under the trade names Cylan® and Cyolane®. Code designations include AC-47031, CL-47031, EI-47031, and ENT-25830. The CAS registry number is 947-02-4.

Physical and Chemical Properties Phosfolan has the empirical formula $C_7H_{14}NO_3PS_2$ and a molecular weight of 255.28. It is a solid with a melting point of 36.5°C and a boiling point of 115–118°C at 0.01 mm Hg. Phosfolan is sparingly soluble in aliphatic hydrocarbons but soluble in water and many organic solvents.

History and Uses Synthesized in 1963 by the American Cyanimid Company, phosfolan is a systemic insecticide which is known to persist in soil.

16.7.18.2 Toxicity to Laboratory Animals

Basic Findings Phosfolan is highly toxic to mammals with an acute oral LD 50 in rats of about 9 mg/kg; Kenaga and Allison (1969) determined the dermal LD 50 for rabbits to be 23 mg/kg.

16.7.18.3 Toxicity to Humans

Use Experience Soliman *et al.* (1979) calculated the total dermal exposure to phosfolan spray among workers using the pesticide on cotton crops in Egypt to range from 11.637 mg/person/day for spraymen to 110.416 mg/person/day for those mixing the pesticide. Reduction of erythrocyte acetylcholinesterase activities in this group ranged from 23.5 to 43.8%. Approximately half of the activity was recovered 48 hr following exposure. However, full recovery of acetylcholinesterase activity required at least 3–4 weeks.

16.8 OTHER DIALKOXY COMPOUNDS OF CATEGORY IV

As discussed in Section 16.1, the last six groups of category IV are diverse and stand in contrast to the first two (dimethoxy and diethoxy compounds), which have many properties in common and include the great majority of organic phosphorus insecticides. Table 16.49 shows the structures of one or more examples of the six diverse groups. The remainder of this chapter is concerned with compounds belonging to these miscellaneous groups that have been investigated in humans.

16.8.1 PROPAPHOS

16.8.1.1 Identity, Properties, and Uses

Chemical Name Propaphos is 4-(methylthio)phenyl dipropyl phosphate.

Structure See Table 16.49.

Synonyms Propaphos (BSI, JMAF, ISO) is the common name. A trade name is Kayaphos® and a code designation of the compound is NK-1,158. The CAS registry number is 7292-16-2.

Table 16.49
Structure of Miscellaneous Organic Phosphorus Pesticides of Category IV

Group and compound	Structure	Group and compound	Structure
Dialkoxy compounds of category IV other than dimethoxy or diethoxy ones		*p*-cresyl saligenin phosphate	CH_3— ⬡ —R
isopropyl paraoxon	$[(CH_3)_2CH-O]_2-P=O$, NO_2—⬡—O	Mixed substituent compounds of category IV cerejin	CH_3-O, O, P, O, S—⬡—Cl
isopropyl parathion	$[(CH_3)_2CH-O]_2-P=S$, NO_2—⬡—O	crufomate	CH_3-O, O, Cl, P, CH_3-NH, S—⬡—$C(CH_3)_3$
propaphos	C_3H_7-O, O, P, C_3H_7-O, O—⬡—$S-CH_3$	cyanofenphos	C_2H_5-O, S, P, ⬡, O—⬡—CN
TIPP	$(C_3H_7-O)_2-P=O$, $(C_3H_7-O)_2-P=O$	DMPA	CH_3-O, S, Cl, P, $(CH_3)_2-CH-NH$, O—⬡—Cl
Diamino compounds of category IV schradan	$(CH_3)_2N$, $N(CH_3)_2$, P—O—P, $(CH_3)_2N$, O, O, $N(CH_3)_2$	edifenphos	C_2H_5-O, O, P, ⬡—S, S—⬡
Chlorinated dialkoxy compounds of category IV O,O-di(2-chloroethyl)-*p*-nitrophenyl phosphate	$(ClCH_2-CH_2-O)_2-P=O$, O_2N—⬡—O	EPBP	C_2H_5-O, S, Cl, P, ⬡, O—⬡—Cl
haloxon	$(ClCH_2-CH_2-O)_2-P=O$	EPN	C_2H_5-O, S, P, ⬡, O—⬡—NO_2
Trithiobutyl compounds of category IV DEF	$(C_4H_9-S)_3P=O$	fonofos	C_2H_5-O, S, P, C_2H_5, S—⬡
merphos	$(C_4H_9-S)_3P$		
Triphenyl compounds of category IV and their derivatives TOCP *o*-cresyl saligenin phosphate		leptiphos	C_2H_5-O, S, Cl, P, ⬡, O—⬡—Br, Cl

(continued)

Table 16.49 (*Continued*)

Group and compound	Structure	Group and compound	Structure
metamidophos		methyl-*O*-ethyl-2,4-dichlorophenyl phosphonothionate	
O-methyl-*O*,*p*-(5-chloro-2,2'-biphenylene) phosphonothioate		trichloronat	

Physical and Chemical Properties Propaphos has an empirical formula $C_{13}H_{21}O_4PS$ and a molecular weight of 304.3. Propaphos is a colorless liquid with a boiling point of 176 ± 1°C. Solubility in water at 25°C is 125 ppm. It is soluble in most organic solvents. Propaphos is stable in neutral and acid media but is slowly decomposed in alkaline media.

History, Formulations, and Uses Propaphos was introduced in 1967 in Japan and first was described in 1970. It is an insecticide used to control rice pests.

16.8.1.2 Toxicity to Laboratory Animals

Acute oral LD 50 values are 70, 90, and 83 mg/kg for rats, mice, and rabbits, respectively. The acute dermal LD 50 for mice is 156 mg/kg. Dietary levels of 100 and 5 ppm were no-effect levels in rats and mice, respectively (Martin and Worthing, 1974).

16.8.1.3 Toxicity to Humans

Use Experience Of 72 workers who cooperated in applying an insecticidal dust, 41 became sick, and one died. The dust contained 2% propaphos and 1.5% carbaryl; 7770 kg was applied to 243.3 ha. Signs and symptoms were nausea, vomiting, abdominal pain, diarrhea, fever, sweating, miosis, increased blood pressure, muscular spasm, fever, and clouding of consciousness. The people were organized into six groups of 12 each. The groups began work between 0600 and 0630 hr and stopped as early as 0930 hr or as late as 1230 hr with or without a recess. Symptoms began in some at 1000 hr but most sickness was delayed until the workers got home. Symptoms tended to be most severe in those who worked the longest. Although he was hospitalized 30 min after he finished work, a 45-year-old man died at 1115 hr the next day. The unusually widespread and severe intoxication with propaphos was attributed to the high ambient temperature of 30°C and to direct contamination of the workers by the dust (Itayama, 1978).

16.9 DIAMINO COMPOUNDS OF CATEGORY IV

It seems likely that all diamino compounds of category IV cause truly irreversible inhibition of cholinesterase, just as schradan does. This, in addition to the obvious chemical difference, is sufficient justification for recognizing the group as separate.

16.9.1 SCHRADAN

16.9.1.1 Identity, Properties, and Uses

Chemical Name Schradan is octamethylpyrophosphoramide.

Structure See Table 16.49.

Synonyms The common name schradan (BSI, ISO) is in general use (in France it is spelled schradane.) Other common names include octamethyldiphosphoramide and OMPA. Trade names include Pestox III®, Pestox 3®, and Sytam®. The CAS registry number is 152-16-9.

Physical and Chemical Properties Schradan has the empirical formula $C_8H_{24}N_4O_3P_2$ and a molecular weight of 286.26. The pure material is a colorless viscous liquid at temperatures above 14–20°C. The boiling point is 118–122°C at 0.3 mm Hg. The vapor pressure is 1×10^{-3} mm Hg at 25°C. The density is 1.09 at 25°C. Schradan is soluble in water and most organic solvents. It is slightly soluble in petroleum oils. Schradan is not hydrolyzed readily, except by acid. Under acid conditions it is converted to dimethylamine and orthophosphoric acid. It is stable in water and alkali.

History, Formulations, Uses, and Production Schradan was discovered about 1942 in Germany. It is a systemic insecticide effective against sap-feeding insects and mites, but it is relatively inert as a contact insecticide. It is nonphytotoxic at insecticidal concentrations. Schradan is available as a 30% aqueous solution or 60–80% solutions in organic solvents.

16.9.1.2 Toxicity to Laboratory Animals

Basic Findings The symptoms produced by schradan in all species are typical of parasympathomimetic drugs, except that symptoms referable to the central nervous system tend to be absent. This is explained by the fact that there is little or no inhibition of brain cholinesterase by a single dose capable of producing severe inhibition of cholinesterase in the blood and other tissues such as skeletal muscles and submaxillary glands. Even after a lethal dose (15 mg/kg) that produced about 90% inhibition of cholinesterase in peripheral tissues, inhibition in the brain was only 7% (DuBois *et al.*, 1950).

Schradan has approximately the same acute toxicity as parathion (see Table 16.50). It is well absorbed from the gastrointestinal tract and the skin.

Repeated intraperitoneal dosages of 1, 1.5, and 2 mg/kg/day produced progressive cholinesterase depletion and cumulative toxic action in rats, but these animals tolerated 0.25 and 0.5 mg/kg/day for at least 60 days without apparent untoward effect (DuBois *et al.*, 1950).

Frawley *et al.* (1952a) found that a dietary level as high as 25 ppm for 4 weeks produced only a 10% reduction of brain cholinesterase activity. Marked inhibition of the red cell cholinesterase of rats was observed at a dietary level of 5 ppm for 8 weeks and slight inhibition at 1 ppm. At twice that dietary level, inhibition of brain cholinesterase was only 16 and 21% in male and female rats, even though their blood cholinesterase values were inhibited 76 and 66%. Red cell enzyme was more sensitive than plasma enzyme (Barnes and Denz, 1954). The findings of Edson (1964) were similar, that is, complete inhibition of red cell cholinesterase at a dietary level of 5 ppm (about 0.25 mg/kg/day) but no effect on brain cholinesterase; a dietary level of 1 ppm caused a substantial reduction in red cell

Table 16.50
Single-Dose LD 50 for Schradan

Species	Route	LD 50 (mg/kg)	Reference
Rat	oral	10	DuBois *et al.* (1950)
Rat, M	oral	13.5	Frawley *et al.* (1952a)
Rat, F	oral	35.5	Frawley *et al.* (1952a)
Rat, M	oral	9.1	Gaines (1969)
Rat, F	oral	42	Gaines (1969)
Rat, M	dermal	15	Gaines (1969)
Rat, F	dermal	44	Gaines (1969)
Rat	intraperitoneal	8	DuBois *et al.* (1950)
Rat, M	intraperitoneal	5.5	Kato *et al.* (1962)
Rat, F	intraperitoneal	24	Kato *et al.* (1962)
Mouse	oral	30.0	Frawley *et al.* (1952a)
Mouse	intraperitoneal	17	DuBois *et al.* (1950)
Guinea pig	oral	15.0	Frawley *et al.* (1952a)
Guinea pig	intraperitoneal	10	DuBois *et al.* (1950)

enzyme activity, and 0.25 ppm (about 0.012 mg/kg/day) gave the first indication of inhibition.

In female pigs, a dietary level of 2.5 ppm reduced red cell cholinesterase to 45% of normal but had only slight action on plasma enzyme activity and none on brain cholinesterase activity. A dietary level of 0.1 ppm produced a statistically insignificant decrease in red cell cholinesterase activity (Edson, 1964).

Dogs were severely poisoned by schradan at 1 mg/kg/day. Over a prolonged period, 0.5 mg/kg/day inhibited red cell cholinesterase activity to practically zero and plasma enzyme activity to about 50% of normal, but there was no clinical toxicity and no pathology (Hazleton, 1955).

Absorption, Distribution, Metabolism, and Excretion Toxicity data cited earlier indicate that schradan is absorbed almost as easily from the gastrointestinal tract as from the peritoneal cavity and almost as easily from the skin as from the gut.

Whereas the liver is most active in metabolizing schradan (DuBois *et al.*, 1950; Cheng, 1951; Frawley *et al.*, 1952b), the microsomal enzymes of the lung, heart, and testes can convert schradan also (O'Brien, 1956).

Evidence that the metabolism necessary for the toxication of schradan depends on microsomal enzymes includes the following. The toxicity of the compound is low in infant rats and increases progressively until the animals are 1–2 months old. Adult male rats are more susceptible than females. The toxicity of schradan is increased by phenobarbital and other inducers and decreased by SKF 525A and other inhibitors of microsomal enzymes (Kato *et al.*, 1967).

At dosages used, pretreatment with several catatoxic steroids had no detectable effect on the toxicity of schradan, even though, at appropriate dosages, they too are inducers of microsomal enzymes. On the contrary, pretreatment with estradiol, estrone, or stilbestrol increased the toxicity of schradan to female rats, whether they were normal or ovariectomized (Selye, 1970). The result is unexpected because untreated male rats are more susceptible than females to schradan. Therefore, the mechanism by which estrogens exerted their effect seems to require further study. Schradan itself is a weak inhibitor of cholinesterase (DuBois *et al.*, 1950; Casida and Stahmann, 1953). The pI 50 of the parent compound is 0.8 for rat brain cholinesterase. It is metabolized by both animals and plants to what is thought to be the same compound with a pI 50 of 6.4 (Casida and Stahmann, 1953). There is still some controversy over the identity of the active compound. The oxidation of schradan to its amide oxide and further conversion to the hydroxymethylamide was first proposed by Casida and Stahmann (1953). The reactions involve only one amide group; $R—N—(CH_3)_2$ (schradan) is oxidized to $R—N(O)—(CH_3)_2$ (amide oxide), which is then rapidly rearranged to form $R—N(CH_3)—CH_2OH$ (hydroxymethylamide). Casida offered reasons for believing that the amide oxide is the active metabolite (Casida *et al.*, 1952; Casida and Stahmann, 1953; Tsuyuki *et al.*, 1955). However, Heath (1961, pp. 227–233) reviewed complex evidence for discounting this interpretation and considering the hydroxymethylamide as the active metabolite.

Biochemical Effects   When schradan is fed to people, the red cell cholinesterase activity is decreased more than that of plasma (Edson, 1964; Rider *et al.*, 1969), whereas the opposite is true in cats (Koelle *et al.*, 1974).

16.9.1.3 Toxicity to Humans

Experimental Exposure   Six men and six women consumed 1.4 mg/day, 5 days/week for 32 doses; taking body weight into account, this amounted to 0.013–0.015 mg/kg/day. One subject took 4.2 mg/day (0.057 mg/kg/day) for 74 days and on two occasions took as much as 12.6 mg. Twelve other adults served as controls. The lower dosage caused a slow fall in whole-blood cholinesterase activity, reaching 80% of normal by day 18 and 75% by day 44. At the higher dosage, red cell cholinesterase activity reached 50% of normal in 2 months and then began to recover, although exposure was continued another 2 weeks. In both series, cholinesterase activity was more inhibited in red cells than in plasma. Symptoms did not develop at any dosage tested (Edson, 1964).

In a completely separate study, schradan was given for 39 days to three groups of five healthy men each. The plasma cholinesterase activity of those who received 0.75 mg/person/day (about 0.01 mg/kg/day) decreased by 11% after 16 days but then increased by the end of the dosing period; the red cell activity decreased 15% by the end of the period. At a dosage of 1.125 mg/person/day there was no effect on plasma cholinesterase activity, but there was a gradual decrease in red cell enzyme activity to 16% below the preexposure mean, the greatest decrease being 4 days after exposure was stopped. The administration of 1.5 mg/person/day (about 0.02 mg/kg/day) produced a decrease of 23.5% in plasma cholinesterase activity after 30 days, with some recovery thereafter in spite of continuing exposure. The red cell cholinesterase had maximal depression of 34% at 5 days after administration of schradan was concluded. Both plasma and red cell levels approached normal during the 19-day postexposure observation period. None of the dosages produced symptoms (Rider *et al.*, 1969). The two studies are consistent with the conclusion that a dosage level of 0.01 mg/kg/day does not produce a statistically significant change in cholinesterase activity but that 0.02 mg/kg/day is what has been called the level of minimal toxicity, that is, the dosage which, over a period of several weeks, will cause an average decrease in cholinesterase activity of 20–25% below control values. However, 0.057 mg/kg/day is tolerated without symptoms.

Therapeutic Use   Schradan is one of several organic phosphorus insecticides that have been used for treating myasthenia gravis. It certainly is more stable in solution than is TEPP, and it has the possible advantage that it has little or no effect on the central nervous system. Some patients were transferred completely from neostigmine to schradan. In an early study it was found that two daily oral doses of 9.5–18 mg resulted in muscular strength that was more uniform throughout the day and often exceeded the peak that could be achieved with neostigmine. However, there was mutual potentiation of the side effects of the two drugs. Because this was most marked in patients with severe disease, it was sometimes difficult or impossible to make the transfer. Strangely enough, there was no correlation between the severity of myasthenia gravis or the patient's requirement for neostigmine on the one hand and the requirement for schradan on the other, except that patients who got their relief from large doses of neostigmine usually received little improvement from schradan (Rider *et al.*, 1951; Gregory *et al.*, 1952).

The prolonged action of schradan was an advantage in patients who were doing well. However, the weakness caused by excessive doses of schradan was difficult to distinguish from the weakness of myasthenic crisis. The slow onset and prolonged effect of schradan were disadvantages, compared to the action of neostigmine, in dealing with patients in crisis. Some patients died while on dosages of 40, 50, and 56 mg/day. Because of these facts, an arbitrary limit of 30 mg/day was suggested for schradan. Patients who could not be managed on this, or preferably a lower dosage, were placed on neostigmine, regardless of the difficulties involved (Schulman *et al.*, 1953). Schradan does not satisfactorily solve the problem of the patient who has become refractory to neostigmine (Grob, 1953; Osserman and Kaplan, 1954). By 1954 some had concluded that the range between toxic and therapeutic levels of schradan is too narrow to warrant its continued use in the treatment of myasthenia gravis (Osserman and Kaplan, 1954).

The treatment of myasthenia gravis is complex whether schradan is employed or not. When it was used, interpretation of its effects tended to be complicated by (*a*) the complex interaction with the effects of prostigmine used simultaneously for the same purpose and the effects of atropine used to mitigate muscarinic side effects and (*b*) the natural progression of the disease. These points are illustrated by a case (Hayes, 1982) of a man who first noted weakness during military service. However, his difficulty was so mild that its true nature was not recognized and he received a regular discharge about 1 year later. In spite of gradual progression and treatment for various complaints, his condition was not diagnosed until 8 years after onset. By this time, he had weakness of his legs, masseter muscles, and voice; fatigue of his arms; and droop of his left eyelid. During hospitalization, a tumor of the thymus was discovered, and it was removed surgically. Unlike some patients with myasthenia gravis, he showed no improvement following this operation. During hospitalization he was maintained only by a combination of large oral and subcutaneous doses of prostigmine. He was discharged on 30 mg orally every 2 hr. A few months later, still on the same medication, he entered another hospital complaining of upper respiratory infection, considerable nasal discharge, slight cough, no fever or chills, but abundant diaphoresis. Physical examination revealed no weakness but, because such frequent doses of prostigmine were required, the patient was started on schradan at 5 mg every 12 hr. This was slowly increased to a final dosage of 15 mg every 12 hr; he also received prostigmine sulfate 120 mg/day and atropine sulfate, 0.4 mg four times a day to control minimal sweating and one episode of slight abdominal cramping. At the time of discharge he had been on this final regimen for 5 weeks with no untoward reaction, and he was discharged on this medication. He said he felt better than at any time since the onset of his illness. However, in about 6 days he began to complain of neck weakness and inability to get air through his nostrils and throat. Eight days after discharge he was readmitted. He failed to respond to intramuscular and intravenous prostigmine; atropine also appeared ineffectual in clearing the airway of moderately excessive secretions, and the patient lapsed into coma. His color remained good. The muscles were flaccid, and the patient soon required artificial respiration, manually at first and later by iron lung. Additional treatment included antibiotics and oxygen by intratracheal tube. Although the lungs were clear as judged by physical examination and X-ray soon after admission, he developed a temperature on the second hospital day and died on the third day with clinical pulmonary edema. Autopsy revealed, in addition to pulmonary congestion and edema, bronchopneumonia in all parts of the lungs except the apices; this was considered the immediate cause of death. There were focal infiltrations of lymphocytes (and in some instances plasma cells and polymorphonuclear leukocytes) in the heart, muscles, thyroid, and the area of the excised thymus.

Schradan was not listed in the third edition of "AMA Drug Evaluations" or in the nineteenth edition of the "United States Pharmacopeia."

Use Experience According to Kagan (1957a), depression of serum cholinesterase activity by 50% or more was common among workers who applied schradan.

Treatment of Poisoning See Section 16.2.2.7.

16.10 TRITHIOALKYL COMPOUNDS OF CATEGORY IV

Only a few of these compounds have been tested for neurotoxicity, but apparently all those tested were positive (see Table 16.14).

16.10.1 MERPHOS

16.10.1.1 Identity, Properties, and Uses

Chemical Name Merphos is tributyl phosphorotrithioite.

Structure See Table 16.49.

Synonyms Merphos has been proposed as a common name. A trade name is Folex®. The CAS registry number is 150-50-5.

Physical and Chemical Properties Merphos has the empirical formula $C_{12}H_{27}PS_3$ and a molecular weight of 298.51. It is a colorless to pale yellow liquid. The technical product is at least 95% pure. The solubility of merphos in water is very low, but the compound is very soluble in most organic solvents. It has a boiling point of 115–134°C at 0.08 mm Hg.

History, Formulations, Uses, and Production Merphos is a defoliant. It is available in a 72% formulation.

16.10.1.2 Toxicity to Laboratory Animals

Basic Findings Merphos is a compound of low toxicity so far as its anticholinesterase effects are concerned. In rats, Gaines (1969) found oral LD 50 values of 1475 and 910 mg/kg in males and females, respectively, and dermal values of 690 and 615 mg/kg, respectively. Martin and Worthing (1974) reported an almost identical oral LD 50 value in male rats (1272 mg/kg) and a dermal value of 4600 mg/kg in rabbits. The similarity of oral and dermal toxicity in the rat is striking. In sheep and cattle, depression of blood cholinesterase activity, loss of weight, and sometimes diarrhea were the most evident effects of single doses at rates as high as 200 mg/kg or of as many as 10 doses at rates as high as 25 mg/kg/day (Palmer and Schlinke, 1973).

Merphos is neurotoxic to hens (see Table 16.14). The compound is a weak inhibitor of cholinesterase. Even a single oral dosage as high as 2000 mg/kg promptly produced only mild illness rapidly relieved by atropine. However, a few hens that received 800 or 2000 mg/kg died abruptly after 23 and 4 days, respectively. Similar illness that was not responsive to atropine was seen beginning on day 4 of oral dosing at a rate of 80 mg/kg/day; this illness, referred to as late acute poisoning, was attributed to n-butylmercaptan and was considered the same as that produced by a single oral dose of the mercaptan at a rate as low as 400 mg/kg. No neurological lesions were detected in birds made ill or killed by the mercaptan. Hens that received single or repeated dermal doses of merphos failed to show late acute poisoning, presumably because they metabolized little or none of it to n-butylmercaptan.

Uncomplicated, delayed neurotoxicity with typical pathology in some birds was produced in hens by oral administration at rates of 0.5–40 mg/kg/day for 3 months or dermal administration at rates of 20 or 40 mg/kg/day for 3 months or by a single dermal application of 1000 mg/kg. Delayed neurotoxicity also appeared following high single or repeated oral doses of merphos, but the condition tended to appear in the course of late acute poisoning (Abou-Donia et al., 1980b).

Absorption, Distribution, Metabolism, and Excretion Merphos is readily absorbed through the skin. When applied to the combs of hens, at a rate of 1000 mg/kg, it caused greater inhibition of brain acetylcholinesterase than when administered orally at a rate of 100 mg/kg. Delayed neurotoxicity was produced in all hens by an dermal dosage of 1000 mg/kg but in only a portion of hens by an oral dosage of 2000 mg/kg (Abou-Donia *et al.*, 1980b).

The three major compounds excreted by hens after ingesting merphos are merphos, DEF, and *n*-butylmercaptan. The *n*-butylmercaptan is produced to a large extent in the intestine by hydrolysis (Abou-Donia *et al.*, 1980b).

16.10.1.3 Toxicity to Humans

Accidental and Intentional Poisoning   While mixing the defoliant, a healthy 28-year-old man accidentally splashed some of the undiluted, 72% formulation on his bare upper arms and his T-shirt, soaking the garment through to the skin. He did not wash or remove the shirt. During the next 2 days, he splashed smaller amounts of merphos on his bare arms. Approximately 4 days after the exposure, he noted that his arms and hands were weak. He did not seek medical attention until 2 days later, when he entered hospital because he was unable to stand, could barely lift his legs while lying in bed, and could not move his hands and arms. He showed no signs of anticholinesterase poisoning; his pupils were at midposition and were reactive, and he was alert. On the presumptive diagnosis of organic phosphorus poisoning, he was given substantial doses of atropine and pralidoxime chloride without producing either improvement or side effect. Because of the fear that paralysis would extend to the muscles of respiration, the patient was moved to another hospital where facilities for assisted respiration were better. Actually, no need for respiratory assistance developed. Examination after transfer revealed an obese, tachypneic, apprehensive, areflexic man totally unable to move his extremities but with cutaneous sensation intact. Vital capacity, arterial blood gases, plasma cholinesterase level, and other measured laboratory findings were normal. Approximately 14 days after the initial exposure, complete facial diplegia developed. A lumbar puncture revealed clear fluid under normal pressure with normal glucose but with 150 mg/dl of protein and four lymphocytes per cubic milliliter. Electromyography demonstrated decreased voltage of muscle action potentials, delayed conduction velocity in motor nerve fibers, increased insertional activity, and denervation potentials. The patient received supportive care and intense physical therapy. At the time of hospital discharge 6 weeks after initial exposure, he had residual facial weakness but could grasp objects and get about with a walker. Fourteen weeks after discharge he had recovered completely (Fisher, 1977).

That a sufficient dosage of merphos would cause polyneuropathy in humans could have been predicted from the test carried out by Gaines (1969) with hens; paralysis began in these birds 3–21 days after a subcutaneous dose at the rate of 600 mg/kg and was still present at the end of a 90-day period of observation.

Fisher (1977) considered the EMG findings in the case he described similar to those in the Guillain–Barré syndrome and also to those described in a high proportion of formulators and agricultural workers, who received this test. However, as discussed in Section 7.4.1 in Hayes (1975), the significance of these EMG changes in healthy workers is unclear. Whatever their meaning in these workers, it is certain that EMG changes have been reported in connection with compounds never demonstrated to have caused polyneuropathy in people or hens. Under these circumstances the changes are reversible in 48 hr. It may be that EMG changes are a relatively nonspecific response to different kinds of injury. Apparently, the occurrence of facial paralysis in this case is unique among cases associated with organic phosphorus compounds. However, because this was the first reported case associated with merphos, there is no way to judge how common it might be in persons with sufficient exposure to this compound.

The appropriateness of designating the condition caused by merphos as Guillain–Barré syndrome is questionable because that syndrome generally is considered identical to or at least a form of acute, infectious polyneuritis.

Use Experience   Seven workers routinely applying an unspecified mixture of DEF and merphos for cotton defoliation were found to be most heavily exposed by the dermal route. Although lymphocyte NTE values in these workers were reduced approximately 50% following total exposure periods of 25–294 hr, erythrocyte and plasma acetylcholinesterase and butyrylcholinesterase activities did not change significantly, and no electrophysiological changes or adverse clinical effects on the peripheral nervous system were observed (Lotti *et al.*, 1983).

Toxiphobia   Although an episode of mass panic associated with merphos (McLeod, 1975) throws no light on any real danger of the compound, it constitutes a classical example of one aspect of toxiphobia.

Treatment of Poisoning   There is no experience in treating cholinergic illness produced by merphos. If such signs and symptoms occurred, the patient should be treated as if some other organic phosphorus compound were involved (see Section 16.2.2.7). Unfortunately, no specific treatment for neurotoxic effects is known, and care of the patient must be symptomatic.

16.10.2 DEF

16.10.2.1 Identity, Properties, and Uses

Chemical Name   DEF is *S,S,S*-tributyl phosphorotrithiolate.

Structure   See Table 16.49.

Synonyms   The common and trade name DEF® is generally accepted. It is also known as butifos. The CAS registry number is 78-48-8.

Physical and Chemical Properties   DEF has the empirical formula $C_{12}H_{27}OPS_3$ and a molecular weight of 314.54. It is a colorless to pale yellow liquid with a boiling point of 150°C at 0.3 mm Hg. DEF is soluble in most organic solvents but insoluble in water.

History, Formulations, and Uses   The Ethyl Corporation first demonstrated the defoliating properties of DEF in 1954. DEF is most frequently used as a defoliant of cotton.

16.10.2.2 Toxicity to Laboratory Animals

Basic Findings   DEF has an oral LD 50 in rats of 325 mg/kg. It is a synergist of malathion and is known to cause delayed neuropathy.

16.10.2.3 Toxicity to Humans

Use Experience   A study of seven workers using a mixture of DEF and merphos for cotton defoliation found heaviest exposures by the dermal route. Following total exposure periods of 25–294 hr, erythrocyte and plasma acetylcholinesterase and butyrylcholinesterase activities were not significantly affected, and no electrophysiological changes or adverse effects on the peripheral nervous system were noted (Lotti *et al.*, 1983).

16.11 MIXED SUBSTITUENT COMPOUNDS OF CATEGORY IV

A substantial proportion of these compounds produce neurotoxicity in hens. However, EPN, to which people have been exposed experimentally, occupationally, and accidentally, has not produced neurotoxicity in humans, even though it has produced severe poisoning. Leptophos has produced neurological changes in persons with heavy occupational exposure, but the conditions described differed significantly from classical polyneuropathy caused by TOCP or mipafox. The other mixed constituent compounds to which people have had substantial exposure failed to produce neurotoxicity.

16.11.1 EPN

16.11.1.1 Identity, Properties, and Uses

Chemical Name   EPN is *O*-ethyl *O*-4-nitrophenyl phenylphosphonothioate.

Structure   See Table 16.49.

Synonyms   EPN are the initials accepted as the common name by ESA and JMAP. EPN-300® has been used as a trade name. Code designations have included ENT-17,798. The CAS registry number is 2104-64-5.

Physical and Chemical Properties   EPN has the empirical formula $C_{14}H_{14}NO_4PS$ and a molecular weight of 323.31. The pure material is a light yellow crystalline powder with a melting point of 36°C. The vapor pressure of EPN is 9.45×10^{-7} mm Hg at 25°C. EPN is practically insoluble in water but soluble in most organic solvents. It is stable in neutral and acidic media, but it is hydrolyzed by alkali and is incompatible with alkaline pesticides.

History, Formulations, and Uses   EPN was introduced in 1949 by E. I. duPont de Nemours and Company, Inc., as a nonsystemic insecticide and acaricide. EPN is available as a 45% emulsifiable concentrate, as granules, and in combination with other insecticides.

16.11.1.2 Toxicity to Laboratory Animals

Toxicity Related to Cholinesterase Inhibition   As shown in Table 16.51, EPN is a compound of high to moderate toxicity, as judged by tests in different species and in rats of both sexes. Hodge *et al.* (1954) noted that the compound was less toxic intraperitoneally than orally, an unusual finding that they attributed to very rapid absorption from the gastrointestinal tract.

Although EPN is an indirect inhibitor of cholinesterase, the commercial product is equally as toxic as the crystalline material.

Young cattle are more susceptible than adults to EPN. The minimal toxic oral dosages for calves and yearling cattle are 2.5 and 25 mg/kg (Palmer, 1974).

In a 2-year study, dietary levels of 450 ppm in male and 225 ppm in female rats caused intermittent tremors and slight retardation of growth; mortality was not greater than in controls. When the rats were first placed on these diets as weanlings, EPN dosage was 86 and 42 mg/kg/day in males and females, respectively, but, because of decreasing feed consumption, was reduced to 29 and 12 mg/kg/day for the same animals as adults. Other groups of rats tolerated oral dosages up to 10 and 4 mg/kg/day in males and females, respectively.

Table 16.51
Single-Dose LD 50 for EPN

Species	Route	LD 50 (mg/kg)	Reference
Rat, M	oral	91.0	Frawley *et al.* (1952a)
Rat, F	oral	14.5	Frawley *et al.* (1952a)
Rat, M	oral	42.0	Hodge *et al.* (1954)
Rat, F	oral	14.0	Hodge *et al.* (1954)
Rat, M	oral	50.0	Shaffer and West (1960)
Rat, M	oral	36.0	Gaines (1960)
Rat, F	oral	7.7	Gaines (1960)
Rat, M	oral	37.5	Suzuki (1973)
Rat, M	dermal	230.0	Gaines (1960)
Rat, F	dermal	25.0	Gaines (1960)
Mouse, M	oral	38	Klassen *et al.* (1959)
Mouse, F	oral	42	Klassen *et al.* (1959)
Mouse, M	intraperitoneal	16	Ohkawa *et al.* (1977)
Guinea pig	oral	79	Frawley *et al.* (1952a)
Dog, M	oral	20–30	Hodge *et al.* (1954)
Dog, F	oral	20–45	Hodge *et al.* (1954)

There were no histological changes, even in those that exhibited tremors and retarded growth (Hodge *et al.*, 1954).

Neurotoxicity EPN produced neurotoxicity when administered subcutaneously to atropine-protected hens at dosages of 40 mg/kg or more. Although this effect was prompt in onset and lasted as little as 6 days in some hens, it persisted over 330 days in others (Gaines, 1969). Thus, the effects of EPN stand midway between those of compounds causing typical reversible neurotoxicity and those causing classical irreversible effects.

EPN is neurotoxic to hens at single oral dosages as low as 25 mg/kg (see Table 16.14). Dosages of 0.1–10 mg/kg/day for 90 days produced delayed neurotoxicity in hens; those receiving 0.01 mg/kg/day showed no effect. The lowest effective dosage produced only ataxia; dosages of 5 or 10 mg/kg/day produced paralysis and some deaths (Abou-Donia and Graham, 1978a).

Although the optical isomers of EPN were equally toxic to mice, a dosage of 40.6 mg/kg of the (−) isomer produced paralysis in hens but the (+) isomer failed to do so at dosages as high as 89.2 mg/kg (Ohkawa *et al.*, 1977). The effects of repeated administration at 5 mg/kg/day were consistent in that the (−) isomer caused the greater effect; however, the (+) isomer did produce a lesser neurotoxicity (Abou-Donia *et al.*, 1978).

Absorption, Distribution, Metabolism, and Excretion EPN is readily absorbed by the skin as well as by the gastrointestinal tract.

In rats, following a single oral dose of ^{14}C-labeled EPN at a rate of 1.5 mg/kg, the highest initial levels of radioactivity were found in the liver, kidney, and lungs (Charles and Farmer, 1979).

In hens, tissue levels peaked 12 hr after an oral dosage of 10 mg/kg of EPN; 33% of the dose was then found in the tissues with the highest concentration in the muscles and lesser concentrations in the skin and liver. The brain, spinal cord, and sciatic nerve had low levels (B. L. Reichert *et al.*, 1978).

EPN undergoes the usual oxidative toxication through desulfuration and detoxication through removal of *p*-nitrophenol (Hitchcock and Murphy, 1967; Bradway *et al.*, 1977). In addition, the nitro group can be reduced to an amino group by enzymes in the liver of mammals, birds, and fish and in the kidneys, spleens, hearts, lungs, and erythrocytes of mammals. The resulting amine is a weak inhibitor of cholinesterase, but the importance of this reduction for detoxication *in vivo* is unknown (Hitchcock and Murphy, 1967).

In rats, urinary excretion of metabolites of [^{14}C]EPN totaled 68.2 and 60.6% of the total dose in males and females, respectively; the corresponding fecal values were 6.7 and 17.2%. Biliary as well as fecal excretion was higher in females (Charles and Farmer, 1979). In hens, most of the excretion was via the cloaca; only 0.39% of the dose was found in the expired air (B. L. Reichert *et al.*, 1978).

Biochemical Effects The great attention that has been given to the potentiation of certain organic phosphorus compounds started with the discovery of the potentiation of malathion by EPN (see Section 16.3.1).

Animals pretreated with phenobarbital are less susceptible to EPN (Welch and Coon, 1964; Kelemen and Volle, 1965; Brodeur, 1967). This finding indicated that the net effect of the metabolism of EPN by microsomal enzymes is detoxication. However, different authors have reported different results in animals pretreated with SKF 525A, some finding them more susceptible (Kelemen and Volle, 1965) and some less susceptible (Welch and Coon, 1964). The basis for the difference is unknown.

The decreased susceptibility of mice pretreated with thiouracil suggests that thiouracil competes with EPN for enzymes leading to desulfuration and the substitution of =O (Kelemen and Volle, 1965).

No cholinesterase inhibition was observed in rats maintained on a dietary level of 25 ppm (about 1.2 mg/kg/day) for 2 weeks (Frawley *et al.*, 1952a), but some inhibition was detected in rats on the same dietary concentration for 13 weeks (DuBois *et al.*, 1968) and even in rats at a dietary level of 5 ppm (about 0.24 mg/kg/day) or higher for 13 weeks or more (DuBois *et al.*, 1968; Suzuki, 1973). No inhibition of cholinesterase occurred at a dietary level of 1 ppm (about 0.05 mg/kg/day), although this dosage did cause some inhibition of other esterases. No effect on any enzymes was detected at a dietary level of 0.2 ppm (about 0.01 mg/kg/day) (DuBois *et al.*, 1968).

Effects on Organs and Tissues EPN was not mutagenic to *Salmonella*, even in the presence of microsomal enzymes (Byeon *et al.*, 1976).

Effects on Reproduction Apparently, the effect of EPN on mammalian reproduction has not been investigated.

The injection of duck eggs with EPN causes deformity of the feet of the ducklings (Khera *et al.*, 1965b, 1966), but this is not necessarily predictive of mammalian teratogenicity.

16.11.1.3 Toxicity to Humans

Experimental Exposure Studies of EPN in volunteers were begun at a dosage of 3 mg/person/day. The threshold of incipient toxicity for EPN appears to be 9 mg/person/day (about 0.13 mg/kg/day). Ten subjects between the ages of 23 and 36 ingested EPN at the rate of 6 mg/person/day for 47 days without any significant effect on plasma or red cell cholinesterase activity (Rider *et al.*, 1959; Moeller and Rider, 1959, 1962a). See also Section 16.6.1.3.

Accidental and Intentional Poisoning Deaths from EPN have followed ingestion (Hosaka and Yamaura, 1976; Shiozaki *et al.*, 1977; Sugaya and Wakatsuki, 1978). A case described in detail showed several unusual features. When first hospitalized, a 73-year-old man showed typical signs of anticholinesterase poisoning, and he was already in coma. Appropriate treatment led to some improvement. However, fibrillary twitching appeared mainly in the arms and legs, and persistent spasms that tended to bend the knees appeared in the legs. While spasms were present, electroencephalograms showed frequent, abrupt occurrences of high-amplitude sharp waves and a combination of these with slow waves. By day 12, the level of consciousness had improved, spasms had stopped, and the EEG had returned to near normal. However, the passage of uncontrollable bloody mucoid feces debilitated the patient, and in spite of intravenous feedings he died on day 14 (Hosaka and Yamaura, 1976).

Use Experience   In spite of its considerable toxicity, there have been few reports of poisoning by EPN. For example, Kawashiro (1959) recorded only one death associated with spraying EPN and only nine deaths associated with suicide with the compound compared to 735 caused by parathion (41 occupational, 21 accidental, and 673 suicidal) during the same period.

Some inhibition of serum cholinesterase and nonspecific symptoms were found among chrysanthemum workers exposed to EPN and a number of other organic phosphorus insecticides. Some of the workers had dermatitis, but patch tests showed that it was caused by the plants (Rikimaru *et al.*, 1972).

Dosage Response   A 73-year-old man survived a surprisingly long time (14 days) following a dosage of EPN estimated at about 1429 mg/kg. His death was the result of bloody diarrhea and debility after the usual effects of poisoning had disappeared (Hosaka and Yamaura, 1976).

The threshold limit value (0.5 mg/m^3) indicates that occupational intake of 0.07 mg/kg/day is considered safe, and this is consistent with the no-effect level of 0.087 mg/kg/day in volunteers who received EPN orally.

Treatment of Poisoning   See Section 16.2.2.7.

16.11.2 LEPTOPHOS

16.11.2.1 Identity, Properties, and Uses

Chemical Name   Leptophos is *O*-4-bromo-2,5-dichlorophenyl-*O*-methyl phenylphosphonothioate.

Structure   See Table 16.49.

Synonyms   The common name leptophos (ANSI, BSI, ISO) is in general use. The term MBCP (JMAF) also is used. Trade names have included Abar® and Phosvel®. Code designations include VCS-506 and VVS-506. The CAS registry number is 21609-90-5.

Physical and Chemical Properties   Leptophos has the empirical formula $C_{13}H_{10}BrCl_2O_2PS$ and a molecular weight of 412.06. The pure material is a white amorphous solid melting at 20.2–20.6°C. Leptophos is stable to acids under long ex-

posure at normal temperatures but hydrolyzes slowly under strongly alkaline conditions. It decomposes at temperatures above 350°C. Leptophos is soluble in water at 25°C to 2.4 ppm. At 25°C its solubility in grams per 100 milliliters is: acetone, 47; benzene, 129.6; cyclohexane, 14.2; heptane, 5.9; and 2-propanol, 2.4.

History, Formulations, and Uses   Leptophos first was introduced in 1969 by the Velsicol Company. It was available as an emulsifiable concentrate containing 3 lb of active ingredient per U.S. gallon. Formulations also included 45% wettable powder, 3% dusts, and 5% granules.

16.11.2.2 Toxicity to Laboratory Animals

Toxicity Related to Cholinesterase Inhibition   Leptophos has a moderate toxicity in species that are relatively immune to the neurotoxic effects of organic phosphorus compounds (see Table 16.52).

Rats tolerated dietary levels as high as 90 ppm (about 4.4 mg/kg/day) for 12 weeks without illness, reduction in body weight, or change in a number of clinical laboratory findings. However, a dietary level of only 30 ppm caused slight inhibition of red cell, plasma, and brain cholinesterase. A dietary level of 10 ppm (about 0.5 mg/kg/day) caused temporary inhibition of red cell enzyme, but activity recovered while dosing continued (Hassan *et al.*, 1977). Ten times that dosage (5 mg/kg/day) for 28 weeks was not neurotoxic to rats but was neurotoxic to hens (Hussain and Olloffs, 1979). Eight oral doses at a rate of 10 mg/kg/day failed to paralyze a monkey (Horiguchi *et al.*, 1977). A dietary level of 500 ppm (about 64 mg/kg) for 12 weeks caused marked inhibition of cholinesterase activity and some retardation of growth but did not affect antibody formation or produce detectable neurotoxicity (Koller *et al.*, 1976).

Neurotoxicity   The neurotoxicity of leptophos should have been suspected because of its structural similarity to EPN, the neurotoxicity of which to hens has been recognized for many years (Table 16.14). Apparently, the first direct evidence for the neurotoxicity of leptophos was the paralysis of about 1300

Table 16.52
Single-Dose LD 50 for Leptophos

Species	Route	LD 50 (mg/kg)	Reference
Rat, M	oral	40	Seizaburo and Takabumi (1978)
Rat, F	oral	33	Seizaburo and Takabumi (1978)
Rat, M	oral	19	Gaines and Linder (1986)
Rat, F	oral	20	Gaines and Linder (1986)
Rat[a]	oral	12	Gaines and Linder (1986)
Rat, M	dermal	103	Gaines and Linder (1986)
Rat, F	dermal	44	Gaines and Linder (1986)
Rabbit	oral	124.7	Kamel *et al.* (1973)
Chicken	oral	4700	Abou-Donia *et al.* (1974)

[a] Male weanling.

water buffaloes in Egypt, which was reported in the *Near East News Roundup,* an FAO regional publication issued in Cairo on November 22, 1971 (Abou-Donia *et al.,* 1974). Pathology of the animals was reported by Hamza (1973). The signs observed in the field were reproduced experimentally in buffaloes by feeding them forage sprayed with leptophos, but the results were not published at once (Abou-Donia and Preissig, 1976a). Later, the ability of the compound to produce typical, delayed, permanent neurotoxicity in hens was demonstrated (Abou-Donia *et al.,* 1974; Abou-Donia and Preissig, 1976a,b) (see Table 16.14). Ataxia never appeared in less than 8 days following a single oral dose. Leptophos also is neurotoxic to mice and sheep (El-Sebae *et al.,* 1977).

Desbromoleptophos and leptophos oxon are approximately three and two times, respectively, more effective than the parent compound as neurotoxic agents in chickens (Sanborn *et al.,* 1977). The results of other investigators (Yatomi *et al.,* 1978) were consistent. However, although Abou-Donia *et al.* (1980a) agreed that desbromoleptophos was more active, they found the oxon only weakly neurotoxic. The reason for the disagreement is unclear.

Absorption, Distribution, Metabolism, and Excretion
The absorption of leptophos is similar to that of other organic phosphorus insecticides (see Section 16.2.2.1). There is some evidence that the compound accumulates in tissue to a greater extent than most other organic phosphorous compounds do. The metabolism of leptophos is generally similar to that of parathion (see Section 16.7.1.2). Far more interesting is the fact that desbromoleptophos has been reported as a minor impurity in technical leptophos and as a product of the compound in the presence of ultraviolet light, either in the laboratory or in plants under field conditions (FAO/WHO, 1976). In an irradiated solution, photocyclization produced a compound believed to be *O*-methyl-*O,P*-(5-chloro-2,2′-biphenylene) phosphonothioate, the structure of which is shown in Table 16.49, which also shows two examples of closely related and highly neurotoxic saligenin phosphates.

In spite of some tendency to storage, leptophos, in the form of water-soluble metabolites, is excreted rapidly by rodents, with virtually complete elimination in 48–72 hr. In mice fed [^{14}C]leptophos at a rate of 25 mg/kg the rate of excretion of the phenoxy moiety was distinctly faster than that of the phenyl moiety; radioactivity was found in the urine as long as 6 days after treatment (Holmstead *et al.,* 1973).

In rats, excretion of radioactive carbon was essentially complete in 72 hr following a single dose or the last of a series of doses of [^{14}C]leptophos. Six days after the last dose, the highest concentration of ^{14}C was in the liver, but it constituted <0.25% of the total dose. More than 97% of the radioactivity in the urine of rats that had received [^{14}C]leptophos was organosoluble. The phenyl moiety was excreted as *O*-methylphenylphosphonic acid (about 90%), phenylphosphoric acid (about 10%), and a trace of *O*-methylphenylthiophosphoric acid. This pattern differs from that of the mouse, in which the latter compound predominates. In

both species, the substituted phenoxy moiety was excreted as the corresponding phenol (Whitacre *et al.,* 1976). Many of these findings were confirmed, and it was shown that a small portion of the methyl carbon is metabolized to carbon dioxide and exhaled (Hassan *et al.,* 1977).

Within 8 days after a single oral dose to a cat, the following percentages of radioactivity derived from leptophos were recovered from feces, urine, expired air, and tissues: 67.42, 27.33, 1.78, and 2.57%, respectively. Whereas most of the metabolites in the urine were water-soluble, most of the radioactivity in the feces and liver was in the form of unchanged parent compound and desbromoleptophos. It was speculated that the susceptibility of the cat to the neurotoxic effects of leptophos might be related to the relative stability of leptophos on the one hand and its conversion to the more neurotoxic desbromo derivative on the other (Abou-Donia and Ashry, 1978).

The stability of leptophos is even more striking in the hen. Following a single oral dose at the rate of 400 mg/kg, only 74% of the dose was recovered in the combined urine and feces in 15 days. Some was excreted in the eggs. The half-life for disappearances of [^{14}C]leptophos form the birds' bodies was 11.55 days. At a dosage of 400 mg/kg, ataxia, paralysis, and death appeared in 9–11, 15–19, and 24–47 days, respectively (Abou-Donia, 1976b). Leptophos tends to persist in the fat of hens. Following oral administration at rates of 50 and 250 mg/kg, the concentration in fat reached peaks of 2.5 and 8.6 ppm, respectively, in 24 hr (Konno and Kinebuchi, 1978b).

Similar pharmokinetic results were found following a single dose of [^{14}C]phenyl leptophos applied to the combs of hens at a subneurotoxic rate of 50 mg/kg. A total of 35.4% of the applied dose was absorbed during a 20-day experiment. Radioactivity reached a peak of 17.1% of the dose 12 hr after application; 5% of the dose still remained after 20 days. The highest ^{14}C concentrations after 20 days were in muscle, brain, spinal cord, contents of the large intestine, and bile, in that order. Combined urinary–fecal excretion accounted for 24.3% of the applied dose; expired carbon dioxide accounted for 1.3%; and egg accounted for 4.5%. The half-life for elimination was 17 days (Abou-Donia, 1979b).

Biochemical Effects   Hens that received repeated doses of leptophos at rates ranging from 0.5 to 20 mg/kg/day showed a decrease in plasma cholinesterase activity and an increase in acid phosphatase activity. It was suggested that these changes may act as an early warning of overexposure (Abou-Donia, 1978). However, there apparently has been no demonstration that the increase in acid phosphatase, much less the decrease in cholinesterase, is characteristic of neurotoxic compounds.

Liver microsomal enzymes tend to protect against leptophos. Whereas all pregnant rats were killed by a dosage of 50 mg/kg, most of those pretreated with phenobarbital survived (Kanoh *et al.,* 1979).

Pathology   Spinal cord lesions produced by leptophos in the hen were more consistent than the peripheral nerve lesions and correlated better with the clinical signs (Preissig and Abou-Donia, 1978).

16.11.2.3 Toxicity to Humans

Accidents and Use Experience   Apparently, the first published mention of human injury from leptophos was an undocumented paragraph in a review discussing, among other things, the use of the compound in Egypt (Shea, 1974). The paragraph concerns six people in Egypt who suffered neurotoxic disease (see Section 16.4.1) first observed long after the spraying season was over, so that no one was able to say how these victims contacted the chemical. It was alleged that traces of the compound were found in their tissues. The review implied that the cases occurred after 1972 and, of course, before the review was published in 1974. El-Sebae *et al.* (1977) also referred to six persons affected by neurotoxic poisoning and in whose tissues traces of leptophos were found; the information was attributed to M. T. Shafik, a distinguished analytical chemist. However, in one study of Egyptian farmers exposed to leptophos by both respiratory and dermal routes in connection with application of the insecticide to cotton, no mention was made of polyneuropathy. Characteristic illness proportional to inhibition of red cell cholinesterase activity was observed (Hassan *et al.,* 1978).

Another set of cases of possible polyneuropathy occurred among workers in Texas engaged in making leptophos. The first news (Anonymous, 1976) was sensational and referred to leptophos only. However, an investigation by the National Institute for Occupational Safety and Health (Xintaras *et al.,* 1978) left doubt that any incapacitating disease had occurred or that leptophos was entirely or even partially responsible. Briefly, nearly all of the 301 current and former workers with potential exposure were notified of the availability of medical examinations, and 155 reported for study of physical, neurological, neuromuscular, ophthalmological, psychological, and biochemical function. Many complaints were recorded and many abnormalities were observed. Although some of the findings were regarded as "serious," the report was simply not clear on whether any of the conditions were incapacitating. The report failed to establish that a single worker had suffered classical polyneuropathy, and it raised the possibility that the diverse complaints might be caused entirely or partially by a variety of chemicals, especially *n*-hexane.

Treatment of Poisoning   Treatment of the cholinergic effects of leptophos is the same as that for other organic phosphorus compounds (see Section 16.2.2.7). Unfortunately, no treatment is known for the neurotoxic effects, whether typical or otherwise.

16.11.3 CAREJIN

Carejin is *O*-methyl-*O*-cyclohexyl-*S*-(parachlorophenyl)thiophosphate. Its structural formula appears in Table 16.49. The compound also has been called MHCP. Hiraki *et al.* (1972) described cases of acute poisoning in a male and a female farmer. In spite of using respirators and full clothing, both became acutely ill less than an hour after applying the material. The signs and symptoms were typical of acute cholinergic poisoning. Although the man was so weak that he was unable to stand, neither patient lost consciousness or suffered serious respiratory difficulty. In fact, both already were beginning to recover when they entered the hospital. Electroencephalographic studies were carried out over a period of 6 days, and the results were described in detail. During the period of observation, nothing to suggest polyneuropathy was seen.

16.11.4 EDIFENPHOS

16.11.4.1 Identity, Properties, and Uses

Chemical Name   Edifenphos is *O*-ethyl *S,S*-diphenyl phosphorodithioate.

Structure   See Table 16.49.

Synonyms   The common name edifenphos (BSI, ISO) is in general use. The trade name Hinosan® has been used. A code designation is BAY-78,418. The CAS registry number is 17109-49-8.

Physical and Chemical Properties   Edifenphos has the empirical formula $C_{14}H_{15}O_2PS_2$ and a molecular weight of 310.36. The pure material is a clear yellow to light brown liquid with a boiling point of 154°C at 0.01 mm Hg. Its density is 1.23 at 20°C. Edifenphos is practically insoluble in water but soluble in acetone and xylene. At 25°C and pH 7 the half-life of edifenphos is 1135 hr. At the same temperature but a pH of 9 edifenphos has a half-life of only 49 hr.

History, Formulations, and Uses   Edifenphos was introduced in 1968 by Bayer Leverkusen. It is a fungicide with specific action against rice blast. It also is effective against sheath blight and ear blight, and it has insecticidal action. Edifenphos is available as 30, 40, and 50% emulsifiable concentrates and as 1.5, 2.0, and 2.5% dusts.

16.11.4.2 Toxicity to Laboratory Animals

Basic Findings   Edifenphos produces typical signs of cholinesterase inhibition. Following intraperitoneal injection, illness appears within 15 min and death occurs within 3 hr. The compound is only moderately toxic, as indicated by intraperitoneal LD 50 values of 66.5 and 25.5 mg/kg in male and female rats, respectively (Chen *et al.,* 1972).

Absorption, Distribution, Metabolism, and Excretion The major degenerative reaction of edifenphos involves cleavage of one of the P—S bonds (Tomizawa *et al.*, 1972). Metabolites formed in this way include *O*-ethyl-*S*-phenyl-hydrogen-phosphorothioate and *O*-conjugates of *m*- and *p*-(hydroxyphenyl) methyl-sulfone. Other metabolites include *S,S*-diphenyl-hydrogen-phosphorodithioate and *S*-phenyl-hydrogen-phosphorodithioate (Ueyama and Takase, 1975). The compound is rapidly absorbed, metabolized, and eliminated by rats and mice following oral administration. From 98.6 to 101.1% of the dose was recovered within 72 hr, at which time 4% was recovered from the tissues. No qualitative difference in metabolic pattern between male and female was found (Ueyama *et al.*, 1978).

Biochemical Effects Edifenphos is a direct inhibitor of cholinesterase; the pI 50 is 6.98. *In vivo*, cholinesterases of the central nervous system and of the peripheral tissues are inhibited about equally. This effect is rapid in onset and of long duration. The compound is also a potent inhibitor of aliesterases, and it potentiates the action of malathion. The toxicity of edifenphos is reduced in rats pretreated with phenobarbital and other inducers of microsomal enzymes, indicating that their net effect is detoxication (Chen *et al.*, 1972).

16.11.4.3 Toxicity to Humans

Use Experience In general, use experience with edifenphos has been good. Two cases of poisoning have been reported that were the result not of an accident but of poor management. A male and a female worker in a manufacturing plant were assigned to clean a bin in which 1.5% dust had been stored. Each wore a mask of considerable porosity plus ordinary work clothing and a cap. Apparently, the mask involved no cannister to remove vapor, and no mention was made of gloves. Ordinarily, supplied-air masks would have been used, but the hoses were not long enough. The sides of the bins were beaten to remove adhering material, and this action released dust into the air. The man developed headache, abdominal pain, vomiting, diarrhea, and numbness of the extremities while at work. The woman developed similar signs and symptoms after she reached home after work. Both responded well to atropine (Section of Labor Hygiene, 1972).

Treatment of Poisoning See Section 16.2.2.7.

16.11.5 FONOFOS

16.11.5.1 Identity, Properties, and Uses

Chemical Name Fonofos is *O*-ethyl *S*-phenyl ethylphosphonothiolothionate.

Structure See Table 16.49.

Synonyms Fonofos is the common name approved by BSI and ISO. A trade name for fonofos is Dyfonate®, and a code designation is N-2,790. The CAS registry number is 944-22-9.

Physical and Chemical Properties Fonofos has the empirical formula $C_{10}H_{15}OPS_2$ and a molecular weight of 246.32. Fonofos is a light yellow liquid with a pungent mercaptan odor. The boiling point is 130°C at 0.1 mm Hg, and the vapor pressure is 2.1×10^{-4} mm Hg at 25°C. The density of the compound is 1.16. Fonofos is practically insoluble in water but is miscible with organic solvents such as kerosene, xylene, and isobutyl methyl ketone. It is stable under normal conditions.

History, Formulations, and Uses Fonofos was introduced in 1967 by the Stauffer Chemical Company and first was described by Menn and Szabo (1965). It is used as a soil insecticide.

16.11.5.2 Toxicity to Laboratory Animals

Fonofos is a toxic compound. The oral LD 50 in rats is 16 mg/kg (Menn and Szabo, 1965).

Although acute administration of fonofos produced 19% inhibition of hen brain neurotoxic esterase, 90 oral doses at rates as high as 8 mg/kg did not produce delayed neurotoxicity (Miller *et al.*, 1979).

Absorption, Distribution, Metabolism, and Excretion In the presence of rat liver microsomal enzymes, fonofos is metabolized to the oxon and also, by a different reaction, to *O*-ethyl-ethylphosphonothiotic acid (ETP) and thiophenol. The oxon, in turn, is hydrolzyed to *O*-ethyl-ethylphosphoric acid (EOP) and thiophenol (McBain *et al.*, 1971b, 1972). Similar metabolites were formed by the intact rat, except that the oxon was not found due to rapid hydrolysis. The other metabolites were much less toxic than the parent compound (McBain *et al.*, 1971c).

"Oxygenated fonofos," a compound thought to have a P—S—O ring structure but no other changes in the molecule, was synthesized in 30% yield in a peracid system. It was considered a metabolic intermediate. In the presence of enzymes, the oxygenated fonofos was converted rapidly to ETP, EOP, and thiophenol, but not to the oxon (McBain *et al.*, 1971a). However, later work showed unequivocally that the compound in question was phenylethoxy(ethyl)phosphinyl disulfide and cast grave doubt on its formation as a metabolic intermediate (Wustner *et al.*, 1972).

After a single oral or intraperitoneal dose of fonofos labeled in the ring position, 98% of the radioactivity was excreted in the urine and feces within 96 hr. Conditioning with unlabeled fonofos did not change the excretion pattern. Excretion of radioactivity from the ^{14}C-ethoxy moiety was essentially complete in 4 days, with about 91% in the urine, 7.4% in the feces, and 0.35% in the expired air. Radioactivity in the bile was an important source of activity in the feces. Tissue residues were very small and had virtually disappeared by day 16 (Hoffman *et al.*, 1972).

The reactions and toxicity of the chiral isomers have been studied in detail (Allahyari *et al.*, 1977; Lee *et al.*, 1976,

1978a,b,c). The mouse oral LD 50 values for the (*S*)*p*- and (*R*) *p* isomers were 32.0 and 9.5 mg/kg, respectively, for fonofos and 6.0 and 38.0 mg/kg, respectively, for the oxon, indicating considerable interconversion during metabolism (Lee *et al.*, 1978a).

16.11.5.3 Toxicity to Humans

Accidental and Intentional Poisoning A 19-year-old woman developed nausea, vomiting, salivation, and sweating soon after breakfast, and she was taken to a local hospital. She suffered cardiorespiratory arrest. Following successful resuscitation she was transferred to a medical center, where she arrived unconscious and without spontaneous respiration; she had muscle fasciculations, blood pressure of 64/0 mm Hg, a pulse rate of 46, pinpoint pupils, and profuse salivary and bronchial secretions. She was maintained on a respirator. In addition to predictable findings, she showed temperature spiking to 40°C and an increase in serum amylase, which decreased rapidly to normal on hospital day 4 and then peaked again between days 9 and 18. On day 9, abdominal distension was noted, and an epigastric mass was palpated. On hospital day 12 a 10-cm pancreatic pseudocyst was drained externally. The postoperative course was stormy, but the patient was discharged 2 months later and was still well when last reported 15 months later. During her illness, she received no specific treatment because it was not until the tenth day in the medical center that investigation by the medical examiner revealed the true cause of illness as an organic phosphorus compound, specifically fonofos, a formulation of which had been used as flour in making pancake batter the night before the cakes were cooked for breakfast (Dressel *et al.*, 1979a). Although not reported in the original paper, three other members of the family were poisoned by the pancakes, and one of them died. A fifth family member who may have mixed the batter but did not eat pancakes remained well.

This case, complicated by a pancreatic cyst, led to extensive research in animals regarding the effects of cholinesterase inhibition in the pancreas (see Section 16.2.2.5).

16.11.6 METAMIDOPHOS

16.11.6.1 Identity, Properties, and Uses

Chemical Name Metamidophos is *O,S*-dimethyl phosphoramidothioate.

Structure See Table 16.49.

Synonyms The common name metamidophos (ANSI, BSI, ISO) is generally accepted. Trade names include Monitor® and Tamaron®. The CAS registry number is 10265-92-6. Code designations include Bayer-71628, ENT-27396, Ortho-9006, and SRA-5172.

Physical and Chemical Properties Metamidophos has the empirical formula $C_2H_8NO_2PS$ and a molecular weight of 141.12. It is a colorless, crystalline solid with a melting point of 54°C. Vapor pressure is 3×10^{-4} mm Hg at 30°C. It is highly soluble in aliphatic hydrocarbons, alcohols, ketones, and water; slightly soluble in ether; and very slightly soluble in petroleum ether.

History, Formulations, and Uses Metamidophos was synthesized by Bayer AG in 1964 and in an independent effort by Chevron Research Company in 1965. It is a broad-spectrum insecticide and acaricide with both contact and systemic action.

16.11.6.2 Toxicity to Laboratory Animals

Basic Findings Metamidophos is a compound of high mammalian toxicity. Gaines and Linder (1986) determined the acute oral LD 50 values in rats to be 31, 32, and 21 mg/kg for males, females, and male weanlings, respectively. The acute dermal LD 50 values for adult rats are 94 mg/kg for males and 85 mg/kg for females (Gaines and Linder, 1986).

16.11.6.3 Toxicity to Humans

Accidental and Intentional Poisoning Although metamidophos has not been previously associated with delayed neuropathy, 10 poisonings involving technical grade Tamaron® (60% methamidofos) (five ingesting 30–80 ml, three ingesting unknown quantities, and two involving dermal and/or inhalation exposures) resulted in signs of delayed neuropathy 2–4 weeks following exposure (see Section 16.4.1) (Senanayake and Johnson, 1982).

Without stating the nature of the exposure or of the illness, Sallam and El-Ghawaby (1980) reported a mortality of 1% among 3000 workers exposed to a mixture of metamidophos and azinphos in Egypt in 1976.

16.11.7 TRICHLORONAT

16.11.7.1 Identity, Properties, and Uses

Chemical Name Trichloronat is ethyl 2,4,5-trichlorophenyl ethylphosphonothionate.

Structure See Table 16.49.

Synonyms The common name trichloronat (BSI, ISO) is generally accepted. The name trichloronate was discontinued in 1984. It is also known by the trade names Agrisil®, Agritox®, and Phytosol®. Code numbers include OMS 412, OMS 578, and ENT 25,712. The CAS registry number is 327-98-0.

Physical and Chemical Properties Trichloronat has the empirical formula $C_{10}H_{12}Cl_3O_2PS$ and a molecular weight of 333.60. The pure material is an amber liquid with a boiling point of 108°C at 0.01 mm Hg. Trichloronat is practically insoluble in water but is soluble in most organic solvents.

History, Formulations, and Uses First synthesized by Bayer AG in 1960 as soil insecticide, trichloronat is a nonsystemic insecticide with a persistent residual.

16.11.7.2 Toxicity to Laboratory Animals

Basic Findings The acute oral LD 50 of trichloronat in rats is 50 mg/kg (Eto, 1979).

16.11.7.3 Toxicity to Humans

Accidental and Intentional Poisoning A 29-year-old male attempted suicide by drinking approximately 2 glasses of Phytosol®. He vomited immediately and was brought to a hospital 10 hr later in an unconscious state with cold, moist, pale skin. Pupils were constricted, muscle twitches were noted, pulse was 90 beats/min, although blood pressure and respiration were normal. Rales and rhonchi were heard in the upper lungs and moist rales were noted in the lower lungs. Blood cholinesterase activity was reduced by 93%, blood glucose was 308 mg/100 ml, and there was 1.2% glycosuria and a leukocytosis of 10,600/mm³. Atropine, cardiac drugs, and antibiotics were administered to treat the initial acute toxicity as well as circulatory failure and pneumonia that occurred in the first week. Although the patient began walking on day 10 following exposure, paresthesia and distal weakness in the lower limbs occurred. Over the next 3 weeks, characteristic signs and symptoms of delayed neuropathy developed (see Section 16.4.1). By 2 months, the patient complained of a burning sensation in the feet, and atrophy of the legs and distal portions of the arms was observed. Signs of polyneuropathy decreased with time and the patient was able to walk with assistance during the seventh month following exposure. However, spastic paraplegia began to develop at this time, confining the patient to a wheelchair by 30 months after exposure (Jedrzejowska *et al.*, 1980).

REFERENCES

Abbasov, T. G. (1971). Effect of chlorophos, phosphamide, trichlorometaphos-3, and methylnitrophos on rabbits following long-term feeding. *Tr. VNIIVS* **39**, 220–227.

Abdel-Aal, A. M. A., El-Hawary, M. F. S., Kamel, H., Abdel-Khalek, M. K., and El-Diwany, K. M. (1970). Blood cholinesterases, hepatic, renal and haemopoietic functions in children receiving repeated doses of "Dipterex." *J. Egypt. Med. Assoc.* **53**, 265–271.

Abou-Donia, M. B. (1976a). Pharmacokinetics of a sub-neurotoxic dose of leptophos. *Fed. Proc., Fed. Am. Soc. Exp. Biol.* **35**, 664.

Abou-Donia, M. B. (1976b). Pharmacokinetics of a neurotoxic oral dose of leptophos in hens. *Arch. Toxicol.* **36**, 103–110.

Abou-Donia, M. B. (1978). Role of acid phosphatases in delayed neurotoxicity induced by leptophos in hens. *Biochem. Pharmacol.* **27**, 2055–2058.

Abou-Donia, M. B. (1979a). Delayed neurotoxicity of phenylphosphonothioate esters. *Science* **205**, 713–714.

Abou-Donia, M. B. (1979b). Pharmacokinetics and metabolism of a topically applied dose of O-4-bromo-2,5-dichlorophenyl O-methyl phenylphosphonothioate in hens. *Toxicol. Appl. Pharmacol.* **51**, 311–328.

Abou-Donia, M. B., and Ashry, M. A. (1978). Pharmacokinetics and metabolism of an oral dose of leptophos in the cat. *Toxicol. Appl. Pharmacol.* **45**, 280.

Abou-Donia, M. B., and Graham, D. G. (1978a). Delayed neurotoxicity of O-ethyl O-4-nitrophenyl phenylphosphonothioate: Subchronic (90 days) oral administration in hens. *Toxicol. Appl. Pharmacol.* **45**, 685–700.

Abou-Donia, M. B., and Graham, D. G. (1978b). Delayed neurotoxicity from long-term low-level administration of leptophos to the comb of hens. *Toxicol. Appl. Pharmacol.* **46**, 199–213.

Abou-Donia, M. B., and Graham, D. G. (1979). Delayed neurotoxicity of O-ethyl O-4-nitrophenyl phenylphosphonothionate: Toxic effects of a single oral dose on the nervous system of hens. *Toxicol. Appl. Pharmacol.* **48**, 57–66.

Abou-Donia, M. B., and Preissig, S. H. (1975). Studies in delayed neurotoxicity produced by leptophos. *Fed. Proc., Fed. Am. Soc. Exp. Biol.* **34**, 810.

Abou-Donia, M. B., and Preissig, S. H. (1976a). Delayed neurotoxicity of leptophos: Toxic effects on the nervous system of hens. *Toxicol. Appl. Pharmacol.* **35**, 269–282.

Abou-Donia, M. B., and Preissig, S. H. (1976b). Delayed neurotoxicity from continuous low-dose oral administration of leptophos to hens. *Toxicol. Appl. Pharmacol.* **38**, 595–608.

Abou-Donia, M. B., Othman, M. A., Khalil, A. Z., Tantawy, G., and Shavier, M. F. (1974). Neurotoxic effect of leptophos. *Experientia* **30**, 63–64.

Abou-Donia, M. B., Nomeir, A. A., and Dauterman, W. C. (1978). Stereospecificity of delayed neurotoxic and cholinergic effects of EPN and EPN oxon optical isomers. *Pharmacologist* **20**, 179.

Abou-Donia, M. B., Graham, D. G., and Komeil, A. A. (1979). Delayed neurotoxicity of O-ethyl O-2,4-dichlorophenyl phenylphosphonothioate: Effects of a single oral dose on hens. *Toxicol. Appl. Pharmacol.* **49**, 293–303.

Abou-Donia, M. B., Graham, D. G., Ashry, M. A., and Timmons, P. R. (1980a). Delayed neurotoxicity of leptophos and related compounds: Differential effects of subchronic oral administration of pure, technical grade and degradation products on the hen. *Toxicol. Appl. Pharmacol.* **53**, 150–163.

Abou-Donia, M. B., Graham, D. G., Timmons, P. R., and Reichert, B. L. (1980b). Late acute delayed neurotoxic and cholinergic effects of S,S,S-tributyl phosphorotrithioite (merphos) in hens. *Toxicol. Appl. Pharmacol.* **53**, 439–457.

Ackerman, H. (1969). Studies concerning inhibition of cholinesterase by phosphorothionates. *Arch. Toxikol.* **24**, 325–331.

Ackerman, H. (1970). Studies on the mechanism of action of thionophosphoric acid esters. Comparative studies between the appearance of PO-analogs after the application of methyl parathion, the intensity of the manifestations of intoxication and esterase inhibition. *Arch. Exp. Veterinaermed.* **24**, 1293–1300.

Agarwal, R., and Matin, M. A. (1981). Effect of oximes and atropine on the concentration of cerebral glycogen and blood glucose in malathion-treated rats. *J. Pharm. Pharmacol.* **33**, 795–796.

Ahdaya, S. M., Shah, P. V., and Guthrie, F. E. (1976). Thermoregulation in mice treated with parathion, cabaryl, or DDT. *Toxicol. Appl. Pharmacol.* **35**, 575–580.

Aizenshtad, V. S., Dolmatova-Guseva, E. G., Perkhurova, V. P., Shtifel'man, A. V., Bogomolova, L. M., and Nerubai, S. M. (1971). Work hygiene and the state of workers' health in the production of carbophos. *Gig. Tr. Prof. Zabol.* **15**, 49–51 (in Russian).

Akimov, G. A., Buchko, V. M., and Kremleva, R. V. (1975). Neurological disorders in chlorophos poisoning. *Klin. Med. (Moscow)* **5**, 65–69 (in Russian).

Akimov, G. A., Buchko, V. M., Kremleva, R. V., and Kolesnichenko, I. P. (1977). Changes in the nervous system in acute peroral intoxications with chlorophos (clinical and pathomorphological data). *Zh. Nevropatol. Psikhiatr. im. S. S. Korsakova* **77**, 204–207 (in Russian).

Alam, M. T., and Kasitiya, S. S. (1974). Chromosomal aberrations induced by an organic phosphate pesticide. *Can. J. Genet. Cytol.* **16**, 701.

Alam, M. T., and Kasitiya, S. S. (1975). Chromosome damage induced by an organic phosphate pesticide in human cells. *Can. J. Genet. Cytol.* **17,** 544.

Alam, M. T., Corbeil, M., Chagnon, A., and Kasitiya, S. S. (1974). Chromosomal anomalies induced by the organic phosphate pesticide Guthion in Chinese hamster cells. *Chromosoma* **49,** 77–86.

Alary, J. G., and Brodeur, J. (1969). Studies on the mechanism of phenobarbital-induced protection against parathion in adult female rats. *J. Pharmacol. Exp. Ther.* **169,** 159–167.

Albert, J. R., and Stearns, S. M. (1974). Delayed neurotoxic potential of a series of alkyl esters of 2,2-dichlorovinyl phosphoric acid in the chicken. *Toxicol. Appl. Pharmacol.* **29,** 136.

Aldridge, W. N. (1954). Tricresyl phosphates and cholinesterase. *Biochem. J.* **56,** 185–189.

Aldridge, W. N., and Barnes, J. M. (1961). Neurotoxic and biochemical properties of some triaryl phosphates. *Biochem. Pharmacol.* **6,** 177–188.

Aldridge, W. N., and Barnes, J. M. (1966a). Further observation on the neurotoxicity of organophosphorus compounds. *Biochem. Pharmacol.* **15,** 541–548.

Aldridge, W. N., and Barnes, J. M. (1966b). Esterases and neurotoxicity of some organophosphorus compounds. *Biochem. Pharmacol.* **15,** 549–554.

Aldridge, W. N., and Barnes, J. M. (1966c). Neurotoxic side effects of certain organophosphorus compounds. *Proc. Eur. Soc. Study Drug Toxic.* **8,** 162–168.

Aldridge, W. N., and Davison, A. N. (1952). The inhibition of erythrocyte cholinesterase by tri-esters of phosphoric acid. *Biochem. J.* **52,** 663–671.

Aldridge, W. N., Barnes, J. M., and Johnson, M. K. (1969). Studies on delayed neurotoxicity produced by some organophosphorus compounds. *Ann. N. Y. Acad. Sci.* **160,** 314–322.

Aldridge, W. N., Miles, J. W., Mount, D. L., and Verschoyle, R. D. (1979). The toxicological properties of impurities in malathion. *Arch. Toxicol.* **42,** 95–106.

Allahyari, R., Lee, P. W., Lin, G. H. Y., Wing, R. M., and Fukuto, T. R. (1977). Resolution and reactions of the chiral isomers of *O*-ethyl *S*-phenyl ethylphosphonodithioate (fonofos) and its analogues. *J. Agric. Food Chem.* **25,** 471–478.

Allison, A. C., and Burn, G. P. (1955). Enzyme activity as a function of age in the erythrocyte. *Br. J. Haematol.* **1,** 291–303.

Amarasingham, R. D., and Ti, T. H. (1976). A review of poisoning cases examined by the Department of Chemistry, Malaysia, from 1968 to 1972. *Med. J. Malay.* **30,** 185–193.

Ambrose, A. M., Larson, P. S., Borzelleca, J. F., and Hennigan, G. R., Jr. (1970). Toxicologic studies on diethyl-1-(2,4-dichlorophenyl)-2-chlorovinylphosphate. *Toxicol. Appl. Pharmacol.* **17,** 323–336.

Amos, W. C., and Hall, A. (1965). Malathion poisoning treated with Protopam. *Ann. Intern. Med.* **62,** 1013–1016.

Anderson, L. S., Warner, D. L., Parker, J. E., Bluman, N., and Page, B. D. (1965). Parathion poisoning from flannelette sheets. *Can. Med. Assoc. J.* **92,** 809–813.

Anderson, P. H., and Machin, A. F. (1969). The organophosphorus warble fly dressings: Some aspects of their toxicity to cattle including antidote therapy. *Vet. Rec.* **85,** 484–487.

Andjelkovic, D., and Milosevic, M. P. (1969). Potassium-stimulated respiration of cerebral cortex of rats poisoned with phosphamidone. *Experientia* **25,** 720.

Andrashko, V. V., Levanyuk, V. F., Kampo, M. A., and Gryzhak, I. P. (1975). The effect of chlorophos on the energy metabolism in the placenta and organs of the intrauterine fetus. *Farmakol. Toksikol.* **2,** 208–210.

Angle, C. R., and Wermers, J. (1974a). Accidental organophosphate poisoning: Even flea-dip needs safety packaging. *N. Engl. J. Med.* **290,** 1031–1032.

Angle, C. R., and Wermers, J. (1974b). Human poisoning with flea-dip concentrate. *J. Am. Vet. Med. Assoc.* **165,** 174–175.

Anonymous (1956). New hurdle for organic pesticides. New insecticides must pass stiffer toxicity tests to gain FDA approval. *Chem. Eng. News* **34,** 5398.

Anonymous (1959). Child dies after bath following fumigation of house. (*Stertz* v. *Briscoe,* 334 p. 2d 357, (Kansas) Supreme Court of Kansas, January 24, 1959). *Public Health Court Dig.* **4,** 5.

Anonymous (1976). Insecticide blamed for nervous disorders. *Chem. Eng. News* **54**(50), 6.

Ariëns, A. T., Cohen, E. M., Meeter, E., and Wolthuis, O. L. (1968). Reversible necrosis in striated muscle fibres of the rat after severe intoxication with various cholinesterase inhibitors. *Ind. Med. Surg.* **37,** 845–847.

Ariëns, A. T., Meeter, E., Wolthuis, O. L., and VanBenthem, R. B. J. (1969). Reversible necrosis at the end-plate region in striated muscles of the rat poisoned with cholinesterase inhibitors. *Experientia* **25,** 57–59.

Aripdzhanov, T. M. (1973a). Effect of pesticides Anthio and milbex on the immunologic reactivity and certain autoimmune processes of the body. *Gig. Sanit.* **38,** 39–42 (in Russian).

Aripdzhanov, T. M. (1973b). Experimental study of the effects of Anthio and milbex on immunobiological reactivity and some autoimmune processes. *Gig. Sanit.* **38,** 101–102 (in Russian).

Arterberry, J. D., Durham, W. F., Elliott, J. W., and Wolfe, H. R. (1961). Exposure to parathion: Measurement by blood cholinesterase level and urinary *p*-nitrophenol excretion. *Arch. Environ. Health* **3,** 476–485.

Arterberry, J. D., Bonifaci, R. W., Nash, E. W., and Quinby, G. E. (1962). Potentiation of phosphorus insecticides by phenothiazine derivatives. *JAMA, J. Am. Med. Assoc.* **182,** 848–850.

Asanuma, N. (1973). Experimental studies on organophosphorus pesticide residues in living organisms. Part 2. *J. Jpn. Assoc. Rural Med.* **22,** 282–283 (in Japanese).

Asanuma, N., Suzuki, A., and Kurosawa, K. (1976). Experimental studies on organophosphorus pesticide residues in living bodies. Part 2. Report of Studies Commissioned by Ministry of Health and Welfare. *Jpn. Soc. Rural Med.* **1–2,** 60–66 (in Japanese).

Asanuma, S., Nakamura, T., Suzuki, A., Hirooka, Y., Kurosawa, K., and Matsushima, S. (1974). An experimental study on the organophosphorus pesticide residues in humans. *Jpn. J. Ind. Health* **16,** 36–37 (in Japanese).

Ashwood-Smith, M. J., Trevino, J., and Ring, R. (1972). Mutagenicity of dichlorvos. *Nature (London)* **240,** 418–420.

Augustinsson, K. (1955). The normal variation of human blood cholinesterase activity. *Acta Physiol. Scand.* **35,** 40–52.

Augustinsson, K., Eriksson, H., and Faijersson, Y. (1978). A new approach to determining cholinesterase activities in samples of whole blood. *Clin. Chim. Acta* **89,** 239–252.

Austin, L., and James, K. A. C. (1970). Rates of regeneration of acetylcholinesterase in rat brain subcellular fractions following DFP inhibition. *J. Neurochem.* **17,** 705–707.

Avrahami, M., and Gernert, I. L. (1973). Distribution, metabolism, and excretion of ^{32}P-labelled fensulfothion in sheep. *N. Z. J. Exp. Agric.* **1,** 197–202.

Avrahami, M., and White, D. A. (1975). Residues in milk of cows after spot treatment with ^{32}P-fenthion. *N. Z. J. Exp. Agric.* **3,** 309–311.

Awad, O., and Karczmar, A. G. (1960). Anticholinesterase actions of thiophosphate compounds (EPN and malathion). *Fed. Proc., Fed. Am. Soc. Exp. Biol.* **19,** 276.

Axelsson, U. (1969). Glaucoma, miotic therapy, and cataract. *Acta Ophthalmol., Suppl.* **102,** 1–37.

Axelsson, U., and Nyman, K. G. (1970). Side effects from use of long-acting cholinesterase inhibitors in young persons. *Acta Ophthalmol.* **48,** 396–400.

Babchina, I. P. (1972). Nervous system damage in trichlorfon poisoning. *Vrach. Delo* **2,** 137–139 (in Russian).

Baetjer, A. M. (1973). Dehydration and susceptibility to toxic chemicals. *Arch. Environ. Health* **26,** 61–63.

Baker, E. L., Jr., Zack, M., Miles, J. M., Alderman, L., Warren, M., Dobbin, R. D., Miller, S., and Teeters, W. R. (1978). Epidemic malathion poisoning in Pakistan malaria workers. *Lancet* **1,** 31–34.

Bakhodirov, B. U. (1970). A case of very severe mercaptophos poisoning. *Zdravookhr. Tadzh.* **17,** 47 (in Russian).

Bakke, J. E., Feil, V. J., and Price, C. E. (1976). Rat urinary metabolites from *O,O*-diethyl-*O*-(3,5,6-trichloro-2-pyridyl) phosphorothioate. *J. Environ. Sci. Health, Part B* **11,** 225–230.

Baksi, S. N. (1978). Effect of dichlorvos on embryonal and fetal development on thyro-parathyroidectomized, thyroxine-treated and euthyroid rats. *Toxicol. Lett.* **2,** 213–216.

Balani, S. G., Fernandes, S. O., Lakhani, R. H., and Juthani, V. J. (1968). Diazinon poisoning: A report on 100 cases with particular reference to evaluation of treatment. *J. Assoc. Physicians India* **16,** 911–917.

Balogh, S., Egeto, S., Horvath, Z., Papp, K., Razsa, J., and Szabo, J. (1972). Diagnostic and therapeutic data on accidental and experimental Ekatin poisoning. *Magy. Allatorv. Lapja* **27,** 239–240 (in Hungarian).

Balthrop, J. E. (1966). Ronnel in creeping eruption. *J. Fla. Med. Assoc.* **53,** 820–821.

Banerjee, D. (1967). Pericarditis in acute Diazinon poisoning. A case report. *Armed Forces Med. J. India* **23,** 187–190.

Barabach, V. I. (1971). Neuropsychiatric disorders in chlorphos (trichlorfon) poisoning. *Zh. Nevropatol. Psikhiatr. im. S. S. Korsakova* **71,** 594–598 (in Russian).

Barckow, D., Neuhaus, G., and Erdmann, W. D. (1969). The treatment of parathion (E 605) poisoning with the cholinesterase-reactivating substance obidoxime (Toxogonin). *Arch. Toxikol.* **24,** 133–146.

Barkov, A. M., and Glukhovets, B. I. (1971). A case of acute chlorphos poisoning with fatal outcome. *Ter. Arkh.* **43,** 118–119.

Barna, J., and Simon, G. (1974). Effect of small oral doses of Birlane (chlorfenvinphos) on intestinal resorption. *Kiserl. Orvostud.* **26,** 605–609.

Barnard, E. A., Budd, G. C., and Ostrowski, K. (1970). Autoradiographic methods in enzyme cytochemistry. IV. The cellular and ultrastructural localisation of organophosphate-sensitive esterases in mouse liver and kidney. *Exp. Cell Res.* **60,** 405–418.

Barnes, J. M. (1953). The reactions of rabbits to poisoning by *p*-nitrophenyldiethylphosphate (E600). *Br. J. Pharmacol. Chemother.* **8,** 208–211.

Barnes, J. M., and Davies, D. R. (1951). Blood cholinesterase levels in workers exposed to organo-phosphorus insecticides. *Br. Med. J.* **2,** 1–9.

Barnes, J. M., and Denz, F. A. (1951). The chronic toxicity of *p*-nitrophenyl diethyl thiophosphate (E605). *J. Hyg.* **49,** 430–441.

Barnes, J. M., and Denz, F. A. (1953). Experimental demyelination with organophosphorus compounds. *J. Pathol. Bacteriol.* **65,** 597–605.

Barnes, J. M., and Denz, F. A. (1954). The reaction of rats to diets containing octamethyl pyrophosphoramide (schradan) and *O,O*-diethyl-*S*-ethylmercaptoethanol thiophosphate ("Systox"). *Br. J. Ind. Med.* **11,** 11–19.

Barnes, W. W., Eldridge, B. F., Greenberg, J. H., and Vinona, S. (1962). A field evaluation of malathion dust for the control of body lice. *J. Econ. Entomol.* **55,** 391–394.

Baron, R. L., and Casida, J. E. (1962). Enzymatic and antidotal studies on the neurotoxic effect of certain organophosphates. *Biochem. Pharmacol.* **11,** 1129–1136.

Baron, R. L., and Johnson, H. (1964). Neurological disruption produced in hens by two organophosphorus esters. *Br. J. Pharmacol. Chemother.* **23,** 295–304.

Barquet, A., Davies, J. E., and Davis, J. H. (1968). Death due to parathion? Exhumation of an embalmed body. *Clin. Toxicol.* **1,** 257–263.

Barr, A. M. (1964). Poisoning by anticholinesterase organic phosphates: Its significance in anaesthesia. *Med. J. Aust.* **1,** 792–796.

Barr, A. M. (1966). Further experience in the treatment of organic phosphate poisoning. *Med. J. Aust.* **1,** 490–492.

Barrows, C. H., Jr., Shock, N. W., and Chow, B. F. (1958). Age differences in cholinesterase activity of serum and liver. *J. Gerontol.* **13,** 20–23.

Barsegyan, R. G. (1967). Adaptive changes in the activity of some enzymes in the blood of healthy nursing children. *Zh. Eksp. Klin. Med.* **7,** 66–68.

Bartels, E., and Nachmansohn, D. (1969). Organophosphate inhibitors of acetylcholine-receptor and -esterase tested on the electroplax. *Arch. Biochem. Biophys.* **133,** 1–10.

Bass, S. W., Triolo, A. J., and Coon, J. M. (1972). Effect of DDT on the toxicity and metabolism of parathion in mice. *Toxicol. Appl. Pharmacol.* **22,** 684–693.

Beat, V. B., and Morgan, D. P. (1977). Evaluation of hazards involved in treating cattle with pour-on organophosphate insecticides. *J. Am. Vet. Med. Assoc.* **170,** 812–814.

Bedford, C. T., and Robinson, J. (1972). The alkylating properties of organophosphates. *Xenobiotica* **2,** 307–337.

Beheyti, P., Lebrun, A., Cerf, J., Dierickx, J., and Degroote, V. (1961). Study of the toxicity for man of an organophosphorus insecticide. *Bull. W.H.O.* **24,** 465–473 (in French).

Belenkii, V. M., and Landesman, L. M. (1970). Severe chlorophos poisoning. *Ter. Arkh.* **42,** 99–100 (in Russian).

Bell, A., Barnes, R., and Simpson, G. R. (1968). Cases of absorption and poisoning by the pesticide "Phosdrin." *Med. J. Aust.* **1,** 178–180.

Bello, T. R., Amborski, G. F., and Torbert, B. J. (1974). Effects of organic phosphorus anthelmintics on blood cholinesterase values in horses and ponies. *Am. J. Vet. Res.* **35,** 73–78.

Belyayev, V. I. (1969). Toxicological study of trichlorometaphos-3, trichlorfon, and Trolene in animals. *Veterinariya (Moscow)* **46,** 58–60 (in Russian).

Benes, V., Sram, R. J., and Tuscany, R. (1975). Fenitrothion. I. Study of mutagenic activity in rats. *J. Hyg., Epidemiol., Microbiol., Immunol.* **19,** 163–172.

Benjamini, E., Metcalf, R. L., and Fukuto, T. R. (1959). The chemistry and mode of action of the insecticide *O,O*-diethyl *O*-*p*-methylsulfinyl phenyl phosphorothionate and its analogues. *J. Econ. Entomol.* **52,** 94–98.

Benke, G. M., and Murphy, S. D. (1975). The influence of age on the toxicity and metabolism of methyl parathion and parathion in male and female rats. *Toxicol. Appl. Pharmacol.* **31,** 254–269.

Bennett, B. G., and Best, J. (1962). Successful use of an antidote in phosphorus insecticide poisoning. *Med. J. Aust.* **2,** 150.

Benson, W. W., Marr, T. A., and Bagica, J. (1970). An apparent case of pesticide poisoning. *Public Health Rep.* **85,** 600–602.

Berends, F., Posthumus, C. H., Sluys, I. V. D., and Deierkauf, F. A. (1959). The chemical basis of the "aging process" of DFP-inhibited pseudocholinesterase. *Biochim. Biophys. Acta* **34,** 576–578.

Bermejillo, M. (1971). Occupational poisoning by tri-*ortho*-cresylphosphate. *Med. Segur. Trab.* **19,** 49–58.

Berteau, P. E., and Deen, W. A. (1978). A comparison of oral and inhalation toxicities of four pesticides to mice and rats. *Bull. Environ. Contam. Toxicol.* **19,** 113–120.

Bertoncin, D., Russolo, A., Caroldi, S., and Lotti, M. (1985). Neuropathy target esterase in human lymphocytes. *Arch. Environ. Health* **40,** 139–144.

Bhagwat, V. M., and Ramachandran, B. V. (1975). Malathion A and B esterases of mouse liver. I. Separation and properties. *Biochem. Pharmacol.* **24,** 1713–1717.

Bianchi, P. (1966). Acute pericarditis from parathion (a case report). *Arch. Med. Intern.* **18,** 25–30.

Bidstrup, P. L., and Hunter, D. (1952). Toxic chemicals in agriculture. *Br. Med. J.* **1,** 277.

Bidstrup, P. L., Bonnell, J. A., and Beckett, A. G. (1953). Paralysis following poisoning by a new organic phosphorus insecticide (mipafox). *Br. Med. J.* **1,** 1068–1072.

Biernat, S., and Giermaziak, H. (1974). Pathomorphological lesions of the myocardium and endocardium in rabbits following acute intoxication with intrathion and the action of various detoxifying agents. *Patol. Pol.* **25,** 59–66 (in Polish).

Biernat, S., and Giermaziak, H. (1976). Pathomorphological changes in rat heart after administration of intrathion in toxic doses and after large doses of PAM. *Med. Pr.* **27,** 241–251 (in Polish).

Bignami, G., and Gatti, G. L. (1967). Neurotoxicity of anticholinesterase agents. Antagonistic action of various centrally acting drugs. *Proc. Eur. Soc. Study Drug Toxic.* **8,** 93–106.

Bisby, S. A., and Simpson, G. R. (1975). An unusual presentation of systemic phosphate poisoning. *Med. J. Aust.* **2,** 394–395.

Blaber, L. C., and Creasey, N. H. (1960a). The mode of recovery of cholinesterase activity *in vivo* after organophosphorus poisoning. I. Erythrocyte cholinesterase. *Biochem. J.* **77,** 591–596.

Blaber, L. C., and Creasey, N. H. (1960b). The mode of recovery of cholinesterase activity *in vivo* after organophosphorus poisoning. 2. Brain cholinesterase. *Biochem. J.* **77,** 597–604.

Blair, D., Hoadley, E. C., and Hutson, D. H. (1975). The distribution of dichlorvos in the tissues of mammals after its inhalation or intravenous administration. *Toxicol. Appl. Pharmacol.* **31,** 243–253.

Blair, D., Dix, K. M., Hunt, P. F., Thorpe, E., Stevenson, D. E., and Walker, A. I. T. (1976). Dichlorvos—a 2-year inhalation carcinogenesis study in rats. *Arch. Toxicol.* **35,** 281–294.

Blakey, D. L., Ochs, M. O., Rye, W., Philp, J. R., Redmond, R. B., and Townsend, W. (1977). Insecticide-associated illness—Mississippi, California. *Morbid. Mortal. Wkly. Rep.* **26,** 37–38.

Blesdoe, F. H., and Seymour, E. Q. (1972). Acute pulmonary oedema associated with parathion poisoning. *Radiology* **103,** 53–56.

Blinn, R. C. (1969). Metabolic fate of Abate insecticide in the rat. *J. Agric. Food Chem.* **17,** 118–122.

Bloch, H. (1941). The action of Coramine on the failing rabbit heart. *Helv. Med. Acta* **7,** 51–57 (in German).

Bockel, P. (1957). Poisonings with a phosphoric acid ester formulation of the Diazinon group. *Dtsch. Med. Wochenschr.* **82,** 1230–1231 (in German).

Boelcke, G., and Erdmann, W. D. (1969). The effect of E-605 poisoning and specific antidote therapy on the liver function of rabbits *Naunyn-Schmiedebergs Arch. Pharmakol.* **263,** 198–199.

Boelcke, G., and Gaaz, J. W. (1970). The question of the hepatic toxicity of nitrostigmine (E 605 forte) and obidoxime (Toxogonin) in dogs. *Arch. Toxikol.* **26,** 93–101.

Boelcke, G., and Kamphenkel, L. (1970). The effect of nitrostigmine poisoning and specific antidotal therapy with obidoxime on the bilirubin clearance and bile flow in rats. *Arch. Toxikol.* **26,** 210–219.

Boelcke, G., Butigan, N., Davar, H., Erdmann, W. D., Gaaz, J. W., and Nenner, M. (1970). Recent experiences in the toxicologically controlled therapy of an unusually severe poisoning with nitrostigmine (E 605 forte). *Dtsch. Med. Wochenschr.* **95,** 2516–2521.

Bonderman, R. P., and Bonderman, D. P. (1971). A titrimetric method for differentiating between atypical and inhibited human serum pseudocholinesterase. A titrimetric method for differentiation. *Arch. Environ. Health* **22,** 578–581.

Bondy, H. F., Field, E. J., Worden, A. N., and Hughes, J. P. W. (1960). A study on the acute toxicity of the tri-aryl phosphates used as plasticizers. *Br. J. Ind. Med.* **17,** 190–200.

Bordiug, O. F. (1968). The blood gases in acute poisonings with barbiturates and organophosphate insecticides. *Vrach. Delo* **11,** 124–125 (in Russian).

Borowitz, S. M. (1988). Prolonged organophosphate toxicity in a twenty-six-month-old child. *J. Pediatr.* **112,** 302–304.

Bossen, F., Karlog, O., and Rasmussen, F. (1973). The cholinesterase activity in red blood cells and blood plasma after oral intake of Atgard vet. R. (dichlorvos) in pigs. *Nord. Veterinaermed.* **25,** 584–587 (in Danish).

Botescu, M., Pastia, Al., and Scripcaru, Gh. (1970). Some aspects of the mechanism of intoxication with parathion: Experimental data. *Rev. Med.-Chir.* **74,** 707–712.

Bouilliat, G., and Duperray, J. N. (1964). Considerations on the blood cholinesterase levels of subjects handling organophosphorus insecticides. I. Practical methods of measurement. *Arch. Mal. Prof. Med. Trav. Secur. Soc.* **25,** 589–595.

Bouldin, T. W., and Cavanagh, J. B. (1979a). Organophosphorus neuropathy. I. A teased-fiber study of the spatio-temporal spread of axonal degeneration. *Am. J. Pathol.* **94,** 241–252.

Bouldin, T. W., and Cavanagh, J. B. (1979b). Organophosphorus neuropathy. II. A fine-structural study of the early stages of axonal degeneration. *Am. J. Pathol.* **94,** 253–270.

Bourke, J. B., Broderick, E. J., Hackler, L. R., and Lippold, P. C. (1968). Comparative metabolism of carbon-labeled malathion in plants and animals. *J. Agric. Food Chem.* **16,** 585–589.

Bourne, J. G., Collier, H. O. J., and Somers, G. F. (1952). Succinylcholine (succinoylcholine). Muscle relaxant of short action. *Lancet* **1,** 1225–1229.

Bourne, J. R., and Arthur, B. W. (1967). Diazinon residues in the milk of dairy cows. *J. Econ. Entomol.* **60,** 402–405.

Bowman, J. S., and Casida, J. E. (1957). Metabolism of the systemic insecticide *O,O*-diethyl-*S*-ethylthiomethyl phosphorodithioate (Thimet) in plants. *J. Agric. Food Chem.* **5,** 192–197.

Bowman, J. S., and Casida, J. E. (1958). Further studies on the metabolism of Thimet by plants, insects, and mammals. *J. Econ. Entomol.* **51,** 838–843.

Boyd, E. M., and Krupa, V. (1969). The acute oral toxicity of demeton in albino rats fed from weaning on diets of varying protein content. *Can. J. Pharm. Sci.* **4,** 35–40.

Boyd, E. M., and Muis, L. F. (1970). Acute oral toxicity of dimethoate in albino rats fed a protein-deficient diet. *J. Pharm. Sci.* **59,** 1098–1102.

Boyd, E. M., and Tanikella, T. K. (1969). The acute oral toxicity of malathion in relation to dietary protein. *Arch Toxikol.* **24,** 292–303.

Boyd, E. M., Chen, C. P., and Liu, S. J. (1969). The acute oral toxicity of parathion in relation to dietary protein. *Arch. Toxikol.* **25,** 238–253.

Boyd, E. M., Krijinen, C. J., and Tanikella, T. K. (1970). The influence of a wide range of dietary protein concentration on the acute oral toxicity of malathion. *Arch. Toxikol.* **26,** 125–132.

Brachfeld, J., and Zavon, M. R. (1965). Organic phosphate (Phosdrin) intoxication. Report of a case and the results of treatment with 2-PAM. *Arch. Environ. Health* **11,** 859–862.

Bradway, D. E., and Shafik, T. M. (1977). Malathion exposure studies. Determination of mono- and dicarboxylic acids and alkyl phosphates in urine. *J. Agric. Food Chem.* **25,** 1342–1344.

Bradway, D. E., Shafik, T. M., and Lores, E. M. (1977). Comparison of cholinesterase activity, residue levels, and urinary metabolite excretion of rats exposed to organophosphorus pesticides. *J. Agric. Food Chem.* **25,** 1353–1358.

Brady, U. E., and Arthur, B. W. (1961). Metabolism of *O,O*-dimethyl-*O*-[4-(methylthio)*m*-tolyl] phosphorothioate by white rats. *J. Econ. Entomol.* **54,** 1232–1236.

Braid, P. E., and Nix, M. (1969). The kinetic constants for the inhibition of acetylcholinesterase by Phosdrin, Sumioxon, DDVP and phosphamidon. *Can. J. Biochem.* **47,** 1–6.

Braito, E. (1959). Case reports on poisonings by phosphoric acid esters. *Riv. Infort. Mal. Prof.* **46,** 1232–1239 (in Portuguese).

Brglez, J., and Skubic, T. (1971). Contribution to knowledge of the activity of dichlorvos anthelmintics ("Atgard," "Equigard," and "Task"). *Vet. Glas.* **25,** 351–360.

Briggs, C. J., and Simons, K. J. (1986). Recent advances in the mechanism and treatment of organophosphorus poisoning. *Pharm. Int.* **7,** 155–159.

Bris, E. J., Dyer, I. A., Howes, A. D., Schooley, M. A., and Todd, A. (1968). Anthelmintic activity of 2,2-dichlorovinyl dimethyl phosphate in cattle. *Vet. Med. Assoc. J.* **152,** 175–181.

Brodeur, J. (1967). Studies on the mechanism of phenobarbital-induced protection against malathion and EPN. *Can. J. Physiol. Pharmacol.* **45,** 1061–1069.

Brodeur, J., and DuBois, K. P. (1963). Comparison of acute toxicity of anticholinesterase insecticides to weanling and adult male rats. *Proc. Soc. Exp. Biol. Med.* **114,** 509–511.

Brodeur, J., and DuBois, K. P. (1964). Ali-esterase activity and sex difference in malathion activity. *Fed. Proc., Fed. Am. Soc. Exp. Biol.* **23,** 200.

Brown, D. R., and Murphy, S. D. (1971). Factors influencing dimethoate and triethyl phosphate-induced narcosis in rats and mice. *Toxicol. Appl. Pharmacol.* **18,** 895–906.

Brown, H. R., and Sharma, R. P. (1975). Inhibition of neural membrane adenosinetriphosphatases by organophosphates. *Toxicol. Appl. Pharmacol.* **33,** 140.

Bruaux, P. (1957). Toxicity of two organophosphorus insecticides (Diazinon and malathion) among workers using these insecticides. *Ann. Soc. Belg. Med. Trop.* **37,** 789–799 (in French).

Bruce, R. B., Howard, J. W., and Elsea, J. R. (1955). Toxicity of *O,O*-diethyl *O*-(2-isopropyl-6-methyl-4-pyrimidyl)phosphorothioate (Diazinon). *J. Agric. Food Chem.* **3**(12), 1017–1021.

Bruener, H., Gandawidjaja, L., Hettwer, H., and Oldiges, H. (1977). Possibilities of a combination antidote therapy in rats poisoned by phosphoric acid esters. *Arzneim.-Forsch.* **27,** 1983–1988 (in German).

Brzezicka-Bak, M., and Bojanowska, A. (1969). The subacute toxicity of the organophosphorus insecticides: Naled, ethoate-methyl and Supracide. *Rocz. Panstw. Zakl. Hig.* **20,** 463–469 (in Polish).

Brzezinski, J. (1969). Catecholamines in urine of rats intoxicated with phosphorganic insecticides. *Diss. Pharm. Pharmacol.* **21**, 381–385.

Buchthal, F., and Engbaek, L. (1948). On the neuromuscular transmission in normal and myasthenic subjects. *Acta Psychiatr. Neurol.* **23**, 3–11.

Budreau, C. H., and Singh, R. P. (1973a). Teratogenicity and embryotoxicity of demeton and fenthion in CF-1 mouse embryos. *Toxicol. Appl. Pharmacol.* **24**, 324–332.

Budreau, C. H., and Singh, R. P. (1973b). Effect of fenthion and dimethoate on reproduction in the mouse. *Toxicol. Appl. Pharmacol.* **26**, 29–38.

Budreau, C. H., and Singh, R. P. (1973c). Transplacental passage of demeton in CF-1 mice. *Arch. Environ. Health* **26**, 161–163.

Bull, D. L. (1968). Metabolism of O,O-dimethyl phosphorodithioate S-ester with 4-(mercaptomethyl)-2-methyl-Δ^2-1,3,4-thiadazolin-5-one (Geigy GS-13005) in plants and animals. *J. Agric. Food Chem.* **16**, 610–616.

Bull, D. L., and Lindquist, D. A. (1964). Metabolism of 3-hydroxy-N,N-dimethyl-crotonamide dimethyl phosphate by cotton plants, insects, and rats. *J. Agric. Food Chem.* **12**, 310–317.

Bull, D. L., and Lindquist, D. A. (1966). Metabolism of 3-hydroxy-N-methyl-cis-crotonamide dimethyl phosphate (Azodrin) by insects and rats. *J. Agric. Food Chem.* **14**, 105–109.

Burgen, A. S. V., Keele, C. A., and McAlpine, D. (1948). Tetraethylpyrophosphate in myasthenia gravis. *Lancet* **254**, 519–521.

Burnstein, S., and Sampson, J. (1955). Severe hypotensive reaction to oral chlorpromazine therapy. *J. Calif. Med.* **82**, 45–47.

Bus, J. S., and Gibson, J. E. (1974). Bidrin: Perinatal toxicity and effect on the development of brain acetyltransferase in mice. *Food Cosmet. Toxicol.* **12**, 313–322.

Buselmaier, W., Roerhrborn, G., and Propping, P. (1973). Comparative investigations on the mutagenicity of pesticides in mammalian test systems. *Mutat. Res.* **21**, 25–26.

Butt, H. R., Comfort, M. W., Dry, T. J., and Osterberg, H. E. (1942). Values for acetylcholine esterase in blood serum of normal persons and patients with various diseases. *J. Lab. Clin. Med.* **27**, 649–655.

Bwibo, N. O. (1971). Accidental poisoning with Diazinone—an organophosphorus insecticide. *East Afr. Med. J.* **48**, 601–605.

Bychkovskiy, V. N., and Pisarchik, K. I. (1972). Clinical course and treatment of organophosphorus poisoning (carbophos) in children. *Vopr. Okhr. Materin. Det.* **17**, 63–67 (in Russian).

Byeon, W., Hyun, H. H., and Lee, S. Y. (1976). Mutagenicity of pesticides in the *Salmonella* microsomal enzyme activation system. *Korean J. Microbiol.* **14**, 128–134.

Cabejszek, I., Rybak, M., and Szulinski, S. (1967). Effects of thiometon (S-(2-(ethylthio)ethyl) O,O-diethyl phosphorodithioate) in drinking water on warm-blooded animals. *Rocz. Panstw. Zakl. Hig.* **18**, 257–266 (in Polish).

Callaway, S., and Davies, D. R. (1957). The association of blood cholinesterase levels with the susceptibility of animals to sarin and ethyl pyrophosphate poisoning. *Br. J. Pharmacol. Chemother.* **12**, 382–387.

Callaway, S., Davies, D. R., and Rutland, J. P. (1951). Blood cholinesterase levels and range of personal variation in a healthy adult population. *Br. Med. J.* **2**, 812–816.

Camargo, L. A. A., Saad, W. A., and Larini, L. (1970a). Acute toxicity of fenitrothion (= Sumithion, Folithion). *Arq. Inst. Biol., Sao Paulo* **35**, 219–222.

Camargo, L. A. A., Saad, W. A., and Larini, L. (1970b). Acute toxicity of O,O dimethyl-O-(3-methyl-4-nitrophenyl) phosphorothioate. Determination of the oral LD50 in the rat. *Rev. Fac. Farm. Odontol. Araraquara* **4**, 53–60.

Camp, H. B., Fukuto, T. R., and Metcalf, R. L. (1969). Selective toxicity of isopropyl parathion—metabolism in the housefly, honey bee, and white mouse. *J. Agric. Food Chem.* **17**, 249–254.

Casale, G. P., Cohen, S. D., and DiCapua, R. A. (1984). Parathion-induced suppression of humoral immunity in inbred mice. *Toxicol. Lett.* **23**, 239–247.

Casida, J. E. (1955). Isomeric substituted-vinyl phosphates as systemic insecticides. *Science* **122**, 597–598.

Casida, J. E. (1961). Specificity of substituted phenyl phosphorus compounds for esterase inhibition in mice. *Biochem. Pharmacol.* **5**, 332–342.

Casida, J. E., and Sanderson, D. M. (1961). Toxic hazard from formulating the insecticide dimethoate in methyl "Cellosolve." *Nature (London)* **189**, 507–508.

Casida, J. E., and Sanderson, D. M. (1963). Solvent effects on toxicity: Reaction of certain phosphorothionate insecticides with alcohols and potentiation by breakdown products. *J. Agric. Food Chem.* **11**, 91–96.

Casida, J. E., and Stahmann, M. A. (1953). Metabolism and mode of action of schradan. *J. Agric. Food Chem.* **1**, 883–888.

Casida, J. E., Allen, T. C., and Stahmann, M. A. (1952). Reaction of certain octamethylpyrophosphoramide derivatives with chymotrypsin. *J. Am. Chem. Soc.* **74**, 5548.

Casida, J. E., Eto, M., and Baron, R. L. (1961). Biological activity of a tri-o-cresyl phosphate metabolite. *Nature (London)* **191**, 1396–1397.

Casida, J. E., McBride, L., and Niedermeier, R. P. (1962). Metabolism of 2,2-dichlorovinyl dimethylphosphate in relation to residues in milk and mammalian tissues. *J. Agric. Food Chem.* **10**, 370–377.

Casida, J. E., Baron, R. L., Eto, M., and Engel, J. L. (1963). Potentiation and neurotoxicity induced by certain organophosphates. *Biochem. Pharmacol.* **12**, 72–83.

Castedo, C., and Bruno, O. (1966). Clinical picture and neurotoxicity of parathion poisoning. *Prensa Med. Argent.* **53**, 1532–1535.

Casterline, J. L., Jr., and Williams, C. H. (1969). The effect of pesticide administration on serum and tissue esterases of rats fed diets of varying casein, calcium, and magnesium content. *Toxicol. Appl. Pharmacol.* **15**, 532–539.

Casterline, J. L., Jr., and Williams, C. H. (1971). The effect of 28-day pesticide feeding on serum and tissue enzyme activities of rats fed diets of varying casein content. *Toxicol. Appl. Pharmacol.* **18**, 607–618.

Casterline, J. L., Jr., Williams, C. H., and Keys, J. E. (1969). Effect of pesticide administration upon esterase activities in serum and tissues of rats fed variable casein diets. *Toxicol. Appl. Pharmacol.* **14**, 266–275.

Casterline, J. L., Jr., Brodie, R. E., and Sobotka, T. (1971). Effect of Banol and parathion on operant learning behavior of rats fed adequate and inadequate casein diets. *Bull. Environ. Contam. Toxicol.* **6**, 297–393.

Cavagna, G., Locati, G., and Vigliani, E. C. (1969). Clinical effects of exposure to DDVP (Vapona) insecticide in hospital wards. *Arch. Environ. Health* **19**, 112–123.

Cavagna, G., Locati, G., and Vigliani, E. C. (1970). Exposure of newborn babies to Vapona insecticide. *Eur. J. Toxicol.* **3**, 49–57.

Cavanagh, J. B. (1954). The toxic effects of tri-*ortho*-cresyl phosphate on the nervous system. *J. Neurol., Neurosurg. Psychiatry* **17**, 163–172.

Cavanagh, J. B. (1964). The significance of the "dying back" process in experimental and human neurological disease. *Int. Rev. Pathol.* **3**, 219–267.

Cavanagh, J. B. (1973). Peripheral neuropathy caused by chemical agents. *CRC Crit. Rev. Toxicol.* **2**, 365–417.

Cecconello, D. (1968). Acute poisoning from organo-phosphoric esters. *Minerva Anestesiol.* **34**, 1258–1260.

Célice, J., Fournel, J., Hillion, P., Barthelme, P., and Roger, S. (1961). Treatment of human intoxications by organophosphorus compounds by classical methods plus pralidoxime methylsulfate (7676 RP). *Arch. Mal. Prof. Med. Trav. Secur. Soc.* **22**, 108–119 (in French).

Cerf, J., Lebrun, A. S., and Dierichx, J. (1962). A new approach to helminthiasis controls: The use of an organophosphorus compound. *Am. J. Trop. Med. Hyg.* **11**, 514–517.

Cervoni, W. A., Gonzalez, J. O., Kaye, S., and Slomka, M. B. (1968). Evaluation of dichlorvos as single dose gastrointestinal anthelmintic therapy for man—a preliminary report. *Pharmacologist* **10**, 171.

Cervoni, W. A., Oliver-Gonzalea, J., Kaye, S., and Slomka, M. B. (1969). Dichlorvos as a single-dose intestinal anthelmintic therapy for man. *Am. J. Trop. Med. Hyg.* **18**, 912–919.

Chadli, A., Kchouk, M., and Dvoracek, G. (1970). Morphological study of parathion intoxication. *Arch. Inst. Pasteur Tunis* **47**, 89–102 (in French).

Chakraborty, D., Bhattacharyya, A., Majumdar, K., Chatterjee, K., Chatterjee, S., Sen, A., and Chatterjee, G. C. (1978). Studies on L-ascorbic acid metabolism in rats under chronic toxicity due to organophosphorus insecticides: Effects of supplementation of L-ascorbic acid in high doses. *J. Nutr.* **108**, 973–980.

Chamberlain, W. F., Gatterdam, P. E., and Hopkins, D. E. (1960). Metabolism of P32-Delnav in cattle. *J. Econ. Entomol.* **53**, 642–675.

Chamberlin, H. R., and Cooke, R. E. (1953). Organic phosphate insecticide poisoning. *Am. J. Dis. Child.* **85**, 164–172.

Chapman, S. K., and Leibman, K. C. (1971). The effects of chlordane, DDT, and 3-methylcholanthrene upon the metabolism and toxicity of diethyl-4-nitrophenyl phosphorothionate (parathion). *Toxicol. Appl. Pharmacol.* **18**, 977–987.

Charles, J. M., and Farmer, J. (1979). Disposition of an oral dose of *O*-ethyl-*O*-*p*-nitrophenyl phenylphosphonothioate (EPN) in the rat. *Toxicol. Appl. Pharmacol.* **48**, A38.

Chattopadhyay, D. P., Dighe, S. K., Nashikkar, A. B., and Dube, D. K. (1986). Species differences in the *in vitro* inhibition of brain acetylcholinesterase and carboxylesterase by mipafox, paraoxon and soman. *Pestic. Biochem. Physiol.* **26**, 202–208.

Chen, T. S., Kinoshita, F. K., and DuBois, K. P. (1972). Acute toxicity and antiesterase action of *O*-ethyl-*S*-*S*-diphenyl phosphorodithioate (Hinosan). *Toxicol. Appl. Pharmacol.* **23**, 519–527.

Cheng, K. K. (1951). A technique for total hepatectomy in the rat and its effect on toxicity of octamethyl pyrophosphoramide. *Br. J. Exp. Pathol.* **32**, 444–447.

Chhabra, M. L., Sepaha, G. C., Jain, S. R., Bhagwat, R. R., and Khandekar, J. D. (1970). E.C.G. and necropsy changes in organophosphorus compound (malathion) poisoning. *Indian J. Med. Sci.* **24**, 424–429.

Chiantera, A., Brienza, A., and DeBlasi, S. (1968). Serum cholinesterase behavior in relation to oxime treatment in a cause of acute Rogor intoxication. *Rass. Int. Clin. Ter.* **48**, 843–850 (in Italian).

Christensen, C. B. (1959). Parathion poisoning. *Ugeskr. Laeg.* **121**, 2028–2030.

CIBA (1967). "Dimecron." CIBA Agrochemical Division, Basel, Switzerland.

Cichecki, Z. (1971). Hallucinosis following intoxication with phoschlorine R-20. *Psychiatr. Pol.* **5**, 607–609 (in Polish).

Claborn, H. V., Mann, H. D., Younger, R. L., and Radeleff, R. D. (1963). Diazinon residues in the fat of sprayed cattle. *J. Econ. Entomol.* **56**, 858–859.

Clark, D. E., Younger, R. L., and Ayala, C. H. (1966). Toxicosis and residues in bromophos-dipped sheep. *J. Agric. Food Chem.* **14**, 608–609.

Clement, J. G. (1979). Efficacy of pro-PAM (*N*-methyl-1,6-dihydropyridine-2-carbaldoxime hydrochloride) as a prophylaxis against organophosphate poisoning. *Toxicol. Appl. Pharmacol.* **47**, 305–311.

Clemons, G. P., and Menzer, R. E. (1968). Oxidative metabolism of phosphamidon in rats and a goat. *J. Agric. Food Chem.* **16**, 312–318.

Cleveland, J. P., and Treon, J. F. (1961). Response of experimental animals to Phosdrin insecticide in their daily diets. *J. Agric. Food Chem.* **9**, 484–488.

Clothier, B., and Johnson, M. K. (1979). Rapid aging of neurotoxic esterase after inhibition by di-isopropyl phosphorofluoridate. *Biochem. J.* **177**, 549–558.

Cohen, S. D. (1984). Mechanisms of toxicological interactions involving organophosphate insecticides. *Fundam. Appl. Toxicol.* **4**, 315–324.

Cohen, S. D., and Murphy, S. D. (1971a). Malathion potentiation and inhibition of hydrolysis of various carboxylic esters by tri-orthotolyl phosphate (TOTP) in mice. *Biochem. Pharmacol.* **20**, 575–587.

Cohen, S. D., and Murphy, S. D. (1971b). Carboxylesterase inhibition as an indicator of malathion potentiation in mice. *J. Pharmacol. Exp. Ther.* **176**, 733–742.

Cohen, S. D., Callaghan, J. E., and Murphy, S. D. (1972). Investigation of multiple mechanisms for potentiation of malaoxon (MX) by triorthotolyl phosphate. *Toxicol. Appl. Pharmacol.* **22**, 300.

Cole, M. M., Clark, P. H., and Weidhass, D. E. (1958). Sleeve tests with malathion powders against DDT-resistant body lice. *J. Econ. Entomol.* **51**, 741–742.

Colinese, D. L., and Terry, H. J. (1968). Phosalone—a wide spectrum organophosphorus insecticide. *Chem. Ind. (London)* **44**, 1507–1511.

Collins, J. A., Schooley, M. A., and Singh, V. K. (1971). The effect of dietary dichlorvos on swine reproduction and viability of their offspring. *Toxicol. Appl. Pharmacol.* **19**, 377.

Comer, S. W., Ruark, H. E., and Robbins, A. L. (1976). Stability of parathion metabolites in urine samples collected from poisoned individuals. *Bull. Environ. Contam. Toxicol.* **16**, 618–625.

Comroe, J. H., Jr., Todd, J., Gammon, G. D., Leopold, I. H., Koelle, G. B., Bodansky, O., and Gilman, A. (1946a). The effect of di-isopropyl fluorophosphate (DFP) upon patients with myasthenia gravis. *Am. J. Med. Sci.* **212**, 641–651.

Comroe, J. H., Jr., Todd, J., and Koelle, G. B. (1946b). Pharmacology of di-isopropyl fluorophosphate (DFP) in man. *J. Pharmacol. Exp. Ther.* **87**, 281–290.

Conyers, R. A. J., and Goldsmith, L. E. (1971). A case of organophosphorus-induced psychosis. *Med. J. Aust.* **1**, 27–29.

Cook, J. W., and Yip, G. (1958). Malathionase. II. Identity of a malathion metabolite. *J. Assoc. Off. Agric. Chem.* **41**, 407–411.

Cook, J. W., Blake, J. R., Yip, G., and Williams, M. (1958). Malathionase. I. Activity and inhibition. *J. Assoc. Off. Agric. Chem.* **41**, 399–407.

Cooney, D. P., and Fawley, D. E. (1968). The use of ^{32}di-isopropylfluorophosphate (^{32}DFP) as a platelet label: Evidence of reutilization of this isotope in man. *Blood* **31**, 791–805.

Copcland, F., Cranmer, M., Carroll, J., and Ollner, W. (1971). Fate of 14-C-ring and 14-C-ethyl labeled parathion in the rhesus monkey. *Toxicol. Appl. Pharmacol.* **19**, 400.

Coulombe, P. A., Lortie, S., Cote, M. G., and Chevalier, G. (1986). Pulmonary toxicity of the insecticide fenitrothion in the rat following a single field exposure. *J. Appl. Toxicol.* **6**, 317–323.

Cranmer, J. S., Avery, D. L., Grady, R. R., and Kitay, J. I. (1978). Postnatal endocrine dysfunction resulting from prenatal exposure to carbofuran, Diazinon, or chlordane. *J. Environ. Pathol. Toxicol.* **2**, 357–369.

Crawford, C. R., and Dull, J. (1970). Antagonism of the lethal effects of Dipterex and Guthion with atropine and related drugs. *Fed. Proc., Fed. Am. Soc. Exp. Biol.* **29**, 349.

Croft, P. G., and Richter, D. (1943). Muscular activity and choline esterase. *J. Physiol. (London)* **102**, 155–169.

Cronce, P. C., and Alden, H. S. (1968). Flea-collar dermatitis. *JAMA, J. Am. Med. Assoc.* **206**, 1563–1564.

Crowley, W. J., Jr., and Johns, T. R. (1966). Accidental malathion poisoning. *Arch. Neurol. (Chicago)* **14**, 611–616.

Culvert, D., Caplan, P., and Batchelor, G. S. (1956). Studies on human exposure during aerosol application of malathion and clorthion. *AMA Arch. Ind. Health* **13**, 37–50.

Cupp, C. M., Kleiber, G., Reigart, R., and Sandifer, S. H. (1975). Hypothermia in organophosphate poisoning and response to PAM. *JSC Med. Assoc.* **71**, 166–168.

Dagli, A. J., and Shaikh, W. A. (1983). Pancreatic involvement in malathion-anticholinesterase insecticide intoxication, a study of 75 cases. *Br. J. Clin. Pract.* July/August, pp. 270–272.

Dalvi, R. R., and Howell, C. D. (1978). Interaction of parathion and malathion with hepatic cytochrome P-450 from rats treated with phenobarbital and carbon disulfide. *Drug Chem. Toxicol.* **1**, 191–202.

Danilow, V. B. (1968). Hygienic evaluation of atmospheric air pollution by carbophos used in agriculture in Uzbekistan. *Med. Zh. Uzb.*, pp. 23–26 (in Russian).

Dauterman, W. C. (1971). Biological and nonbiological modifications of organophosphorus compounds. *Bull. W.H.O.* **44**, 133–150.

Dauterman, W. C., Casida, J. E., Knaak, J. B., and Kowalczyk, T. (1959). Bovine metabolism of organophosphorus insecticides. Metabolism and residues associated with oral administration of dimethoate to rats and three lactating cows. *J. Agric. Food Chem.* **7**, 188–193.

Davies, D. R., and Green, A. L. (1956). The kinetics of reactivation, by oximes, of cholinesterase inhibited by organophosphorus compounds. *Biochem. J.* **63**, 529–535.

Davies, D. R., and Holland, P. (1972). Effects of oximes and atropine upon the development of delayed neurotoxic signs in chickens following poisoning by DFP and sarin. *Biochem. Pharmacol.* **21**, 3145–3151.

Davies, D. R., Holland, P., and Rumens, M. J. (1960). The relationship between the chemical structure and neurotoxicity of alkyl organophosphorus compounds. *Br. J. Pharmacol. Chemother.* **15**, 271–278.

Davies, J. E. (1975). "Occupational and Environmental Pesticide Exposure Study in South Florida," Natl. Tech. Inf. Study, PB-243, 826. U.S. Govt. Printing Office, Washington, D.C.

Davies, J. E., Davis, J. H., Frazier, D. E., Mann, J. B., Reich, G. A., and Tocci, P. M. (1967). Disturbances of metabolism in organophosphate poisoning. *Ind. Med. Surg.* **36**, 58–62.

Davies, J. E., Barquet, A., Freed, V. H., Haque, R., Morgade, C., Sonneborn, R. E., and Vaclavek, C. (1975). Human pesticide poisonings by a fat-soluble organophosphate insecticide. *Arch. Environ. Health* **30**, 608–613.

Davies, R. O., Marton, A. V., and Kalow, W. (1960). The action of normal and atypical cholinesterase of human serum upon a series of esters of choline. *Can. J. Biochem. Physiol.* **38**, 545–551.

Davis, F. (1957). Insecticide toxicity. Fatality from ingestion of tetraethylphosphate (TEPP). *Northwest Med.* **56**, 435–437.

Davis, K. K., Yesavage, J. A., and Berger, P. A. (1978). Possible organophosphate-induced parkinsonism. *J. Nerv. Ment. Dis.* **166**, 222–225.

Davison, A. N. (1953). Some observations on the cholinesterases of the central nervous system after the administration of organophosphorus compounds. *Br. J. Pharmacol. Chemother.* **8**, 212–216.

Davison, A. N. (1955a). Return of cholinesterase activity in the rat after inhibition by organophosphorus compounds. 2. A comparative study of true and pseudo cholinesterase. *Biochem. J.* **60**, 339–346.

Davison, A. N. (1955b). The conversion of shradan (OMPA) and parathion into inhibitors of cholinesterase in mammalian liver. *Biochem. J.* **61**, 203–209.

Dean, B. J. (1972a). The mutagenic effects of organophosphorus pesticides on micro-organisms. *Arch. Toxikol.* **30**, 67–74.

Dean, B. J. (1972b). The effect of dichlorvos on cultured human lymphocytes. *Arch. Toxikol.* **30**, 75–85.

Dean, B. J., and Blair, D. (1976). Dominant lethal assay in female mice after oral dosing with dichlorvos or exposure to atmospheres containing dichlorvos. *Mutat. Res.* **40**, 67–72.

Dean, B. J., and Thorpe, E. (1972a). Cytogenetic studies with dichlorvos in mice and Chinese hamsters. *Arch. Toxikol.* **30**, 39–49.

Dean, B. J., and Thorpe, E. (1972b). Studies with dichlorvos vapour in dominant lethal mutation tests on mice. *Arch. Toxikol.* **30**, 51–59.

Dean, B. J., Doak, S. M. A., and Funnell, J. (1972). Genetic studies with dichlorvos in the host-mediated assay and in liquid medium using *Saccharomyces cerevisiae. Arch. Toxikol.* **30**, 61–66.

Dean, G., Coxon, J., and Brereton, D. (1967). Poisoning by an organophosphorus compound: A case report. *S. Afr. Med. J.* **41**, 1017–1019.

DeBaun, J. R., and Menn, J. J. (1975). Sulfoxide reduction in relation to organophosphorus insecticide detoxication. *Science* **191**, 187–188.

Dedek, W., and Schwarz, H. (1969). The behavior of the slightly toxic insecticide P-32-bromophos after cutaneous application to the cow. *Z. Naturforsch., B: Anorg. Chem., Org. Chem., Biochem., Biophys., Biol.* **24**, 744–747 (in German).

Dedek, W., and Schwarz, H. (1970a). Formation of residues of ^{32}P-labeled dimethoate after back-washing of cattle. *Monatsh. Veterinaermed.* **25**, 963–964 (in German).

Dedek, W., and Schwarz, H. (1970b). Studies of the percutaneous resorption of 32-*P*-trichlorfon and 32-*P*-dimethoate in sheep. *Z. Naturforsch., B: Anorg. Chem., Org. Chem., Biochem., Biophys., Biol.* **25**, 1193–1194 (in German).

Dedek, W., Scheufler, H., and Fisher, G. W. (1975). On the mutagenicity of desmethyl trichlorphon in the dominant lethal test in the house mouse. *Arch. Toxikol.* **33**, 163–168 in (German).

Degraeve, N., Chollet, M.-C., and Moutschen, J. (1984). Cytogenetic effects induced by organophosphorus pesticides in mouse spermatocytes. *Toxicol. Lett.* **21**, 315–319.

Deichmann, W. B., and Lampe, K. (1955). Dipterex, its pharmacological action. *Bull., Univ. Miami Sch. Med. Jackson Meml. Hosp.* **9**, 7–12.

Deichmann, W. B., and Rakoczy, R. (1953). Buscopan in treatment of experimental poisoning by parathion, methyl parathion, and Systox. *Arch. Ind. Hyg. Occup. Med.* **7**, 152–156.

Deichmann, W. B., and Rakoczy, R. (1955). Toxicity and mechanism of action of Systox. *Arch. Ind. Health* **11**, 324–331.

Deichmann, W. B., Brown, P., and Downing, C. (1952). Unusual protective action of a new emulsifier for the handling of organic phosphates. *Science* **116**, 221.

DeKay, D. E., Stanton, H. C., Brown, L. J., Mersmann, H. J., and Siers, D. G. (1974). Cold stress and the dichlorvos litter response. *J. Anim. Sci.* **39**, 181.

Delons, S., Leverque, J., and Berbich, A. (1964). Intoxication by parathion-like organophosphorus insecticides. *Maroc Med.* **43**, 749–751 (in French).

Demidenko, N. M., and Mirgiyazova, M. G. (1974). Combined effect of high air temperature and Anthio pesticide on the body. *Gig. Sanit.* **39**, 18–21 (in Russian).

DePalma, A. E., Kwalick, D. S., and Zukerberg, N. (1970). Pesticide poisoning in children. *JAMA, J. Am. Med. Assoc.* **211**, 1979–1981.

de Potas, G. M., and de D'Angelo, A. M. P. (1987). Perturbation effect of organophosphate insecticides on human erythrocyte. *Bull. Environ. Contam. Toxicol.* **39**, 802–806.

Dequeker, R. (1964). Detection of parathion (E 605) in parts of a cadaver buried for more than 6 months. *Verh. K. Vlaam. Acad. Geneeskd. Belg.* **26**, 395–412.

Derbyshire, J. C., and Murphy, R. T. (1962). Diazinon residues in treated silage and milk of cows fed powdered Diazinon. *J. Agric. Food Chem.* **10**, 384–386.

DeReuck, J., and Willems, J. (1975). Acute parathion poisoning. Myopathic changes in the diaphragm. *J. Neurol.* **208**, 309–314.

Desi, I., Farkas, I., Simon, G., and Czieleszky, V. (1971a). Neurotoxicological examination of bromophos, a phosphate ester. *Egeszsegtudomany* **15**, Suppl., 48–63 (in Hungarian).

Desi, I., Farkas, I., Simon, G., and Czieleszky, V. (1971b). Investigation of the neurotoxic effects of the phosphate ester, bromophos. *Int. Arch. Arbeitsmed.* **28**, 203–222 (in German).

Devens, B. H., Grayson, M. H., Imamura, T., and Rodgers, K. E. (1985). *O,O,S*-Trimethyl phosphorothioate effects on immunocompetence. *Pestic. Biochem. Physiol.* **24**, 251–259.

Diggle, W. M., and Gage, J. C. (1950). Cholinesterase inhibition *in vitro* by *O,O*-diethyl *O-p*-nitrophenyl thiophosphate (parathion, E 605). *Biochem. J.* **49**, 491–494.

Diggory, H. J. P., Landrigan, P. J., Latimer, K. P., Ellington, A. C., Kimbrough, R. D., Liddle, J. A., Cline, R. E., and Smrek, A. L. (1977). Fatal parathion poisoning caused by contamination of flour in international commerce. *Am. J. Epidemiol.* **106**, 145–153.

Dikshith, T. S. S., Behari, J. R., Datta, K. K., and Mathur, A. K. (1975). Effect of Diazinon on male rats. Histopathological and biochemical studies. *Environ. Physiol. Biochem.* **5**, 293–299.

Dikshith, T. S. S., Datta, K. K., Kushwah, H. S., Chandr, P., and Raizada, R. D. (1980). Effect of methyl demeton on vital organs and cholinesterase in male rats. *Indian J. Exp. Biol.* **18**, 163–166.

DiModugno, G., Albano Annicchino, G., Perrone, C., and Renna, P. (1973). Acute poisoning by phosphate esters in laying hens. *Acta Med. Vet.* **19**, 137–144.

Dinerman, A. A., Lavrent'eva, N. A., and Il'inskaia, N. A. (1970). The embryo-toxic action of some pesticides. *Gig. Sanit.* **35**, 39–42 (in Russian).

Dinman, B. D. (1964). Acute combined toxicity due to DDVP and chlordane. *Arch. Environ. Health* **9**, 765–769.

Dishovski, K., and Kotev, G. (1972). Electron microscopic examination of synaptic structures of n. caudatus in rat cerebrum during experimental poisoning with dimethyldichlorovinylphosphate and its treatment with TMB-4. *Eksp. Med. Morfol.* **11**, 141–145.

Dixon, E. M. (1957). Dilatation of the pupils in parathion poisoning. *JAMA, J. Am. Med. Assoc.* **163**, 444–445.

Dmochowska-Mroczek, H., Lebensztejn, W., and Tolwinski, K. (1972). Severe intoxication with Dipterex in a pregnant woman. *Pol. Tyg. Lek.* **27**, 1406–1407 (in Polish).

Dobbins, P. K. (1967). Organic phosphate insecticides as teratogens in the rat. *J. Fla. Med. Assoc.* **54**, 542–546.

Dobson, K. J. (1976). Trichlorfon toxicity in pigs. *Aust. Vet. J.* **53**, 115–117.

Dressel, T. D., Goodale, R. L., Jr., Arneson, M. A., and Borner, J. W. (1979a). Pancreatitis as a complication of anticholinesterase insecticide intoxication. *Ann. Surg.* **189**, 199–204.

Dressel, T. D., Goodale, R. L., Jr., Hunninghake, D. B., and Borner, J. W. (1979b). Sensitivity of the canine pancreatic intraductal pressure to subclinical reduction in cholinesterase activity. *Ann. Surg.* **190**, 6–12.

Drudge, J. H., and Lyons, E. T. (1972). Critical tests of a resin-pellet formulation of dichlorvos against internal parasites of the horse. *Am. J. Vet. Res.* **33**, 1365–1375.

DuBois, K. P. (1958). Potentiation of the toxicity of insecticidal organic phosphates. *Arch. Ind. Hyg. Occup. Med.* **6**, 9–13.

DuBois, K. P. (1961). Potentiation of the toxicity of organophosphorus compounds. *Adv. Pest Control Res.* **4**, 117–151.

DuBois, K. P., and Coon, J. M. (1952). Toxicology of organic phosphorus-containing insecticides to mammals. *Arch. Ind. Hyg. Occup. Med.* **6**, 9–13.

DuBois, K. P., and Cotter, G. J. (1955). Studies on the toxicity and mechanism of action of Dipterex. *AMA Arch. Ind. Health* **11**, 53–60.

DuBois, K. P., and Kinoshita, F. (1964a). Acute toxicity and anticholinesterase action of *O,O*-diethyl-*O-p*- (methylsulfinyl)phenyl phosphorothioate (DMSP) and some related compounds. *Toxicol. Appl. Pharmacol.* **6**, 78–85.

DuBois, K. P., and Kinoshita, F. (1964b). Acute toxicity and anticholinesterase action of *O,O*-dimethyl-*O*-[4-methylthio)-*m*-tolyl]phosphorothioate (DMTP; Baytex) and related compounds. *Toxicol. Appl. Pharmacol.* **6**, 86–95.

DuBois, K. P., and Plzak, G. J. (1962). The acute toxicity and anticholinesterase action of *O,O*-diethyl *S*-ethyl-2- sulfenylethyl phosphorothioate (Meta-Systox®) and related compounds. *Toxicol. Appl. Pharmacol.* **4**, 621–630.

DuBois, K. P., Doull, J., Salerno, P. R., and Coon, J. M. (1949). Studies on the toxicity and mechanism of action of *p*-nitrophenyl diethyl thionophosphate (parathion). *J. Pharmacol. Exp. Ther.* **95**, 79–91.

DuBois, K. P., Doull, J., and Coon, J. M. (1950). Studies on the toxicity and pharmacological action of octamethyl pyrophosphoramide (OMPA, Pestox III). *J. Pharmacol. Exp. Ther.* **99**, 376–393.

DuBois, K. P., Doull, J., Deroin, J., and Cummings, O. K. (1953). Studies on the toxicity and mechanism of action of some new insecticidal thionophosphates. *Arch. Ind. Hyg. Occup. Med.* **8**, 350–358.

DuBois, K. P., Murphy, S. D., and Thursh, D. R. (1956). Toxicity and mechanism of action of some metabolites of Systox. *AMA Arch. Ind. Health* **13**, 606–612.

DuBois, K. P., Thursh, D. R., and Murphy, S. D. (1957). Studies on the toxicity and pharmacological actions of the d methoxy ester of benzotriazine dithiophosphoric acid (DBD, Guthion). *J. Pharmacol. Exp. Ther.* **119**, 208–218.

DuBois, K. P., Kinoshita, F. K., and Frawley, J. P. (1968). Quantitative measurement of inhibition of aliesterases, acylamidase, and cholinesterase by EPN and Delnav. *Toxicol. Appl. Pharmacol.* **12**, 273–284.

Dudek, B. R., and Richardson, R. J. (1982). Evidence for the existence of neurotoxic esterase in neural and lymphatic tissue of the adult hen. *Biochem. Pharmacol.* **31**, 1117–1121.

Dudek, B. R., Barth, M. Gephart, L., Huggins, J., and Richardson, R. J. (1979). Correlation of brain and lymphocyte neurotoxic esterase inhibition in the adult hen following dosing with neurotoxic compounds. *Toxicol. Appl. Pharmacol.* **48**, A198.

Dugl'nyy, G. A. (1971). Labor expertise on eye disease and trauma occurring among agricultural equipment operators and workers exposed directly to poisonous compounds. *Oftal'mol. Zh.* **26**, 458–460.

Duggan, R. E. (1968). Residues in food and feed. *Pestic. Monit. J.* **2**, 2–46.

Duke-Elder, S., and Weale, R. A. (1968). Visual perceptions. *In* "System of Ophthalmology. Vol. IV. The Physiology of the Eye and of Vision" (S. Duke-Elder, ed.). Mosby, St. Louis, Missouri.

Durham, W. F., and Wolfe, H. R. (1963). An additional note regarding measurement of the exposure of workers to pesticides. *Bull. W.H.O.* **29**, 279–281.

Durham, W. F., Gaines, T. B., and Hayes, W. J., Jr. (1956). Paralytic and related effects of certain organic phosphorus compounds. *AMA Arch. Ind. Health* **13**, 326–330.

Durham, W. F., Gaines, T. B., McCauley, R. H., Sedlak, V. A., Mattson, A. M., and Hayes, W. J., Jr. (1957). Studies on the toxicity of *O,O*-dimethyl-2,2-dichlorovinyl phosphate (DDVP). *AMA Arch. Ind. Health* **15**, 340–349.

Durham, W. F., Hayes, W. J., Jr., and Mattson, A. M. (1959). Toxicological studies of *O,O*-dimethyl-2,2-dichlorovinyl phosphate (DDVP) in tobacco warehouses. *AMA Arch. Ind. Health* **20**, 202–210.

Durham, W. F., Wolfe, H. R., and Quinby, G. E. (1965). Organophosphorus insecticides and mental alertness. *Arch. Environ. Health* **10**, 55–66.

Dyer, K. F., and Hanna, P. J. (1973). Comparative mutagenic activity and toxicity of triethylphosphate and dichlorvos in bacteria and *Drosophila*. *Mutat. Res.* **21**, 175–177.

Earl, C. J., Thompson, R. H. S., and Webster, G. R. (1953). Observations on the specificity of the inhibition of cholinesterases by tri-*ortho*-cresyl phosphate. *Br. J. Pharmacol. Chemother.* **8**, 110–114.

Earl, F. L., Melveger, B. E., Reinwall, J. E., Bierbower, G. W., and Curtis, J. M. (1968). Diazinon toxicity—comparative studies in dogs and miniature swine. *Toxicol. Appl. Pharmacol.* **12**, 287.

Earl, F. L., Melveger, B. E., Reinwall, J. E., Bierbower, G. W., and Curtis, J. M. (1971). Diazinon toxicity—comparative studies in dogs and miniature swine. *Toxicol. Appl. Pharmacol.* **18**, 285–295.

Ecobichon, D. J., and Comeau, A. M. (1973). Pseudocholinesterases of mammalian plasma: Physicochemical properties and organophosphate inhibition in eleven species. *Toxicol. Appl. Pharmacol.* **24**, 92–100.

Ecobichon, D. J., Myatt, G. L., and Greenhalgh, R. (1975). Mammalian toxicity and degradation of fenitrooxon and *S*-methyl fenitrooxon. *Toxicol. Appl. Pharmacol.* **33**, 143–144.

Ecobichon, D. J., Ozere, R. L., Reid, E., and Crocker, J. F. S. (1977). Acute fenitrothion poisoning. *Can. Med. Assoc. J.* **116**, 377–379.

Edmundson, W. F., and Davies, J. E. (1967). Occupational dermatitis from naled. A clinical report. *Arch. Environ. Health* **15**, 89–91.

Edson, E. F. (1955). "The Effect of Prolonged Ingestion of Low Dosages of Schradan in Humans," Mimeographed report from the Medical Department, Fisons Pest Control Ltd., Chesterford Park Research Station, Nr. Saffron Walden, Essex, UK.

Edson, E. F. (1956). "The Effects of Prolonged Administration of Small Daily Doses of Dimefox in the Rat, Pig, and Man," Mimeographed report from the Medical Department, Fisons Pest Control Ltd., Chesterford Park Research Station, Nr. Saffron Walden, Essex, UK.

Edson, E. F. (1957). "The Effects of Prolonged Administration of Small Daily Doses of Parathion in the Rat, Pig, and Man," Mimeographed report from the Medical Department, Fisons Pest Control Ltd., Chesterford Park Research Station, Nr. Saffron Walden, Essex, UK.

Edson, E. F. (1958). Blood tests for users of O.P. insecticides. *World Crops* **40**, 49–51.

Edson, E. F. (1964). No-effect levels of three organophosphates in the rat, pig, and man. *Food Cosmet. Toxicol.* **2**, 311–316.

Edson, E. F., and Noakes, D. N. (1960). The comparative toxicity of six organophosphorus insecticides in the rat. *Toxicol. Appl. Pharmacol.* **2**, 523–539.

Edson, E. F., Sanderson, D. M., Watson, W. A., and Noakes, D. N. (1962). The stability of blood cholinesterase after death. *Med. Sci. Law* **2**, 258–267.

Edson, E. F., Jones, K. H., and Watson, W. A. (1967). Safety of dimethoate insecticide. *Br. Med. J.* **4**, 554–555.

Efendiev, T. M. (1961). The clinical aspect of mercaptophos (demeton) poisoning. *Klin. Med. (Moscow)* **39**, 126–130.

Egyed, M. N., Malkinson, M., Eilat, A., and Shlosberg, A. (1974). Basudin (Diazinon) poisoning in goslings. *Refuah Vet.* **31**, 22–26.

Ekin, F. H. (1971). Accidental poisoning with malathion. *Br. Med. J.* **3**, 47.

El-Achrafi, T. A. (1963). On twelve deaths due to an anticholinesterase insecticide: Parathion. Pharmacological description, symptoms and treatment. *Recl. Med. Moyen Orient.* **20**, 429–436 (in French).

Elaikis, E. C., Elaikis, A. C., and Coutselinis, A. S. (1966). Influence of putrefaction on the toxicological analysis of parathion. *Ann. Med. Leg.* **46**, 106–107.

Eliason, D. A., Cranmer, M. F., von Windeguth, D. L., Kilpatrick, J. W., Suggs, J. E., and Schoof, H. F. (1969). Dursban premises applications and their effect on the cholinesterase levels in spraymen. *Mosq. News* **29**, 591–595.

Eljasz, L., and Krzyszton-Przkop, T. (1975). Polyneuropathy as the result of Foschlor poisoning. *Pol. Tyg. Lek.* **30**, 1841–1842.

Elliott, J. W., Walker, K. C., Penick, A. E., and Durham, W. F. (1960). A sensitive procedure for urinary *p*-nitrophenol determination as a measure of exposure to parathion. *J. Agric. Food Chem.* **8**, 111–113.

Elliott, R., and Barnes, J. M. (1963). Organophosphorus insecticides for the control of mosquitos in Nigeria. *Bull. W.H.O.* **28**, 35–54.

El-Sebae, A. H., Soliman, S. A., Elamayem, M. A., and Ahmed, N. S. (1977). Neurotoxicity of organophosphorus insecticides leptophos and EPN. *J. Environ. Sci. Health, Part B* **12**, 269–288.

El-Sebae, A. H., Ahmed, N. S., and Soliman, S. A. (1978). Effect of pre-exposure on acute toxicity of organophosphorus insecticides to white mice. *J. Environ. Sci. Health, Part B* **13**, 11–14.

Endo, T., Kimura, Y., Masuyama, E., Yazaki, H., and Kusunoki, F. (1974). A case of acute intoxication caused by swallowing fenthion by mistake. *J. Jpn. Assoc. Rural Med.* **23**, 142 (in Japanese).

Engbaek, L., and Jensen, O. S. (1951). Toxic and cholinesterase inhibitory action of diethyl *p*-nitrophenyl thiophosphate (parathion). *Acta Pharmacol. Toxicol.* **7**, 189–200.

England, D. C. (1974). Husbandry components in prenatal and perinatal development in swine. *J. Anim. Sci.* **35**, 1045–1049.

English, T., Ellis, E. F., and Ackerman, J. (1970). Organic phosphate poisoning—Cleveland, Ohio. *Morbid. Mortal. Wkly. Rep.* **19**, 397–404.

Erdmann, W. D., and Clarmann, M. V. (1963). A new esterase reactivator for treating poisoning by alkylphosphates. *Dtsch. Med. Wochenschr.* **88**, 2201–2206 (in German).

Esser, H. O., Muchke, W., and Alt, K. O. (1968). The degradation of the insecticide GS 13005 in the rat. Elucidation of the structure of the more important metabolites. *Helv. Chim. Acta* **51**, 513–517 (in German).

Eto, M. (1979). "Organophosphorus Pesticides: Organic and Biological Chemistry." CRC Press, Boca Raton, Florida.

Eto, M., Casida, J. E., and Eto, T. (1962). Hydroxylated and cyclization reactions involved in the metabolism of tri-*o*-cresyl phosphate. *Biochem. Pharmacol.* **11**, 337–352.

Evans, F. T., Gray, P. W. S., Lehmann, H., and Silk, E. (1952). Sensitivity to succinylcholine in relation to serum cholinesterase. *Lancet* **1**, 1229–1230.

Evans, F. T., Gray, P. W. S., Lehmann, H., and Silk, E. (1953). Effect of pseudocholinesterase level on action of succinylcholine in man. *Br. Med. J.* **1**, 136–138.

Faber, M. (1943). The relationship between serum choline esterase and serum albumin. *Acta Med. Scand.* **114**, 72–91.

Faerman, I. S. (1967). Aftereffects of acute poisoning with organo-phosphorus insecticides. *Gig. Tr. Prof. Zabol.* **4**, 39–41.

Faerman, I. S., Pongard, E. M., Zhalnina, L. V., Shapkina, T. G., and Sonia, A. (1961). Some characteristics of the clinical picture of acute mercaptophos poisoning. *Gig. Tr. Prof. Zabol.* **95**, 45–47.

Fahrig, R. (1973). Detection of a genetic action of organophosphorus insecticides. *Naturwissenschaften* **60**, 50–51 (in German).

Fallscheer, H. O., and Cook, J. W. (1956). Report on enzymatic methods for insecticides. Studies on the conversion of some thionophosphates and a dithiophosphate to *in vitro* cholinesterase inhibitors. *J. Assoc. Off. Agric. Chem.* **39**, 691–697.

Farago, A. (1967). Fatal suicidal malathion poisonings. *Arch. Toxikol.* **23**, 11–16.

Fazekas, I. G. (1971). Macroscopic and microscopic changes in Wofatox (parathion-methyl) intoxication. *Z. Rechtsmed.* **68**, 189–194 (in German).

Feldmann, R. J., and Maibach, H. I. (1970). Pesticide percutaneous penetration in man. *J. Invest. Dermatol.* **54**, 435–436.

Feldmann, R. J., and Maibach, H. I. (1974). Percutaneous penetration of some pesticides and herbicides in man. *Toxicol. Appl. Pharmacol.* **28**, 126–132.

Felsenstein, W. C., Staiff, D. C., and Miller, G. C. (1976). Acute demeton poisoning in a child. *Arch. Environ. Health* **31**, 266–269.

Felthous, J. M. (1978). Pesticide poisoning fatality. *Chem. Eng. News.* **56**, 67–68.

Fenichel, G. M., Dettbarn, W. D., and Newman, T. M. (1974). An experimental myopathy secondary to excessive acetylcholine release. *Neurology* **24**, 41–45.

Fenton, J. C. B. (1955). The nature of the paralysis in chickens following organophosphorus poisoning. *J. Pathol. Bacteriol.* **69**, 181–189.

Fish, S. A. (1966). Organophosphorus cholinesterase inhibitors and fetal development. *Am. J. Obstet. Gynecol.* **96**, 48–54.

Fisher, J. R. (1977). Guillain-Barré syndrome following organophosphate poisoning. *JAMA, J. Am. Med. Assoc.* **238**, 1950–1951.

Flesch, R. (1958). On poisoning by the phosphoric acid ester, Wofatox. *Z. Gesamte Inn. Med. Ihre Grenzgeb.* **13**, 375 (in German).

Flockhart, I. R., and Casida, J. E. (1972). Relationship of the acylation of membrane esterases and proteins to the teratogenic action of organophosphorus insecticides and Eserine in developing hen eggs. *Biochem. Pharmacol.* **21**, 2591–2603.

Flugel, M., and Geldmacher-von Mallinckrodt, M. (1978). On the kinetics of parathion-splitting enzymes in human serum (EC 3.1.1.2). *Klin. Wochenschr.* **56**, 911–916 (in German).

Fogg, T. J., Schooley, M. A., Brown, L. J., Chai, E. Y., and Keasling, H. H. (1974). Factors affecting the litter dichlorvos response. *J. Anim. Sci.* **39**, 182.

Foll, C. V., and Pant, C. P. (1964). "A Large-Scale Field Trial with Dichlorvos as a Residual Fumigant Insecticide in Kankiya District, Northern Nigeria," prelim. rep., WHO/Mal/451. World Health Organ., Geneva.

Food and Agriculture Organization/World Health Organization (FAO/WHO) (1965). "Evaluation of the Toxicity of Pesticide Residues in Food." Monograph prepared by the Joint Meeting of the FAO Committee on Pesticides in Agriculture and the WHO Expert Committee on Pesticide Residues, which met in Rome, 15–22 March 1965, WHO/Food Add./27.65. Food Agric. Organ., Rome.

Food and Agriculture Organization/World Health Organization (FAO/WHO) (1967). "Evaluation of Some Pesticide Residues in Food." Monograph prepared by the Joint Meeting of the FAO Working Party and the WHO Expert Committee on Pesticide Residues, which met in Geneva, 14–21 November 1966, WHO/Food Add./67.32. World Health Organ., Geneva.

Food and Agriculture Organization/World Health Organization (FAO/WHO) (1969). "1968 Evaluations of Some Pesticide Residues in Food." Monograph prepared by the Joint Meeting of the FAO Working Party of Experts and the WHO Expert Committee on Pesticide Residues, which met in Geneva, 9–16 December 1968, WHO/Food Add./69.35. World Health Organ., Geneva.

Food and Agriculture Organization/World Health Organization (FAO/WHO) (1970). "1969 Evaluations of Some Pesticide Residues in Food." Monograph prepared by the Joint Meeting of the FAO Working Party of Experts and the WHO Expert Group on Pesticide Residues, which met in Rome, 8–15 December 1969, WHO/Food Add./70.38. Food Health Organ., Rome.

Food and Agriculture Organization/World Health Organization (FAO/WHO) (1972). "1971 Evaluations of Some Pesticide Residues in Food." Monograph prepared by the Joint Meeting of the FAO Working Party of Experts on Pesticide Residues and the WHO Expert Committee on Pesticide Residues that met in Geneva from 22 to 29 November 1971, WHO Pestic. Residue Ser., No. 1. World Health Organ., Geneva.

Food and Agriculture Organization/World Health Organization (FAO/WHO) (1973). "1972 Evaluations of Some Pesticide Residues in Food." Monograph prepared by the Joint Meeting of the FAO Working Party of Experts on Pesticide Residues and the WHO Expert Committee on Pesticide Residues that met in Rome from 20 to 28 November 1972, WHO Pestic. Residue Ser., No. 2. World Health Organ., Geneva.

Food and Agriculture Organization/World Health Organization (FAO/WHO) (1974). "1973 Evaluations of Some Pesticide Residues in Food." Monograph prepared by the Joint Meeting of the FAO Working Party of Experts on Pesticide Residues and the WHO Expert Committee on Pesticide Residues that met in Geneva from 26 November to 5 December 1973, WHO Pestic. Residue Ser., No. 3. World Health Organ., Geneva.

Food and Agriculture Organization/World Health Organization (FAO/WHO) (1975). "1974 Evaluations of Some Pesticide Residues in Food." Monograph prepared by the Joint Meeting of the FAO Working Party of Experts on Pesticide Residues and the WHO Expert Committee on Pesticide Residues that met in Rome from 2 to 11 December 1974, WHO Pestic. Residue Ser., No. 4. World Health Organ., Geneva.

Food and Agriculture Organization/World Health Organization (FAO/WHO) (1976). "1975 Evaluations of Some Pesticide Residues in Food." Monograph prepared by the Joint Meeting of the FAO Working Party of Experts on Pesticide Residues and the WHO Expert Committee on Pesticide Residues that met in Geneva from 24 November to 3 December 1975, WHO Pestic. Residue Ser., No. 5. World Health Organ., Geneva.

Forsyth, D. M., and Rashid, C. (1967). Treatment of urinary schistosomiasis. *Lancet* **1,** 130–133.

Fournier, E., Dally, S., and Cambier, J. (1976). Peripheral neuropathy probably due to anticholinesterase insecticides. *Nouv. Presse Med.* **5,** 718 (in French).

Fowler, J. L., Warne, R. J., Furusho, Y., and Sugiyama, M. (1970). Testing fenthion, dichlorvos, and diethylcarbamazine for prophylactic effects against developing stages of *Dicrofilaria immitis. Am. J. Vet. Res.* **31,** 903–906.

Francis, J. I., and Barnes, J. M. (1963). Studies on the mammalian toxicity of fenthion. *Bull. W.H.O.* **29,** 205–212.

Frawley, J. P. (1976). Test protocols and limitations for detection of neurotoxicity. *In* "Pesticide Induced Delayed Neurotoxicity" (R. L. Baron, ed.), pp. 234–252. Environ. Health Eff. Res. Ser., EPA-600/1-76-025. Environ. Prot. Agency, Research Triangle Park, North Carolina.

Frawley, J. P., and Fuyat, H. N. (1957). Pesticide toxicity. Effect of low dietary levels of parathion and Systox on blood cholinesterase of dogs. *J. Agric. Food Chem.* **5,** 346–348.

Frawley, J. P., Hagan, E. C., and Fitzhugh, O. G. (1952a). A comparative pharmacological and toxicological study of organic phosphate-anticholinesterase compounds. *J. Pharmacol. Exp. Ther.* **105,** 156–165.

Frawley, J. P., Laug, E. P., and Fitzhugh, O. G. (1952b). Effect of liver damage on toxicity of octamethylpyrophosphate (OMPA). *Fed. Proc., Fed. AM. Soc. Exp. Biol.* **11,** 347.

Frawley, J. P., Zwickey, R. E., and Fuyat, H. N. (1956). Myelin degeneration in chickens with subacute administration of organic phosphorus insecticides. *Fed. Proc., Fed. Am. Soc. Exp. Biol.* **15,** 424.

Frawley, J. P., Fuyat, H. N., Hagan, E. C., Blake, J. R., and Fitzhugh, O. G. (1957). Marked potentiation in mammalian toxicity from simultaneous administration of two anticholinesterase compounds. *J. Pharmacol. Exp. Ther.* **121,** 96–106.

Frawley, J. P., Weir, R., Tusing, T., DuBois, K. P., and Calandra, J. C. (1963). Toxicologic investigations in Delnav. *Toxicol. Appl. Pharmacol.* **5,** 605–624.

Fredriksson, T. (1961). Percutaneous absorption of parathion and paraoxon. *Arch. Environ. Health* **3,** 185–188.

Fredriksson, T., and Bigelow, J. K. (1961). Tissue distribution of P32-labeled parathion. *Arch. Environ. Health* **2,** 633–667.

Freed, V. H., Matin, M. A., Fang, S. C., and Kar, P. P. (1976). Role of striatal dopamine in delayed neurotoxic effects of organophosphorus compounds. *Eur. J. Pharmacol.* **35,** 229–232.

Freedman, A. M., and Himwich, H. E. (1948). Effect of age on lethality of diisopropyl fluorophosphate. *Am. J. Physiol.* **153,** 121–126.

Freeman, G., and Epstein, M. A. (1955). Therapeutic factors in survival after lethal cholinesterase inhibition by phosphorus insecticides. *N. Engl. J. Med.* **253,** 266–271.

Freemon, F. R. (1975). Causes of polyneuropathy. *Acta Neurol. Scand.* **51,** Suppl. 59, 1–43.

Fremont-Smith, K., Volwiler, W., and Wood, P. A. (1952). Serum acetylcholinesterase: Its close correlation with serum albumin, and its limited usefulness as a test of liver function. *J. Lab. Clin. Med.* **40,** 692–702.

Freundlich, A., and Steinlauf, I. (1964). Malathion poisoning of a 40-day old infant. *Harefuah* **67,** 346–347.

Friis, H. (1966). Parathion mortality in Denmark. *Bibl. Laeg.* **158,** 137–199.

Frugoni, G., Tatarelli, G. F., and Bardelli, A. (1959). Behavior of some serum enzyme activities during protracted physical effort. *Arch. Ital. Sci. Med. Trop. Parassitol.* **40,** 491–497.

Fryer, J. H., Steel, R. G. D., and Williams, H. H. (1955). Cholinesterase activity levels in normal human subjects. *AMA Arch. Ind. Health* **12,** 406–411.

Fuchs, V., Golbs, S., Kuhnert, M., and Osswald, F. (1976). Studies into prenatal toxic action of parathion methyl on Wistar rats and comparison with prenatal toxicity of cyclophosphamide and trypan blue. *Arch. Exp. Veterinaermed.* **30,** 343–350.

Fuhremann, T. W., Lichtenstein, E. P., Zahlten, R. N., Stratman, F. W., and Schnoes, H. K. (1974). Metabolism of ^{14}C-parathion and ^{14}C-paraoxon in isolated perfused rat livers. *Pestic. Sci.* **5,** 31–39.

Fukel'man, L. D., and Afonin, A. V. (1971). Acute chlorophos poisoning. *Voen.-Med., Zh.* **11,** 68–69.

Fukuhara, N., Hoshi, M., and Mori, S. (1977). Core targetoid fibres and multiple cytoplasmic bodies in organophosphate neuropathy. *Acta Neuropathol.* **40,** 137–144 (in Russian).

Fukuto, T. R., Metcalf, R. L., March, R. B., and Maxon, M. G. (1955). Chemical behavior of Systox isomers in biological systems. *J. Econ. Entomol.* **48,** 347–354.

Fukuto, T. R., Wolf, J. P., III, Metcalf, R. L., and March, R. B. (1956). Identification of the sulfoxide and sulfone plant metabolites of the thiol isomer of Systox. *J. Econ. Entomol.* **49,** 147–151.

Fukuto, T. R., Wolf, J. P., III, Metcalf, R. L., and March, R. B. (1957). Identification of the sulfone plant metabolite of the thiono isomer of Systox. *J. Econ. Entomol.* **50,** 399–401.

Funckes, A. J., Hayes, G. R., Jr., and Hartwell, W. F. (1963a). Urinary excretion of paranitrophenol by volunteers following dermal exposure to parathion at different ambient temperatures. *J. Agric. Food Chem.* **11,** 455–457.

Funckes, A. J., Miller, S., and Hayes, W. J., Jr. (1963b). Initial field studies in Upper Volta with dichlorvos. *Bull. W.H.O.* **29,** 243–246.

Furuno, J., Sugawara, N., and Funatsu, H. (1975). Cholinesterase activity in the blood of a person fatally intoxicated by an organophosphorus pesticide. *Yamaguchi Med. J.* **24,** 27–31 (in Japanese).

Futenma, M. (1973). A screening of the visual field on 13,357 school children. *J. Jpn. Ophthalmol. Soc.* **77,** 719–730.

Gaddum, J. H., and Wilson, A. (1947). Treatment of myasthenia gravis with diisopropylfluorophosphonate. *Nature (London)* **159,** 680–681.

Gadoth, N., and Fisher, A. (1978). Late onset of neuromuscular block in organophosphorus poisoning. *Ann. Intern. Med.* **88,** 654–655.

Gage, J. C. (1953). A cholinesterase inhibition derived from O,O-diethyl O-p-nitrophenyl thiophosphate *in vivo. Biochem. J.* **54,** 426–430.

Gage, J. C. (1955). Blood cholinesterase values in early diagnosis of excessive exposure to phosphorus insecticides. *Br. Med. J.* **1,** 1370.

Gage, J. C. (1967). The significance of blood cholinesterase activity measurements. *Residue Rev.* **18,** 159–173.

Gagne, J., and Brodeur, J. (1972). Metabolic studies on the mechanisms of increased susceptibility of weanling rats to parathion. *Can. J. Physiol. Pharmacol.* **59,** 902–915.

Gaines, T. B. (1960). The acute toxicity of pesticides to rats. *Toxicol. Appl. Pharmacol.* **2,** 88–99.

Gaines, T. B. (1962). Poisoning by organic phosphorus pesticides potentiated by phenothiazine derivatives. *Science* **138,** 1260–1261.

Gaines, T. B. (1969). Acute toxicity of pesticides. *Toxicol. Appl. Pharmacol.* **14,** 515–534.

Gaines, T. B., and Linder, R. E. (1986). Acute toxicity of pesticides in adult and weanling rats. *Fundam. Appl. Toxicol.* **7,** 299–308.

Gaines, T. B., Hayes, W. J., Jr., and Linder, R. E. (1966). Liver metabolism of anticholinesterase compounds in live rats: Relation to toxicity. *Nature (London)* **209,** 88–89.

Gaines, T. B., Kimbrough, R., and Laws, E. R., Jr. (1967). Toxicology of Abate in laboratory animals. *Arch. Environ. Health* **14**, 283–288.

Gal, G., Simon, L., Rengei, B., Mindszentry, L., and Ember, M. (1970). Hemodialysis in the treatment of poisoning by methylparathion. *Res. Commun. Chem. Pathol. Pharmacol.* **1**, 553–560.

Galdney, W. J., Ernst, S. E., Dawkins, C. C., Drummond, R. O., and Graham, O. H. (1972). Feeding systemic insecticides to cattle for control of the tropical horse tick. *J. Med. Entomol.* **9**, 439–442.

Gallo, M. A. (1975). Studies in the toxicity of phosalone. *Toxicol. Appl. Pharmacol.* **33**, 144.

Gallo, M. A. (1976). Chronic toxicologic investigations of phosalone in the dog and rat. *Toxicol. Appl. Pharmacol.* **36**, 561–568.

Gallo, M. A., Knaak, J. B., Little, D. T., and Maddy, K. T. (1976). Workers safety reentry study involving phosalone on citrus. *Toxicol. Appl. Pharmacol.* **37**, 167.

Galzon, Y., and Levin, S. (1968). A case of poisoning by malathion as a result of its use as a rinse in the hair. *Harefuah* **74**, 261.

Ganelin, R. S. (1964). Measurement of cholinesterase activity of the blood. *Ariz. Med.* **21**, 710–714.

Ganz, J. W., Poser, W., and Erdmann, W. D. (1974). Investigation of the liver toxicity of nitrostigmine (parathion, E 605) in the perfused rat liver. *Arch. Toxicol.* **33**, 31–40 (in German).

Gar, K. A., Sazonova, N. A., Fadeev, Y. N., Vladimirova, I. L., and Golubeva, Z. Z. (1958). Incorporation and excretion of dimethyl 4-nitrophenyl thiophosphate in guinea pigs. *Org. Insektofungitsidy Gerbitsidy*, pp. 93–105.

Gardner, A. L., and Iverson, R. E. (1968). The effect of aerially applied malathion on an urban population. *Arch. Environ. Health* **16**, 823–826.

Gardocki, J. F., and Hazleton, L. W. (1951). Urinary excretion of the metabolic products of parathion following its intravenous injection. *J. Am. Pharm. Assoc.* **40**, 491–494.

Garlick, N. L. (1971). Intravenous and oral medication for the elimination of heartworms (*Dirofilaria immitis*). *J. Am. Vet. Med. Assoc.* **159**, 1435–1443.

Gasser, R. (1953). Regarding a new insecticide with a broad spectrum of action. *Z. Naturforsch., B: Anorg. Chem., Org. Chem., Biochem., Biophys., Biol.* **8**, 225–232 (in German).

Gassmann, R. (1957). Poisoning by anticholinesterase insecticides in the period 1950–1956. *Praxis (Bern)* **46**, 393–402, 416–424 (in German).

Gaultier, M., Bismuth, C., and Conso, F. (1975). Severe organophosphate intoxication—five cases. *Bull. Med. Leg. Toxicol.* **18**, 349–356.

Gazzard, B. G., Weston, M. J., Murray-Lyon, I. M., Flax, H., Record, C. D., Portmann, B., Langley, P. G., Dunlop, E. H., Mellou, P. J., Ward, M. B., and Williams, R. (1974). Charcoal haemoperfusion in the treatment of fulminant hepatic failure. *Lancet* **1**, 1301–1307.

Gehlbach, S. H., and Williams, W. A. (1975). Pesticide containers—their contribution to poisoning. *Arch. Environ. Health* **30**, 49–50.

Gejewski, D. (1974). Effect of diazepam on the antidotal action of atropine sulfate and Toxogonin in phosphamidon poisoning of rats. *Med. Weter.* **30**, 484–487.

Gelbke, H. P., and Schlicht, H. J. (1978). Fatal poisoning with a plant protective containing monocrotophos, dodine, and dinocap. *Toxicol. Eur. Res.* **1**, 181–184.

Geldmacher-von Mallinckrodt, M., and Deinzer, K. (1966). Rapid determination of *p*-nitrophenol in the urine as an indication of E-605 poisoning. *Dtsch. Med. Wochenschr.* **9**, 1381–1382.

Gembitskii, E. V., Moshkin, E. A., and Maksimov, G. V. (1970). Antidote therapy of acute chlorophos poisonings. *Voen.-Med. Zh.* **10**, 49–53 (in Russian).

Genina, S. A. (1974). Dynamics of blood cholinesterase activity in workers exposed to some organophosphorus insecticides during aerochemical application. *Gig. Tr. Prof. Zabol.* **12**, 42–44 (in Russian).

Geoffroy, H., Slomic, A., Bebebadji, M., and Pascal, P. (1960). Tricresyl phosphate myelo-polyneuropathy. Moroccan poisoning outbreak of September–October 1959. *World Neurol.* **1**, 244–315 (in French).

Georgian, L. (1975). The comparative cytogenic effects of aldrin and phosphamidon. *Mutat. Res.* **31**, 103–108.

Gershon, S., and Shaw, F. H. (1961). Psychiatric sequelae of chronic exposure to organophosphorus insecticides. *Lancet* **1**, 1371–1374.

Gerstengarbe, S. (1975). Mutagenicity of dimethoate investigated by the dominant lethal test in the house mouse (*Mus musculus* L.). *Wiss. Z.—Martin-Luther-Univ. Halle-Wittenberg, Math.-Naturwiss. Reihe* **24**, 87–88 (in German).

Ghachem, A., and Hassen, M. (1973). Some circumstances of observation of acute intoxications by parathion in Tunisia. *Med. Leg. Dommage Corpor.* **6**, 365–366 (in French).

Ghadiri, M., Greenwood, D. A., and Binns, W. (1967). Feeding of malathion and carbaryl to laying hens and roosters. *Toxicol. Appl. Pharmacol.* **10**, 392.

Gibel, W., Lohs, K., Wildner, G. P., and Ziebarth, D. (1971). Experimental animal investigation of the hepatotoxic and carcinogenic action of organophosphorus compounds. I. Trichlorfon. *Arch. Geschwulstforsch.* **37**, 303–312 (in German).

Gibel, W., Lohs, K., Wildner, G. P., Ziebarth, D., and Stieglitz, R. (1973). On the carcinogenic, hemotoxic, and hepatotoxic action of pesticidal organophosphorus compounds. *Arch. Geschwulstforsch.* **41**, 311–328 (in German).

Giermaziak, H. (1973). Studies on the effect of organophosphorus compounds on the body as exemplified by "Intrathion." *Med. Pr.* **24**, 487–494.

Giermaziak, H. (1977). Evaluation of the cytotoxic action of phosphorothioaliphatic pesticides on the basis of intoxication with intrathion. *Med. Pr.* **27**, 253–257 (in Polish).

Giermaziak, H., and Andrzejewski, S. (1976). Comparative studies of the effect of acute intrathion intoxication and treatment on the record of electrocardiographic curves in rats and rabbits. *Med. Pr.* **27**, 377–383.

Ginsberg, G. L., Placke, M. E., Wyand, D. S., and Cohen, S. D. (1982). Protection against acetaminophen-induced hepatotoxicity by prior treatment with fenitrothion. *Toxicol. Appl. Pharmacol.* **66**, 383–399.

Gitelson, S., Davidson, J. T., and Werczberger, A. (1965). Phosphamidon poisoning. *Br. J. Ind. Med.* **22**, 236–239.

Gitelson, S., Aladjemoff, L., Ben-Hadar, S., and Katznelson, R. (1966). Poisoning by malathion–xylene mixture. *JAMA, J. Am. Med. Assoc.* **197**, 819–821.

Glazer, E. (1976). The neuropathology of organophosphorus toxicity at the cat soleus neuromuscular junction. *Anat. Rec.* **184**, 411–412.

Glow, P. H. (1969). Incidence of chromophobe adenoma after chronic di-isopropylfluorophosphate poisoning. *Nature (London)* **221**, 1265.

Gnadt, J. W., Pegram, G. V., and Baxter, J. F. (1985). The acetylcholinesterase inhibitor di-isopropyl-fluorophosphate increases REM sleep in rats. *Physiol. Behav.* **35**, 911–916.

Gnadt, J. W., Atwood, C. W., Meighen, G. A., and Pegram, G. V. (1986). Di-isopropyl-fluorophosphate (DFP): Acute toxicity and sleep. *Neurotoxicology* **7**, 165–172.

Goebel, R., Zeichen, R., and Giessauf, W. (1969). Severe Meta-Systox R poisoning. *Wien. Med. Wochenschr.* **119**, 649–651.

Gofmekler, V. A., and Tabakova, S. A. (1970). The effect of chlorphos on rat embryogenesis. *Farmakol. Toksikol. (Moscow)* **33**, 735–737 (in Russian).

Goldberg, A. M., and Hanin, I. (1976). "Biology of Cholinergic Function." Raven Press, New York.

Goldblatt, M. W. (1950). Organic phosphorus insecticides and the antidotal action of atropine. *Pharmacol. J.* **164**, 229–233.

Goldin, A. R., Rubenstein, A. H., Bradlow, B. A., and Elliott, G. A. (1964). Malathion poisoning with special reference to the effect of cholinesterase inhibition on erythrocyte survival. *N. Engl. J. Med.* **271**, 1289–1293.

Goldman, H., and Teitel, M. (1958). Malathion poisoning in a 34-month-old child following accidental ingestion. *J. Pediatr.* **52**, 76–81.

Golubeva, A. V., and Guglin, E. R. (1964). Clinical features of mercaptophos poisoning. *Gig. Tr. Prof. Zabol.* **8**, 46–47.

Golz, H. H. (1959). Controlled human exposures to malathion aerosols. *AMA Arch. Ind. Health* **19**, 516–523.

Goncharenko, N. G. (1975). Toxicity of Abate during inhalation entrance into the organism. *Vrach. Delo* **9**, 130–133.

Gonzalez Laprat, J. A., Migliaro, J. P., Ferrari Fourcade, A., Saavedra, M., and Tugentman, A. (1966). Intoxication with organo-phosphate inhibitors of cholinesterase. Three cases of simultaneous accidental intoxication with Phosdrin. *An. Fac. Med. Montevideo* **50**, 255–268 (in Spanish).

Goodale, R. H., and Humphreys, M. B. (1931). Jamaica ginger paralysis. Autopsy observations. *JAMA, J. Am. Med. Assoc.* **86**, 14–16.

Gough, B. J., and Shellenberger, G. L. (1971). Rabbit whole blood cholinesterase inhibition and reactivation after intravenous infusion of Azodrin. *Toxicol. Appl. Pharmacol.* **19**, 398–399.

Goulding, R. (1968). Toxicological case records. *Practitioner* **200**, 599–600.

Grant, W. M. (1948). Miotic and antiglaucomatous activity of tetraethyl pyrophosphate in human eyes. *Arch. Ophthalmol. (Chicago)* **39**, 576–586.

Grant, W. M. (1950). Additional experiences with tetraethyl pyrophosphate in treatment of glaucoma. *Arch. Ophthalmol. (Chicago)* **44**, 362–364.

Gratz, N. G., Bracha, P., and Carmichael, A. (1963). A village-scale trial with dichlorvos as a residual fumigant insecticide in southern Nigeria. *Bull. W.H.O.* **29**, 251–270.

Great Britain Ministry of Agriculture, Fisheries and Food (1969). "Report on the Use of Poisonous Substances in Agriculture and on the Working of the Agriculture (Poisonous Substances) Regulations during 1969." H. M. Stationary Office, London.

Grech, J. L. (1965). Alterations in serum enzymes after repeated exposure to malathion. *Br. J. Ind. Med.* **22**, 67–71.

Greenberg, J., and LaHam, Q. N. (1969). Malathion-induced teratisms in the developing chick. *Can. J. Zool.* **47**, 539–542.

Greenberg, J., and LaHam, Q. N. (1970). Reversal of malathion-induced teratisms and its biochemical implications in the developing chick. *Can. J. Zool.* **48**, 1047–53.

Gregory, L., Futch, E. D., and Stone, C. T. (1952). Octamethyl pyrophosphoramide in the therapy of myasthenia gravis. *Am. J. Med.* **13**, 423–427.

Griffin, T. B., Coulston, F., and McCollister, D. D. (1976). Studies of the relative toxicities of chlorpyrifos and chlorpyrifosmethyl in man. *Toxicol. Appl. Pharmacol.* **37**, 105.

Grigorowa, R. (1960). On the health hazard from Wolfatox (dimethyl-*p*-nitrophenylthiophosphate) in the manufacture of a pesticide. *Z. Gesamte Hyg. Ihre Grenzgeb.* **6**, 556–560 (in German).

Grob, D. (1953). Course and management of myasthenia gravis. *JAMA, J. Am. Med. Assoc.* **153**, 529–532.

Grob, D., and Harvey, A. M. (1949). Observations on the effects of tetraethyl pyrophosphate (TEPP) in man and on its use in the treatment of myasthenia gravis. *Bull. Johns Hopkins Hosp.* **84**, 532–567.

Grob, D., Lilienthal, J. L., Jr., Harvey, A. M., and Jones, B. F. (1947a). The administration of di-isopropyl fluorophosphate (DFP) to man. I. Effect on plasma and erythrocyte cholinesterase; general systemic effects; use in study of hepatic function and erythropoiesis; and some properties of plasma cholinesterase. *Bull. John Hopkins Hosp.* **81**, 217–244.

Grob, D., Lilienthal, J. L., Jr., and Harvey, A. M. (1947b). The administration of di-isopropyl fluorophosphate (DFP) to man. II. Effect on intestinal motility and the use in the treatment of abdominal distention. *Bull. Johns Hopkins Hosp.* **81**, 245–256.

Grob, D., Harvey, A. M., Langworthy, O. R., and Lilienthal, J. L., Jr. (1947c). The administration of di-isopropyl fluorophosphate (DFP) to man. III. Effect on the central nervous system with special reference to the electrical activity of the brain. *Bull. Johns Hopkins Hosp.* **81**, 257–266.

Grob, D., Garlick, W. L., and Harvey, A. M. G. (1950). The toxic effects in man of the anticholinesterase insecticide parathion. *Bull. Johns Hopkins Hosp.* **87**, 106–129.

Groblewski, G. E., Vitorovic, S. L., Ngatia, J., Wills, J. H., and Coulston, F. (1975). The effects of fenthion and some of its metabolites on enzymic functional activities of the cat. *Toxicol. Appl. Pharmacol.* **33**, 139.

Guenther, R., Doenhardt, A., Altland, K., Jensen, M., and Goedde, H. W. (1972). Alkylphosphate intoxication. History of a severe case and use of a purified human cholinesterase preparation. *Med. Klin. (Munich)* **66**, 785–788 (in German).

Guiti, N., and Sadeghi, D. J. (1969). Acute toxicity of malathion in the mongrel dog. *Toxicol. Appl. Pharmacol.* **15**, 244–245.

Gundu Rao, H. R., and Anders, M. W. (1973). Inhibition of microsomal drug metabolism by anticholinesterase insecticides. *Bull. Environ. Contam. Toxicol.* **9**, 4–9.

Gunner, H. B., and Zuckerman, B. M. (1968). Degradation of "Diazinon" by synergistic microbial action. *Nature (London)* **217**, 1183–1184.

Gupta, O. P., and Patel, D. D. (1968). Diazinon poisoning. A study of sixty cases. *J. Assoc. Physicians India* **16**, 457–463.

Gupta, P. K. (1976). Duration of phenthoate-induced changes in blood and brain cholinesterase and the toxicity of phenthoate in rats. *Chemosphere* **5**, 201–205.

Gupta, P. K., and Paul, B. S. (1971). Effect of malathion on blood cholinesterase and its toxicity in *Gallus domesticus*. *Indian J. Exp. Biol.* **9**, 455–457.

Gupta, R. C., Patterson, G. T., and Dettbarn, W.-D. (1985). Mechanisms involved in the development of tolerance to DFP toxicity. *Fundam. Appl. Toxicol.* **5**, 17–28.

Gutentag, P. J. (1959). "Cutaneous Application of 1.1% Malathion Powder to Volunteers," U. S. Army Chem. Warfare Lab. Tech. Rep., CWLR 2290. U.S. Govt. Printing Office, Washington, D.C.

Guyot, H. (1958). Changes in plasma and erythrocyte cholinesterase activity in the guinea pig during prolonged inhalation of O,O-dimethyl-2,2-dichlorovinylphosphate (DDVP). *C. R. Seances Soc. Biol. Ses Fil.* **152**, 1532–1534 (in French).

Gysin, H., and Margot, A. (1958). Chemistry and toxicological properties of O,O-diethyl-O-isopropyl-4-methyl-6-pyrimidinyl) phosphorothioate (Diazinon). *J. Agric. Food Chem.* **6**, 900–903.

Haavik, T. K., and Ihlen, H. (1974). Alkyl phosphate poisoning. A case of Lebaycid (fenthion) poisoning. *Tiddskr. Nor. Laegeforen.* **94**, 1251–1253 (in Norwegian).

Hagan, E. C., Jenner, P. M., and Fitzhugh, O. G. (1961). Acute oral toxicity and potentiation studies with anticholinesterase compounds. *Fed. Proc., Fed. Am. Soc. Exp. Biol.* **20**, 432.

Hagan, E. C., Jenner, P. M., and Jones, W. I. (1971). Increased lethal effects of acutely administered anticholinesterases in female rats prefed with similar agents. *Toxicol. Appl. Pharmacol.* **18**, 235–237.

Haley, T. J., Farmer, J. H., Harmon, J. R., and Dooley, K. L. (1975a). Estimation of the LD 1 and extrapolation of the LD 0.1 for five organothiophosphate pesticides. *J. Eur. Toxicol.* **8**, 229–235.

Haley, T. J., Farmer, J. H., Dooley, K. L., and Harmon, J. R. (1975b). Comparison of low dose acute oral toxicity of trichlorfon and fospirate. *Fed. Proc., Fed. Am. Soc. Exp. Biol.* **34**, 245.

Haley, T. J., Farmer, J. H., Harmon, J. R., and Dooley, K. L. (1975c). Estimation of the LD 1 and extrapolation of the LD 0.1 for five organophosphate pesticides. *Arch. Toxicol.* **34**, 103–109.

Haley, T. J., Reichert, E. R., and Klemmer, H. W. (1978). Acute human poisoning with parathion and mevinphos. *Fed. Proc., Fed. Am. Soc. Exp. Biol.* **37**, 247.

Hall, G. E., and Lucas, C. C. (1937). Choline-esterase activity of normal and pathological human sera. *J. Pharmacol. Exp. Ther.* **59**, 34–42.

Hamada, H. (1955). Detection of parathion from organs of a cadaver, by the diazotization method together with paper chromatography. *Shikoku Acta Med.* **7**, 389–394.

Hamada, H. (1956). Spectrophotometrical detection of parathion (Folidol) from organs of a cadaver. *Shikoku Acta Med.* **8**, 1–6.

Hamlin, D. O., and Marchand, J. F. (1951). Parathion poisoning. *Am. Pract.* **2**, 1–12.

Hammond, P. S., Braunstein, H., Kennedy, J. M., Badawy, S. M. A., and Fukuto, T. R. (1982). Mode of action of the delayed toxicity of O,O,S-trimethyl phosphorothioate in the rat. *Pestic. Biochem. Physiol.* **18**, 77–89.

Hamza, S. M. (1973). Relationship between depression of blood cholinesterase and paralysis in Egyptian buffaloes by an organic phosphorus compound. *Egypt. J. Vet. Sci.* **10**, 53–63.

Hanna, N. F., Clay, J. C., and Harris, J. R. W. (1978). *Sarcoptes scabiei* infestation treated with malathion liquid. *Br. J. Vener. Dis.* **54**, 354.

Hanna, S., Basmy, K., Selim, O., Shoeb, S. M., and Awny, A. Y. (1966). Effects of administration of an organo-phosphorus compound as an anti-biharzial agent, with special reference to plasma cholinesterase. *Br. Med. J.* **1**, 1390–1392.

Hansen, D., Schaum, E., and Wasserman, O. (1968). Serum level and excretion of diisopropylfluoro-phosphate (DFP) in cats. *Biochem. Pharmacol.* **17,** 1159–1162.

Hanyu, I., and Tsuji, T. (1974). Results of investigation on the effects of agricultural chemicals especially organophosphorus pesticides on farmers' health. *Jpn. Public Health Inf.* **4,** 20 (in Japanese).

Hara, S., Inoue, T., and Tsuda, R. (1977). Autopsy in a case of gastromalacia due to ingestion of dichlorvos. *Jpn. J. Leg. Med.* **31,** 72 (in Japanese).

Harbison, R. D. (1975a). Comparative toxicity of some selected pesticides in neonatal and adult rats. *Toxicol. Appl. Pharmacol.* **32,** 443–446.

Harbison, R. D. (1975b). Parathion-induced toxicity and phenobarbital-induced protection against parathion during prenatal development. *Toxicol. Appl. Pharmacol.* **32,** 482–493.

Harned, W. H., and Casida, J. E. (1976). Dioxathion metabolites, photoproducts, and oxidative degradation products. *J. Agric. Food Chem.* **24,** 689–699.

Harris, H., and Whittaker, M. (1962). The serum cholinesterase variants. Study of twenty-two families selected via the "intermediate" phenotype. *Ann. Hum. Genet.* **26,** 59–72.

Harris, L. W., Fleisher, J. H., Clark, J., and Cliff, W. J. (1966). Dealkylation and loss of capacity for reactivation of cholinesterase inhibited by sarin. *Science* **154,** 404–406.

Harris, L. W., Innerebner, T. A., Fleisher, J. H., and Cliff, W. J. (1968). Reactivation of cholinesterase in rats poisoned with *O,O*-diethyl *O*-(2-isopropyl-6-methyl-4-pyrimidyl) phosphorothioate (Diazinon). *Fed. Proc., Fed. Am. Soc. Exp. Biol.* **27,** 472.

Hartwell, W. V., and Hayes, G. R. (1965). Respiratory exposure to organic phosphorus insecticides. *Arch. Environ. Health* **11,** 564–568.

Hartwell, W. V., Hayes, G. R., Jr., and Funckes, A. J. (1964). Respiratory exposure of volunteers to parathion. *Arch. Environ. Health* **8,** 820–825.

Harvey, A. M., Jones, B. F., Talbot, S., and Grob, D. (1946). The effect of diisopropyl fluorophosphate (DFP) on neuromuscular transmission in normal individuals and in patients with myasthenia gravis. *Fed. Proc., Fed. Am. Soc. Exp. Biol.* **5,** 182.

Harvey, A. M., Lilienthal, J. L., Jr., Grob, D., Jones, B. F., and Talbot, S. A. (1947). The administration of di-isopropylfluorophosphate to man. *Bull. Johns Hopkins Hosp.* **81,** 267–292.

Hass, D. K. (1973). Critical evaluation of dichlorvos tablets in puppies. *VM/SAC, Vet. Med. Small Anim. Clin.* **68,** 900–901.

Hass, D. K., Collins, J. A., and Kodama, J. K. (1972). Effects of orally administered dichlorvos in rhesus monkeys. *J. Am. Vet. Med. Assoc.* **16,** 714–719.

Hassan, A., Zayed, S. M. A. D., and Bahig, M. R. E. (1969). Metabolism of organophosphorus insecticides. XI. Metabolic fate of dimethoate in the rat. *Biochem. Pharmacol.* **18,** 2429–2438.

Hassan, A., Abdel-Hamid, F. M., and Afifi, L. M. (1977). Chemistry and toxicology of pesticide chemicals. V. Some pharmacological aspects of leptophos exposure in the rat. *Bull. Environ. Contam. Toxicol.* **18,** 640–647.

Hassan, A., Abdel-Hamid, F. M., Abou-Zeid, A., Mokhtar, O. A., Abdel-Razek, A. A., and Ibrahim, M. S. (1978). Clinical observations and biochemical studies on humans exposed to leptophos. *Chemosphere* **7,** 283–290.

Hattori, J., Oizumi, K., Sato, Y., Tsuda, K., Abe, T., and Harada, M. (1976). Biological properties of Sumithion. *Residue Rev.* **60,** 39–82.

Hayes, G. R., Funckes, A. J., and Hartwell, W. V. (1964). Dermal exposure of human volunteers to parathion. *Arch. Environ. Health* **8,** 829–833.

Hayes, W. J., Jr. (1961). Diagnostic problems in toxicology (agriculture). *Arch. Environ. Health* **3,** 49–56.

Hayes, W. J., Jr. (1963). "Clinical Handbook on Economic Poisons. Emergency Information for Treating Poisoning," Public Health Serv. Publ. No. 476. U. S. Govt. Printing Office, Washington, D.C.

Hayes, W. J., Jr. (1967). The 90-dose LD50 and a chronicity factor as measures of toxicity. *Toxicol. Appl. Pharmacol.* **11,** 327–335.

Hayes, W. J., Jr. (1975). "Toxicology of Pesticides." Williams & Wilkins, Baltimore, Maryland.

Hayes, W. J., Jr. (1976). Mortality in 1969 from pesticides, including aerosols. *Arch. Environ. Health* **31,** 61–72.

Hayes, W. J., Jr., and Durham, W. (1954). Studies of organic phosphorus insecticide poisoning. *Congr. Int. Patol. Comp.* [Actas Commun.], *6th, 1952* pp. 231–240.

Hayes, W. J., Jr., Dixon, E. M., Batchelor, G. S., and Upholt, W. M. (1957). Exposure to organic phosphorus sprays and occurrence of selected symptoms. *Public Health Rep.* **72,** 787–794.

Hayes, W. J., Jr., Mattson, A. M., Short, J. G., and Witter, R. F. (1960). Safety of malathion dusting powder for louse control. *Bull. W.H.O.* **22,** 503–514.

Hazleton, L. W. (1955). Review of current knowledge of toxicity of cholinesterase inhibitor insecticides. *J. Agric. Food Chem.* **3,** 312–319.

Hazleton, L. W., and Holland, E. G. (1950). Pharmacology and toxicology of parathion. *Adv. Chem. Ser.* **1,** 31–38.

Hazleton, L. W., and Holland, E. G. (1953). Toxicity of malathion. Summary of mammalian investigations. *Arch. Ind. Hyg. Occup. Med.* **8,** 399–405.

Healy, J. K. (1959). Reports of cases. Ascending paralysis following malathion intoxication: A case report. *Med. J. Aust.* **1,** 765–767.

Hearn, C. E. D. (1961). Trithion poisoning. *Br. J. Ind. Med.* **18,** 231–233.

Hearn, C. E. D. (1973). A review of agricultural pesticide incidents in man in England and Wales, 1952–71. *Br. J. Ind. Med.* **30,** 253–258.

Heath, D. F. (1961). "Organophosphorus Poisons: Anticholinesterase and Related Compounds." Pergamon, New York.

Heath, D. F., and Vandekar, M. (1957). Some spontaneous reactions of *O,O*-dimethyl *S*-ethylthioethyl phosphorothiolate and related compounds in water and storage, and their effects on the toxicological properties of the compounds. *Biochem. J.* **67,** 187–201.

Heering, H. (1970). The ECG of the rat in paraoxon intoxication under the effect of atropine and pralidoxime (2-PAM). *Arch. Int. Pharmacodyn. Ther.* **186,** 321–328.

Hegazy, M. R. (1965). Poisoning by a metaisosystox in spraymen and accidentally exposed patients. *Br. J. Ind. Med.* **22,** 230–235.

Hemsworth, B. A., and Cholakis, J. M. (1972). Some actions of a new organophosphorus compound and one of its major metabolites at the neuromuscular junction. *Toxicol. Appl. Pharmacol.* **22,** 287.

Hendrichova, E., Mayer, J., and Kortus, J. (1972). Distribution of radioactive phosphorus after application of ^{32}P-labeled fenitrothion on the skin of rats. *Cesk. Hyg.* **17,** 172–176 (in Slovakian).

Heyndrickx, A., VanHoof, F., DeWolf, L., and VanPeteghem, C. (1974). Fatal Diazinon poisoning in man. *J. Forensic Sci. Soc.* **14,** 131–133.

Hierons, R., and Johnson, M. K. (1978). Clinical and toxicological investigations of a case of delayed neuropathy in man after acute poisoning by an organophosphorus pesticide. *Arch. Toxicol.* **40,** 279–284.

Hillarp, N. A. (1960). Peripheral autonomic mechanisms. *In* "Handbook of Physiology" (J. Field, H. W. Magoun, and V. E. Hall, eds.), Sect. 1, Vol. II, Chapter 38, p. 979. Am. Physiol. Soc., Washington, D.C.

Hine, C. H., and Slomka, M. B. (1968). Human tolerance to the acute and subacute oral administration of a polyvinylchloride formulation of dichlorvos (V-3 and V-12). *Pharmacologist* **10,** 222.

Hine, C. H., and Slomka, M. B. (1970). Human toxicity studies on polyvinyl chloride formulation of dichlorvos. *Toxicol. Appl. Pharmacol.* **17,** 304–305.

Hine, C. H., Dunlap, M. K., Rice, E. G., Coursey, M. M., Gross, R. M., and Anderson, H. H. (1956). The neurotoxicity and anticholinesterase properties of some substituted phenyl phosphates. *J. Pharmacol. Exp. Ther.* **116,** 227–236.

Hiraki, K., Iwasaki, I., and Namba, M. (1972). Electroencephalograms in pesticide poisoning cases. *Clin. Electroencephalogr.* **14,** 333–340.

Hirschy, I. D., Minette, H., Matsuura, H., Reichert, E., Klemmer, H., Yauger, W., and Short, W. B. (1970). Diazinon poisoning—Hawaii. *Morbid. Mortal. Wkly Rep.* **19,** 130–131.

Hitchcock, M., and Murphy, S. D. (1967). Enzymatic reduction of *O,O*(4-nitrophenyl) phosphorothioate, *O,O*-diethyl *O*-(4-nitrophenyl) phosphate, and *O*-ethyl *O*-(4-nitrophenyl) benzene thiophosphorate by tissues from mammals, birds, and fishes. *Biochem. Pharmacol.* **16,** 1801–1811.

Hladka, A. (1977). Evaluation of the influence of accompanying impurities on the toxic effect of fenitrothion. *Prac. Lek.* **29,** 173–176.

Hladka, A., Batora, V., Kovacicova, J., and Rosival, L. (1977). Occupational health hazards and significance of technical fenitrothion and its contaminant S-methyl fenitrothion in toxicology of formulations. *Natl. Res. Counc. Can., NRC Assoc. Comm. Sci. Criter. Environ. Qual. [Rep.]* NRCC **NRCC/CNRC-16073**, 415–449.

Hobbiger, F. (1955). Effect of nicotinhydroxamic acid methoxide on human plasma cholinesterase inhibited by organophosphates containing a dialkylphosphate group. *Br. J. Pharmacol. Chemother.* **10**, 356–362.

Hobbiger, F. (1956). Chemical reactivation of phosphorylated human and bovine true cholinesterase. *Br. J. Pharmacol. Chemother.* **11**, 295–303.

Hoberman, A. M., Cranmer, J. S., Avery, D. L., and Cranmer, M. F. (1979). Transplacental inhibition of esterases in fetal brain following exposure to the organophosphate Diazinon. *Teratology* **19**, 30A–31A.

Hodge, H. C., Maynard, E. A., Hurwitz, L., DiStefano, V., Downs, W. L., Jones, C. K., and Blanchet, H. J. (1954). Studies of the toxicity and of the enzyme kinetics of ethyl *p*-nitrophenyl thionobenzene phosphonate (EPN). *J. Pharmacol. Exp. Ther.* **112**, 29–39.

Hodgson, E., and Casida, J. E. (1962). Mammalian enzymes involved in the degradation of 2,2-dichlorovinyl dimethyl phosphate. *J. Agric. Food Chem.* **10**, 208–214.

Hodgson, M. J., and Parkinson, D. (1985). Diagnosis of organophosphate intoxication. *N. Engl. J. Med.* **313**, 329.

Hoffman, D. G., Worth, H. M., and Anderson, R. C. (1968). Stimulation of hepatic microsomal drug-metabolizing enzymes by *a,a*-bis(*p*-chlorophenyl)-3-pyridine methanol and a method for determining no-effect levels in rats. *Toxicol. Appl. Pharmacol.* **12**, 464–472.

Hoffman, F., Schramm, T., and Lohs, K. (1973). Test of trichlorfon and dimethoate for tumor inhibitory effects in mice. *Arch. Geschwulstforsch.* **42**, 54–57 (in German).

Hoffman, L. J., Ford, I. M., and Menn, J. J. (1972). Dyfonate metabolism studies. I. Absorption, distribution, and excretion of *O*-ethyl-*S*-phenylethylphosphonothioate in rats. *Pestic. Biochem. Physiol.* **1**, 349–355.

Hollingworth, R. M., Fukuto, T. R., and Metcalf, R. L. (1967a). Selectivity of Sumithion compared with methyl parathion. Influence of structure on anticholinesterase activity. *J. Agric. Food Chem.* **15**, 235–241.

Hollingworth, R. M., Metcalf, R. L., and Fukuto, T. R. (1967b). The selectivity of Sumithion compared with methyl parathion. Metabolism in the white mouse. *J. Agric. Food Chem.* **15**, 242–249.

Hollingworth, R. M., Alstott, R. L., and Littenberg, R. D. (1973). Glutathione *S*-aryl transferase in the metabolism of parathion and its analogs. *Life Sci.* **13**, 191–199.

Hollwich, F., and Diekhues, B. (1974). Ocular light perception and metabolic activity of the liver. *Klin. Monatsbl. Augenheilkd.* **264**, Suppl., 449–452 (in German).

Holmes, J. H., and Gaon, M. D. (1956). Observations on acute and multiple exposure to anticholinesterase agents. *Trans. Am. Clin. Climatol. Assoc.* **68**, 86–101.

Holmes, J. H., Starr, H. G., Jr., Hanisch, R. C., and von Kaulla, K. N. (1974). Short-term toxicity of mevinphos in man. *Arch. Environ. Health* **29**, 84–89.

Holmstead, R. L., Fukuto, T. R., and March, R. B. (1973). The metabolism of *O*-(4-bromo-2,5-dichlorophenyl) *O*-methyl phenylphosphonothioate (leptophos) in white mice and cotton plants. *Arch. Environ. Contam. Toxicol.* **1**, 133–147.

Holmstedt, B. (1959). Pharmacology of organophosphorus cholinesterase inhibitors. *Pharmacol. Rev.* **11**, 567–588.

Holmstedt, B. (1963). Structure–activity relationship of the organophosphorus anticholinesterase agents. *Handb. Exp. Pharmacol.* **15**, Suppl., 428–485 (in German).

Holmstedt, B. (1971). Distribution and determination of cholinesterases in mammals. *Bull. W.H.O.* **44**, 99–107.

Holmstedt, B., Nordgren, I., Sandoz, M., and Sundwall, A. (1978). Metrifonate, summary of toxicological and pharmacological information available. *Arch. Toxicol.* **41**, 3–29.

Holtz, P., and Westermann, E. (1959). Poisoning and detoxication involving parathion and paraoxon. *Arch. Exp. Pathol. Pharmakol.* **23**, 211–221.

Hopmann, G., and Wanke, H. (1974). Maximum dose atropine treatment in severe organophosphate poisoning. *Dtsch. Med. Wochenschr.* **99**, 2106–2108.

Horiguchi, Y., Asanuma, N., Abe, E., Kurosawa, K., Sasaki, K., Suzuki, A. (1977). Effects of leptophos administered orally to mammals. *J. Jpn. Assoc. Rural Med.* **26**, 322–323.

Horiguchi, Y., Asanuma, N., Abe, E., Kurosawa, K., Sasaki, K., Suzuki, A., and Yanagisawa, T. (1978). Studies on the effects of organophosphorus pesticides to the central nerve system. Second report. *J. Jpn. Assoc. Rural Med.* **27**, 782–790.

Hosaka, Y., and Yamaura, A. (1976). Electroencephalograms in a case of acute fatal intoxication due to an organophosphorus pesticide. *Clin. Electroencephalogr.* **18**, 655–656.

Hosokawa, S., and Miyamoto, J. (1975). Effects of subchronic feeding of Sumithion, Sumioxon, and *p*-nitrocresol on rat liver oxidative phosphorylation and mixed function oxidases. *Bochu Kagaku* **40**, 33–38.

Hristic, B., and Milenkovic, D. (1961). Accidental poisonings by parathion introduced by the dermal route. *Arh. Hig. Rada Toksikol.* **12**, 185–189 (in French).

Huang, C. C. (1973). Effect on growth but not on chromosomes of the mammalian cells after treatment with three organophosphorus insecticides. *Proc. Soc. Exp. Biol. Med.* **142**, 36–40.

Huelse, M., and Federspil, P. (1975). Disturbances of equilibrium due to poisoning by organophosphorus insecticides. *HNO* **23**, 185–189 (in German).

Hughes, H. C., Jr., and Lang, C. M. (1973). Effect of orally administered dichlorvos on demodectic mange in the dog. *J. Am. Vet. Med. Assoc.* **163**, 142–143.

Hunter, C. G. (1969). Dermal toxicity of chlorfenvinphos (FVP). *Ind. Med. Surg.* **38**, 49–51.

Hunter, C. G., Robinson, J., Bedford, C. T., and Lawson, J. M. (1972). Exposure to chlorfenvinphos by determination of a urinary metabolite. *J. Occup. Med.* **14**, 119–122.

Husain, K., and Matin, M. A. (1986a). Cerebral glycolysis and glycogenolysis in Diazinon treated animals. *Arh. Hig. Rada Toksikol.* **37**, 29–34.

Husain, K., and Matin, M. A. (1986b). Changes in the level of glycogen and certain enzymes in malathion treated hyperglycaemic rats. *Adv. Biosc.* *(Muzaffarnagar, India)* **5**, 87–90.

Hussain, M. A., and Olloffs, P. C. (1979). Neurotoxic effects of leptophos (Phosvel) on chickens and rats following chronic low-level feeding. *J. Environ. Sci. Health* **14**, 367–382.

Hutson, D. H., and Hathway, D. E. (1967). Toxic effects of chlorfenvinphos in dogs and rats. *Biochem. Pharmacol.* **16**, 949–962.

Hutson, D. H., and Hoadley, E. C. (1972a). The comparative metabolism of (¹⁴C-vinyl) dichlorvos in animals and man. *Arch. Toxikol.* **30**, 9–18.

Hutson, D. H., and Hoadley, E. C. (1972b). The metabolism of (¹⁴C-methyl) dichlorvos in the rat and the mouse. *Xenobiotica* **2**, 107–116.

Hutson, D. H., Akintonwa, D. A. A., and Hathway, D. E. (1967). The metabolism of 2-chloro-1-(2,4′-dichlorophenyl) vinyldiethyl phosphate (chlorfenvinphos) in the dog and rat. *Biochem. J.* **102**, 133–142.

Hutson, D. H., Hoadley, E. C., and Pickering, B. A. (1971). The metabolic fate of (vinyl-1-¹⁴C) dichlorvos in the rat after oral and inhalation exposure. *Xenobiotica* **1**, 593–611.

Ikuta, S. (1973). A case of acute intoxication by an organophosphorus pesticide. *J. Jpn. Assoc. Rural Med.* **22**, 113 (in Japanese).

Imai, H. (1974a). Toxicity of organophosphorus pesticides (fenthion) on the retina. Electroretinographic and biochemical study. *J. Jpn. Ophthalmol. Soc.* **78**, 1–10 (in Japanese).

Imai, H. (1974b). Studies on the ocular toxicity of organophosphorus pesticides. Part I. Electroretinographic and biochemical study on rats after a single administration of fenthion. *J. Jpn. Ophthalmol. Soc.* **78**, 163–172 (in Japanese).

Imai, H., Miyata, M., and Ishikawa, T. (1973). Retinal disturbances in rats due to single-dose administration of an organophosphate pesticide, fenthion. *Prog. Med. (Tokyo)* **86**, 28–30 (in Japanese).

Imaizumi, K., Atsumi, K., Hatano, M., Ohara, Y., and Miyashita, H. (1973). Biochemical examination of eyes of rabbits intoxicated by organophosphorus pesticides. *Clin. Ophthalmol.* **27**, 1163 (in Japanese).

Imo, K. (1959). Management of a E605 poisoning with atropin and PAM. *Medizinische* No. 44, pp. 2114–2115 (in German).

Inoue, T., Horiue, T., Akiyama, K., Uehara, M., and Kuroda, M. (1979). An experience on treatment with hemoperfusion in intoxication due to thiometon. *J. Jpn. Soc. Int. Med.* **68**, 202.

International Union for Pure and Applied Chemistry (IUPAC) (1970). IUPAC tentative rules for the nomenclature of organic chemistry. Section E. Fundamental stereochemistry. *J. Org. Chem.* **35**, 2849–2867.

Introna, F. (1959). Acute poisoning by percutaneous absorption of E605. *Riv. Infort. Mal. Prof.* **46**, 1222–1231.

Irányi, J. (1975). Organophosphate-induced polyneuropathy. *Orv. Hetil.* **116**, 1572–1575.

Ishihara, O., Onuma, T., and Fukushima, H. (1974). A case of peripheral neuropathy by intoxication due to pesticide, trichlorfon. *Clin. Neurol. (Tokyo)* **14**, 57 (in Japanese).

Ishikawa, S. (1970). Ophthalmopathy by pesticides and its treatment with special reference to "Saku strange disease." *J. Ther.* **52**, 1840–1848.

Ishikawa, S., and Oto, K. (1970). On strange disease found among children in Saku district (Nagano Prefecture, Japan) with chief complaint of amblyopia. *Med. Bull. Wkly.* No. 2425, Oct. 17, pp. 8–15.

Ising, E. (1971). Residues of the thiophosphoric acid ester, bromophos (Cela) in guinea pig feces after oral administration. *Z. Angew. Zool.* **58**, 465–473 (in German).

Isoshima, T. (1960). Cholinesterase activity of blood in several mental disorders. *Shikoku Igaku Zasshi* **16**, Suppl., 839–854.

Itayama, T. (1978). On an accidental intoxication due to cooperative pesticide application in Nagasaki Prefecture. *Plant Prot. (Tokyo)* **32**, 525–526.

Ito, R., Kawamura, H., Chang, H. S., Toida, S., Matsu-ura, S., Sasaki, T., and Tanihata, T. (1972). Acute, subchronic, and chronic toxicity of *O,O,O',O'*-tetramethyl-*O,O'*-thio-di-*para*-phenylene phosphorothioate (Abate). *J. Med. Soc. Toho Univ.* **19**, 363–367 (in Japanese).

Iverson, F., Grant, D. L., and Lacroix, J. (1975). Diazinon metabolism in the dog. *Bull. Environ. Contam. Toxicol.* **13**, 611–618.

Ivey, M. C., Mann, H. D., Oehler, D. D., Claborn, H. V., Eschle, J. L., and Hogan, B. F. (1972). Chlorpyrifos and its oxygen analogue: Residues in the body tissues of dipped cattle. *J. Econ. Entomol.* **65**, 1647–1649.

Jablecki, C., Tisdale, W., and Schultz, P. (1983). Delayed organophosphorous neurotoxicity. *Muscle Nerve* **6**, 534.

Jackson, J. (1822). On a peculiar disease resulting from the use of ardent spirits. *N. Engl. J. Med. Surg.* **11**, 351–353.

James, K. A. C., and Austin, L. (1970). The effect of DFP on axonal transport of protein in chicken sciatic nerve. *Brain Res.* **18**, 192–194.

James, N. F., Machin, A. F., Quick, M. P., Rogers, H., Mundy, D. E., and Cross, A. J. (1973). Toxic metabolites of Diazinon in sheep. *J. Agric. Food Chem.* **21**, 121–124.

Jaques, R. (1964). The protective effect of pyridine-2-aldoxime methiodide (P₂AM), bis-[4-hydroxyimino-methyl-pyridinium-1-methyl]-ether dichloride (Toxogonin®) and atropine in experimental DDVP poisoning. *Helv. Physiol. Pharmacol. Acta* **22**, 174–183.

Jaques, R., and Bein, H. J. (1960). Toxicology and pharmacology of a new systemically acting insecticide of the phosphoric acid ester group. Phosphamidon (2-chloro-2-diethylcarbomyl-1-methylvinyl dimethyl phosphate). *Arch. Toxikol.* **18**, 316–330 (in German).

Jaros, F., and Kratinova, R. (1973). Acute poisoning by Birlan 24 EC with serious course cured after the application of TMB4. *Prac. Lek.* **25**, 152–155.

Jax, W., Eimermacher, H., Sturm, A., Jr., Eben, A., Hofmann, K., and Grabensee, B. (1977). New point of view in the treatment of alkylphosphate poisoning. *Intensivmedizin* **14**, 75–82 (in German).

Jedrzejowska, H., Rowinska-Marcinska, K., and Hoppe, B. (1980). Neuropathy due to phytosol (agitox): Report of a case. *Acta Neuropathol.* **49**, 163–168.

Jensen, J. A., Flury, V. P., and Schoof, H. F. (1965). Dichlorvos vapour disinfection of aircraft. *Bull. W.H.O.* **32**, 175–180.

Johannsen, F. R., and Knowles, C. (1970). Metabolism of *O*-(2,5-dichloro-4-iodophenyl) *O,O*-dimethyl phosphorothioate in rats and tomato plants. *J. Econ. Entomol.* **63**, 693–697.

Johns, R. J., Bales, P. D., and Himwich, H. E. (1951). The effects of DFP on the convulsant dose of theophylline, theophylline-ethylenediamine, and 8-chloro-theophylline. *J. Pharmacol. Exp. Ther.* **101**, 237–242.

Johnson, M. K. (1969a). A phosphorylation site in brain and the delayed neurotoxic effect of some organophosphorus compounds. *Biochem. J.* **111**, 487–495.

Johnson, M. K. (1969b). The delayed neurotoxic effect of some organophosphorus compounds: Identification of the phosphorylation site as an esterase. *Biochem. J.* **114**, 711–717.

Johnson, M. K. (1970). Organophosphorus and other inhibitors of brain "neurotoxic esterase" and the development of delayed neurotoxicity in hens. *Biochem. J.* **120**, 523–531.

Johnson, M. K. (1974). The primary biochemical lesion leading to the delayed neurotoxic effects of some organophosphorus esters. *J. Neurochem.* **23**, 785–789.

Johnson, M. K. (1975a). Structure–activity relationship for substrates and inhibitors of hen brain neurotoxic esterase. *Biochem. Pharmacol.* **221**, 797–805.

Johnson, M. K. (1975b). The delayed neuropathy caused by some organophosphorus esters: Mechanism and challenge. *CRC Crit. Rev. Toxicol.* **3**, 289–316.

Johnson, M. K. (1975c). Organophosphorus esters causing delayed neurotoxic effects. Mechanism of action and structure/activity studies. *Arch. Toxicol.* **34**, 259–288.

Johnson, M. K. (1977). Improved assay of neurotoxic esterase for screening organophosphates for delayed neurotoxicity potential. *Arch. Toxicol.* **37**, 113–115.

Johnson, M. K. (1978). The anomalous behavior of dimethyl phosphates in the biochemical test for delayed neurotoxicity. *Arch. Toxicol.* **41**, 107–110.

Johnson, M. K. (1981). Initiation of organophosphate neurotoxicity. *Toxicol. Appl. Pharmacol.* **61**, 480–481.

Johnson, M. K. (1987). Receptor or enzyme: The puzzle of NTE and organophosphate-induced delayed neuropathy. *Trends Pharmacol. Sci.* **8**, 174–179.

Johnson, M. K., and Barnes, J. M. (1970). Age and the sensitivity of chicks to the delayed neurotoxic effects of some organophosphorus compounds. *Biochem. Pharmacol.* **19**, 3045–3047.

Johnson, M. K., and Lauwerys, R. (1969). Protection by some carbamates against the delayed neurotoxic effects of diisopropyl phosphorofluoridate. *Nature (London)* **222**, 1066–1067.

Jonecko, U., and Jonecko, A. (1973). Histochemical and histological studies of severe experimental poisoning with organophosphoric compound Metasystox (Bayer). *Folia Histochem. Cytochem.* **10**, 201.

Jordanova, E., Dochovskiy, D., Mishkova, R., Perfanov, K., and Kapralov, G. (1974). Hematologic and enzyme examinations in agricultural workers with acute intrathion intoxication. *Vutr. Boles.* **13**, 59–62 (in Bulgarian).

Jordi, A. W. (1952). Acute poisoning by tricresylphosphate. *J. Aviat. Med.* **23**, 623–625.

Jorgenson, T. A., Rushbrook, C. J., and Newell, G. W. (1976). *In vivo* mutagenesis investigations of ten commercial pesticides. *Toxicol. Appl. Pharmacol.* **37**, 109.

Joubert, J., and Joubert, P. H. (1984). Acute organophosphate poisoning presenting with choreo-athetosis. *Clin. Toxicol.* **22**, 187–191.

Jovic, R., Bachelard, H. S., Clark, A. G., and Nicholas, P. C. (1971). Effects of soman and DFP *in vivo* and *in vitro* on cerebral metabolism in the rat. *Biochem. Pharmacol.* **20**, 519–527.

Juhl, E. (1971). Deaths from phosphostigmine poisoning in Denmark. An analysis of the medico-social and medico-legal aspects. *Dan. Med. Bull.* **18**, Suppl. 1, 1–112.

Jusic, A., and Milic, S. (1978). Neuromuscular synapse testing in two cases of suicidal organophosphorus pesticide poisoning. *Arch. Environ. Health* **33**, 240–243.

Kabrawala, V. N., Shah, R. M., and Oza, G. G. (1965). Diazinon poisoning (a study of 25 cases). *Indian Pract.* **18**, 711–717.

Kadota, T., Koda, H., and Miyamoto, J. (1975a). Subchronic toxicity studies of Sumithion, Sumioxon, and *p*-nitrocresol in rats, and 92-week feeding study of Sumithion with special reference to change of cholinesterase activity. *Sci. Pest Control* **40**, 38–48.

Kadota, T., Okuna, Y., and Miyamoto, J. (1975b). Acute oral toxicity and delayed neurotoxicity of 5 organophosphorus compounds, Salithion, Cyanox, Surecide, Sumithion, and Sumioxon in adult hens. *Sci. Pest Control* **40**, 49–53.

Kagan, Y. S. (1956). Problems of industrial health in connection with the use of the new organic phosphorus derivative "mercaptophos" as an insecticide in agriculture. *Kiev (Ser. 'Obmen Opytom')* No. 55.

Kagan, Y. S. (1957a). Work hygiene in the use of systemic organophosphorus insecticides. First communication. *Gig. Sanit.* 22(7), 15–22.

Kagan, Y. S. (1957b). Experimental data on the toxicology of organophosphorus insecticides and on the therapy of poisonings with them. *Farmakol. Toksikol.* 2, 49–52.

Kagan, Y. S., Kundiev, Y. I., and Trotsenko, M. A. (1958). Work hygiene in the use of systemic organophosphorus insecticides. Second communication. *Gig. Sanit.* 23(6), 25–32.

Kaiser, H. (1953). The first fatal "Systox" poisoning. *Dtsch. Apoth.-Ztg.* 93, 41–42 (in German).

Kalas, D. (1978). Light group poisoning by metathion E-50 inhalation when spraying by means of aircraft. *Prac. Lek.* 30, 145–147.

Kalow, W., and Davies, R. O. (1958). The activity of various esterase inhibitors towards atypical serum cholinesterase. *Biochem. Pharmacol.* 1, 183–192.

Kalow, W., and Genest, K. (1957). A method for the detection of atypical forms of human serum cholinesterases. Determination of dibucaine numbers. *Can. J. Biochem. Physiol.* 35, 339–346.

Kalow, W., and Marton, A. (1961). Second-generation toxicity of malathion in rats. *Nature (London)* 192, 464–465.

Kalow, W., and Staron, N. (1957). On the distribution and inheritance of atypical forms of human serum cholinesterase as indicated by dibucaine numbers. *Can. J. Biochem. Physiol.* 35, 1305–1320.

Kaloyanova-Simenova, F. P. (1970). Prevention of intoxication by pesticides in Bulgaria. *In* "Rural Medicine—Whither Rural Medicine?" (H. Kuroiwa *et al.,* eds.), pp. 35–37. Jpn. Assoc. Rural Med., Tokyo.

Kamataki, T., and Neal, R. A. (1976). Metabolism of diethyl *p*-nitrophenol phosphorothionate (parathion) by a reconstituted mixed-function oxidase enzyme system: Studies of the covalent binding of the sulfur atom. *Mol. Pharmacol.* 12, 933–944.

Kamataki, T., Lee Lin, M. C. M., Belcher, D. H., and Neal, R. A. (1976). Studies of the metabolism of parathion with an apparently homogenous preparation of rabbit liver cytochrome P-450. *Drug Metab. Dispos.* 4, 180–189.

Kamath, P. G., Dagli, A. J., and Patel, B. M. (1964). Diazinon poisoning, a report of 25 cases. *J. Assoc. Physicians India* 12, 477–481.

Kamel, S. H., E-Gruindi, M. M., and Shaban, F. E. (1973). Toxicological studies of phosvel (V.C.S.) in mammals). *Eur. J. Toxicol.* 6, 70–80.

Kanagaratnam, K., Boon, W. H., and Hoh, T. K. (1960). Parathion poisoning from contaminated barley. *Lancet* 1, 538–542.

Kanda, M., and Matsushima, S. (1974). A case of acute fenthion poisoning. *Annu. Rep. Jpn. Inst. Rural Med.* 3, 50–53.

Kane, P. F. (1958). "The Normal Variation in the Interpretation of Blood Cholinesterase Activity," Rep. No. 2662. Chemagro Corporation Research Dept. (cited by Gage, 1967).

Kanoh, S., Ema, M., and Itami, T. (1979). Studies on the relationship between fetal toxicity and maternal functions. 2. Effect of P-450. *Teratology* 20, 172–173.

Kaplanis, J. N., Louloudes, S. J., and Roan, C. C. (1962). The distribution and excretion of P^{32}-labeled diazinon in guinea pigs. *Trans. Kans. Acad. Sci.* 65, 70–75.

Kar, P. P., and Matin, M. A. (1971). Duration of diazinon induced changes in the brain acetylcholine of rats. *Pharmacol. Res. Commun.* 3, 351–354.

Karalliedde, L., and Senanayake, N. (1988). Acute organophosphorous insecticide poisoning in Sri Lanka. *Forensic Sci. Int.* 36, 97–100.

Karimov, A. M. (1979). A case of toxiderma induced by the pesticide Anthio. *Vestn. Dermatol. Venerol.* 6, 40–41 (in Russian).

Karimov, V. A. (1974). Role of vitamin C and B1 in therapy of chronic poisoning with pesticides. *Med. Zh. Uzb.* 2, 6–12 (in Russian).

Karlog, O., Nimb, M., and Poulsen, E. (1958). Parathion (Bladan) poisoning treated with 2-PAM (pyridyl-(2)-aldoxime-*N*-methyliodide. *Ugeskr. Laeg.* 120, 177–183 (in German).

Karnik, V. M., Ichaporia, R. N., and Wadis, R. S. (1970). Cholinesterase levels in diazinon poisoning. I. Relation to severity of poisoning. *J. Assoc. Physicians India* 18, 337–344.

Karzcmar, A. G., Awad, O., and Blachut, K. (1962). Toxicity arising from joint intravenous administration of EPN and malathion to dogs. *Toxicol. Appl. Pharmacol.* 4, 133–147.

Kashlan, K. M., and Wagih, I. M. (1969). Patterns of deaths due to toxic agents in Cairo. *J. Egypt. Med. Assoc.* 52, 407–420.

Kashyap, S. K., and Gupta, S. K. (1976). Effect of ultra low-volume aerial spray of phosphamidon (organophosphorus insecticide) on human volunteers: A field surveillance study. *Indian J. Med. Res.* 64, 579–583.

Katja, W., Pleština, R., and Svetličoć, B. (1973). Blood cholinesterase activity of workers exposed to the organophosphorus insecticide Ekatin. *Arh. Hig. Rada Toksikol.* 24, 107–116 (in Serbo-Croatian).

Kato, R., Chiesara, E., and Frontino, G. (1962). Influence of sex difference on the pharmacological action and metabolism of some drugs. *Biochem. Pharmacol.* 11, 221–227.

Kato, R., Takanaka,. A., and Omori, Y. (1967). Factors affecting toxicity and metabolism of OMPA (octamethylpyrophosphoramide) in rats. *Jpn. J. Pharmacol.* 17, 509–518.

Kato, S. (1971). Summary on the ophthalmologic examinations among pupils in Nagano Prefecture. *Nagano Med. Gaz.* Feb. 15, pp. 1–4.

Kats, P. D., and Gabuchiya, A. K. (1964). Activity of cholinesterase in the blood of healthy children. *Izv. Akad. Nauk Az. SSR, Ser. Biol. Nauk* 5, 109–111.

Kaufman, K. (1954). Serum cholinesterase activity in the normal individual and in people with liver disease. *Ann. Intern. Med.* 41, 533–545.

Kaufman, L., Lehmann, H., and Silk, E. (1960). Suxamethonium apnoea in an infant. Expression of familial pseudocholinesterase deficiency in three generations. *Br. Med. J.* 1, 166–167.

Kaufman, P. L., and Axelsson, U. (1975). Induction of subcapsular cataracts in aniridic vervet monkeys by echothiopate. *Invest. Ophthalmol.* 14, 863–866.

Kawai, M., and Naito, M. (1974). Experimental studies on ocular disturbances due to organophosphorus pesticide. *J. Jpn. Assoc. Rural Med.* 23, 543–544 (in Japanese).

Kawamura, A., Ogata, S., Shigeno, K., Nishimura, M., Someya, N., and Ueda, K. (1974). On the effects of long term administration of an organophosphorus pesticide to male beagles. *Jpn. J. Hyg.* 29, 216 (in Japanese).

Kawashiro, I. (1959). Organophosphorus compounds. *WHO Inf. Circ. Toxic. Pestic. Man* No. 3, p. 4.

Kay, K., Monkman, L., Windish, J. P., Doherty, T., Pare, J., and Racicot, C. (1952). Parathion exposure and cholinesterase response of Quebec apple growers. *Arch. Ind. Hyg. Occup. Med.* 6, 252–262.

Kaye, S. (1970). Patterns of poisoning in Puerto Rico. *Bol. Asoc. Med. P. R.* 62, 18–21.

Kazakevich, R. L., and Shamrai, L. M. (1977). State of the nervous system after acute chlorphos poisoning. *Zh. Nevropatol. Psikhiatr.* 77, 207–210.

Kazakevich, R. L., Parkhomov, A. A., and Gorenshteyn, G. S. (1972). On complications occurring following acute poisoning with trichlorfon. *Vrach. Delo* 10, 134–136 (in Russian).

Keasling, H. H., Schooley, M. A., Collins, J. A., and Brown, L. J. (1974). Dichlorvos and the litter weight response. *J. Anim. Sci.* 39, 184.

Kelemen, M. H., and Volle, R. L. (1965). Protective action of thiouracil against the acute toxicity to mice of *O*-ethyl *O*-(4-nitrophenyl) phenylphosphonothioate (EPN). *Toxicol. Appl. Pharmacol.* 7, 418–424.

Kenaga, E. E., and Allison, W. E. (1969). Commercial and experimental organic insecticides. *Bull. Entomol. Soc. Am.* 15, 85–148.

Kennedy, G. L., Frawley, J. P., and Calandra, J. C. (1973). Multigeneration reproductive effects of three pesticides in rats. *Toxicol. Appl. Pharmacol.* 25, 589–596.

Kessler, H., and Mracek, J. F. (1973). Nonfatal accidental organophosphate pesticide intoxication in seven inmates of a correctional institution. *J. Med. Assoc. State Ala.* 42, 775–781.

Kewitz, H. (1957). A specific antidote against lethal alkyl phosphate intoxication. III. Repair of chemical lesion. *Arch. Biochem. Biophys.* 66, 263–270.

Khaitov, R. K., Baymuradov, T. B., and Kadyrov, U. S. (1971). The toxic effect of organophosphorus pesticides on animals. *Veterinariya (Moscow)* 47(4), 81–82.

Khaitov, R. K., Shevchenko, N. K., Baymuradov, T. B., and Khaitov, V. R. (1976). Sanitary-toxicological appraisal of products from cattle poisoned by Anthio. *Veterinariya (Moscow)* **3**, 105–107 (in Russian).

Khandekar, J. D. (1971). Organophosphate poisoning. *JAMA, J. Am. Med. Assoc.* **217**, 1864.

Khasanov, V. K., and Li, A. P. (1970). Experience in studying blood cholinesterase activities as an index of the effect of organophosphorus compounds on the population's health. *Med. Zh. Uzb.* **7**, 12–13 (in Russian).

Khera, K. S. (1979). Teratogenicity evaluation of commercial formulation of dimethoate (Cygon 4E) in the cat and rat. *Toxicol. Appl. Pharmacol.* **48**, A34.

Khera, K. S., and Bedok, S. (1967). Effects of thiol phosphates on notochordal and vertebral morphogenesis in chick and duck embryos. *Food Cosmet. Toxicol.* **5**, 359–365.

Khera, K. S., La Ham, Q. N., and Grice, H. C. (1965a). Toxic effects induced by inoculation of EPN and Systox into duck eggs. *Toxicol. Appl. Pharmacol.* **7**, 488.

Khera, K. S., La Ham, Q. N., and Grice, H. C. (1965b). Toxic effects in ducklings hatched from embryos inoculated with EPN or Systox. *Food Cosmet. Toxicol.* **3**, 581–586.

Khera, K. S., La Ham, Q. N., Ellis, C. F. G., Zawidzka, Z. Z., and Grice, H. C. (1966). Foot deformity in ducks from injection of EPN during embryogenesis. *Toxicol. Appl. Pharmacol.* **8**, 540–549.

Khera, K. S., Whalen, C. Angers, G., and Trivett, G. (1979a). Assessment of the teratogenic potential of piperonyl butoxide, biphenyl, and phosalone in the rat. *Toxicol. Appl. Pharmacol.* **47**, 353–358.

Khera, K. S., Whalen, C., Trivett, G., and Angers, G. (1979b). Teratogenicity studies on pesticidal formulations of dimethoate, diuron and lindane in rats. *Bull. Environ. Contam. Toxicol.* **22**, 522–529.

Kidd, J. G., and Langworthy, O. R. (1933). Jake paralysis. Paralysis following the ingestion of Jamaica ginger extract adulterated with tri-*ortho*-cresyl phosphate. *Bull. Johns Hopkins Hosp.* **52**, 39–66.

Kim, A. S., Aminov, K. A., and Zaitsev, A. A. (1967). Psychosis with poisoning by fenthion and hexachlorane. *Nauchn. Tr., Samark. Med. Inst.* **37**, 282–287.

Kim, J. S., Lee, H. H., Kim, H. Y., Hong, W. P., and Lee, B. H. (1970). Clinical observations on parathion intoxication in 52 cases. *Korean J. Intern. Med.* **13**, 73–79.

Kim, Y. I., Whang, D. W., Nam, Y. I., Lee, C. H., Lee, H. C., Park, M. H., and Park, H. S. (1977). Study on liver injury in acute drug intoxication. *Korean J. Intern. Med.* **20**, 146–152.

Kimbrough, R. D., and Gaines, T. B. (1968). Effect of organic phosphorus compounds and akylating agents on the rat fetus. *Arch. Environ. Health* **16**, 805–808.

Kimmerle, G. (1976). Subchronic inhalation toxicity of azinphos-methyl in rats. *Arch. Toxicol.* **35**, 83–89.

Kinebuchi, H., and Konno, N. (1977). Neurotoxicity of leptophos administered at intervals in a divided threshold dose. *J. Jpn. Assoc. Rural Med.* **26**, 320–321.

Kinebuchi, H., and Konno, N. (1978). Increase and decrease of the neurotoxicity of leptophos, caused by administration of a critical dose in divided amounts. *Jpn. J. Public Health* **25**, 393–397.

Kinebuchi, H., Konno, N., and Yamauchi, T. (1976). Ascending paralysis in domestic fowls due to Phosvel, an organophosphorus pesticide. *J. Jpn. Assoc. Rural Med.* **25**, 514–515.

Kinebuchi, H., Konno, N., Yamauchi, T., Kaneda, M., and Sasaki, K. (1977). Delayed neurotoxicity caused by divided administration of critical doses of an organophosphorus insecticide, Phosvel (leptophos). *Prog. Med. (Tokyo)* **101**, 837–838.

Kinkel, J., Muacevic, G., Sehring, R., and Bodenstein, G. (1966). Toxicity of bromophos (*O,O*-dimethyl-*O*-(4-bromo-2,5-dichlorophenyl)-phosphorothioate). *Arch. Toxikol.* **22**, 36–57.

Kirichek, L. T., and Kharchenko, N. S. (1968). The cumulative properties of chlorophos. *Farmakol. Toksikol. (Moscow)* **31**, 497–500 (in Russian).

Kirkland, V. L., Albert, J. R., and VanKampen, K. (1974). Studies on dichlorvos-induced intestinal enteritis in the dog. *Toxicol. Appl. Pharmacol.* **29**, 136.

Kito, S. (1970). Neurological observation of children with complaints of visual disorders. *Prog. Med. (Tokyo)* **75**, 303–304.

Klein, H. (1956). The special glands in E605 poisoning. *Dtsch. Z. Gesamte Gerichtl. Med.* **45**, 510–515 (in German).

Kleinman, G. D. (1960). Occupational disease in California attributed to pesticides and agricultural chemicals. *Arch. Environ. Health* **1**, 118–124.

Klemmer, H. W., Reichert, E. R., Yauger, W. L., and Haley, T. J. (1978). Five cases of intentional ingestion of 25 percent diazinon with treatment and recovery. *Clin. Toxicol.* **12**, 435–444.

Kligman, A. M. (1966). The identification of contact allergens by human assay. III. A maximization test: A procedure for screening and rating contact sensitizers. *J. Invest. Dermatol.* **47**, 393–409.

Klimková-Deutschová, E. (1959). Neurological troubles resulting from insecticides. *Prakt. Lek.* **39**, 976.

Klimmer, O. R., and Pfaff, W. (1955). Comparative investigations of the toxicity of organic thiophosphate esters. *Arzneim.-Forsch.* **5**, 626–630.

Klimmer, O. R., and Pfaff, W. (1958). Toxicological investigation involving the practical application of the systemic insecticide, *O,O*-dimethyl-(ethylthioethyl)-thiophosphate. *Arzneim.-Forsch.* **8**, 365–369 (in German).

Klonglan, E. D., Denny, G. H., and Morris, J. F. (1956). "A Study of the Variation of Human Blood Cholinesterases," Res. Rep. No. 109. Dugway Proving Ground, Utah.

Klose, R., and Gutensohn, G. (1976). Treatment of an alkylphosphate poisoning with purified serum cholinesterase. *Prakt. Anaesth.* **11**, 1–7.

Klotzsche, C. (1955). On the toxicology of the newer insecticidal phosphoric acid esters. *Arzneim.-Forsch.* **5**, 436–439 (in German).

Klotzsche, C. (1958a). New insecticides. Phosphoric and phosphonic acid esters. *Nachr. Deutsch. Pflanzenschutzd.* **10**, 60–63 (in German).

Klotzsche, C. (1958b). Thiometon, a new systemic phosphoric acid ester. *Mitt. Geb. Lebensmittelunters. Hyg.* **49**, 72–77 (in German).

Klotzsche, C. (1961). Formothion, a new systemic organic phosphorus ester of low toxicity. *Mitt. Geb. Lebensmittelunters. Hyg.* **52**, 340–349.

Klotzsche, C. (1966). Toxicologic studies with a systemic phosphoric acid ester, formothion. *Int. Arch. Gewerbepathol. Gewerbehyg.* **22**, 246–261.

Klotzsche, C. (1970). Teratological and embryotoxic studies with formothion and thiometon. *Pharm. Acta Helv.* **45**, 434–440 (in German).

Klugman, H. B. (1959). Parathion poisoning. *S. Afr. Med. J.* **33**, 899–901.

Knaak, J. B., and O'Brien, R. D. (1960). Effect of EPN on *in vivo* metabolism of malathion by the rat and dog. *J. Agric. Food Chem.* **8**, 198–203.

Knaak, J. B., Maddy, K. T., Gallo, M. A., Lillie, D. T., Craine, E. M., and Serat, W. F. (1978a). Worker reentry study involving phosalone application to citrus groves. *Toxicol. Appl. Pharmacol.* **46**, 363–374.

Knaak, J. B., Peoples, S. A., Jackson, T. J., Fredrickson, A. S., Enos, R., Maddy, K. T., Bailey, J. B., Duesch, M. E., Gunther, F. A., and Winterlin, W. L. (1978b). Reentry problems involving the use of dialifor on grapes in the San Joaquin valley of California. *Arch. Environ. Contam. Toxicol.* **7**, 465–481.

Knolle, J. (1970). Suicidal poisoning by subcutaneous injection of a mixture of parathion and demcton-*O*-methylsulfoxide (E 605 MR). *Arch. Toxikol.* **26**, 29–39 (in German).

Knowles, C. O., and Arthur, B. W. (1966). Metabolism of and residues associated with dermal and intramuscular application of radiolabeled fenthion to diary cows. *J. Econ. Entomol.* **59**, 1346–1352.

Knox, B., Askaa, J., Basse, A., Bitsch, V., Eskildsen, M., Mandrup, M., Ottosen, H. E., Overby, E., Pedersen, K. B., and Rasmussen, F. (1978). Congenital ataxia and tremor with cerebellar hypoplasia in piglets borne by sows treated with Neguvon® vet. (*Metrifonate, Trichlorfon*) during pregnancy. *Nord. Veterinaermed.* **30**, 538–545.

Kobayashi, O., Ohishi, I., and Kume, S. (1964). Anthelmintic effect of the organophosphorus preparation JSR-381 on intestinal parasites of dogs. *J. Jpn. Vet. Med. Assoc.* **17**, 465–471.

Kocher, C., and Treboux, J. (1957). The insecticidal effect of diazinon and its dependence on concentration. *Ans. Schadlingskd.* **30**, 104.

Kodama, J. K., Horse, M. S., Anderson, H. H., Dunlap, M. K., and Hine, C. H. (1954). Comparative toxicity of two vinyl-substituted phosphates. *Arch. Ind. Hyg. Occup. Med.* **9**, 45–61.

Koeffler, H. (1958). Acute E605 poisoning by percutaneous absorption of the poison. *Med. Klin. (Munich)* **53**, 749–751.

Koelle, G. B., ed. (1963). Cholinesterases and anticholinesterase agents. *Handb. Exp. Pharmacol.* **15** (in German).

Koelle, G. B., and Gilman, A. (1946). The chronic toxicity of diisopropyl fluorophosphate (DFP) in dogs, monkeys, and rats. *J. Pharmacol. Exp. Ther.* **87**, 435–447.

Koelle, G. B., Davis, R., Diliberto, E. J., Jr., and Koelle, W. A. (1974). Selective, near-total, irreversible inactivation of peripheral pseudocholinesterase and acetylcholinesterase in cats *in vivo. Biochem. Pharmacol.* **23**, 175–188.

Kohli, J. D., Hasan, M. Z., and Gupta, B. N. (1974). Dermal absorption of fenitrothion in rat. *Bull. Environ. Contam. Toxicol.* **11**, 285–290.

Kohn, F. E. (1962). "Research Report on Dibrom." Report to the Ortho Division, California Chemical Company.

Koller, L. D., Exon, J. H., and Roan, J. G. (1976). Immunological surveillance and toxicity in mice exposed to the organophosphate pesticide, leptophos. *Environ. Res.* **12**, 238–242.

Kolosovskaya, V. M. (1971). Alterations of some indices of serotonin metabolism and of cholinesterase activity under conditions of a curative effect of different doses of chlorophos. *Zdravookhr. Beloruss.* **17**, 54–56 (in Russian).

Kondo, K., Korokuma, M., and Takahasi, K. (1973). A case of acute intoxication by a pesticide. *J. Jpn. Assoc. Rural Med.* **22**, 123 (in Japanese).

Konno, N., and Kinebuchi, H. (1978a). Residues of phosvel in plasma and in adipose tissues of hens after single oral administration. *Toxicol. Appl. Pharmacol.* **45**, 541–547.

Konno, N., and Kinebuchi, H. (1978b). Phosvel level in blood and adipose tissue of hens after a single oral dose. *Jpn. J. Public Health* **25**, 1–5.

Konno, N., Kinebuchi, H., Yamauchi, T., Kaneda, M., and Sasaki, K. (1977). Effects of aging on residues of phosvel (leptophos) in adipose tissue. *Prog. Med. (Tokyo)* **101**, 896–898 (in Japanese).

Konno, N., Fukuto, T. R., and Imamura, T. (1984). Lung injury and delayed toxicity produced by *O,O,S*-trimethyl phosphorodithioate, an impurity of malathion. *Toxicol. Appl. Pharmacol.* **75**, 219–228.

Kono, K., Ishikawa, S., and Uga, S. (1975). Impairment of optic nerve and peripheral nerve in chronic organophosphorus intoxication. *Jpn. J. Clin. Ophthalmol.* **69**, 969–971 (in Japanese).

Konyukhov, A. F., Poloz, D. D., and Kokhtyuk, F. P. (1974). Metabolism of formothion in chickens. *Veterinariia* **4**, 108–109.

Koopman, J. P., Henderson, P. T., Cools, A. R., and Braak, G. J. (1977). Possible side effects of the use of diazinon to control insects in a central animal laboratory. *Z. Versuchstierkd.* **19**, 253–259.

Kosik, V. N. (1968). Chlorphos poisoning at home complicated by polyneuritis. *Vrach. Delo* **8**, 133–134 (in Russian).

Kotlarek-Haus, S., Dzierzkowa-Borodej, W., and Lawinska, B. (1971). Autoimmune hemolytic anemia after handling insecticides and herbicides with simultaneous detection of the Australia antigen (Au I) in the serum. *Folia Haematol. (Leipzig)* **95**, 249–253 (in German).

Kramer, J. P. (1972). Acute parathion poisoning in an adolescent. *Del. Med. J.* **44**, 31–35.

Krause, W., and Homola, S. (1972). The influence of DDVP (dichlorvos) on spermatogenesis. *Arch. Dermatol. Forsch.* **244**, 439–441 (in German).

Krause, W., and Homola, S. (1974). Alterations of the seminiferous epithelium and the Leydig cells of the rat testis after the application of dichlorvos (DDVP). *Bull. Environ. Contam. Toxicol.* **11**, 429–433.

Krivoy, W. A., and Wills, J. H. (1956). Adaptation to constant concentrations of acetylcholine. *J. Pharmacol. Exp. Ther.* **116**, 220–226.

Kronevi, T. (1977). Neguvon treatment of pregnant sows as a possible cause of cerebellar hypoplasia in piglets. *Sven. Vet. Tidn.* **29**, 931–932.

Kubistova, J. (1959). Parathion metabolism in female rat. *Arch. Int. Pharmacodyn. Ther.* **118**, 308–315.

Kur, D. A. (1974). Biological action of organophosphorus pesticides as a function of their chemical structures. *Med. Zh. Uzb.* **2**, 3–6 (in Russian).

Kutty, K. M., Jacob, J. C., Hutton, C. J., Davis, P. J., and Peterson, S. C. (1975). Serum beta-lipoproteins: Studies in a patient and in guinea pigs after the ingestion of organophosphorus compounds. *Clin. Biochem. (Ottawa)* **8**, 379–383.

Kutz, F. W., and Strassman, S. C. (1977). Human urinary metabolites of organophosphate insecticides following mosquito adulticiding. *Mosq. News* **37**, 211–218.

Kutz, N. (1977). Chemotherapy of schistosomiasis mansoni. *Adv. Pharmacol. Chemother.* **14**, 1–70.

Lalli, G., and Cascino, L. (1961). Modification of plasma and erythrocyte cholinesterase activity in subjects undergoing muscular effort carried to exhaustion. *World Aviat. Space Med. Congr., 2nd, 1959*, Part 1, Relaz., pp. 173–180.

Lancaster, M. C. (1960). A note on the demyelination produced in hens by dialkylfluoridates. *Br. J. Pharmacol. Chemother.* **15**, 279–281.

Lanyi, I., and Horvath, L. (1966). The treatment of Wofatox poisoning in children. *Orv. Hetil.* **107**, 2004–2006 (in Hungarian).

Lapushkov, A. G. (1973). Treatment of trichlorfon poisoning in animals. *Veterinarria* **11**, 96–97.

Larini, L., Camargo, L. A. A., Saad, W. A., and Bareicha, I. (1970). Determination of the dermal LD50 of *O,O*-dimethyl-*O*-(3-methyl-4-nitrophenyl) phosphorthioate in the rat. *Rev. Fac. Farm. Odontol. Araraquara* **4**, 61–71 (in Portuguese).

Laskowski, M. B., and Dettbarn, W.-D. (1977). The pharmacology of experimental myopathies. *Annu. Rev. Pharmacol. Toxicol.* **17**, 387–409.

Laskowski, M. B., Olson, W. H., and Dettbarn, W.-D. (1976). Motor endplate degeneration coincident with cholinesterase inhibition and increased frequency of miniature end-plate potentials. *Fed. Proc., Fed. Am. Soc. Exp. Biol.* **35**, 800.

Lawley, P. D., Shah, S. A., and Orr, D. J. (1974). Methylation of nucleic acids by 2,2-dichlorovinyl dimethyl phosphate (dichlorvos, DDVP). *Chem.-Biol. Interact.* **8**, 171–182.

Laws, E. R., Jr. (1966). Route of absorption of DDVP after oral administration to rats. *Toxicol. Appl. Pharmacol.* **8**, 193–196.

Laws, E. R., Jr., Morales, F. R., Hayes, W. J., Jr., and Joseph, C. R. (1967). Toxicology of Abate in volunteers. *Arch. Environ. Health* **14**, 289–291.

Laws, E. R., Jr., Sedlak, V. A., Miles, J. W., Joseph, C. R., Lacomba, J. R., and Rivera, A. D. (1968). Field study of the safety of Abate for treating potable water and observations on the effectiveness of a control programme involving both Abate and malathion. *Bull. W.H.O.* **38**, 439–445.

Leary, J. S., Hirsch, L., Lavor, E. M., Feichtmeir, E., Schulta, D., Koos, B., Roan, C. R., Fontenot, C., and Hine, C. H. (1971). An evaluation of the safety of NO-PEST® Strip insecticide with special reference to respiratory and dietary exposure of occupants of homes in Arizona. *Toxicol. Appl. Pharmacol.* **19**, 379.

Leary, J. S., Keane, W. T., Fontenot, C., Feichmier, E. F., Schultz, D., Koos, B. A., Hirsch, L., Lavor, E. M., Roan, C. C., and Hine, C. H. (1974). Safety evaluation in the home of polyvinyl chloride resin strip containing dichlorvos (DDVP). *Arch. Environ. Health* **29**, 308–314.

LeBlanc, F. N., Benson, B. E., and Gilg, A. D. (1986). A severe organophosphate poisoning requiring the use of an atropine drip. *Clin. Toxicol.* **24**, 69–75.

Lebrun, R., and Cerf, C. (1960). Preliminary note on the toxicity for man of an organophosphorus insecticide (Dipterex). *Bull. W.H.O.* **22**, 579–582 (in French).

Lee, P. W., Allahyari, R., and Fukuto, T. R. (1976). Stereospecificity in the metabolism of the chiral isomers of fonofos by mouse liver microsomal mixed function oxidase. *Biochem. Pharmacol.* **25**, 2671–2674.

Lee, P. W., Allahyari, R., and Fukuto, T. R. (1978a). Studies on the chiral isomers of fonofos and fonofos oxon. I. Toxicity and antiesterase activities. *Pestic. Biochem. Physiol.* **8**, 146–157.

Lee, P. W., Allahyari, R., and Fukuto, T. R. (1978b). Studies on the chiral isomers of fonofos and fonofos oxon. II. *In vitro* metabolism. *Pestic. Biochem. Physiol.* **8**, 158–169.

Lee, P. W., Allahyari, R., and Fukuto, T. R. (1978c). Studies on the chiral isomers of fonofos and fonofos oxon. III. *In vivo* metabolism. *Pestic. Biochem. Physiol.* **9**, 23–32.

Lehman, A. J. (1951). Chemicals in foods: A report to the Association of Food and Drug Officials on current developments. *Q. Bull.—Assoc. Food Drug Off.* **15**(I), 122–125.

Lehman, A. J. (1952). Chemicals in foods: A report to the Association of Food and Drug Officials on current developments. *Q. Bull.—Assoc. Food Drug Off.* **16**(II), 3–9; (III), 47–53; (IV), 85–91; (V), 126–132.

Lehman, A. J. (1965). "Summaries of Pesticide Toxicity." Association of Food and Drug Officials of the United States, Topeka, Kansas.

Lehman, H., and Liddell, J. (1969). Human cholinesterase (pseudocholinesterase): Genetic variants and their recognition. *Br. J. Anaesth.* **41**, 235–244.

Leonard, A. (1976). Heritable chromosome aberrations in mammals after exposure to chemicals. *Radiat. Environ. Biophys.* **13**, 1–8.

Leopold, I. H. (1965). Cholinergic and anticholinesterase agents in glaucoma therapy. *Trans. Pac. Coast Oto-Ophthalmol. Soc.* **49**, 25–42.

Leopold, I. H., and Comroe, J. H. (1946). Effect of diisopropyl fluorophosphate ("DFP") on the normal eye. *Arch. Ophthalmol. (Chicago)* **36**, 17–32.

Leopold, I. H., and McDonald, P. R. (1948). Diisopropyl fluorophosphate (DFP) in treatment of glaucoma. *Arch. Ophthalmol. (Chicago)* **40**, 176–188.

Leshev, V. V., Kan, P. T., and Talanov, G. A. (1972). Excretion of Dursban and diazinon in milk. *Veterinarria* **10**, 114–115.

Levine, B. S., and Murphy, S. D. (1977a). Esterase inhibition and reactivation in relation to piperonyl butoxide–phosphorothionate interactions. *Toxicol. Appl. Pharmacol.* **40**, 379–391.

Levine, B. S., and Murphy, S. D. (1977b). Effect of piperonyl butoxide on the metabolism of dimethyl and diethyl phosphorothionate insecticides. *Toxicol. Appl. Pharmacol.* **40**, 393–406.

Levinskas, G. J., and Shaffer, C. B. (1970). Toxicity of Abate, a mosquito larvicide, and its sulfoxide. *Toxicol. Appl. Pharmacol.* **17**, 301.

Lewin, J. F., and Love, J. L. (1974). A death caused by the ingestion of mevinphos. *Forensic Sci.* **4**, 253–255.

Leybovich, D. L. (1973). Assessment of embryotropic action of small doses of phosphororganic pesticides chlorophos, metaphos, and carbophos. *Gig. Sanit.* **38**, 21–24 (in Russian).

Lieben, J., Waldman, R. K., and Krause, L. (1953). Urinary excretion of paranitrophenol following exposure to parathion. *Arch. Ind. Hyg. Occup. Med.* **7**, 93–98.

Limaye, M. R. (1966). Acute organophosphorus compound poisoning. A study of 76 necropsies. *J. Indian Med. Assoc.* **47**, 492–498.

Lin, T. (1974). Toxicological study of Baythion and Cythion on rat feeding test. *J. Taiwan Agric. Res.* **23**, 149–154.

Lippi, M. (1950). Changes in serum cholinesterase during 24 hours in normal subjects. *Minerva Med.* **41**, 301–306.

Lloyd, J. E., and Matthysse, J. G. (1971). Residues of dichlorvos, diazinon and dimetilan in milk of cows fed PVC–insecticide feed additives. *J. Econ. Entomol.* **64**, 821–822.

Lobzin, V. S., and Tsinovoi, P. E. (1969). Neurological disorders in chlorphos poisoning. *Zh. Nevropatol. Pskhiatr. im. S.S. Korsakova* **69**, 679–683 (in Russian).

Loeffler, J. E., DeVries, D. M., Young, R., and Page, A. C. (1971). Metabolic fate of inhaled dichlorvos in pigs. *Toxicol. Appl. Pharmacol.* **19**, 378.

Loeffler, J. E., Potter, J. C., Scordelis, S. L., Hendrickson, H. R., Huston, C. K., and Page. A. C. (1976). Long-term exposure of swine to a [^{14}C]dichlorvos atmosphere. *J. Agric. Food Chem.* **24**, 367–371.

Löfroth, G. (1970). Alkylation of DNA by dichlorvos. *Naturwissenschaften* **57**, 393–394.

Löfroth, G., Kim, C., and Hussain, S. (1969). Alkylating property of 2,2-dichlorovinyl dimethyl phosphate: A disregarded hazard. *Newsl.—Environ. Mutagen. Soc.* **2**, 21–27.

Lohs, Kh., and Gibel, W. (1971). On the hepatotoxic and carcinogenic action of trichlorfon. *Ernaehrungsforschung* **16**, 515–517 (in German).

Lopez, C. (1970). Therapy with corticosteroid compounds in acute poisoning with carbamate and organophosphate pesticides. *Int. Arch. Arbeitsmed.* **26**, 51–62.

Lores, E. M., Bradway, D. E., and Moseman, R. F. (1978a). Organophosphorus pesticide poisonings in humans: Determination of residues and metabolites in tissues and urine. *Arch. Environ. Health* **33**, 270–276.

Lores, E. M., Sovocool, G. W., Harless, R. L., Wilson, N. K., and

Moseman, R. F. (1978b). A new metabolite of chlorpyrifos: Isolation and identification. *J. Agric. Food Chem.* **26**, 118–122.

Lorot, C. (1899). Creosote preparations in the treatment of pulmonary tuberculosis. Thesis, Paris (cited by D. Hunter, in "Industrial Toxicology." Oxford Univ. Press 1944 (Clarendon), London and New York (in French).

Lotti, M. (1986). Biological monitoring for organophosphate-induced delayed polyneuropathy. *Toxicol. Lett.* **33**, 167–172.

Lotti, M. (1987). Organophosphate-induced delayed polyneuropathy in humans: Perspectives for biomonitoring. *Trends Pharmacol. Sci.* **8**, 176–177.

Lotti, M., and Johnson, M. K. (1978). Neurotoxicity of organophosphorus pesticides: Predictions can be based on *in vitro* studies with hen and human enzymes. *Arch. Toxicol.* **41**, 215–221.

Lotti, M., Becker, C. E., Aminoff, M. J., Woodrow, J. E., Seiber, J. N., Talcott, R. E., and Richardson, R. J. (1983). Occupational exposure to the cotton defoliants DEF and Merphos. *J. Occup. Med.* **25**, 517–522.

Loveless, A. (1969). Possible relevance of O-6 alkylation of desoxyguanosine to the mutagenicity and carcinogenicity of nitrosamines and nitrosamides. *Nature (London)* **223**, 206–207.

Lowndes, H. E. (1973). Alterations in neuromuscular function in delayed organophosphate toxicity. *Proc. Can. Fed. Biol. Soc.* **16**, 8.

Lowndes, H. E., Riker, W. F., Jr., and Baker, T. (1973). Alterations in neuromuscular function in delayed organophosphate toxicity. *Proc. Can. Fed. Biol. Soc.* **16**, 8.

Lowndes, H. E., Baker, T., and Riker, W. F., Jr. (1975). Motor nerve terminal response to endrophonium in delayed DFP neuropathy. *Eur. J. Pharmacol.* **30**, 69–72.

Lu, F. C., Jessup, D. C., and Lavallee, A. (1965). Toxicity of pesticides in young versus adult rats. *Food Cosmet. Toxicol.* **3**, 591–596.

Lucier, G. W., and Menzer, R. E. (1970). Nature of oxidation metabolites of dimethoate formed in rats, liver microsomes, and bean plants. *J. Agric. Food Chem.* **18**, 698–704.

Lucier, G. W., and Menzer, R. E. (1971). Nature of neutral phosphorus ester metabolites of phosphamidon formed in rats and liver microsomes. *J. Agric. Food Chem.* **19**, 1249–1255.

Luederitz, B., Boelke, G., Gaaz, J. W., Schmidt, H., and Reicker, G. (1974). Repeated poisoning with nitrostigmine (E 605 forte). *Dtsch. Med. Wochenschr.* **99**, 529–533 (in German).

Lusk, E. E., Womeldorf, D. J., Washino, R. K., Akesson, N. B., and Whitesell, K. G. (1976). Effects of nonthermal aerosol applications of chlorpyrifos on nontarget arthropods and people in an urban area. *Proc. Pap. Annu. Conf. Calif. Mosq. Control Assoc.* **44**, 78–85.

Lutterotti, A. (1961). Liver injury in poisoning by cholinesterase blocking insecticides. *Med. Welt* No. 46, pp. 2430–2433 (in German).

Luzhnikov, E. A. (1966). Some problems of clinical picture and treatment in acute poisoning with organophosphorus insecticides. *Gig. Tr. Prof. Zabol. 1966*, 36–42 (in Russian).

Luzhnikov, E. A., and Kosarev, V. A. (1971). Clinical features of acute poisoning with organo-phosphate insecticides. *Ter. Arkh.* **43**, 106–108 (in Russian).

Luzhnikov, E. A., and Pankov, A. G. (1969). Experience in the use of cholinesterase reactivators in acute poisoning with organophosphoric compounds. *Klin. Med. (Moscow)* **47**, 134–136 (in Russian).

Luzhnikov, E. A., Yaroslavsky, A. A., Molodenkov, M. N., Shurkalin, B. K., Evseev, N. G., and Barsukov, U. F. (1977). Plasma perfusion through charcoal in methyl parathion poisoning. *Lancet* **1**, 38–39.

Lynch, W. T., and Coon, J. M. (1972). Effect of tri-o-tolyl phosphate pretreatment on the toxicity and metabolism of parathion and paraoxon in mice. *Toxicol. Appl. Pharmacol.* **21**, 153–165.

Lyubetskii, K. Z., and Vengerskaya, K. Y. (1961). Comparative evaluation of working conditions in the treatment of cotton with mercaptophos (demeton), methyl Systox, and preparation M-81. *Gig. Sanit.* **26**, 36–39.

MacDonald, W. E., MacQueen, J., Deichmann, W. B., Hamill, T., and Copsey, K. (1970). Effect of parathion on liver microsomal enzyme activities induced by organochlorine pesticides and drugs in female rats. *Int. Arch. Arbeitsmed.* **26**, 31–44.

Machin, A. F., Quick, M. P., Rogers, H., and Anderson, P. H. (1971). The conversion of diazinon to hydroxydiazinon in the guinea pig and sheep. *Bull. Environ. Contam. Toxicol.* **6,** 26–27.

Maddock, D. R., and Sedlak, V. A. (1961). Dosage–mortality response of *Anopheles quadrimaculatus* exposed to DDVP vapour. *Bull. W.H.O.* **24,** 644–646.

Maddock, D. R., Sedlak, V. A., and Schoof, H. F. (1961). Dosage–mortality response of *Musca domestica* exposed to DDVP vapour. *Bull. W.H.O.* **24,** 643–644.

Maddy, K. T. (1976). Worker reentry safety. IV. The position of the California Department of Food and Agriculture on pesticide reentry safety intervals. *Residue Rev.* **62,** 21–34.

Maebashi, H., Nishimura, M., Veda, K., Ogata, S., and Kawamura, A. (1972). Experimental chronic intoxication caused by organophosphorus insecticides on beagles. *Jpn. J. Ind. Health* **14,** 411 (in Japanese).

Man'ko, N. N. (1970). Establishing the maximum permissible concentration of phosalone in the air of a work zone. *Gig. Tr. Prof. Zabol.* **14,** 46–48 (in Russian).

Marchenko, L. I. (1973). Trichlorfon poisoning complicated by polyneuritis. *Vrach. Delo* **4,** 116–117 (in Russian).

Maresch, W. (1957). On Systox poisoning. *Wien. Klin. Wochenschr.* **69,** 774–776 (in German).

Margot, A., and Gysin, H. (1957). Diazinon. Decomposition products and their properties. *Helv. Chim. Acta* **40,** 1562 (in German).

Maric, M. (1970). Toxic exanthema caused by Ekatin. *Med. Pregl.* **23,** 51–52 (in Serbo-Croatian).

Marliac, J. P., and Mutchler, M. K. (1963). Use of the chick embryo technique for detecting potentiating effects of chemicals. *Fed. Proc., Fed. Am. Soc. Exp. Biol.* **22,** 188.

Maroni, M., and Bleecker, M. L. (1986). Neuropathy target esterase in human lymphocytes and platelets. *J. Appl. Toxicol.* **6,** 1–7.

Marquardt, W. C., and Lovelace, S. A. (1961). A comparison of dimethoate administered by injection and in supplementary feed for control of cattle grubs. *J. Econ. Entomol.* **54,** 252–254.

Marr, W. G. (1947). The clinical use of di-isopropyl fluorophosphate (D.F.P.) in chronic glaucoma. *Am. J. Ophthalmol.* **30,** 423–426.

Marr, W. G., and Grob, D. (1950). Some ocular effects of a new anticholinesterase agent: Tetraethyl pyrophosphate (TEPP) and its use in the treatment of chronic glaucoma. *Am. J. Ophthalmol.* **33,** 904–908.

Marsden, A. T. H., and Reid, H. A. (1961). Pathology of sea-snake poisoning. *Br. Med. J.* **1,** 1290–1293.

Marsh, W. H., Vukov, G. A., and Conradi, E. C. (1988). Acute pancreatitis after cutaneous exposure to an organophosphate insecticide. *Am. J. Gastroenterol.* **83,** 1158–1160.

Martin, H., and Worthing, C. R., eds. (1974). "Pesticide Manual." British Crop Prot. Counc., Malvern, Worchestershire, England.

Martson, I. V., and Badayeva, L. N. (1975). Functional–morphological characteristic of the gonadotoxic effect of chlorophos. *Dopov. Akad. Nauk Ukr. RSR, Ser. B: Geol., Khim. Biol. Nauki* No. 4, pp. 361–367.

Martynov, A. A. (1970). On the clinical picture and the treatment of poisonings with trichlorfon. *Uch. Zap. Petrozavodsk. Gos. Univ. im. O. V. Kuusinena* **17,** 136–140 (in Russian).

Masiak, M., and Olajossy, M. (1973). Depressive reaction following intoxication with an organophosphorus preparation, Rogor (Bi 58). *Wiad. Lek.* **26,** 1933–1936 (in Polish).

Mathewson, I., and Hardy, E. A. (1970). Treatment of malathion poisoning. *Anaesthesia* **25,** 265–271.

Matin, M. A., and Hussain, K. (1984). The effect of certain drugs on glycogen and acetylcholine levels in cerebral and peripheral tissues in rats with malathion induced hyperglycemia. *Origins Sci. Pap., UDC* **615** (917:57.085.1), 325–332.

Matin, M. A., and Hussain, K. (1987). Cerebral glycogenolysis and glycolysis in malathion-treated hyperglycaemic animals. *Biochem. Pharmacol.* **36,** 1815–1817.

Matsueda, S., Mikami, M., Ohtaki, Y., and Kudo, N. (1972a). Interrelations between blood glutathione and cholinesterase activity in methyl parathion poisoning. *J. Jpn. Biochem. Soc.* **44,** 299–302.

Matsueda, S., Nagaki, H., Tsukada, N., Kudo, N., and Uchiyama, M.

(1972b). On the variation of GSH and ChE in organophosphorus pesticide intoxicated pigs' serum. *J. Jpn. Biochem. Soc.* **44,** 722.

Matsueda, S., Ohtaki, Y., Mikami, M., and Kudo, N. (1973a). Relationship between human blood glutathione and serum cholinesterase activity. *J. Jpn. Biochem. Soc.* **45,** 88–90.

Matsueda, S., Ohtaki, Y., Mikami, M., and Kudo, N. (1973b). Inhibition of rat blood cholinesterase activity by ethyl parathion. *J. Jpn. Biochem. Soc.* **45,** 91–93.

Matsueda, S., Nagaki, M., Tsukada, N., Sato, M., Ishida, S., and Sasaki, K. (1974). Therapeutic effect of chlorella extract (crude drug) and enzyme-histochemical findings on human blood cell cholinesterase inhibited by agricultural drugs. *Sci. Rep. Hirosaki Univ.* **20,** 14–22.

Matsumura, F., and Ward, C. T. (1966). Degradation of insecticides by the human and the rat liver. *Arch. Environ. Health* **13,** 257–261.

Matsushima, S. (1972). On disturbances of the nervous system induced by organophosphorus pesticides. *J. Jpn. Assoc. Rural Med.* **21,** 94–95 (in Japanese).

Matsushima, S., Abe, E., Kurosawa, K., Yanagisawa, T., Sasaki, K., Yamazaki, H., and Shimazaki, K. (1972). Experimental study on subacute toxicity of fenitrothion. *J. Jpn. Assoc. Rural Med.* **21,** 310–311 (in Japanese).

Matsushima, S., Abe, E., Sasaki, K., Asanuma, N., Nakano, T., and Fujita, K. (1976). Long-term administration test in dogs and monkeys with fenitrothion at a minute dose rate. Part I. Interim Report. *J. Jpn. Assoc. Rural Med.* **25,** 510–511.

Matsushima, S., Abe, E., Sasaki, K., and Kurosawa, K. (1978). Long-term low-dose administration of fenitrothion to dogs and monkeys. Part II. *Jpn. J. Rural Med.* **27,** 624–625.

Mattson, A. M., and Sedlak, V. A. (1960). Measurement of insecticide exposure. Ether-extractable urinary phosphates in man and rats derived from malathion and similar compounds. *J. Agric. Food Chem.* **8,** 107–110.

Mattson, A. M., Spillane, J. T., and Pearce, G. W. (1955). Dimethyl 2,2-dichlorovinyl phosphate (DDVP), an organic phosphorus compound highly toxic to insects. *J. Agric. Food Chem.* **3,** 319–321.

Mayer, R. T., and Himel, C. M. (1972). Dynamics of fluorescent probe–cholinesterase reactions. *Biochemistry* **11,** 2082–2090.

McBain, J. B., Yamamoto, I., and Casida, J. E. (1971a). Mechanism of activation and deactivation by Dyfonate (O-ethyl S-phenyl ethylphosphonodithioate) by rat liver microsomes. *Life Sci.* **10** (Part 2), 947–954.

McBain, J. B., Yamamoto, I., and Casida, J. E. (1971b). Oxygenated intermediate in peracid and microsomal oxidations of the organophosphothionate insecticide Dyfonate. *Life Sci.* **10** (Part 2), 1311–1319.

McBain, J. B., Hoffman, L. J., Menn, J. J., and Casida, J. E. (1971c). Dyfonate metabolism studies. II. Metabolic pathway of O-ethyl S-phenyl ethyl phosphonodithioate in rats. *Pestic. Biochem. Physiol.* **1,** 356–365.

McCarthy, R. T., Haufler, M., and McBeth, C. A., Jr. (1968). Toxicological effects of a phosphorothioic acid insecticide in sheep. *J. Am. Vet. Med. Assoc.* **152,** 279–381.

McCollister, S. B., Kociba, R. J., Humiston, C. G., McCollister, D. D., and Gehring, P. J. (1974). Studies of the acute and long-term oral toxicity of chlorpyrifos (O,O-diethyl-O-3,5,6-trichloro-2 pyridyl) phosphorothioate. *Food Cosmet. Toxicol.* **12,** 45–61.

McDonald, B. E., Costa, L. G., and Murphy, S. D. (1988). Spatial memory impairment and central muscarinic receptor loss following prolonged treatment with organophosphates. *Toxicol. Lett.* **40,** 47–56.

McGehee, H., Jones, B. F., Talbot, S., and Grob, D. (1946). The effect of diisopropyl fluorophosphate (DFP) on neuromuscular transmission in normal individuals and in patients with myasthenia gravis. *Fed. Proc., Fed. Am. Soc. Exp. Biol.* **5,** 182.

McLaughlin, J. T., and Sonnenschein, R. R. (1960). Action of paraoxon (diethyl 4-nitrophenyl phosphate) on human sweat glands and the sympathetic axone reflex. *Acta Pharmacol. Toxicol.* **17,** 7–17.

McLaughlin, L. A., Jr., and Snyder, C. H. (1956). Encephalopathy in a child following exposure to malathion. *Ochsner Clin. Rep.* **2,** 37–40.

McLeod, W. R. (1975). Merphos poisoning or mass panic? *Aust. N.Z. J. Psychiatry* **9,** 225–229.

McNamara, B. P., Bergner, A. D., Robinson, E. M., Murtha, E. F., Bender,

C. W., and Wills, J. H. (1954). Mechanism of DFP and TEPP action. *J. Pharmacol. Exp. Ther.* **110**, 232–240.

McPhillips, J. J., and Coon, J. M. (1966). Adaptation to octamethyl pyrophosphoramide in rats. *Toxicol. Appl. Pharmacol.* **8**, 66–76.

Meeter, E. (1969). Desensitization of the end-plate membrane following cholinesterase inhibition, an adjustment to a new working situation. *Acta Pharmacol. Neerl.* **15**, 243–258.

Meeter, E., and Wolthuis, O. L. (1968a). The spontaneous recovery of respiration and neuromuscular transmission in the rat after anticholinesterase poisoning. *Eur. J. Pharmacol.* **2**, 377–386.

Meeter, E., and Wolthuis, O. L. (1968b). The effects of cholinesterase inhibitors on the body temperature of the rat. *Eur. J. Pharmacol.* **4**, 18–24.

Meeter, E., Wolthuis, O. L., and van Benthem, R. M. J. (1971). The anticholinesterase hypothermia in the rat: Its practical application in the study of the central effectiveness of oximes. *Bull. W.H.O.* **44**, 251–257.

Mehta, A. B., Shah, A. C., Joshi, L. G., Kale, A. K., and Vora, D. D. (1971). Clinical features and plasma acetylcholinesterase activity in poisoning with insecticidal organophosphorus compounds. *J. Assoc. Physicians India* **19**, 181–184.

Meier, E. P., Dennis, W. H., Rosencrance, A. B., Randall, W. F., Cooper, W. J., and Warner, M. C. (1979). Sulfotepp, a toxic impurity in formulations of diazinon. *Bull. Environ. Contam. Toxicol.* **23**, 158–164.

Meleney, W. P., and Peterson, H. O. (1964). The relationship of shelf age to toxicity of dimethoate to sheep. *J. Am. Vet. Med. Assoc.* **144**, 756–758.

Mello, D., Rodrigues Puga, F., and Benintendi, R. (1972). Intoxications produced by degradation products of diazinon in its use as a tick killer. *Biologico* **38**, 136–139.

Melnikov, N. N. (1971). "Chemistry of Pesticides," Residue Rev., Vol. 36. Springer-Verlag, New York.

Meneses de Almeida, L., and Pedrosos de Lima, A. (1964). Concerning intoxication of an infant by parathion. *Opusc. Med.* **31**, 306–317 (in Portuguese).

Menn, J. J., and McBain, J. B. (1974). New aspects of organophosphorus pesticides. IV. Newer aspects of the metabolism of phosphonate insecticides. *Residue Rev.* **53**, 35–51.

Menn, J. J., and Szabo, K. (1965). The synthesis and biological properties of new *O*-alkyl *S*-aryl alkylphosphonodithioates. *J. Econ. Entomol.* **58**, 734–739.

Menz, M., Luetkemeier, H., and Sachsse, K. (1974). Long-term exposure of factory workers to dichlorvos (DDVP) insecticide. *Arch. Environ. Health* **28**, 72–76.

Menzer, R. E., and Best, N. H. (1968). Effect of phenobarbital on the toxicity of several organophosphorus insecticides. *Toxicol. Appl. Pharmacol.* **13**, 37–42.

Menzer, R. E., and Casida, J. E. (1965). Nature of toxic metabolites formed in mammals, insects, and plants from 3-(dimethoxyphosphinyloxy)-*N-N*-dimethyl-*cis*-crotonamide and its *N*-methyl analog. *J. Agric. Food Chem.* **13**, 102–112.

Metcalf, D. R., and Holmes, J. H. (1969). EEG, psychological and neurological alterations in humans with organophosphorus exposure. *Ann. N.Y. Acad. Sci.* **160**, 357–365.

Metcalf, R. A., and Metcalf, R. L. (1973). Selective toxicity of analogs of methyl parathion. *Pestic. Biochem. Physiol.* **3**, 149–159.

Metcalf, R. L., Fukuto, T. R., and March, R. B. (1957). Plant metabolism of dithio-Systox and Thimet. *J. Econ. Entomol.* **50**, 338–345.

Metcalf, R. L., Branch, C. E., Swift, T. R., and Sikes, R. K. (1985). Neurologic findings among workers exposed to fenthion in a veterinary hospital—Georgia. *Morbid. Mortal. Wkly. Rep.* **34**, 402–403.

Meyer, L. M., Sawitsky, A., Ritz, N. D., and Fitch, H. M. (1948). A study of cholinesterase activity of the blood of patients with pernicious anemia. *J. Lab. Clin. Med.* **33**, 189–202.

Michaelek, H., and Stavinoha, W. B. (1977). Differential dose-dependent inhibition of acetylcholine and butyrylcholine hydrolysis in rat brain by dichlorvos: Potentiation of dichlorvos effects by chlorpromazine. *Proc. Eur. Soc. Toxicol.* **18**, 258–261.

Michaelek, H., and Stavinoha, W. B. (1978). Effect of chlorpromazine pretreatment on the inhibition of total cholinesterases and butyryl cho-

linesterase in brain of rats poisoned by physostigmine or dichlorvos. *Toxicology* **9**, 205–218.

Michel, H. O. (1940). An electrometric method for the determination of red blood cell and plasma cholinesterase activity. *J. Lab. Clin. Med.* **34**, 1564–1568.

Michelsen, R. (1958). Insecticide poisoning: A case of suicide with Systox. *Tidsskr. Nor. Naegeforen.* **78**, 356–357.

Mick, D. L., Gartin, T. D., and Long, K. R. (1970). A case report: Occupational exposure to the insecticide naled. *J. Iowa Med. Soc.* **60**, 395–396.

Midtling, J. E., Barnett, P. G., Coye, M. J., Velasco, A. R., Romero, P., Clements, C. L., O'Malley, M. A., Tobin, M. W., Rose, T. G., and Monosson, I. H. (1985). Clinical management of field worker organophosphate poisoning. *West. J. Med.* **142**, 514–518.

Milby, T. H., and Epstein, W. L. (1964). Allergic contact sensitivity to malathion. *Arch. Environ. Health* **9**, 434–437.

Miles, J. W., Mount, D. L., Staiger, M. A., and Teeters, W. R. (1979). *S*-Methyl isomer content of stored malathion and fenitrothion water-dispersible powders and its relationship to toxicity. *J. Agric. Food Chem.* **27**, 421–425.

Miller, J. L., Sandvik, L., Sprague, G. L., Bickford, A. A., and Castles, T. R. (1979). Evaluation of delayed neurotoxic potential of chronically administered dyfonate in adult hens. *Toxicol. Appl. Pharmacol.* **48**, A197.

Milman, H. A., Ward, J. M., and Chu, K. C. (1978). Pancreatic carcinogenesis and naturally occurring pancreatic neoplasms of rats and mice in the NCI carcinogenesis testing program. *J. Environ. Pathol. Toxicol.* **1**, 829–840.

Milthers, E., Clemmeson, C., and Nimb, M. (1963). Poisoning with phosphostigmines treated with atropine, pralidoxime methiodide and diacetyl monoxime. *Dan. Med. Bull.* **10**, 122–129.

Mirer, F. E., Levine, B. S., and Murphy, D. (1977). Parathion and methyl parathion toxicity and metabolism in piperonyl butoxide and diethyl maleate pretreated mice. *Chem.-Biol. Interact.* **17**, 99–112.

Mirza, A. M., Schaub, N., Samler, L., and Reichelderfer, T. E. (1972). Organophosphate insecticide diazinon poisoning in children. *Med. Ann. D. C.* **41**, 559–560.

Misu, Y., Segawa, T., Kuruma, I., Kojima, M., and Takagi, H. (1966). Subacute toxicity of *O,O*-dimethyl *O*-(3-methyl-4-nitrophenyl) phosphorothioate (Sumithion) in the rat. *Toxicol. Appl. Pharmacol.* **9**, 17–26.

Mitra, P. (1966). Electrocorticographic observations on cats and rabbits after experimental poisoning with phosphoric acid esters (parathion). *Pisani* **90**, 3–19.

Miyamoto, J. (1964a). Studies on the mode of action of organophosphorus compounds. III. Activation and degradation of Sumithion and methyl parathion in mammal *in vivo*. *Agric. Biol. Chem.* **28**, 411–421.

Miyamoto, J. (1964b). Studies on the mode of action of organophosphorus compounds. IV. Penetration of Sumithion, methyl parathion and their oxygen analogs into guinea pig brain and inhibition of cholinesterase *in vivo*. *Agric. Biol. Chem.* **28**, 422–430.

Miyamoto, J. (1969). Mechanism of low toxicity of Sumithion toward mammals. *Residue Rev.* **25**, 251–264.

Miyamoto, J., Sato, Y., Kadota, T., and Fujinami, A. (1963). Studies on the mode of action of organophosphorus compounds. Part II. Inhibition of mammalian cholinesterase *in vivo* following administration of Sumithion and methylparathion. *Agric. Biol. Chem.* **27**, 669–676.

Miyamoto, J., Mihara, K., and Hosokawa, S. (1975). Comparative metabolism of *m*-methyl-^{14}C-Sumithion in several species of mammals *in vivo*. *J. Pestic. Sci.* **1**, 9–21.

Miyata, M., Imai, H., and Ishikawa, S. (1973). Electroretinographic study of the rat after fenthion intoxication. *Jpn. J. Ophthalmol.* **17**, 335–343.

Miyata, M., Imai, H., and Ishikawa, S. (1974). Cholinesterase in rat retina, and the effects of an organophosphorus compound, fenthion, on it. *Jpn. J. Ophthalmol.* **25**, 89–93 (in Japanese).

Miyazaki, S., and Hodgson, G. C. (1972). Chronic toxicity of Dursban and its metabolite, 3,5,6-trichloro-2-pyridinol, in chickens. *Toxicol. Appl. Pharmacol.* **22**, 391–398.

Modak, A. T., Stavinoha, W. B., and Weintraub, S. T. (1975). Dichlorvos and the cholinergic system: Effects on cholinesterase and acetylcholine and choline contents of rat tissues. *Arch. Int. Pharmacodyn. Ther.* **217,** 293–301.

Moeller, H. C., and Rider, J. A. (1959). The effects of various organic phosphate insecticides on RBC and plasma cholinesterase in humans. *Fed. Proc., Fed. Am. Soc. Exp. Biol.* **18,** 424.

Moeller, H. C., and Rider, J. A. (1961). Studies on the anticholinesterase effect of parathion and methyl parathion in humans. *Fed. Proc., Fed. Am. Soc. Exp. Biol.* **20,** 434.

Moeller, H. C., and Rider, J. A. (1962a). Plasma and red blood cell cholinesterase activity as indications of the threshold of incipient toxicity of ethyl-*p*-nitrophenyl thionobenzenephosphonate (EPN) and malathion in human beings. *Toxicol. Appl. Pharmacol.* **4,** 123–130.

Moeller, H. C., and Rider, J. A. (1962b). Threshold of incipient toxicity to Systox and methyl parathion. *Fed. Proc., Fed. Am. Soc. Exp. Biol.* **21,** 451.

Moeller, H. C., and Rider, J. A. (1963). Further studies on the toxicity of Systox and methyl parathion. *Fed. Proc., Fed. Am. Soc. Exp. Biol.* **22,** 189.

Moeller, H. C., and Rider, J. A. (1965). Further studies on the anticholinesterase effect of Systox and methyl parathion in humans. *Fed. Proc., Fed. Am. Soc. Exp. Biol.* **24,** 641.

Molander, D. W., Friedman, M. M., and LaDue, J. S. (1954). Serum cholinesterase in hepatic and neoplastic diseases: A preliminary report. *Ann. Intern. Med.* **41,** 1139–1151.

Molphy, R., and Rathus, E. M. (1964). Organic phosphorus poisoning and therapy. *Med. J. Aust.* **2,** 337–340.

Monseur, J. (1963). Poisoning by a mixture of chlorine and phosphorus insecticides. A fatal case. *Ann. Soc. Belg. Med. Trop.* **43,** 143–150 (in French).

Moore, C. B., Birchall, R., Horack, H. M., and Batson, H. M. (1957). Changes in serum pseudo-cholinesterase levels in patients with diseases of the heart, liver or musculoskeletal systems. *Am. J. Med. Sci.* **234,** 538–546.

Mootoo, C. L. (1965). Poisoning from pesticides. *N. Engl. J. Med.* **273,** 1226.

Morelli, M. A., and Nakatsugawa, T. (1978). Inactivation *in vitro* of microsomal oxidases during parathion metabolism. *Biochem. Pharmacol.* **27,** 293–299.

Morelli, M. A., and Nakatsugawa, T. (1979). Sulfuroxyacid production as a consequence of parathion desulfuration. *Pestic. Biochem. Physiol.* **10,** 243–250.

Moretto, A., Fassina, A., and Lotti, M. (1983). Neurotoxic esterase in extranervous tissue of man. *In* "Cholinesterases: Fundamental and Applied Aspects" (M. Brazin, E. A. Barnard, and D. Sket, eds.), 2nd Int. Meet. Cholinesterases, Bled. Yugoslavia. de Gruyter, New York.

Morgan, D. P., Hetzler, H. L., Slach, E. F., and Lin, L. I. (1977). Urinary excretion of paranitrophenol and alkyl phosphates following ingestion of methyl or ethyl parathion by human subjects. *Arch. Environ. Contam. Toxicol.* **6,** 159–173.

Morgan, J. P., and Penvich, P. (1978). Jamaica ginger paralysis. Forty-seven year follow-up. *Arch. Neurol. (Chicago)* **35,** 530–532.

Mori, S., Onishi, Y., Hoshi, M., Fukuhara, N., and Tsubaki, T. (1976). A case of polyneuropathy due to trichlorfon intoxication with abnormal muscle tissue. *Clin. Neurol. (Tokyo)* **16,** 594.

Mozes, I. A. (1977). Morphological changes in respiratory organs in fatal poisoning with organophosphorus compounds and their significance for forensic medicine. *Sud. Med. Ekspert.* **20,** 37–39.

Muacevic, G., Dirks, E., Kinkel, H. J., and Leuschner, F. (1970). Anticholinesterase activity of bromophos in rats and dogs. *Toxicol. Appl. Pharmacol.* **16,** 585–596.

Muecke, W., Alt, K. O., and Esser, H. O. (1970). Degradation of ^{14}C-labeled diazinon in the rat. *J. Agric. Food Chem.* **18,** 208–212.

Mukhamedshin, R. A. (1969). Histochemical changes in the organs in Nuvan poisoning. *Farmakol. Toksikol. (Moscow)* **32,** 740–742 (in Russian).

Mukhamedshin, R. A. (1970a). The histochemical characteristics of intoxication of the organism with Dibrom. *Farmakol. Toksikol. (Moscow)* **33,** 625–627 (in Russian).

Mukhamedshin, R. A. (1970b). Toxic effect of Nuvan (DDVP) on hens. *Veterinariya (Moscow)* **46,** 83–86 (in Russian).

Muller, G. H. (1970). Flea collar dermatitis in animals. *J. Am. Vet. Med. Assoc.* **157,** 1616–1626.

Munkner, T., Matzke, J., and Videbaek, A. (1961). Cholinesterase activity of human plasma after intramuscular diisopropyl fluorophosphonate. *Acta Pharmacol. Toxicol.* **18,** 170–174.

Muramatsu, M., and Kuriyama, K. (1976). Effect of organophosphorus compounds on acetylcholine synthesis in brain. *Jpn. J. Pharmacol.* **26,** 249–254.

Muratore, F., Faiolo, H., and Ponzetta, G. (1960). On four cases of poisoning by organophosphorus acid esters (antiparasitic) with recovery, with special reference to hepatic involvement. *Minerva Med.* **51,** 3342–3345.

Murphy, S. D. (1966). Liver metabolism and toxicity of thiophosphate insecticides in mammalian, avian and piscine species. *Proc. Soc. Exp. Biol. Med.* **123,** 392–398.

Murphy, S. D. (1967). Malathion inhibition of esterases as a determinant of malathion toxicity. *J. Pharmacol. Exp. Ther.* **156,** 352–365.

Murphy, S. D., and Cheever, K. L. (1968). Effect of feeding insecticides. *Arch. Environ. Health* **17,** 749–758.

Murphy, S. D., and Cheever, K. L. (1972). Carboxylesterase and cholinesterase inhibition in rats. *Arch. Environ. Health* **24,** 107–114.

Murphy, S. D., and DuBois, K. P. (1957). Quantitative measurement of inhibition of the enzymatic detoxification of malathion by EPN (ethyl *p*-nitrophenyl thionobenzenephosphonate). *Proc. Soc. Exp. Biol. Med.* **96,** 813–818.

Murphy, S. D., Anderson, R. L., and DuBois, K. P. (1959). Potentiation of toxicity of malathion by triorthotolyl phosphate. *Proc. Soc. Exp. Biol. Med.* **100,** 482–487.

Mutalik, G. S., Wadia, R. C., and Pai, V. R. (1962). Poisoning by diazinon an organophosphorus insecticide. *J. Indian Med. Assoc.* **38,** 67–71.

Myers, D. K., Rekel, J. B. J., Veeger, C., Kemp, A., and Simons, E. G. L. (1955). Metabolism of triaryl phosphates in rodents. *Nature (London)* **176,** 259–260.

Nabb, D. P., and Whitfield, F. (1967). Determination of cholinesterase by an automated pH stat method. *Arch. Environ. Health* **15,** 147–154.

Nabb, D. P., Stein, W. J., and Hayes, W. J., Jr. (1966). Rate of skin absorption of parathion and paraoxon. *Arch. Environ. Health* **12,** 501–505.

Najera, J. A., Shidrawi, G. R., Gibson, F. D., and Stafford, J. S. (1967). A large-scale field trial of malathion as an insecticide for antimalarial work in southern Uganda. *Bull. W.H.O.* **36,** 913–935.

Nakatsugawa, T., and Dahm, P. A. (1967). Microsomal metabolism of parathion. *Biochem. Pharmacol.* **16,** 25–38.

Nakatsugawa, T., Tolman, N. M., and Dahm, P. A. (1969a). Oxidative degradation of diazinon by rat liver microsomes. *Biochem. Pharmacol.* **18,** 685–688.

Nakatsugawa, T., Tolman, N. M., and Dahm, P. A. (1969b). Degradation of parathion in the rat. *Biochem. Pharmacol.* **18,** 1103–1114.

Nalin, D. R. (1973). Epidemic of suicide by malathion poisoning in Guyana. *Trop. Geogr. Med.* **25,** 8–14.

Namba, T., and Hiraki, K. (1958). PAM (pyridine-2-aldoxime methiodide) therapy for alkylphosphate poisoning. *JAMA, J. Am. Med. Assoc.* **166,** 1834–1839.

Namba, T., Greenfield, M., and Grob, D. (1970). Malathion poisoning. A fatal case with cardiac manifestations. *Arch. Environ. Health* **21,** 533–541.

Namba, T., Nolte, C. T., Jackrel, J., and Grob, D. (1971). Poisoning due to organophosphate insecticides: Acute and chronic manifestations. *Am. J. Med.* **50,** 475–492.

Nameche, J., and Bartman, J. (1964). Parathion intoxication. *Acta Paediatr. Belg.* **18,** 41–45 (in French).

Nathan, M. B., and Giglioli, M. E. C. (1982). Eradication of *Aedes aegypti* on Cayman Brac and Little Cayman, West Indies, with Abate (Temephos) in 1970–1972. *Bol. Of. Sanit. Panam.* **92,** 18–31 (in Spanish).

National Cancer Institute (NCI) (1977). "Bioassay of Dichlorvos for Possible Carcinogenicity," Carcinogenesis Tech. Rep. Ser. No. 10, DHEW Publ. No. (NIH)77-810. U. S. Govt. Printing Office, Washington, D.C.

National Cancer Institute (NCI) (1978a). "Bioassay of Technical-Grade Azinphosmethyl for Possible Carcinogenicity," U. S. NTIS PB Rep., PB-286, 371. U. S. Govt. Printing Office, Washington, D.C.

National Cancer Institute (NCI) (1978b). "Bioassay of Dioxathion for Possible Carcinogenicity," Tech. Rep. Ser. No. 125. U. S. Govt. Printing Office, Washington, D.C.

Natoff, I. L. (1967). Influence of the route of administration on the toxicity of some cholinesterase inhibitors. *J. Pharm. Pharmacol.* **19**, 612–616.

Natoff, I. L., and Reiff, B. (1970). Differential antagonism of the acutely lethal effects of organophosphates in rats. *Br. J. Pharmacol.* **38**, 433P-x.

Nazardinov, F. V., and Spicin, M. N. (1974). The use of chlorpromazine for the treatment of acute poisoning caused by organophosphorus compounds. *Sov. Med.* **37**, 147 (in Russian).

Neal, R. A. (1967a). Studies on the metabolism of diethyl 4-nitrophenyl phosphorothionate *in vitro. Biochem. J.* **103**, 183–191.

Neal, R. A. (1967b). Enzymic mechanism of the metabolism of diethyl 4-nitrophenyl phosphorothionate by rat liver microsomes. *Biochem. J.* **105**, 289–297.

Nehéz, M., Huszta, E., Mazzag, E., Scheufler, H., Fischer, G. W., and Desi, I. (1986). Cytogenic and embryotoxic effects of bromophos and demethylbromophos. *Regul. Toxicol. Pharmacol.* **6**, 416–421.

Nemec, S. J., Adkisson, P. L., and Dorough, H. W. (1968). Methyl parathion adsorbed on skin and blood cholinesterase levels of persons checking cotton treated with ultra-low-volume sprays. *J. Econ. Entomol.* **61**, 1740–1742.

Nepoklonov, A. A., and Bukshtynov, V. I. (1969). Thermomechanical aerosols of chlorophos against the sheep botfly. *Veterinariia* **6**, 49–50 (in Russian).

Nepoklonov, A. A., and Bukshtynov, V. I. (1971). Chlorophos release time from sheep after aerosol treatment. *Tr. Vses. Nauchno-Issled. Ins. Vet. Sanit.* **39**, 200–202 (in Russian).

Nepoklonov, A. A., and Metelitsa, V. K. (1971a). Excretion of chlorophos in cow milk following external applications. *Tr. VNIIVS* **39**, 149–154 (in Russian).

Nepoklonov, A. A., and Metelitsa, V. K. (1971b). Metabolism and retention of chlorophos in cattle. *Tr. VNIIVS* **39**, 155–164 (in Russian).

Nicholas, A. H., Vienne, M., and Van Den Berghe, H. (1979). Induction of sister-chromatid exchanges in cultured human cells by an organophosphorus insecticide: Malathion. *Mutat. Res.* **67**, 167–172.

Nikolayev, K. A. (1973). The effect of trichlorfon and dimethoate on the enzyme activity of the brain. *Veterinariia* **3**, 105–106 (in Russian).

Nishimura, M., Kaneko, Y., Sakama, H., Tomita, M., Yomeya, N., Ueda, K., Ogata, S., and Kawamura, A. (1974). Experiments on the toxicity of organophosphorus pesticides to beagles. *Jpn. J. Ind. Med.* **16**, 362 (in Japanese).

Nishimura, M., Aoki, M., and Endo, R. (1978). Effect of an organophosphorus insecticide on rat's muscles of mastication. *Jpn. J. Ind. Med.* **20**, 548–549.

Nishiyama, K., Sato, I., and Usuya, S. (1974). Studies on preventing pesticidal injuries in apple growing work: On the amount of exposure to organophosphorus pesticides and their movement in the blood. *Jpn. J. Hyg.* **29**, 205 (in Japanese).

Noda, K., Numata, H., Hirabayashi, M., and Endo, I. (1972). Influence of pesticides on embryos. I. On influence of an organophosphorus pesticide. *Pharmacometrics* **6**, 667–672.

Nolan, R. J., Rick, D. L., Freshour, N. L., and Saunders, J. H. (1984). Chlorpyrifos: Pharmacokinetics in human volunteers. *Toxicol. Appl. Pharmacol.* **73**, 8–15.

Nordgren, I., Bergstrom, N., Holmstedt, B., and Dandoz, M. (1978). Transformation and action of metrifonate. *Arch. Toxicol.* **41**, 31–41.

Norman, B. J., and Neal, R. A. (1974). An examination of the *in vitro* metabolism of parathion in rat lung and brain. *Toxicol. Appl. Pharmacol.* **29**, 125.

Norman, B. J., and Neal, R. A. (1976). Examination of the metabolism *in vitro* of parathion (diethyl *p*-nitrophenyl phosphorothionate) by rat lung and brain. *Biochem. Pharmacol.* **25**, 37–45.

Nosal, M., and Hladka, A. (1968). Determination of the exposure to fenitrothion (*O,O*-dimethyl-*O*[3-methyl-4-nitrophenyl]thiophosphate) on the basis of the excretion of *p*-nitro-*m*-cresol by the urine of the persons tested. *Int. Arch. Gewerbepathol. Gewerbehyg.* **25**, 28–38.

Oarda, M. (1971). Etiological, clinical, and therapeutic considerations concerning 276 cases of parathion poisoning. *Arh. Hig. Rada Toksikol.* **22**, 33–35.

Oberheu, J. C., Soule, R. D., and Wolf, M. A. (1970). The correlation of cholinesterase levels in test animals and exposure levels resulting from thermal fog and aerial spray applications of Dursban insecticide. *Down Earth* **26**, 12–16.

O'Brien, R. D. (1956). Activation of schradan by mammalian tissue homogenates. *Can. J. Biochem. Physiol.* **34**, 1131–1141.

O'Brien, R. D. (1960). "Toxic Phosphorus Esters. Chemistry, Metabolism, and Biological Effects." Academic Press, New York.

O'Brien, R. D. (1967). Effects of induction by pentobarbital upon susceptibility of mice to insecticides. *Bull. Environ. Contam. Toxicol.* **2**, 162–168.

Ochs, S., Sabri, M. I., and Johnson, J. (1969). Fast transport system of materials in mammalian nerve fibers. *Science* **163**, 686–687.

Ogata, S. (1972). Effects of organophosphorus pesticides on beagles in chronic toxicity studies. *J. Jpn. Ophthalmol. Soc.* **76**, 1143–1150 (in Japanese).

Ohela, K., Toivonen, T., and Kaipainen, W. J. (1958). Parathion, a murderous stuff in general use. *Suom. Elainlaakaril.* **13**, 1571–1576.

Ohkawa, H., Mikami, N., Okuno, Y., and Miyamoto, J. (1977). Stereospecificity in toxicity of the optical isomers of EPN. *Bull. Environ. Contam. Toxicol.* **18**, 535–540.

Okinaka, A. J., Doull, J., Coon, J. M., and DuBois, K. P. (1954). Studies on the toxicity and pharmacological actions of bis(dimethylamido) fluorophosphate (BFP). *J. Pharmacol. Exp. Ther.* **112**, 231–245.

Okonek, S. (1976a). Probable progress in the therapy of organophosphate poisoning. Extracorporeal hemodialysis and hemoperfusion. *Arch. Toxicol.* **35**, 221–227.

Okonek, S. (1976b). Detection of paraoxon in the blood of patients with severe suicidal nitrostigmine intoxication. *Naunyn-Schmiedeberg's Arch. Pharmacol.* **293**, R68.

Okonek, S., and Kilbinger, H. (1974). Determination of acetylcholine, nitrostigmine, acetylcholinesterase activity in four patients with severe nitrostigmine (E 605 forte®) intoxication. *Arch. Toxicol.* **32**, 97–108.

Okuyama, A., Arima, T., Toto, Y., Imai, M., and Haraoka, S. (1975). A case of hypocholinesterasemia induced by trichlorfon. *Acta Med. Okayama* **29**, 233–236.

Olajos, E. J., and Rosenblum, I. (1978). Mechanisms of organophosphate axonopathy in hens. *Toxicol. Appl. Pharmacol.* **45**, 271–272.

Olajos, E. J., DeCaprio, A. P., and Rosenblum, I. (1978). Central and peripheral neurotoxic esterase activity and dose–response relationship in adult hens after acute and chronic oral administration of diisopropyl fluorophosphate. *Ecotoxicol. Environ. Saf.* **2**, 383–399.

Older, J. J., and Hatcher, R. L. (1969). Food poisoning caused by carbophenothion. *JAMA, J. Am. Med. Assoc.* **209**, 1328–1230.

Orzel, R. A., and Weiss, L. R. (1966). The effect of various chemicals on rat brain cholinesterase inhibition by parathion. *Arch. Int. Pharmacodyn. Ther.* **164**, 150–157.

Osserman, K. E., and Kaplan, L. I. (1954). Studies in myasthenia gravis: Present status of therapy with octamethyl pyrophosphoramide (OMPA). *Ann. Intern. Med.* **41**, 108–111.

Osterloh, J., Lotti, M., and Pond, S. M. (1983). Toxicologic studies in a fatal overdose of 2,4,0-MCDP, and chlorpyrifos. *J. Anal. Toxicol.* **7**, 125–129.

Osumi, Y., Fujiwara, H., Oishi, R., and Takaori, S. (1975). Central cholinergic activation by chlorfenvinphos, an organophosphate, in the rat. *Jpn. J. Pharmacol.* **25**, 47–54.

Ottevanger, C. F. (1975). Neuromuscular function of persons exposed to resin granules of dichlorvos. Benefit of electromyography. *J. Eur. Toxicol.* **8**, 192–195 (in French).

Overstreet, D. H., Kozar, M. D., and Lynch, G. S. (1973). Reduced hypothermic effects of cholinometric agents following chronic anticholinesterase treatment. *Neuropharmacology* **12**, 1017–1032.

Overstreet, D. H., Russell, R. W., Vasquez, B. J., and Dalglish, F. W. (1974).

Involvement of muscarinic and nicotinic receptors in behavioral tolerance to DFP. *Pharmacol., Biochem. Behav.* **2**, 45–54.

Overstreet, D. H., Schiller, G. D., and Day, T. A. (1977). Failure of cycloheximide to alter rate of recovery of temperature following acute DFP treatment. *Eur. J. Pharmacol.* **44**, 187–190.

Ozgen, T. (1959). Regarding several cases of intoxication by an insecticide based on parathion (Corthion). *Presse Med.* **67**, 680 (in French).

Padgett, G., Bell, T. G., and Farrell, K. (1975). Dichlorvos flea collar ataxia-depression and dermatitis in the laboratory cat. *Fed. Proc., Fed. Am. Soc. Exp. Biol.* **34**, 245.

Page, A. C., Loeffler, J. E., Hendrickson, H. R., Hutson, C. K., and DeVries, D. M. (1972). Metabolic fate of dichlorvos in swine. *Arch. Toxikol.* **30**, 19–27.

Palmer, J. S. (1974). Toxicologic evaluation of *O*-ethyl *O*-ethyl *O*-(*p*-nitrophenyl) phenylphosphonothioate in cattle and sheep. *J. Am. Vet. Med. Assoc.* **164**, 936–938.

Palmer, J. S., and Schlinke, J. C. (1973). Oral toxicity of tributylphosphorotrithioite, a cotton defoliant, to cattle and sheep. *J. Am. Vet. Med. Assoc.* **163**, 1172–1174.

Palut, D., Grzymala, W., and Syrowatka, T. (1969). Study of the metabolism of organophosphorus insecticides in model animal systems. II. Hydrolytic mechanisms. *Rocz. Pantsw. Zakl. Hig.* **20**, 551–555 (in Polish).

Pan'shina, T. N. (1963a). Experimental data on the toxicology of phosphamide—a new organophosphoric insecticide. *Farmakol. Toksikol. (Moscow)* **26**, 476–484.

Pan'shina, T. N. (1963b). Changes in conditioned reflex activity and blood cholinesterase activity in animals under the effect of phosphamide, a phosphoroorganic insecticide. *Byull. Eksp. Biol. Med.* **56**, 56–60.

Parker, G., Jr., and Chattin, W. R. (1955). A case of malathion intoxication in a 10-year-old girl. *J. Indiana State Med. Assoc.* **48**, 491–492.

Pasquet, J., Mazuret, A., Fournel, J., and Koenig, F. H. (1976). Acute oral and percutaneous toxicity of phosalone in the rat, in comparison with azinphosmethyl and parathion. *Toxicol. Appl. Pharmacol.* **37**, 85–92.

Patocka, J., and Bajgar, J. (1971). Affinity of human brain cholinesterase to some organophosphates and carbamates *in vitro*. *J. Neurochem.* **18**, 2545–2546.

Paul, A. H. (1960). Poisoning by organophosphorus insecticide (malathion): Report of a case. *N. Z. Med. J.* **59**, 346–347.

Peiris, J. B., Fernando, R., and De Abrew, K. (1988). Respiratory failure from severe organophosphate toxicity due to absorption through the skin. *Forensic Sci. Int.* **36**, 251–253.

Pellegrini, G., and Santi, R. (1972). Potentiation of toxicity of organophosphorus compounds containing carboxylic ester functions toward warm-blooded animals by some organophosphorus impurities. *J. Agric. Food Chem.* **20**, 944–950.

Peña Chavarría, A., Schwartzwelder, J. C., Villarejos, V. M., Kotcher, E., and Arguedas, J. (1969). Dichlorvos, an effective broad-spectrum anthelmintic. *Am. J. Trop. Med. Hyg.* **18**, 907–911.

Peoples, S. A., and Maddy, K. T. (1978). Organophosphate pesticide poisoning. *West. J. Med.* **129**, 273–277.

Perkow, W. (1954). Reactions with alkylphosphites. I. Rearrangement by reaction with chloral and bromal. *Chem. Ber.* **87**, 755–758 (in German).

Perkow, W., Ullerich, K., and Meyer, F. (1952). New phosphoric acid esters that contract the pupil. *Naturwissenschaften* **39**, 353 (in German).

Perron, R., and Johnson, B. B. (1969). Insecticide poisoning. *N. Engl. J. Med.* **281**, 274–275.

Petrova, E. V., and Arestov, I. G. (1968). Effect of chlorphos on the cardiovascular systems of animals. *Veterinarria* **2**, 83–84 (in Russian).

Petrova, N. I., Kogan, Y. M., Botsyurko, V. I., and Krekhovetskiy, Z. S. (1972). Acute trichlorfon poisoning, complicated by polyneuritis. *Vrach. Delo* **12**, 114–115 (in Russian).

Petry, H. (1951). Polyneuritis from E605. *Zentrabl. Arbeitsmed. Arbeitsschutz* **1**, 86–89 (in German).

Petty, C. S. (1957). Organic phosphate insecticide poisoning: An agricultural occupational hazard. *J. La. State Med. Soc.* **109**, 158–164.

Petty, C. S. (1958a). Organic phosphate insecticide poisoning. Residual effects in two cases. *Am. J. Med.* **24**, 467–470.

Petty, C. S. (1958b). Histochemical proof of organic phosphate poisoning. *AMA Arch. Pathol.* **66**, 458–463.

Petty, C. S., Lovell, M. P., and Moore, E. J. (1958). Organic phosphorus insecticides and post-mortem blood cholinesterase levels. *J. Forensic Sci.* **3**, 226–237.

Petty, C. S., Hedmeg, A., Reinhart, W. H., Moore, E. J., and Dunn, L. F. (1959). Organic phosphate insecticides—a survey of blood cholinesterase activity of exposed agricultural workers in Louisiana—1957. *Am. J. Public Health* **49**, 62–69.

Pietsch, R. L., Bobo, C. B., Finklea, J. F., and Vallotton, W. W. (1972). Lens opacities and organophosphate cholinesterase inhibiting agents. *Am. J. Ophthalmol.* **73**, 236–242.

Pilat, L., Moscovici, B., and Georgescu, A. M. (1961). Parathion poisoning (clinical observations). *Med. Interna* **13**, 1567–1573.

Pitts, C. W., and Hopkins, T. L. (1964). Toxicological studies on dichlorvos feed-additive formulations to control houseflies and face flies in cattle feces. *J. Econ. Entomol.* **57**, 881–884.

Plapp, F. W., and Casida, J. E. (1958). Hydrolysis of the alkyl-phosphate bond in certain dialkyl aryl phosphorothioate insecticides by rats, cockroaches, and alkali. *J. Econ. Entomol.* **51**, 800–803.

Pleasure, D. E., Mishler, K. C., and Engel, W. K. (1969). Axonal transport of proteins in experimental neuropathies. *Science* **166**, 524–525.

Pleština, R., and Piukovič-Pleština, M. (1978). Effect of anticholinesterase pesticides on the eye and on vision. *CRC Crit. Rev. Toxicol.* **6**, 1–23.

Pleština, R., Davis, A., and Bailey, D. R. (1972). Effect of metrifonate on blood cholinesterases in children during the treatment of schistosomiasis. *Bull. W.H.O.* **46**, 747–759.

Poehlmann, E., and Schwerd, W. (1976). Analysis of E605 in a corpse exhumed after 21 months. *Z. Rechtsmed.* **77**, 149–155 (in German).

Polan, C. E., and Chandler, P. T. (1971). Metabolism of ^{14}C-carbonyl labeled Supracide by lactating cows. *J. Dairy Sci.* **54**, 847–853.

Pollinger, B., Cozma, V., and Oprisan, C. (1973). Clinical and electromyographic study of two cases of severe polyneuritis following acute poisoning with Neguvon (organophosphoric pesticide). *Electroencephalogr. Clin. Neurophysiol.* **35**, 433.

Poloz, D. D., and Nikolayev, K. A. (1973). Biochemical mechanism of action of organophosphorus compounds on animals. *S-kh. Biol.* **8**, 219–223 (in Russian).

Popendorf, W. J., Spear, R. C., Leffingwell, J. T., Yager, J., and Kahn, E. (1979). Harvester exposure to Zolone (phosalone) residues in peach orchards. *J. Occup. Med.* **21**, 189–194.

Posada, B., and Valencia, J. P. (1966). Poisoning with parathion. A study of 44 cases. *Antioquia Med.* **16**, 837–852.

Potter, J. C., Loeffler, J. E., Collins, R. D., Young, R., and Page, A. C. (1973a). Carbon-14 balance and residues of dichlorvos and its metabolites in pigs dosed with dichlorvos-^{14}C. *J. Agric. Food Chem.* **21**, 163–166.

Potter, J. C., Boyer, A. C., Marxmiller, R. L., Young, R., and Loeffler, J. E. (1973b). Radioisotope residues and residues of dichlorvos and its metabolites in pregnant sows and their progeny dosed with dichlorvos-^{14}C or dichlorvos-^{36}Cl formulated as PVC pellets. *J. Agric. Food Chem.* **21**, 734–738.

Preissig, S. H., and Abou-Donia, M. B. (1978). The neuropathology of leptophos in the hen: A chronological study. *Environ. Res.* **17**, 242–250.

Prellwitz, W., Schuster, H. P., Schylla, G., Baum, P., Schoenborn, H., von Ungern-Sternberg, A., Brodersen, H. C., and Peoplau, W. (1970). Differential diagnosis of organ involvement in exogenous intoxications with the aid of clinical and clinical-chemical examinations. *Klin. Wochenschr.* **48**, 51–53.

Preussman, R. (1968). Direct alkylating agents as carcinogens. *Food Cosmet. Toxicol.* **6**, 576–577.

Prineas, J. (1969). The pathogenesis of dying-back polyneuropathies. Part I. An ultrastructural study of experimental triortho-cresyl phosphate intoxication in the cat. *J. Neuropathol. Exp. Neurol.* **28**, 571–597.

Prinz, H. J. (1969). A severe percutaneous poisoning with parathion (E 605®). *Arch. Toxikol.* **25**, 318–328.

Pritchard, J. A., and Weisman, R., Jr. (1956). Erythrocyte cholinesterase activity in normal pregnancy and in megaloblastic and other anemias of pregnancy and the puerperium. *J. Lab. Clin. Med.* **47,** 98–107.

Przezdziak, J., and Wisniewska, W. (1975). A case of acute organophosphate poisoning. *Wiad. Lek.* **28,** 1093–1095.

Pugh, W. S. (1975). An outbreak of organophosphate poisoning (Thimet) in cattle. *Can. Vet. J.* **16,** 56–58.

Pukach, L. P., and Shakov, V. D. (1971). Epileptoform seizures during acute poisoning with organophosphorus insecticides. *Voen.-Med. Zh.* **10,** 67–68.

Pulfrich, C. (1922). Stereoscopy in the service of isochromatic and heterochromatic photometry. *Naturwissenschaften* **10,** 553–564, 569–574, 596–601, 714–722, 735–743, 751–761 (in German).

Quinby, G. E. (1964). Further therapeutic experience with pralidoximes in organic phosphorus poisoning. *JAMA, J. Am. Med. Assoc.* **187,** 202–206.

Quinby, G. E., and Clappison, G. B. (1961). Parathion poisoning: A near-fatal pediatric case treated with 2-pyridine aldoxime methiodide (2-PAM). *Arch. Environ. Health* **3,** 538–542.

Quinby, G. E., and Doornink, G. M. (1965). Tetraethyl pyrophosphate poisoning following airplane dusting. *JAMA, J. Am. Med. Assoc.* **191,** 1–6.

Quinby, G. E., and Lemmon, A. B. (1958). Parathion residues as a cause of poisoning in crop workers. *JAMA, J. Am. Med. Assoc.* **166,** 740–746.

Quinby, G. E., Walker, K. C., and Durham, W. F. (1958). Public health hazards involved in the use of organic phosphorus insecticides in cotton culture in the Delta area of Mississippi. *J. Econ. Entomol.* **51,** 831–838.

Quinby, G. E., Loomis, T. A., and Brown, H. W. (1963). Oral occupational parathion poisoning treated with 2-PAM iodide (2-pyridine aldoxime methiodide). *N. Engl. J. Med.* **268,** 639–643.

Radeleff, R. D. (1958). The toxicity of insecticides and herbicides to livestock. *Adv. Vet. Sci.* **4,** 265–276.

Radeleff, R. D. (1964). "Veterinary Toxicology." Lea & Febiger, Philadelphia, Pennsylvania.

Ramade, F., and Roffi, J. (1976). Effect of two insecticides, lindane and DDVP (dichlorvos), on mouse adrenal glands. *C. R. Hebd. Seances Acad. Sci., Ser. D* **282,** 1067–1070 (in French).

Ramakrishna, N., and Ramachandran, B. V. (1977). Potentiation of malathion toxicity by parathion. *Indian J. Biochem. Biophys.* **14,** 53.

Ramakrishna, N., and Ramachandran, B. V. (1978). Malathion A and B esterases of mouse liver. III. *In vivo* effect of parathion and related PNP-containing insecticides on esterase inhibition and potentiation of malathion toxicity. *Biochem. Pharmacol.* **27,** 2049–2054.

Ramazzini, B. (1713). "Diseases of Workers" (translated by Wilmer Cave Wright. Hafner, New York, 1964).

Rampelberg, J. (1975). Purpura in organophosphorus poisoning—two cases brought to the attention of the Intensive Care Unit of Brussels. *Bull. Med. Leg., Toxicol.* **18,** 285–287.

Ramu, A., Slonim, A. E., London, M., and Eyal, F. (1973). Hyperglycemia in acute malathion poisoning. *Isr. J. Med. Sci.* **9,** 631–634.

Rao, A. Y. (1965). An unusual case of diazinon poisoning. *Indian J. Med. Sci.* **19,** 768–770.

Rashev, Z. (1972). Cytopathogenic and cytotoxic action of some pesticides on embryonal cell cultures. *Eksp. Med. Morfol.* **11,** 35–39 (in Bulgarian).

Rasmussen, W. A., Jensen, J. A., Stein, W. J., and Hayes, W. J., Jr. (1963). Toxicological studies of DDVP for disinsection of aircraft. *Aerosp. Med.* **34,** 594–600.

Rasuleva, M. A. (1970). On the effect of organophosphorus insecticides used in cotton processing on otolaryngological organs. *Med. Zh. Uzb.* **3,** 48–50.

Ravin, H. A., and Altschule, M. D. (1952). Serum cholinesterase activity in mental disease. *Arch. Neurol. Psychiatry* **68,** 645–650.

Readhead, I. H. (1968). Poisoning on the farm. Report of a case of organophosphorus poisoning. *Lancet* **1,** 686–688.

Reeder, D. H. (1961). Organic phosphate insecticide poisoning. *J. Occup. Med.* **3,** 129–130.

Reichert, B. L., and Abou-Donia, M. B. (1979). Inhibition of axoplasmic transport by delayed neurotoxic organophosphorus esters: A possible mode of action. *Toxicol. Appl. Pharmacol.* **48,** A196.

Reichert, B. L., Ashry, M. A., Timmons, P., and Abou-Donia, M. B. (1978).

Toxicokinetics and metabolism of a sub-neurotoxic dose of ^{14}C-EPN. *Pharmacologist* **20,** 178.

Reichert, E. R., Yauger, W. L., Hattis, R. P., Rashad, M. N., and Klemmer, H. W. (1977). Diazinon poisoning in eight members of related households. *Clin. Toxicol.* **11,** 5–11.

Reichert, E. R., Klemmer, H. W., and Haley, T. J. (1978). A note on dermal poisoning from mevinphos and parathion. *Clin. Toxicol.* **12,** 33–35.

Reiff, B., Lambert, S. M., and Natoff, I. L. (1971). Inhibition of brain cholinesterase by organophosphorus compounds in rats. *Arch. Int. Pharmacodyn. Ther.* **192,** 48–60.

Reiner, E., and Pleština, R. (1979). Regeneration of cholinesterase activities in humans and rats after inhibition by *O,O*-dimethyl-2,2-dichlorovinyl-phosphate. *Toxicol. Appl. Pharmacol.* **49,** 451–454.

Reiner, E., Krauthacker, B., Simeon, V., and Skrinjaric-Spoljar, M. (1975). Mechanism of inhibition *in vitro* of mammalian acetylcholinesterase and cholinesterase in solutions of *O,O*-dimethyl 2,2,2-trichloro-1-hydroxy-ethylphosphonate (trichlorphon). *Biochem. Pharmacol.* **24,** 717–722.

Reinhold, J. G., Tourigny, L. G., and Yonan, V. L. (1953). Measurement of serum cholinesterase activity by a photometric indicator method, together with a study of the influence of sex and race. *Am. J. Clin. Pathol.* **23,** 645–653.

Reinl, W. (1949). Poisoning by a new insecticide. *Neiderschr. Wiss. Tag. Staat. Gewerbearz. Deutschlands,* pp. 125–144.

Reiter, L., Talens, G., and Woolley, D. (1973a). Effects of parathion administration on cholinesterase activities and visual discrimination in monkeys. *Fed. Proc., Fed. Am. Soc. Exp. Biol.* **32,** 250.

Reiter, L., Talens, G., and Woolley, D. (1973b). Acute and subacute parathion treatments: Effects on cholinesterase activities and learning in mice. *Toxicol. Appl. Pharmacol.* **25,** 582–588.

Revzin, A. M. (1976a). Effects of mevinphos (Phosdrin) on unit discharge patterns in avian hippocampus. *Aviat. Space Environ. Med.* **47,** 608–611.

Revzin, A. M. (1976b). Effects of organophosphate pesticides and other drugs on subcortical mechanisms of visual integration. *Aviat. Space Environ. Med.* **47,** 627–629.

Rice, W. B., and Lu, F. C. (1963). The effect of sodium fluoride on the actions of succinylcholine, parathion, and demeton in rats. *Acta Pharmacol.* **20,** 39–42.

Richards, A. G. (1964). Malathion poisoning successfully treated with large doses of atropine. *Can. Med. Assoc. J.* **91,** 82–83.

Richardson, R. J., Davis, C. S., and Johnson, M. K. (1979). Subcellar distribution of marker enzyme and of neurotoxic esterase in adult hen brain. *J. Neurochem.* **32,** 607–615.

Rider, J. A., and Moeller, H. C. (1960). Effects of various organic phosphate anticholinesterase agents on serum and red cell cholinesterase and their relation to the treatment of myasthenia gravis. *In* "Myasthenia Gravis" (H. R. Viets, ed.), pp. 556–580. Thomas, Springfield, Illinois.

Rider, J. A., and Moeller, H. C. (1964). Studies on the anticholinesterase effects of Systox and methyl parathion in humans. *Fed. Proc., Fed. Am. Soc. Exp. Biol.* **23,** 176.

Rider, J. A., and Puletti, E. J. (1969). Studies on the anticholinesterase effects of Gardona, methyl parathion and Guthion in human subjects. *Fed. Proc., Fed. Am. Soc. Exp. Biol.* **28,** 479.

Rider, J. A., Schulman, S., Richter, R. B., Moeller, H. C., and DuBois, K. P. (1951). Treatment of myasthenia gravis with octamethyl pyrophosphoramide. *JAMA, J. Am. Med. Assoc.* **145,** 967–972.

Rider, J. A., Ellinwood, L. E., and Coon, J. M. (1952). Production of tolerance in the rat to octamethyl pyrophosphoramide (OMPA). *Proc. Soc. Exp. Biol. Med.* **81,** 455–459.

Rider, J. A., Hodges, J. L., Swader, J., and Wiggins, A. D. (1957). Plasma and red cell cholinesterase in 800 "healthy" blood donors. *J. Lab. Clin. Med.* **50,** 376–383.

Rider, J. A., Moeller, H. C., Swader, J., and Weilerstein, R. W. (1958). The effect of parathion on human red blood cell and plasma cholinesterase. Section II. *AMA Arch. Ind. Health* **18,** 441–445.

Rider, J. A., Moeller, H. C., Swader, J., and Devereaux, R. G. (1959). A study of the anticholinesterase properties of EPN and malathion in human volunteers. *Clin. Res.* **7,** 81–82.

Rider, J. A., Moeller, H. C., and Puletti, E. J. (1966). Continuing studies on anticholinesterase effect of methyl parathion in humans and determination of level of incipient toxicity of OMPA. *Fed. Proc., Fed. Am. Soc. Exp. Biol.* **25**, 687.

Rider, J. A., Moeller, H. C., and Puletti, E. J. (1967). Continuing studies on anticholinesterase effect of methyl parathion, initial studies with Guthion, and determination of incipient toxicity level of dichlorvos in humans. *Fed. Proc., Fed. Am. Soc. Exp. Biol.* **26**, 427–x.

Rider, J. A., Moeller, H. C., Puletti, E. J., and Swader, J. (1968). Studies on the anticholinesterase effects of methyl parathion, Guthion, dichlorvos, and Gardona in human subjects. *Fed. Proc., Fed. Am. Soc. Exp. Biol.* **27**, 597.

Rider, J. A., Moeller, H. C., Puletti, E. J., and Swader, J. I. (1969). Toxicity of parathion, Systox, octamethyl pyrophosphoramide and methyl parathion in man. *Toxicol. Appl. Pharmacol.* **14**, 603–611.

Rider, J. A., Swader, J. I., and Puletti, E. J. (1970). Methyl parathion and Guthion anticholinesterase effects in human subjects. *Fed. Proc., Fed. Am. Soc. Exp. Biol.* **29**, 349.

Rider, J. A., Swader, J. I., and Puletti, E. J. (1971). Anticholinesterase toxicity studies with methyl parathion, Guthion, and Phosdrin in human subjects. *Fed. Proc., Fed. Am. Soc. Exp. Biol.* **30**, 443.

Rider, J. A., Swader, J. I., and Puletti, E. J. (1972). Anticholinesterase toxicity studies with guthion, phosdrin, di-syston, and trithion in human subjects. *Fed. Proc., Fed. Am. Soc. Exp. Biol.* **31**, 520.

Rider, J. A., Puletti, E. J., and Swader, J. I. (1975). The minimal oral toxicity level for mevinphos in man. *Toxicol. Appl. Pharmacol.* **32**, 97–100.

Rikimaru, T., Goto, T., Ezaki, H., and Takamatsu, M. (1972). Status of pesticide application and injuries in cultivators of illuminated chrysanthemum. *Nippon Noson Igakkai Zasshi* **21**, 236–237 (in Japanese).

Rishikesh, N., Mathis, H. L., Ramasamy, M., and King, J. S. (1977a). "A Field Trial of Chlorphoxim for the Control of *Anopheles gambiae* and *An. funestus* in Nigeria," WHO/VBC/77.661. World Health Organ., Geneva.

Rishikesh, N., Mathis, H. L., King, J. S., and Nambiar, R. V. (1977b). "A Field Trial of Pirimiphos-Methyl for the Control of *Anopheles gambiae* and *Anopheles funestus* in Nigeria," WHO/VBC/77.671. World Health Organ., Geneva.

Rivett, K., and Potgieter, P. D. (1987). Diaphragmatic paralysis after organophosphate poisoning: A case report. *S. Afr. Med. J.* **72**, 881–882.

Roan, C. C., Morgan, D. P., Cook, N., and Paschal, E. H. (1969). Blood cholinesterases, serum parathion concentrations and urine *p*-nitrophenol concentrations in exposed individuals. *Bull. Environ. Contam. Toxicol.* **4**, 362–369.

Robbins, W. E., Hopkins, T. L., and Eddy, G. W. (1957). Metabolism of insecticides. Metabolism of excretion of phosphorus-32-labeled diazinon in a cow. *J. Agric. Food Chem.* **5**, 509–513.

Robens, J. F. (1969). Teratologic studies of carbaryl, diazinon, Norea, disulfiram and thiram in small laboratory animals. *Toxicol. Appl. Pharmacol.* **15**, 152–163.

Robens, J. F. (1970). Teratogenic activity of several phthalimide derivatives in the golden hamster. *Toxicol. Appl. Pharmacol.* **16**, 24–35.

Roberts, D. V. (1977). A longitudinal electromyographic study of six men occupationally exposed to organophosphorus compounds. *Int. Arch. Occup. Environ. Health* **38**, 221–229.

Robinson, E. M., Beck, R., McNamara, B. P., Edberg, L. J., and Wills, J. H. (1954). The mechanism of action of anticholinesterase compounds on the patellar reflex. *J. Pharmacol. Exp. Ther.* **110**, 385–391.

Roche, L., LeJeune, E., and Madonna, R. J. M. (1961). Four poisonings with Phosdrin. *Arch. Mal. Prof. Med. Trav. Secur. Soc.* **22**, 52–55.

Rodgers, K. E., Imamura, T., and Devens, B. H. (1986a). Organophosphorus pesticide immunotoxicity: Effects of *O,O,S*-trimethyl phosphorothioate on cellular and humoral immune response systems. *Immunopharmacology* **12**, 193–202.

Rodgers, K. E., Leung, N., Ware, C. F., Devens, B. H., and Imamura, T. (1986b). Lack of immunosuppressive effects on acute and subacute administration of malathion on murine cellular and humoral immune responses. *Pestic. Biochem. Physiol.* **25**, 358–365.

Rodgers, K. E., Leung, N., Ware, C. F., and Imamura, T. (1987). Effects of

O,O,S-trimethyl phosphorodithioate on immune function. *Toxicology* **43**, 201–216.

Rodnitzky, R. L., Levin, H. S., and Morgan, D. P. (1978). Effects of ingested parathion on neurobehavioral functions. *Clin. Toxicol.* **13**, 347–359.

Roger, J. C. (1964). Nicotinic acid analogs: Effects on response of chick embryos and hens to organophosphate toxicants. *Science* **144**, 539–540.

Roger, J. C., Upshall, D. G., and Casida, J. E. (1969). Structure–activity and metabolism studies on organophosphate teratogens and their alleviating agents in developing hen eggs with special reference to Bidrin. *Biochem. Pharmacol.* **18**, 373–392.

Rogers, A. W., Darzynkiewicz, Z., Salpeter, M. M., Ostrowski, K., and Barnard, E. A. (1969). Quantitative studies on enzymes in structures in striated muscles by labeled inhibitor methods. I. The number of acetylcholinesterase molecules and of other DFP-reactive sites at motor endplates, measured by radioautography. *J. Cell Biol.* **41**, 665–685.

Rose, J. A., and Voss, G. (1971). Anticholinesterase activity and enzymatic degradation of phosphamidon and gamma-chlorophosphamidon: A comparative study. *Bull. Environ. Contam. Toxicol.* **6**, 205–208.

Rosen, F. S. (1960). Toxic hazards, parathion. *N. Engl. J. Med.* **262**, 1243–1244.

Rosenberg, P., and Coon, J. M. (1958). Potentiation between cholinesterase inhibitors. *Proc. Soc. Exp. Biol. Med.* **97**, 836–839.

Rosival, L., Vargova, M., Szokolayova, J., Cerey, K., Hladka, A., Batora, V., Kovacicova, J., and Truchlik, S. (1976). Contribution to the toxic action of *S*-methyl fenitrothion. *Pestic. Biochem. Physiol.* **6**, 280–286.

Rowntree, D. W., Nevin, S., and Wilson, A. (1950). The effects of diisopropylfluorophosphonate in schizophrenia and manic depressive psychosis. *J. Neurol., Neurosurg. Psychiatry* **13**, 47–62.

Rozin, D. G. (1969). A case of acute poisoning with the preparation "Antio." *Gig. Tr. Prof. Zabol.* **13**, 41.

Rump, S., Faff, J., Borkowska, G., Ilozuk, I., and Rabsztyn, T. (1978). Central therapeutic effects of dihydro derivative of pralidoxime (pro-2-PAM) in organophosphate intoxication. *Arch. Int. Pharmacodyn. Ther.* **232**, 321–332.

Russell, R. W., Vasquez, B. J., Overstreet, D. H., and Dalglish, F. W. (1971). Effects of cholinolytic agents on behavior following development of tolerance to low cholinesterase activity. *Psychopharmacologia* **20**, 32–41.

Russell, R. W., Overstreet, D. H., Cotman, C. W., Carson, V. G., Churchhill, L., Dalglish, F. W., and Vasquez, B. J. (1975). Experimental tests of hypotheses about neurochemical mechanisms underlying behavioral tolerance to the anticholinesterase, diisopropylfluorophosphate. *J. Pharmacol. Exp. Ther.* **192**, 73–85.

Ryback, M. (1973). The effect of Foschlor administered in water on the ontogenetic development of white rats and their offspring. *Rocz. Panstw. Zakl. Hig.* **24**, 465–475 (in Polish).

Sachs, A., Cameron, G. R., Cruikshank, J. D., Collumbine, H., Holford, J. M., Evans, C. L., Potter, P. B. L., and Muir, A. (1956). "Medical Manual of Chemical Warfare." Chem. Publ. Co., New York.

Sachsse, K. R., and Hess, R. (1973). Exposure of volunteers and animals in aerial application tests of phosphamidon (Dimecron 100) in India. *Proc. Eur. Soc. Study Drug. Toxic.* **14**, 247–253.

Sachsse, K. R., and Voss, G. (1971). Toxicology of phosphamidon. *Residue Rev.* **37**, 61–88.

Safiulina, S. K., Varlamova, V. P., and Zefirov, Y. N. (1962). Cholinesterase activity in the whole blood, serum, and erythrocytes of normal children. *Vopr. Gematol. Pediatrii, Leningr., Sb.* **2**, 27–32.

Safonov, N. M. (1968). Toxicological characteristics of the new organophosphorus insecticide phosalone: Preliminary data. *Gig. Tr. Prof. Zabol.* **12**, 43–44 (in Russian).

St. John, L. E., Jr., and Lisk, D. J. (1974). Feeding studies with Supracide in the dairy cow. *Bull. Environ. Contam. Toxicol.* **12**, 594–598.

Sakama, H., Nishimura, M., Someya, N., and Ueda, K. (1975). An improved spray inhalation apparatus and inhalation toxicity of organophosphorus pesticides to rats. *Proc. 18th Annu. Meet. Jpn. Soc. Ind. Med.*, pp. 68–69 (in Japanese).

Salazar Mallen, M., Gonzales Barranco, D., and Jurado Mendoze, J. (1971).

Trichlorphone treatment of onchocerciasis. *Ann. Trop. Med. Parasitol.* **65**, 393–398.

Salibaev, N. V. (1966). Arterial pressure in poisoning with organophosphorus insecticides. *Med. Zh. Uzb.* **4**, 23–25 (in Russian).

Salibaev, N. V. (1969). Some hemodynamic indices and cholinesterase activity in persons poisoned by organophosphorus insecticides. *Med. Zh. Uzb.* **8**, 67 (in Russian).

Sallam, M., and El-Ghawaby, S. H. (1980). Safety in the use of pesticides. *J. Environ. Sci. Health, Part B* **B15**, 677–681.

Salpeter, M. M., Kasprzak, H., Feng, H., and Fertuck, H. (1979). Endplates after esterase inactivation *in vivo*: Correlation between esterase concentration, functional response and fine structure. *J. Neurocytol.* **8**, 95–115.

Sanborn, J. R., Metcalf, R. L., and Hansen, L. G. (1977). The neurotoxicity of *O*-(2,5-dichlorophenyl) *O*-methyl phenylphosphonothioate, an impurity and photoproduct of leptophos (Phosvel) insecticide. *Pestic. Biochem. Physiol.* **7**, 142–145.

Sanderson, D. M., and Edson, E. F. (1959). Oxime therapy in poisoning by six organophosphorus insecticides in the rat. *J. Pharm. Pharmacol.* **11**, 721–728.

Sanderson, D. M., and Edson, E. F. (1964). Toxicological properties of the organophosphorus insecticide dimethoate. *Br. J. Ind. Med.* **21**, 52–64.

Santolucito, J. A., and Morrison, G. (1971). EEG of rhesus monkeys following prolonged low-level feeding of pesticides. *Toxicol. Appl. Pharmacol.* **19**, 147–154.

Santolucito, J. A., and Whitcomb, E. (1971). Effect of paraoxon on erythrocyte metabolism as measured by oxygen uptake *in vitro. Br. J. Pharmacol.* **42**, 298–302.

Sare, W. W. (1972). Chronic poisoning by a phosphate ester insecticide, malathion. *N. Z. Med. J.* **75**, 93–94.

Sato, I. (1959). Studies on organic phosphorus Gusathion (Guthion) and Phosdrin. I. The toxicity of Gusathion and Phosdrin. *Kumamoto Med. J.* **12**, 312–317.

Satoh, T., and Moroi, K. (1973). Comparative studies on the inhibition of liver amidases, aminopeptidase and serum cholinesterase by EPN. *Toxicol. Appl. Pharmacol.* **25**, 553–559.

Sauter, E. A., and Steele, E. E. (1972). The effect of low level pesticide feeding on the fertility and hatchability of chicken eggs. *Poult. Sci.* **51**, 71–76.

Sawitsky, A., Fitch, H. M., and Meyer, L. M. (1948). A study of cholinesterase activity in the blood of normal subjects. *J. Lab. Clin. Med.* **33**, 203–206.

Saxena, R. K., Mishra, N. P., and Gupta, S. S. (1974). Experimental study of Tik-Z poisoning and its treatment. *Indian J. Physiol. Pharmacol.* **18**, 212.

Schaffer, N. K., May, S. C., Jr., and Summerson, W. H. (1954). Serine phosphoric acid from diisopropylphosphoryl derivative of eel cholinesterase. *J. Biol. Chem.* **206**, 201–207.

Schiemann, S. (1975). Investigation of the mutagenic action of trichlorfon in the house mouse under different aspects of the dominant lethal test. *Wiss. Z.—Martin-Luther-Univ. Halle-Wittenberg, Math. Naturwiss. Reihe* **24**, 85–86 (in German).

Schiller, G. D., and Overstreet, D. H. (1979). Altered sensitivity of the muscarinic acetylcholine receptor induced by chronic administration of the anticholinesterase agent di-isopropyl fluorophosphate (DFP). *Clin. Exp. Pharmacol. Physiol.* **6**, 228.

Schlinke, J. C. (1970). Chronic toxicity of Dursban in chickens, 1969. *J. Econ. Entomol.* **63**, 319.

Schmidt, G., Schmidt, M., and Nenner, M. (1975). Inhibition of acetylcholinesterase in the bronchial system of rats caused by inhalation of dichlorvos (DDVP). *Naunyn-Schmiedebergs Arch. Pharmacol.* **287**, Suppl, R97.

Scholz, R. O., and Wallen, L. J. (1946). Effects of di-isopropyl fluorophosphate on normal human eyes. *J. Pharmacol. Exp. Ther.* **88**, 238–245.

Schoof, H. F., Jensen, J. A., Porter, J. E., and Maddock, D. R. (1961). Disinsection of aircraft with a mechanical dispenser of DDVP vapour. *Bull. W.H.O.* **24**, 623–628.

Schorn, D. (1972). Parathion poisoning: A case report. *S. Afr. Med. J.* **46**, 262–265.

Schrader, G. (1963a). "The Development of Phosphoric Acid Esters." Verlag Chemie, Weinhein, West Germany (in German).

Schrader, G. (1963b). Construction and action of organic phosphorus compounds. *Z. Naturforsch., B: Anorg. Chem., Org. Chem., Biochem., Biophys., Biol.* **18**, 965–975 (in German).

Schrader, G. (1975). Insecticidal phosphoric acid esters. *Angew. Chem.* **69**, 86 (in German).

Schubert, W. (1970). Investigation of the activity of dimethoate against the migratory stage of *Ascaris suum* (Linné, 1758) in experimentally infested mice and rabbits. *Arch. Exp. Veterinaermed.* **24**, 1263–1268.

Schulman, S., Rider, J. A., and Richter, R. B. (1953). Use of octamethyl pyrophosphoramide in treatment of myasthenia gravis. Further observations. *JAMA, J. Am. Med. Assoc.* **152**, 1707–1711.

Schuppon, R. (1961). Recent acquisitions in the domain of insecticides. *Chim. Ind. (Paris)* **85**, 421–436 (in French).

Schwarz, H. (1965). Investigation on the decomposition and separation of ^{32}P-labeled trichlorfon in swine. *Zentralbl. Veterinaermed., Reihe B* **17**, 653–660 (in German).

Scudamore, H. H., Vorhaus, L. J., and Kark, R. M. (1951). Observations on erythrocyte and plasma cholinesterase activity in dyscrasias of the blood. *Blood* **6**, 1260–1273.

Sealey, J. L. (1951). "Organic Phosphate Study of the Environmental Research Laboratory, University of Washington, Dec. 1951" (cited by Wolfsie and Winter, 1952).

Section of Labor Hygiene, Division of Safety and Hygiene, Japan Ministry of Labor (1972). Case histories of occupational disease. Poisoning ascribed to an organophosphorus pesticide. *Rodo Eisel* **13**, 52–54.

Seizaburo, K., and Takabumi, I. (1978). Studies on the relationship between enzyme inhibition and fetal toxicity by organophosphorus insecticides. *Congenital Anom.* **18**, 164–165.

Selye, H. (1970). Estrogen sensitization to toxic effect of octamethyl pyrophosphorimide. *Arzneim.-Forsch.* **20**, 1488–1490.

Senanayake, N., and Johnson, M. K. (1982). Acute polyneuropathy after poisoning by a new organophosphate insecticide. *N. Engl. J. Med.* **306**, 155–157.

Senanayake, N., and Karalliedde, L. (1987). Neurotoxic effects of organophosphorus insecticides: An intermediate syndrome. *N. Engl. J. Med.* **316**, 761–763.

Seume, F. W., and O'Brien, R. D. (1960a). Potentiation of the toxicity to insects and mice of phosphorothionates containing carboxyester and carboxyamide groups. *Toxicol. Appl. Pharmacol.* **2**, 495–503.

Seume, F. W., and O'Brien, R. D. (1960b). Metabolism of malathion by rat tissue preparations and its modification by EPN. *J. Agric. Food Chem.* **8**, 36–47.

Seume, F. W., Casida, J. E., and O'Brien, R. D. (1960). Effects of parathion and malathion separately and jointly upon rat esterases *in vivo. J. Agric. Food Chem.* **8**, 43–47.

Seybold, R., and Braeutigam, K. H. (1968). Prolonged succinyl apnea as an indication of alkyl phosphate poisoning. *Dtsch. Med. Wochenschr.* **93**, 1405–1406.

Shaffer, C. B., and West, B. (1960). The acute and subacute toxicity of technical *O,O*-diethyl *S*-2 diethylaminoethyl phosphorothioate hydrogen oxalate (Tetram®). *Toxicol. Appl. Pharmacol.* **2**, 1–13.

Shafik, T. M. (1973). The determination of pentachlorophenol and hexachlorophene in human adipose tissue. *Bull. Environ. Contam. Toxicol.* **10**, 57–63.

Shankar, P. S. (1966). Pralidoxime chloride in diazinon poisoning. A report of six cases. *J. Indian Med. Assoc.* **46**, 263–264.

Shankar, P. S. (1967). Diazinon poisoning. *Antiseptic* **64**, 155–162.

Shanor, S. P., Baart, N., van Hees, G. R., Erdos, E. E. G., and Foldes, F. F. (1956). Sex variation in human plasma cholinesterase activity. *Fed. Proc., Fed. Am. Soc. Exp. Biol.* **15**, 482.

Shanor, S. P., van Hees, G. R., Baart, N., Erdos, E. E. G., and Foldes, F. F. (1961). The influence of age and sex on human plasma and red cell cholinesterase. *Am. J. Med. Sci.* **242**, 357–361.

Sharkey, S. J. (1896). On peripheral neuritis. *Br. Med. J.* 456–458.

Sharma, R. P., Shupe, J. L., and Potter, J. R. (1973). Tissue cholinesterase inhibition by 2-carbomethoxyl-1-methylvinyldimethyl phosphate (mevinphos). *Toxicol. Appl. Pharmacol.* **24**, 645–652.

Shawarby, A. A., El-Rafai, A. R., El-Hawary, M. F. S., and El-Essawi, M. (1963). Field and laboratory studies on the use of malathion for control of body-lice in Egypt. *Bull. W.H.O.* **28**, 111–120.

Shea, K. P. (1974). Nerve damage—the return of "ginger jake." *Environment* **16**(9), 6–10.

Sherman, M., and Herrick, R. B. (1973). Fly control and chronic toxicity from feeding Dursban (*O,O*-diethyl-*O*-3,5,6-trichloro-2-pyridylphosphorothioate) to laying hens. *Poult. Sci.* **52**, 741–747.

Sherman, M., and Ross, E. (1961). Acute and subacute toxicity of insecticides to chicks. *Toxicol. Appl. Pharmacol.* **3**, 521–533.

Sherman, M., Ross, E., and Chang, M. T. Y. (1965). Acute and subacute toxicity of several insecticides to chicks. *Toxicol. Appl. Pharmacol.* **7**, 606–608.

Sherman, M., Herrick, R. B., Ross, E., and Chang, M. T. Y. (1967). Further studies on the acute and subacute toxicity of insecticides to chicks. *Toxicol. Appl. Pharmacol.* **11**, 49–67.

Sherman, M., Beck, J., and Herrick, R. B. (1972). Chronic toxicity and residues from feeding Nemacide [*O*-(2,4-dichlorophenyl)-*O,O*-diethyl phosphorothioate] to laying hens. *J. Agric. Food Chem.* **20**, 617–624.

Shimamoto, K., and Hattori, K. (1968). Chronic feeding of Baytex (*O,O*-dimethyl-*O*-(4-methyl-mercapto-3 methyl)phenyl-thiophosphate) in rats. *Acta Sch. Med. Univ. Kioto* **40**, 163–171.

Shinoda, H., Ito, K., Matsunaga, T., Takada, T., and Nomura, T. (1972). Two suicides by acute pesticide intoxication. *J. Jpn. Assoc. Rural Med.* **21**, 242 (in Japanese).

Shiozaki, H., Kuwahara, R., Tsujita, E., Taraka, A., Kihira, Y., Inoue, S., and Takasaki, H. (1977). Two cases of autopsies of victims of acute intoxication by organophosphorus pesticides, EPN and dichlorvos. *Med. Treatment* **31**, 161–163.

Shivanandappa, T., Joseph, P., and Krishnakumari, M. K. (1988). Response of blood and brain cholinesterase to dermal exposure of bromophos in the rat. *Toxicology* **48**, 199–208.

Shrivastava, S. P., and Knowles, C. O. (1972). Stability studies of iodofenphos insecticide. *J. Econ. Entomol.* **65**, 1488–1490.

Shutov, A. A., and Varavkina, T. T. (1969). Neurological disorders in acute chlorophos poisoning. *Klin. Med. (Moscow)* **47**, 140–142 (in Russian).

Siers, D. G., Brown, L. J., Chai, E. Y., and Schooley, M. A. (1974). Components of the dichlorvos litter weight effect. *J. Anim. Sci.* **39**, 189.

Siers, D. G., Mersmann, H. J., Brown, L. J., and Stanton, H. C. (1976). Late gestation feeding of dichlorvos: A physiological characterization of the neonate and a growth–survival response. *J. Anim. Sci.* **42**, 381–392.

Silver, A. (1960). Ataxia in hens poisoned by triparaethylphenyl phosphate. *Nature (London)* **185**, 247–248.

Simkin, A. Z., and Mironov, Y. P. (1971). Acute poisoning with chlorphos. *Klin. Med. (Moscow)* **49**, 133–134 (in Russian).

Simmon, V. P., Poole, D. C., and Newell, G. W. (1976). *In vitro* mutagenic studies of twenty pesticides. *Toxicol. Appl. Pharmacol.* **37**, 109.

Simpson, G. R., and Penney, D. J. (1974). Pesticide poisoning in the Namoi and Macquare valleys. *Med. J. Aust.* **1**, 258–260.

Simson, R. E., Simpson, G. R., and Penney, D. J. (1969). Poisoning with monocrotophos, an organophosphorus pesticide. *Med. J. Aust.* **2**, 1013–1016.

Singh, S., Balkrishan, Singh, S., and Malhotra, V. (1969). Parathion poisoning in Punjab: A clinical and electrocardiographic study of 20 cases. *J. Assoc. Physicians India* **17**, 181–187.

Slott, V., and Ecobichon, D. J. (1984). An acute and subacute neurotoxicity assessment of trichlorfon. *Can. J. Physiol. Pharmacol.* **62**, 513–518.

Smerling, M. (1976). A case of nonfatal criminal E605 forte poisoning. Forensic, clinical, toxicological, and juristic aspects. *Z. Rechtsmed.* **77**, 149–155 (in German).

Smith, G. N. (1966). Basic studies of Dursban insecticide. *Down Earth* **22**, 3–7.

Smith, G. N., Watson, B. S., and Fischer, F. S. (1967). Investigations on Dursban insecticide. Metabolism of (^{36}Cl) *O,O*-diethyl *O*-3,5,6-trichloro-2-pyridyl phosphorothioate in rats. *J. Agric. Food Chem.* **15**, 132–138.

Smith, H. V., and Spalding, J. M. K. (1959). Outbreak of paralysis in Morocco due to *ortho*-cresyl phosphate poisoning. *Lancet* **2**, 1019–1021.

Smith, K. F., Volwiler, W., and Wood, P. A. (1952). Serum acetyl cholinesterase, its close correlation with serum albumin and its limited usefulness as a test of liver function. *J. Lab. Clin. Med.* **40**, 692–702.

Smith, M. I., and Lillie, R. D. (1931). The histopathology of triorthocresyl phosphate poisoning. The etiology of so-called ginger paralysis. *Arch. Neurol. Psychiatry* **26**, 976–992.

Smith, M. I., Elvove, E., Uglaer, P. J., Jr., Frazier, W. H., and Mallory, G. E. (1930a). Pharmacological and chemical studies on the cause of so-called ginger paralysis. *Public Health Rep.* **45**, 1703–1716.

Smith, M. I., Elvove, E., and Frazier, W. H. (1930b). The pharmacological action of certain phenol esters with special reference to the etiology of so-called ginger paralysis. *Public Health Rep.* **45**, 2509–2524.

Smith, M. I., Engel, E. W., and Stohlman, E. F. (1932). Further studies on the pharmacology of certain phenol esters with special reference to the relation of chemical constitution and physiological action. *Natl. Inst. Health Bull.*, **160**, 1–53.

Smith, P. W., Stavinoha, W. B., and Ryan, L. C. (1968). Cholinesterase inhibition in relation to fitness to fly. *Aerosp. Med.* **39**, 754–758.

Smith, P. W., Mertens, H., Lewis, M. F., Funkhouser, G. E., Higgins, E. A., Crane, C. R., Sanders, D. C., Endecott, B. R., and Flux, M. (1972). Toxicology of dichlorvos at operational aircraft cabin altitudes. *Aerosp. Med.* **43**, 473–478.

Smith, R. C., Kimura, M., and Ibsen, M. (1955). Poisoning by organic phosphate insecticides. *Calif. Med.* **83**, 240–243.

Snow, D. H. (1971). The effects of dichlorvos on several blood enzyme levels in the greyhound. *Aust. Vet. J.* **47**, 468–471.

Snow, D. H. (1974). Studies on the action of an anthelmintic preparation of dichlorvos in horses. *Vet. Rec.* **95**, 231–233.

Sobels, F. H., and Todd, N. K. (1979). Absence of a mutagenic effect of dichlorvos in *Drosophila melanogaster*. *Mutat. Res.* **67**, 89–92.

Soliman, S. A., El-Sebae, A. M., and El-Fiki, S. (1979). Occupational effect of phosfolan insecticide on spraymen during field exposure. *J. Environ. Sci. Health, Part B* **14**, 27–37.

Solly, S. R. B., and Harrison, D. L. (1971). Fensulfothion. I. Toxicity to sheep and rats, residues in sheep and persistence on pasture. *N. Z. J. Agric. Res.* **14**, 66–78.

Sonejee, S. L., Manghani, K. K., and Mehta, J. M. (1969). A study of 23 cases of organophosphate poisoning. *Antiseptic* **66**, 161–167.

Sorokin, M. (1969). Orthocresyl phosphate neuropathy: Report of an outbreak in Fiji. *Med. J. Aust.* **1**, 506–509.

Spear, R. C., Popendorf, W. J., Leffingwell, J. T., and Jenkins, D. (1975). Parathion residues on citrus foliage, decay and composition as related to worker hazard. *J. Agric. Food Chem.* **23**, 808–810.

Spear, R. C., Popendorf, W. J., Leffingwell, J. T., Milby, T. H., Davies, J. E., and Spencer, W. J. (1977a). Fieldworkers' response to weathered residues of parathion. *J. Occup. Med.* **19**, 406–410.

Spear, R. C., Popendorf, W. J., Spencer, W. F., and Milby, T. H. (1977b). Worker poisonings due to paraoxon residues. *J. Occup. Med.* **19**, 411–414.

Spencer, P. S., and Schaumburg, H. H. (1976). Feline nervous system response to chronic intoxication with commercial grades of methyl *n*-butyl ketone, methyl *iso*-butyl ketone, and methyl ethyl ketone. *Toxicol. Appl. Pharmacol.* **37**, 301–311.

Spiers, F., and Juul, P. (1964). Cholinesterase activity in plasma and erythrocytes. *Acta Ophthalmol.* **42**, 696–712.

Spyker, J. M., and Avery, K. L. (1977). Neurobehavioral effects of prenatal exposure to the organophosphate diazinon in mice. *J. Toxicol. Environ. Health* **3**, 989–1002.

Sram, R. (1974). Evaluation of the genetic danger of chemical substances. *Gig. Sanit.* **4**, 80–83 (in Russian).

Stanton, H. C., Albert, J. R., and Mershmann, H. J. (1979). Studies on the pharmacology and safety of dichlorvos in pigs and pregnant sows. *Am. J. Vet. Res.* **40**, 315–320.

Staples, R. E., and Goulding, E. H. (1979). Dipterex teratogenicity in the rat, hamster, and mouse when given by gavage. *Environ. Health Perspect.* **30**, 105–113.

Stavinoha, W. B., Modak, A. T., and Weintraub, S. T. (1976). Rate of accumulation of acetylcholine in discrete regions of the rat brain after dichlorvos treatment. *J. Neurochem.* **27**, 1375–1378.

Steen, J. A., Hannemann, G. D., Nelson, P. L., and Folk, E. D. (1976). Acute toxicity of mevinphos to gerbils. *Toxicol. Appl. Pharmacol.* **36**, 195–198.

Stein, W. J., Miller, S., and Fetzer, L. E., Jr. (1966). Studies with dichlorvos residual fumigant as a malaria eradication technique in Haiti. III. Toxicological studies. *Am. J. Trop. Med. Hyg.* **15**, 672–675.

Steinberg, M., Cole, M. M., Miller, T. A., and Godke, R. A. (1972). Toxicological and entomological field evaluation of Mobam and Abate powders used as body louse toxicants (Anoplura: Pediculidae). *J. Med. Entomol.* **9**, 73–77.

Stenger, E. G. (1960). Contribution to the antidotal effect of pyridine-2-aldoxime-N-methiodide (PAM). *Med. Exp.* **3**, 143–149.

Stevens, J. T. (1972). The effects of anticholinesterase insecticides on hepatic microsomal metabolism. *Diss. Abstr. Int. B* **33**, 1707B–1708B.

Stevens, J. T. (1973). The effect of parathion on the metabolism of ^{3}H-testosterone by hepatic microsomal enzymes from the male mouse. *Pharmacology* **10**, 220–225.

Stevens, J. T. (1974). The role of binding in inhibition of hepatic microsomal metabolism by parathion and malathion. *Life Sci.* **14**, 2215–2229.

Stevens, J. T., and Greene, F. E. (1974). Alteration of hepatic microsomal metabolism of male mice by certain anticholinesterase insecticides. *Bull. Environ. Contam. Toxicol.* **11**, 538–544.

Stevens, J. T., Greene, F. E., and Passananti, G. T. (1973). Binding of malathion, parathion, and their oxygenated analogs to cytochrome P-450 in the rat. *Fed. Proc., Fed. Am. Soc. Exp. Biol.* **32**, 761.

Stevenson, D. E., and Blair, D. (1977). The uptake of dichlorvos during long-term inhalation studies. *Proc. Eur. Soc. Toxicol.* **18**, 215–217.

Stiasni, M., Rehbinder, D., and Deckers, W. (1967). Absorption, distribution, and metabolism of O-(4-bromo-2,5-dichlorophenyl)-O,O-dimethyl-phosphorothioate (bromophos) in the rat. *J. Agric. Food Chem.* **15**, 474–478.

Stieglitz, R., Gibel, W., Werner, W., and Stobbe, H. (1974). Experimental study of haemototoxic and leukaemogenic effects of trichlorophone and dimethoate. *Acta Haematol.* **52**, 70–76.

Stoeckel, H., and Meinecke, K. H. (1966). An occupational poisoning by mevinphos. *Arch. Toxikol.* **21**, 284–288 (in German).

Stoller, A., Krupinski, J., Christophers, A. J., and Blanks, G. K. (1965). Organophosphorus insecticides and major mental illness. An epidemiological investigation. *Lancet* **1**, 1387–1388.

Stone, C. T., and Rider, J. A. (1949). Treatment of myasthenia gravis. *JAMA, J. Am. Med. Assoc.* **141**, 107–111.

Stone, W. C. (1950). Use of di-isopropyl fluorophosphate (DFD) in treatment of glaucoma. *Arch. Ophthalmol. (Chicago)* **43**, 36–42.

Stoner, H. B., and Wilson, A. (1943). The effect of muscular exercise on the serum cholinesterase level in normal adults and in patients with myasthenia gravis. *J. Physiol. (London)* **102**, 1–4.

Stuneyeva, G. I. (1974). Toxicity of mixtures of Kelthane, trichlorfon, and copper chloride. *Gig. Sanit.* **39**, 102–103 (in Russian).

Su, M. Q., Kinoshita, F. K., Frawley, J. P., and DuBois, K. P. (1971). Comparative inhibition of aliesterases and cholinesterase in rats fed 18 organophosphorus insecticides. *Toxicol. Appl. Pharmacol.* **20**, 241–249.

Sugahara, N., and Oki, S. (1976). A case of suicide by fenitrothion and the cholinesterase levels in the blood of the corpse. *Jpn. J. Leg. Med.* **30**, 46.

Sugaya, H., and Wakatsuki, S. (1978). Countrywide investigation of clinical cases of pesticide intoxication (collected during 1970–1977). *Jpn. J. Rural Med.* **27**, 436–437.

Sumerford, W. T., Hayes, W. J., Jr., Johnston, J. M., Walker, K., and Spillane, J. (1953). Cholinesterase response and symptomatology from exposure to organic phosphorus insecticides. *Arch. Ind. Hyg. Occup. Med.* **7**, 383–398.

Suplain, Supratman, Shaw, R. F., Pradhan, G. D., Bang, Y. H., Fleming, G. A., and Fanara, D. N. (1979). "A Village-Scale Trial of Primiphos-Methyl (OMS-1424) Emulsifiable Concentrate at the Reduced Dosage of 1 g/m² for Control of the Malaria Vector *Anopheles aconitus* in Central Java, Indonesia," WHO/BVC, 79.752. World Health Organ., Geneva.

Suzuki, S. (1970). Fenitrothion (Sumithion). *Pestic. Tech.* **22**, 57–69 (in Japanese).

Suzuki, Y. (1973). Toxicological study of ethyl-p-nitrophenyl phosphonothionate (EPN) in rats, with special reference to the toxicity criteria for the determination of its residual toxicity in food. *J. Med. Soc. Toho Univ.* **20**, 126–144 (in Japanese).

Suzuki, Y., Kikuchi, H., and Uchiyama, M. (1975). The release of β-glucuronidase from rat liver by the administration of diazinon, the organophosphorus insecticide. *Chem. Pharm. Bull.* **23**, 886–890.

Svetličić, B., and Vandekar, M. (1960). Therapeutic effect of pyridine-2-aldoxime methiodide in parathion poisoned animals. *J. Comp. Pathol. Ther.* **70**, 257–271.

Svetličić, B., and Wilhelm, K. (1968). Accidental poisoning due to the dermal application of the organo-phosphorus insecticide Neguvon. *Arh. Hig. Rada Toksikol.* **19**, 241–243 (in Serbo-Croatian).

Szutowski, M. M. (1975). Effect of carbon tetrachloride on activation and detoxication of organophosphorus insecticides in the rat. *Toxicol. Appl. Pharmacol.* **33**, 350–355.

Tabershaw, I. R., and Cooper, W. C. (1966). Sequelae of acute organic phosphate poisoning. *J. Occup. Med.* **8**, 5–20.

Tajima, S., and Todoriki, I. (1955). Detection of parathion from dead bodies, especially buried for 10 months. *Sci. Crime Detect.* **8**, 32–36.

Takade, D. Y., Allsup, T., Khasawinah, A., Kao, T. S., and Fukuto, T. R. (1976). Metabolism of O,O-dimethyl 5a(carboethoxy)benzyl phosphorodithioate (phenthoate) in the white mouse and house flies. *Pestic. Biochem. Physiol.* **6**, 367–376.

Takahashi, K., Nakamura, H., and Iwata, K. (1975). On the ultrafine structure of peripheral nerves in toxic polyneuropathy due to trichlorfon. *Clin. Neurol. (Tokyo)* **15**, 430–435 (in Japanese).

Talaat, S. M. (1964). "The Treatment of Schistosomiasis and Other Intestinal Parasites with Dipterex." United Arab Republic, Cairo.

Talcott, R. E., Mallipudi, N. M., Umetsu, N., and Fukuto, T. R. (1979a). Inactivation of esterases by impurities isolated from technical malathion. *Toxicol. Appl. Pharmacol.* **49**, 107–112.

Talcott, R. E., Denk, H., and Mallipudi, N. M. (1979b). Malathion carboxylesterase activity in human liver and its inactivation by isomalathion. *Toxicol. Appl. Pharmacol.* **49**, 373–376.

Talcott, R. E., Mallipudi, N. M., and Fukuto, T. R. (1979c). Malathion carboxylesterase titer and its relationship to malathion toxicity. *Toxicol. Appl. Pharmacol.* **50**, 501–504.

Talens, G., and Woolley, D. (1973). Effects of parathion administration during gestation in the rat on development of the young. *Proc. West. Pharmacol. Soc.* **16**, 141–145.

Taneda, M., and Hara, T. (1975). Narcoleptic-like symptoms in organophosphorus poisoning, a case report. *Brain Nerve* **27**, 211–218.

Tanimura, T., Katsuya, T., and Nishimura, H. (1967). Embryotoxicity of acute exposure to methyl parathion in rats and mice. *Arch. Environ. Health* **15**, 609–613.

Taraschyuk, V. V. (1966a). The clinical picture of intoxication with methyl-mercaptophos. *Sov. Med.* **29**, 80–82.

Taraschyuk, V. V. (1966b). Poisoning with methylsystox. *Klin. Med. (Moscow)* **44**, 40–43.

Taya, T., Sugiura, K., Fukuda, M., Ishibara, K., and Niwa, T. (1976). Intoxication of an entire family by fenitrothion. *J. Jpn. Assoc. Rural Med.* **25**, 330–331.

Taylor, A. (1963). Observations on human exposure to the organophosphorus insecticide fenthion in Nigeria. *Bull. W.H.O.* **29**, 205–212.

Teichert-Kuliszewska, K., and Szymczyk, T. (1979). Changes in rat carbohydrate metabolism after acute and chronic treatment with dichlorvos. *Toxicol. Appl. Pharmacol.* **47**, 323–330.

Teichmann, B., and Hauschild, F. (1978). Testing of the carcinogenic action of O,O-dimethyl-(1-hydroxy-2,2,2-trichloroethyl)-phosphate (trichlorfon) in mice by oral (stomach tube), intraperitoneal, and dermal application. *Arch. Geschwulstforsch.* **48**, 301–307 (in German).

Teichmann, B., and Schmidt, A. (1978). Testing of the carcinogenic action of *O,O*-dimethyl-(1-hydroxy-2,2,2-trichloroethyl) phosphate (trichlorfon) in the Syrian golden hamster (*Mesocricetus auratus* Waterhouse) by intraperitoneal injection. *Arch. Geschwulstforsch.* **48**, 718–721 (in German).

Teichmann, B., Hauschild, F., and Ecklemann, A. (1978). Testing of the carcinogenic action of *O,O*-dimethyl-(1-hydroxy-2,2,2-trichloroethyl) phosphate (trichlorfon) in the rat by oral (stomach tube) and intraperitoneal administration. *Arch. Geschwulstforsch.* **48**, 112–119 (in German).

Teitelman, U., Adler, M., Levy, L., and Dikstein, S. (1975). Treatment of massive poisoning by the organophosphate pesticide methidathion. *Clin. Toxicol.* **8**, 277–282.

Tenhet, J. N., Bare, C. O., and Childs, D. P. (1957). "Studies of DDVP for Control of Cigarette Beetles in Tobacco Warehouses," Publ. AMS-214. U. S. Dept. Agric., Washington, D.C.

Thomas, J. A., and Mawhinney, M. G. (1974). Failure of parathion to alter male mouse reproductive organ activity. *Toxicol. Appl. Pharmacol.* **29**, 134–135.

Thomas, J. A., and Schein, L. G. (1974). Effect of parathion on the uptake and metabolism of androgens in rodent sex accessory organs. *Toxicol. Appl. Pharmacol.* **29**, 53–58.

Thorpe, E., Wilson, A. B., Dix, K. M., and Blair, D. (1972). Teratological studies with dichlorvos vapour in rabbits and rats. *Arch. Toxikol.* **30**, 29–38.

Tilsner, V. (1966). Case history of a patient with delayed onset of poisoning by a plant-protection agent. *Aerztl. Forsch.* **20**, 272–273 (in German).

Timmons, E. H., Chaklos, R. J., Bannister, T. M., and Kaplan, H. M. (1975). Dichlorvos effects on estrus cycle onset in the rat. *Lab. Anim. Sci.* **25**, 45–47.

Titova, N. N., and Badiugin, I. S. (1970). Acute chlorphos poisoning. *Kazan. Med. Zh.* **1**, 37–40.

Tomizawa, C., Uesugi, Y., and Murai, T. (1972). Fate and significance of fungicides in rice. *In* "Radiotracer Studies of Chemical Residues in Food and Agriculture." Int. At. Energy Agency, Vienna.

Tracy, R. L. (1960). Insecticidal and toxicological properties of DDVP. *Soap Chem. Spec.* **36**, 74–76.

Tracy, R. L., Woodcock, J. G., and Chodroff, S. (1960). Toxicological aspects of 2,2-dichlorovinyl dimethyl phosphate (DDVP) in cows, horses, and white rats. *J. Econ. Entomol.* **53**, 593–601.

Trefilov, V. N., Faerman, I. S., and Skanavi, M. D. (1968). The hygiene characteristics of working conditions and the health status of workers engaged in the manufacture of carbophos. *Gig. Tr. Prof. Zabol.* **12**, 7–11 (in Russian).

Tsumuki, H., Saito, T., Miyata, T., and Kisabu, I. (1970). Acute and subacute toxicity of organophosphorus insecticides to mammals. *In* "Biochemical Toxicology of Insecticides" (R. D. O'Brien and I. Yamamoto, eds.). Academic Press, New York.

Tsuyuki, H., Stahmann, M. A., and Casida, J. E. (1955). Preparation, purification, isomerization, and biological properties of octamethyl-pyrophosphoramide *N*-oxide. *J. Agric. Food Chem.* **3**, 922–932.

Tumbleson, M. E., and Wescott, R. B. (1969). Serum biochemic values in piglets from sows fed dichlorvos prior to farrowing. *J. Comp. Lab. Med.* **3**, 67–70.

Tuthill, J. W. G. (1958). Toxic hazards: Malathion poisoning. *N. Engl. J. Med.* **258**, 1018–1019.

Tzoneva-Maneva, M. T., Kaloianova, F., and Georgieva, V. (1971). Influence of diazinon and lindane on the mitotic activity and the caryotype of human lymphocytes, cultivated *in vitro*. *Bibl. Haematol.* **38**, 344–347.

Uchida, T., and O'Brien, R. D. (1967). Dimethoate degradation by human liver and its significance for acute toxicity. *Toxicol. Appl. Pharmacol.* **10**, 89–94.

Uchida, T., Dauterman, W. C., and O'Brien, R. D. (1964). The metabolism of dimethoate by vertebrate tissues. *J. Agric. Food Chem.* **12**, 48–52.

Uchida, T., Zschintzsch, J., and O'Brien, R. D. (1966). Relation between synergism and metabolism of dimethoate in mammals and insects. *Toxicol. Appl. Pharmacol.* **8**, 259–265.

Uchiyama, M., Yoshida, T., and Homma, K. (1973). Persistence of organophosphorus insecticides in animals and changes in detoxifying activity. *J. Jpn. Biochem. Soc.* **45**, 551 (in Japanese).

Uchiyama, M., Yoshida, T., Homma, K., and Hongo, T. (1974). Inhibition of hepatic drug-metabolizing enzymes by thiophosphate insecticides and its drug toxicological implications. *Biochem. Pharmacol.* **24**, 1221–1225.

Ueyama, I., and Takase, I. (1975). Metabolic behavior of *O*-ethyl S,S-diphenyl phosphorodithioate (edifenphos) in female goat. *Agric. Biol. Chem.* **39**, 1719–1727.

Ueyama, I., Takase, I., and Tomizawa, C. (1978). Metabolism of edifenphos (*O*-ethyl diphenyl phosphorodithioate) in mouse and rat. *Agric. Biol. Chem.* **42**, 885–887.

Umetsu, N., Grose, F. H., Allahyari, R., Abu-El-Haj, S., and Fukuto, T. R. (1977). Effect of impurities on the mammalian toxicity of technical malathion and acephate. *J. Agric. Food Chem.* **25**, 946–953.

Umetsu, N., Mallipudi, N. M., Toia, R. F., March, R. B., and Fukuto, T. R. (1981). Toxicological properties of phosphorothioate and related esters as impurities in technical organophosphorus insecticides. *J. Toxicol. Environ. Health* **7**, 481.

Upholt, W. M., Quinby, G. E., and Batchelor, G. S. (1954). Eating Systox-treated fruit under controlled conditions. *Proc. 50th Annu. Meet. Washington State Horticult. Assoc.* pp. 217–220.

Upholt, W. M., Quinby, G. E., Batchelor, G. S., and Thompson, J. P. (1956). Visual effects accompanying TEPP induced miosis. *Arch. Ophthalmol. (Chicago)* **56**, 128–134.

Urban, E., and Sando, M. J. W. (1965). Organic phosphate poisoning. *Med. J. Aust.* **2**, 313–316.

U.S. Department of Health, Education, and Welfare (USDHEW) (1969). Uses and benefits (Chapter 1). *In* "Report of the Secretary's Commission on Pesticides and Their Relationship to Environmental Health," Part 2, pp. 43–46. U. S. Dept. Health, Educ., Welfare, Washington, D.C.

Vahlquist, B. (1935). On the esterase activity of human blood plasma. *Skand. Arch. Physiol.* **72**, 113–160.

Vaidya, V. G., and Patankar, N. (1980). Studies on the cytogenetic effects of oxydemetonmethyl in the human leukocyte and mouse micronucleus test systems. *Mutat. Res.* **78**, 385–387.

Vajda, A., Schmid, H., Groll-Knapp, E., and Haider, M. (1974). EEG changes and changes in evoked potentials, caused by insecticides. *Electroencephalogr. Clin. Neurophysiol.* **37**(4), 442.

Vale, J. A., Rees, A. J., Widdop, B., and Goulding, R. (1975). Use of charcoal haemoperfusion in the management of severely poisoned patients. *Br. Med. J.* **1**, 5–9.

Valero, A., and Golan, D. (1967). Accidental organic phosphorus poisoning: The use of propranolol to counteract vagolytic cardiac effects of atropine. *Isr. J. Med. Sci.* **3**, 582–584.

Van Asperen, K., and Dekhuijzen, H. M. (1958). A quantitative analysis of the kinetics of cholinesterase inhibition in tissue homogenates of mice and houseflies. *Biochim. Biophys. Acta* **28**, 603–613.

Vandekar, M. (1957). Anaesthetic effect produced by organophosphorus compounds. *Nature (London)* **179**, 154–155.

Vandekar, M. (1958). The toxic properties of demeton-methyl ("Metasystox") and some related compounds. *Br. J. Ind. Med.* **15**, 158–167.

Vandekar, M. (1965). "Observations of the Toxicity of Two Organophosphorus and One Carbamate Insecticide in a Village Trial Performed by WHO Insecticide Testing Unit in Lagos During 1964," WHO Work. Doc. 65/Tox/2.64. U.S. Govt. Printing Office, Washington, D.C.

Vandekar, M., and Heath, D. F. (1957). The reactivation of cholinesterase after inhibition *in vivo* by some dimethyl phosphate esters. *Biochem. J.* **67**, 202–208.

Vandekar, M., and Svetličić, B. (1966). Observations on the toxicity of three anticholinesterase insecticides in a village-scale trial and comparison of methods used for determining cholinesterase activity. *Arh. Hig. Rada Toksikol.* **17**, 135–150.

Varnai, L. (1971). Data on the pathological anatomy and pathological histology of malathion poisoning. *Orv. Hetil.* **112**, 1651–1653 (in Hungarian).

Vashkov, V. I., Volkova, A. P., Tsetlin, V. M., and Yankovsky, E. Y. (1966). Assessment of the use of dimethyldichlorvinylphosphate (DDVP) in insecticide mixtures. *Gig. Sanit.* **31**, 15–17 (in Russian).

Vasilescu, C. (1972). Motor nerve conduction velocity and electromyogram in triorthocresyl-phosphate poisoning. *Rev. Roum. Neurol.* **9**, 345–350.

Vasilescu, C., Alexianu, M., and Dan, A. (1984). Delayed neuropathy after organophosphorus insecticide (Dipterex) poisoning: A clinical, electrophysiological and nerve biopsy study. *J. Neurol., Neurosurg. Psychiatry* **47**, 543–548.

Vatulin, N. T., Goncharov, V. P., and Malyutina, L. M. (1971). Acute poisoning with chlorphos. *Vrach. Delo* **9**, 140–141 (in Russian).

Velbinger, H. H. (1949). On the different action of modern insecticides DDT, Gammexane, and E605. *Pharmazie* **4**, 165–176 (in German).

Verberk, M. M. (1977). Incipient cholinesterase inhibition in volunteers ingesting monocrotophos or mevinphos for one month. *Toxicol. Appl. Pharmacol.* **42**, 345–350.

Verberk, M. M., and Salle, H. J. A. (1977). Effects on nervous function in volunteers ingesting mevinphos for one month. *Toxicol. Appl. Pharmacol.* **42**, 351–358.

Vercruysse, A., and Deslypere, P. (1967). Acute parathion poisoning. *MD. J.* **16**, 21–33.

Verhulst, H. L., and Crotty, J. J. (1965). Di-isopropyl fluorophosphate. *Natl. Clearinghouse Poison Control Cent. Bull.*, May–June.

Vernik, A. Y. (1971). Polyneuritis from chlorophos. *Sov. Med.* **9**, 44–45.

Veronesi, B., and Padilla, S. (1985). Phenylmethylsulfonyl fluoride protects rats from mipafox-induced delayed neuropathy. *Toxicol. Appl. Pharmacol.* **81**, 258–264.

Vesileva, R., and Abrasheva, P. (1960). Experimental studies on a possibility of determining E-605 in exhumed cadavers and chemical and legal determination of poisoning. *Nauchn. Tr. Vissh. Med. Inst., Sofia* **39**, 189–202.

Vethanayagam, A. V. (1962). Folidol poisoning. *Ceylon Med. J.* **7**, 209–211.

Villares, E. J. (1968). The pesticides problem in Puerto Rico. *Ind. Med. Surg.* **37**, 518.

Villeneuve, D. C., Phillips, W. E. J., and Syrotiuk, J. (1970). Modification of microsomal enzyme activity and parathion toxicity in rats. *Bull. Environ. Contam. Toxicol.* **5**, 125–132.

Villeneuve, D. C., Willes, R. F., Lacroix, J. B., and Phillips, W. E. J. (1972). Placental transfer of ^{14}C-parathion administered intravenously to sheep. *Toxicol. Appl. Pharmacol.* **21**, 542–548.

Vinopal, J. H., and Fukuto, T. R. (1971). Selective toxicity of phoxim. *Pestic. Biochem. Physiol.* **1**, 44–60.

Viyevskiy, N. A. (1974). Comparative experimental characterization of the allergenic effect of some pesticides. *Vrach. Delo* **5**, 126–130 (in Russian).

Vogin, E. E., Carson, S., and Slomka, M. B. (1971). Teratology studies with dichlorvos in rabbits. *Toxicol. Appl. Pharmacol.* **19**, 377–378.

Voiculescu, V., Gheorghiu, M., Cioran, C., Dumitrescu, C., and Plaiasu, D. (1971). Polyneuritis due to organophosphate insecticide (parathion and Dipterex) poisoning. *Neurol., Psihiatr., Neurochir.* **16**, 535–539 (in Romanian).

von Clarmann, M., and Gelmacher-von Mallinckrodt, M. (1966). A successfully treated case of acute oral poisoning by fenthion and its demonstration in the gastric contents and urine. *Arch. Toxikol.* **22**, 2–11.

Voogd, C. E., Jacobs, J. J. J. A. A., and Van Der Stel, J. J. (1972). On the mutagenic action of dichlorvos. *Mutat. Res.* **16**, 413–416.

Vorhaus, L. J., II, and Kark, R. M. (1953). Serum cholinesterase in health and disease. *Am. J. Med.* **14**, 707–719.

Vorob'yeva, N. M., and Lapchenko, V. S. (1970). Indexes of the functional state of the liver during poisoning with the preparation Anthio. *Vopr. Ratsion. Pitan.* **6**, 141–144.

Vorob'yeva, N. M., and Lapchenko, V. S. (1973). Toxicological characteristics of the new pesticide Anthio. *Farmakol. Toksikol. (Moscow)* **6**, 104 (in Russian).

Vrbovský, L., Selecký, F. V., and Rosival, L. (1959). Toxicological and pharmacological studies of phosphoric acid ester insecticides. *Naunyn-Schmiedebergs Arch. Exp. Pathol. Pharmakol.* **236**, 202–204 (in German).

Vukovich, R. A., Triolo, A. J., and Coon, J. M. (1971). The effect of chlorpromazine on the toxicity and biotransformation of parathion in mice. *J. Pharmacol. Exp. Ther.* **178**, 395–401.

Vyas, S. P., Vijayargiya, R., Sharma, K. S., and Saxena, M. (1977). Reversal by L-histidine of phosphamidon-inhibited cholinesterase activity of brain and liver of rats. *Indian J. Physiol. Pharmacol.* **21**, 280.

Wadia, R. S., Karnik, V. M., and Ichaporia, R. N. (1971). Cholinesterase levels in diazinon poisoning. *J. Assoc. Physicians India* **19**, 185–191.

Wadia, R.S., Sadagopan, C., Amin, R. B., and Sardesai, H. V. (1974). Neurological manifestations of organophosphorus insecticide poisoning. *J. Neurol., Neurosurg. Psychiatry* **37**, 841–847.

Wadia, R. S., Bhirud, R. H., Gulavani, A. V., and Amin, R. B. (1977). Neurological manifestations of three organophosphate poisons. *Indian J. Med. Res.* **66**, 460–468.

Wagner, J. E., and Johnson, D. R. (1970). Toxicity of dichlorvos for laboratory mice—LD50 and effect on serum cholinesterase. *Lab. Anim. Care* **20**, 45–47.

Wakasuki, S. (1976). Animal experiments on pesticide residues in living organisms and on the occurrence of intoxication symptoms. *J. Jpn. Assoc. Rural Med.* **25**, 48.

Waldman, R. K., and Krouse, L. A. (1952). A rapid routine method for determination of paranitrophenol in urine. *Occup. Health* **12**, 37–38.

Walker, C. M., and Mackness, M. I. (1987). "A" esterases and their role in regulating the toxicity of organophosphates. *Arch. Toxicol.* **60**, 30–33.

Walker, N. E. (1971). The effect of malathion and malaoxon on esterases and gross development of the chick embryo. *Toxicol. Appl. Pharmacol.* **19**, 590–601.

Wallach, J. D., and Frueh, R. (1968). Pilot study of an organophosphate anthelmintic in camels and primates. *J. Am. Vet. Med. Assoc.* **153**, 798–799.

Walters, M. N. I. (1957). Malathion intoxication. *Med. J. Aust.* **44**, 876–877.

Ward, F. P., and Glicksberg, C. L. (1971). Effects of dichlorvos on blood cholinesterase activity in dogs. *J. Am. Vet. Med. Assoc.* **158**, 457–461.

Ware, G. W., Morgan, D. P., Estesen, B. J., and Cahill, W. P. (1975). Establishment of reentry intervals for organophosphate-treated cotton fields based on human data. III. 12 to 72 hours post-treatment exposure to monocrotophos, ethyl- and methyl parathion. *Arch. Environ. Contam. Toxicol.* **3**, 289–306.

Warren, M. C., Conrad, J. P., Bocian, J. J., and Hayes, M. (1963). Clothing-borne epidemic. *JAMA, J. Am. Med. Assoc.* **184**, 266–268.

Warriner, R. A., III, Nies, A. S., and Hayes, W. J., Jr. (1977). Severe organophosphate poisoning complicated by alcohol and turpentine ingestion. *Arch. Environ. Health* **32**, 203–205.

Waser, P. G., ed. (1975). "Cholinergic Mechanisms." Raven Press, New York.

Watanabe, H., Shirai, O., and Ebata, N. (1974). A case report of organophosphorus insecticide (DDVP) intoxication with respiratory intensive care. *Sapporo Med. J.* **43**, 334–337.

Watanabe, S. (1972a). Acute organophosphate poisoning detected in plasma, and its significance. *Prog. Med.* **80**, 696–697 (in Japanese).

Watanabe, S. (1972b). Detection of organophosphate pesticides in sera from diagnosed cases of acute or chronic organophosphate poisoning. *J. Jpn. Soc. Intern. Med.* **61**, 953–954 (in Japanese).

Watanabe, S. (1972c). Poisoning by parathion used in apple orchards. *Biotechnol. Bioeng. Symp.* **3**, 268–274.

Webb, R. E., Bloomer, C. C., and Miranda, C. L. (1973). Effects of casein diets on the toxicity of malathion and parathion and their oxygen analogues. *Bull. Environ. Contam. Toxicol.* **9**, 102–107.

Weber, R. P., Coon, J. M., and Triolo, A. J. (1974). Effect of organophosphate insecticide parathion and its active metabolite paraoxon on the metabolism of benzo(a)pyrene in the rat. *Cancer Res.* **34**, 947–952.

Weiner, A. (1961). Bronchial asthma due to the organic phosphate insecticides. *Ann. Allergy* **19**, 397–401.

Welch, R. M., and Coon, J. M. (1964). Studies on the effect of chlorcyclinizine and other drugs on the toxicity of several organo-phosphate anticholinesterases. *J. Pharmacol. Exp. Ther.* **144**, 192–198.

Welsch, F., and Dettbarn, W. D. (1972). Inhibition of rat diaphragm muscle by organophosphates and spontaneous recovery of enzyme activity *in vitro*. *Biochem. Pharmacol.* **21**, 1039–1049.

Wender, M., and Owsianowski, M. (1969). On a successfully treated acute oral paraoxon (E 600) poisoning. *Arch. Toxikol.* **25**, 329–332.

Wenger, B. S., and Wenger, E. (1973). Prevention of malathion-induced malformations in chick embryos by nicotinamide and tryptophan. *Proc. Can. Fed. Biol. Soc.* **16**, 61.

Wennerberg, R., and Löfroth, G. (1974). Formation of 7-methylguanine by dichlorvos in bacteria and mice. *Chem.-Biol. Interact.* **8**, 339–348.

Wenzel, K. D., and Dedek, W. (1971). Isolation and identification of eye-irritating byproducts of dimethoate synthesis. *Z. Chem.* **11**, 461–462 (in German).

Wenzl, J. E., and Burke, E. C. (1962). Poisoning from a malathion–aerosol mixture. A case report. *JAMA, J. Am. Med. Assoc.* **182**, 495–497.

Wescoe, W. C., Hunt, C. C., Riker, W. F., and Litt, I. C. (1947). Regeneration rates of serum cholinesterase in normal individuals and in patients with liver damage. *Am. J. Physiol.* **149**, 549–551.

West, B., Vidone, L. B., and Shaffer, C. B. (1961). Acute and subacute toxicity of dimethoate. *Toxicol. Appl. Pharmacol.* **3**, 210–223.

Wetstone, H. J., and LaMotta, R. V. (1965). The clinical stability of serum cholinesterase activity. *Clin. Chem. (Winston-Salem, N.C.)* **11**, 653–663.

Wetstone, H. J., LaMotta, R. V., Bellucci, A., Tennant, R., and White, B. V. (1960). Studies of cholinesterase activity. V. Serum cholinesterase in patients with carcinoma. *Ann. Intern. Med.* **52**, 102–125.

Whitacre, D. M., Badie, M., Schwemmer, B. A., and Diaz, L. T. (1976). Metabolism of ^{14}C-leptophos and ^{14}C-4-bromo-2,5-dichlorophenol in rats: A multiple dosing study. *Bull. Environ. Contam. Toxicol.* **16**, 689–696.

Wilhelm, K., Pleština, R., and Svetličić, B. (1974). The toxicity of Ekatin and its action on occupationally exposed workers. *Arh. Hig. Rada Toksikol.* **25**, 319 320 (in Serbo-Croatian).

Williams, C. H. (1970). *Beta*-glucuronidase activity in the serum and liver of rats treated with parathion. *Toxicol. Appl. Pharmacol.* **16**, 533–539.

Williams, M. W. (1961). Acute and subacute toxicity of Trithion® and the dimethyl homolog. *Toxicol. Appl. Pharmacol.* **3**, 500–508.

Williams, M. W., Fuyat, H. N., and Fitzhugh, O. G. (1954). The subacute toxicity of four organic phosphates to dogs. *Toxicol. Appl. Pharmacol.* **1**, 1–7.

Williams, M. W., Fitzhugh, O. G., and Cook, J. W. (1957). Serum protein changes following feeding of parathion to dogs. *Proc. Soc. Exp. Biol. Med.* **96**, 539–540.

Williams, M. W., Fitzhugh, O. G., and Cook, J. W. (1958a). Parathion-induced changes in the serum proteins of the dog. *J. Pharmacol. Exp. Ther.* **122**, 83A.

Williams, M. W., Fitzhugh, O. G., and Cook, J. W. (1958b). The effect of parathion on human red blood cell and plasma cholinesterase. *AMA Arch. Ind. Health* **18**, 441–445.

Williams, M. W., Fuyat, H. N., Frawley, J. P., and Fitzhugh, O. G. (1958c). *In vivo* effects of paired combinations of five organic phosphate insecticides. *J. Agric. Food Chem.* **6**, 514–516.

Williams, M. W., Fuyat, H. N., and Fitzhugh, O. G. (1959). The subacute toxicity of four organic phosphates to dogs. *Toxicol. Appl. Pharmacol.* **1**, 1–7.

Williams, M. W., Baker, R. D., and Covill, R. W. (1962). Blood cholinesterase inhibition after dermal absorption of two organophosphorus agents. *Toxicol. Appl. Pharmacol.* **4**, 271–275.

Williams, R. L., and Pearson, J. E., Jr. (1970). Functional study of the renal effect of the anticholinesterase paraoxon. *Arch. Int. Pharmacodyn. Ther.* **184**, 195–208.

Wills, J. H., and Chalakis, J. (1968). Neuromuscular block by a new organophosphorus compound. *Fed. Proc., Fed. Am. Soc. Exp. Biol.* **27**, 407.

Wills, J. H., McNamara, B. P., and Fine, E. A. (1950). Ventricular fibrillation in delayed treatment of TEPP poisoning. *Fed. Proc., Fed. Am. Soc. Exp. Biol.* **9**, 136.

Wills, J. H., Bradley, J. D., Russell, J. C., and Coulston, F. (1971). The safety for man of small daily doses of an organophosphate acaricide. *Toxicol. Appl. Pharmacol.* **19**, 399.

Wilson, I. B. (1951). Acetylcholinesterase. XI. Reversibility of tetraethylpyrophosphate inhibition. *J. Biol. Chem.* **190**, 111–117.

Winterlin, W., Kilgore, W., Mourer, C., Mull, R., Walker, G., Knaak, J., and Maddy, K. (1978). Dislodgeable residue of dialifor and phosalone and their oxygen analogs following a reported worker-injury incident in San Joaquin Valley, California. *Bull. Environ. Contam. Toxicol.* **20**, 255–260.

Wirth, W. (1956). Detection of E-605 intoxication: Research on ChE activity in the brain. *Arch. Toxicol.* **16**, 125–128.

Wirth, W. (1958). On the action of systemic phosphoric acid ester insecticides on the metabolism of warm blooded animals. *Naunyn-Schmiedebergs Arch. Exp. Pathol. Pharmakol.* **234**, 352–363 (in German).

Witherup, S., Jolley, W. J., Stemmer, K., and Pfitzer, E. A. (1971). Chronic studies with 2,2-dichlorvinyl dimethyl phosphate (DDVP) in dogs and rats including observations on rat reproduction. *Toxicol. Appl. Pharmacol.* **19**, 377.

Witter, R. F. (1960). Effect of DDVP aerosols on blood cholinesterase of fogging machine operators. *AMA Arch. Ind. Health* **21**, 7–9.

Witter, R. F. (1963). Measurement of blood cholinesterase. *Arch. Environ. Health* **6**, 537–563.

Witter, R. F., and Gaines, T. B. (1963a). Relationship between depression of plasma cholinesterase and paralysis in chickens caused by certain organic phosphorus compounds. *Biochem. Pharmacol.* **12**, 1377–1386.

Witter, R. F., and Gaines, T. B. (1963b). Rate of formation *in vivo* of the unreactivable form of brain cholinesterase in chickens given DDVP or malathion. *Biochem. Pharmacol.* **12**, 1421–1427.

Witter, R. F., Gaines, T. B., Short, J. G., Sedlak, V. A., and Maddock, D. R. (1961). Studies on the safety of DDVP for the disinsection of commercial aircraft. *Bull. W.H.O.* **24**, 635–642.

Wojcik, J. (1975). The effect of Foschlor present in drinking water on the organs of three rat generations. *Rocz. Panstw. Zakl. Hig.* **26**, 383–391 (in Polish).

Wolfe, H. R., Durham, W. F., and Armstrong, J. F. (1970). Urinary excretion of insecticide metabolites: Excretion of paranitrophenol and DDA as indicators of exposure to parathion and DDT. *Arch. Environ. Health* **21**, 711–716.

Wolfe, H. R., Armstrong, J. F., and Durham, W. F. (1974). Exposure of mosquito control workers to fenthion. *Mosq. News* **34**, 263–267.

Wolfsie, J. H., and Winter, G. D. (1952). Statistical analysis of normal human red blood cell and plasma cholinesterase activity values. *Arch. Ind. Hyg. Occup. Med.* **6**, 43–49.

Wolthuis, O. L., and Meeter, E. (1968). Cardiac failure in the rat caused by diisopropyl fluorophosphate (DFP). *Eur. J. Pharmacol.* **2**, 387–392.

Wood, J. R. (1950). Medical problems in chemical welfare. *JAMA, J. Am. Med. Assoc.* **144**, 606–609.

Woodard, G., Woodard, M., and Cronin, M. T. I. (1968). Safety evaluation of the pesticide diazinon by a two-year feeding trial in rhesus monkeys. *Fed. Proc., Fed. Am. Soc. Exp. Biol.* **27**, 597.

Wooder, M. F., Wright, A. S., and King, L. J. (1977). *In vivo* alkylation studies with dichlorvos at practical use concentrations. *Chem.-Biol. Interact.* **19**, 25–46.

Worden, A. N., Wheldon, G. H., Noel, P. R. B., and Mawdesley-Thomas, I. E. (1973). Toxicity of gusathion for the rat and dog. *Toxicol. Appl. Pharmacol.* **24**, 405–412.

World Health Organization (WHO) (1967). "Sixteenth Report of the WHO Expert Committee on Insecticides: Safe Use of Pesticides in Public Health," Tech. Rep. Ser. No. 356. World Health Organ., Geneva.

World Health Organization (WHO) (1968). "Studies on the Safety of OMS-708 (Mobam) and OMS-214 (dicapthon) Sprayed as Adulticides in Stage V in Northern Nigeria," VBC/ETI/68.6 Add. 1. World Health Organ., Geneva.

World Health Organization (WHO) (1969). "Studies on the Safety of Two Organophosphorus Insecticides Tested in a Village Scale Trial by Anopheles Control Research Unit No. 1 in Northern Nigeria," VBC/ETI/69.9. World Health Organ., Geneva.

World Health Organization (WHO) (1973). "Twentieth Report of the WHO Expert Committee on Insecticides: Safe Use of Pesticides," Tech. Rep. Ser. No. 513. World Health Organ., Geneva.

World Health Organization (WHO) (1977). "Programme for Evaluating and Testing New Insecticides: Stage I, II and III Test Results on Insects and Mammals Obtained from 1960 through 1977. Pesticide Development and Safe Use Unit," VBC/77.3. World Health Organ., Geneva.

World Health Organization (WHO) (1985). "Report of a WHO Expert Committee: The Control of Schistosomiasis," Tech. Rep. Ser. No. 728. World Health Organ., Geneva.

World Health Organization/Food and Agriculture Organization (WHO/FAO)

(1982a). "Draft of WHO/FAO Data Sheet on Pesticides: Phenthoate," No. 48. World Health Organ./Food Agric. Organ., Geneva.

World Health Organization/Food and Agriculture Organization WHO/FAO) (1982b). "Draft of WHO/FAO Data Sheet on Pesticides: Pirimiphosmethyl," No. 49. World Health Organ./Food Agric. Organ., Geneva.

World Health Organization/Food and Agriculture Organization (WHO/FAO) (1984a). "First Draft of WHO/FAO Data Sheet on Pesticides: Azinphosethyl," No. 72. World Health Organ., Food Agric. Organ., Geneva.

World Health Organization/Food and Agriculture Organization (WHO/FAO) (1984b). "First Draft of WHO/FAO Data Sheet on Pesticides: Bromophos," No. 76. World Health Organ./Food Agric. Organ., Geneva.

Worrell, C. L. (1975). The management of organophosphate intoxication. *South. Med. J.* **68**, 335–339.

Wright, F. C., and Riner, J. C. (1979). Biotransformation and deposition of residues of fenthion and oxidative metabolites in the fat of cattle. *J. Agric. Food Chem.* **27**, 576–577.

Wustner, D. A., Desmarchelier, J., and Fukuto, T. R. (1972). Structure for the oxygenated product of peracid oxidation of Dyfonate insecticide (*O*-ethyl-*S*-phenyl ethylphosphonodithioate). *Life Sci.* **11**, (Part 2), 583–588.

Wyckoff, D. W., Davies, J. E., Barquet, A. C., and Davis, J. H. (1968). Diagnostic and therapeutic problems of parathion poisoning. *Ann. Intern. Med.* **68**, 875–882.

Xintaras, C., Burg, J. R., Tanaka, S., Lee, S. T., Johnson, B. L., Cottrill, C. A., and Bender, J. (1978). "NIOSH Health Survey of Velsicol Pesticide Workers; Occupational Exposure to Leptophos and Other Chemicals." U. S. Govt Printing Office, Washington, D.C.

Yamanaka, S., and Nishimura, M. (1979). Effect of cholinesterase inhibitors on isoenzyme. *Jpn. J. Hyg.* **34**, 187 (in Japanese).

Yamashita, K. (1962). Toxicity of Dipterex and its vinyl derivative (DDVP). *Ind. Med. Surg.* **31**, 170–173.

Yašnova, G. P., Abbasov, T. G., and Tsaregorodtseva, G. N. (1971). Pathomorphological and histochemical changes in organs and tissues of calves following prolonged addition of organophosphorus insecticides to their feed. *Tr. VNIIVS* **39**, 228–233 (in Russian).

Yatomi, T., Ueda, K., Oikawa, K., and Kawai, M. (1978). Delayed neurotoxicity of organophosphorus compounds. Part II. *Jpn. J. Rural Med.* **27**, 622–623.

Yoshihara, S., and Neal, R. A. (1977). Comparison of the metabolism of parathion by a rat liver reconstituted mixed-function oxidase enzyme system and by a system containing cumene hydroperoxide and purified rat liver cytochrome P-450. *Drug Metab. Dispos.* **5**, 191–197.

Young, R., Jr., Hass, D. K., and Brown, L. J. (1979a). Effect of late gestation feeding of dichlorvos in non-parasitized sows. *J. Anim. Sci.* **48**, 45–51.

Young, R., Jr., Jung, F. P., and Ayer, H. E. (1979b). Phorate intoxication at an insecticide formulation plant. *Am. Ind. Hyg. Assoc. J.* **40**, 1013–1016.

Younger, R. L., Radleff, R. D., and Weidenbach, C. P. (1962). Toxicological studies of compound VCl-13 in livestock. *J. Econ. Entomol.* **55**, 249–252.

Yushkevich, L. B. (1958). Blood changes in workers suffering from chronic exposure to mercaptophos. *Probl. Gematol. Pereliv. Krovi* **6**, 35–36.

Zaratzian, V. L., Fuyat, H. V., and Fitzhugh, O. G. (1960). Effects of combinations of Systox and methyl parathion in the dog. *Fed. Proc., Fed. Am. Soc. Exp. Biol.* **19**, 275.

Zavon, M. R. (1962). Insecticides and other pesticides of home and garden. *Mod. Med. (Minneapolis)* **30**, 90.

Zavon, M. R. (1965). Blood cholinesterase levels in organic phosphate intoxication. *JAMA, J. Am. Med Assoc.* **192**, 51.

Zavon, M. R., and Kindel, E. A. (1966). Potential hazard in using dichlorvos insecticide resin. *Adv. Chem. Ser.* **60**, 177–186.

Zhabin, V. A., and Litvishchenko, F. I. (1971). A case of chlorophos poisoning. *Vrach. Delo* **3**, 143–144 (in Russian).

Zhivoglyadova, L. M. (1968). A characterization of the toxicity of chlorphos for animals of various age-groups. *Sb. Nauchn. Rab. Kirg. Nauchno-Issled Inst. Okhr. Materin. Det.* **6**, 265–268.